Transitions Theory

Middle-Range and Situation-Specific Theories in Nursing Research and Practice

Afaf Ibrahim Meleis, PhD, DrPS (hon), FAAN, is the Margaret Bond Simon Dean of Nursing at the University of Pennsylvania School of Nursing, Professor of Nursing and Sociology, and Director of the School's WHO Collaborating Center for Nursing and Midwifery Leadership. Prior to coming to Penn, she was a professor on the faculty of nursing at the University of California, Los Angeles, and the University of California, San Francisco, for 34 years. She is a Fellow of the Royal College of Nursing in the UK, the American Academy of Nursing, and the College of Physicians of Philadelphia. She is a member of the Institute of Medicine and its Committee on Transforming the Case for American Commitment to Global Health as well as the Robert Wood Johnson Foundation Nurse Faculty Scholar National Advisory Committee, a Trustee of the National Health Museum, and a Board Member of CARE, Institute for the Advancement of Multicultural and Minority Medicine and Life Science Career Alliance. She is Council General of ICOWHI, the International Council on Women's Health Issues, an international nonprofit association dedicated to the goal of promoting health, health care, and the well-being of women throughout the world through participation, empowerment, advocacy, education, and research. She is also a Global Ambassador for the Girl Child Initiative of the International Council of Nurses.

Dr. Meleis's research scholarship is focused on the structure and organization of nursing knowledge, transitions and health, and international nursing, as well as global health, immigrant and women's health, and the theoretical development of the nursing discipline. She has mentored hundreds of students, clinicians, and researchers from Thailand, Brazil, Egypt, Jordan, Israel, Columbia, Korea, and Japan. She is the author of more than 150 articles in social sciences, nursing, and medical journals; and has written 40 book chapters, 6 books, and numerous monographs and proceedings.

Dr. Meleis is the recipient of numerous honors and awards, as well as honorary doctorates and distinguished and honorary professorships around the world. In 1990, Egyptian President Hosni Mubarak presented her the Medal of Excellence for professional and scholarly achievements; in 2000 she received the Chancellor's Medal from the University of Massachusetts, Amherst. In 2007, she received three distinguished awards: an Honorary Doctorate of Medicine from the Linköping University, Sweden; the Global Citizenship Award from the United Nations Association of Greater Philadelphia; the Sage Award from the University of Minnesota; and The Dr. Gloria Twine Chisum Award for Distinguished Faculty at University of Pennsylvania, which is awarded for community leadership and commitment to promoting diversity. She is the first Dean at the University of Pennsylvania to receive this award. Dr. Meleis also received the 2008 Commission on Graduates of Foreign Nursing Schools (CGFNS) International Distinguished Leadership Award based on her outstanding work in the global health care community; she recently received the Take the Lead 2009 Award from the Girl Scouts of Eastern Pennsylvania.

Dr. Meleis graduated Magna Cum Laude from the University of Alexandria (1961), earned an MS in nursing (1964), an MA in sociology (1966), and a PhD in medical and social psychology (1968) from the University of California, Los Angeles.

TRANSITIONS THEORY

MIDDLE-RANGE AND SITUATION-SPECIFIC THEORIES IN NURSING RESEARCH AND PRACTICE

AFAF IBRAHIM MELEIS, PhD, DrPS (HON), FAAN

EDITOR

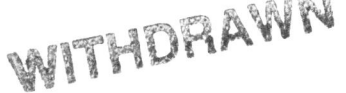

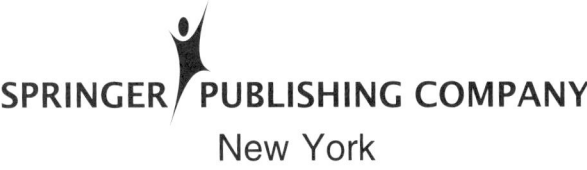

Copyright © 2010 Springer Publishing Company, LLC

All rights reserved.

No part of this publication may be reproduced, stored in a retrieval system, or transmitted in any form or by any means, electronic, mechanical, photocopying, recording, or otherwise, without the prior permission of Springer Publishing Company, LLC, or authorization through payment of the appropriate fees to the Copyright Clearance Center, Inc., 222 Rosewood Drive, Danvers, MA 01923, 978-750-8400, fax 978-646-8600, info@copyright.com or on the Web at www.copyright.com.

Springer Publishing Company, LLC
11 West 42nd Street
New York, NY 10036
www.springerpub.com

Acquisitions Editor: Margaret Zuccarini
Production Editor: Pamela Lankas
Cover design: Steve Pisano
Composition: International Graphic Services

Ebook ISBN: 978-0-8261-0535-6

10 11 12 13/ 5 4 3 2

The author and the publisher of this Work have made every effort to use sources believed to be reliable to provide information that is accurate and compatible with the standards generally accepted at the time of publication. Because medical science is continually advancing, our knowledge base continues to expand. Therefore, as new information becomes available, changes in procedures become necessary. We recommend that the reader always consult current research and specific institutional policies before performing any clinical procedure. The author and publisher shall not be liable for any special, consequential, or exemplary damages resulting, in whole or in part, from the readers' use of, or reliance on, the information contained in this book. The publisher has no responsibility for the persistence or accuracy of URLs for external or third-party Internet Web sites referred to in this publication and does not guarantee that any content on such Web sites is, or will remain, accurate or appropriate.

Library of Congress Cataloging-in-Publication Data

Transitions theory : middle-range and situation-specific theories in nursing research and practice / [edited by] Afaf Ibrahim Meleis.
   p. ; cm.
  Includes bibliographical references and index.
  ISBN 978-0-8261-0534-9 (alk. paper)
  1. Nursing models. 2. Life change events. I. Meleis, Afaf Ibrahim. [DNLM: 1. Nursing Theory. 2. Life Change Events. 3. Nursing Care—psychology. WY 86 T772 2009]
  RT84.5.T733 2009
  610.73—dc22
                                  2009045573

Printed in the United States of America by Hamilton Printing

> Special discounts on bulk quantities of our books are available to corporations, professional associations, pharmaceutical companies, health care organizations, and other qualified groups.
> If you are interested in a custom book, including chapters from more than one of our titles, we can provide that service as well.
>
> **For details, please contact:**
> Special Sales Department, Springer Publishing Company, LLC
> 11 West 42nd Street, 15th Floor, New York, NY 10036-8002
> Phone: 877-687-7476 or 212-431-4370; Fax: 212-941-7842
> Email: sales@springerpub.com

*To Amani Paulina, Karim Salvatore,
and Samir Alexander Meleis,
for coaching me in my transition to grandparenthood.*

CONTENTS

Contributors   *xi*
Foreword by Patricia Benner   *xiii*
Preface   *xv*
Acknowledgments   *xvii*
Permissions   *xix*

Part I	Transitions From Practice to Evidence-Based Models of Care	1
Part II	Transitions as a Nursing Theory	11
Chapter 1	Theoretical Development of Transitions	13
1.1	Role Insufficiency and Role Supplementation: A Conceptual Framework *Afaf Ibrahim Meleis*	13
1.2	Transitions: A Nursing Concern *Norma Chick and Afaf Ibrahim Meleis*	24
1.3	Transitions: A Central Concept in Nursing *Karen L. Schumacher and Afaf Ibrahim Meleis*	38
Chapter 2	Transition Theory	52
2.1	Experiencing Transitions: An Emerging Middle-Range Theory *Afaf Ibrahim Meleis, Linda M. Sawyer, Eun-Ok Im, DeAnne K. Hilfinger Messias, and Karen Schumacher*	52
2.2	Facilitating Transitions: Redefinition of the Nursing Mission *Afaf Ibrahim Meleis and Patricia A. Trangenstein*	65
2.3	Transition: A Literature Review *Debbie Kralik, Kate Visentin, and Antonia van Loon*	72
Part III	The Experience of and Responses to Transitions	85
Chapter 3	Developmental Transitions	87
3.1	Developmental Transitions *Marianne Hattar-Pollara*	87
3.2	Becoming a Mother Versus Maternal Role Attainment *Ramona T. Mercer*	94
3.3	The Conceptual Structure of Transition to Motherhood in the Neonatal Intensive Care Unit *Hyunjeong Shin and Rosemary White-Traut*	104
3.4	Nursing Practice Model for Maternal Role Sufficiency *Kathleen Flynn Gaffney*	114
3.5	A Situation-Specific Theory of Korean Immigrant Women's Menopausal Transition *Eun-Ok Im and Afaf Ibrahim Meleis*	121

viii   CONTENTS

3.6	Helping Elderly Persons in Transition: A Framework for Research and Practice *Karen L. Schumacher, Patricia S. Jones, and Afaf Ibrahim Meleis*	129
3.7	Geriatric Sexual Conformity: Assessment and Intervention *Merrie J. Kaas and G. Kay Rousseau*	145
Chapter 4	Situational Transitions: Discharge and Relocation	153
4.1	Perceived Readiness for Hospital Discharge in Adult Medical-Surgical Patients *Marianne E. Weiss, Linda B. Piacentine, Lisa Lokken, Janice Ancona, Joanne Archer, Susan Gresser, Sue Baird Holmes, Sally Toman, Anne Toy, and Teri Vega-Stromberg*	153
4.2	Transition Experiences of Stroke Survivors Following Discharge Home *Maude Rittman, Craig Boylstein, Ramon Hinojosa, Melanie Sberna Hinojosa, and Jolie Haun*	170
4.3	Assessing Older Persons' Readiness to Move to Independent Congregate Living *Eileen K. Rossen*	182
4.4	Women's Well-Being After Relocation to Independent Living Communities *Eileen K. Rossen and Kathleen A. Knafl*	187
4.5	Women in Transition: Being Versus Becoming or Being and Becoming *Afaf Ibrahim Meleis in association with Sandra Rogers*	198
4.6	Meleis's Theory of Nursing Transitions and Relatives' Experiences of Nursing Home Entry *Sue Davies*	209
Chapter 5	Situational Transitions: Immigration	226
5.1	Migration Transitions *DeAnne K. Hilfinger Messias*	226
5.2	A Model of Psychological Adaptation to Migration and Resettlement *Karen J. Aroian*	232
5.3	Immigrant Transitions and Health Care: An Action Plan *Afaf Ibrahim Meleis*	241
5.4	Primary Health Care Nurses' Conceptions of Involuntarily Migrated Families' Health *Kerstin Samarasinghe, Bengt Fridlund, and Barbro Arvidsson*	242
5.5	Transnational Health Resources, Practices, and Perspectives: Brazilian Immigrant Women's Narratives *DeAnne K. Hilfinger Messias*	250
5.6	Employed Mexican Women as Mothers and Partners: Valued, Empowered and Overloaded *Afaf Ibrahim Meleis, Marilyn K. Douglas, Carmen Eribes, Fujin Shih, and DeAnne K. Messias*	271
Chapter 6	Situational Transitions: Education	283
6.1	Exploring the Transition and Professional Socialisation From Health Care Assistant to Student Nurse *Graeme Brennan and Rob McSherry*	283
6.2	Clinical Transition of Baccalaureate Nursing Students During Preceptored, Pregraduation Practicums *Diane M. Wieland, Geralyn M. Altmiller, Mary T. Dorr, and Zane Robinson Wolf*	292
6.3	There Really Is a Difference: Nurses' Experiences With Transitioning From RNs to BSNs *Colleen Delaney and Barbara Piscopo*	300
6.4	A Qualitative Study of How Experienced Certified Holistic Nurses Learn to Become Competent Practitioners *Leighsa Sharoff*	310

Chapter 7	Health and Illness Transitions	320
7.1	Self-Care of Heart Failure: A Situation-Specific Theory of Health Transition *Barbara Riegel and Victoria Vaughan Dickson*	320
7.2	Health–Illness Transition Experiences Among Mexican Immigrant Women With Diabetes *Marylyn Morris McEwen, Martha Baird, Alice Pasvogel, and Gwen Gallegos*	326
7.3	Transitions in Chronic Illness: Rheumatoid Arthritis in Women *Muriel P. Shaul*	338
7.4	Recurrence of Ovarian Cancer—Living in Limbo *Ewa Ekwall, Britt-Marie Ternestedt, and Bengt Sorbe*	347
7.5	Admitted With a Hip Fracture: Patient Perceptions of Rehabilitation *Lars-Eric Olsson, Anne E. M. Nyström, Jòn Karlsson, and Inger Ekman*	358
7.6	Taiwanese Patients' Concerns and Coping Strategies: Transition to Cardiac Surgery *Fu-Jin Shih, Afaf Ibrahim Meleis, Po-Jui Yu, Wen-Yu Hu, Meei-Fang Lou, and Guey-Shiun Huang*	366
7.7	Suffering in Silence: The Experience of Early Memory Loss *Petra Robinson, Sirkka-Liisa Ekman, Afaf Ibrahim Meleis, Bengt Winblad, and Lars-Olof Wahlund*	386
7.8	Transition Towards End of Life in Palliative Care: An Exploration of Its Meaning for Advanced Cancer Patients in Europe *Philip J. Larkin, Bernadette Dierckx de Casterlé, and Paul Schotsmans*	396
7.9	Towards a Conceptual Evaluation of Transience in Relation to Palliative Care *Philip J. Larkin, Bernadette Dierckx de Casterlé, and Paul Schotsmans*	410
Chapter 8	Organizational Transitions	423
8.1	On Becoming a Flexible Pool Nurse: Expansion of the Meleis Transition Framework *Victoria L. Rich*	423
8.2	The Experience of Role Transition in Acute Care Nurse Practitioners in Taiwan Under the Collaborative Practice Model *Wei-Chin Chang, Pei-Fan Mu, and Shiow-Luan Tsay*	430
8.3	Guiding the Transition of Nursing Practise From an Inpatient to a Community-Care Setting: A Saudi Arabian Experience *Elaine Simpson, Mollie Butler, Shayda Al-Somali, and Mary Courtney*	439
8.4	Implementing an Interdisciplinary Governance Model in a Comprehensive Cancer Center *Patricia Reid Ponte, Anne H. Gross, Eric Winer, Mary J. Connaughton, and James Hassinger*	445
Part IV	Nursing Therapeutics	455
Chapter 9	Transitional Care Model	459
9.1	The Transitional Care Model for Older Adults *Mary D. Naylor and Janet Van Cleave*	459
9.2	Transitional Environments *Dorothy Brooten and Mary Duffin Naylor*	465
9.3	Transitional Care of Older Adults Hospitalized With Heart Failure: A Randomized, Controlled Trial *Mary D. Naylor, Dorothy A. Brooten, Roberta L. Campbell, Greg Maislin, Kathleen M. McCauley, and J. Sanford Schwartz*	480
9.4	Adolescents With Type 1 Diabetes: Transition Between Diabetes Services *Kate Visentin, Tina Koch, and Debbie Kralik*	494

9.5	Advanced Practice Nurse Strategies to Improve Outcomes and Reduce Cost in Elders With Heart Failure *Kathleen M. McCauley, M. Brian Bixby, and Mary D. Naylor*	505
Chapter 10	Role Supplementation Models	514
10.1	Preventive Role Supplementation: A Grounded Conceptual Framework *Afaf Ibrahim Meleis, Leslee Swendsen, and Deloras Jones*	514
10.2	Role Supplementation for New Parents—A Role Mastery Plan *Leslee A. Swendsen, Afaf Ibrahim Meleis, and Deloras Jones*	523
10.3	A Role Supplementation Group Pilot Study: A Nursing Therapy for Potential Parental Caregivers *Margaret H. Brackley*	531
10.4	Role Supplementation: An Empirical Test of a Nursing Intervention *Afaf Ibrahim Meleis and Leslee A. Swendsen*	539
10.5	Group Counseling in Cardiac Rehabilitation: Effect on Patient Compliance *Kathleen Dracup, Afaf Ibrahim Meleis, Suzanne Clark, Arline Clyburn, Linda Shields, and Marilyn Staley*	552
10.6	Family-Focused Cardiac Rehabilitation: A Role Supplementation Program for Cardiac Patients and Spouses *Kathleen Dracup, Afaf Ibrahim Meleis, Katherine Baker, and Patricia Edlefsen*	563
10.7	Role Supplementation as a Nursing Intervention for Alzheimer's Disease: A Case Study *Lisa Skemp Kelley and Jean A. Lakin*	571
10.8	Transition Entry Groups: Easing New Patients' Adjustment to Psychiatric Hospitalization *Karen Aroian and Marita Prater*	579
Chapter 11	Debriefing Models	582
11.1	A Survey of Postnatal Debriefing *Anne-Marie Steele and Mary Beadle*	582
11.2	The Longitudinal Effects of Midwife-Led Postnatal Debriefing on the Psychological Health of Mothers *Rosemary Selkirk, Suzanne McLaren, Alison Ollerenshaw, Angus J. McLachlan, and Julie Moten*	590
11.3	Perceived Effectiveness of Critical Incident Stress Debriefing by Australian Nurses *Jillian O'Connor and Sue Jeavons*	603
11.4	Critical Incident Stress Debriefing: Application for Perianesthesia Nurses *Maureen Iacono*	612
Part V	Epilogue (Frequently Asked Questions)	617
Epilogue		619
Index		625

CONTRIBUTORS

Victoria Vaughan Dickson, PhD, CRNP
Assistant Professor
New York University College of Nursing
New York, NY

Marianne Hattar-Pollara, DNSc, RN, FAAN
Professor
Azusa Pacific University School of Nursing
Azusa, CA

DeAnne K. Hilfinger Messias, PhD, RN, FAAN
Associate Professor
College of Nursing and Women's and Gender Studies Program
University of South Carolina
Columbia, SC

Mary D. Naylor, PhD, FAAN, RN
Marian S. Ware Professor in Gerontology
Director, New Courtland Center for Transitions and Health
University of Pennsylvania School of Nursing
Philadelphia, PA

Victoria L. Rich, PhD, RN, FAAN
Chief Nurse Executive
University of Pennsylvania Medical Center
Associate Executive Director
Hospital of the University of Pennsylvania
Associate Professor of Nursing Administration
University of Pennsylvania School of Nursing
Philadelphia, PA

Barbara Riegel, DNSc, RN, FAAN, FAHA
Professor
University of Pennsylvania School of Nursing
Philadelphia, PA

Janet Van Cleave, MSN, PhD
Research Fellow
University of Pennsylvania School of Nursing
Philadelphia, PA

FOREWORD

Some have remarked with truth-laden humor that it is not change that is so difficult but the transition. This volume illustrates that truth. The stress experienced and the new coping required when one is in transition are amply documented in this stunning research- and theory-based volume. This book brings together and integrates other middle-range theories about transitions in self-understanding and in one's situation and situated possibilities. The theorizing begins within role theory but soon expands to focus on the process of transition with all of its demands for new concerns, habits, skills, practices, and new coping capacities across many aspects of one's lifeworld and human development.

Transitions Theory: Middle-Range and Situation-Specific Theories in Nursing Research and Practice provides a remarkable intellectual history of the evolution of the concept of transitions in the lifeworld of persons and the universal human experience of transitions that evoke personal and community change. A transition may begin with enchantment and excitement or fear and grieving. Transition occupies a space between what went before and what is evolving. The place most bereft of equanimity is that period of protest and holding on to a no-longer-tenable past. Transitions can be empowering and growth producing, or they may end in self- and world diminishment. This is what makes transitions such a pivotal time for coaching and supporting growth and resilience.

Transitions Theory will be a classic and must-read for anyone doing research on transitions in relation to developmental and situational health and illness, organizational, and therapeutic transitions. The work of nurses in coaching and supporting persons through major life transitions is comprehensively articulated and examined theoretically. Dr. Meleis provides the scaffolding and anchoring of this work in her own scholarly career as a faculty member, nursing leader, and researcher. Many of the readings come out of her work with doctoral and postdoctoral students and her faculty colleagues. This book exemplifies the work of a scholarly community.

Transitions Theory addresses a core problem in nursing, psychology, and social sciences in which the person is unwittingly decontextualized and rendered ahistorical in many research methods, theories, and human science studies. Technical rationality typically focuses on frozen moments in time and yields an unplanned presentism while ignoring changes *in* the situation and *over time*. This theory and research offers a corrective focus that can enrich our understanding of development, formation, as well as stressful responses to both predictable and unpredictable change in human life. Nursing is concerned with growth and development, health promotion, coping with the demands of the human experience of illness and recovery. Transition theory introduces a broader view of rationality that includes relationships, change over time, and the person *in* particular situations and contexts. Giving birth; becoming parents; growing up; coping with chronic illnesses; recovering from injury or acute illness; changes in jobs and family structures, communities, or cultures all demand studying persons in their social relationships, context, and their experience of transitioning into new self-understandings and new lifeworlds.

This work is to be commended for the development of strategies to help people come to terms with new situations, demands, resources, and relationships in their lives. A cutting edge of this work involves studying migration and immigrant health. Role supplementation programs examined new sets of skills and capacities that would be required for becoming a parent or moving into new work roles. Coming to terms with the transformed situated possibilities of evolving heart disease and other chronic illness is also a cutting edge in this work. There are many commonalities in transitions that are identified here. Discovering what aspects of these commonalities matter most and are the most challenging for particular individuals and groups are rich areas for creating new support programs and services for persons in transition. Social support, whether it is informational, emotional, or tangible, matters in different ways, in different transitions, to different people. So although much has been accomplished in articulating the particular challenges and opportunities of social transitions, this is still a field with large potential and vast horizons in this era of globalization and increasing cultural exchanges.

Finally, this book is exemplary in tracing the intellectual history of theory and research in social transitions and for identifying new directions and gaps in the field. It demonstrates a coherent and evolving body of research and thinking that will be informative for any graduate student and faculty member embarking on a career of research and scholarship. I recommend it as essential reading for all graduate students learning to do literature reviews, interpretation, and synthesis and for inspiring them in developing coherent and integrated programs of research. I also recommend it for clinicians who work on facilitating transitions toward well-being and policy developers who want to reform the health care systems.

Patricia Benner, PhD, FAAN

PREFACE

Ever since I became interested in understanding the theoretical underpinnings of our discipline of nursing, learning that nursing practice is a rich resource for theory development, and finding out that advancing nursing science is the key to providing quality nursing care, I became convinced that "transitions" were central to the mission of nursing. Developing transitions as a theoretical construct, which then led to the development of theories, models, and research, is an example of the microcosm of how we can bring coherence to other central thoughts, concepts, and propositions in nursing. Theoretical coherence leads to sound nursing science, which in turn leads to evidence-based practice.

To the readers of this volume, I present to you what I have been thinking and writing about for 40 years. The articles and writings selected for inclusion in this book also represent the thinking and writing of many prominent colleagues. The collection of writings reflects the depth and breadth of what nurse scientists produced to advance theory and research related to "transitions." What we know about transitions is the result of answers to many significant questions: the hows and whys of experiencing and responding to events that trigger a transitional process; it is these questions and answers that make up the substance of this volume.

Many scientists in many disciplines have addressed life transitions of individuals and families and they developed theories to describe the experiences that occur during transitions, as well as the different strategies proposed to cope with the events that caused the changes in the lives of people. The divorce transition is one example of an event that has attracted much discussion and many scientific and popular books read by scientists and the lay public. Organizational transitions as well as the transition to adolescence have also commanded the attention of many different scientists.

Similarly, nurses have always cared for individuals, families, and communities experiencing changes that trigger new roles, losses of networks and support systems; these periods of disequilibrium are marked by turning points and a short or a long transitional process. These changes required the attention and the caring of nurses with or without the theory and the research to back their caring interventions.

Therefore, it is with pride in the progress nurses have made in advancing knowledge about caring for people in transition that I put together writings that bring theoretical coherence to an area in nursing that is giving more centrality to anticipating, experiencing, responding to, coping with, and providing nursing care to people who are in "transition." People in transition may be individuals, groups, families, partners, organizations, students, nurses, faculty members, or administrators. What makes their transition a nursing concern is the potential risk that the transitional experience may place on them. Preventing these risks, enhancing well-being, maximizing functioning, and mastering self-care activities are outcomes that nurses strive for in their interventions.

There are several goals attempted in producing this book of readings. First, because of the increasing interest in transitions as a scientific area of inquiry, there are global requests for writings for those who are interested in using transitions as a framework in their practice or research. Many of these requests are for the early publications about transitions. For that reason I have republished these hard-to-locate writings in this volume. Second, with the establishment of the New Courtland Center for Transitions and Health Research at the University of Pennsylvania, we anticipate an increasing interest in the transitional care model, which is based on much researched evidence and is cost-effective in enhancing the well-being for elders and those with heart failure. Third, by bringing to the discipline of nursing more theoretical and research coherence, this volume could be an example for those who may wish to bring together other theory, research, practice, education, and policy writings related to other central concepts.

Who should be using this book? Here are examples of potential readers of this book: undergraduate and graduate students who are studying the philosophical and epistemological underpinnings of the nursing discipline as well as advanced graduate students who are interested in theory development. This book will be useful to clinicians who use theory, who translate theory, and who plan to use the evidence to support their practice of clients in transition. One of the central goals for this book is to inspire researchers to ask new research questions, to continue to advance nursing theory and science related to transitions, and to translate and evaluate models of care in practice. This book could also be used by policymakers who want to develop and implement transitional care models in practice. Finally, faculty members who want to develop syllabi related to theory, research, and practice will find this book very useful.

Readers of this book can study the different sections and chapters sequentially, starting with the comprehensive introduction in Part I, proceeding to the theoretical development of transitions and then reviewing each category of transitions: developmental transitions, situational transitions, health–illness, and organizational transitions, followed by the three models of nursing therapeutics outlined in Part IV. Or, they may select a particular category of transition to focus on. In Part V, I conclude the book with the most frequently asked questions about transitions. These questions are a microcosm of the many questions that we have received over the years. The answers to these questions, as incomplete as they may be, are offered to challenge the readers to ask other questions and to offer their own answers.

The selection of the articles included in this volume is only a fraction of all that is written about transitions. I hope readers will be inspired to find other pertinent examples, to develop their own research programs, and to revise and extend the theories and models reviewed in this book.

ACKNOWLEDGMENTS

There are many people to acknowledge in the writing of this book. First and foremost, I thank my theoretical guru who inspired my interest in role theory in particular, and in theoretical development of disciplines in general, Dr. Ralph Turner. I continue to owe him so much debt. My second sense of debt is to my mentees, who became collaborators, then became scientists who are making many contributions to our discipline—Drs. Karen Schumacher, Eun-Ok Im, DeAnne Messias, Marianne Hattar-Pollara, Siriorn Sindhu, Ameporn Ratinthorn, Linda Sawyer, Norma Chick, and Leslee Swendsen. I am most grateful for their collaboration and for their contributions. I am also grateful to many mentees, colleagues, and strangers who have used transitions as a framework all over the world. It is their letters, e-mails, questions, and requests that have prompted me to complete this book.

Dr. Mary Naylor, who is the Director of the Center of The New Courtland Center for Transitions and Health, is leading the future of the transitional care model, which is the intervention of choice for many populations in transitions as well as the elders and the chronically ill. I also acknowledge my friend and colleague, Dr. Patricia Benner, who wrote the foreword to this book. In teaching theory together as well as spending time in Golden Gate Park during the cherry blossom season, we enjoyed many theoretical dialogues that affirmed our mutual intellectual fascination and commitment to advancing our nursing discipline.

In addition to the inspiring mentors, mentees, and colleagues, completing a book is a project that requires daily attention to details, managing correspondence, identifying materials, and meeting deadlines. Without Caroline Glickman and her organizational expertise and superb project oversight, I would not have been able to complete this book. Chenjuan Ma, my research assistant, has been eager to learn as well as to contribute her expertise in library research, bringing her newly acquired library research skills to this project. In the process she absorbed a great deal about theoretical nursing and working on a book project.

Finally, I am so pleased to be working with my editor from past projects, Margaret Zuccarini. She continues to inspire me with her vision and technical skills.

Afaf Ibrahim Meleis, PhD, DrPS (hon), FAAN

PERMISSIONS

Each of the following articles has been reprinted with the permission of the publisher:

CHAPTER 1:

1.1 Meleis, A. I. (1975). Role insufficiency and role supplementation: A conceptual framework. *Nursing Research, 24*, 264–271.

1.2 Chick, N., & Meleis, A. I. (1986). Transitions: A nursing concern. In P. L. Chinn (Ed.), *Nursing research methodology* (pp. 237–257). Boulder, CO: Aspen Publication.

1.3 Schumacher, K. L., & Meleis, A. I. (1994). Transitions: A central concept in nursing. *Journal of Nursing Scholarship, 26*(2), 119–127.

CHAPTER 2:

2.1 Meleis, A. I., Sawyer, L. M., Im, E. O., Hilfinger Messias, D. K., & Schumacher, K. (2000). Experiencing transitions: An emerging middle range theory. *Advances in Nursing Science, 23*(1), 12–28.

2.2 Meleis, A. I., & Trangenstein, P. A. (1994). Facilitating transitions: Redefinition of a nursing mission. *Nursing Outlook, 42*(6), 255–259.

2.3 Kralik, D., Visentin, K., & van Loon, A. (2006). Transition: A literature review. *Journal of Advanced Nursing, 55*(3), 320–329.

CHAPTER 3:

3.2 Mercer, R. T. (2004). Becoming a mother versus maternal role attainment. *Nursing Scholarship, 36*(3), 226–232.

3.3 Shin, H., & White-Traut, R. (2007). The conceptual structure of transition to motherhood in the neonatal intensive care unit. *Journal of Advanced Nursing, 58*(1), 90–98.

3.4 Gaffney, K. F. (1992). Nursing practice-model for maternal role sufficiency. *Advances in Nursing Sciences, 15*(2), 76–84.

3.5 Im, E. O., & Meleis, A. I. (1999). A situation-specific theory of Korean immigrant women's menopausal transition. *Journal of Nursing Scholarship, 31*(4), 333–338.

3.6 Schumacher, K. L., Jones, P. S., & Meleis, A. I. (1999). Helping elderly persons in transition: A framework for research and practice. In E. A. Swanson & T. Tripp-Reimer (Eds.), *Life transitions in the older adult: Issues for nurses and other health professionals* (pp. 1–26). New York: Springer.

3.7 Kaas, M. J., & Rousseau, G. K. (1983). Geriatric sexual conformity: Assessment and intervention. *Clinical Gerontologist, 2*(1), 31–44.

CHAPTER 4:

4.1 Weiss, M. E., Piacentine, L. B., Lokken, L., Ancona, J., Archer, J., Gresser, S., et al. (2007). Perceived readiness for hospital discharge in adult medical-surgical patients. *Clinical Nurse Specialist, 21*(1), 31–42.

4.2 Rittman, M., Boylstein, C., Hinojosa, R., Hinojosa, M. S., & Haun, J. (2007). Transition experiences of stroke survivors following discharge home. *Topics in Stroke Rehabilitation, 14*(2), 21–31.

4.3 Rossen, E. (2007). Assessing older persons' readiness to move to independent congregate living. *Clinical Nurse Specialist, 21*(6), 292–296.

4.4 Rossen, E., & Knafl, K. (2007). Women's well-being after relocation to independent living communities. *Western Journal of Nursing Research, 29*(2), 183–199.

4.5 Meleis, A. I., & Rogers, S. (1987). Women in transition: Being versus becoming or being and becoming. *Healthcare for Women International, 8*(4), 199–217.

4.6 Davies, S. (2005). Meleis' theory of nursing transitions and relatives' experiences of nursing home entry. *Journal of Advanced Nursing, 52*(6), 658–671.

CHAPTER 5:

5.2 Aroian, K. J. (1990). A model of psychological adaptation to migration and resettlement. *Nursing Research, 39*(1), 5–10.

5.3 Meleis, A. I. (1997). Immigrant transitions and health care: An action plan. *Nursing Outlook, 45*(1), 42.

5.4 Samarasinghe, K., Fridlund, B., & Arvidsson, B. (2006). Primary health care nurses' conceptions of involuntarily migrated families' health. *International Nursing Review, 53*(4), 301–307.

5.5 Messias, D. K. H. (2002). Transnational health resources, practices, and perspectives: Brazilian immigrant women's narratives. *Journal of Immigrant Health, 4*(4), 183–200.

5.6 Meleis, A. I., Douglas, M. K., Eribes, C., Shih, F., & Messias, D. K. (1996). Employed Mexican women as mothers and partners: Valued, empowered and overloaded. *Journal of Advanced Nursing, 23*, 82–90.

CHAPTER 6:

6.1 Brennan, G., & McSherry, R. (2007). Exploring the transition and professional socialization from health care assistant to student nurse. *Nurse Education in Practice, 7*(4), 206–214.

6.2 Wieland, D., Altmiller, G. M., Dorr, M. T., & Wolf, Z. R. (2007). Clinical transition of baccalaureate nursing students: During preceptored, pregraduation practicums. *Nursing Education Perspectives, 28*(6), 315–321.

6.3 Delaney, C., & Piscopo, B. (2007). There really is a difference: Nurses' experiences with transitioning from RNs to BSNs. *Journal of Professional Nursing, 23*(3), 167–173.

6.4 Sharoff, L. (2006). A qualitative study of how experienced certified holistic nurses learn to become competent practitioners. *Journal of Holistic Nursing, 24*(2), 116–124.

CHAPTER 7:

7.2 McEwen, M. M., Baird, M., Pasvogel, A., & Gallegos, G. (2007). Health-illness transition experiences among Mexican immigrant women with diabetes. *Family and Community Health, 30*(3), 201–212.

7.3 Shaul, M. P. (1997). Transitions in chronic illness: Rheumatoid arthritis in women. *Rehabilitation Nursing, 22*(4), 199–205.

7.4 Ekwall, E., Ternestedt, B. M., & Sorbe, B. (2007). Recurrence of ovarian cancer—living in limbo. *Cancer Nursing, 30*(4), 270–277.

7.5 Olsson, L. E., Nyström, A., Karlsson, J., & Ekman, I. (2007). Admitted with a hip fracture: Patient perceptions of rehabilitation. *Journal of Clinical Nursing, 16*(5), 853–859.

7.6 Shih, F. J., Meleis, A. I., Yu, P. J., Hu, W. Y., Lou, M. F., & Huang, G. S. (1998). Taiwanese patients' concerns and coping strategies: Transitions to cardiac surgery. *Heart and Lung, 27*(2), 82–98.

7.7 Robinson, P., Ekman, S. L., Meleis, A. I., Winblad, B., & Wahlund, L. O. (1997). Suffering in silence: The experience of early memory loss. *Health Care in Later Life, 2*(2), 107–120.

7.8 Larkin, P. J., Dierckx de Casterlé, B., & Schotsmans, P. (2007). Transition towards end of life in palliative care: An exploration of its meaning for advanced cancer patients in Europe. *Journal of Palliative Care, 23*(2), 69–79.

7.9 Larkin, P. J., Dierckx de Casterlé, B., & Schotsmans, P. (2007). Towards a conceptual evaluation of transience in relation to palliative care. *Journal of Advanced Nursing, 59*(1), 86–96.

CHAPTER 8:

8.2 Chang, W. C., Mu, P. F., & Tsay, S. L. (2006). The experience of role transition in acute care nurse practitioners in Taiwan under the collaborative practice model. *Journal of Nursing Research, 14*(2), 83–91.

8.3 Simpson, E., Butler, M., Al-Somali, S., & Courtney, M. (2006). Guiding the transition of nursing practice from an inpatient to a community-care setting: A Saudi Arabian experience. *Nursing and Health Sciences, 8*(2), 120–124.

8.4 Ponte, P., Gross, A. H., Winer, E., Connaughton, M. J., & Hassinger, J. (2007). Implementing an interdisciplinary governance model in a comprehensive cancer center. *Oncology Nursing Forum, 34*(3), 611–616.

CHAPTER 9:

9.2 Brooten, D., & Naylor, M. D. (1999). Transitional environments. In A. S. Hinshaw, S. L. Feetham, & J. L. F. Shaver (Eds.), *Handbook of clinical nursing research* (pp. 641–653). Thousand Oaks, CA: Sage Publications, Inc.

9.3 Naylor, M., Brooten, D. A., Campbell, R. L., Maislin, G., McCauley, K. M., & Schwartz, J. S. (2004). Transitional care of older adults hospitalized with heart failure: A randomized, controlled trial. *Journal of the American Geriatrics Society, 52*(5), 675–684.

9.4 Visentin, K., Koch, T., & Kralik, D. (2006). Adolescents with type 1 diabetes: Transition between diabetes services. *Journal of Clinical Nursing, 15*(6), 761–769.

9.5 McCauley, K., Bixby, M. B., & Naylor, M. D. (2006). Advanced practice nurse strategies to improve outcomes and reduce cost in elders with heart failure. *Disease Management, 9*(5), 302–310.

CHAPTER 10:

10.1 Meleis, A. I., Swendsen, L., & Jones, D. (1980). Preventive role supplementation: A grounded conceptual framework. In M. H. Miller & B. Flynn (Eds.), *Current perspectives in nursing: Social issues and trends* (Vol. 2, pp. 3–14). St. Louis, MO: C.V. Mosby.

10.2 Swendsen, L., Meleis, A. I., & Jones, D. (1978). Role supplementation for new parents: A role mastery plan. *American Journal of Maternal Child Nursing, 3*(2), 84–91.

10.3 Brackley, M. H. (1992). A role supplementation group pilot study: A nursing therapy for potential parental caregivers. *Clinical Nurse Specialist,* 6(1), 14–19.

10.4 Meleis, A. I., & Swendsen, L. (1978). Role supplementation: An empirical test of a nursing intervention. *Nursing Research,* 27, 11–18.

10.5 Dracup, K., Meleis, A. I., Clark, S., Clyburn, A., Shields, L., & Staley, M. (1985). Group counseling in cardiac rehabilitation: Effect on patient compliance. *Patient Education and Counseling,* 6(4), 169–177.

10.6 Dracup, K., Meleis, A. I., Baker, K., & Edlefsen, P. (1985). Family-focused cardiac rehabilitation: A role supplementation program for cardiac patients and spouses. *Nursing Clinics of North America,* 19(1), 113–124.

10.7 Kelley, L. S., & Lakin, J. A. (1988). Role supplementation as a nursing intervention for Alzheimer's disease: A case study. *Public Health Nursing,* 5(3), 146–152.

10.8 Aroian, K., & Prater, M. (1988). Transitions entry groups: Easing new patients' adjustment to psychiatric hospitalization. *Hospital and Community Psychiatry,* 39, 312–313.

CHAPTER 11:

11.1 Steele, A. M., & Beadle, M. (2003). A survey of postnatal debriefing. *Journal of Advanced Nursing,* 43(2), 130–136.

11.2 Selkirk, R., McLaren, S., Ollerenshaw, A., McLachlan, A., & Moten, J. (2006). The longitudinal effects of midwife-led postnatal debriefing on the psychological health of mothers. *Journal of Reproductive and Infant Psychology,* 24(2), 133–147.

11.3 O'Connor, J., & Jeavons, S. (2003). Perceived effectiveness of critical incident stress debriefing by Australian nurses. *Australian Journal of Advanced Nursing,* 20(4), 22–29.

11.4 Iacono, M. (2002). Critical incident stress debriefing: Application for perianesthesia nurses. *Journal of PeriAnesthesia Nursing,* 17(6), 423–426.

I

Transitions From Practice to Evidence-Based Models of Care

In a world that is in constant change as a result of economic upheavals, political shifts, geographical relocations, environmental challenges, resurgence of microbes, bird and H1N1 influenzas, and new medical discoveries, human beings are experiencing periods of transition that may or may not lead to an ability to cope with these changes. How, when, why, and in what ways people experience and respond to these changes are questions for which some answers are found in this book. The human experiences, the responses, the consequences to transitions on the well-being of people are an area of scholarship that has become even more central to the discipline of nursing. Equally as important are the strategies that nurses may use to care for and support people to achieve healthy transition processes as well as outcomes.

There are several reasons why transition is the business of nursing. *First,* nurses spend a great deal of their clinical time caring for individuals who are experiencing one or more changes in their lives that affect their health. Examples of transitions requiring nurses' attention are the hospital admission transition, the discharge transition, the postpartum transition, the rehabilitation transition, and the transition toward recovery, among many others.

Second, when the nursing literature of 1986 to 1992 was reviewed, we found 310 citations that identified "transitions" as the framework for the discussion demonstrating nurse authors' interest in transitions. *Third*, because of the increased use of technology, insurance-driven policies related to hospitalization and discharge, and increasing costs of hospitalization worldwide, patients tend to leave hospitals earlier and continue their recovery and rehabilitation transition at home. The transition to recovery is somewhat more protracted, and patients need expert and competent care until they complete their recovery transition. When patients and their families are not cared for during these transitions they experience many complications and possible readmissions.

Fourth, there are many world events that trigger a transition period which affect the well-being of people. Examples of such events are the movement of people between countries and within countries through immigration and migration. These movements put people at risk of illness, render them more vulnerable to stress, and may profoundly influence health care and outcome of populations as they cope with and adjust to the new environments.

Fifth, the increase in the graying populations in the world brings with it a different set of health care challenges that require different patterns of long-term caring by nurses. Nurses are expected to help individuals and families to live and cope with the multiplicity of changes the elders face, whether these are physical, geographical, spatial, emotional, and/or mental.

Sixth, people are living longer with chronic illness, and premature babies are being saved with modern science even when born before their organs are fully developed. Living with chronic illness and maintaining well-being initiate a series of transitions that requires nursing interventions at different stages and at critical points. *Finally*, there have been many natural disasters (earthquakes and floods) and human-made disasters (wars, nuclear plant explosions, and bombings) that not only require the immediate involvement of nurses, but also require nurses' long-term attention while people are learning to cope with the aftermath of these situations and to cope with their healing and recovery processes (Taylor & Frazer, 1982). The earthquakes in Kobe City, Japan, in 1994, in San Francisco (Loma Prieta) in 1989, and in Italy in 2009 prompt reflections about ways in which nurses may support and care for individuals, families, and communities that have experienced such devastating events. The questions that these events raise for nurses are, who are the target populations for their care and support, how do they respond to these events at different times, who gets neglected, who gets marginalized, and what processes do people go through as they begin to heal from the effects of these experiences? Other questions include what strategies do nurses use to create a healing environment and to enhance people's well-being in the process toward healing? And what are the milestones and critical periods in the long recovery process that nurses need to be aware of? Similar questions could be asked about many other transitional situations that, I believe, require nurses' thoughtful analyses, understanding, and actions.

My interest in transitions dates back to the mid-1960s when many support groups were formed to help people deal with a variety of developmental experiences or with health problems through teaching and/or support. These support groups were initiated by nurses or by lay members of communities to help individuals and families deal with the demands of such events as new parenting responsibilities, losing a family member, receiving a devastating diagnosis, undergoing such surgeries as a mastectomy or a colostomy, as well as with other events or experiences in a person's life that were deemed out of the ordinary. As a new graduate from a doctoral program, I found myself practicing what I had learned in theory and research courses. I asked questions about these support groups' similarities and differences, omissions and commissions, processes and outcomes, as well as what if the groups were not formed or were formed differently? With my colleagues, I looked for common and uncommon themes, experiences, responses, group agendas, and strategies nurses used in these support groups. We became aware of the need to consider that there were some universal features in creating and conducting these support and educational group meetings and in considering the nature of outcomes to be gained from the group work.

This awareness of the common threads woven throughout the groups was part of the quest to uncover some order in what appeared to be seemingly unrelated sets of events, experiences, and responses. This quest to uncover order was also driven by the growing interest in theory and theorizing about nursing that was the hallmark of the 1960s in the United States. This awareness was also nurtured by my interest in the phenomena surrounding planning pregnancies, the processes involved in becoming a new parent, and in mastering the parenting roles. I had studied the process of decision making in family planning and discovered the significance of spousal communication and interaction in effective or ineffective planning of the number of children in families (Meleis, 1971). Thus, family and support groups became a primary focus in any investigation or theoretical development. Then I asked similar questions about the processes involved in becoming parents. Although there were minimal data and interest at the time in processes and responses to transitions, I assumed that the knowledge area to be advanced was not about transitions but rather that it was about how nurses can make a difference in helping people achieve healthy outcomes after their transitions (Meleis & Swendsen, 1978).

My next set of research questions concerned what happens to people who do not make healthy transitions, how do nurses care for these people, and what nursing interventions do nurses use in facilitating clients' progress to achieve healthy transitions? This was where my clinical observations of parenting and chronically ill groups came in. So, first I defined unhealthy transitions or ineffective transitions as leading to role insufficiency and defined role insufficiency as any difficulty in the cognizance and/or performance of a role or of the sentiments and goals associated with the role behavior as perceived by the self or by significant others. Role insufficiency is characterized by behaviors and sentiments affiliated with the perception of disparity in fulfilling role obligations or expectations (Meleis, 1975). Role insufficiency may be manifested in assuming any new roles that range from an at-risk role, recovery role, parenting role, and/

or new-graduate-student or new-faculty roles. All these different groups that are undergoing a change had certain things in common—some losses and gains in their different roles and in support systems.

I then moved to define the goal of healthy transitions as mastery of behaviors, sentiments, cues, and symbols associated with new roles and identities as nonproblematic transitions. Although the nature of transitions and the nature of responses to different transitions were still a mystery, at the time they were not a mystery I felt compelled to uncover! I believed that knowledge development in nursing should be geared toward the development of nursing therapeutics and not toward understanding the phenomena related to responses to health and illness situations. In retrospect, I think that it is this belief in the need for developing nursing therapeutics and in finding out the difference that nursing makes may have been the driving force toward my development of role supplementation as a nursing therapeutic and for the research that occupied me during all of the 1970s, which is presented here in Part II and Part IV (Meleis, 1975; Meleis & Swendsen, 1978).

Backtracking from a focus on intervention to the questions about the nature of transition and the human experiences of transitions became the new focus in the 1980s. I believe this awareness, that we need knowledge related to how people tend to interpret their experiences, was prompted by many developments in nursing and by my growing interest in immigrants and their health. Inspired by better definitions of nursing as dealing with human processes and experiences related to health and illness, I began to ask questions about the transition experience as a concept. Dr. Norma Chick of Massey University, Palmerston North, New Zealand, came to work with me during her sabbatical and agreed to collaborate with me in developing transition as a concept. In 1985 we compiled and published the results of our findings in an article that we entitled "Transitions: A Nursing Concern" (Chick & Meleis, 1986). Ten years later, with Dr. Karen Schumacher, then a doctoral student at the University of California at San Francisco, we wondered about the extent to which transitions were used as a concept or a framework in nursing literature. A search of the literature yielded 310 articles that focused on transitions. We then analyzed the findings in these articles and identified transitions as a central concept in nursing (Schumacher & Meleis, 1994). Our interest in transitions was solidified and our conviction that transitions matter in advancing nursing knowledge was affirmed. From all these research and theoretical explorations, we identified four major categories of transitions that nurses tend to be involved in. This textbook is organized around these four major transitions, which are developmental, situational, health-illness, and organizational transitions.

In the article that I coauthored with Dr. Karen Schumacher (1994), we found out that among developmental transitions there are a wide variety of events that trigger a transitional process. Among these events, the process of becoming a parent has received the most attention in the nursing literature. More specifically, we found out that nurse scientists examined the transitions of pregnancy, motherhood, and fatherhood (Imle, 1990; Imle & Atwood, 1988), analyzed mothers' postpartum transitions (Brouse, 1988; Pridham & Chang, 1992; Pridham, Lytton, Change, & Rutledge, 1991; Tomlinson, 1987), and extended the postpartum transition up to 18 months after an infant's birth (Majewski, 1986, 1987). Although it is the mother's transition to parenthood that is most often studied, transition to fatherhood has also been addressed (Battles, 1988), and subsequently other transitions commanded much attention of nurse scientists such as the menopausal transition (Im, 2003; Im & Meleis, 2001).

In this textbook, we include in chapter 3 an analysis and synthesis of developmental transitions as a category and three examples of developmental transitions that nurses frequently encounter: the transition into motherhood, the menopausal transition, as well as the aging transition. Chapter 4 is devoted to situational transitions as a category. In reviewing the literature in our earlier article (Schumacher & Meleis, 1994), we found out that situational transitions include changes in family situations, for example, widowhood as a transition has been addressed by Poncar (1989) and by Adlersberg and Thorne (1990). The transition of an elderly family member from home to a nursing home has been conceptualized as a series of transitions (Brown & Powell-Cope, 1991). Situational transitions are exemplified by geographical changes, discharge from hospitals, and relocation to rehabilitation or elder care homes. Therefore, in this text, I included six articles in chapter 4 that address different aspects of this transition.

However, globalization has driven nurses' interest to another important situational transition. Although this transition is geographical as well, it is more complex and requires adding a component of cultural sensitivity and competence. Chapter 5 is devoted to immigration as a situational transition. The six articles in this chapter reflect nursing science's focus on patients' and nurses' immigration, beginning with an article that introduces immigration as a situational transition. It includes chapters about Brazilians, Mexicans, and Swedes.

Because nursing educators created opportunities for nursing students to move from one educational level to the next, nurse researchers found these transitions to be fertile areas for investigation. Therefore, chapter 6 is devoted to nursing education as a trigger for situational transition.

In addition to the examples provided in this book about situational transitions, there are other changes that begin a long transition experience that appear in the nursing literature such as homelessness (Gonzales-Osler, 1989), near-death experiences (Dougherty, 1990), and leaving abusive relationships (Henderson, 1989). All of these receive nurses' attention at one point or another, and require different nursing interventions and strategies in the transition process. The divorce transition is also another transition with many health and illness consequences (Sakraida, 2005; Sandfield, 2006).

The impact of illness-related transitions on individuals and families has been explored within the context of several illnesses such as myocardial infarction (Christman et al., 1988), postoperative recovery (Wild, 1992), HIV infection (Thurber & DiGiamarino, 1992), spinal cord injury (Selder, 1989), advanced cancer (Reimer, Davies, & Martens, 1991), and chronic illness (Catanzaro, 1990; Loveys, 1990). E. J. Bridges (1992) conceptualized weaning from mechanical ventilation as a transition in the process of recovery from critical illness. The progression from tube feeding to oral nutrition was also described as a rehabilitation transition by De Bonde and Hamilton (1991). In this volume, chapter 7 is devoted to the health and illness transition. The chapter is introduced with a situation-specific theory that describes the transition of patients with heart failure toward self-care, which has been developed by Dr. Barbara Riegel. The health–illness experiences are profoundly influenced by cultural diversity (Chinese, Mexican, and Taiwanese experiences), illness diversity (acute and chronic illness), differences in fields (mental health, surgical care, and palliative care), and depends on which stage in a person's lifespan (different ages) the transition occurs. Therefore, we have included in this text articles that demonstrate this rich variety. Together these articles provide a comprehensive framework for understanding the experiences and responses of diverse patients and a beginning interpretation of coping with these events in their lives within a cultural context.

The reviews of nursing literature helped us uncover another important category of transitions that nurses deal with. That is organizational transition, which represents changes in environments that pertain to nurses. These may be driven by the larger context and by the wider social, political, or economic environment, as well as by changes in the structure and dynamics of the organization itself (Schumacher & Meleis, 1994). Changes in leadership have been described as transitional periods in the life of organizations with consequences that influence different groups in the organization (Gilmore, 1990; Hegyvary & de Tornyay, 1991; Kerfoot, Serafin-Dickson, & Green, 1988; Losee & Cook, 1989; Tierney, Grant, Cherrstrom, & Morris, 1990), and may also affect the qualitative dimensions of the leadership roles (Ehrat, 1990). Instituting new policies, procedures, and practices has been identified as triggering a process of organizational transition. Several examples were offered in the literature such as introducing "restraint-free" care in a nursing home (Blakeslee, Goldman, Papougenis, & Torell, 1991), new staffing patterns (Rotkovitch & Smith, 1987), implementation of new models of nursing care (Main, Mishler, Ayers, Poppa, & Jones, 1989; Vezeau & Hallsten, 1987; Walker & deVooght, 1989), and the introduction of new technology (Shields, 1991; Turley, 1992). Another organizational transition described is the structural reorganization of facilities and the introduction of new programs, creating a period of upheaval in organizations (Condi, Oliver, & Williams, 1986; Harper, 1989; Swearingen, 1987; Walker & Devooght, 1989). The technology revolution and the introduction of computerization, robotic care, and the electronic health records initiate transition processes of many constituents requiring different answers about best practices for best outcomes (Brokel & Harrison, 2009; Moody, Scocumb, Berg, & Jackson, 2004)

In this text, I have included articles that reflect the general category of organizational transitions within a global theme that includes studies of Taiwanese and Saudi Arabian transitional experiences. All these are transitions that nurses anticipate, assess, diagnose, deal with, or help others to deal with. It is clearly an area that requires more systematic, scholarly attention for nurses.

During transitions, there are losses of networks, social supports, meaningful objects, and changes in familiar objects. There are also periods of uncertainty requiring different skills and competencies. Advancing knowledge about phases and milestones may require modification in strategies that have been used to cope with situations and events before transitions may have to be modified. Transitions may marginalize people (Hall, Stevens, & Meleis, 1994) and render them more vulnerable (Stevens, Hall, & Meleis, 1992); living with the effects and consequences of transitions may be exacerbated for marginalized populations. Transitional problems may result from not being able to separate from past identities and ways of functioning. Problems may also result from the inability to make decisions as to which path or route to take, from difficulties in abilities to make decisions, or from living through the adjustment periods (Golan, 1981). All of these processes require the attention of clinical scholars in ways that relate findings to their results to advance knowledge related to experiences and responses during transitions.

Populations also experience different consequence of transitions. There may be a physical debilitation, lowered immune system, a period of grief, a period of elation, an emergence of spirituality, and discovering of newfound meanings, and/or the experience of traumatic stress syndromes. Transitions are multidimensional and the means associated with them are important in shaping the intensity and nature of the consequences that clients experience. Indicators of healthy transitions include subjective well-being, role mastery, and well-being of relationships. Understanding the experiences embedded in transitions requires uncovering the experiences of individuals within the context of their significant others, family members, friends, or coworkers. It also includes uncovering the meanings attached to the transition experiences within the particular society, as well as the facilitating and constraining forces that help or hinder individuals in achieving healthy transitions. Coping with transition is a dynamic process that includes different processes, some of which are creatively and dynamically constructed while learning and acquiring expertise as exemplified by family members acquiring and developing expertise in caregiving (Schumacher, 1995).

Having established the significance of transitions to nursing and having demonstrated the extent to which nurses participate in patients' transitions led to extensive dialogues with Dr. Trish Trangenstein. Together we decided that a primary goal of the nursing mission may be to help people go through healthy transitions to enhance healthy outcomes. Therefore with this in mind we defined nursing as the art and science of facilitating the transition of populations' health and well-being. We also defined it as "being concerned with the processes and the experiences of human beings undergoing transitions where health and perceived well-being is the outcome" (Meleis & Trangenstein, 1994, p. 257). Within this definition, areas for knowledge development that have some universality and that could support a more systematic effort in knowledge development were identified. Examples are knowledge related to the processes and experiences of human beings undergoing transitions; the nature of emerging life patterns that result from transitions; the nature of environments that support or constrain healthy transitions; and the models that could be used to prevent unhealthy transitions, to augment healthy transitions, or to promote wellness during transitions (Meleis, 1993).

In spite of some progress in defining models of care during transitions, the most important question remains: What are the different strategies that nurses use to prevent unhealthy transitions, to support people's and families' well-being during transitions, and to promote healthy outcomes at the end of a major transition? William Bridges (1980, 1991), the guru of transitions and author of two significant books, *Making Sense of Life's Changes: Transitions* and *Managing Transitions: Making the Most of Change*, describes three phases experienced when going through transitions. These are: an ending phase characterized by disenchantment, a neutral phase characterized by disintegration and disequilibrium, and a beginning phase characterized by anticipations and taking on new roles. Each one of these phases would require different coping strategies and congruent nursing therapeutics. Perhaps through different research programs in nursing, phases of transition and milestones can be uncovered leading to more specific interventions congruent with each phase and milestone. Part IV of this book is devoted to introducing three well-conceptualized and investigated models of care during transitions. Although these models of care are used most often, there may be others that could be uncovered, or they may even already exist. The transitional care model is introduced and discussed as a model of choice for older adults and those with chronic illness. Creating healthy transitional environments is the crux of the transitional care model. Another model for enhancing healthy transitions is role supplementation, which was used for helping new parents, enhancing positive outcomes during cardiac rehabilitation, as a nursing intervention for patients with Alzheimer's, and in easing the transition of new patients into a psychiatric hospital.

The third care model selected for this volume is debriefing. Nurses have used this model of allowing patients to process critical events through dialogue, recreating situations, and/or through reminiscing. Several articles were selected to describe this model and to demonstrate its strengths and weaknesses.

Having a focus on transitions promotes a coherent use of different theories. In fact, different theories could guide the analyses of transitions and the development of nursing therapeutics to facilitate the transitions that people go through. Examples of theories that could be used are psychoanalysis, ecology, problem solving, and task orientations (Golan, 1981). For example, when we consider the transition experience from a psychoanalytic approach, we tend to ask questions related to early childhood experiences, personality changes, personality formation, and ego structures in dealing with transitions. An adaptation framework drives questions of coping with an outside situation, and on individual capacity to adapt. A problem-solving model of transitions relies on the cognitive abilities of clients to assess and plan for dealing with the process and consequences of transitions. Crisis theories are also useful for helping clients and communities deal with the crises that initiated the transition and the aftermath of a crisis.

Another useful theory is role theory, which provides a framework to describe and anticipate roles lost, modified, or acquired, and the processes, the behaviors, and the sentiments attached to them. In addition, a theory that is based on structural and psychosocial resources can add to nurses' repertoires in describing clients' transitions. A feminist postcolonialist framework will drive different sets of questions that incorporate the effects of inequality and societal oppressions on differential treatment of individuals experiencing transitions (Kirkham & Anderson, 2001). Each of these theories drives different questions and approaches to research, but all could lead to a more coherent whole and a focus on knowledge developments. With the establishment of the New Courtland Center for Transitions and Health at the University of Pennsylvania, under the leadership of Dr. Mary Naylor and its endowment by New Courtland, transitions and health will continue to grow and new models of care will emerge.

Identifying "transitions" as a central concern for nursing and developing coherent frameworks to describe transition may provide the impetus for uncovering the mechanisms used by diverse populations to experience different changes in their lives that lead to health–illness consequences (some are healthy and others are not), and to advance knowledge about nursing therapeutics that facilitate the transition experience and enhance healthy coping and healing.

This textbook is offered to provide clinicians and scientists with the knowledge and the impetus to continue to ask and answer critical questions and provide the knowledge base to enhance the transition experience, to prevent unhealthy transitions, and to promote well-being of patients, families, organizations, and communities. It is a testament to how clinical practice informs theory development, how theory drives programs of research, and how programs of research can influence policies that change practice. Although the focus may be on the concept of transitions, which is considered central in the discipline of nursing, the selection of chapters for inclusion reflects the connection between a central concept and how it is connected to research, practice, education, and policies. Similar collections focused on a nursing concept can help bring more coherence and integration to our discipline.

Though so much has been written, researched, and defined about transitions, transitions as a focal area of inquiry for nurse scientists is still wide open. Advancing nursing knowledge about the experience and the responses of the many transitions that individuals, families, and communities tend to encounter as well as the experiences, the responses, and the therapeutics that nurses tend to use will ultimately be translated to evidence-based practice and better quality care in the 21st century.

REFERENCES

Adlersberg, M., & Thorne, S. (1990). Emerging from the chrysalis: Older widows in transition. *Journal of Gerontological Nursing, 16,* 4–8.

Battles, R. S. (1988). Transition entry groups: Easing new patients' adjustment to psychiatric hospitalization. *Hospital and Community Psychiatry, 39*(3), 312–313.

Blakeslee, J. A., Goldman, B. D., Papougenis, D., & Torell, C. A. (1991). Making the transition to restraint-free care. *Journal of Gerontological Nursing, 17,* 4–8.

Bridges, E. J. (1992). Transition from ventilatory support: Knowing when the patient is ready to wean. *Critical Care Nursing Quarterly, 15*(1), 14–20.

Bridges, W. (1980). *Transitions: Making sense of life's changes.* New York: Da Capo Press.

Bridges, W. (1991). *Managing transitions: Making the most of change.* New York: Da Capo Press.

Brokel, J. M., & Harrison, M. I. (2009). Redesigning care processes using an electronic health record: A system's experience. *Joint Commission Journal on Quality and Patient Safety, 35*(2), 82–92.

Brouse, A. J. (1988). Easing the transition to the maternal role. *Journal of Advanced Nursing, 13,* 167–172.

Brown, M. A., & Powell-Cope, G. M. (1991). AIDS family caregiving: Transitions through uncertainty. *Nursing Research, 40,* 338–345.

Catanzaro, M. (1990). Transitions in midlife adults with long-term illness. *Holistic Nursing Practice, 4*(3), 65–73.

Chick, N., & Meleis, A. I. (1986). A nursing concern. In P. L. Chinn (Ed.), *Nursing research methodology: Issues and implementation* (pp. 237–257). Rockville, MD: Aspen.

Christman, N. J., McConnell, E. A., Pfeiffer, C., Webster, K. K., Schmitt, M., & Ries, J. (1988). Unverainty, coping, and distress following myocardial infarction: Transition from hospital to home. *Research in Nursing and Health, 11,* 71–82.

Condi, J. K., Oliver, A., & Williams, E. (1986). Managing the transition to a neuroscience unit. *Journal of Neuroscience Nursing, 18,* 200–205.

De Bonde, K., & Hamilton, R. (1991). Dysphagia: A staged transition to oral nutrition. *Australian Nurses Journal, 20*(7), 12–13.

Dougherty, C. M. (1990). The near-death experience as a major life transition. *Holistic Nursing Practice, 4*(3), 84–90.

Ehrat, K. S. (1990). Leadership in transition. *Journal of Nursing Administration, 20,* 6–7.

Gilmore, T. N. (1990). Effective leadership during organizational transitions. *Nursing Economics, 8,* 135–141.

Golan, N. (1981). *Passing through transitions.* New York: Free Press.

Gonzales-Osler, E. (1989). Coping with transition. *Journal of Psychosocial Nursing and Mental Health Services, 27*(6), 29, 32–35.

Hall, J. M., Stevens, P. E., & Meleis, A. I. (1994). Marginalization: A guiding concept for valuing diversity in nursing knowledge development. *Advances in Nursing Science, 16*(4), 23–41.

Harper, W. (1989). Transition. *Canadian Nurse, 85*(9), 32–34.

Hegyvary, S. T., & de Tornyay, R. (1991). Transition in the deanship. *Journal of Professional Nursing, 7*, 41–44.

Henderson, A. D. (1989). Use of social support in a transition house for abused women. *Health Care for Women International, 10*, 61–73.

Im, E. O. (2003). Symptoms experienced during the menopausal transition: Korean women in South Korea and the U.S. *Journal of Transcultural Nursing, 14*(4), 321–328.

Im, E. O., & Meleis, A. I. (2001). Women's work and symptoms during menopausal transition: Korean immigrant women. *Women and Health, 33*(1/2), 93–103.

Imle, M. A. (1990). Third trimester concerns of expectant parents in transition to parenthood. *Holistic Nursing Practice, 4*(3), 25–36.

Imle, M. A., & Atwood, J. R. (1988). Retaining qualitative validity while gaining quantitative reliability and validity: Development of the transition to parenthood concerns scale. *Advances in Nursing Science, 11*(1), 61–75.

Kerfoot, K., Serafin-Dickson, F., & Green, S. (1988). Managing transition: Resigning with style from the nurse manager position. *Nursing Economics, 6*, 200–202.

Kirkham, S. R., & Anderson, J. M. (2001). Postcolonial nursing scholarship: From epistemology to method. *Advances in Nursing Science, 25*(1), 1–17.

Losee, R. H., & Cook, J. W. (1989). Managing organizational transition. *Nursing Management, 20*(9), 82–83.

Loveys, B. (1990). Transitions in chronic illness: The at-risk role. *Holistic Nursing Practice, 4*(3), 54–64.

Main, S., Mishler, S., Ayers, B., Poppa, L. D., & Jones, T. (1989). Easing transitions in care delivery with a core training group. *Nursing Connections, 2*(4), 5–15.

Majewski, J. (1986). Conflicts, satisfactions, and attitudes during transition to the maternal role. *Nursing Research, 35*, 10–14.

Majewski, J. (1987). Social support and the transition to the maternal role. *Health Care for Women International, 8*, 397–407.

Meleis, A. I. (1971). Self concept and family planning. *Nursing Research, 20*, 29–36.

Meleis, A. I. (1975). Role insufficiency and role supplementation: A conceptual framework. *Nursing Research, 24*, 264–271.

Meleis, A. I. (1993, June). *A passion for substance revisited: Global transitions and international commitments.* Published Keynote Speech given at the 1993 National Doctoral Forum, St. Paul, MN.

Meleis, A. I., & Swendsen, P. A. (1978). Role supplementation: An empirical test of a nursing intervention. *Nursing Research, 27*, 11–18.

Meleis, A. I., & Trangenstein, P. A. (1994). Facilitating transitions: Redefinition of a nursing mission. *Nursing Outlook, 42*(6), 255–259.

Moody, L. E., Scocumb, E., Berg, B., & Jackson, D. (2004). Electronic health records documentation in nursing: Nurses' perceptions, attitudes, and preferences. *Computers, Informatics, Nursing, 22*(6), 337–344.

Poncar, P. J. (1989). The elderly widow: Easing her role transition. *Journal of Psychosocial Nursing and Mental Health Services, 27*(2), 6–11, 39–40.

Pridham, K. F., & Chang, A. S. (1992). Transition to being the mother of a new infant in the first three months: Maternal problem solving and self-appraisals. *Journal of Advanced Nursing, 17*, 204–216.

Pridham, K. F., Lytton, D., Chang, A. S., & Rutledge, D. (1991). Early postpartum transition: Progress in maternal identity and role attainment. *Research in Nursing and Health, 14*, 321–327.

Reimer, J. C., Davies, B., & Martens, N. (1991). Palliative care: The nurse's role in helping families through the transition of "fading away." *Cancer Nursing, 14*, 321–327.

Rotkovitch, R., & Smith, C. (1987). ICON I—The future model; ICON II—The transition model. *Nursing Management, 18*(11), 91–92, 94–96.

Sakraida, T. (2005). Divorce transition differences of midlife women. *Issues in Mental Health Nursing, 26*(2), 225–249.

Sandfield, A. (2006). Talking divorce: The role of divorce in women's constructions of relationship status. *Feminism & Psychology, 16*(2), 155–173.

Schumacher, K., & Meleis, A. I. (1994). Transitions: A central concept in nursing. *Image: Journal of Nursing Scholarship, 26*(2), 119–127.

Schumacher, K. L. (1995). Family caregiver role acquisition: Role-making through situated interaction. *Scholarly Inquiry for Nursing Practice, 9*(3), 211–226; discussion 227–229.

Selder, F. (1989). Life transition theory: The resolution of uncertainty. *Nursing and Health Care, 10*, 437–451.

Shields, N. A. (1991). The transition to video: Considerations for the GI laboratory manager. *Gastroenterology Nursing, 14*(1), 44–47.

Stevens, P. E., Hall, J. M., & Meleis, A. I. (1992). Examining vulnerability of women clerical workers from five ethnic racial groups. *Western Journal of Nursing Research, 14*(6), 754–774.

Swearingen, L. (1987). Transitional day treatment: An individualized goal-oriented approach. *Archives of Psychiatric Nursing, 1,* 104–110.

Taylor, A. J. W., & Frazer, A. G. (1982). The stress of post disaster body handling and victim identification work. *Journal of Human Stress, 8,* 4–22.

Thurber, F., & DiGiamarino, L. (1992). Development of a model of transitional care for the HIV-positive child and family. *Clinical Nurse Specialist, 6,* 142–146.

Tierney, M. J., Grant, L. M., Cherrstrom, P. L., & Morris, B. L. (1990). Clinical nurse specialists in transition. *Clinical Nurse Specialist, 4,* 103–106.

Tomlinson, P. S. (1987). Spousal differences in marital satisfaction during transition to parenthood. *Nursing Research, 36,* 239–243.

Turley, J. P. (1992). A framework for the transition from nursing records to a nursing information system. *Nursing Outlook, 40,* 177–181.

Vezeau, T. M., & Hallsten, D. A. (1987). Making the transition to mother–baby care. *Maternal–Child Nursing, 12,* 193–198.

Walker, K., & deVooght, J. (1989). Invasion: A hospital in transition following the 1983 Grenadian intervention. *Journal of Psychosocial Nursing and Mental Health Services, 27*(1), 27–30.

Wild, L. (1992). Transition from pain to comfort: Managing the hemodynamic risks. *Critical Care Nursing Quarterly, 15*(1), 46–56.

II

Transitions as a Nursing Theory

Transitions are triggered by critical events and changes in individuals or environments. The transition experience begins as soon as an event or change is anticipated. Though human beings always face many changes throughout the lifespan that trigger internal processes, nurses come face to face with people going through a transition when and if it relates to their health, well-being, and their ability to take care of themselves. In addition, nurses deal with the environments that support or hamper personal, communal, familial, or population transitions. To capture the definition, meaning, conditions, and outcomes of transitions, it helps to have frameworks that provide coherence and direction from which to ask questions and develop research programs.

Transitions have been defined many different ways. A common definition used in this text is that it is a passage from one fairly stable state to another fairly stable state, and it is a process triggered by a change. Transitions are characterized by different dynamic stages, milestones, and turning points and can be defined through processes and/or terminal outcomes.

This section presents theoretical articles that were published to describe transition, define transition as a central concept in nursing, and detail the emerging middle-range theory of the transition experience. I trace the beginning of the theory of transitions from conceptualizing the potential problems that individuals may suffer from if they are not properly prepared for a transitional experience (role insufficiency), and describe the development of preventative as well as therapeutic intervention (role supplementation). The emergence of transition as a nursing concern, the supporting centrality of the concept in nursing through an extensive literature review, as well as the evolution of transition theory from concept to theory over 3 decades of thinking and writing about transitions are all reflected here. The chapters in this section represent the development of transition theory over 3 decades. Therefore, the sequence of the articles in these two chapters reflects the historical evolution of the theory ending with an integrative review of literature related to transitions.

Chapter 1 Theoretical Development of Transitions

1.1 ROLE INSUFFICIENCY AND ROLE SUPPLEMENTATION: A CONCEPTUAL FRAMEWORK

AFAF IBRAHIM MELEIS

Abstract

A theoretical basis for the diagnosis of nursing problems, centered on the concepts of role insufficiency and role supplementation, is offered. Role insufficiency is anticipated and experienced by clients during role transitions with developmental, situational, and health–illness implications. The conceptual basis of nursing intervention is role supplementation, and components, strategies, and processes of role supplementation are described. Conditions that predispose clients in the health setting to undergo role transition, conditions under which aspects of role transition may become nursing problems, and the role of the nurse in dealing with clients' role transition problems are described. A predictive and prescriptive paradigm, showing the interaction of construct components, is presented.

A theoretical construct and propositions for nursing care, utilizing concepts of roles and role transitions (Burr, 1972; Cottrell, 1942) designed to stimulate the development and pursuit of researchable problems that add to a body of nursing knowledge, while also providing a systematic framework for nursing diagnosis and intervention, are proposed.

Role as a sociopsychological construct is particularly useful in assessing nursing problems and in planning nursing intervention modalities. Because professional nurses deal with clients as biopsychosocial beings, the ability to understand the behavior of clients is imperative for making appropriate diagnosis and intervention. Nurses and other health workers can no longer separate psychosocial influences on clients' health and well-being. In caring for patients, nurses encounter numerous situations of role change, such as the transition from wellness to illness, birth, or death. Nurses, therefore, are in the most opportune position to assess the client's psychosocial needs during role transitional periods and provide the necessary interventions based upon the individual's needs and deprivations created by role transitions.

Although such nursing assessments and ensuing interventions during role transition are essential nursing contributions in all cultures, the need is more acute in more stressful, dynamic, and mobile societies. The dynamic changes that have happened, and are happening, in the structure of the family and the community in Western society intensify the effects of even the most natural and simple role transitions. The network of available social resources that are an integral part of the structure of the less mobile, less developed societies provide for some of the components of the role supplementation intervention modality.

Social conditions also affect the behavior of the role incumbent during role changes. When social conditions permit congruent role definitions, role transitions—being more or less predictable and well defined (Glaser & Strauss, 1971)—are accomplished with relatively little friction and psychosocial discomfort. When, however, definitions and role norms are not widely shared and supported within a given society, personal and interpersonal role enactment problems are created. This situation can result from many factors; social mobility, technological change, cultural differences are examples of intermingling sources of tension and misunderstanding. The resulting anomic stage, termed "role insufficiency," becomes prevalent.

The Concept of Role and Its Relevance to Nursing

By role is meant following not "merely a set of behaviors or expected behaviors, but a sentiment or goal which provides unity to a set of potential actions" (Turner, 1959, p. 26). Turner (1968) suggested that:

> [I]n any interactive situation, behavior, sentiments, and motives tend to be differentiated into units, which can be called roles; once roles are differentiated, elements of behavior, sentiments, and motives which appear in the same situation tend to be assigned to the existing roles. (p. 4)

Thus, role as discussed in this study refers to the symbolic interactionist use of the concept, one developed by George Herbert Mead (1934) and elaborated in contemporary literature. Role in this sense is conceptualized as a way of coping with an imputed other role (Cottrell, 1942; Turner, 1962). Role in this conception does not deny the importance of the situation but considers it as an additional factor in defining roles.

Role, as a concept, is useful in interpreting personal behavior vis-à-vis significant others and in understanding the context in which behavior takes place. Through this concept such interpretations can be made without losing sight of the standardized effects of society's demands on an individual. Role theory emphasizes the notion that human behavior is not a simple matter of stimulus–response reaction, but the result of a complex interaction between ego and society. It synthesizes the culture, the social structure, and the self by considering culture and social structure from the individual's level.

There are three major schools of thought in role theory. The first is the Lintonian approach which views roles as culturally given prescriptions (Linton, 1936, 1945), whereas the second defines role in terms of the actions and expectations of individual members of a society (Parsons, 1951; Parsons & Fox, 1952; Sarbin, 1954, 1968).

The third school of thought, the one adopted in this chapter, conceives of role as stemming from interaction with actors in a social system. In this school, role emerges in a designated reciprocity in which an interaction or a social exchange occurs and is seen in terms of relevant other roles. The role that the actor elects to play is a derivative of his voluntary actions that are motivated by the returns expected, and, indeed, received from others. In addition, the role assumed by an interactant in a given situation is validated when others indicate acceptance of that role allocation. Thus, roles chosen by the patient are validated by the acceptance of his significant others such as the nurse and members of his family. Once a role evolves, the need to reciprocate in role behaviors becomes actually a need for benefits received in order to continue receiving them. As Gouldner (1960, p. 176) pointed out, reciprocation acts as a starting mechanism in the interaction process. The exchange process and the rewards and losses and the ratio between them continue to influence the development of the role played by the ego in the significant alter's presence (Blau, 1964, pp. 145–146).

Through interaction and the role-taking processes with the significant other, each person's roles are discovered, created, modified, and defined. These roles are thus incorporated in the ego's self-conception. In general terms, then, self-conception is actually a conception of how one relates to major significant other roles.

Effective health care requires a broader perspective than that circumscribed by the emergency room, the outpatient department, and/or the hospital. Davis (1963) emphasized that

> there certainly seems a need for a broader definition of a therapeutic activity by treatment personnel. Such a definition would not be confined to the routine, neatly bounded tasks of diagnosis, prescription, and physical treatment but would seek to embrace in addition the many problematic issues of communication, motivation, and social circumstances that also play a part in the state of the patient's health and in the meaning his illness has for him and his family. (p. 173)

Given the strategic position of the nursing staff vis-à-vis the patient, and given the theoretic and dynamic promise of role theory, it seems apparent that role theory can provide an excellent basis for the diagnosis of nursing problems related to the psychosocial dimensions of role and role transitions—a diagnosis which should prove to be of the utmost value in planning for appropriate intervention.

Conditions Predisposing to Problematic Role Transition

Role transition denotes a change in role relationships, expectations, or abilities. Role transitions require the person to incorporate new knowledge, alter his behavior, and thus change his definition of himself in his social context. A number of role transitions are related to the health and illness cycle and should be taken into account by health care personnel—most appropriately, because of her strategic position, by the nurse. Probable manifestations of role insufficiency in each category are depicted in Table 1.1.1. These include developmental, situational, and health–illness transitions.

Developmental Transitions

Numerous role transitions are encountered in the normal course of growth and development. Two significant transitions may be associated with significant health problems (both mental and physiologic): (a) from childhood to adolescence, associated with well-recognized problems of identity formation and with ensuing problems such as drug misuse, venereal diseases, sexuality problems, and unwed motherhood; and (b) from adulthood to old age, accompanied by gerontologic problems relating to identity, retirement, and chronic illness.

Because it is inconceivable that a role can exist without a counterrole to reinforce and complement it, changes in one role necessitate complementary adjustments in the counterrole. In other words, changes have to be made in the behavior of one or more other persons in ego's social circle. Conversely, while ego may not have personally induced role transition, any role transition by a spouse, a parent, a child, or close friend may force a change reciprocally.

Hence, developmental changes undergone by the patient himself and by a significant other should be considered by the health team. Reciprocal changes should be anticipated, explored, and considered when plans for intervention are being considered.

Situational Transitions

These transitions involve the addition or the subtraction of persons in a preexisting constellation of roles and complements. Examples are addition or loss of a member of the family through birth or death. Each such situation requires definition and redefinition of the roles involved in the constellation of interactions. A nurse is a key figure in such situations.

That there is a marked difference in the pattern and quality of interpersonal relationships according to whether a dyad or a triad is involved has been meticulously analyzed in terms of its psychosocial implications of these differences by Georg Simmel (1964).

The transition from nonparental to a parental status is of well-recognized cultural and psychoso-

TABLE 1.1.1 Components of Role Insufficiency and Probable Manifestations

Predisposing areas to role insufficiency	Probable Manifestations		
	Role loss	Role acquisition	Concomitant loss and acquisition
Developmental	Grief and mourning, powerlessness	Anxiety, depression, withdrawal	Combinations[1]
Situational Health–illness	↓	Combinations[1] ↓	↓

[1]Most probably combinations of manifestations of role insufficiency are present at the same time.

cial importance. This situation not only involves major shifts in personal and interpersonal conceptions vis-à-vis the larger society but also requires the adjustments of the smaller systems when the addition of a third person (the infant) shifts the structure of the group from dyad to triad with significant role and complementary role changes that may cause conflict if they are unanticipated, unrecognized, and ignored.

Health–Illness Transitions

This category includes such transitions as sudden role changes that result from moving from a well state to an acute illness; gradual role changes from well to sick (the quality of this transition is significantly different from that of sudden role changes because its gradual nature allows time for gradual incorporation of the behavior and sentiments of the new role); role changes from sickness to wellness; sudden or gradual role transition from wellness to chronic illness.

Each such role transition should be considered in terms of pairs of roles or in the context of a system. For health purposes, therefore, the patient cannot be considered as an isolated unit, but changes in his condition must be explored and considered in terms of his relationship in a network of significant others.

Complementary Nature of the Transitions

Inherent in each of the transitions just described is the other component of the matrix being developed, that of role acquisition, role loss, or the simultaneous loss of one role and gain of another (Table 1.1.1). Role acquisition can be manifested in the changes from a dyadic to a triadic constellation in a situation such as the birth of a baby. Role loss is tied to the loss of some person or of a counterrole. Examples of the simultaneous loss of one role and acquisition of another are numerous. Even the last situation might illustrate loss and acquisition. Other examples are a fashion model who has undergone an amputation, an expectant mother who has lost her first baby and undergone a hysterectomy at the same time, a geriatric client who in becoming old has lost his sense of independence, a primipara who in acquiring the mothering role has lost a number of cosmopolitan roles, the acutely sick person who while in the sick role has lost some roles such as father or executive, or the chronically ill person who acquired a crippled role and lost his role as a sportsman (Davis, 1963).

Role Insufficiency

Role insufficiency is any difficulty in the cognizance and/or performance of a role or of the sentiments and goals associated with the role behavior as perceived by the self or by significant others. The perceived arduousness might result from incongruity between role behavior and the role expectations of the self or of significant others. It is characterized by behaviors and sentiments affiliated with the perception of disparity in fulfilling role obligations or expectations.

Role insufficiency denotes the behavior and sentiments affiliated with any felt disparity in fulfilling role obligations or expectations of self and/or significant others in a health-illness situation. It denotes the incongruency of the self-concept and the role anticipations of others as seen by self or others. It further characterizes an ego confronted with a number of expectations that in its own perception cannot be articulated (Stryker, 1959, pp. 117–119).

In other words, the perception of role performance as inadequate by the self and/or by a significant other, and the behavior and sentiment associated with such perception, in any of the following situations may be called role insufficiency:

- Moving in or out of roles in a social system (more specifically for purposes of this paper, a health system).
- Voluntary or involuntary additions or terminations of roles with or without changes in other roles.
- The concomitant termination of a role or set of roles and beginning of a new role or set of roles.

Role insufficiency may also result from poor role definition, the inner dynamics of role relationships, or simply from lack of knowledge of role behaviors, sentiments, and goals. It may also be generated when perceptions or interpretation of role behavior cues are impaired or absent.

On the other hand, an individual might possibly totally refuse to enact a specific role. Role motivation is a function of the rewards to be derived, the cost the role taken incurs, and the balance between rewards and costs. When a person refuses to enact a specific role, he has made a decision that the costs outweigh the gains. In such a case, role insufficiency is voluntary, self-initiated, and reinforced by a significant other. Thus, a role that an individual decides to assume is a derivative of his voluntary action motivated by the rewards expected and achieved. It also derives from appropriate reinforcements and role clarity. If ego misperceives and, hence, misperforms a role, and alter adjusts his complementary role accordingly, deleterious consequences most probably will not develop.

On the other hand, involuntary role insufficiency may be demonstrated in a variety of ways. Among these are anxiety, depression, apathy, frustrations, grief, powerlessness, unhappiness and/or aggression, and hostility (Table 1.1.1). Any of these could impede a person's maintenance or progression toward health, well-being, and his comfortable adaptation to role transition and should be subjected to empirical exploration, testing, and verification.

Role Supplementation: A Nursing Intervention

In the course of a lifetime an individual passes through many transitional phases that entail extensive mobilization of personal resources to cope with the stresses any change initiates. Changes in roles, loss of some roles, and acquisition of new ones are of particular significance to nurses, because, as noted, health and illness (acute and chronic), situational transformations, and developmental stages directly initiate a number of important role changes.

Role supplementation is defined as any deliberative process whereby role insufficiency or potential role insufficiency is identified by the role incumbent and significant others, and the conditions and strategies of role clarification and role taking are used to develop a preventive or therapeutic intervention to decrease, ameliorate, or prevent role insufficiency. Role supplementation is further defined as the conveying of information or experience necessary to bring the role incumbent and significant others to full awareness of the anticipated behavior patterns, units, sentiments, sensations, and goals involved in each role and its complement. It includes necessary knowledge and experience that emphasizes heightened awareness of one's own roles and other's role and the dynamics of the interrelationships. It encompasses the informal roles and informal role conception (or unofficial roles) as well as the formal or official role systems.

Role supplementations may be both preventive and therapeutic. When role supplementation is used as a way of clarifying roles for persons anticipating transition, it acts as a preventive measure. Public health nurses have been involved mainly in preventive role supplementation in their work with expectant mothers. However, these efforts have not always been made early enough nor systematically enough to hinder role insufficiency from developing.

Therapeutic role supplementation, on the other hand, is resorted to when role insufficiency has become manifest. A client, for example, experiencing apathy and alienation with suicidal fantasies after retirement, may benefit from therapeutic role supplementation. In this case, reminiscence groups, alternative new roles, and new groups might make up an appropriate role supplementation program.

Components, Strategies, and Processes

Role supplementation is operationalized into components, strategies, and processes. Components that comprise the role supplementation nursing intervention construct are those of role clarification and role taking. Strategies used to achieve the goals of heightened role clarification and role taking are role modeling, role rehearsal, and reference group interactions. Communication is the process that both facilitates the implementation of the strategies and enhances the achievement of mastery over the role supplementation components (i.e., role clarification and role taking).

> *The patient cannot be effectively considered as an isolated unit, but changes in his condition must be explored and considered in terms of his relationship in a network of significant others.*

The conception of role supplementation as such was reduced to a number of components, strategies, and processes to subject it to research questions and hypotheses, and for pragmatic clinical use. Such reduction permits the selection of appropriate research tools from corresponding fields. For example, to explore hypotheses that refer to the significance of reference groups, tools could be adapted from previous research on group research from the fields of psychology, sociology, and psychiatric nursing, among others. The area of psychodrama contains tools for practice and research related to role taking and communication. Many research tools are adaptable for the exploration of the communication component in the nursing intervention construct presented here.

As a conceptual basis for a nursing intervention process, role supplementation is operationalized to incorporate role clarification, role taking, role modeling, and role rehearsal, reference group, and communication and interaction.

Role Clarification

Mastery of the knowledge or the specific information and cues needed to perform a role is known as role clarification. It is the identification of role-linked behaviors, sentiments, and goals associated with a role vis-à-vis significant others in the context of the situation. In the course of a lifetime a person discards old roles, assumes new ones, modifies existing roles, or simultaneously manages several—in terms of their demands—incompatible roles. Thus, role clarification becomes essential to the role incumbent.

To enact a role, the individual ego needs a sense of the social boundaries of role as a unit, a clear idea about the sort of role behavior his significant others expect him to enact, and an awareness of mutual expectations in the complementary role. Role clarification requires that the person reduce the ambiguity and conflict involved in meeting and transmitting role expectations.

An evolvement and understanding of a role supplementation program and its essential component, role clarification, could be enhanced through a knowledge of how roles are learned.

Roles are learned and incorporated in a variety of ways. One way is through interactions with relevant others singly or in groups. In this instance, roles may be analyzed and broken down into units of behavior based on reciprocal interaction. Although expectations and previous experience influence the identification of roles, the actual analysis must focus on behavior in an interactive situation.

Role learning may be motivated by certain rewards—positive, negative, or threatening. Role modeling is another means of learning; by observing significant others enacting and playing a certain role, an individual is able to understand and emulate the intricacies of behaviors in a particular role. The fourth mode of role learning is intentional role instruction which occurs in socializing children or adults to specific new roles, but particularly in adult socializing experiences where role learning is made more explicit and pursued deliberately. Examples are numerous of the need for further role instruction guided by the definition of role as offered here, such as in nursing, in which nursing students are taught different roles involved in their profession. However, couples getting married, acquiring partner roles, becoming mothers and fathers, and encountering among similar situations receive, in most cases, very little intentional preparation. Similarly, and even more important in its implication for nursing, is the complete lack of intentional formal instruction in role expectations for patients in the process of changing roles from sick to well, well to sick, or any point between (Davis, 1963, pp. 109–134).

Thus, the individual acquires and masters the behaviors and the sentiments of new roles and transitional roles through gaining knowledge of:

- what the role entails in terms of behavior;
- what the role entails in terms of sentiments and goals; and
- costs and rewards, whether a significant other reinforces the roles negatively or positively.

Thus, role supplementation may become the means for achievement of role mastery.

The strategies for role clarification and role taking are role modeling, role rehearsal, and reference group interaction. The processes utilized for role learning and role clarification are communication and social interaction.

Role Taking

The second essential component, role taking, involves the empathic abilities of ego, both cognitively and affectively. Lindesmith and Strauss (1968) defined role taking as "imaginatively assuming the position or point of view of another person" (p. 282). The ability to take the role of the other is the sine qua non of smooth social interaction and smooth role transition. Role taking is a key concept in the social theory of George Herbert Mead (1934). The self plans and enacts his role by vicariously assuming the role of the other. This further suggests that individuals learn roles in pairs and not singly (Turner, 1970). As with role clarification, key strategies of role taking are those of role modeling, role rehearsal, and reference group interaction. This suggestion leads to the first proposition.

Role transition is less difficult for the ego who has learned to enact a role and counterrole imaginatively and if the significant other understands the salient components of the transitions as it involves ego and the significant other.

Role Modeling

When the significant other is observed enacting and playing a certain role so that an individual is able to understand and emulate the intricacies of behaviors in that role, role modeling occurs (Bandura, 1963). Attributes imitation or role modeling is the most prevalent type of social role learning, and even more so for the child. The process is defined by Mowrer (1960) as imitation, learned through a process of trial-and-error learning, without direct or extrinsic reinforcement for imitation. Thus, role modeling proceeds without direct tuition, or clear learning goals delineated by the models or by the learners.

In a face-to-face society, role modeling is intensive and ensures accurate and relatively smooth role transitions. However, in a highly developed, mobile, technical society intensive role modeling is reduced to a minimum. For example, frequently children are removed from grandparents as significant role models for aging and dying. Or with the small nuclear family, children may not see their parents as role models for child rearing. The impact of role modeling is further reduced in a nontraditional culture, since the role modeling provided by the previous generation is too discontinuous with the new realities. The way mother or grandparents reared children is not considered up-to-date or is incongruent with current cultural values and expectations. Because most acute illness occurs in the institutional setting and the very ill are seldom cared for in the home, the patient role is seldom modeled and becomes isolated from the family's or significant others' perception of how one acts when one is very ill, or what it means to be very ill.

Role Rehearsal

As a concept, role rehearsal refers to a phase in the variable career of interaction (Blumer, 1969). This phase is characterized by internal activity, preceding overt interaction, in which the individual fantasizes, imagines, and mentally enacts how an encounter might take place and how a role might evolve. In other words, the individual mentally enacts his role, anticipating in imagination the responses of significant others.

Role rehearsal, thus, has a crucial function in anticipating and planning the course of future actions and is an important prelude to role taking.

Role rehearsal does not proceed on the assumption that roles will be rigidly structured. The roles that will finally evolve in actual enactment may be quite different from those rehearsed in fantasy. However, rehearsal enables the individual and the significant other to anticipate behavior and sentiments associated with the roles rehearsed. Or, as stated in Proposition 2:

Role rehearsal enables the individual and others in a health–illness situation to master the behavior and sentiments associated with the transitional roles and thus decrease the experience and manifestations of role insufficiency.

Reference Group

A viable role supplementation program should capitalize on the importance of a significant other and/or others in reinforcing new roles and counterroles. Role supplementation should be provided in the context of an appropriately designated reference group involving the self and appropriate significant others as an essential strategy.

To design a role supplementation program, the significant others must be identified. Appropriate strategies and processes of social learning, that is, role modeling, role rehearsal, intentional role instruction, and communication and interaction opportunities, must be designed to prepare or assist persons with role clarification and role taking before or during a role transition. Such programs would have to be outlined and made specific so that persons participating could shape and influence their own role learning.

The literature is rich with examples of the importance and appropriateness of utilizing the reference group media in transitional situations. For example, in anticipation of parental roles, both husband and wife should be in a group with others in a similar situation. Other examples are a colostomy group, a reminiscence group, a single mothers' group.

A postcoronary discussion group with coronary patients and their wives, for example, could be conducted on a postcoronary unit in a hospital setting. Program components should allow for: role modeling; a successfully rehabilitated coronary patient could come and speak; films might be used; role-play situations in which the actor practices limiting his/her schedule in areas identified as stressful and overloading; and an information-giving component where exercise, diet, preventive aspects of managing coronary disease are presented. As noted in Proposition 3:

The peer group, which is an essential strategy of role supplementation, provides the appropriate locus to facilitate role transition.

Communication and Interaction

Communication, the mechanism by which meaning is constructed, is a key process in role supplementation and is the central concept of symbolic interactionist theory, particularly as elaborated by George Herbert Mead (1934). Human communication is a behavioral process based on a system of shared symbols whereby meanings are conveyed and interpreted among social interactants. "Meanings arise…out of group activities, and they come to stand for relationships between actors and object" (Lindesmith & Strauss, 1968, p. 70). Meaning is possible, according to Mead (1934), because the human being possesses, biologically, the ability to create objects.

Human communication, according to Mead, depends upon the sharing of significant symbols. Because the individual can anticipate the interpretation others will put upon his symbolic gestures, a pattern of meaning can be established and lines of intended action can be forged. This interpretation process is possible because human beings can, in the process of using and sharing symbols, create a world of meaningful objects and, the most salient point, the individual can become an object to himself and, thus, view himself in imagination as others view him.

As Mead said, "Gestures become significant symbols when they implicitly arouse in the individual making them the same responses they explicitly arouse, or are supposed to arouse in other individuals" (1934, p. 47). Because the human being can anticipate the response that his gesture (verbal or nonverbal) will produce in others, he is able to communicate meaning (Deutsch & Krauss, 1965, pp. 183–189).

Communication and interaction are central processes of role clarification and role taking and are thus central to role supplementation because it is through open and clear communication of symbols that roles evolve.

Role Supplementation as an Independent Variable

Role supplementation as a construct for a deliberative and planned nursing intervention that incorporates the component mastery[1] based on its strategies and processes can prevent and ameliorate or decrease role insufficiency during role transitions. Role supplementation, as an independent variable, may be explored in relationship to a number of variables. Explorations may involve its relationship with its components, strategies, and processes, or its relationship to the behavioral and physiologic manifestations of role insufficiency in the context of simple, difficult, or disjunctive role transitions.

The central question is whether the component mastery, using the strategies and processes of the role supplementation construct, can prevent, decrease, or ameliorate the degree or amount of role insufficiency experienced during a role transition. This broad question lends itself to the development of testable hypotheses in conditions that predispose to problematic role transitions.

Descriptive research is needed to identify and describe further the behavioral manifestations of role insufficiency syndrome, particularly as they are demonstrated in physiologic responses. Anger, hostility, withdrawal, confusion, depression, fatigue, and anxiety are some of the probable manifestations of role insufficiency that are diagnosed as such only when associated with special role transition's predisposing conditions. As the behaviors and variables that comprise role insufficiency are further delineated, more sophisticated tools and research designs for measuring the impact of role supplementation programs on role insufficiency can be developed.

Tools need to be developed, tested, and validated for testing hypotheses generated from the conceptual framework presented here. A number of research tools utilized in other fields, however, could be modified for the particular goals of nursing research. For example, until new tools are designed and refined, it is possible to measure the role taking as one component of empathic abilities (Feshbach & Kuchenbecker, 1974) of a person during a role transition using Dymond's (1949) Empathic Ability scale (Hobart & Fahlberg, 1965) or the Barrett and Lennard (1967) Relationship inventory. In the meantime, the current tools could be evaluated to assess their sensitivity to isolate and identify role insufficiency and its relationship to the components of role supplementation.

The ability to forecast accurately and realistically the salient and dynamic features of a new futuristic role, behaviors, demands, and the sentiments associated with it vis-à-vis a number of significant others as an indicator of role clarity is a fertile area for tool development. For example, if couples are asked to predict role changes after the birth of a child before the child is born and to measure changes after the child is born, a comparison between the realism of the forecast and the perception after the child is born can be made and considered an indication of the ambiguity or clarity of the role transition process.

Research tools used previously in other fields could be utilized for data related to the process and strategies of role supplementation, much in the same way as is proposed for the components, for example, for communication the Laing et al. (1966) Interpersonal Perception Method or the Hill (1961) Interaction Matrix could be used, depending on the nature of the research question. A number of broad research areas are delineated for the development of testable hypotheses. These areas may be summarized as the need for:

- The clinical definition of the role insufficiency syndrome and its relationship with a variety of

---

[1] Component mastery refers to role-taking and role-clarification mastery, role taking and role clarification being the two components of role supplementation.

role transitions by observing clients during role transitions, describing and collating their behaviors, reactions, and interactions surrounding the transition. (Previous research in this area could be used.)
- The development and adaptation of valid tools for the components, strategies, and processes of role supplementation.
- Studies to explore the relationship between role insufficiency and role supplementation.

Relationship Among Role Insufficiency, Role Mastery, and Role Supplementation

In addition to the three propositions already presented, at least two additional major propositions with important implications for the timing and nature of nursing interventions may be derived from the preceding analysis. The propositions are general and could be subjected to reduction into researchable hypotheses. Proposition 4 is stated positively:

The earlier preventive role supplementation is offered, the lower the probability of role insufficiency.

Temporarily, early preventive role supplementation allows an individual time to synthesize and incorporate anticipated role behavior into his repertoire (Table 1.1.2). Early supplementation also allows more time for significant others to evolve. Role modeling and role playing facilitate the process of role evaluation for ego and for significant others. Proposition 5 is stated negatively:

The later therapeutic role supplementation is provided, the higher the probability that role insufficiency will be manifested.

Therapeutic role supplementation after role insufficiencies have evolved decreases the probability of further role insufficiencies. However, personal and interpersonal conflicts are likely to have developed. Consequently, role supplementation should also deal with existing insufficiencies.

Table 1.1.2 illustrates the relationships among role insufficiency, role supplementation, and role mastery. Degrees of insufficiency are rank-ordered

TABLE 1.1.2 A Rank Order of Nursing Diagnoses According to None, Early, and Late Preventive and Therapeutic Role Supplementation

Preventive role supplementation	Therapeutic Role Supplementation		
	None	Early	Late
None	Highest insufficiency and lowest mastery (Rank 5)	Medium insufficiency and medium mastery (Rank 2)	Higher insufficiency and lower mastery (Rank 4)
Early	Medium insufficiency and medium mastery (Rank 2)	Lowest insufficiency and highest mastery (Rank 1)	Medium insufficiency and medium mastery (Rank 2)
Late	Higher insufficiency and lower mastery (Rank 4)	Medium insufficiency and medium mastery (Rank 2)	High insufficiency and low mastery (Rank 3)

in Table 1.1.2 in relation to early and late role supplementation and early therapeutic role supplementation. Insufficiency is manifested to the greatest degree when neither preventive nor late therapeutic role supplementations are offered (rank 5). The next highest degree of role insufficiency (rank 4) is manifested when only late therapeutic or only late preventive role supplementation is offered. When both preventive and early supplementation are offered late, role insufficiency is still somewhat high while mastery remains low (rank 4).

Role insufficiency is still manifested, but to a lesser degree, when early preventive and late therapeutic supplementation are offered (rank 2), only early therapeutic supplementation is offered (rank 2), only early preventive supplementation is offered (rank 2), or late preventive and early therapeutic supplementation are offered (rank 2).

Minimal role insufficiency is manifested when both early preventive and early therapeutic supple-

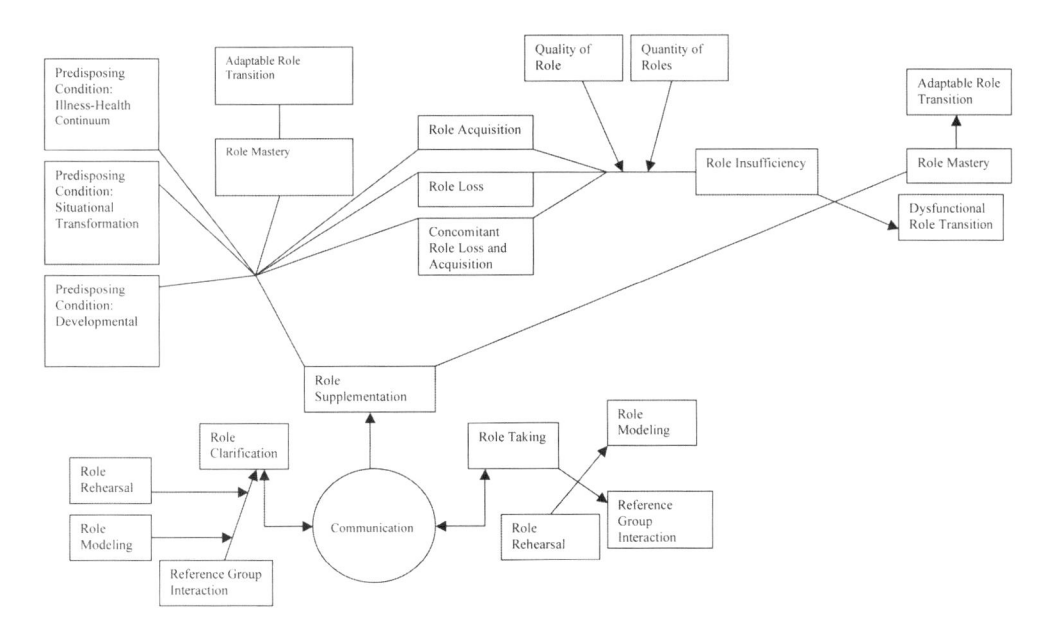

FIGURE 1.1.1 Role insufficiency and role supplementation: A predictive and prescriptive paradigm.

mentation are offered without interruption before role transition occurs and during the early stages of the transition (rank 1).

The concepts, variables, and predisposing conditions of role supplementation and its use in intervention of role insufficiency are presented in a flow chart in a predictive and prescriptive paradigm (see Figure 1.1.1), which depicts the general propositions set forth in this chapter.

REFERENCES

Bandura, A. The role of imitation in personality development. J Nurs Educ 18:207–215, Apr. 1963.

Barrett, H., and Lennard, G. T. Dimensions of therapist response as causal factors in therapeutic change. Psychol Monogr 76(43):1–36, 1967.

Blau, P. M. Exchange and Power in Social Life. New York, John Wiley and Sons, 1964.

Blumer, Herbert. Symbolic Interactionism: Perspective and Method. Englewood Cliffs, N.J., Prentice-Hall, 1969.

Burr, W. R. Role transition: A reformulation of theory. J Marriage Fam 34:407–416, Aug. 1972.

Cottrell, L. S., Jr. The adjustment of the individual to his age and sex roles. Am Sociol Rev 7:617–620, Oct. 1942.

Davis, Fred. Passage Through Crisis: Polio Victims and Their Families. Indianapolis, Ind., Bobbs-Merrill Co., 1963.

Deutsch, Morton, and Krauss, R. M. Theories in Social Psychology. New York, Basic Books, 1965.

Dymond, Rosalind. Measurement of empathic ability. J Consult Psychol 13:127–133, Apr. 1949.

Feshbach, Norma, and Kuchenbecker, Shari. A Three Component Model of Empathy. Paper presented at a meeting of the American Psychological Association, held at New Orleans, La., Sept. 1974. (Unpublished)

Glaser, B. G., and Strauss, A. L. Status Passage. Chicago, Aldine-Atherton, 1971.

Gouldner, A. W. The norm of reciprocity: A preliminary statement. Am Sociol Rev 25:161–178, Apr. 1960.

Hill, W. F. Hill Interaction Matrix Scoring Manual. Los Angeles. Youth Studies Center, University of Southern California, 1961.

Hobart, C. W., and Fahlberg, Nancy. The measurement of empathy. Am J Sociol 70:595–603, Mar. 1965.

Laing, R. D., and others. Interpersonal Perception: A Theory and Method of Research. New York, Springer Publishing Co., 1966.

Lindesmith, A. R., and Strauss, A. L. Social Psychology. 3d ed. New York, Holt, Rhinehart and Winston, 1968.

Linton, Ralph. The Study of Man. New York, D. Appleton-Century, 1936.
Cultural Background of Personality. New York, D. Appleton-Century, 1945.
Mead, G. H. Mind, Self and Society, introduction by C. W. Morris. Chicago, University of Chicago Press, 1934.
Mowrer, O. H. Learning Theory and the Symbolic Process. New York, John Wiley and Sons, 1960.
Parsons, Talcott. The Social System. Glencoe, Ill., Free Press, 1951.
Parsons, Talcott, and Fox, Renee. Illness, therapy and the modern urban American family. J Soc Issues 8:31–44, 1952.
Sarbin, Theodore. Role theory. In Handbook of Social Psychology, ed. by Gardner Lindzey. Cambridge, Mass., Addison Wesley Publishing Co., 1954, vol. 1, pp. 223–258.
Role theory. In The Handbook of Social Psychology. 2d edition edited by Gardner Lindzey and Elliott Aronson. Cambridge, Mass., Addison Wesley Publishing Co., 1968, vol. 1, pp. 488–567.
Simmel, Georg. The Sociology of Georg Simmel, translated and edited by K. H. Wolff. New York, Free Press, 1964.
Stryker, Sheldon. Symbolic interaction as an approach to family research. Marriage Fam Living 21:111–119, May 1959.
Turner, R. H. Role Taking as Process. Los Angeles, University of California, 1959. (Unpublished manuscript)
Turner, R. H. Role taking: Process vs. conformity. In Human Behavior and Social Processes, ed. by Arnold Rose. Boston, Houghton-Mifflin Co., 1962, pp. 20–40.
Turner, R. H. The self-conception in social interaction. In Self in Social Interaction, ed. by Chad Gordon and K. J. Gergen, New York, John Wiley and Sons, 1968.

Reprinted with permission from: Meleis, A. I. (1975). Role insufficiency and role supplementation: A conceptual framework. *Nursing Research, 24,* 264–271.

1.2 TRANSITIONS: A NURSING CONCERN

NORMA CHICK AND AFAF IBRAHIM MELEIS

Analysis is a methodological option in the development of knowledge in nursing. It is defined as a process of identifying parts and components, examining them against a number of identified criteria. Analysis includes both concept and theory analysis.

Concept analysis is a useful process in the cycle of theory development and testing and may occur at many points in the process. A number of structures have been provided in the literature as guidelines for concept analysis.[1-4] Strategies for analysis depend on levels of knowledge development within disciplines. As the boundaries of nursing domain develop and are sharpened, analysis takes on new dimensions. The use of multidimensional components of analyses that are more congruent with level of development in nursing would help in further developing nursing knowledge. The components used in analysis of transition are presented below. These may be used sequentially or nonsequentially.

1. Definition, identification, and description of the different dimensions and components of the concept. In defining different dimensions, a description of some of the antecedents to the concept and some of the consequences is essential, matching some of these descriptions with what occurs in nursing practice.
2. Examination and analysis of concept congruency with existing nursing theories and other domain concepts.
3. Development, description, and analysis of exemplars of model cases. This step may include clinical or empirical results that are related to the concept.
4. Comparison with other concepts with similar properties and dimensions to establish its boundaries.
5. Development, description, and analysis of contrary cases to the normal cases. Situations in which the concept appears sometimes or under a new set of conditions are called borderline cases and are also useful in analyzing concepts.
6. Analysis of the research potential related to the concept by consideration of its properties as dependent and independent variables. This component is completed when measurement issues are considered.

Each of these processes has a methodology of its own and could be used as a test of the occurrence of a concept. These tests are both conceptual and clinical. When these processes are complemented by testing through empirically valid and reliable research instruments, the cycle of theory-research-theory is complete.

The purpose of this chapter is twofold: To articulate an argument for the centrality of transitions as a concept within the domain of nursing by using the guidelines of concept analysis identified earlier and to provide an analysis of transition as an exemplar for concept analysis.

Definition, Dimensions, and Components of Transition

Transition is a familiar concept in developmental theories and in stress and adaptation theories. It accommodates both the continuities and discontinuities in the life processes of human beings. Transitions are invariably related to change and development, both of which are highly pertinent themes for nursing. Superimposed on developmental transitions are other forms of transition that are linked more directly to situational and health-illness events. One example of the latter is hospitalization for acute illness or injury, which automatically precipitates the person into contact with nurses and nursing. In some instances, transition is initiated by events beyond the individual's control; in other cases, it may be sought deliberately through events such as marriage, migration, career change, or cosmetic surgery.

Transitions are those periods in between fairly stable states. Transitions fall within the domain of nursing when they pertain to health or illness or when responses to the transition are manifested in health-related behaviors. It is conceivable that in the first instance, the health–illness condition is the independent variable and the transition, the dependent variable. An acutely ill patient who is hospitalized, a patient who is discharged from a health care institution, or a patient undergoing surgery are all examples of conditions or situations with an impending state of transition. In the second instance, exemplified by immigration, transition is the independent variable that may predispose human beings to health problems. The transition may also influence responses to health problems and types of action taken because of potential or actual health problems.

A number of writers have argued that there is now sufficient consensus about the discipline's central concerns—human beings, environment, and health—for these concepts to be accepted as summarizing nursing's domain.[5] While each of these, singly or in various combinations, is the concern of scholars and researchers from many disciplines, nursing's concern lies in their interrelatedness as the irreducible minimum from which knowledge for nursing practice can evolve. Given that this triad forms the basic structure for nursing knowledge, it is conceivable that additional concepts will be required before we can identify all the intricate patterns that make up the whole of nursing. Transition is one such concept. It offers a key to interpreting person-environment interactions in terms of their actual and potential effects on health. In the wake of sound empirically based descriptions of transition, both as process and as outcome, more prescriptive theory can be generated to impact on practice. Nursing practice stands to gain from careful conceptualization of transition and its consequences in all the biopsychosociocultural variations.

Definition

The noun transition is derived from the Latin verb *transire*, meaning to go across. That sense is reflected in the first meaning given in Webster's Third International Dictionary[6]; "a passage or movement from one state, condition, or place to another." Because there are connotations of both time and movement, transition can be thought of as linking change with experienced time.

As conceptualized in this chapter, transition, as passage from one life phase, condition, or status to another, is a multiple concept embracing the elements of process, time span, and perception.

Process suggests phases and sequence; time span indicates an ongoing but bounded phenomenon; and perception has to do with the meaning of the transition to the person experiencing it. The process involves both the disruption that the transition occasions and the person's responses to this interference. The time span extends from the first anticipation of transition until stability in the new status has been achieved. Perception of the transition will reflect how the associated role ambiguity and threat to self-concept are experienced. In summary, transition refers to both the process and the outcome of complex person–environment interactions. It may involve more than one person and is imbedded in the context and the situation. (J. Benoliel, personal communication, 1985).

One important characteristic of transition is that it is essentially positive. The completion of a transition implies that the person has reached a period of greater stability relative to what has gone before. Even if overall, by comparison with a pre-transition state, the changes seem more decremental than incremental, this does not mean that the transition outcome cannot be positive. The completed transition would then signify that the potential for disruption and disorganization associated with the precipitating circumstances had been countered. As Hall noted, "A theory focused on transition could deal with decreases as well as increases."[7] [p. 3] Defining characteristics of transition include process, disconnectedness, perception, and patterns of response.

Process. Whether the event that causes the transition is anticipated or not, and whether the event is short or long term, transition is a process. Its beginning and end do not occur simultaneously; there is a sense of movement, a development, a flow associated with it. The distance between the beginning and the end may be short or long, and its end may or may not have the same characteristics as its beginning. Certain boundaries imply limits to the process. Although Bridges conceptualized the structure of life transitions a little differently, referring to "(1) an ending, followed by (2) a period of confusion and distress, leading to (3) a new

TABLE 1.2.1 Events Leading to a Process of Transition

Illness	Loss	Pregnancy
Recovery	Immigration	Retirement
Birthing	Migration	Maturation
Death	Hospitalization	

beginning,"[8(p9)] there is still the same sense of transition being an ongoing and bounded phenomenon.

Although certain aspects of an individual's life will be affected more than others by the transition that he or she is currently experiencing, the extent and intensity of this influence may vary over time. Further, the boundaries of transition-related behavior are not fixed, but may expand and recede in accordance with other happenings in the total context of the person's life. Events and circumstances that are likely to be precursors to the process of transition are listed in Table 1.2.1.

Disconnectedness. Perhaps the most pervasive characteristic of transition is disconnectedness associated with disruption of the linkages on which the person's feelings of security depend. It is interesting in this regard to note that the authors of an extensive review of factors related to health commented that all the findings they described have "as a common element the importance to health of being 'connected'.... These connections are not passive, but require that people actively relate to one another and with the environment" (p. 354). Other characteristics allied to disconnectedness are loss of familiar reference points, incongruity between expectations based on the past and perceptions dictated by the present, and discrepancy between needs and the availability of, as well as access to, means for their satisfaction.

Perception. Meanings attributed to transition events vary between persons, communities, and societies, and thus influence the outcome. Hospitalization is considered necessary for healing by some and as a step toward dying by those from another culture.[11] A patient describing her hemiparesis after a stroke—"I feel like I have a dead body in bed with me" (N. Doolittler, personal communication, February 1985)—aptly illustrates the individuality of perception. This characteristic suggests that differences in perception of transition events may influence reactions and responses to such events, thus making them less predictable.

Awareness. Transition is a personal phenomenon, not a structured one. Processes and outcomes of transitions are related to definitions and redefinitions of self and situation. Such defining and redefining may be done by the person experiencing the transition or by others in the environment. However, it is contended here that to be in transition, a person must have some awareness of the changes that are occurring. In the event that the changes have not yet reached the level of awareness, or are being denied either totally or in terms of their implications (irrespective of whether the denial is conscious or unconscious), then that person is not yet in transition. He or she is still in a pretransition phase. In such cases, it would be necessary to resolve barriers to awareness of transition before attempting to facilitate the transition itself.

Patterns of Response. Patterns of response arise out of the observable and nonobservable behaviors during the process of transition that, however disturbed or dysfunctional they may appear, are not random occurrences. The behaviors embody patterns that reflect both intrapsychic structure and processes as well as those of the wider sociocultural context.[11] Pattern recognition would be an important part of developing a taxonomy of transitions. Table 1.2.2 shows the labels commonly applied to some of these patterns. Examples are disorientation, distress, and perhaps elation and happiness.

Dimensions

Transitions are not experienced uniformly by different people even when the circumstances, such as first-time parenting, are similar. However, there are some commonalities. First of all, there is a general

TABLE 1.2.2 Patterns of Response to Transition Events

Disorientation	Changes in self-concept
Distress	Changes in role performance
Irritability	Changes in self-esteem
Anxiety	(And others)
Depression	

structure consisting of at least three phases: entry, passage, and exit. It may be, too, that research will reveal some general dimensions that can be used to categorize transitions across different types of events: life cycle, situational, and health-illness.

The sequence is invariant, but the duration of each phase and associated degree of disruption are not. Impediments to the passage can occur at any point. Phases are more likely to merge into one another than to be discrete. Research would yield information on which to base a typology of transitions. This knowledge in turn would open up the possibility of prediction about general forms and specific phases most likely to generate stress. Such understanding would provide a useful background against which to interpret an individual's perception of a particular transition. Some of the possible dimensions by which transitions can be described are duration, scope, magnitude, reversibility, effect, and the extent to which the transition is anticipated and voluntary and has clear boundaries. Some of the dimensions along which it is proposed that transitions may vary are listed in Table 1.2.3 as a set of polar opposites.

Knowledge of general patterns would be useful for guiding nursing assessment, but planning and implementation, to be effective, must take account of how the transition and associated events are perceived by the person experiencing them. In recognition of the likely degree of individual variation, one aspect of theory development in this area would concern instrument construction. The dimensions described earlier could provide the starting point for an instrument that would allow the nurse to generate a profile of how the individual perceives the transition of which he or she is the

TABLE 1.2.3 Dimensions of Transitions

Single transition *v* multiple transitions
Clear entry and exit *v* ambiguous entry and exit
Impeded passage *v* unimpeded passage
Minor disruption *v* major disruption
Particular disruption *v* pervasive disruption
Brief duration *v* extended duration
Temporary *v* permanent
Positive value *v* negative value
Pleasant *v* unpleasant
Desired *v* undesired
Planned/predicted *v* unplanned/unpredicted

---

center. Its further development would depend on feedback from research and conceptual analysis. Cues from such a profile would help the nurse to more accurately infer the meaning that the situation has for the patient, this latter being the only valid data base from which to plan intervention. The transition event, the meaning and the consequences, are depicted in Figure 1.2.1.

Congruence With Nursing Theories and Relationship to Domain Concepts

There are strong threads of congruence among the many current theories in nursing. Each theorist appears to be working with different parts of the whole rather than with entirely different entities. The concept of transition has the potential for both accommodating and being accommodated by these various theoretical schemes.

Nursing theories, almost by definition, must address change in one form or another. The rationale for that assertion is that nursing's focus—responses to health–illness events—and instability for the person concerned, and the achievement of nursing's health-related goals generally depends on initiation of changes in interaction between person and environment.

An early nursing theory such as that of Peplau,[12] with its emphasis on illness as an opportunity for personal growth and development, could be restated in terms of transition, as could the later work of Travelbee[13] which focuses on the evolution of a therapeutic relationship between nurse and patient and on the need for the patient to find meaning in the illness experience. Transition is also compatible with those theories that emphasize adaptation, such as the Roy Adaptation Model.[14,15]

Transition involves patterns as well. Both Rogers[16,17] and Newman[18,19] see patterning as crucial to their theories. In Rogers's formulation, transitions would mark phases in the person's evolving unitary organization. In Orem's theory, self-care is the key concept[20,21] and transitions are inextricably linked to shifts in self-care capability.

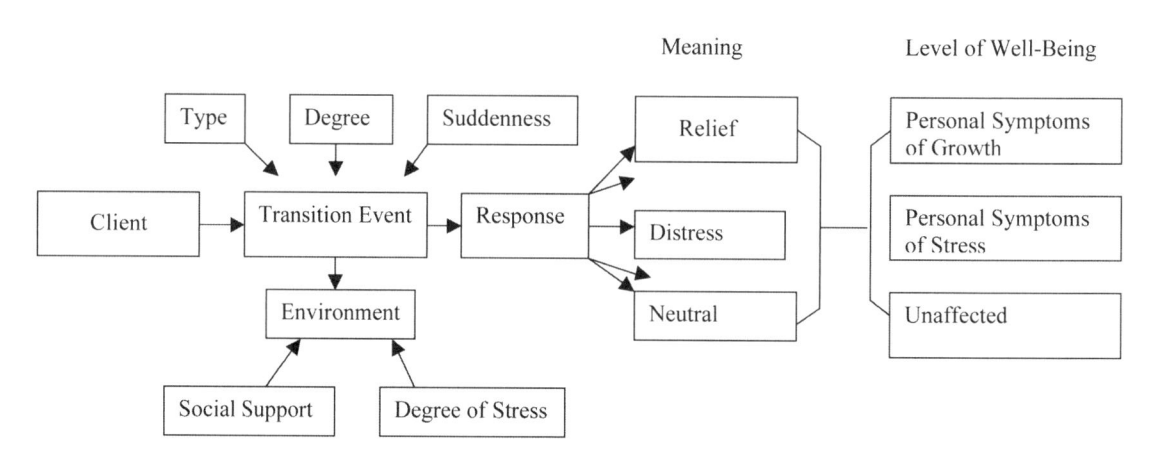

FIGURE 1.2.1 Factors related to response to a transition event.

Transition and Nursing Therapeutics

The most important raison d'être for nursing is the care of patients. This is based on knowledge related to care strategies—i.e., the nursing therapeutics that would enable nurses to select the most fruitful kinds of action and optimal intervention points for achieving the desired health maintenance or health promotion goals. Nursing therapeutics could be conceptually considered in relationship to transitions, antecedents, and consequences. To develop knowledge related to nursing therapeutics, the dimensions of time, pattern, type of transition, and timing of intervention should be considered. These dimensions will lead in the effective development of theoretical and researchable questions. Specifying other components of therapeutic or preventive clinical therapeutics may be useful to further the development of transition specific clinical therapeutics. For example, therapeutic intervention is conceptualized as occurring after the transition consequences have been experienced, and preventive intervention as occurring before the transition or before the consequences.[22]

Examples of existing studies that can be viewed from this perspective are numerous in the nursing literature. Lindeman's[23,24] work on preoperative teaching exemplifies preventive clinical therapeutics. Other examples are work related to patient compliance adherence with treatment regimens[25], such as the work of Johnson,[26] which is geared toward strategies for reducing the stress associated with certain treatment procedures; and a study of role supplementation in the postnatal transition and in a cardiac rehabilitation program.[27,28] These are all instances in which nurses have been concerned with facilitating, either preventively or therapeutically, the transition processes that clients experience. Some of the domain concepts and their relationship to the transition process are depicted in Figure 1.2.2.

Transition and Environment

Transition and environment are related in two main ways. On the one hand, changes in the environment may constitute, or be part of, the events that make the process of transition necessary. Adjustment to slowly occurring change may be so gradual as to be almost imperceptible. There is little, if any, sense of transition. More rapidly occurring environmental changes, whether they be natural, as in the occurrance of an earthquake, or man-made, in the form of urban redevelopment, call for a larger response. Such events not only require adjustment to a new environment, but at the same time severely disrupt the usual sources of support that the individual draws upon from the environment. This leads to a second way in which transition and environment are linked. Irrespective of the source of the initiating conditions for the transition, its course may be mediated by what the environment offers in the way of support. The particular nature of the environment in which it occurs may either impede or facilitate a transition. In the transition from disabled person to able person, an example of a facilitating environment would be one that gives high priority to ensuring wheelchair access for the physically handicapped.

Another factor that may influence how smoothly a transition is experienced is the extent to which the environment in which the transition is occurring is itself stable or in flux. Concurrently occurring transitions compound one another. For instance, it has been commonly observed, although perhaps not so well documented, that in clinical units in which staff are rotated and a large proportion change at one time, the ensuing unsettled period is reflected in patient states. Implications of this observation offer a source of pertinent questions for nursing research.

Transition and the Nursing Client

As with all person-environment interactions, neither processes nor outcomes are ever determined entirely by individual or environmental variables. Different sets of factors may be dominant at various points in time, but mostly what eventuates results from complex interplay between individual and environmental characteristics.

Unfortunately, the concept of transition is not immune to stereotyped thinking, so a note of caution needs to be sounded. There is a danger that we will impose explanation rather than allow understanding of the concept to emerge from evidence

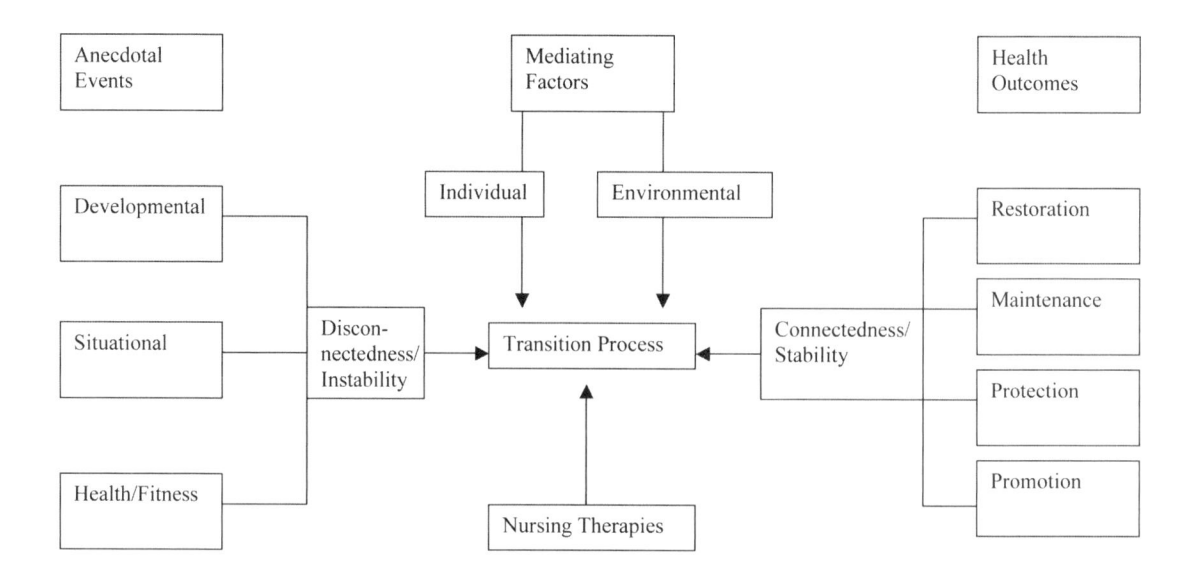

FIGURE 1.2.2 Relationship of transitions to other domain concepts.

of how transitions are actually experienced by those undergoing them. There may be a tendency to use one's own experience or feelings as a frame of reference rather than elicit meanings from the client. Thus, on the basis of personal experience and societal values, the transition to motherhood may be assumed always to be experienced positively. Negative connotations are simply not perceived. To take a further example, for most of us, colostomy poses a threat to autonomy over a natural bodily function, and hence is viewed negatively. Such a conclusion ignores the possibility that, for a particular individual, the colostomy and associated transition may be experienced as a positive resolution to a prolonged distressing and anxiety provoking condition.

Technological advances in medicine are now subjecting people to transitions not dreamed of a few decades ago. At the moment, it is the associated ethical dilemmas that are attracting attention. In the meantime, nurses, by their very "thereness" (compared with the intermittent contacts of other caregivers), are ideally placed to be in the vanguard to help patients and their families with these unprecedented situations.

Exemplars

The critical question for the proposed conceptualization linking transitions with health is what utility it would have for nursing practice. Most currently used assessment guides and other documentation associated with the nursing process model are intended to alert nurses to life context variables relevant to the person's current health-illness status. Therefore, it is germane to ask if the concept of transition adds anything. We suggest that it does. For instance, as a focus for nursing intervention, it helps us to incorporate the "at risk" status that accompanies many forms of transition not directly related to health-illness events. However, even when it is too late for preventive measures, nursing assessment done with the aim of highlighting the kinds of personal and social transitions in which the client is involved has much to offer. It will help to ensure that interventions are maximally relevant, and therefore genuinely therapeutic rather than merely being palliative.

Viewing transition as both process and outcome means that focus can be readily shifted between end result and process. Either can be the subject of assessment. In the first instance, comparisons would be made between present characteristics and those exhibited (or reported to have been present) at a pretransition phase. Some may have been lost, others modified, and some entirely new ones may have emerged. The values (both social and personal) placed on these characteristics will influence the degree of stress associated with such losses and gains. So the notion of transition is likely to be useful in formulating goals for nursing practice. It can also be applied retrospectively to help the nurse understand how a person feels about the outcome of a transition and the process that has led to it.

The concept of transition is consistent with the philosophy of holistic health, which is central to nursing practice. It is unavoidable that at a given point in time, attention will be focused on some aspects of the person more than on others. In practice, there is no way that we can attend to the whole person simultaneously, but we can recognize the coextensiveness of the many dimensions of the person. Thinking in terms of transition promotes continuity not only across time, but also across dimensions of the person.

With transition viewed as a process, the aim would be to anticipate points at which the person is most likely to reach peaks of vulnerability with respect to health. Efforts could then be directed toward establishing and reinforcing defenses as well as modifying hazards. As knowledge accumulates concerning the likely course or trajectory of different types of transition, it will become increasingly possible to plan interventions according to the optimum moment and manner.

Nursing practice based on a transition model would run counter to therapeutic interventions aimed only at cure. Return to a disease-free state may not be possible, and even the premorbid level of health may be unattainable. A goal for nursing is that the client emerge from any nursing encounter not only more comfortable and better able to deal with the present health problem, but also better equipped to protect and promote health for the future.

Sometimes in the drama of a life-threatening event such as might be associated with admission to an intensive care unit or a cardiac care unit, the important point is lost, which is that for the ill person and significant others, the episode is part (perhaps just the beginning) of transition. By definition, crisis care is present-oriented. Yet the questions going through the minds of patient and family are likely to be future-oriented. First of all, "Is there a future? Is this the end?" Then, "If I do recover, what will I be like?" Even the questions themselves indicate a transition, from a time when such doubts and anxieties were nonexistent or peripheral to the moment of their present compelling impact. In other instances, the tendency may be for the person to be fixed in the past as a defense against both present and future. Here the nurse has to work at starting the transition process. The earlier that these doubts and uncertainties are recognized and worked through, the sooner the transition to recovery will be achieved. Once the person perceives himself or herself as an invalid (i.e., as being invalidated as a normal person), it may be difficult to eradicate this perception, even in the presence of seemingly good physical recovery. The difficulty will increase the longer the perception persists.

For some time now, acute care hospitals have been examining their admission procedures in terms of how this transition to inpatient might be facilitated. Currently, too, discharge planning is receiving much attention. Generally, these processes have not been explicitly conceptualized as transition, but there could well be a gain in doing so. Tornberg, McGrath, and Benoliel are quite specific in describing their transition services "as a model of nursing practice designed to offer personalized services and continuity of care to patients and families living with changing demands of progressive, deteriorating illness."[29] (p. 131)

We know of another facility that, without labeling itself as a transition service, functions as one for people who have undergone plastic surgery. Such patients, especially in the case of cosmetic surgery, are often elderly. After the immediate postoperative period, they do not require the complex services of an acute care hospital (in fact, such an atmosphere may not be inductive to their recovery). Nor are they always ready for the full independence of returning home, particularly if they live alone. A short stay in an intermediate facility helps to smooth the multiple facets of this kind of transition.

Analysis of Transition in Relation to Other Concepts

Transition, Change, and Other Change-Related Concepts

Part of the process of concept analysis is to compare the concept to others with comparable properties and dimensions in order to establish its boundaries.[30,31] Although Hall[7] saw certain risks in nursing's present emphasis on change concepts (principally, that we may come to equate understanding change with understanding people), it can still be argued that, for nursing, change is both a raison d'être and a means of goal achievement. Just as it is change in health status that brings about the need for health care, so the goal of intervention usually is to facilitate changes that will restore health to a premorbid level or better. Yet to say that nursing is about managing change is little more than a truism.

A broad concept such as change contains too much ambiguity for it to be effective in guiding either nursing conceptualizations or therapeutics. That is why Becker[32] suggested that nursing might gain more from the exploration of microconcepts. Transition, although not quite micro in the sense intended by Becker, has similar advantages. It can be differentiated from the general concept of change sufficiently to make it useful in alerting nurses to relevant aspects of the life context of clients. In this instance, transition is seen as a special case of the general phenomenon of change.

When looking at the broader social science literature, one cannot but be struck by similarities between our thinking about transitions and other change-related phenomena being discussed by psychologists and sociologists. For instance, *Uprooting and Development* is a volume of essays described in the foreword as having to do with "one of the fundamental properties of human life—the need to change—and with the personal and social mechanisms for dealing with the need[33] (p. xi). The author of the foreword goes on to emphasize dislocation as a distinguishing feature of uprooting events that range from self-imposed relocations and migrations to natural and man-made disasters. Another contributor to the volume offers the following metaphorical description of what the experience of being uprooted is:

> The closest human counterpart to the root structure by which a plant nourishes itself is, I suggest, the structure of meaning by which each of us sustains the relationships to people, work, and the physical and social circumstances on which our lives depend. Like roots, these structures of meaning are at once generic and sensitively adapted to the particular setting in which they are embedded; like roots, too, they transplant from this established setting only at the risk of wilting and stunting.[34] (p.101)

The concern with meaning is germane to our approach, which lends itself well to interpretive research methodologies. Preserving continuity of meaning, either by reestablishing disrupted connections or by substituting new ones, is an essential part of the transition process, and hence the ways of doing these things are of vital concern to nurses. Our sense of transition makes the latter concept complementary to notions such as uprooting. Transition is a response to the disrupting events. It takes up the developmental theme of the book title just cited.

As well as the focus on transition as a response, another difference from these other writings is provided by the health emphasis that emanates from our nurse-scientist perspective. Admittedly, the difference is largely one of emphasis. Writers in other disciplines are sensitive to the health hazards associated with change. Since the research of the 1960s and 1970s, we have been aware of the deleterious effects of accumulated stress from sequential and contiguous life changes.[35,36] Some, such as Coelho and Stein,[37] refer specifically to health risks associated with rural to urban migrations. In all these instances, however, health risks are seen as consequents or dependent variables, that is, they are effects of the change phenomena. Perhaps subtler relationships emerge when, as from our health-cen-

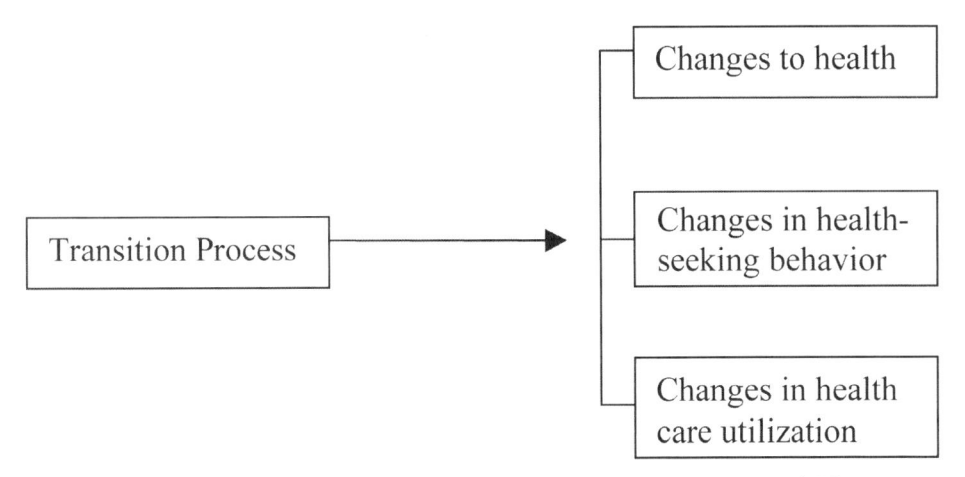

FIGURE 1.2.3 Transition as an independent variable.

tered focus, illness and injury are viewed as antecedent or independent variables that initiate the need for transition and, by their characteristics, help to determine the trajectory that the transition will follow. In this sense, the illness, injury, or "at-risk" status becomes analogous to the uprooting events described earlier.

Research Potential

Transition may enter the formulation of a research question as either an independent or a dependent variable, as indicated in Figures 1.2.3 and 1.2.4.

Transition as an Independent Variable

A transition resulting from such events as immigration, migration, relocation, pregnancy, birthing, and loss may lead to health-related consequences in the form of biophysical symptoms or psychosocial symptoms and may lead to ineffective health-seeking or help-seeking behavior. It may also lead to overutilization of health care services. Studies of transition as an independent variable may consider several relationships. These relationships are discussed and demonstrated in Figure 1.2.3.

Transitions and Health. Some transitions reflect movement along the health illness continuum more directly than others. For instance, catastrophic illness, a diagnosis of chronic or degenerative disease, and discharge from hospital after a severe illness are all clearly related to health status. Certain developmental transitions, such as childbirth, aging, and dying, also come within the orbit of health–illness services because of the way in which they have been institutionalized in Western societies.

In other circumstances, the relationships are less clear-cut. Instead of figuring directly in the situation, the transition provides the ground against which the health–illness episode or period of increased vulnerability to risk occur. McKinlay[38] supports the view that ethnographic studies, historical epidemiology, and observations in societies where rapid increase of technology has occurred indicate that people who are in a state of physical and cultural transition have higher risk of illness. All too often the contribution of a concurrent transition is recognized only after a crisis, for example, acute depression, has occurred.

Although the foregoing discussion has emphasized the tendency for transition to increase vulnerability to health hazards, transitions can also be viewed as opportunities. Transition can mean gain or loss. The perturbations associated with the beginning of the transition process may create fertile ground for new learning. In this sense, the concept of transition is consistent with eudaimonistic and self-actualizing views of health.[31]

Transitions and Health-Seeking Behaviors. For someone in transition, health-seeking behavior may be inhibited simply because the appropriate course of action is no longer obvious. For instance, a new immigrant still operating within the norms of the culture of origin may not perceive the physician as a satisfactory substitute for the traditional healer and, in the absence of the latter, may delay taking any action until forced to do so by a crisis. Not knowing the available options, or even how to initiate entry into the health care system, is a further cause of inaction. Choosing a new physician in a strange city can be a daunting task for anyone. For a person unfamiliar with the customs and perhaps not fluent in the language, it may seem an insurmountable obstacle. One can only conjecture how often people in this situation are labeled by health care providers as irresponsible with respect to their children's health.

Retirement is another event that launches people into a period of transition. Particularly when involuntary, it is an outward sign of growing old. One effect of this transition on older persons is that, because of prevailing confusion between the effects of aging and symptoms of illness, they tend to accept distressing symptoms such as decreased sensory acuity and urinary incontinence as inevitable aspects of aging, and therefore are reluctant to seek advice or treatment. Thus to fully understand a person's response to being in transition, it is important to understand how they perceive the transition process and what expectations they have for the outcome.

Transitions and Health Care Utilization. Even if the transition does not prevent the person from seeking health care, it may result in changes in utilization of health services.[38] A familiar example is the new immigrant's utilization of the hospital emergency department when what is needed is a regular office visit. There are at least two possible reasons for this behavior. One is the visibility of the service and relative case of access as compared with visiting a physician's office or other facility that operates on an appointment basis. Another is that the strangeness of the new environment and lack of familiar resources may result in a high level of uncertainty and anxiety, which leaves the person unable to make judgments about the severity and seriousness of symptoms. Consequently, there may be a tendency to overrely on professionals for reassurance.

Transition as a Dependent Variable

In this case, transition occurs as a result of illness and changes in health status as is presented in Figure 1.2.4. People who experience life-threatening illnesses pass through a transition. Although we have some insightful descriptive accounts,[40,41] there is still much that is unknown about the meanings that are constructed out of these events and why—irrespective of the actual amount of pathology involved—they are more devastating for some people than for others. Rehabilitation and reablement programs assume a transition. The effectiveness of such programs depends on congruence between the goals of the client and those of the therapist. This in turn presumes knowledge about the transition process and the client's perception of it.

In approaching measurement issues associated with developing the concept of transition, it is likely that we will be able, in part, to build on existing work. The conclusion of a recent review paper was that "there are currently at least 27 published scales that measure various aspects of social functioning and that have been reasonably well developed and tested" (p. 1257).[42] No doubt some of these overlap with the dimensions that we deem especially pertinent to the transition process. The growing literature on coping strategies is another likely source of material.

Summary and Conclusions

This chapter illustrates one of the options for theory development—concept analysis and clarification. The broad concept of transition, a period of change

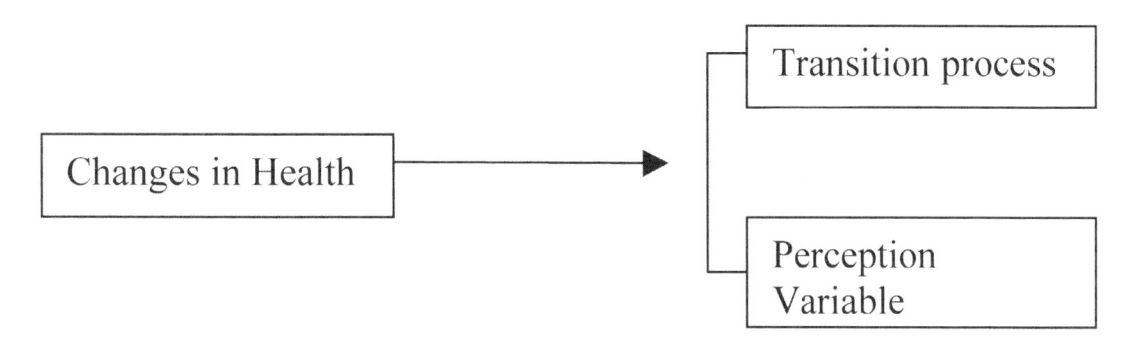

FIGURE 1.2.4 Transition as a dependent variable.

between two relatively stable states that comes to be associated with some degree of self-redefinition, has been explored specifically within a nursing context, a context in which the central domains are person-client, health, and environment. Ramifications of the definition were traced. It was argued that a theory with transition as its central concept would provide continuity with directions evident from historical analysis of the work of other nurse theorists, meet nursing's present needs, and at the same time be congruent with trends in knowledge development in related fields. We see such a framework as conducive to more integrated and effective theoretical and research programs for nursing. It is contended that the kind of theoretical development proposed would have at least the following three advantages that will have implications for further knowledge development.

1. Nurses sometimes tend to view clients historically, and therefore, they fail to recognize or meet the client's needs at the point where the client presently is in his or her perception of the situation. Conceptualizations that encompass flexible time orientation incorporating past, present, and future, as does transition, promote greater synchrony between the time orientations of nurse and client, and therefore provide a basis from which to more accurately define client needs.
2. Although the trend toward adopting "models of nursing practice" may be useful in alerting nurses to sets of problems associated with particular diagnostic categories, there is much that we still need to learn about how to set priorities in individual cases. There is a commonly held view that inadequacies in nursing care are due less to paucity of data than they are to failure by nurses to appreciate the relevance of data that are available. A transition framework would have the heuristic value of prompting researchers to pose questions pertinent to cue recognition and utilization.
3. An integrating and organizing conceptual framework makes it easier for a nurse to capitalize on what he or she knows already and to use existing knowledge more insightfully. This is not to deny the need for nurses to continually update their knowledge, which is a basic requirement in any practice discipline. But most nurses—through both education and experience—have already acquired a good deal of knowledge about human development and person-environment interactions. Unfortunately, such knowledge is not always well articulated and so made maximally available to benefit practice. Transition theory could be the key to changing this situation. This, broadly, has been the intent of this chapter: to analyze the concept of transition for the purpose of knowledge development in nursing.

We are aware that, in suggesting transition as a focus for theory development and research in nursing, the concept is not an entirely new one. Other disciplines are already working with it. However, analysis from a nursing perspective with the further development of theoretical and empirical linkages with nursing's other central domain concepts does signify an original approach with significant implications for knowledge development.

A theory linking transitions and health would meet Johnson's[43] three criteria for evaluating nursing theory: social congruence, social significance, and social utility. The ubiquity of the term transition in the recent nursing literature is evidence of its congruence with current orientations to change held by health care users and providers. That transition is a concept relevant to many of nursing's immediate concerns is evident from the frequency with which the term has appeared in recent nursing literature in the context of transition and nursing practice;[29,44,45] transition, education, and service;[46] research in transition;[47] and theory development.[48]

Significance must be judged, finally, on empirical evidence. That the concept of transition already pervades much of the current thinking about nurses and nursing suggests that it is not a trivial notion or passing fad. In the body of this chapter, we have endeavored to show how the concept has potential application in a wide spectrum of nursing practice settings. It follows that the utility value of the concept is expected to be high. We see applications transculturally, for all age groups, and independent of clinical speciality. Yet, having micro aspects, it avoids the limitations of grand theory. Some general concepts that appear insightful in the broad scene have little to say in the individual case. So utility may in fact be this concept's major strength. Certainly nursing needs new knowledge, but it also needs tools and strategies that assist nurses to make best use of existing knowledge and to use it in a uniquely nursing way. Part of the work of theories is to generate new knowledge. They also serve to organize extant knowledge and make it more accessible. It may be that the concept of transitions will be a catalyst in the task of uncovering the knowledge embedded in clinical practice.[29,49,50]

Finally, in order to meet the challenge of the American Nurses' Association policy statement that defines nursing as the "diagnosis and treatment of human responses to actual and potential health problems" (p. 9),[51] a plurality of theories is needed. A theory linking health, illness, and nursing with transition would not supercede the variety of theoretical formulations that now inform nursing research and practice. Certainly there would be some overlap (this speaks to the issue of validity), but transition theory offers a framework and a perspective for organization of knowledge related to events and responses to transitions. The realization of such a theory would depend on a program of inquiry aimed at clarifying theoretical and operational linkages between transition and a broad spectrum of health-illness states. The next stage would be the empirical testing of several kinds of propositions, such as those linking the transition process with health-illness states and those linking it with nursing therapeutics.

REFERENCES

1. Wilson J: *Thinking with Concepts.* London, Cambridge University Press, 1983.
2. Chinn PL, Jacub M: *Theory and Nursing: A Systematic Approach.* St Louis, CV Mosby, 1983.
3. Walker LO, Avant KC: *Strategies for Theory Construction in Nursing.* Norwalk, CT, Appleton-Century-Crofts, 1983.
4. Norris CM: *Concept Classification in Nursing.* Rockville, MD, Aspen Systems, 1982.
5. Stevens B: *Nursing Theory: Analysis, Application and Evaluation*, ed. 2. Boston, Little, Brown, 1984.
6. *Webster's Third International Dictionary.* Springfield, Mass, G & C Merriam, 1971.
7. Hall B: The change paradigm in nursing: Growth versus persistence. *Adv Nurs Sci* 1981:116.
8. Bridges W: *Transitions.* Reading, MA, Addison-Wesley, 1980.
9. Lyndheim R, Syme L: Environment, people and health. *Ann Rev Public Health* 1981, 4:335–359.
10. Lipson, JG, Meleis AI: Issues in health care of middle eastern patients. *West J Med* 1981, 149: 854–861.
11. Newman MA. The Newman model. Overview. Paper presented at the Nurse Theorist Conference, Edmonton, Alberta, Canada, 1984.

12. Peplau H. *Interpersonal Relations in Nursing.* New York, G Putnam's Sons, 1952.
13. Travelbee J: *Interpersonal Aspects of Nursing.* ed 2. Philadelphia, FA Davis, 1971.
14. Roy C: *Introduction to Nursing: An Adaptation Model.* Englewood Cliffs, NJ. Prentice Hall, 1984.
15. Roy C. Roberts S: *Theory Construction in Nursing.* Englewood Cliffs, NJ. Prentice Hall, 1981.
16. Rogers M: *An Introduction to a Theoretical Basis of Nursing.* Philadelphia, FA Davis. 1970.
17. Rogers M: Nursing: A science of unitary man, in Riehl JP, Roy C (eds): *Conceptual Models for Nursing Practice,* ed 2. New York. Appleton-Century-Crafts, 1980.
18. Newman MA: *Theory Development in Nursing.* Philadelphia, FA Davis, 1979.
19. Newman MA: Newman's health theory, in Clements I. Roberts F (eds): *Family Health: A Theoretical Approach to Nursing Care.* New York. John Wiley, 1983.
20. Orem D: *Nursing: Concepts of Practice.* New York. McGraw-Hill, 1971.
21. Orem D: *Nursing: Concepts of Practice,* ed 3. New York. McGraw-Hill, 1985.
22. Meleis AI: Role insufficiency and role supplementation: A conceptual framework. *Nurs Res* 24:264–271.
23. Lindeman CA: The challenge of nursing research in the 1980s, in *Communicating Nursing Research: Directions for the 1980s.* Boulder Col. Western Interstate Commission for Higher Education, 1980.
24. Lindeman CA. Van Aernam B: Nursing intervention with the presurgical patient: The effects of structured and unstructured preoperative teaching, in Downs F. Newman M (eds): *A Source Book in Nursing Research.* Philadelphia, FA Davis, 1973.
25. Dracup KA. Meleis AI: Compliance: An interactionist approach. *Nurs Res* 1982;31:31–36.
26. Johnson JE: Effects of structuring patients' expectations on their reactions to threatening events. *Nurs. Res.* 1972;21:499–504.
27. Dracup K, Meleis AI, Baker C, Edlefsen P: Family focused cardiac rehabilitation: A role supplementation program for cardiac patients and spouses. *Nurs Clin North Am* 1984;19:112–124.
28. Meleis AI, Swendsen L: Role supplementation: An empirical test of nursing intervention. *Nurs Res* 1978;27:11–18.
29. Tornberg M, McGrath B, Benoliel J: Oncology transition services. *Cancer Nurs* April 1984, pp 131–137.
30. Norris C. *Concept Clarification in Nursing.* Rockville, MD. Aspen Publishers, 1982.
31. Walker LD, Avant KC: *Strategies for Theory Construction in Nursing.* Norwalk, Conn, Appleton-Century-Crofts, 1983.
32. Becker C: A conceptualization of a concept. *Nursing Papers: Perspectives on Nursing* 1983;15:51–57.
33. Bryant JH: Foreword, in Coelho CV, Ahmed PI (eds). *Uprooting and Development.* New York. Plenum Press, 1980.
34. Marris P. The uprooting of meaning, in Coelho CV, Ahmed PI (eds): *Uprooting and Development.* New York. Plenum Press, 1980.
35. Holmes TH, Rahe RH: The social readjustment rating scale. *J. Psychosom Med* 1967; 11:211–218.
36. Holmes TH, Masuda M. Life change and illness susceptibility, in Dohrendwend BP (ed), *Stressful Life Events: Their Nature and Effect.* New York, John Wiley, 1974.
37. Coelho CV. Stein JJ: Change, vulnerability, and coping: Stresses of uprooting and overcrowding, in Coelho CV. Ahmed PI (eds): *Uprooting and Development.* New York. Plenum Press. 1980.
38. McKinley J: Some issues associated with migration, health status, and use of human services. *J Chronic Dis* 1975;28:579–592.
39. Smith JA: The idea of health: A philosophical inquiry. *Adv in Nurs Sci* 1981;3:43–50.
40. Smith DW: *Survival of Illness: Implications for Nursing.* New York, Springer, 1981.
41. Schwartz D: Catastrophic illness: How it feels. *Geriatr Nurs* 1982;3:303–306.
42. Weissman M, Sholomskas D, John K: The assessment of social adjustment. *Arch Gen Psychiatry* 1981;38:1250–1258.
43. Johnson D. Development of theory. *Nurs Res* 1974;23:372–377.
44. Benoliel JQ: Dying is a family affair, in Prichard ER, Collard J, Start J, Lockwood JA, Kutscher AH. Beland I (eds): *Home Care: Living with Dying.* New York, Columbia University Press, 1979.
45. Norris C: Restlessness: A nursing phenomenon in search of meaning. *Nurs Outlook* 1975;23:103–107.
46. Weiss S: The effect of transition modules on new graduate adaptation. *Res Nurs Health* 1984;7:51–59.
47. Gortner S: Nursing science in transition. *Nurs Res* 1980;29:180–183.
48. Meleis AI: *Theoretical Nursing: Development and Progress.* Philadelphia, JB Lippincott, 1985.
49. Benner P: Uncovering the knowledge embedded in clinical practice. *Image* 1983;15:36–41.
50. Benner P, Wrubel J: Skilled clinical knowledge: The value of perceptual awareness. *Nurse Educator* 1982;7:11–17.
51. American Nurses' Association: *Nursing: A Social Policy Statement.* Kansas City, MO, American Nurses' Association. 1980.

Reprinted with permission from: Chick, N., & Meleis, A. I. (1986). Transitions: A nursing concern. In P. L. Chinn (Ed.),

Nursing research methodology (pp. 237–257). Boulder, CO: Aspen Publication.

1.3 TRANSITIONS: A CENTRAL CONCEPT IN NURSING

KAREN L. SCHUMACHER
AFAF IBRAHIM MELEIS

Abstract

Transition is a concept of interest to nurse researchers, clinicians, and theorists. This chapter builds on earlier theoretical work on transitions by providing evidence from the nursing literature. A review and synthesis of the nursing literature (1986–1992) supports the claim of the centrality of transitions in nursing. Universal properties of transitions are process, direction, and change in fundamental life patterns. At the individual and family levels, changes occurring in identities, roles, relationships, abilities, and patterns of behavior constitute transitions. At the organizational level, transitional change is that occurring in structure, function, or dynamics. Conditions that may influence the quality of the transition experience and the consequences of transitions are meanings, expectations, level of knowledge and skill, environment, level of planning, and emotional and physical well-being. Indicators of successful transitions are subjective well-being, role mastery, and the well-being of relationships. Three types of nursing therapeutics are discussed. A framework for further work is described.

Meleis (1975; 1985; 1986; 1991) has proposed that transition is one of the concepts central to the discipline of nursing. Nurse–client encounters often occur during transitional periods of instability precipitated by developmental, situational, or health illness changes. Such changes may produce profound alterations in the lives of individuals and their significant others and have important implications for well-being and health.

In an earlier article, Chick and Meleis (1986), approached theory development for the concept of transition through concept analysis. They defined transition as a passage or movement from one state, condition, or place to another; they proposed an array of properties and dimensions of transition; and they examined its relationship to nursing therapeutics, environment, client, and health. In this chapter, we extend this work through a review of the nursing literature published since 1986.

Articles were identified through a MEDLINE search of the nursing literature from 1986 to 1992 using the key word *transition*. The search was limited to English language publications; 310 citations were identified. We then limited our review to publications in which the word *transition* appeared in the title to capture articles in which transition was a major focus.

The initial overview of this body of literature revealed that nurses have used a wide variety of publication modes to communicate their ideas about transitions. Transitions were addressed in an editorial (O'Brien, 1990), a letter to the editor (Schwartz, 1989), regular columns or features (Grady, 1992; Scherting, 1988), and accounts of personal experience (Rice, 1988; Shea, Adamzczak, & Flanagan, 1987), as well as in full-length articles on practice, theory, or research. Entire issues of two journals have been devoted to exploring transitions (Fought, 1992; Murphy, 1990b), as have publications of major professional organizations (Ryan, 1988; Watson, 1988).

Two instruments have been developed (Flandermeyer, Kenner, Spaite, & Hostiuck, 1992; Imle & Atwood, 1988). Such variety produced a wealth of ideas and reflects the interest in transitions. Although theory development was the stated intent of only a small subset of these publications, the descriptions of transitions and the many ideas about transitions discussed in the literature can be used as a basis for theory development. This review exemplifies an approach to theory development in which the nursing literature is used as "data" to address three questions: What are the types of transitions addressed in the nursing literature? What conditions influence transitions? What constitutes a healthy transition?

Types of Transitions

The literature reveals that nurses think of many diverse situations as transitions. Previously, three types of transitions relevant to nursing were identified: Developmental, situational, and health–illness (Chick & Meleis, 1986). This review allowed us to add subcategories to each of these types and to identify an additional category of organizational transitions. We present these categories as a typology of transitions to demonstrate the scope of phenomena that can be conceptualized as transitions and to stimulate the reader to think of additional phenomena to further expand the typology.

Developmental Transitions

Among developmental transitions, becoming a parent is the transition that has received the most attention. Nurse researchers and theorists have examined the transition to parenthood as it occurs during pregnancy (Imle, 1990; Imle & Atwood, 1988), during the postpartum period (Brouse, 1988; Pridham & Chang, 1992; Pridham, Lytton, Chang, & Rutledge, 1991; Tomlinson, 1987), and up to 18 months after an infant's birth (Majewski, 1986; 1987). Although it is the mother's transition to parenthood that is most often studied, transition to fatherhood has also been addressed (Battles, 1988).

Other stages in the life cycle have been identified as transitions, but have received less attention. Lauer (1990) conceptualized adolescence as a developmental period encompassing a number of transitions, one of which is the transition in body image. Midlife also has been conceptualized in terms of multiple transitions for women (Frank, 1991), one of which is menopause (Fishbein, 1992). Mercer, Nichols, and Doyle (1988) described the transitions experienced by women from childhood to old age, contrasting the transitions of mothers and non-mothers.

Most of the work on developmental transitions has focused on the individual. However, several writers have addressed developmental transitions in relationships such as the mother–daughter dyad (Martell, 1990; Patsdaughter & Killien, 1990) and the childbearing family (Imle, 1990). Hollander and Haber (1992) described the developing awareness of a gay or lesbian identity as an ecological transition in that change occurs in the individual and in the social environment.

Situational Transitions

Transitions in various educational and professional roles are situational transitions that have received a great deal of attention. Many writers have addressed transitions into and throughout educational programs (Klaich, 1990; Lengacher & Keller, 1992; Myton, Allen, & Baldwin, 1992; Pullen, 1988; Wuest, 1990). The transition to staff nurse at the completion of an educational program also has received a great deal of attention (Alex & MacFarlane, 1992; Andersen, 1991; Cassells, Redman, & Jackson, 1986; Hindman, 1986; Jairath, Costello, Wallace, & Rudy, 1991; Lathlean, 1987; Paterniti, 1987; Talarczyk & Milbrandt, 1988). Subsequent transitions in clinical practice roles occur throughout the career. Among these transitions are changes in practice setting (Ceslowitz & Loreti, 1991; Dunn, 1992; Kane, 1992; Shea et al., 1987), return to clinical practice (Brautigan, Bryson, & Doster, 1989), changes in function and scope of practice (Reed-McKay, 1989), changes the role transitions required of nurses who simultaneously care for patients with strikingly different needs (Samarel, 1989). The transition from clinician to administrator has been addressed by several writers (Gardner & Gander, 1992; Rice, 1988; Scherting, 1988; Starke & Rempel, 1990). And, in a series of columns Blouin and Brent (1992a; 1992b; 1992c; 1992d; 1992e; 1992f) discussed the transitions experienced by nurses upon leaving executive positions. Hegyvary and de Tornyay (1991) described the transitions into and out of the role of dean.

Other writers have conceptualized changes in family situations as transitions. For example, widowhood as a transition has been addressed by Poncar (1989) and by Adlersberg and Thorne (1990). The transition of an elderly family member from home to a nursing home has been explored by Johnson, Morton, and Knox (1992) and Young (1990). Finally, family caregiving has been conceptualized as a series of transitions (Brown & Powell-Cope, 1991).

Other situations that have been conceptualized as transitions are immigration (Meleis, 1987), homelessness (Gonzales-Osler, 1989), near-death experiences (Dougherty, 1990), and moving out of abusive relationships (Henderson, 1989).

Health–Illness Transitions

The impact of illness-related transitions on individuals and families has been explored in a number of illness contexts, including myocardial infarction (Christman, McConnell, Pfeiffer, Webster, Schmitt, & Ries, 1988), post-operative recovery (Wild, 1992), HIV infection (Thurber & DiGiamarino, 1992); spinal cord injury (Selder, 1989), advanced cancer (Reimer, Davies, & Martens, 1991), and chronic illness (Catanzaro, 1990; Loveys, 1990). Bridges (1992) conceptualized weaning from mechanical ventilation as a transition in the process of recovery from critical illness. Similarly, De Bonde and Hamilton (1991) described the progression from tube feeding to oral nutrition as a transition in the process of rehabilitation.

Many articles addressed transitions among levels of care within the health care system over the course of an illness. A prominent concern is the transition from hospital to outpatient care and to the home environment (Brooten et al., 1988; Chielens & Herrick, 1990; Christman et al., 1988; Cohen, Arnold, Brown, & Brooten, 1991; Howard-Glenn, 1992; Kenner & Lott, 1990; Ladden, 1990; Michels, 1988; Salitros, 1986; Wong, 1991). Other transitions within the health care system that have been addressed by nurses are the transition from hospital to rehabilitation center (Swarczinski & Graham, 1990), home follow-up care for persons traditionally seen in out-patient clinics (Thurber & DiGiamarino, 1992) and the transition from psychiatric hospital to community (Robinson & Pinkney, 1992; Staples & Schwartz, 1990). Models in which nurses provide transitional care services have been proposed and implemented to increase continuity of care across the health care system and to promote cost effective utilization of health services (Brooten et al., 1988; Cohen et al., 1991; Ritz & Walker, 1989; Thurber & DiGiamarino, 1992).

Organizational Transitions

The transitions described thus far have been those occurring at the individual, dyadic, or family level. Organizations can also experience transitions that affect the lives of persons who work within them and their clients. Organizational transitions represent transitions in the environment. They may be precipitated by changes in the wider social, political, or economic environment or by intraorganizational changes in structure or dynamics.

Changes of incumbents in leadership positions have been described as transitional periods in the life of organizations with far-reaching effects (Gilmore, 1990; Hegyvary & de Tornyay, 1991; Kerfoot, Serafin-Dickson, & Green, 1988; Losee & Cook, 1989; Tierney, Grant, Cherrstrom, & Morris, 1990), as have changes in the qualitative dimensions of leadership roles (Ehrat, 1990). The adoption of new policies, procedures, and practices also has been conceptualized as a transition. Exemplifying this kind of transition are the introduction of restraint-free care in a nursing home (Blakeslee, Goldman, Papougenis, & Torell, 1991), new staffing patterns (Rotkovitch & Smith, 1987), implementation of new models of nursing care (Main, Mishler, Ayers, Poppa, & Jones, 1989; Vezeau & Hallsten, 1987; Walker & DeVooght, 1989), and the introduction of new technology (Shields, 1991; Turley, 1992). Finally, structural reorganization of facilities and the introduction of new programs constitute organizational transitions (Condi, Oliver, & Williams, 1986; Harper, 1989; Swearingen, 1987; Walker & DeVooght, 1989).

Transitions experienced by the nursing profession have interested several writers. According to

Allen (1986) the history of nursing is a story of transition. Transitions have been described in educational preparation in nursing (Schwartz, 1989), in curricular content (Clifford, 1989), in modes of thinking (O'Brien, 1990), and in research methods (Clarke & Yaros, 1988). The transition of nursing from an occupation to a profession was the subject of an essay by van Maanen (1990).

Communities in transition were addressed by one writer. Bushy (1990) examined recent transitions in rural communities, the stressors engendered by such transitions, and the consequences for the health of women.

It should be noted that the types of transitions we present are not mutually exclusive. Transitions are complex processes and multiple transitions may occur simultaneously during a given period of time. For example, Catanzaro (1990) explored developmental transitions in midlife in people with progressive neurological disease, demonstrating the complex challenges that occur when developmental and health/illness transitions overlap. Young (1990) also described the way in which situational, health/illness, and developmental transitions may occur concurrently for elderly people. Furthermore, a major transition may encompass a number of discrete transitions. As conceptualized by Lauer (1990), adolescence comprises a number of discrete transitions, one of which is the transition in body image. And according to Wild (1992) the transition from pain to comfort postoperatively must be managed within the context of multiple physiologic transitions; understanding these can lead to improved patient outcomes. Finally, a major transition, such as entering graduate school, may have a "ripple effect," precipitating concurrent transitions in familial relationships and social networks (Klaich, 1990).

Universal Properties of Transitions

Despite the diversity of transitions, some commonalities across categories are evident and support properties that were identified earlier (Chick & Meleis, 1986). These commonalities may be thought of as universal properties of transitions. One such universal property, manifested in definitions of transitions (Table 1.3.1) and supported by the literature, is that transitions are processes that occur over time. Further, the process involves development, flow, or movement from one state to another (Chick & Meleis, 1986). Many writers have advanced our understanding of the development and flow of transitions by dividing the process into stages or phases (Blakeslee et al., 1991; De Bonde & Hamilton, 1991; Fishbein, 1992; Gilmore, 1990; Hegyvary & de Tornyay, 1991; Reimer et al., 1991; Wong, 1991).

Another universal property is found in the nature of change that occurs in transitions. Examples in individuals and families include changes in identities, roles, relationships, abilities, and patterns of behavior (Brown & Powell-Cope, 1991; Catanzaro, 1990; Imle, 1990; Klaich, 1990; Pridham et al., 1991). Examples at the organizational level include changes in structure, function, or dynamics (Condi et al., 1986; Tierney et al., 1990; Walker & De-Vooght, 1989). These properties help to differentiate transitions from nontransitional change. For example, brief, self-limiting illness has not been characterized as a transition, whereas chronic illness has (Catanzaro, 1990; Loveys, 1990). Similarly, phenomena such as mood changes, that are dynamic but do not have a sense of movement or direction have not been conceptualized as transitions. Internal processes usually accompany the process of transition, while external processes tend to characterize change (Bridges, 1980; 1986).

Transition Conditions

Wide variation occurs among individuals, families, or organizations in transition and nurses must have a framework for assessment that allows them to capture this variation if they are to understand the transition experience of individual clients. In the Chick and Meleis (1986) model, personal and environmental factors that affected the transition process were identified. The nursing literature since then has provided substance and specificity to our understanding of what constitutes important influencing factors. Transition conditions include meanings, expectations, level of knowledge and skill, the environment, level of planning, and emotional and physical well-being (Table 1.3.1). Across the four types of transitions, we found considerable consensus that these were important factors influencing transitions. Future research might identify additional factors and amplify our understanding of conditions which are conducive to a smooth transition and conditions which place the client at risk for a difficult transition.

Meanings

Meaning refers to the subjective appraisal of an anticipated or experienced transition and the evaluation of its likely effect on one's life. Meanings attached to transitions may be positive, neutral, or negative. The transition may be desired or not and it may or may not be the result of personal choice. Awareness of the meaning of a transition for clients is essential for understanding their experience of it as well as its health consequences.

The inclusion of meanings in a theory of transition draws attention to the importance of understanding a transition from the perspective of those experiencing it. The importance of the perspective of the person undergoing transition has been emphasized by several writers (Adlersberg & Thorne, 1990; Kenner & Lott, 1990; Pridham & Chang, 1992). For example, Adlersberg and Thorne (1990) studied widowhood and found that rather than being a uniformly negative experience of loss, many experienced a sense of relief and new opportunities for personal growth. Meanings must also be understood from the perspective of the cultural context of the transition. For example, the meaning of the transition of menopause varies across cultures (Fishbein, 1992).

Meaning also has an existential connotation such as searching for meaning during the family transition of losing a member through death as described by Reimer et al. (1991). Brown and Powell-Cope (1991) found that time was needed to make meaning of events and experiences when caring for loved ones with AIDS.

TABLE 1.3.1 Definitions of Transition in the Nursing Literature

Bridges (1980, 1986): A process that involves three phases: An ending phase (disengagement, disidentification, disenchantment), a neutral phase (disorientation, disintegration, discovery), and a new beginning phase (finding meaning and future, experiencing control and challenge).

Chick and Meleis (1986): A passage from one life phase, condition, or status to another....transition refers to both the process and the outcome of complex person–environment interactions. It may involve more than one person and is embedded in the context and the situation. Defining characteristics of transition include process, disconnectedness, perception, and patterns of response.

Chiriboga (1979): Marker events with discrete entries and exits.

Golan (1981): A period of moving from one state of certainty to another, with an interval of uncertainty and change in between.

Meleis (1986): The period in which a change is perceived by a person or others, as occurring in a person or in the environment. Commonalities that characterize a transition period: 1) disconnectedness from usual social network and social support systems; 2) temporary loss of familiar reference points of significant objects or subjects; 3) new needs that may arise or old ones not met in a familiar way; and 4), old sets of expectations no longer congruent with changing situations. A transition denotes a change in health status, in role relations, in expectations, or in abilities.

Meleis (1991): A transition denotes a change in health status, in role relations, in expectations, or in abilities. It denotes changes in needs of all human systems. Transition requires the person to incorporate new knowledge, to alter behavior, and therefore to change the definition of self in social context, of a healthy or ill self, or of internal and external needs, that affects the health status.

Morris (1979): A process of change from one activity or from of activity to another.

Murphy (1990a): Common themes in definitions of transition: Disruption in routine, emotional upheaval, and adjustment required of individuals undergoing life changes.

Parkes (1971): Processes of change that are lasting in their effects, force one to give up how one views the world and his or her place in it, and necessitates the development of new assumptions and skills to enable the individual to cope with a new altered life space (Paraphrased by Murphy, 1990a).

Schlossberg (1981): An event or nonevent that results in changes in relationships, routines, assumptions, and/or roles within the settings of self, work, family, health, and economics.

Tyhurst (1957): A passage or change from one place or state or act or set of circumstances to another. Features common to all transitions: 1) a phase of turmoil; 2) disturbances in bodily function, mood, and cognition; 3) symptoms of psychologic distress; and 4) altered time perspective.

Webster (1981): The passage from one state, condition, or place to another.

Expectations

Expectations are other subjective phenomena that collectively influence the transition experience (Imle, 1990; Selder, 1989). People undergoing transition may or may not know what to expect and their expectations may or may not be realistic (Kane, 1992; Kenner & Lott, 1990; Rice, 1988). When one knows what to expect, the stress associated with transition may be somewhat alleviated (Hollander & Haber, 1992).

Expectations are influenced by previous experience (Reimer et al., 1991). However, the frame of reference created through previous experience may or may not be applicable to a new transition. When it is not applicable, expectations for the new transition may be unclear or unrealistic (Kenner & Lott, 1990).

As a transition proceeds, expectations may prove to be incongruent with unfolding reality. Shea and colleagues (1987) described surprise when reality differed from expectations. Incongruity also may occur between expectations of self and those of others such as one's colleagues (Rice, 1988). High performance expectations may be unrealistic during a transition (Kane, 1992; Rice, 1988).

Level of Knowledge/Skill

The level of knowledge and skill relevant to a transition is another condition that influences health outcomes and may be insufficient to meet the demands of the new situation.

Several researchers and clinicians have documented the need for new knowledge and skill during a transition. Parents of premature infants (Kenner & Lott, 1990; Ladden, 1990), chronically ill children (Howard-Glenn, 1992; Wong, 1991), and adult patients and their caregivers (Michels, 1988) need information during the transition from hospital to home or from inpatient to outpatient care (Chielens & Herrick, 1990). Families need information when a member is moving to a nursing home (Johnson et al., 1992) or dying (Reimer et al., 1991). The transition to new professional roles also necessitates new knowledge and skill (Dunn 1992; Shea et al., 1987; Starke & Rempel, 1990).

In the literature reviewed, uncertainty was interwoven with the need for new knowledge and skill development as a significant aspect of transition. Brown and Powell-Cope (1991) found uncertainty to be such a strong theme in interviews with caregivers of persons with AIDS that they called this experience "transition through uncertainty." Uncertainty is a similarly central focus of Selder's (1989) Life Transition Theory. Other transitions characterized by uncertainty are the transition from hospital to home (Christman et al., 1988; Michels, 1988), from home to nursing home (Johnson et al., 1992), and leadership transitions (Gilmore, 1990).

Environment

A prominent theme in many articles was the importance of resources within the environment during a transition (Battles, 1988; Chielens & Herrick, 1990; Ladden, 1990; Loveys, 1990; Meleis, 1987). In a grounded theory study of the transition to parenthood, Imle (1990) conceptualized environment as external facilitative resources. External facilitative resources were defined as the cyclic process of perceiving, building, and evaluating the helpfulness and supportiveness of support outside the person that may help during transition.

Social support from family members, partners, and friends has received a great deal of attention (Battles, 1988; Frank, 1991; Henderson, 1989; Hollander & Haber, 1992; Kenner & Lott, 1990; Majewski, 1987). Support from nurses (Pridham et al., 1991; Wong, 1991) and therapeutic groups (Robinson & Pinkney, 1992; Staples & Schwartz, 1990) also was identified as important. When support was lacking or communication with professional staff was less than optimal, clients in transition experienced feelings of powerlessness, confusion, frustration, and conflict (Johnson et al., 1992; Kenner & Lott, 1990).

Personal transitions that occur within the context of formal organizations also are shaped by the environment. The presence of a supportive preceptor, mentor, or role model was identified as an important resource during professional transitions. Preceptors facilitate clinical role transitions (Brautigan et al., 1989; Ceslowitz & Loreti, 1991; Dunn, 1992; Hindman, 1986; Shea et al., 1987) and an experienced teacher/mentor can smooth a transition by serving as a guide, role model, and sounding board (Grady, 1992; Rice, 1988; Wuest, 1990). Furthermore, in the relationship between person and organization it is important to take into account many legal and ethical considerations (Blouin & Brent 1992a, 1992b, 1992c, 1992d, 1992e, 1992f).

When an organization is in transition, interaction among persons and subsystems within the organization facilitates or impedes the process. Collaboration, team work, effective communication, and support from key persons and groups all contribute to an environment in which the transition can be managed effectively (Condi et al., 1986; Harper, 1989; Losee & Cook, 1989; Main et al., 1989; Vezeau & Hallsten, 1987).

The wider sociocultural environment is another factor that shapes the transition experience. Mercer, Nichols, and Doyle (1988) emphasized the importance of the sociocultural context in understanding transitions. Awareness of the sociocultural context of a transition enables nurses to develop therapeutics at the group, community, and societal level (Lauer, 1990). For example, lack of institutional support and flexibility, such as lack of paternity leave and inflexible work hours, impedes the transition to fatherhood (Battles, 1988).

Clearly, nurses are concerned with the effect of environment on transitions at many levels. Hollander and Haber (1992) used Bronfenbrenner's ecological model to conceptualize multiple levels of environment and showed how each level influences individual transitions. In the specific transition they addressed—the coming out process experienced by gay and lesbian persons—they noted that there is an ecological as well as identity transition.

Level of Planning

The level of planning that occurs before and during a transition is another condition that influences the success of the transition. Extensive planning helps to create a smooth and healthy transition (Kerfoot et al., 1988). Even when precipitated by an unplanned or crisis event, such as a catastrophic injury, planning can occur during the ensuing transition process so that optimal preparation for each phase is achieved.

Effective planning requires comprehensive identification of the problems, issues, and needs which may arise during a transition (Howard-Glenn, 1992; Ladden, 1990; Vezeau & Hallsten, 1987; Wong, 1991). Key people must be identified including those making the transition and those in a position to provide support. Communication among all these people is a key element in planning (Blakeslee et al., 1991; Condi et al., 1986; Kerfoot et al., 1988; Salitros, 1986; Vezeau & Hallsten, 1987). Planning takes place over time in concert with ongoing assessment and evaluation (Howard-Glenn, 1992; Wong, 1991). Developing a time line that shows stages of the transition facilitates an organized approach to planning (Vezeau & Hallsten, 1987).

Emotional and Physical Well-Being

Transitions are accompanied by a wide range of emotions, many of which attest to the difficulties encountered during transition. Several writers have noted that stress and emotional distress occur during transition (Christman et al., 1988; Fishbein, 1992; Kerfoot et al., 1988; Ladden 1990; Meleis, 1987; Shea et al, 1987)—specifically, anxiety, insecurity, frustration, depression, apprehension, ambivalence, and loneliness (Chielens & Herrick, 1990; Kerfoot et al., 1988; Rice, 1988; Salitros, 1986; Shea et al., 1987; Tierney et al., 1990). Role conflict and low self-esteem also may be present (Condi et al., 1986; Majewski, 1986; Rice, 1988). Some of the most vivid descriptions of the distress that may be experienced during transition were found in personal accounts of transitions (Rice, 1988; Shea et al., 1987). Fear of failure and unwarranted self-criticism were described as well as feeling overwhelmed, defeated, and isolated which can result in an inability to concentrate, unwillingness to take risks, and avoidance of the unknown.

Physical well-being is also important during a transition. When physical discomfort accompanies transition, it may interfere with the assimilation of new information (Kenner & Lott, 1990). Bodily unpredictability may be distressing, whereas energy, bodily predictability, and normal operation facilitate transition (Imle, 1990). Profound bodily changes are inherent in some developmental transitions (Fishbein, 1992; Lauer, 1990) and the level of comfort with these changes in the body influences well-being during the transition.

Indicators of Healthy Transitions

We found that more emphasis has been placed on the process of transition than on the identification of factors which indicate a positive transition outcome. It is critical that nurses identify healthy transition outcomes in order to facilitate research on transitions and the evaluation of clinical interventions. We have identified three indicators of healthy transition that appear relevant across all types of transition: A subjective sense of well-being, mastery of new behaviors, and the well-being of interpersonal relationships (Table 1.3.1). Although we have used the term outcome in describing these indicators of successful transition, we do so with the caveat that these "outcomes" may occur at any point in the transition process. For example, mastery may occur early in the transition for some and later for others. Thus, the assessment of these indicators of healthy transition is appropriate periodically throughout the transition and not simply at the end of the transition period.

Subjective Well-Being

When a successful transition is occurring feelings of distress give way to a sense of well-being. Subjective well-being during transition includes effective coping (Hollander & Haber, 1992; Kane, 1992) and managing one's emotions (Johnson et al., 1992) as well as a sense of dignity (Robinson & Pinkney, 1992), personal integrity (Myton et al., 1992), and quality of life (Robinson & Pinkney, 1992). Job, marital, or other role satisfactions are other subjective responses indicative of a successful transition (Cassells et al., 1986; Main et al., 1989; Majewski, 1986; Rice, 1988; Rotkovitch & Smith, 1987). Growth, liberation, self-esteem, and empowerment also may occur during a transition (Fishbein, 1992; Kane, 1992).

Role Mastery

Another indicator of healthy transition is role mastery, which denotes achievement of skilled role performance and comfort with the behavior required in the new situation. Mastery has several components, including competence (Alex & MacFarlane, 1992; Chielens & Herrick, 1990; Dunn, 1992; Meleis, 1987; Salitros, 1986), which entails knowledge or cognitive skill, decision-making, and psychomotor skills, and self-confidence (Alex & MacFarlane, 1992; Brautigan et al., 1989; Flandermeyer et al., 1992; Grady, 1992; Lathlean, 1987; Robinson & Pinkney, 1992; Salitros, 1986). Transitions of particular interest to nurses may require competence with complex skills in self care (Chielens & Herrick, 1990; Thurber & DiGiamarino, 1992) and in the care of others (Imle, 1990; Pridham et al., 1991).

Mastery is indicative of successful transition at the organizational as well as individual level. In this context, the components are high quality care and efficient work performance (Condi et al., 1986; Main et al., 1989; Rotkovitch & Smith; 1987; Turley, 1992).

Well-Being of Relationships

Well-being in one's relationships indicates that a successful transition is occurring. Transitions that ostensibly involve one or two family members must be evaluated in terms of the whole family (Wong, 1991). Disagreements or family disruption may occur during a transition (Johnson et al., 1992; Tomlinson, 1987), but when the process moves toward a successful conclusion, the well-being of family relationships is restored or promoted. Relationship well-being has been conceptualized in terms of family adaptation (Patsdaughter & Killien, 1990), family integration (Salitros, 1986), enhanced appreciation and closeness (Reimer et al., 1991), and meaningful interaction (Battles, 1988). Integration with broader social networks and the community are also indicators of healthy transition (Meleis, 1987; Robinson & Pinkney, 1992; Staples & Schwartz, 1990; Swearingen, 1987) and are crucial in preventing social isolation as a result of transition. Intervention during a transition should be aimed at mitigating disruption in relationships and promoting the development of new relationships (Hollander & Haber, 1992).

At the organizational level, undesirable transition outcomes include lack of cohesiveness, increased absenteeism and turnover, rumors, suspicion, an increase in fighting, a decrease in cooperation, resignations, and failure to recruit and retain new people (Kerfoot et al., 1988). On the other hand, cooperation among staff, effective communication, team work, and trust reflect a healthy transition (Condi et al., 1986; Losee & Cook, 1989; Scherting, 1988).

Nursing Therapeutics

We have identified three nursing measures that are widely applicable to therapeutic intervention during transitions. The first is assessment of readiness, which is a multidisciplinary endeavor and requires a comprehensive understanding of the client (Battles, 1988; Bridges, 1992; Brooten et al., 1988; Wong, 1991). In some instances, a trial transition may be possible and provides a means for assessing readiness (Wong, 1991). We suggest that assessment of readiness should include each of the conditions identified above to create individual profiles of client readiness and enable clinicians and researchers to identify various patterns of the transition experience.

Preparation for transition is another nursing therapeutic that has been widely discussed in the literature. Education is the primary modality for creating optimal conditions in preparation for transition. Approaches to education have been described by many (Brautigan et al., 1989; Condi et al., 1986; Howard-Glenn, 1992; Kane, 1992; Vezeau & Hallsten, 1987; Wong, 1991). Adequate preparation requires sufficient time for the gradual assumption of new responsibilities and implementation of new skills (Ladden, 1990; Paterniti, 1987).

Several nurses have described environments that have been specially created for preparing clients or colleagues for transition. Included are Transitional Infant Care (Salitros, 1986), the Transitional Treatment Program (Swearingen, 1987), the Transitional Orientation Nursing Unit (Paterniti, 1987), Project Adventure (Losee & Cook, 1989), and a transition house for abused women (Henderson, 1989). Many other formal programs designed to facilitate transition include orientation programs for new nurses (Lathlean, 1987; Talarczyk & Milbrandt, 1988), inservice programs, seminars, and preceptorships for nurses entering new professional roles (Andersen, 1991; Dunn, 1992; Jairath et al., 1991; Reed-McKay, 1989; Rotkovitch & Smith, 1987), transition courses (Pullen, 1988), and support groups (Kane, 1992). Educational programs to provide skill development and rehearsal are needed during organizational transition to prepare staff (Blakeslee et al., 1991; Condi et al., 1986).

The third nursing therapeutic is role supplementation which was initially introduced theoretically and empirically by Meleis (1975) and used for first time parents (Meleis & Swendsen, 1978), and patients recovering from myocardial infarction (Dracup, Meleis, Baker, & Edlefsen, 1984). More recently it has been used with family caregivers (Brackley, 1992) and battered children (Gaffney, 1992). A variation on role supplementation is the Transition Model used by Brooten and colleagues to decrease cost and enhance quality of care for people being discharged from acute care settings (Brooten et al., 1988).

Discussion and Conclusions

The literature review presented here demonstrates that transition is a concept relevant to a wide range of phenomena across many clinical and substantive areas in nursing. Most of the transition literature to date consists of clinical descriptions and personal ideas and experiences which provide many thought-provoking ideas for clinically relevant research. Descriptions of transitions in additional clinical areas are needed as well as additional research on transitions.

Transitions are of distinctive interest to nurses because of their health consequences. The literature suggests a conceptualization of transition health outcomes that incorporates subjective, behavioral, and interpersonal dimensions. Nursing therapeutics are aimed at promoting and restoring these dimensions of individual, family, and organizational health. Furthermore, the literature reveals a holistic understanding of the conditions that influence transition experiences. Nursing intervention is aimed at assisting clients to create conditions conducive to a healthful transition. The broad range of subjective, cognitive, behavioral, environmental, emotional, and physical conditions suggests a comprehensive approach to intervention, taking into account a holistic experience of transition.

The findings of our review extend the original Chick and Meleis (1986) model of transitions. Substance and specificity are added in the domains of types of transitions, transition conditions (called mediators in the earlier model), and indicators of healthful transition (called outcomes) (Figure 1.3.1). The expansion and clarification of transition conditions and outcomes provided by the recent literature is significant for research and clinical practice alike. By specifying successful and healthful outcomes, clinicians can evaluate their clinical assessments and researchers can provide an understanding of useful and effective transitions. We expect further elaboration of conditions and indicators of successful transitions to be a major focus of research and practice in the future.

We believe that this review provides support for the argument that transition is a central concept in nursing. It has documented that nurses give attention to the process and consequences of transitions in the lives of clients.

By articulating transition as a central concept and acknowledging its significance in nursing, researchers can continue to develop knowledge related to transitions, focus on gaps in knowledge, and build on each other's work. Furthermore, attention could be given to the development of methodologies that go beyond a single event. To use transition as a central concept with its universal features of processes, identities, and roles prompts nurses to

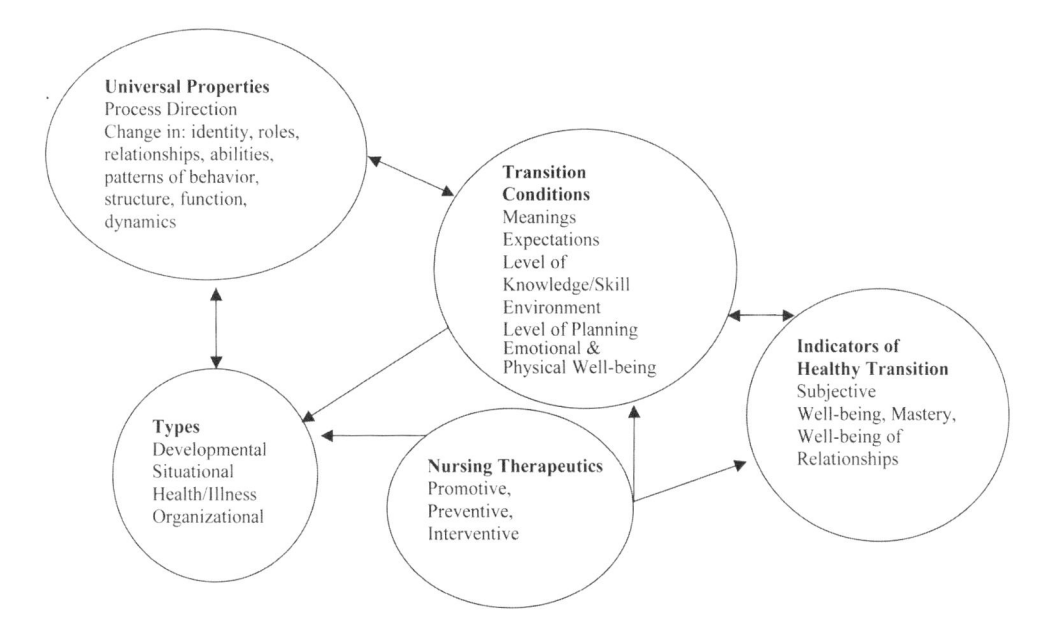

FIGURE 1.3.1 A nursing model of transitions.

consider patterns of responses rather than single responses, and to identify vulnerable and critical points during transitions for preventive work. The centrality of transitions may also have implications for nursing practice by providing clinicians with a framework to describe the critical needs of patients during admission, discharge, recovery, and transfer. Acknowledging the centrality of transitions may help focus research on types of transitions and conditions, each of which may have a different effect on responses and consequences. Finally, because transitions have profound health-related effects on clients, there is a need for nursing therapeutics designed to prevent negative consequences and enhance health outcomes (Meleis, 1991).

REFERENCES

Adlersberg, M., & Thorne, S. (1990). Emerging from the chrysalis: Older widows in transition. *Journal of Gerontological Nursing, 16,* 4–8.

Alex, M. R., & MacFarlane, M. E. (1992). The transition process: Joint responsibility of nurse educators and employers. *Canadian Journal of Nursing Administration, 5*(4), 23–26.

Allen, A. (1986). Transitions. *Journal of Post Anesthesia Nursing, 1,* 2–4.

Andersen, S. L. (1991). Preceptor teaching strategies: Behaviors that facilitate role transition in senior nursing students. *Journal of Nursing Staff Development, 7,* 171–175.

Battles, R. S. (1988). Factors influencing men's transition into parenthood. *Neonatal Network, 6*(5), 63–66.

Blakeslee, J. A., Goldman, B. D., Papougenis, D., & Torell, C. A. (1991). Making the transition to restraint-free care. *Journal of Gerontological Nursing, 17,* 4–8.

Blouin, A. S., & Brent, N. J. (1992a). Nurse administrators in job transition: Defining the issues. *Journal of Nursing Administration. 22*(1), 10–11.

Blouin, A. S., & Brent, N. J. (1992b). Nurse administrators in job transition: Evolution of the issue. *Journal of Nursing Administration. 22*(3), 19–20, 60.

Blouin, A. S., & Brent, N. J. (1992c). Nurse administrators in job transition: Contractual considerations. *Journal of Nursing Administration. 22*(5), 8–10.

Blouin, A. S., & Brent, N. J. (1992d). Nurse administrators in job transition: Negotiated resignations and severance agreements. *Journal of Nursing Administration. 22*(7/8), 16–17.

Blouin, A. S., & Brent, N. J. (1992e). Nurse administrators in job transition: Managing the exit. *Journal of Nursing Administration. 22*(10), 12–13, 24.

Blouin, A. S., & Brent, N. J. (1992f). Nurse administrators in job transition: Stories from the front. *Journal of Nursing Administration. 22*(12), 13–14, 27.

Brackley, M. H. (1992). A role supplementation group pilot study: A nursing therapy for potential parental caregivers. *Clinical Nurse Specialist, 6*(1), 14–19.

Brautigan, R., Bryson, J., & Doster, S. (1989). Returning nurses: Easing the transition. *Nursing 89, 19*(8), 32K, 32N, 32R.

Bridges, E. J. (1992). Transition from ventilatory support: Knowing when the patient is ready to wean. *Critical Care Nursing Quarterly, 15*(1), 14–20.

Bridges, W. (1980). *Transitions.* Reading, MA: Addison-Wesley.

Bridges, W. (1986). Managing organizational transitions. *Organizational Dynamics, 14,* 24–33.

Brooten, D., Brown, L. P., Munro, B. H., York, R., Cohen, S. M., Roncoli, I., & Hollingsworth, A. (1988). Early discharge and specialist transitional care. *IMAGE: Journal of Nursing Scholarship, 20,* 64–68.

Brouse, A. J. (1988). Easing the transition to the maternal role. *Journal of Advanced Nursing, 13,* 167–172.

Brown, A. M., & Powell-Cope, G. M. (1991). AIDS family caregiving: Transitions through uncertainty. *Nursing Research, 40,* 338–345.

Bushy, A. (1990). Rural U.S. women: Traditions and transitions affecting health care. *Health Care for Women International, 11,* 503–513.

Cassells, J. M., Redman, B. K., & Jackson, S. S. (1986). Student choice of baccalaureate nursing programs, their perceived level of growth and development, career plans, and transition into practice: A replication. *Journal of Professional Nursing, 2,* 186–196.

Catanzaro, M. (1990). Transitions in midlife adults with long-term illness. *Holistic Nursing Practice, 4*(3), 65–73.

Ceslowitz, S. B., & Loreti, S. T. (1991). Easing the transition from hospital nursing to home care: A research study. *Home Healthcare Nurse, 9*(4), 32–35.

Chick, N., & Meleis, A. I. (1986). Transitions: A nursing concern. In P. L. Chinn (Ed.), *Nursing research methodology: Issues and implementation* (pp. 237–257). Rockville, MD: Aspen.

Chielens, D., & Herrick, E. (1990). Recipients of bone marrow transplants: Making a smooth transition to an ambulatory care setting. *Oncology Nursing Forum, 17,* 857–862.

Chiriboga, D. A. (1979). Conceptualizing adult transitions: A new look at an old subject. *Generations, 4*(3), 4–6.

Christman, N. J., McConnell, E. A., Pfeiffer, C., Webster, K. K., Schmitt, M., & Ries, J. (1988). Uncertainty, coping, and distress following myocardial infarction: Transition from hospital to home. *Research in Nursing and Health, 11,* 71–82.

Clarke, P. N., & Yaros, P. S. (1988). Research blenders: Commentary and response. Transitions to new methodologies in nursing sciences. *Nursing Science Quarterly, 1,* 147–151.

Clifford, C. (1989). An experience of transition from a medical model to a nursing model in nurse education. *Nurse Education Today, 9,* 413–418.

Cohen, S. M., Arnold, L., Brown L., & Brooten, D. (1991). Taxonomic classification of transitional follow-up care nursing interventions with low birthweight infants. *Clinical Nurse Specialist, 5,* 31–36.

Condi, J. K., Oliver, A., & Williams, E. (1986). Managing the transition to a neuroscience unit. *Journal of Neuroscience Nursing, 18,* 200–205.

De Bonde, K., & Hamilton, R. (1991). Dysphagia: A staged transition to oral nutrition. *Australian Nurses Journal, 20*(7), 12–13.

Dougherty, C. M. (1990). The near-death experience as a major life transition. *Holistic Nursing Practice, 4*(3), 84–90.

Dracup, K., Meleis, A., Baker, K., & Edlefsen, P. (1984). Family-focused cardiac rehabilitation. *Nursing Clinics of North America, 19,* 113–124.

Dunn, S. V. (1992). Orientation: The transition from novice to competent critical care nurse. *Critical Care Nursing Quarterly, 15*(1), 69–77.

Ehrat, K. S. (1990). Leadership in transition. *Journal of Nursing Administration, 20,* 6–7.

Fishbein, E. G. (1992). Women at midlife: The transition to menopause. *Nursing Clinics of North America, 27,* 951–957.

Flandermeyer, A., Kenner, C., Spaite, M. E., & Hostiuck, J. (1992). Transition from hospital to home, Part II. *Neonatal Network: Journal of Neonatal Nursing, 11*(5), 62–63.

Fought, S. G. (Ed.). (1992). Transitions in critical care. *Critical Care Nursing Quarterly, 15*(1), 1–90.

Frank, M.E. (1991). Transition into midlife. *NAACOG's Clinical Issues in Perinatal and Women's Health Nursing, 2,* 421–428.

Gaffney, K. F. (1992). Nursing practice model for maternal role sufficiency. *Advances in Nursing Science, 15*(2), 76–84.

Gardner, K. L., & Gander, M. (1992). Transition: From clinician to administrator. *Nursing Management, 23*(1), 38–39.

Gilmore, T. N. (1990). Effective leadership during organizational transitions. *Nursing Economics, 8,* 135–141.

Golan, N. (1981). *Passing through transitions.* New York: Free Press.

Gonzales-Osler, E. (1989). Coping with transition. *Journal of Psychosocial Nursing and Mental Health Services, 27*(6), 29, 32–35.

Grady, J. L. (1992). SN to GN to RN: Facilitating the transition. *Nurse Educator, 17*(4), 36, 40.

Harper, W. (1989). Transition. *Canadian Nurse, 85*(9), 32–34.

Hegyvary, S. T., & de Tornyay, R. (1991). Transitions in the deanship. *Journal of Professional Nursing, 7,* 41–44.

Henderson, A. D. (1989). Use of social support in a transition house for abused women. *Health Care for Women International, 10,* 61–73.

Hindman, B. (1986). Role transition. *Nursing Success Today, 3*(11), 4–7.

Hollander, J., & Haber, L. (1992). Ecological transition: Using Bronfenbrenner's model to study sexual identity change. *Health Care for Women International, 13,* 121–129.

Howard-Glenn, L. (1992). Transition to home: Discharge planning for the oxygen-dependent infant with bronchopulmonary dysplasia. *Journal of Perinatal and Neonatal Nursing, 6*(2), 85–94.

Imle, M. A. (1990). Third trimester concerns of expectant parents in transition to parenthood. *Holistic Nursing Practice, 4*(3), 25–36.

Imle, M. A., & Atwood, J. R. (1988). Retaining qualitative validity while gaining quantitative reliability and validity: Development of the Transition to Parenthood Concerns Scale. *Advances in Nursing Science, 11*(1), 61–75.

Jairath, N., Costello, J., Wallace, P., & Rudy, L. (1991). The effect of preceptorship upon diploma program nursing students' transition to the professional nursing role. *Journal of Nursing Education, 30,* 251–255.

Johnson, M. A., Morton, M. K., & Knox, S. M. (1992). The transition to a nursing home: Meeting the family's needs. Family members face their own transition when a loved one enters a nursing home. *Geriatric Nursing, 13,* 299–302.

Kane, J. J. (1992). Allowing the novice to succeed: Transitional support in critical care. *Critical Care Nursing Quarterly, 15*(3), 17–22.

Kenner, C., & Lott, J. W. (1990). Parent transition after discharge from the NICU. *Neonatal Network, 9*(2), 31–37.

Kerfoot, K., Serafin-Dickson, F., & Green, S. (1988). Managing transition: Resigning with style from the nurse manager position. *Nursing Economics, 6,* 200–202.

Klaich, K. (1990). Transitions in professional identity of nurses enrolled in graduate educational programs. *Holistic Nursing Practice, 4*(3), 17–24.

Ladden, M. (1990). The impact of preterm birth on the family and society. Part 2: Transition to home. *Pediatric Nursing, 16,* 620–622, 626.

Lathlean, J. (1987, September 16). The staff nurse: Prepared transition. *Nursing Times, 83*(37), 42, 44, 47.

Lauer, K. (1990). Transition in adolescence and its potential relationship to bulimic eating and weight control patterns in women. *Holistic Nursing Practice, 4*(3), 8–16.

Lengacher, C. A., & Keller, R. (1992). Comparison of role conception and role deprivation in LPN-transition students and traditional ADN students in a specially designed associate program. *Journal of Nursing Education, 31,* 79–84.

Losee, R. H., & Cook, J. W. (1989). Managing organizational transition. *Nursing Management, 20*(9), 82–83

Loveys, B. (1990). Transitions in chronic illness: The at-risk role. *Holistic Nursing Practice, 4*(3), 56–64.

Main, S., Mishler, S., Ayers, B., Poppa, L. D., & Jones, T. (1989). Easing transitions in care delivery with a core training group. *Nursing Connections, 2*(4), 5–15.

Majewski, J. (1986). Conflicts, satisfactions, and attitudes during transition to the maternal role. *Nursing Research, 35,* 10–14.

Majewski, J. (1987). Social support and the transition to the maternal role. *Health Care for Women International, 8,* 397–407.

Martell, L. K. (1990). The mother-daughter relationship during daughter's first pregnancy: The transition experience. *Holistic Nursing Practice, 4*(3), 47–55.

Meleis, A. I. (1975). Role insufficiency and role supplementation: A conceptual framework. *Nursing Research, 24,* 264–271.

Meleis, A. I. (1985). *Theoretical nursing: Development and progress.* Philadelphia: J. B. Lippincott.

Meleis, A. I. (1986). Theory development and domain concepts. In P. Moccia (Ed.), *New approaches to theory development* (pp. 3–21). New York: National League for Nursing.

Meleis, A. I. (1987). Women in transition: Being versus becoming or being and becoming. *Health Care for Women International, 8,* 199–217.

Meleis, A. I. (1991). *Theoretical nursing: Development and progress* (2nd ed.). Philadelphia: J.B. Lippincott.

Meleis, A. I., & Swendsen, L. A. (1978). Role supplementation: An empirical test of a nursing intervention. *Nursing Research, 27,* 11–18.

Mercer, R. T., Nichols, E. G., & Doyle, G. C. (1988). Transitions over the life cycle: A comparison of mothers and nonmothers. *Nursing Research, 37,* 144–151.

Michels, N. (1988). The transition from hospital to home: An exploratory study. *Home Health Care Services Quarterly, 9*(1), 29–44.

Morris, W. (1979). *American heritage dictionary of the English language.* Boston: Houghton Mifflin.

Murphy, S. A. (1990a). Human responses to transitions: A holistic nursing perspective. *Holistic Nursing Practice, 4*(3), 1–7.

Murphy, S. A. (Ed.). (1990b). Nursing care of clients in transition. *Holistic Nursing Practice, 4*(3), 1–90.

Myton, C. L., Allen, J. K., & Baldwin, J. A. (1992). Students in transition: Services for retention and outplacement. *Nursing Outlook, 40,* 227–230.

O'Brien, D. D. (1990). Transitions…continued. *Journal of Post Anesthesia Nursing, 5*(2), 73–74.

Parkes, C. M. (1971). Psychosocial transitions: A field for study. *Social Science and Medicine, 5,* 101–115.

Paterniti, A. P. (1987). Using Montessori's concepts on a transitional orientation nursing unit. *Journal of Nursing Staff Development, 3*(2), 71–75.

Patsdaughter, C. A., & Killien, M. (1990). Developmental transitions in adulthood: Mother-daughter relationships. *Holistic Nursing Practice, 4*(3), 37–46.

Poncar, P. J. (1989). The elderly widow: Easing her role transition. *Journal of Psychosocial Nursing and Mental Health Services, 27*(2), 6–11, 39–40.

Pridham, K. F., & Chang, A. S. (1992). Transition to being the mother of a new infant in the first three months: Maternal problem solving and self-appraisals. *Journal of Advanced Nursing, 17,* 204–216.

Pridham, K. F., Lytton, D., Chang, A. S., & Rutledge, D. (1991). Early postpartum transition: Progress in maternal identity and role attainment. *Research in Nursing and Health, 14,* 21–31.

Pullen, C. H. (1988). Are we easing the transition from LPN to ADN? *American Journal of Nursing, 88,* 1129.

Reed-McKay, K. L. (1989). Role transition for school nurses in the Spokane Public Schools. *Journal of School Health, 59,* 444–445.

Reimer, J. C., Davies, B., & Martens, N. (1991). Palliative care: The nurse's role in helping families through the transition of "fading away." *Cancer Nursing, 14,* 321–327.

Rice, J. M. (1988). Transition from staff nurse to head nurse: A personal experience. *Nursing Management, 19*(4), 102.

Ritz, L. J., & Walker, M. K. (1989). Transitional care services and chronicity: Oncology as a case in point. *Hospice Journal, 5,* 55–66.

Robinson, G. M., & Pinkney, A. A. (1992). Transition from the hospital to the community: Small group program. *Journal of Psychosocial Nursing and Mental Health Services, 30*(5), 33–38.

Rotkovitch, R., & Smith, C. (1987). ICON I—The future model; ICON II—The transition model. *Nursing Management, 18*(11), 91–92, 94–96.

Ryan, S. (1988). Transition from institutional to home and ambulatory care. *American Nurses Association Publications, (American Nurse CH-18),* 41–45.

Salitros, P.H. (1986). Transitional infant care: A bridge to home for high-risk infants. *Neonatal Network, 4*(4), 35–41.

Samarel, N. (1989). Caring for the living and dying: A study of role transition. *International Journal of Nursing Studies, 26,* 313–326.

Scherting, D. G. (1988). Making the transition from staff nurse to nurse manager. *ANNA Journal, 15,* 369.

Schlossberg, N. K. (1981). A model for analyzing human adaptation to transition. *The Counseling Psychologist, 9*(2), 2–18.

Schwartz, D. (1989). A long transition [Letter to the editor]. *Nursing Outlook, 37,* 146.

Selder, F. (1989). Life transition theory: The resolution of uncertainty. *Nursing and Health Care, 10,* 437–451.

Shea, L. E., Adamzczak, P., & Flanagan, T. J. (1987). Transition to flight nursing: Three experiences. *Journal of Emergency Nursing, 13*(4), 31A–35A.

Shields, N. A. (1991). The transition to video: Considerations for the GI laboratory manager. *Gastroenterology Nursing, 14*(1), 44–47.

Staples, N. R., & Schwartz, M. (1990). Anorexia nervosa support group: Providing transitional support. *Journal of Psychosocial Nursing and Mental Health Services, 28*(2), 6–10, 36–37.

Starke, F., & Rempel, E. (1990). From nursing to nursing administration: Making the transition easier. *Canadian Journal of Nursing Administration, 3,* 6–11.

Swarczinski, C., & Graham, P. (1990). From ICU to rehabilitation: A checklist to ease the transition for the spinal cord injured. *Journal of Neuroscience Nursing, 22*(2), 89–91.

Swearingen, L. (1987). Transitional day treatment: An individualized goal-oriented approach. *Archives of Psychiatric Nursing, 1,* 104–110.

Talarczyk, G., & Milbrandt, D. (1988). A collaborative effort to facilitate role transition from student to registered nurse practitioner. *Nursing Management, 19*(2), 30–32.

Thurber, F., & DiGiamarino, L. (1992). Development of a model of transitional care for the HIV-positive child and family. *Clinical Nurse Specialist, 6,* 142–146.

Tierney, M. J., Grant, L. M., Cherrstrom, P. L., & Morris, B. L. (1990). Clinical nurse specialists in transition. *Clinical Nurse Specialist, 4,* 103–106.

Tomlinson, P. S. (1987). Spousal differences in marital satisfaction during transition to parenthood. *Nursing Research, 36,* 239–243.

Turley, J. P. (1992). A framework for the transition from nursing records to a nursing information system. *Nursing Outlook, 40,* 177–181.

Tyhurst, J. (1957). *The role of transition states—including disasters—in mental illness.* In Symposium on Preventive and Social Psychiatry (pp. 149–169). Washington, DC: Walter Reed Army Institute of Research.

van Maanen, H. M. T. (1990). Nursing in transition: An analysis of the state of the art in relation to the conditions of practice and society's expectations. *Journal of Advanced Nursing, 15,* 914–924.

Vezeau, T. M., & Hallsten, D. A. (1987). Making the transition to mother-baby care. *MCN: Maternal-Child Nursing, 12,* 193–198.

Walker, K., & DeVooght, J. (1989). Invasion: A hospital in transition following the 1983 Grenadian intervention. *Journal of Psychosocial Nursing and Mental Health Services, 27*(1), 27–30.

Watson, J. (1988). A case study: Curriculum in transition. *NLN Publications,* (15–2224), 1–8.

Webster's third new international dictionary. (1981). Springfield, MA: C.G. Merriam.

Wild, L. (1992). Transition from pain to comfort: Managing the hemodynamic risks. *Critical Care Nursing Quarterly, 15*(1), 46–56.

Wong, D. L. (1991). Transition from hospital to home for children with complex medical care. *Journal of Pediatric Oncology Nursing, 8,* 3–9.

Wuest, J. (1990). Trying it on for size: Mutual support in role transition for pregnant teens and student nurses. *Health Care for Women International, 11,* 383–392.

Young, H. M. (1990). The transition of relocation to a nursing home. *Holistic Nursing Practice, 4*(3), 74–83.

Reprinted with permission from: Schumacher, K. L., & Meleis, A. I. (1994). Transitions: A central concept in nursing. *Journal of Nursing Scholarship, 26*(2), 119–127.

Chapter 2   Transition Theory

2.1 EXPERIENCING TRANSITIONS: AN EMERGING MIDDLE-RANGE THEORY

AFAF IBRAHIM MELEIS
LINDA M. SAWYER
EUN-OK IM
DEANNE K. HILFINGER MESSIAS
KAREN SCHUMACHER

Abstract

Changes in health and illness of individuals create a process of transition, and clients in transition tend to be more vulnerable to risks that may in turn affect their health. Uncovering these risks may be enhanced by understanding the transition process. As a central concept of nursing, transition has been analyzed, its components identified, and a framework to articulate and to reflect the relationship between these components has been defined. In this chapter, the previous conceptual analysis of transitions is extended and refined by drawing on the results of five different research studies that have examined transitions using an integrative approach to theory development. The emerging middle-range theory of transitions consists of types and patterns of transitions, properties of transition experiences, facilitating and inhibiting conditions, process indicators, outcome indicators, and nursing therapeutics. The diversity, complexity, and multiple dimensionality of transition experiences need to be further explored and incorporated in future research and nursing practice related to transitions.

Changes in health status may provide opportunities for enhanced well-being and expose individuals to increased illness risks, as well as trigger a process of transition. Vulnerability may be conceptualized as a quality of daily lives uncovered through an understanding of clients' experiences and responses during times of transition. In this sense, vulnerability is related to transition experiences, interactions, and environmental conditions that expose individuals to potential damage, problematic or extended recovery, or delayed or unhealthy coping. Clients' daily lives, environments, and interactions are shaped by the nature, conditions, meanings, and processes of transition experiences. Transitions are both a result of, and result in, change in lives, health, relationships, and environments.

Nurses often are the primary caregivers of clients and their families who are undergoing transition. They attend to the changes and demands that transitions bring into the daily lives of clients and their families. Furthermore, nurses tend to be the caregivers who prepare clients for impending transitions and who facilitate the process of learning new skills related to clients' health and illness experiences. Examples of transitions that may make clients vulnerable are *illness experiences* such as diagnosis, surgical procedures, rehabilitation and recovery; *developmental and lifespan transitions* such as pregnancy, childbirth, parenthood, adolescence, menopause, aging, and death; and *social and cultural transitions* such as migration, retirement, and family caregiving.[1,2]

As a central concept in nursing, transition has been analyzed and a framework has been defined to articulate and reflect the relationships among the components of a transition.[1,3] Transition has been used both as a perspective and as a framework.

The purpose of this chapter is: (a) to continue the conceptual analysis of transition from a nursing perspective, extending and refining the existing framework by drawing on the results of five nursing studies that were based on a transition framework,[4-8] and (b) to identify future directions for nursing research and theory building regarding transitions and a transition framework. In the process, the findings across studies were compared and contrasted, emerging properties were identified, the literature from 1993 to 1997 was reviewed, and respective clinical and research experiences and perspectives were integrated into the analyses. Using an integrative concept analysis strategy,[9] a middle-range theory was developed. In presenting the analysis, each study will be introduced briefly and then the emerging theoretical framework and the conceptual modifications that were developed from the analysis of this collective research will be outlined.

Studies Using Transitions as a Framework

The frameworks articulated by Chick and Meleis[3] and Schumacher and Meleis[1] were used to guide the development of each of the following studies and the analysis of data. The intent of each study was to uncover emerging themes that may not have been originally a part of the framework. The process of using inductive and deductive reasoning not only enabled evaluation of the utility of the different components of the framework, but also identified additional emerging components.

The studies reflect cultural diversity in vulnerable populations including African Americans, Brazilian immigrants, and Korean immigrants. They also reflect a variety of transitions that may lead to heightened vulnerability, including pregnancy, motherhood, menopause, work, migration, caregiving, and diagnostic processes. Although different approaches were used for data analysis, each study used a qualitative research design with the goal of theory development. In addition, each study reflected a feminist perspective in the design and in the interpretation of data, allowing an examination of the data within the context of race, class, culture, and gender.

Becoming an African-American Mother

Using grounded theory methodology, 17 first-time African-American mothers were interviewed to elicit their experiences of pregnancy and motherhood.[4,10] This transition spanned the time period between the woman's decision to get pregnant or to continue a pregnancy and the time when mothering was incorporated into her identity. Women were interviewed both individually and in focus groups from one to three times during the postpartum period. *Engaged mothering* was identified as the core category, denoting the active, involved, and mutual process in which African-American mothers get ready to be a mother, deal with the reality involved, settle in with their babies, and dream and plan for a good life for themselves and their children and families. The outcome of engaged mothering is incorporation of mothering into the woman's identity and a healthy, happy, strong, safe, and secure child. In this study, all women demonstrated engaged mothering. However, the environment for this group of women increased their stress during pregnancy. Women frequently anticipated and dealt with incidents of racism, stereotyping, and negativity in their daily lives. The environment mediated the transition both by providing support and by increasing stress. Two conditions affected transition experiences and responses: First, the level of planning for motherhood was influenced by the degree to which the pregnancy was intentional, with women who were actively trying to get pregnant proceeding through the transition more easily. Second, prior miscarriage or history of health problems of the mother diminished the woman's sense of emotional and physical well-being and inhibited the transition.[10]

Neglecting and Ignoring the Menopausal Transition

The purpose of this study was to describe the perceived meanings that low-income Korean immigrant women had about their menopausal transition, to describe their perceived symptoms during this transition, and to analyze their responses within a context of immigration and their work situations.[5] The study was cross-sectional, utilizing methodological triangulation.[11] For the qualitative portion of the study, semi-structured in-depth interviews were conducted with 21 perimenopausal or postmenopausal women. Data were analyzed using thematic analysis. A major conceptual category that emerged was *neglecting and ignoring the menopausal transition* because of other imminent demands in the women's lives such as immigration, new work experiences, and the patriarchal cultural heritage that makes women's experiences invisible and inaudible. The number, seriousness, and priority of transitions that these women were experiencing contributed to neglect of their menopausal transition.[12] In addition, the participants relayed stories of neglect because of their experiences within the context of gender, low-income status, and attitudes toward health and illness. Participants related these conditions to their menopausal transitions.

Parents and Diagnostic Transitions

Messias et al.[6] examined the experiences of parents of children diagnosed with congenital heart defects (CHD). The analysis was part of a larger exploratory investigation[13-15] of the transitions in health, social relations, and development experienced by adolescents and young adults with CHD and their families. The stories collected from eight parents about the birth and diagnosis of a child with CHD revealed the superimposition of an unanticipated transition with possible negative outcomes (becoming the parent of a child with CHD) on an anticipated transition with an expected positive outcome (becoming the parent of a normal, healthy newborn). As the parents observed health care providers and environments and their own infants, they began to gather evidence that something was wrong. They frequently became confused with the *illusiveness of normality*, as they tried to sort out the sometimes paradoxical meanings and appearances of "normal pregnancies," "normal, healthy babies," and the di-

agnosis of CHD. For some, the diagnostic event per se came as an abrupt shock. For others, coming to know the diagnosis was a gradual process over time, characterized more by ambivalence and unknowing. The process of coming to know, recognize, and acknowledge the congenital condition in the child was characterized as a *rude awakening*. Eventually, parents' acknowledgment and understanding of the reality of CHD became the *work of managing uncertainty*, which would become one of the hallmarks of their parenting in the ensuing years. As parents reflected back on their experiences, they told of how they *created new meanings* in their own and their children's lives and talked about *taking stock of costs and benefits* of having a child with CHD.

Migration, Work, and Health: Complex, Multidimensional Transitions

In another study, Messias[7] explored the lived experiences of transnational migration, work, employment, and health. Embedded in the narratives of 26 Brazilian women who had migrated to the United States were stories of *multiple transitions, fluid identities, constant comparisons,* and *changing perspectives on class, culture, and women's work.* All of the women in the study experienced some form of work or occupational transition in conjunction with their transnational migration. For some, migration signified the transition from being a Brazilian professional, student, or middle-class housewife to immigrant domestic worker. Domestic work was one of the limited employment options for many, particularly for the newly arrived and the undocumented. Women viewed this occupational transition from different perspectives and found different meanings in the experience. Over time, domestic or food service work was a temporary stepping stone for some; for others, domestic work signified a long-term career change. Such migratory occupational transitions were embedded in social transitions, which in many cases translated into perceived downward social mobility. However, for some of the women who had been employed as domestic workers in Brazil, migration was perceived as an upward social and economic transition. Within the narratives of the women, there were both strong support and interesting challenges for the use of a transition framework to understand and explain migration experiences. What characterized their experiences as transitions was not so much the movement across national borders but the resulting passages between different life phases, conditions, and statuses, accompanied by some degree of self-redefinition.[3] The results of this research support the concept of migration as a transnational transition. However, the study suggested that transnational migration transitions are characterized by movement that is ongoing, recurring, and multidirectional and is between multiple places, spaces, situations, and identities, rather than movement that is linear or unidirectional.

> *The results of this research support the concept of migration as a transnational transition.*

The Family Caregiving Study

The purpose of this study was to generate a grounded theory of family caregiver role acquisition among caregivers of persons receiving chemotherapy for cancer.[8] Specifically, the study sought to identify patterns of role acquisition and conditions influencing these patterns, using an interactionist perspective. Thus, the study included both family caregivers and the persons for whom they were providing care. A longitudinal design in which participants were interviewed three times across the course of chemotherapy was consistent with a transition perspective.[1] The sample consisted of 19 caregivers and 20 patients with solid tumors or lymphoma. Semi-structured interviews addressed illness care experiences, strategies, and interactions. Although the original intent of the study was to explore caregivers' transitions into the caregiving role, it quickly became apparent that caregiving could not be isolated analytically from self-care by the ill person. Thus, self-care and caregiving by the dyad became the focus for analysis. Patterns of self-care and caregiving were quite fluid and shifted often over the course of chemotherapy as conditions for care changed, leading to the identification of *shifting patterns of self-care and caregiving* as the core concept of the grounded theory. The study revealed the fluidity of care involvement during the transition into illness care roles and the need to study complementary role transitions together.

Emerging Framework

Through our collective research, an expanded theoretical framework emerged consisting of:

- types and patterns of transitions
- properties of transition experiences
- transition conditions: facilitators and inhibitors
- process indicators
- outcome indicators
- nursing therapeutics

In this chapter, the first five components of the framework are addressed. Concurrently with the analysis presented here, implications for nursing therapeutics are addressed; however, a full exposition of this part of the framework is beyond the scope of this chapter. The relationships between the six components of the framework are illustrated in Figure 2.1.1. These components were identified through a collaborative process of dialogue, constant comparison of the findings across the five studies, and analysis. In the following sections each of the components is discussed, focusing in particular on the extensions and modifications of previous frameworks and on the emerging framework.

Types and Patterns of Multiple and Complex Transitions

Types of transitions that nurses encounter in working with patients and families have been identified as developmental, health and illness, situational, and organizational.[1,3,16] The results of our research supported this typology as representative of the transitions central to nursing practice. However, the research also supported the notion of transitions as

Nature of Transitions
Types
 Developmental
 Situational
 Health/Illness
 Organizational

Patterns
 Single
 Multiple
 Sequential
 Simultaneous
 Related
 Unrelated

Properties
 Awareness
 Engagement
 Change and Difference
 Transition Time Span
 Critical Points and Events

Transition Conditions: Facilitators & Inhibitors
Personal
 Meanings
 Cultural Beliefs & Attitudes
 Socioeconomic status
 Preparation & knowledge

Community   Society

Patterns of Response
Progress Indicators
 Feeling Connected
 Interacting
 Location and Being Situated
 Developing Confidence and Coping

Outcome Indicators
 Mastery
 Fluid Integrative Identities

Nursing Therapeutics

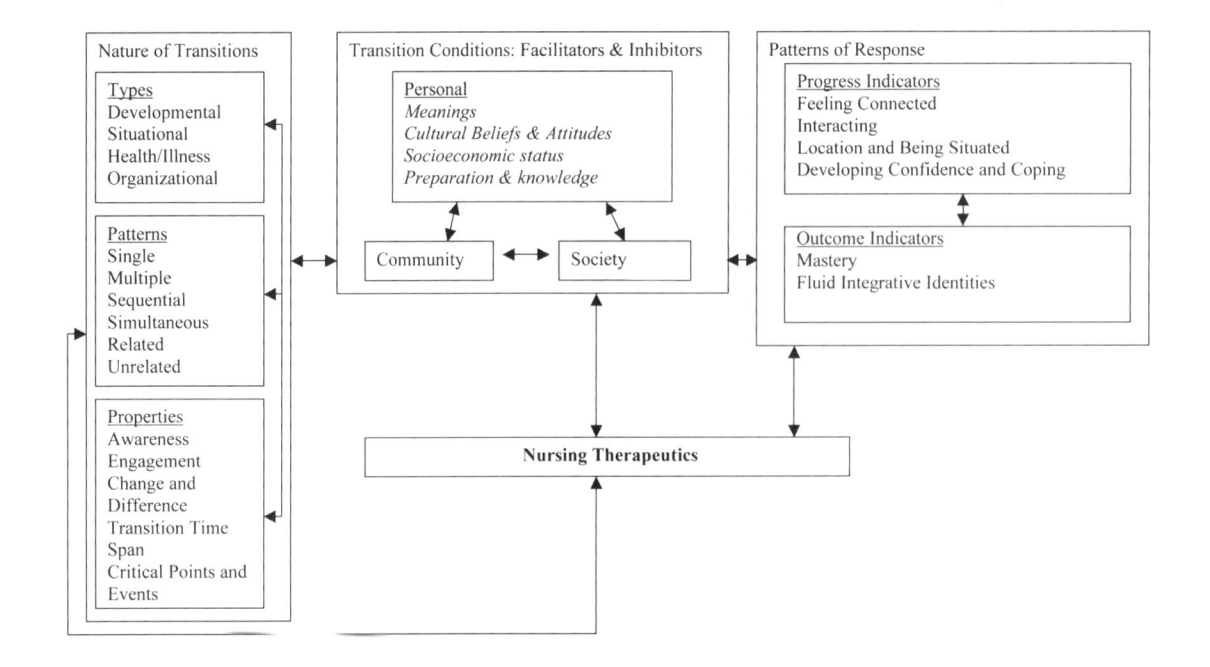

FIGURE 2.1.1 Transitions: A middle-range theory.

patterns of multiplicity and complexity.[7] For example, each of the previously described studies involved individuals who were experiencing at least two types of transitions, indicating that transitions are not discrete or mutually exclusive. Migration scholars have called attention to the multiple structural transitions involved in migration, such as transitions in employment, socioeconomic status, culture, and social networks.[17] Messias[7] noted that the migration experiences of Brazilian women were multiple and complex in nature and did not occur in isolation, but rather in conjunction with other situational, developmental, and health-illness transitions. As the women talked about their migration, work, and health experiences, the interrelations and connections of multiple transitions were woven throughout their narratives. Similarly, Im[5] found that the Korean women were not only dealing with the developmental transition of menopause, but also situational transitions related to migration and work. In fact, for these women, the menopausal transition was found to be less of a priority than the other transitions they were experiencing.

Messias et al.[6] found that the diagnosis of CHD in newborns or infants created an unexpected transition superimposed on other personal and family transitions related to childbirth and parenting. Schumacher[18] found that the transition into the caregiving role could not be understood in isolation from the health and illness transition experienced by the family member with cancer.

At the same time the caregiver was experiencing the transition to the caregiving role, the care receiver was experiencing the transition to having a life-threatening illness.

In light of the results of these studies, our analyses of the nature of transitions suggest that nurses need to consider the patterns of all significant transitions in an individual or family's life rather than focusing only on one specific type of transition. Patterns of transition would include whether the client is experiencing a single transition or multiple transitions. Important considerations are whether multiple transitions are sequential or simultaneous, the extent of overlap among transitions, and the nature of the relationship between the different events that are triggering transitions for a client.

Properties of the Transition Experience

Transitions are complex and multidimensional, but several essential properties of transition experiences have been identified. These include:

- awareness
- engagement
- change and difference
- time span
- critical points and events

These properties are not necessarily discrete. Rather, they are interrelated properties of a complex process.

Awareness

Awareness is related to perception, knowledge, and recognition of a transition experience. Level of awareness is often reflected in the degree of congruency between what is known about processes and responses and what constitutes an expected set of responses and perceptions of individuals undergoing similar transitions. Chick and Meleis[3] included awareness as a defining characteristic of transition, and they purported that to be in transition, a person must have some awareness of the changes that are occurring. They posited that an absence of awareness of change could signify that an individual may not have initiated the transition experience. We propose that although awareness appears to be an important property of transition, the lack of manifestation of such awareness does not preclude the onset of a transition experience. For example, some of the Korean women in Im's[5] study did not recognize that they were experiencing a menopausal transition; others recognized the experience only at the cessation of menstruation. However, although the changes related to menopause were not fully recognized, there was evidence that the women were going through a transition related to menopause.

We do not believe that our analysis of these studies has completely resolved the tension between *transition awareness by clients* and *nurses knowledge of whether clients are in transition*. Thus, the question remains: Whose awareness (nurses or clients) triggers the beginning of the process? These studies provide a context for discussion but do not resolve the paradox.

Engagement

Another property of transitions is the level of engagement in the process. Engagement is defined as the degree to which a person demonstrates involvement in the processes inherent in the transition. Examples of engagement are seeking out information, using role models, actively preparing, and proactively modifying activities. The level of awareness influences the level of engagement in that engagement may not happen without awareness. The level of engagement of a person who is aware of physical, emotional, social, or environmental changes will differ from that of a person unaware of such changes. Sawyer[1] found various instances of differing levels and types of engagement in the transition to motherhood among the participants in her study. For example, a woman in the early months of pregnancy who is unaware of changes in her body may not be as careful about potentially harmful medications or balancing her diet.

Change and Difference

Change and difference are essential properties of transitions. Although similar, these properties are not interchangeable, nor are they synonymous with transition. All transitions involve change, whereas not all change is related to transition.[19] An example from the study of parents' diagnostic transitions illustrates the difference between change and transition. One of the fathers described the impact of the diagnosis of CHD as having resulted in an abrupt *change* in family focus. However, the *transition* was a long-term process, which involved the father adapting to new roles and situations, coming to terms with the diagnosis, and eventually resulting in new meanings and a sense of mastery when he understood the "whole picture."[6] Transitions are both the result *of change* and result *in change*.

To fully understand a transition process it is necessary to uncover and describe the effects and meanings of the changes involved. Dimensions of change that should be explored include the nature, temporality, perceived importance or severity, and personal, familial, and societal norms and expectations. Change may be related to critical or disequilibrating events, to disruptions in relationships and routines, or to ideas, perceptions, and identities. For example, some parents of infants with CHD perceived the "diagnostic event" itself as the critical disequilibrating event, but for others cardiac surgery was more forcefully disequilibrating. Sawyer[4] noted that the African-American women understood that any changes they experienced in their bodies could affect the development of their babies.

Confronting difference is another property of transitions, exemplified by unmet or divergent expectations, feeling different, being perceived as different, or seeing the world and others in different ways. Messias[7] noted that immigrant women confronted difference on many different levels. Those who had expectations of facile, abundant opportunities and easy money frequently were confronted upon arrival in the United States with the very different reality of restricted and sometimes demeaning employment. However, expectations were varied and individualized, and the disjuncture between expectations, and reality was not always for the worse. Whereas some immigrants were stunned, shocked, or disappointed with the reality they encountered, others were pleasantly surprised. Immigrant women also found differences in the food, supermarkets, health care system, social patterns and beliefs, landscape, language, and the way Americans show affection. One woman remarked that it involved a lot of work *"not to be affected by all of these differences."* Some immigrants admitted that they themselves had changed, that they were now different because they had become *"more American,"* more impersonal, and less socially engaged. Others identified themselves as more independent, responsible, and autonomous. Migration often resulted in a blurring of previously perceived differences such as social class or gendered employment. However, such blurring did not necessarily signify that the differences had been erased. Perceived difference sometimes resulted in changed behaviors or perceptions, but not all differences affected women in the same way or held the same meanings. In examining transition experiences, it may be useful for nurses to consider a client's level of comfort and mastery in dealing with change and difference.

Time Span

All transitions are characterized by flow and movement over time.[2] Bridges[19,20] characterized transition as a time span with an identifiable end point, extending from the first signs of anticipation, perception, or demonstration of change; through a period of instability, confusion, and distress; to an eventual "ending" with a new beginning or period of stability. However, the results of the research examined here suggest that it may be difficult or impossible, and perhaps even counterproductive, to put boundaries on the time span of certain transition experiences.[6] The stories told by parents of infants with CHD indicated that their transition did not always follow the same chronological trajectory. Migration provided another case in point.[7] Immigrants may consider their transition as "temporary" even though they may live in another country for an extended period. Even for those who settle permanently, the migration experience may best be characterized as an ongoing, undulating, unending transition. This does not necessarily mean that immigrants or others experiencing long-term transitions are constantly in a state of disconnectedness, flux, or change. However, such states may periodically surface, reactivating a latent transition experience. In evaluating transition experiences, it is important to consider the possibility of flux and variability over time, which may necessitate reassessment of outcomes.

> *All transitions are characterized by flow and movement over time.*

Critical Points and Events

Some transitions are associated with an identifiable marker event; such as birth, death, the cessation of menstruation, or the diagnosis of an illness; whereas in other transitions, specific marker events are not as evident.[19,20] The various studies involving multiple transitions provided evidence that most transition experiences involved critical turning points or events. Critical points were often associated with increasing awareness of change or difference or more active engagement in dealing with the transition experience. In addition, there were final critical points, which were characterized by a sense of stabilization in new routines, skills, lifestyles, and self-care activities. In each study there was a period of uncertainty marked with fluctuation, continuous change, and disruption in reality. Symptoms related to the transition might also occur. During a period of uncertainty there were a number of critical points depending on the nature of the transition. Each critical point requires the nurse's attention, knowledge, and experience in different ways.

For example, in the family caregiving study,[8] four critical periods were identified:

1. the diagnostic period
2. the side-effect–intensive periods of chemotherapy cycles
3. the junctures between treatment modalities
4. the completion of treatment

These were periods of heightened vulnerability during which participants encountered difficulties with self-care and caregiving. Illness care conditions were changing, self-care and caregiving patterns were shifting, access to health care providers was changing, and participants experienced uncertainty and anxiety.

Transition Conditions: Facilitators and Inhibitors

In the discipline of nursing, humans are defined as active beings who have perceptions of and attach meanings to health and illness situations. These perceptions and meanings are influenced by and in turn influence the conditions under which a transition occurs. Thus, to understand the experiences of clients during transitions, it is necessary to uncover the personal and environmental conditions that facilitate or hinder progress toward achieving a healthy transition. Personal, community, or societal conditions may facilitate or constrain the processes of healthy transitions and the outcomes of transitions.

Personal Conditions

Meanings. The meanings attributed to events precipitating a transition and to the transition process itself may facilitate or hinder healthy transitions. In the Korean menopause study,[5] although the participants had ambivalent feelings toward menopause, menopause itself did not have special meaning attached to it. Most of the women did not relate any special problems they were having to their menopausal transition. Furthermore, some participants indicated that they went through their menopause without experiencing or perceiving any problems. Therefore, in a sense, "no special meanings" may have facilitated the women's menopausal transition.[5] On the other hand, the African-American women attributed intense enjoyment to their roles as mothers and described motherhood in terms of being responsible, protecting, supporting, and being needed.[4] In these two examples neutral and positive meanings may have facilitated menopause and motherhood.

Cultural Beliefs and Attitudes. When stigma is attached to a transition experience, such as menopause in Korean culture, the expression of emotional states related to the transition may be inhibited. Because women in Korean culture tend to regard menopause as shameful to discuss in public,[21] they silently go through menopause on their own, and their menopausal experience becomes a lonely experience. Symptoms then get attributed to their emotional state and become stigmatized. Their psychological symptoms were noted only when expressed physically, through headaches, muscle aches, and exhaustion. Perhaps Asian and Middle-Eastern cultures express psychological symptoms through somatization because of the fear of stigma.[22]

Socioeconomic Status. Another inhibitor to healthy menopausal transition was the women's low socioeconomic status. The women's experience of psychological symptoms was significantly affected by their socioeconomic status rather than their menopausal states. As other studies have shown,[23-27] participants who have low socioeconomic status were more likely to experience psychological symptoms.

Preparation and Knowledge. Anticipatory preparation facilitates the transition experience, whereas lack of preparation is an inhibitor. Inherently related to preparation is knowledge about what to expect during a transition and what strategies may be helpful in managing it. For one immigrant Brazilian woman, lack of preparation was particularly stark.[7] The woman's limited knowledge and understanding of geography, language, and culture were transparent, and upon her arrival in the United States, the consequences of her lack of preparation and understanding immediately became evident. She was shocked culturally, physically, and emotionally. The woman had brought only summer clothes and the cold April weather in New York took her by surprise. Crammed into a room with 10 people, she looked out the window on a strange, unknown world and thought she was losing her mind. Her nightmares were a reflection of what life itself had become. Immigration was not only a move to a different place, a different city, a different country, or a different hemisphere; she found herself literally in a different world, a world she had no idea existed.

The transition to motherhood provides another example of the importance of preparation and expectations.[4] When a pregnancy was not planned, or when the mother had a history of either miscarriage or illness, the transition through the stages toward developing a maternal identity was delayed. In the menopause study, lack of knowledge about menopause was found to inhibit the menopausal transition. Women who lacked knowledge often visited clinics because of changes in their menstruation. When their physicians recommended surgical treatment, the women silently followed the physicians' suggestions because they rarely knew about other alternatives.

Community Conditions

Community resources also facilitate or inhibit transitions. For example, to deal with their immigration transition, Korean immigrants turned to restaurants, laundries, and/or grocery shops in the Korean community seeking the support of other immigrants.[5] However, because of the need for privacy and the mistrust within the Korean immigrant community, women rarely used these readily available community resources for issues related to health and illness. Thus, distrust within immigrant communities may prevent women from using familiar resources to support their various transitions. Until they become familiar with and have access to host country resources, they may get inadequate community support during critical times in their transitions.[5]

African-American women also described community-level conditions that both facilitated and inhibited their transitions to motherhood.[4] Facilitators included:

- support from partners and families, especially from the woman's mother and other significant women in her life
- relevant information obtained from trusted health care providers and from classes, books, and other written materials
- advice from respected sources
- role models
- answers to questions

Inhibitors of a healthy transition for these mothers included insufficient resources to support pregnancy and motherhood. Planning and offering classes that were inconvenient for the women was also an inhibitor. As one woman said, "Well, actually, all the classes were at the hospital, and I don't have a car. And they're at night. And I didn't have a coach." Other inhibitors of a healthy transition for these mothers included inadequate support, unsolicited or negative advice, insufficient or contradictory information, and the hassles of being stereotyped, facing negativity from others, or being treated like "public property."[4]

Societal Conditions

Society at large could also be a facilitator or inhibitor for transitions. Viewing a transitional event as stigmatized and with stereotyped meanings tends to interfere in the process of healthy transition. For example, gender inequity is a constraint at the societal level that influences a woman's menopausal transition. In patriarchal Korean culture, the position of women in the family structure is well known.[28] Women's position in the family explains why their own health care needs are put behind other family members' needs, and why they sacrifice time for themselves. Therefore, viewing the menopausal transition alone without considering gender inequities embedded in the daily experiences of women cannot be adequate.

Marginalization was another societal inhibitor to the Korean immigrant women's menopausal experience. Because they were in the margin both in the host society and in their own culture, they neglected and ignored their menopausal experiences. They rarely recognized menopause as a health problem. Rather, they gave priority to their family matters and made their own needs secondary. Cultural attitudes toward women's bodies and experiences were yet another societal inhibitor to a healthy menopausal transition.[21]

Patterns of Response

Process Indicators

Meleis and Trangenstein[2] state that

> nursing...is concerned with the process and the experiences of human beings undergoing transitions where health and perceived well-being is the outcome. (p. 257)

Based on the studies described in this chapter, a healthy transition is characterized by both process and outcome indicators. Because transitions unfold over time, identifying process indicators that move clients either in the direction of health or toward vulnerability and risk allows early assessment and intervention by nurses to facilitate healthy outcomes.[24] In each of the studies, methods were used to uncover the processes inherent in healthy transitions. Some of the observations about the indicators or patterns of response that characterized healthy transitions are discussed below. These patterns of response included feeling connected, interacting, being situated, and developing confidence and coping.

Feeling Connected

The need to feel and stay connected is a prominent theme in many transition narratives.[29] For example, making new contacts and continuing old connections with extended family and friends were an important part of Brazilian women's migration experiences.[7] Similar to what has been documented by other researchers,[30-34] the immigrant women in this study utilized social and kinship networks as important sources of information, housing, transportation, employment, and social support.

> The need to feel and stay connected is a prominent theme in many transition narratives.

Personal contacts and connections were a primary source of information about health care services and resources. Feeling connected to health care professionals who could answer questions and with whom they felt comfortably connected was another important indicator of a positive transition experience.[7] This emerging dimension of transition supports the clinical evidence that providing culturally competent care in hospitals requires continuity in relationships between health care providers and patients.[35]

Interacting

Among people with cancer and their family caregivers,[8] intra-dyadic interaction was a critical dimension of the transition experience. Through interaction, the meaning of the transition and the behaviors developed in response to the transition were uncovered, clarified, and acknowledged. Although the diagnosis of cancer was seen by all as a crisis event, the meaning of self-care and caregiving varied from one dyad to another. In some dyads, the involvement of the caregiver was resisted as the person with the diagnosis of cancer struggled to maintain self-care. In other dyads, the involvement of the caregiver was welcomed as a supportive gesture. These strategies were clarified through interaction and reflection about the new and emerging relationship. Through interaction, dyads created a context in which self-care and caregiving could take place effectively and harmoniously.

Location and Being Situated

Location is important to most transition experiences, although it may be more obvious in some than in others, such as migration, where location often implies a unidirectional movement from one place to another. For immigrants, there is a constant actual or imaginary migration back and forth between home and host country, between their pre- and postmigration lives.[7] In their stories, the Brazilian women constantly made comparisons. They compared their lives, experiences, practices, and attitudes pre– and postmigration, from when they first arrived, and after they had lived in the United States for a while. They compared almost anything: Health care, food, diet, nutrition, family relationships, child rearing, prices, domestic work, climate, weather, employment and work opportunities, and gender and class relations. The women also brought diverse perspectives to their migration experiences. One of the characteristics of transitions is the creation of new meanings and perceptions. Comparisons were one of the ways the immigrant women presented, examined, and made meaning of their experiences. They understood their new life by comparing it to the old.

Making comparisons was also a way of "situating" themselves in terms of time, space, and relationships; a way to explain and perhaps justify how or why they came, where they are and where they have been, and who and what they are. The comparisons were multidirectional in the sense that some were favorable toward Brazil or the premigration experience, and others were favorable toward the United States or the postmigration experience. Such comparisons most certainly served different purposes for different women at different times, but they highlight the multiplicity of perspectives in immigrants' experiences, something that nonmigrants may find difficult to understand or may misinterpret as criticism or condemnation.[7]

Developing Confidence and Coping

Another dimension that reflects the nature of the transition process is the extent to which there is a pattern indicating that the individuals involved are experiencing an increase in their level of confidence. Developing confidence is manifested in the level of understanding of the different processes inherent in diagnosis, treatment, recovery, and living with limitations; in the level of resource utilization; and in the development of strategies for managing. The dimensions of developing and manifesting confidence are progressive from one point to the next in the transition trajectory. As one participant in the African-American pregnancy study[4] put it, "So I figured…I guess he's getting enough milk. He's gaining weight. It must be OK. So I didn't worry." Another participant in the same study was more confident because, as she put it, "I have a schedule, and I'm just so in tune with his schedule." Participants demonstrated cumulative knowledge of situations, more understanding of critical and turning points, and a sense of wisdom resulting from their lived experiences.

Outcome Indicators

Two outcome indicators emerged from the studies examined in this analysis: Mastery of new skills needed to manage a transition and the development of a fluid yet integrative identity. The levels at which these outcomes are experienced may reflect by proxy the quality of life for those who are experiencing transitions. The determination of when a transition is complete must be flexible and variable depending on the type of change or the event initiating the transition, as well as the nature and patterns of transition. If outcomes are considered too soon in a transition process, they may be process indicators. If they are examined too long after a transition is complete, they may be related to other events in the client's life. In some transitions, it is easier to determine a beginning and an ending point. In all transitions, there is a subjective element of achieving a sense of balance in one's life. In the studies reported here, mastery and having a new sense of identity reflected healthy outcomes of the transition process.

Mastery

A healthy completion of a transition is determined by the extent to which individuals demonstrate mastery of the skills and behaviors needed to manage their new situations or environments.[36] In the motherhood study,[4] one participant described mastery by indicating that "At about 2 months I started making my own decisions." Another described mastery as taking charge of her care: "I had to ask for that test you know. I would think that the doctors would know...she had forgotten." Skills needed to achieve mastery in the caregiving situation included monitoring and interpreting symptoms, making decisions, taking action, providing hands-on care, making adjustments, accessing resources, working collaboratively with the care receiver, and negotiating the health care system.[37] The results of the family caregiving study suggest that mastery results from blending previously established skills with skills newly developed during the transition process. Also, skill develops over time with experience. Thus, mastery is unlikely to be seen early in a transition experience. However, by the time clients are experiencing a new sense of stability near the completion of a transition, their level of mastery will indicate the extent to which they have achieved a healthy transition outcome.

Fluid Integrative Identities

Transition experiences have been characterized as resulting in identity reformulation.[3,38] The results of Messias's[7] research support the conceptualization of immigrants' reformulated identities as *fluid* rather than static, as dynamic rather than stable. Some degree of ambiguity is also a part of the notion of a fluid migrant identity. The concept of fluid migrant identities as identified in the stories of these Brazilian immigrant women also supports the incorporation of a transnational perspective within a transition framework of migration. For the women in this study, one of the characteristics of the "new identity" that came with migration was that their perspectives were now bicultural, rather than monocultural.

In moving to, settling in, working, and interacting within another social, political, economic, and cultural environment and context, the migrant acquires added baggage, in that she begins to carry around the baggage of two (or more) cultures, two (or more) different ways of being. At different times and in different spaces in a migrant's life, she may carry more baggage from the home or host country or culture. In terms of space, she may have more home country baggage in her domestic or social arena, in contrast to the workplace where she may have adapted more to the host country. However, there is no set pattern or formula. Because the migration transition is dynamic and ongoing, over time an immigrant may periodically pick up or leave behind different pieces of this identity baggage. Situations that may trigger a change in focus or perspective include developmental, situational, or health-illness transitions such as marriage, pregnancy, personal or family illness, or a change in employment. These transitions are then likely to be viewed from a bifocal perspective.[7]

Conclusion

Knowledge is empowering to those who develop it, those who use it, and those who benefit from it. Understanding the properties and conditions inherent in a transition process will lead to the development of nursing therapeutics that are congruent with the unique experiences of clients and their families, thus promoting healthy responses to transition.

Theories provide frameworks for understanding complex situations such as vulnerable clients' processes and responses to transitions. A middle-range theory of transitions emerged from the analyses of the studies presented here.

Middle-range theories are characterized by more limited scope and less abstraction than grand theories. Also, they address specific phenomena or concepts and reflect practice.[9] Because diverse types and patterns of transitions were considered in this theoretical development, we believe that the emerging framework gives a more comprehensive view of transitions, providing more specific guidelines for practice and driving more systematic and coherent research questions.

As the studies presented in this chapter indicate, transition experiences are not unidimensional. Rather, each transition is characterized by its own uniqueness, complexities, and multiple dimensions. Future endeavors should be directed toward defining the diversities and complexities in transition experiences through research with diverse populations in diverse types and patterns of transitions. Each concept proposed here needs to be further developed and refined. Similarly, research to discover the levels and nature of vulnerability at different points during transitions could be driven by this middle-range theory. Finally, nursing therapeutics that reflect the diversities and complexities of the transition experiences need to be identified, clarified, developed, tested, and evaluated.

REFERENCES

1. Schumacher KL. Meleis AI. Transitions: a central concept in nursing. *Image J Nurs Scholarship.* 1994:26(2): 119–127.
2. Meleis AI. Trangenstein PA. Facilitating transitions: redefinition of the nursing mission. *Nurs Outlook.* 1994:42:255–259.
3. Chick N. Meleis AI. Transitions: a nursing concern. In: Chinn PL. ed. *Nursing Research Methodology: Issues and Implantation.* Gaithersburg, MD: Aspen Publishers: 1986.
4. Sawyer LM. *Engaged Mothering Within a Racist Environment: The Transition to Motherhood for a Group of African American Women.* San Francisco: University of California, San Francisco: 1997. Doctoral dissertation.
5. Im EO. *Neglecting and Ignoring Menopause Within a Gendered Multiple Transitional Context: Low Income Korean Immigrant Women.* San Francisco: University of California, San Francisco: 1997. Doctoral dissertation.
6. Messias DKH. Gilliss CL. Sparacino PSA. Tong EM. Foote D. Stories of transition: parents recall the diagnosis of congenital heart defects. *Fam Systems Med.* 1995: 3(3/4):367–377.
7. Messias DKH. *Narratives of Transnational Migration. Work, and Health: The Lived Experiences of Brazilian Women in the United States.* San Francisco: University of California, San Francisco: 1997. Doctoral dissertation.
8. Schumacher KL. *Shifting Patterns of Self-Care and Caregiving During Chemotherapy.* San Francisco: University of California, San Francisco: 1994. Doctoral dissertation.
9. Meleis AI. *Theoretical Nursing: Development and Progress.* 3rd ed. New York: JB Lippincott: 1997.
10. Sawyer LM. Engaged mothering: the transition to motherhood for a group of African American women. *J Transcultural Nurs.* 1999:1:14–21.
11. Denzin NK. *Sociological Methods; A Source Book.* 2nd ed. New York: McGraw-Hill: 1978.
12. Im EO. Meleis AI. A situation specific theory of menopausal transition of Korean immigrant women. *Image J Nurs Scholarship.* 1999:31: 333–338.
13. Gudmundsdottir M. Gilliss CL. Sparacino PSA. Tong EM. Messias DK. Foote D. Congenital heart defects in parent-adolescent coping. *Fam Systems Health.* 1996: 14:245–255.
14. Sparacino PSA. Tong EM. Messias DKH. Chesla CA. Gilliss CL. The dilemmas of parents of adolescents and young adults with congenital heart disease. *Heart Lung.* 1997:26:187–195.
15. Tong EM. Sparacino PSA. Messias DKH. Foote D. Chesla C. Gilliss CL. Growing up with congenital heart disease: the dilemmas of adolescents and young adults. *Cardiovas Diseases Young.* 1998: 8:303–309.
16. George LK. Models of transition in middle and later life. *Ann Am Acad Political Social Sci.* 1982: 464:22–37.
17. Rogler L. International migrations: a framework for directing research. *Am Psychologist.* 1994:49(8): 701–708.
18. Schumacher KL. Reconceptualizing family caregiving: family-based illness care during chemotherapy. *Res Nurs Health.* 1996:19:261–271.
19. Bridges W. *Managing Transitions: Making the Most of Change.* Menlo Park, CA: Addison Wesley: 1991.

20. Bridges W. *Transitions.* Reading, MA: Addison Wesley: 1980.
21. Im EO. An analytical study of the relationship between menopausal symptoms and the stress of life events. *J Korea Community Health Nurs Acad Society.* 1994:8(2): 1–34.
22. Spector RE. Health and illness in the Asian-American community. In: Spector RE. ed. *Cultural Diversity in Health and Illness.* Norwalk, CT: Appleton Century Crofts: 1985:127–110.
23. Abe T. Moritsuka T. A case-control study on menopausal symptoms and complaints of Japanese women by symptomatic type for psychosocial variables. *Maturitas.* 1986:8(3):255–265.
24. Ballinger SE. Psychosocial stress and symptoms of menopause: a comparative study of menopause clinic patients and non-patients. *Maturitas.* 1985:7:315–327.
25. Greene JG. Bereavement and social support at the menopausal. *Maturitas.* 1983:5:115–124.
26. Schneider M. Brotherton P. Physiological, psychological and situational stresses in depression during the menopausal. *Maturitas.* 1979:1:153–158.
27. Uphold C. Susman E. Self-reported menopausal symptoms as a function of the relationship between marital adjustment and childrearing stage. *Nurs Res.* 1981:30:166–220.
28. Cho O. Women in transition: the low income family. In: Yu EY. Phillips EH. eds. *Korean Women in Transition: at Home and Abroad.* Los Angeles: Center for Korean-American and Korean Studies. California State University. Los Angeles: 1987: 71–84.
29. Schumacher KL. Jones PS, Meleis AI. Helping elderly persons in transition: a framework for research and practice. In: Swanson EA. Tripp-Reimer T. eds. *Life Transitions in the Older Adult: Issues for Nurses and Other Health Professionals.* New York: Springer Publishing Company: 1999:1–26.
30. Hondagneu-Sotel P. *Gendered Transitions: Mexican Experiences of Immigration.* Berkeley, CA: University of California Press: 1994.
31. Hondagneu-Sotel P. Regulating the unregulated? Domestic workers' social networks. *Social Problems.* 1994:41(1):50–64.
32. Margolis MS. *Little Brazil: An Ethnography of Brazilian Immigrants in New York City.* Princeton, NJ: Princeton University Press: 1994.
33. Salzinger L. A maid by any other name. In: Burawoy M. et al. eds. *Ethnography Unbound: Power and Resistance in the Modern Metropolis.* Berkeley, CA: University of California Press: 1991: 189–160.
34. Segura DA. *Chicanas and Mexican Immigrant Women in the Labor Market: A Study of Occupational Mobility and Stratification.* Berkeley, CA: University of California Berkeley: 1986. Doctoral dissertation.
35. Lipson JG, Meleis AI. Research with immigrants and refugees. In: Hinshaw A. Feetham S. Shaver J. eds. *Hand-book of Clinical Nursing Research.* Thousand Oaks, CA: Sage Publications: 1999: 87–106.
36. Meleis AI. Swendsen L. Role supplementation: an empirical test of a nursing intervention. *Nurs Res.* 1978:27: 11–18.
37. Schumacher KL. Stewart BJ. Archbold PG. Dodd MJ. Dibble SL. Family caregiving skill: development of the concept. *Res Nurs Health.* 2000 Jun; 23(3):191–203.
38. Meleis AI. Lipson JG. Paul SM. Ethnicity and health among five Middle Eastern immigrant groups. *Nurs Res.* 1992:41(2):98–103.

Reprinted with permission from: Meleis, A. I., Sawyer, L. M., Im, E. O., Hilfinger Messias, D. K., & Schumacher, K. (2000). Experiencing transitions: An emerging middle range theory. *Advances in Nursing Science, 23*(1), 12–28.

2.2 FACILITATING TRANSITIONS: REDEFINITION OF THE NURSING MISSION

AFAF IBRAHIM MELEIS
PATRICIA A. TRANGENSTEIN

There have been numerous dialogues in nursing about its mission and definition, but a refinement of existing definitions has yet to be offered. This chapter is written with the goal of maintaining a vigorous discourse.

The phenomena of concern to the discipline of nursing that have been described by various theorists, and generally accepted by members of the discipline, are health, person, environment, and nursing therapeutics. Yet the multiplicity of viewpoints regarding these concepts and the paucity in their systematic development has prompted many to question their utility in providing the discipline with a coherent definition. The extent to which the mere identification of these concepts as central has helped in furthering the development of nursing knowledge is also questionable. The challenge members of the discipline face is to define the mission of nursing. The mission, then, could give more substance to these central concepts.

Recently, defining the mission has been advocated by many in nursing. For example, Newman[1] has stated that the challenge before nursing is to identify and agree on the central focus of nursing. Similarly, one of us (Meleis) has pleaded for substantive knowledge development in nursing and has identified constraints to knowledge development as the multiplicity of educational preparations, the multiplicity of driving theories, the lack of an organizing concept, the focus on process rather than substance, the devaluation of clinical focus and valuation of science, and the rise of ethnocentricity.[2] What is needed is an organizing concept that allows for a variety of viewpoints and theories within the discipline of nursing. Such a concept should not be culturally bound, and it should help in identifying the focus of the discipline. *We submit that the transition experience of clients, families, communities, nurses, and organizations, with health and well-being as a goal and an outcome, meets these criteria.*

Previously, Chick and Meleis[3]; Meleis[4]; and Schumacher and Meleis[5] argued that transition is a central concept to nursing. Unlike the other identified central concepts in nursing, transition is not a concept that is inherent in the writings of many of the nurse theorists. However, the concept of transition may be thought of as being congruent with or related to such concepts as adaptation[6]; self-care[7]; unitary human development[8]; expanding consciousness[9]; and human becoming.[10] Therefore the purpose of this chapter is to propose that facilitating transitions is a focus for the discipline of nursing. We argue that the mission of nursing should be redefined in terms of facilitating and dealing with people who are undergoing transitions, and we provide a framework that clarifies aspects of clients, health, and environment. We further argue that such a focus is not being imposed on the discipline; rather, it is a focus that reflects the practice of nursing as demonstrated by clients' nursing care needs, by actions of clinicians, and by the choices of investigators of nursing research questions.

The challenge members of the discipline face is to define the mission of nursing.

The Mission of Nursing

Attempts at articulating a substantive focus in nursing have been made by a number of metatheorists, as well as by the authors of the 1980 ANA Social Policy Statement that defined nursing as "the diagnosis and treatment of human responses to actual and potential health problems."[11] This definition, used by members of the discipline, has been instrumental in providing nursing with a focus. However, further development of the mission of nursing has been limited. In addition, the definition of nursing practice as described in this important document has lent itself to the development of topologies or listings of human responses without an equal emphasis on the nursing therapeutics needed. Moreover, there is a lack of a framework that may help nurses decide what is a health problem and what are the health care priorities from a nursing perspective.

Such a focus is not a focus that is being imposed on the discipline; it reflects the practice of nursing.

More recently, Newman et al.[12] proposed that the focus of the discipline of nursing is "caring in the human health experience." Some questions emanating from this focus: (a) Is it possible to study caring using empiricism as a framework? (b) If caring is universal and not limited to one discipline, what aspects of caring are unique to nursing?[1] and (c) Which human health experiences require nurses' unique contributions? Furthermore, because of the impersonal nature of bureaucratic systems, caregivers in institutions are often unable to provide personalized care, because of limitation in defining the scope of care, the diffusion in their daily responsibilities, their limited power, and the expectations that bedside caregivers compensate for deficiencies in the resources of the system through their caring process. Without an expectation of mutuality and reciprocity in the caring relationship, exploitation and oppression of the caregiver at the individual and institutional level may occur.[13] And without the identification of some defining boundaries for the human health experience, priorities of care may not be clear.

The scope of nursing was also defined. According to Fawcett,[14] who utilized the work of Donaldson and Crowley[15] and Gortner,[16] four propositions that define the scope of nursing are as follows:

- The discipline of nursing is concerned with the principles and laws that govern the life process, well-being, and optimal functioning of human beings, sick or well.
- The discipline of nursing is concerned with the patterning of human behavior in interaction with the environment in normal life events and critical life situations.
- The discipline of nursing is concerned with the nursing actions or processes by which positive changes in health status are affected.
- The discipline of nursing is concerned with the wholeness or health of human beings recognizing that they are in continuous interaction with their environment.

While these definitions and scope of nursing practice have been instrumental in promoting constructive dialogues about the mission of nursing, we believe that using transitions as a framework adds an important dimension to identifying boundaries of nursing, to refining phenomenon of the discipline, to establishing priorities, and to developing congruent nursing therapeutics.

Transitions: The Mission of Nursing Redefined

In previous work by Chick and Meleis[3] and Schumacher and Meleis[5] a framework with which to view the concept of transitions was identified. *Transition has been defined as "a passage from one life phase, condition, or status to another..... Transition refers to both the process and outcome of complex person-environment interactions. It may involve more than one person and is embedded in the context and the situation."*[3] A transition denotes a change in health status, in role relations, in expectations, or in abilities. It denotes a unique constellation of patterns of responses over a span of time.

In general, the structure of a transition consists of three phases: Entry, passage, and exit.[17] Commonalities that characterize a transition period include process, disconnectedness, perception, and patterns of response. One important consideration of transition is that the completion of a transition implies that a person has reached a period of less disruption or greater stability through growth relative to what has occurred before. Increments, as well as decrements, may be viewed as positive, as the potential for disruption and disorganization associated with pretransitional states is countered on successful completion of the transition.[3]

Additional support for transitions as the focus of the discipline of nursing comes from the extensive literature review provided by Schumacher and Meleis.[5] Three hundred-ten citations with the word "transition" appearing in the nursing literature between 1986 and 1992 were reviewed. The identified articles crossed specialty areas and professional roles (educator, practitioner, administrator, and researcher). In the analysis, several categories emerged. These categories, emerging from research and clinical article reviews, lend support to the theoretical categories identified earlier.[3] Types of transitions that nurses deal with are as follows:

Individual developmental transitions, such as adolescence, becoming aware of sexual identity and going into midlife.
Family developmental transitions, such as mother–daughter relationship, parenthood, and childbearing family.
Situational transitions, such as educational transitions, changing professional roles, widowhood, relocation to nursing home, family caregiving, and immigration.

Health/illness transitions, such as the recovery process, hospital discharge, and diagnosis of chronic illness.

Organizational transitions, such as changes in leadership, implementation of new policies or practices, implementation of a new curriculum, changes in nursing as a profession, and changes in communities.

In the review of these articles, three indicators of successful transitions were described: emotional well-being, mastery, and well-being of relationships.

> *Nursing's unique contribution is its goal of a sense of well-being.*

Given the unique focus of nursing on health, additional indicators identified included quality of life, adaptation, functional ability, self-actualization, expanding consciousness, and personal transformation.[5] Theoretically, there is support that an additional outcome indicator that should be addressed is purposeful and mobilized energy.[18,19] Although some outcomes have been identified from existing literature, it is most likely that emphasis on selected outcomes will be dictated by the profession's social commitment and responsibility within a given culture and not only by the theoretical nature of the discipline.

Other disciplines may also focus on transition; however, nursing's unique contribution is its goal of a sense of well-being. Defining *nursing* as "facilitating transitions to enhance a sense of well-being" gives nursing a unique perspective. Only nursing facilitates transitions toward health and a perception of well-being. No other discipline has this process orientation to the transition experience. No other discipline needs as much of a knowledge base to help clients achieve a sense of mastery, a level of functioning, and a knowledge of ways by which their energy can be mobilized. Within the transition framework, *caring* would be seen as a process that facilitates successful transitions that is not bound by a medically determined beginning and ending of an event. Admission and discharge of patients are events that could be considered either at a point of time or as transitional experiences. The former limits nursing actions to that slice of time; the latter allows preparation for continuity of care, a process of coping within, and a longer time framework.

The development of nursing therapeutics could be focused on the prevention of unhealthy transitions, promoting perceived well-being and dealing with the experience of transitions. Theory development should aim to provide greater understanding and insight into the transitional experiences. Within this focus, then, the goals of knowledge development in nursing are to enhance an understanding of[2]:

The processes and experiences of human beings who are in transition.

The nature of emerging life patterns and new identities.

The processes or conditions that promote healthy outcomes, such as mastery, perceived well-being, energy mobilization, quality of life, self-actualization, expanding consciousness, personal transformation, and functional ability.

Environments that constrain, support, or promote healthy transitions.

Structure and components of nursing therapeutics that deal with transitions.

A focus on transitions provides a framework that:

Acknowledges universal aspects of nursing;

Enhances nurses' potential in supporting emerging identities and life patterns;

Supports nurses' concerns about changing systems and societies;

Challenges nurses to develop therapeutics supportive of positive experiences and healthy outcomes.

It provides nurses with a framework to understand variations in the recovery transition, the hospital admission transition, the immigration transitions, the discharge transition, the rehabilitation transition, as well as the experiences of clients who are in multiple transitions. It highlights the need for knowledge related to transitions into new roles and new skills. The transition experienced by people during the modernization process of societies becomes an important focus within the discipline. The birthing transition, the transition into home care, and the caregiving transition would also receive more attention internationally. None of these events, experiences, and responses becomes ahistorical or isolated. When considering transition as an organizing framework, the events, experiences, and responses are recognized as processes that require a longitudinal and multidimensional approach and a focus on patterns of response over time, all of which are more congruent with nursing than viewing any of their transitional experiences as events creating change. Such consideration limits the events to singular responses in a single slice of time.

Transition Versus Change

Transitions are processes that occur over time and that have a sense of flow and movement. *Change*, on the other hand, is defined "to take instead of, substitute one thing for another, put, adopt a thing in place of another, and tends to be abrupt."[20] Transition incorporates some aspects of change but extends the concept to incorporate flow and movement. Another universal property is found in the nature of change that occurs in transitions. At the individual and family levels, changes occur in identities, roles, relationships, abilities, and patterns of behaviors. At the organizational level, changes occur in structure, function, and of the dynamics of the organization. These properties help to differentiate transitions from nontransitional change. For example, brief, self-limiting illness has not been characterized as a transition, whereas chronic illness has been viewed as requiring a process of transition.[21,22] Similarly, phenomena such as mood changes that are dynamic but do not have a sense of movement or direction are not conceptualized as transitions. Finally, internal processes usually accompany the process of transition, while external processes tend to characterize change.[17]

> *Only nursing facilitates transitions toward health and a perception of well-being.*

A Clinical Example

One of the challenging clinical problems is the treatment and management of breathing difficulties. Conceptually, breathing difficulties are similar to other problems in that they are not merely a reflection of a physiologic event but evolve out of a complex interaction of personal, environmental, and health status factors.[23,24] Currently, three major approaches to the study and treatment of breathing difficulties have emerged. These are the biomedical/physiologic approaches, with an emphasis on medication and oxygen therapy, breathing retraining, smoking cessation, exercise conditioning, and nutritional evaluation.[25-30] A second approach has been the exploration of various psychologic and personal characteristics associated with dyspnea primarily in clients with chronic obstructive pulmonary disease (COPD). Findings from this approach have led to the use of psychotropic agents and relaxation methods.[26,31-37] The third approach has focused on coping strategies used by clients with dyspnea.[24,38-40]

Few interventions have been proposed or clinically tested to relieve breathing difficulties.[41] Some nursing interventions, such as teaching breathing techniques, energy-conservation measures, exercise programs, desensitization and guided imagery, and environmental temperature control, have been applied in a clinical setting. However, one of the most challenging and frustrating dilemmas for the nurse at the bedside is the experience of caring for a frightened client sitting up at bedside unable to catch his or her breath. The focus on symptom control rather than viewing this as a transitional experience may contribute to the lack of long-term, intermittent, and only hospital bound nursing interventions. If the experience of the client with breathing difficulties was viewed as a transitional experience with desired outcomes being mastery, improved functional ability, or improved quality of life, and with the goal of achieving a period of less disruption or greater stability through growth, the nursing approach to the problem would be qualitatively different. It could transcend hospitalization and strategies that are biomedically driven. The lived experiences, the daily life events, and lifestyles will more accurately drive nursing therapeutics. A variety of research methods could be used to study which groups of clients do better with selected interventions at different phases of the transitional experience and to identify which kinds of environments support or hinder a healthy transition. Levels of mastery in coping with the transitional phases will need to be explored. Similarly, the cumulative nature of knowledge related to breathing difficulties will be taken into consideration when conceptualizing breathing ease as a transition.

Conclusions

There are multiple paradigms and viewpoints that guide and inform the discipline of nursing. This multiplicity has prompted many analyses and critiques and polarized some to prefer and espouse the adaption of one view, one theory, or one paradigm over another. Our intention is not to reconcile the differences between these different viewpoints. As Skrtic[42] has stated:

> the point is not to accommodate or reconcile the multiple paradigms; *and to recognize them for what they are—ways of seeing that simultaneously reveal and conceal.*

Rather, our intent is to suggest that by considering transitions as focal and central to the discipline of nursing a more focused dialogue and debate that advances knowledge development could occur.

What advantages does transition offer for the development of nursing? First, it offers an organizing framework that emphasizes processes that are longitudinal and multidimensional in nature and patterns of responses over time. All are more congruent with nursing. An integrating and organizing conceptual framework makes it easier for a nurse to capitalize on what he or she already knows and to use existing knowledge more insightfully. Second, it provides a common language that can encompass all specialty areas, professional roles, and theoretical and methodologic camps. Both the received viewers and perceived viewers can equally find questions to consider and contributions to make. Better articulation across specialties and professional roles is made possible. Third, because transitions are not bounded by current nursing theories but encompass them, nursing theories could compete to answer critical questions in nursing. For example, what nursing therapeutics are effective in treating the frightful experience of shortness of breath? Are certain nursing therapeutics more successful with different groups of clients, in a particular sequence, or at selected stages? The challenge is for nurses to develop and test therapeutics supportive of healthy experiences and outcomes and not only events. In addition, transitions acknowledge the universal aspects of nursing, and this is not limited by a particular cultural viewpoint.

Without an organizing framework such as transitions, the focus of the discipline may be lost; advances in nursing knowledge may be slow and erratic; nurses' expertise may go unacknowledged and staffing patterns may be limited to caring for events, rather than processes of becoming. Last, using the facilitation of transitions as a defining mission for nursing allows nurses to demonstrate their expertise in supporting admission, recovery, discharge, birthing, parenting, menopausing, and battering as processes that are not bound by time and space. The experience of transitions is longer, multidimensional, and far more multilayered than each of the situations when conceptualized as events. Transitions could be utilized to turn the tide to the advantage of our clients with an emphasis on the process of achieving healthy outcomes.

The concept of transition already pervades much of current thinking about nursing, and this suggests it is not a trivial notion or passing fad. We see applications cross-culturally, for all age groups, and independent of clinical specialty or professional role. Certainly nursing needs new knowledge, but it also needs tools and strategies to make the best use of existing knowledge and to use it in a way unique to nursing.

REFERENCES

1. Newman MA. Prevailing paradigms in nursing. Nurs Outlook 1990;40: 10–13, 32.
2. Meleis AI. A passion for substance revisited: global transitions and international commitments. Keynote paper at the 1993 National Nursing Doctoral Forum, St. Paul, Minn., June 1993.
3. Chick N, Meleis AI. Transitions: a nursing concern. In: Chinn PL, ed. Nursing research methodology: issues and implementation. Rockville, Maryland: Aspen, 1986:237–57.
4. Meleis AI. Theoretical nursing: development and progress. 2nd ed. Philadelphia: JB Lippincott, 1991.
5. Schumacher KL, Meleis AI. Transitions: a central concept in nursing. *Journal of Nursing Scholarship 1994: 26*(2):119–127.
6. Roy C. The Roy adaptation model. In: Riehl-Sisca J, ed. Conceptual models for nursing practice. 3rd ed. Norwalk, Connecticut: Appleton & Lange, 1989.
7. Orem D. Nursing: concepts of practice. 2nd ed. New York: McGraw-Hill, 1980.
8. Rogers ME. Nursing: a science of unitary human beings. In: Riehl-Sisca J, ed. Conceptual models for nursing practice. 3rd ed. Norwalk, Connecticut: Appleton & Lange, 1989.
9. Newman MA. Health as expanding consciousness. St. Louis: CV Mosby, 1986.
10. Parse RR. Man-living-health: a theory of nursing. In: Riehl-Sisca J, ed. Conceptual models for nursing practice. 3rd ed. Norwalk, Connecticut: Appleton & Lange, 1989.
11. American Nurses Association. Nursing: a social policy statement. Kansas City: American Nurses Association, 1980.
12. Newman MA, Sime AM, Corcoran-Perry SA. The focus of the discipline of nursing. Adv Nurs Sci 1991;14:1–6.
13. Condon EH. Nursing and the caring metaphor: gender and political influences on the ethics of care. Nurs Outlook 1992;40: 14–19.
14. Fawcett J. Analysis and evaluation of nursing theories. Philadelphia: FA Davis, 1993.
15. Donaldson SK, Crowley DM. The discipline of nursing. Nurs Outlook 1978;26:13–120.
16. Gortner S. Nursing science in transition. Nurs Res 1980;29:180–183.
17. Bridges W. Managing transitions: making the most of change. Reading, Massachusetts: Addison-Wesley, 1991.
18. Newman MA. Health conceptualizations. Annu Rev Nurs Res 1991;221–243.
19. Levine M. The four conservation principles of nursing. Nurs Forum 1967;6:1, 45–59.
20. Webster Universal Dictionary. New York: Harver Educational Services, 1970.
21. Catanzaro M. Transitions in midlife adults with long-term illness. Holistic Nurs Pract 1990;4:65–73.
22. Loveys B. Transitions in chronic illness: the at-risk role. Holistic Nurs Pract 1990;4:56–64.
23. Carrieri VK, Janson-Bjerklie S, Jacobs S. The sensation of dyspnea. Heart Lung 1984; 13:436–447.
24. Carrieri-Kolhman V, Douglas MK, Gormley JM, Stulbarg MS. Desentization and guided mastery: treatment approaches for the management of dyspnea. Heart Lung 1993;22:226–334.
25. Adams L, Chronos N, Lane R, Guz A. The measurement of breathlessness induced in normal subjects: validity of two scaling techniques. Clin Sci 1985;69:7–16.
26. Agle DP, Baum GL, Chester EH, Wendt M. Multi-discipline treatment of chronic pulmonary insufficiency: psychologic aspects of rehabilitation. Psychosom Med 1973;35:41–49.
27. Gift AG, Plaunt M, Jacax A. Psychologic and physiologic factors related to dyspnea in subjects with chronic obstructive pulmonary diseases. Heart Lung 1986;15:595–601.
28. Guyatt GH, Townsend M, Berman LB, Pugsley SO. Quality of life in patients with chronic airflow limitation. Br J Dis Chest 1987;81:45–54.
29. Weaver TE, Narsavage GL. Physiological and psychological variables related to functional status in chronic obstructive pulmonary disease. Nurs Res 1992;41:286–291.
30. Wolkove N, Dajczman E, Colacone A, Kriesman H. The relationship between pulmonary function test and dyspnea in obstructive lung disease. Chest 1989;6:1247–1251.
31. Agle DP, Baum GL. Psychological aspects of chronic obstructive pulmonary disease. Med Clin North Am 1977;61:749–758.
32. Dudley DL, Glaser EM, Jorgenson BN, Logan DL. Psychosocial concomitants to rehabilitation in chronic obstructive pulmonary disease, 1: psychosocial and psychological considerations. Chest 1980;77:413–420.
33. Fishman DB, Petty TL. Physical, symptomatic and psychological improvement in patients receiving comprehensive care for chronic airway obstruction. J Chron Dis 1971;24:775–785.
34. Fishman DB, Plaunt M, Jacox A. Psychologic and physiologic factors related to dyspnea in subjects with chronic obstructive pulmonary disease. Heart Lung 1986;15:595–601.
35. Light RW, Merrill EJ, Despars J, Gordon GH, Mutalipassi LR. Prevalence of depression and anxiety in patients with COPD. Chest 1985;87:35–38.

36. Rutter B. Some psychological concomitants of chronic bronchitis. Psychol Med 1977; 7:459–464.
37. Rutter B. The prognostic significance of psychological factors in the management of chronic bronchitis. Psychol Med 1979;9:63–70.
38. Carrieri VK, Janson-Bjerklie S. Strategies patients use to manage the sensation of dyspnea. West J Nurs Res 1986;8:284–305.
39. Janson-Bjerklie S, Fahy J, Geaghan S, Golden J. Disappearance of eosinophile from bronchoalveolar lavage fluid after patient education and high dose inhaled corticosteroids. Heart Lung 1993;22:235–238.
40. Parsons EJ. Coping and well-being strategies in individuals with COPD. Health Values 1990;14:9(3): 17–23.
41. Moody L, McCormick K, Williams AR. Psychophysiologic correlates of quality of life in chronic bronchitis and emphysema. West J Nurs Res 1991;13:336–352.
42. Skrtic TM. Social accommodation: toward a dialogical discourse in educational inquiry. In: Guba EG, ed. The paradigm dialogue. Newbury Park, California: Sage, 1990.

Reprinted with permission from: Meleis, A. I., & Trangenstein, P. A. (1994). Facilitating transitions: Redefinition of a nursing mission. *Nursing Outlook, 42*(6), 255–259.

2.3 TRANSITION: A LITERATURE REVIEW

DEBBIE KRALIK
KATE VISENTIN
ANTONIA VAN LOON

Abstract

Aim: This chapter reports a comprehensive literature review exploring how the term 'transition' has been used in the health literature. *Background*: The meaning of transition has varied with the context in which the term has been used. The last 3 decades have seen altered understandings in the concept of transition in the social science and health disciplines, with nurses contributing to more recent understandings of the transition process as it relates to life and health. *Method*: The CINAHL, Medline, Sociofile and Psychlit databases were accessed and papers published between 1994 and 2004 were retrieved to answer the questions 'How is the word transition used?' and 'What is the concept of transition informing?' Transition theoretical frameworks were also explored. *Findings*: Widespread use of the word 'transition' suggests that it is an important concept. Transitional definitions alter according to the disciplinary focus, but most agree that transition involves people's responses during a passage of change. Transition occurs over time and entails change and adaptation, for example developmental, personal, relational, situational, societal or environmental change, but not all change engages transition. Reconstruction of a valued self-identity is essential to transition. Time is an essential element in transition and therefore longitudinal studies are required to explore the initial phase, midcourse experience, and outcome of the transition experience. *Conclusion*: Transition is the way people respond to change over time. People undergo transition when they need to adapt to new situations or circumstances in order to incorporate the change event into their lives. Transition is a concept that is important to nursing; however, to further develop understandings, research must extend beyond single events or single responses. Longitudinal comparative and longitudinal cross-sectional inquiries are required to further develop the concept.

Introduction

Facilitating transition has been identified as being a central concept for nursing (Schumacher & Meleis, 1994). It was considered important to review the relevant literature to guide theoretical development of our research programme, in which the aim has been to describe transition and identify the role of nurses in facilitating transition (Koch & Kralik,

2001; Kralik, 2002). Our research focus has been to develop and consolidate our understanding of what transition means by revising and validating emerging knowledge grounded in the stories of research participants. We have developed a working definition of transition that has evolved from findings of several of our research inquiries. We define it as a process of convoluted passage during which people redefine their sense of self and redevelop self-agency in response to disruptive life events (van Loon & Kralik, 2005).

Theoretical development is ongoing within our research programme, however, and so a review of current literature and theoretical frameworks was undertaken to guide our theoretical deliberations and to develop our position in the debates and issues surrounding transition. We had observed in the literature that the precise meaning of transition has varied with the context in which the term has been used. We were aware that, during the last 3 decades, the concept has evolved in the social sciences and health disciplines, with nurses contributing to more recent understandings of the transition process as it relates to life and health (Cantanzaro, 1990; Chick & Meleis, 1986; van Loon, 2001; Kralik, 2002; Loveys, 1990; Meleis et al., 2000; Meleis & Trangenstein, 1994; Schumacher & Meleis, 1994). While we recognized the complexity of finding a universally acceptable and applicable definition of transition, it was felt that a clearer understanding of the term could be achieved by critically reviewing the health literature. We were also interested in determining the contexts or settings in which the term transition had been used.

Background

This review builds on a previous review of the nursing literature on transition published by Schumacher and Meleis (1994). The questions asked by these authors were: What were the types of transitions addressed in the nursing literature? What conditions influence transitions?

The types of transitions discussed in the earlier nursing literature were developmental, situational, health-illness and organizational (Schumacher & Meleis, 1994). Developmental transitions were those related to the responses of individuals when they experience the changes that occur during the life cycle, such as becoming a parent. Situational transitions were concerned with various educational and professional roles, such as the transitions of graduate nurses. Health–illness transitions explored the responses of individuals and families in illness contexts. A prominent concern was cost effectiveness during the transition of people between types of healthcare services, such as hospital to outpatient care. Organizational transitions represent those that occur in the environment and are precipitated by changes in the social, political, or economic context. Changes in leadership have been described as creating transitional periods within an organization (Schumacher & Meleis, 1994).

The conditions that influence transitions were found to vary widely among individuals, families and organizations. Schumacher and Meleis (1994) concluded that the meanings of change that people have, expectations of events, level of knowledge and skill, availability of new knowledge about a change event, resources available in the environment, capacity to plan for change, and emotional and physical well-being all have an impact on transitions. A successful transition is one where feelings of distress are replaced with a sense of well-being and mastery of a change event (Schumacher & Meleis, 1994). The transitions framework provided by Schumacher and Meleis (1994) has been very useful for our research; however, we considered it important to update the literature review to explore new understandings.

Aim

The aim of the review was to explore how the term 'transition' had been used in the health literature. The research questions guiding analysis of the literature were: How is the word "transition" used in the literature? and What is the concept of transition informing?

Search Methods

The Search

Databases (Medline, CINAHL, Sociofile, Psychlit) were searched using the keyword 'transition' and a large volume of work from diverse professional fields was retrieved. The limits set were:

- articles dated between 1994 and 2004;
- transition as a central concept; and
- health or social focus.

The searches were refined with the query string of *social, life events, illness, crisis, identity, and self*. These terms were taken from keywords identified in relevant papers. The focus of transition in many articles in Medline was molecular or biological in nature and hence these articles were excluded. There was overlap with the papers extracted from the CINAHL search but further articles were located particularly with the illness combination. Sociofile and Psychlit retrieved a number of articles that had a social focus. The reference lists of reviewed articles were also searched for relevant citations.

We were interested in exploring how the word transition was used in the wider health literature. Other disciplines may use different terms to describe transition; hence, it was this understanding that prompted the use of search terms such as disruption, continuity, and self identity. These search terms when combined with transition highlighted a new body of work from psychiatry, social work and the social sciences. Full papers ($n = 45$) were located. We independently reviewed each paper and answered the following questions:

- How is the word transition used?
- What is the concept of transition informing?
- What are the assumptions about transition?
- What were the before and after? (movement to and from)
- What research method was used?

Informed by the findings of our own research, our focus was the disruptions that required the person to reshape their sense of self (Kralik, 2002). We were interested in how transition occurred after forced change, for example in chronic illness, where one's reality and one's sense of self were threatened or disrupted. Consensus on relevance was reached by team debate, focusing on papers where transition was central to the change event/issue, or where the discussions informed our understanding of the transition process. A total of 23 primary studies were appraised and analysed, in addition to identifying and discussing the major theories of transition.

Twenty-three research primary studies were included in the review, and these all used qualitative methodologies. Qualitative methods employ processes that involve the description and interpretation of human experience so that a holistic picture of social and human issues can be explored (Powers & Knapp, 1990; Creswell, 1998). Transition is human experience; therefore, it seems appropriate that qualitative methods have been used to understand the concept of transition.

Criteria for Exclusion

Twenty-two ($n = 22$) papers were excluded from the final review. Non-research-based were excluded but informed the discussion on theoretical frameworks. Papers that did not describe the transition experience or have transition as a central concept were also excluded. Four ($n = 4$) focused on life stages or developmental stages such as the role of mothering or fathering, and these were excluded (Draper, 2003; Mann, Abercrombie, DeJoseph, Norbeck, & Smith, 1999; Nelson, 2003; Sawyer, 1999) because we considered that such life stage transitions are normative and anticipated. Many quantitative research studies ($n = 18$) that used the term transition as indicating a passage of movement failed to define the concept (Brouwer-Dudokdewit, Savenije, Zoeteweij, Maat-Kievit, & Tibben, 2002; Brudenell, 1996; Forss, Tishelman, Widmark, & Sachs, 2004; Gwilliam & Bailey, 2001; Montenko & Greenberg, 1995; Vaartio & Kiviniemi, 2003; White, 1995; White, 2003). Transition was not defined in these papers, although the term had been listed as a key word or included in the title or abstract. Discussions were limited to descriptions of movement or change from one point to another, rather than a transitional process of inner re-orientation (Gwilliam & Bailey, 2001; Vaartio & Kiviniemi, 2003; White, 1995; White, 2003).

Findings

Transition is derived from the Latin word "transition" meaning going across, passage over time, stage, subject, or place to another; that is, to change (Lexico, 2005: http://dictionary.reference.com/search?q=transition). The term *transition* has been used in diverse ways in the literature of disciplines as varied as musicology, history, metallurgy, geography, anthropology, science and health, with discussions ranging from change at the molecular level, to personal and developmental changes, to countries in transition. The literature frequently uses the word transition to describe a process of change in life's developmental stages, or alterations in health and social circumstances rather than people's responses to change. Transition is not just another word for change (Bridges, 2004), but rather connotes the psychological processes involved in adapting to the change event or disruption.

The broader research literature on transition employs a variety of methodologies and theoretical frameworks. All studies included in this review, however, used qualitative methodologies and usually generated data from relatively small, selective, nonrandom sample of participants. Data collection periods were usually of a short time frame and focused on a specified event, with only one inquiry adopting a longitudinal approach (Kralik, 2002). Ethnic and cultural differences were rarely identified in this body of literature.

Theoretical Frameworks

Transition theory has a long history within other disciplines, particularly anthropology. The work of Van Gennep (1960) early in the 20th century was further developed by Turner (1969) and then Sheehy (1977), highlighting the way that *rites of passage* throughout the stages of human life are marked by sociocultural rituals. Martin-McDonald and Biernoff (2002, p. 347) state

> that rites of passage occur when there is a transition in cultural expectations, social roles, and status and/or condition or position, interpersonal relations, and developmental or situational changes to being in the world.

Thus, social transition can be viewed as movement through life. Van Gennep's theory describes the way people move through life's stages in three distinct phases. First, preliminal rites (rites of separation) are characterized by removal of the individual from their *normal* social life, which may occur through the use of customs and taboos. Liminal rites (rites of transition) refer to customs and rituals of the individual when they are in a liminal state, perhaps feeling confused and alienated, in a state of *limbo* or, as (Draper, 2003, p. 63) prefers, "in no man's land."

Last, postliminal rites (rites of incorporation) occur where the individual is brought back into society and takes up their new status (reincorporation). Van Gennep's (1960) three-phase approach to transition continues to influence current transition thinking in the social and health literature.

Three phases of transition are also proposed by Bridges (2004, p. 17), composed of an "ending, then a beginning, and an important empty or fallow time in between." What these models have in common is an almost linear trajectory to transition that involves distinct start and finish points. Kralik (2002), however, proposes that transition does not follow a chronological trajectory. Likewise, Paterson (2001), who performed a metasynthesis of 292 qualitative research studies, describes a *shifting perspectives* model of chronic illness that also challenges the notion of a linear trajectory in transition. Kralik (2002) and Patterson (2001) both propose that learning to live with chronic illness is an ongoing process involving movement in many directions.

Defining Transition

Five varying senses or meanings to the word transition were retrieved from the online lexical reference system *Wordnet* (developed by Princeton University):

- Sense 1: Passage (act of passing from one state to another). Changing something into something. Something performed (as opposed to something said).
- Sense 2: Conversion, transformation, alteration, shift.
- Sense 3: Happening, occurrence, change.
- Sense 4: Modulation (change in tone).
- Sense 5: Connects to what follows, extracting common features.

Transitional definitions alter according to the disciplinary focus, but most agree that transition involves a passage of change. A common definition of transition cited in health disciplines is:

> A passage from one life phase, condition, or status to another...transition refers to both the process and the outcome of complex person-environment interactions. It may involve more than one person and is embedded in the context and the situation. Defining characteristics of transition include process, disconnectedness perception, and patterns and response. (Chick & Meleis, 1986, pp. 239–240)

Transition is not an event, but rather the "inner reorientation and self-redefinition" that people go through in order to incorporate change into their life (Bridges, 2004, p. xii). A concept analysis was presented by Meleis, Sawyer, Im, Hilfinger, Messias, and Schumacher (2000) that provided both a perspective and a framework for creating meaning of the concept of transition such as developmental, health, sociocultural, situational, relational, critical events, and organizational changes. It was proposed that people may undergo more than one transition at any given time; hence, it is important for the person to be aware of the changes taking place and to engage with them (Meleis et al., 2000). Indicators that transition is occurring include the individual feeling connected to, and interacting with, their situation and other people. The person feels located or situated so they can reflect and interact, and develop increasing confidence in coping with change and mastering new skills and new ways of living, while developing a more flexible sense of identity in the midst of these changes (Meleis et al., 2000).

Transition occurs when a person's current reality is disrupted, causing a forced or chosen change that results in the need to construct a new reality (Selder, 1989). It can only occur if the person is aware of the changes that are taking place (Chick & Meleis, 1986). This awareness is followed by engagement, where the person is immersed in the transition process and undertakes activities such as seeking information or support, identifying new ways of living and being, modifying former activities, and making sense of the circumstances. Therefore, level of awareness will influence level of engagement. Lack of awareness signifies that an individual may not be ready for transition (Meleis et al., 2000). Bridges (2004) and Selder (1989) highlight the importance of a person's need to acknowledge that a prior way of living/being has ended, or a current reality is under threat, and that change needs to occur before the transition process can begin. When this acknowledgment has occurred, it is possible to make sense of what is happening and reorganize a new way to live, respond and be in the world. The process of surfacing awareness involves noticing what has changed and how things are different (Meleis et al., 2000, Kralik, 2002). Dimensions of difference that can be explored include the nature of the changes, how long it may take for changes to occur, what trajectory they may follow, the perceived impact of changes, and the personal, familial, and societal influences having an impact on the changes (Meleis et al., 2000). Kralik (2002) notes that people with chronic illness in transition feel different, may be perceived by others as different, and view their world in a changed way as a result of the movement that occurs during transition.

How Has Transition Been Used in the Literature?

Most authors describe transition as not only a passage or movement but also a time of inner reorientation and/or transformation. Fifteen (n = 15) articles have a health-illness focus. Some reports discuss the transition from health to illness (Arman & Rehnsfeldt, 2003; Elmberger, Bolund, & Lutzen, 2002; Fraser 1999; Glacken, Kernohan, & Coates, 2001; Hilton, 2002; Kralik, 2002; Neil & Barrell, 1998; Powell-Cope, 1995; Shaul, 1997; Skarsater, Dencker, Bergbom, Haggstrom, & Fridlund, 2003), whereas others focus on a change within the course of illness, such as commencing dialysis (Kralik, Koch, & Eastwood, 2003; Martin-McDonald & Biernoff, 2002). The transition experience within an institution is explored by three authors (Bertero, 1998; Froggatt, 1997; Walker, 2001). Others focus on life transitions such as motherhood (Bailey, 1999; Miller, 2000); retirement (Luborsky, 1994); relocation (Rossen, 1998); and midlife (Banister, 1999).

If we use the five senses of transition developed by Princeton University, we note that the last two senses have not been included in the papers reviewed. Sense 4 refers to modulation (change in tone), which we interpreted as related to a need for people to have control and balance, much like a musician playing an instrument. Sense 5 refers to transition being a way to connect to what follows and we interpreted this as a process of sense-making.

The focus of papers was that transition involves a movement or passage between two points. Second, a transitional process involves transformation or alteration, whether it is incorporation, integration, or adaptation. Third, transition involves a process of inner-reorientation as the person learns to adapt and incorporate the new circumstances into their life. We suggest that transition needs to be viewed on all these levels if nurses are to take a holistic approach to client care.

Themes involving loss of self or shifts in self-identity as a result of the uncertainty and turmoil that follow a crisis event or disruption emerged from several inquiries (Elmberger et al., 2002; Glacken et al., 2001; Hilton, 2002; Kralik, 2002; Martin-McDonald & Biernoff, 2002; Neil & Barrell, 1998). Participants sought to regain control following the disruptive event, and reconstruction of self-identity was observed through themes of mastery. The experience of transition was a process that involved disruptions in close relationships and daily living (Arman & Rehnsfeldt, 2003; Powell-Cope, 1995). Helping people to make a transition toward a sense of mastery involves the acquisition of information (Fraser, 1999; Hilton, 2002) and social support systems (Rossen, 1998). This was a point that Powell-Cope (1995) also found in his study with homosexual couples living with HIV, and Martin-McDonald and Biernoff (2002) found in their study with people starting renal dialysis.

Assisting people to transition toward a sense of mastery involves the acquisition of information (Hilton, 2002); social support systems (Glacken, Bolund, & Lutzen, 2002); maintaining or developing strong connections with others (Arman & Rehnsfeldt, 2003); and learning ways to adapt to change through a heightened awareness of self (Fraser, 1999; Hilton, 2002; Kralik, 2002; Kralik et al., 2003; Martin-McDonald & Biernoff, 2002; Shaul, 1997). It is evident in these papers that transition is not simply change, but rather the process that people go through to incorporate the change or disruption into their lives.

What Does the Concept of Transition Inform?

The literature review identified a number of areas in which the concept of transition informs practice. The most striking finding is the challenge to self-identity that occurs during the transition process. Self-identity and transition appear to be concepts that are closely linked. The importance of relationships and connections was identified in the literature, as these were seen to be an integral part of successful transition. Furthermore, authors agree that it is important for healthcare professionals to have an understanding of the transition process in order to assist people to move through it.

Transition can be viewed as a process during which suffering may be reduced or alleviated. The suffering invoked by the forced change may be the central driving force for transformation and transition. For example, older women who have survived a stroke may experience a process of transition/

transformation that results in reconstruction of the sense of self (Hilton, 1998). They seek new roles, identify ways of coping, and reconcile with the limitations that the stroke imposes. Arman and Rehnsfeldt (2003) add that the illness experiences change one's notion of self, which Elmberger et al. (2002) claim may be "processed" to "master" the changing sense of identity and family relations imposed by the illness trajectory. Our research reveals that disruption can lead to suffering when it is difficult to become reconciled with the altered sense of self, but this may be ameliorated during the reclaiming process that occurs during transition (Kralik 2002; van Loon, Koch, & Kralik, 2004).

The idea that the suffering experienced during transition may be viewed positively is challenged by Arman and Rehnsfeldt (2003). They use examples of studies where women are classified as *stuck* in the transformation process because they are not able to adapt and integrate cancer into their lives. Other authors assume that all people transition successfully through the illness period because they provide little or no discussion around people who have not readily transitioned (Hilton, 2002; Skarsater et al., 2003).

Healthy transitions are often linked to the development of relationships and connections with others. Rossen (1998) notes that the level of support gained from personal relationships may influence transition, and that women with strong family and friend connections transitioned more readily than those who did not have support. The influence of relationships on transition is supported by Kralik et al. (2003) when researching shifts in sexual self-identity in women with multiple sclerosis: Women in supportive relationships found it easier to adapt to the consequences of intrusive illness.

In some studies, the participants themselves identify transition as an important part of the healing or recovery process (Glacken et al., 2001; Kralik, 2002). They describe the process of reconstructing and incorporating change as essential to transition, whether it be in the context of their relationships, their roles, or new strategies for coping (Hilton, 2002; Skarsater et al., 2003). Further to this, Glacken et al. (2001) suggests that the concept of transition is one way in which to conceptualize human responses to change. However, we have found transition to involve a complex interplay of adaptive activities to manage situational alterations, as well as a deeper psychological and spiritual incorporation of changes that aid reorientation of the sense of self (van Loon & Kralik, 2005).

In all of the studies reviewed, researchers concluded that it is through understanding the transition process that healthcare professionals will be better equipped to aid clients through processes of adaptation. Glacken et al. (2001) highlights the factors that hinder and facilitate transition, and suggests that healthcare professionals can address these factors as part of their care. It has been argued that the planning and implementation of nursing activities could be informed by the concept of transition (Shaul, 1997). Glacken et al. (2001) suggests that a tool be developed that assists healthcare professionals to assess where the person is within the transition process, thus ensuring that appropriate strategies are implemented at the right times. We have begun preliminary work on development of such a therapeutic intervention tool with women survivors of child sexual abuse (van Loon & Kralik, 2005). The aim of this tool will be to build capacity by planning strategies that assist sense-making, which can be employed during the various stages of the transition process (van Loon & Kralik, 2005).

Transition as a Process

The literature review highlights a lack of consensus among researchers as to whether the dynamic transition process has a definite beginning and end, is linear or cyclical, and how we can help people to *move on*. Papers framed by van Gennep's rites of passage theory (Froggatt, 1997; Luborsky, 1994; Martin-McDonald & Biernoff, 2002) tend to assume that transition is linear and unidirectional, even suggesting that the three phases are somehow distinct and readily separated for examination. Many authors propose that transition has a beginning and an end (Bridges, 2004; Elmberger et al., 2002; Fraser, 1999). For example, Elmberger et al.

(2002) describes how men with cancer start the health-illness transition at diagnosis and how it lasts for several years following a spiral movement. Our research challenges these notions, suggesting that transition is a more intricate and convoluted process with forward and backward movement (Kralik, 2002; van Loon & Kralik, 2005).

There was reference by Arman and Rehnsfeldt (2003) to the course of change associated with breast cancer as a type of *transition, transformation,* or *transcendence* encompassing a search for *meaning* as the person traveled a path that aimed to regain *integrity, balance,* and *wholeness*. The authors suggest that women could be in different phases of that transition process and move between them simultaneously while they incorporate various aspects of transition.

Glacken et al. (2001) proposes that living with Hepatitis C is an ongoing transitional process that is neither linear nor time-bound. In their study some of the participants were restructuring their lives, while others remained in the early stages of incorporation. Powell-Cope (1995, p. 54) stated that the transition process is

> not linear but recurring, so that at any given time new losses require ongoing readjustments and thus transition continues throughout life.

It has also been proposed that, although life transitions may have a distinct beginning and end, transition for people with chronic illness may not be complete, as their health and well-being status fluctuates (Shaul, 1997).

Time is an essential element in transition and therefore longitudinal studies are required to explore experiences during the initial phase, the liminal period or midcourse, and the reincorporating period that results in new ways of living and being as the outcome of the transition experience (the ending) (Fraser, 1999; Hilton, 2002; Kralik, 2002; Kralik et al., 2003; Martin-McDonald & Biernoff, 2002; Powell-Cope, 1995; Rossen, 1998; Shaul, 1997). Fraser (1999) conducted multiple interviews over time to describe transition, and given that transition occurs over time, we suggest that researchers consider carrying out longitudinal studies. Kralik (2002) used correspondence as a longitudinal data generation strategy in a study with women with chronic illness to reveal that women move through a phase of 'extraordinariness' in which they are in turmoil and distress. They may then move back into a sense of ordinariness, where life becomes familiar. However, this is never a series of steps; rather, it is movement that is nonlinear, perhaps even cyclical and recurring in nature (Kralik, 2002). Similarly, women recovering from addiction who move from supported accommodation to independent housing find that transition in their recovery involves many movements forward and sometimes slipping back as new issues loom to threaten their progress, and ongoing changes need to be incorporated into new ways of living and being without alcohol and drugs (van Loon et al., 2004).

Other Terms Used to Describe the Transition Process

Transition is clearly linked to the notion of self and identity and how it is affected by disruption (Boeijea, Duijnsteeb, Grypdonckb, & Pool, 2002; Kralik, 2002; Young, Dixon-Woods, Findlay, & Heney, 2002). Self-identity is threatened during disruption and there is a need for reconstruction of identity based on new roles and responsibilities (Boeijea et al., 2002; Luborsky, 1994; Young et al., 2002). Other authors exploring life transitions also focus on the process of shifts in identity and redefining of self (Bailey, 1999; Banister, 1999; Miller, 2000). Although all of these papers have limited discussion about transition, their value lies in the understanding they bring about the forces that influence and shape transition. An exhaustive analysis of this body of work is not within the scope of this review, but we highly recommend that such a review be carried out to better inform our understanding of transition.

Biographical disruption is used by some authors to describe the changes to self-identity that require redefinition in the face of adversity (Boeijea et al., 2002; Gravelle, 1997; Young et al., 2002).

Interestingly, these papers have striking similarity to those describing transition—Young et al. (2002) make reference to transition, whereas Boeijea et al. (2002) focus solely on the notion of biographical disruption. These concepts arose from the work of Bury (1982), which centers on the importance of restructuring meaning during illness. This literature informed our work facilitating transition for women with a history of child sexual abuse and addiction and our research with men and women with chronic illness, because people who have experienced profound disruption often have a diminished sense of identity. Thus restoring their biography has been integral to healing during the transition process (Kralik, Koch, & Brady, 2000; Kralik, van Loon, & Visentin, 2006; van Loon & Kralik, 2005).

Illness trajectory is another term that may be used to describe transition. For example, Gravelle (1997) describes the trajectory that parents caring for a child with a progressive illness travel, raising similar issues to the transition literature, namely adversity, acceptance, living with loss, gaining strength, and normalization.

Review Limitations

The primary studies included in this review used diverse qualitative methods. Data were collected from people in diverse situations, circumstances and environments, using diverse analytical approaches and theoretical perspectives. Clearly, a tension exists between the analytical and systematic approach required to conduct a literature review, where the intention is to undertake a secondary synthesis of knowledge, and the diversity of method and human circumstance and experience that is indicative of qualitative research. In addition, the studies reviewed used small, selective, nonrandom samples of participants; therefore, we decided to broaden the discussion by incorporating theoretical frameworks of transition.

Implications for Nursing

Nurses in diverse practice settings assist people to navigate transitions (LeVasseur, 2002) as illness and change disrupts their lives. Meleis and Trangenstein (1994) suggest that the central focus of nursing is to facilitate clients, families and communities through life transitions, because nursing

> is concerned with the process and the experiences of human beings undergoing transitions where health and perceived well-being is the outcome. (Meleis & Trangenstein, 1994, p. 257)

Transition is the movement and adaptation to change, rather than a return to a pre-existing state. Bridges (2004, p. 11) states "every transition begins with an ending," meaning that people have to let go of familiar ways of being in the world that defines who they are. This is particularly important for nurses, who often support people through forced disruptions such as illness (Kralik, 2002). Transitional processes require time as people gradually disengage from old behaviors and ways of defining self. Nurses working alongside people can help them identify changes forced by illness and seek new possibilities from disruptive experiences. Understanding transition enables nurses to move towards a more holistic approach to the provision of care (Kralik, Koch, & Wotton, 1997; Kralik, 2002).

What is already known about this topic:

Transition is a concept that is widely used in the health literature.
The precise meaning of transition has varied with the context in which the term has been used.
A central focus of nursing is to assist people through transitional processes.

What this chapter adds:

Transition is a central concept to nursing and further longitudinal research is required to inform practice.
Transition occurs over time and entails personal, developmental, relational, situational, societal, or environmental change, but not all change involves transition.
Reconstruction of a valued sense of self-identity is essential to transition.

Implications for Nursing Research

Transition is a concept central to nursing (Meleis et al., 2000) that is in need of further research;

however, we believe that consideration must be given to methodologies that extend beyond a single event or inquire about a single response. Transition is recognized as a process that occurs over time; hence, to understand transition experiences, longitudinal comparative, and longitudinal cross-sectional inquiries are required. Gaps in the transition literature that need to be addressed to firm up the link with nursing are: Why is it that some people experience transition and others do not? What are the structures and processes of transition? What are the gendered experiences of transition? What are the cultural experiences of transition? Is transition experienced differently by people who have experienced disruption at different points across the lifespan? Does age influence the transition experience? How do intrapersonal factors such as personality characteristics, attitudes, beliefs, values, marital expectations, and degree of idealization affect experiences of transition?

Conclusion

Merging understandings from the literature reviewed and the theoretical frameworks reveal that transition processes occur when life's circumstances or relationships change. Transition entails change and adaptation, in areas such as developmental (for example, child to adolescent, adolescent to adult, etc.), personal, relationships, situations, sociocultural, or environmental changes, but not all change results in transition. Life crises and loss experiences may force change and adaptation. Common to these experiences, is the dislocation, disorientation and disruption caused to the person's life and the need for them to locate new ways of living and being in the world that incorporate the changes. We hope that this literature review is a useful beginning point to facilitate communication and discussion that will stimulate further research into transition.

REFERENCES

Arman, M., & Rehnsfeldt, A. (2003). The hidden suffering among breast cancer patients: a qualitative meta-synthesis. *Qualitative Health Research 13*(4), 510–527.

Bailey, L. (1999). Refracted selves? A study of changes in self-identity in the transition to motherhood. *Sociology 33*(2), 335–352.

Banister, E. (1999). Women's midlife experience of their changing bodies. *Qualitative Health Research 9*(4), 520–537.

Bertero, C. (1998). Transition to becoming a leukemia patient: or putting up barriers which increase patient isolation. *European Journal of Cancer Care, 7*(1), 40–46.

Boeijea, H., Duijnsteeb, M., Grypdoncka M., & Pool A. (2002). Encountering the downward phase: Biographical work in people with multiple sclerosis living at home. *Social Science and Medicine, 55*(6), 881–893.

Bridges, W. (2004). *Transitions: Making sense of life's changes.* Cambridge, MA: Da Capo Press.

Brouwer-Dudokdewit, A., Savenije A., Zoeteweij M., Maat-Kievit A., & Tibben A. (2002). A hereditary disorder in the family and the family life cycle: Huntington disease as a paradigm. *Family Process, 41*(4), 677–692.

Brudenell, I. (1996). A grounded theory of balancing alcohol recovery and pregnancy. *Western Journal of Nursing Research, 18*(4), 429–440.

Bury, M. (1982). Chronic illness as biographical disruption. *Sociology of Health and illness 4*, 167–182.

Cantanzaro, M. (1990). Transitions in midlife adults with long-term illness. *Holistic Nurse Practitioner, 4*(3), 65–73.

Chick, N., & Meleis, A. (1986). Transitions: A nursing concern. In P. L. Chinn (Ed.), *Nursing research methodology: Issues and implemenation* (Chap. 18, pp. 237–257). Rockville, MD: Aspen,

Creswell, J. (1998). *Qualitative inquiry and research design: Choosing among the five traditions.* London: Sage.

Draper, J. (2003). Men's passage to fatherhood: An analysis of the contemporary relevance of transition theory. *Nursing Inquiry, 10*(1), 66–77.

Elmberger, E., Bolund, C., & Lutzen, K. (2002). Men with cancer: Changes in attempts to master the self-image as a man and as a parent. *Cancer Nursing, 25*(6), 477–485.

Forss, A., Tishelman, C., Widmark, C., & Sachs, L. (2004). Women's experiences of cervical cellular changes: An unintentional transition from health to liminality. *Sociology of Health and Illness, 26*(3), 306–325.

Fraser, C. (1999). The experience of transition for a daughter caregiver of a stroke survivor. *Journal of Neuroscience Nursing, 31*(1), 9–16.

Froggatt, K. (1997). Signposts on the journey: The place of ritual in spiritual care. *International Journal of Palliative Nursing, 3*(1), 42–46.

Glacken, M., Kernohan, G., & Coates, V. (2001). Diagnosed with Hepatitis C: A descriptive exploratory study. *International Journal of Nursing Studies, 38*(1), 107–116.

Glacken, M., Bolund, C., & Lutzen, K. (2002). Men with Hepatitis C: A man and as a parent. *Cancer Nursing, 25*(6), 477–485.

Gravelle, A. (1997). Caring for a child with a progressive illness during the complex phase: Parents' experience of facing adversity. *Journal of Advanced Nursing, 25*(4), 738–745.

Gwilliam, B., & Bailey, C. (2001). The nature of terminal malignant bowel obstruction and its impact on patients with advanced cancer. *International Journal of Palliative Nursing, 7*(10), 474–476.

Hilton, E. (1998). The meaning of stroke in elderly women: A phenomenological investigation. *Journal of Gerontological Nursing, 28*(7), 19–26.

Hilton, E. (2002). The meaning of stroke in elderly women: A phenomenological investigation. *Journal of Gerontological Nursing, 28*(7), 19–26.

Koch, T., & Kralik, D. (2001). Chronic illness: Reflections on a community-based action research programme. *Journal of Advanced Nursing, 36*(1), 23–31.

Kralik, D. (2002). The quest for ordinariness: Transition experienced by midlife women living with chronic illness. *Journal of Advanced Nursing, 39*(2), 146–154.

Kralik, D., Koch, T., & Wotton, K. (1997). Engagement and detachment: Understanding patients' experiences with nursing. *Journal of Advanced Nursing, 26*(2), 399–407.

Kralik, D., Koch T., & Brady B. (2000). Pen pals: Correspondence as a method for data generation in qualitative research. *Journal of Advanced Nursing, 31*(4), 909–917.

Kralik, D., Koch, T., & Eastwood, S. (2003). The salience of the body: Transition in sexual self-identity for women living with multiple sclerosis. *Journal of Advanced Nursing, 42*(1), 11–20.

Kralik, D., van Loon, A., & Visentin, K. (2006). Resilience in the chronic illness experience. *Educational Action Research, 14*(2), 187–201.

LeVasseur, J. (2002). A phenomenological study of the art of nursing: Experiencing the turn. *Advances in Nursing Science, 24*(4), 14–26.

van Loon, A. (2001). Assessing the spiritual needs of older persons. In S. Koch & S. Garrett (Eds.), *Assessing older people—A work book* (pp. 51–73). Melbourne: MacLennan & Petty.

van Loon, A., & Kralik, D. (2005). *A Self-help companion for the healing journey of survivors of child sexual abuse*. Royal District Nursing Service Foundation Research Unit, Catherine House Inc., Centacare, Adelaide (in press).

van Loon, A., Koch, T., & Kralik, D. (2004). Care for female survivors of child sexual abuse in emergency departments. *Accident and Emergency Nursing Journal, 12*(2), 208–214.

Loveys, B. (1990). Transitions in chronic illness: The at-risk role. *Holistic Nursing Practice, 4*, 45–64.

Luborsky, M. (1994). The retirement process: Making the Person and Cultural Meanings Malleable. *Medical Anthropology Quarterly, 8*(4), 411–429.

Mann, R., Abercrombie, P., DeJoseph J., Norbeck, J., & Smith, R. (1999). The personal experience of pregnancy for African–American women. *Journal of Transcultural Nursing, 10*(4), 297–305.

Martin-McDonald, K., & Biernoff, D. (2002). Initiation into a dialysis-dependent life: An examination of rites of passage...including commentary by Frauman AC with author response. *Nephrology Nursing Journal, 29*(4), 347–353.

Meleis, A., & Trangenstein, P. (1994). Facilitating transitions: Redefinition of the nursing mission. *Nursing Outlook, 42*(6), 255–259.

Meleis, A., Sawyer, L., Im, E.-O., Messias, D. H., & Schumacher, K. (2000). Experiencing transitions: An emerging middle-range theory. *Advances in Nursing Science, 23*(1), 12–28.

Miller, T. (2000). Losing the plot: Narrative construction and longitudinal childbirth research. *Qualitative Health Research, 10*(3), 309–323.

Montenko, A., & Greenberg, S. (1995). Reframing dependence in old age: A positive transition for families. *Social Work, 40*(3), 382–390.

Neil, J., & Barrell, L. (1998). Transition theory and its relevance to patients with chronic wounds. *Rehabilitation Nursing, 23*(6), 295–299.

Nelson, A. (2003). Transition to motherhood. *JOGNN–Journal of Obstetric; Gynecologic and Neonatal Nursing, 32*(4), 465–477.

Paterson, B. (2001). The shifting perspectives model of chronic illness. *Journal of Nursing Scholarship, 33*(1), 21–26.

Powell-Cope, G. (1995). The experiences of gay couples affected by HIV infection. *Qualitative Health Research, 5*(1), 36–62.

Powers, B., & Knapp, T. (1990). *A dictionary of nursing theory and research*. London: Sage.

Rossen, E. (1998). *Older women in relocation transition*. Unpublished doctoral thesis. University of Illinois at Chicago, Health Sciences Center, Chicago, IL.

Sawyer, L. (1999). Engaged mothering: The transition to motherhood for a group of African American women. *Journal of Transcultural Nursing, 10*(1), 14–21.

Schumacher, K., & Meleis, A. (1994). Transitions: A central concept in nursing. *IMAGE: Journal of Nursing Scholarship, 26*(2), 119–127.

Selder, F. (1989). Life transition theory: The resolution of uncertainty. *Nursing and Health Care, 10*(8), 437–451.

Shaul, M. (1997). Transitions in chronic illness: Rheumatoid arthritis in women. *Rehabilitation Nursing, 22*(4), 199–205.

Sheehy, G. (1977). *Passages predictable: Crisis of adult life.* Toronto: Bantam Books.

Skarsater, I., Dencker, K., Bergbom, I., Haggstrom, L., & Fridlund, B. (2003). Women's conceptions of coping with major depression in daily life: A qualitative, salutogenic approach. *Issues in Mental Health Nursing, 24,* 419–439.

Turner, V. (1969). *The ritual process: Structure and antistructure.* Middlesex: Penguin.

Vaartio, H., & Kiviniemi, K. (2003). Men's experiences and their resources from cancer diagnosis to recovery. *European Journal of Oncology Nursing, 7*(3), 182–190.

Van Gennep, A. (1960.) *The rites of passage.* London: Routledge and Kegan Paul.

Walker, A. (2001). Trajectory, transition and vulnerability in adult medical–surgical patients: A framework for understanding in-hospital convalescence. *Contemporary Nurse, 11*(2/3), 206–216.

White, K. (1995). The transition from victim to victor: Application of the theory of mastery. *Journal of Psychosocial Nursing and Mental Health Services, 33*(8), 41–44.

White, A. (2003). Interactions between nurses and men admitted with chest pain. *European Journal of Cardiovascular Nursing, 2*(1), 47–55.

Young, B., Dixon-Woods, M., Findlay, M., & Heney, D. (2002). Parenting in a crisis: Conceptualising mothers of children with cancer. *Social Science and Medicine, 55*(10), 1835–1847.

Reprinted with permission from: Kralik, D., Visentin, K., & van Loon, A. (2006). Transition: A literature review. *Journal of Advanced Nursing, 55*(3), 320–329.

III

The Experience of and Responses to Transitions

To uncover the different experiences of people going through changes and the many different ways they respond to these changes, we categorized the triggers for change that nurses deal with. We first developed the categories based on observing nurses' clinical experiences, we then reviewed the literature to support or refute these categories, after which we used the emerging categorical framework of the triggers to study the experiences and responses to events and situations. Each of these approaches further supported the types of transitions individuals face. Four types of transitions are considered in this volume. These are reflected and represented in this section with chapters that shed more light on the particular type of change being considered. Some of these chapters are reviews, but the majority report research studies.

It is important to note that these transition types are neither pure nor mutually exclusive, because transitions are complex processes and may overlap or occur simultaneously. For example, while experiencing a developmental transition (becoming a mother) a person may also be going through a situational transition (being discharged from a hospital). Chapter 3 in Part III is devoted to the first transition type—those transitions triggered by developmental changes. Among the types of developmental transitions that nurses tend to deal with are those related to the process of becoming a parent, experiencing menopause, and growing old. Others may involve becoming an adolescent, experiencing menarche, and dying. Each of these is a major developmental life event that has been described or researched by nurse scientists. Each of these triggers responses that should be uncovered and may require interventions to ensure healthy outcomes. I have selected articles to represent some of these developmental transitions—parenting, menopause, and growing old.

The second major transition type is situational transition, which is presented in chapter 4. Situational transitions are triggered by events that require spacial or geographic changes such as discharge and relocation (of elders) and/or relationship changes such as divorce. All of these may have health consequences and may affect levels of well-being. Examples of situational transitions are divorce or homelessness.

Immigration is another example of a situational transition (chapter 5) that affects health, health- and illness-seeking behaviors, as well as the immigrant's ability to cope with other life changes. Understanding the immigration experience is usually enhanced by learning about the immigrants in their own homeland, therefore, I have included articles about Brazilians in their homeland as well as Brazilians as immigrants in the U.S.A.

Nurses also go through educational transitions that are situational (chapter 6). Among the events that trigger transitional responses in nurses are their transition from nursing student to nurse, to becoming a competent practitioner, as well as such events as moving up the educational ladder from a diploma or associate degree to a baccalaureate degree. Each of these advancements up the educational ladder creates the need for transitional intervention.

The third type of transition is that which is instigated by a health and illness situation (chapter 7). These we called "health and illness transitions." As individuals receive a diagnosis, undergo surgery, or realize that they will live the rest of their lives at risk for a particular new condition, they go through various processes and they require care during these processes that matches their varying needs during the different stages and milestones in this process. What are these processes, what are the responses to the diagnosis and treatment processes, and how do these responses influence the outcomes for the person, family, and community? These are questions that nurses must uncover, understand, and deal with in planning quality care for those who are undergoing such experiences. These transitions may be compounded by other biobehavorial, sociocultural, or genetic conditions. Being an immigrant and living alone, having a stigmatizing disease, or facing the end of life may affect one's transition experiences and responses. Chapter 7 includes findings from studies that reflect different triggers—diagnosis of acute or chronic disease, beginning rehabilitation, experiencing memory loss, or making a decision to start palliative care. This chapter also reflects studies completed nationally and internationally.

The last type of transition discussed in Part III is the organizational transition (chapter 8). Organizational transitions are triggered by changes in policies, leadership, practices, as well as models of care. The focus in organizational transitions is on uncovering and intervening in the experiences and responses of the members of the group undergoing the transition, either individually or collectively. Technological changes, introduction of electronic health records, robotic caregivers, new Chief Nurse Officers, new leadership models, and staffing patterns create disruptions and the need for strategies that enhance healthy adoption of the new changes. Several articles have been selected to reflect this category, however, many more can be identified in the nursing literature.

Chapter 3 Developmental Transitions

3.1 DEVELOPMENTAL TRANSITIONS

MARIANNE HATTAR-POLLARA

Normative and Nonnormative Developmental Transitions

Human developmental transitions are complex and dynamic phenomena involving a predictable series of biologically determined stages of growth (i.e., physical, cognitive) and of normatively governed psychosocial maturations. Developmental transitions also involve unpredictable events and transitions, which precipitate changes that are likely to influence adult men and women's health and well-being in an adverse manner.

Nursing researchers paid specific attention to adult developmental transitions, particularly those that articulate with health and intersect with nursing, and offered a comprehensive theoretical model of transitions, delineating the nature and types of transitions, the conditions of transitions (which include meanings, expectations, level of knowledge/skills, environment, and level of planning) and the patterns and mediating factors of human responses to transitions (Chick & Meleis, 1986; Meleis, 1975; Schumacher & Meleis, 1994). Meleis and colleagues have conducted empirical studies examining a range of transition experiences including becoming a mother (Sawyer, 1999), experiencing menopause (Im & Meleis, 1999), transitions of Jordanian adolescents and their mothers (Hattar-Pollara & Meleis, 1995), developing chronic illness (Messias, 1997), and taking on a family caregiving role (Schumacher, 1996). Based on the nursing framework of transitions, situation-specifics theories, and specific nursing therapeutics are evident in the work of Mercer (2004) on becoming a mother and maternal role attainment, Gaffney (1992) on maternal role sufficiency, Shin and White-Traut (2007) on transition to motherhood in the neonatal intensive care, Im and Meleis (1999) on menopausal transition of low-income Korean immigrant mothers, Schumacher, Jones, and Meleis (1999) on helping elderly person in transitions, and Kaas and Rousseau (1983) on geriatric sexual conformity.

Until the 1950s, multidisciplinary investigations of developmental transition were exclusively focused on the preadult years. Stage theorists from various disciplines focused their attention on the normative, predictable, linear (hierarchical), and universal developmental processes that all humans go through as they progress in age from the prenatal phase through infancy, early childhood, middle childhood, and pubescence, to the adolescence phase (e.g., Erikson, 1950; Freud, 1955; Piaget, 1967). For example, Freud and Piaget assumed that developmental transitions are largely completed at the end of adolescence, and those who thought that development progresses beyond adolescence paid less attention to adult development (Levinson, 1986). Levinson (1986), Galinsky (1981), and Atchley (1989), through retrospective cohort studies, offered descriptive frameworks detailing the normative phases and corresponding behavior adult men and women are expected to go through as they move through the cycle, through parenthood and into retirement. Transitions that are less predictable, and therefore nonnormative or universal, are those developmental transitions that are concentrated during the different phases of adulthood and are those that are more likely to articulate with health and intersect with nursing. Currently, the knowledge base on developmental transitions of adult men and women is descriptive rather than explanatory. The units of analysis for describing the transitional changes adult men and women go through as they progress in life reflect the investigator's unique disciplinary focus and are non-integrative of the complex individual and environmental variables affecting adult transitions. Most of the knowledge on adult developmental transitions draws on role-theory research (Ebaugh, 1988; Hagestad & Neugarten, 1985), and life-course research (Elder, 1985a).

Investigating the specific attributes of normal and/or disruptive, and predictable or unpredictable developmental transitions so as to understand and explain the mechanisms by which they influence health and well-being is crucial for the development of specific nursing therapeutics that would effectively assist individuals and their families through disruptive developmental transitions and promote their health and well-being.

This chapter examines the literature on adult developmental transitions. Initially, a brief review of current theoretical frameworks on adult transitions is presented, emphasizing the conditions, patterns, and consequences of adult developmental transitions. The subsequent sections examine the process of adult transitions through the lenses of role theory and life-course research, followed by a summary and discussion of the future directions for nursing research.

Theories on Adult Developmental Transitions

Stage theories and research on child and adolescent developmental transitions are important to understand the issues surrounding human developmental transitions of the early life period and the consequence of delayed or disruptive development on later adult years. The focus of this chapter, however, is on exploring the developmental transitions of adulthood. The issues that accompany adult developmental transitions are identified through examinations of theories and research evidence that paid particular attention to the process of adult transitions and the underlying mechanism accompanying such transitions.

Transitions during the adult years have been examined through various lenses including transition through the life cycles, transition to parenthood, continuity theory, role theory, and life-course perspectives. Each of these disciplines offers a unique approach to conceptualizing transitions, and to some degree or another offers a description of the underlying processes of transitions.

Markers of Life Transitions

Among the notable theories on adult development are Levinson's "seasons of a man's life" (1978) and Levinson and Levinson's "seasons of a woman's life" (1996) theories. Focusing his attention on adult development through a series of intensive interviews with men and women, Levinson (1978, 1986) set out to determine the nature and extent of possible personality changes during the ages 17 to 65 years. According to Levinson (1978), personality development takes place during the life span within a specific framework, which he calls "life structure." An individual's life structure is shaped by the social and physical environment, which include family and work, and to some degree or another, other variables such as religion, race, and economic status, among others.

Levinson proposed a series of stages that are clustered around four "seasonal life cycles" that people go through as they develop. Adult series of stages cluster around pre-adulthood, early adulthood, middle adulthood, and late adulthood, with stage-specific markers requiring acquisition of new experience and tasks, and the incorporation of new knowledge and skills. Early adult transition (17–22) is characterized by leaving adolescence and by making preliminary choices for adult life. Entering the adult world (22–28) signifies making initial choices in love, occupation, friendship, values, and lifestyle. The age 30 transition (28–33) is a time when changes occur in life structure, with either a moderate change or, more often, with a severe and stressful crisis. Settling down (33–40) is characterized by establishing a niche in society, and by progressing on a timetable, in both family and career accomplishments. During this period adults are expected to think and behave like a parent, so they are facing more demanding roles and expectations.

During the mid-life transition (40–45), life structure usually comes into question and becomes a time of crisis in the meaning, direction, and value of each person's life. Also, during this period of developmental transition, neglected parts of the self (talents, desires, aspirations) take the forefront and seek expression. Becoming more aware of how short life is and of death, individuals during this period become involved in trying to leave a legacy, and this usually forms the core of the second half of life.

Entering middle adulthood (45–50) signifies making the choices that must be made, which may lead to forming a new life structure and a commitment to new tasks. Late adulthood (50–65) is a period during which individuals spend time reflecting on past achievements and regrets, and making peace with oneself and with others.

Levinson (1986) distinguished the periods of developmental transitions and non-transitions in a person's life and classified them as either stable or transitional. A stable period is a time when a person makes crucial choices in life, while a transitional period signifies the end of one stage and the beginning of a new one. Life during these transitions can be either rocky or smooth, but the quality and significance of one's life commitment often change between the beginning and end of a period.

Levinson's theory, although comprehensive and logical, is heavily descriptive and fails to account for the wide individual, socio-cultural, and socio-economic variations. His theory was widely criticized for the research method used for its initial development, especially with regard to using a small sample of men and for generalizing the findings to both men and women. In response, Levinson (1986) conducted another study with a small sample of 45 women, which included housewives, academic instructors, and businesswomen. His findings show that women go through the same types of transitions as men do, however, gender differences were noted with regard to the meanings and responses women attach to their life transitions, with women tending to be tied closer to family life.

Markers of Transition to Parenthood

Focusing on the psychosocial aspects of transitioning to parenthood, Galinsky (1981) offers a theory of parenthood. She focused her studies on the developmental stages of parenting and described how adults develop through the interaction with their children. Based on interviews with over 200 parents, she identified six stages including the parental image stage, the nurturing stage, the authority stage, the integrative stage, the independent teen stage, and the departure stage. Galinsky (1981) points out that husband and wife become father and mother at the birth of their first baby, which forms the beginning of the first stage, the *parental image stage*, and during which the mother and father form their image of themselves as parents. Father and mother usually have a desire to be perfect, but often experience heavy demands that were unexpected. The *nurturing stage* occurs during infancy, when attachment occurs, and relationships with spouse, infant, and other people are challenged and determined. Often heavy demands are made upon parents at this time, as they establish their roles. During the *authority stage*, between two and four years of age, adults face questions of their effectiveness as parents. The young child is beginning to develop independence, and more demands are made on a parent's time. Often a second child is born, adding to the stress of the family.

The *integrative stage* extends from preschool through middle childhood. As children develop more autonomy and social skills, parents are required to set realistic goals, motivate their children, develop effective communication skills, and establish authority. The fifth stage, the *independent teenage stage*, is the time when adolescents wrestle with identification, responsibility, and maturity. Parents must provide support for their adolescents, while maintaining authority and responsibility. Finally, the *departure stage* occurs when the adolescent leaves home. At this time, parents evaluate past performance and prepare for the future relationship with their offspring.

The important points of Galinsky's theory are that parenthood develops as the children grow and that the adult's self-concepts are shaped through interactions with their children at each stage. When parents are aware of and can achieve their goals, they will be happy and satisfied. If not, they will be frustrated, stressed, and depressed. Galinsky's theory serves a useful framework for the assessment of the psychosocial transition to parenthood.

Markers of Retirement's Transition

Using a framework of continuity, Atchley (1989, 1999) proposed a model of retirement that includes six phases, the preretirement phase, the honeymoon phase, the disenchantment phase, the reorientation phase, the stability phase, and the terminal phase. In the *preretirement phase*, the worker becomes aware that retirement is approaching. In the years prior to retirement, money is saved for funding the dream vacation or to plan for the things that are not possible to do while working. The *honeymoon phase* occurs immediately after the actual event and is normally characterized by enjoyment of one's free time. Now the retiree can paint the garage, do gardening, take a trip, or do other things he or she has wanted to do for years. During the *disenchantment phase*, the retiree begins to feel depressed about life and the lack of things to do. After the traveling, cleaning, and doing the things most desired, the person gets tired and bored. Often the person then goes through a *reorientation phase* of developing a more realistic attitude toward the effective use of time. Here he or she reevaluates these activities and makes some decisions about what is most important. These priorities then set the stage for the next phase. During the *stability phase*, the retirement routine is established and enjoyed. Perhaps volunteer work, visiting, or some other routine is developed that keeps the retiree happy and feeling important. The *terminal phase* (end of retirement) occurs when illness or disability prevents the retiree from actively caring for self, or when retirees regain employment. According to Atchley (1999), there is considerable continuity in identity and self-concept over the retirement transition and this continuity contributes to the retirement adjustment process. He observed that "middle-aged and older adults attempt to preserve and maintain existing structure...and tend to apply familiar strategies in familiar arenas of life" (Atchley, 1989, p.183). However, Wang (2007) found that retirees do not follow a uniform adjustment pattern during retirement and that retirees' patterns of responses have important consequence on their psychological well-being.

Role Theory

As opposed to age-based theories of development, which generally emphasize the maturational aspects of development and associated unique themes, tasks, and difficulties (e.g., Erikson, 1950; Levinson, 1978), social role-based theories view life transition through role entry and exit. Transition is viewed as progressing smoothly if role entry and role exit occur "on time." Conversely, personal lives and social structure are likely to be disruptive if role entry and role exit occur "off time" and are unpredictable or involuntary (e.g., Hagestad & Neugarten 1985; Neugarten, 1976; Neugarten & Datan, 1974).

Ebaugh, (1988, p. 149) defined role-exit as the "departure from any role that is central to one's self-identity." Linking role theory to life transitions and using it to describe both the status and the behaviors associated with role entry and role exit during adult life transitions, Ebaugh (1988) retrospectively investigated the role exits of a diverse group of participants who exited one of nine roles ranging from nuns to transsexuals. Her findings offered a process of four stages in role exit including experiencing doubt, searching for alternative roles, occurrence of a turning point, and creation of a new identity as former role occupant. She also found that three-fourths of her sample experienced "the vacuum" either right before the decision to exit or, in some cases, shortly afterwards. Depending on whether the role exit was voluntary or involuntary,

Ashforth (2001), in his investigation of role exit in organizations and among retirees, found that involuntary exits from push-and-pull forces constitutes a significant threat to one's identity and sense of meaning as well as the sense of control and belonging. The push-and-pull forces leading to involuntary role exit, whether they are located within the life circumstance of the individual, such as failing health, or are extrinsic, tend to be stigmatizing, thus creating the additional burden of coping with the weight of shame and other emotions. Furthermore, involuntary role exit occurs with little or no advance warning, thus shock and distress are additional burdens.

Role theory has been extensively used in studying life events that may or may not accompany life transitions. Gambardella (2008) investigated the effectiveness of applying the concepts of role-exit theory in the counseling of military couples who were experiencing marital discord following extended periods of deployment. Her findings indicate that 60% of her small sample of ten reported improvement in the marital relationship following intervention counseling using a framework approach based on role-exit theory.

Meleis (1975) offered a theoretical base for nursing and introduced role insufficiency and role supplementation for the study and practice of role transitions. She defined role insufficiency as "any difficulty in the cognizance and/or performance of a role or the sentiments and goals associated with role behavior as perceived by self or by significant other." Role supplementation is defined as "a deliberate process that included conveying information or providing experience for the role incumbent to become aware of the anticipated role behaviors and goals, as well as the interrelationships between the new role and the roles of others." Role supplementation is central for nursing in designing specific nursing actions and therapeutics to prevent or ameliorate role insufficiency through role supplementation, which consists of two components: role clarification and role taking.

Role loss can lead to feelings of anxiety or depression, thus leading to low levels of well-being with role exit (Thoits, 1992). When a role is central to one's identity, involuntary role exit may be an especially stressful disruption (Burke, 1991). However, when a role is undesirable, role exit may lead to feeling of relief and well-being (Wheaton, 1990). Therefore both individual and contextual characteristics may influence both the process and the outcomes of role-exit transitions and may have adverse consequences on health and well-being.

Life-Course Perspective

Life-course perspective views transition as a social phenomenon that is distinct from the life-span transitions (Hagestad & Neugarten, 1985). In contrast to the characteristics of life-span developmental transitions, which are normatively governed and predictable across time and space, life-course transition reflects the intersection of social and historical factors with personal biography during the duration of life (Elder, 1985a). Therefore, developmental transitions as viewed through the lens of the life-course perspective are expected to vary across time, space, and populations.

Life-course perspective (Elder, 1995; Elder & Johnson, 2003) draws attention to critical concepts in the life course. Concepts such as transitions and trajectories, contextual embeddedness, interdependence of life spheres, and timing of transitions constitute the essence of theoretical thought and are key concepts in researching life-course transitions (Elder, 1985a; Hagestad, 1990; Shanahan, 2000). These concepts are considered crucial to understanding the well-being of individuals going through developmental transitions. According to Elder (1985a), transitions refer to changes in status over time, which are discrete and bounded in duration, but their consequences may be long term. Trajectories refer to life development during periods of relatively stable status, and often include multiple transitions that can be reliably differentiated from alternate patterns. Transitions and trajectories are interrelated because they are embedded in form and meaning (Elder, 1985a).

Contextual embeddedness implies that the experience of life transitions and developmental trajectories is contingent on the specific circumstances under which transitions occur. These include individual attributes such as health status, coping efforts, current and past status and roles, and family and social context. Independent life spheres emphasizes that experience in one life sphere is influenced by experience in other life spheres (Elder, 1985a, 1995). According to life-course perspective, the experience of life transition is also contingent on its timing in terms of social and cultural deadlines, personal expectations, and occurrences or co-occurrences in other life spheres. Most of the research on life-course transitions focuses on the early adulthood of men and less so on that of women. Barnett & Baruch (1978) recognized that the lives of women follow different patterns and involve somewhat different themes than do the lives of men. For example, whereas men's lives are guided by the development of individuation and autonomy, women's lives are guided by the development of attachment and care (Bardwick, 1980; Gilligan, 1982a, 1982b).

Most of the research on life-course sequence and markers focuses on entry to adulthood. In contrast to Levinson's adult developmental stage of early adulthood, Arnett (2000) distinguished entry to adulthood (18–24) as a period of emerging adulthood that has distinctive features and importance and is characterized by formidable arrays of new experiences and tasks requiring the development of new knowledge and skills to experience a successful transition into adulthood. (Arnett, 2000; Hogan, 1981; Cohen, Kasen, Chen, Hatmark, & Gordon, 2003). Emerging adulthood constitutes a sequence of key transitions for entry into adulthood including leaving school, followed by first-time job, followed by marriage. Studies have found that a disorderly sequence of emerging adulthood transitions resulted in poorer outcomes in life and these were more common among women. (Hogan, 1981; Kerckhoff, 1990). Cohen and colleagues (2003) further note that although, on average, early adult men and women changed roles and assumed responsibility in accordance with the development sequence and expectations of this period, their patterns of doing so were remarkably diverse and most of their study sample had periods during which there was progress and regress in assuming adult roles.

Conclusions and Directions for Future Research

Understanding the complex and dynamic nature of adult developmental transitions requires an understanding of the various variables influencing and mediating the process and its consequences. Adult developmental transitions may be predictable, expected, or even a desirable part of one's life trajectory. They may be anticipated or hoped for (for example, planning for parenthood), or they may be unanticipated or involuntary. While all transitions, by their very nature, expose people to vulnerabilities due to the uncertainties about outcomes, unanticipated or forced transitions are more likely to expose individuals to health risks.

The majority of nursing research is focused on understanding the experiences of men and women undergoing normative single or multiple transitions (for example, becoming a parent, assuming the maternal role, or going through menopause while going through immigration) and on understanding attributes of the developmental transition of motherhood through studies of maternal attachments. However, less attention has been given to investigating processes or consequences of unanticipated or involuntary transitions, or to comparative studies of adult men and women going through similar transitions.

The nursing transition framework integrates the cumulative knowledge on the nature, conditions, and process of transition and offers an organizing framework for both researchers and clinicians to adequately study the variables affecting the process and the variables mediating the positive or negative consequences of transitions. It also serves as a framework for assessing and devising corresponding nursing therapeutics. However, transitions are complex because of the interplay and interweaving of variables situated within individuals and embedded in their context. Depending on the personality, disposition, and coping efforts of individuals, and depending on the significance and meaning of the life-changing event as well as the availability of instrumental support, the impact of the life-changing event on the individual and those in his/her life sphere, the economic resources, the historical factors of the time, and the impact of the life-changing event on the performance of ordinary roles or the emergence of extraordinary hassles affecting ordinary role functions, the process of transition may be smooth or may be hindered by any one of these variables or by the complex interplay of these variables. Such complexity adds difficulty in designing research studies that would take into account all of these variables in theoretically sound and empirically useful studies. Understanding and explaining what exactly accounts for differences between individuals, and sometimes within the same individual at different times of life, or why certain individuals move with ease through life-changing transitions while others suffer severe vulnerabilities and health risks, is challenging and would be impossible without careful investigation and identification of those variables that directly affect the process and those that mediate the process. Future research should focus on explaining the interplay of transition variables so that nursing situation-producing theories aimed toward devising corresponding therapeutics to prevent illness and promote health would be possible.

Furthermore, inquiry into emerging adulthood transitions, particularly as they pertain to women, is needed. A. I. Meleis (personal communication, 2008) asserts that "being women is a risk." In light of the formidable arrays of new experience and knowledge required for successful transitions during this period, and in reference to findings of studies demonstrating that women are faring worse than men on outcomes of emerging adulthood transitions, it is of utmost importance to investigate, understand, and explain the composite effect of being a woman during the emerging adulthood sequence of transitions.

Finally, explicating the distinguishing attributes of the developmental transitions that intersect with nursing and articulate with health and illness, understanding the possible cascade effect of multiple transitions, whether co-occurring or occurring in response to life-changing events, and explaining the health risks and actual health consequences are of importance to building disciplinary knowledge and advancing nursing practice.

REFERENCES

Arnett, J. J. (2000). Emerging adulthood: A theory of development from the late teens through the twenties. *American Psychologist, 55*, 469–480.

Ashforth, B. (2001). *Role transitions in organizational life: An identity-based perspective*. Mahwah, NJ: Erlbaum.

Atchley, R. C. (1989). A continuity theory of normal aging. *The Gerontologist,* 29, 183–190.

Atchley, R. C. (1999). Continuity theory, self, and social structure. In C. D. Ryff & V. W. Marshall (Eds.), *Families and retirement* (pp. 145–158). Newbury Park, CA: Sage.

Bardwick, J. M. (1980). The seasons of a woman's life. In D.G. McGuigan (Ed.), *Women's lives: New theory: Research and policy* (pp. 35–57). Ann Arbor: University of Michigan, Center for Continuing Education of Women.

Barnett, R. C., & Baruch, G. K. (1978). Women in the middle years: A critique of research and theory. *Psychology for Women Quarterly, 3*, 187–197.

Burke, P. J. (1991). Identity processes and social stress. *American Sociological Review, 56,* 836–849.

Chick, N., & Meleis, A. I. (1986). Transitions: A nursing concern. In P. L. Chinn (Ed.), *Nursing research methodology: Issues and implementations* (pp. 237–257). Aspen: Rockville, MD

Cohen, P., Kasen, S., Chen, H., Hatmark, C., & Gordon, K. (2003). Variations in patterns of developmental transitions in the emerging adulthood period. *Developmental Psychology, 39*(4), 657–669.

Ebaugh, H. R. F. (1988). *Becoming an ex: The process of role exit*. Chicago: University of Chicago Press.

Elder, G. H., Jr. (1985a). *Perspectives on the life course*. Ithaca: Cornell University Press.

Elder, G. H., Jr. (1995). The life course paradigm: Social change and individual development. In P. Moen, G. H. Elder, & K. Luscher (Eds.), *Examining lives in context: Perspectives on the ecology of human development* (pp. 101–139). Washington, DC: American Psychological Association.

Elder, G. H., & Johnson, M. K. (2003). The life course and aging: Challenges, lessons, and new directions. In R. A. Settersten, Jr. (Ed.), *Invitation to the life course: Toward new understandings of later life* (pp. 49–81). Amityville, NY: Baywood.

Erikson, E. H. (1950). *Childhood and society*. New York: Norton.

Freud, S. (1955). *Group psychology and the analysis of ego*. London: Hogarth Press.

Gaffney, K. F. (1992). Nursing practice model for maternal role insufficiency. *Advances in Nursing Science, 15*(2), 76–84.

Galinsky, E. (1981). *Between generations: The six stages of parenthood.* New York: Times Books

Gambardella, L. C. (2008). Role-exit theory and marital discord following extended military deployment. *Perspectives in Psychiatric Care, 7*(1), 1–6.

Gilligan, C. (1982a). Adult development and women's development: Arrangements for a marriage. In J. Z. Giele (Ed.), *Women in the middle years: Current knowledge and direction for research and policy* (pp. 89–114). New York: Wiley.

Gilligan, C. (1982b). *In a different voice.* Cambridge, MA: Harvard University Press.

Hagestad, G. O. (1990). Social perspectives on the life course. In H.R. Binstock & L.K. George (Eds.), *Handbook of aging and the social sciences* (3rd ed., pp. 151–168). San Diego: Academic.

Hagestad, G. O., & Neugarten, B. L. (1985). Age and the life course. In H.R. Binstock & E. Shanas (Eds.), *Handbook on aging and the social sciences* (2nd ed., pp. 35–61). New York: Van Nostrand Reinhold.

Hattar-Pollara, M., & Meleis, A. I. (1995). Parenting their adolescents: The experience of Jordanian immigrant women in California. *Health Care for Women International, 16,* 195–211.

Hogan, D. P. (1981). *Transitions and social change: The early lives of American men* (p. 232). New York: Academic Press.

Im, E. O., & Meleis, A. I. (1999). A situation-specific theory for menopausal transition of Korean immigrant women. *Image: Journal of Nursing Scholarship, 31,* 333–338.

Kaas, M. J., & Rousseau, G. K. (1983). Geriatric sexual conformity: Assessment and intervention. *Clinical Gerontologist, 2*(1), 31–44.

Kerckhoff, A. C. (1990). *Getting started: Transition to adulthood in Great Britain.* Boulder, CO: Westview.

Levinson, D. J. (1978). *The seasons of a man's life.* New York: Knopf.

Levinson, D. J. (1986). A conception of adult development. *American Psychologist, 41,* 3–13.

Levinson, D. J., & Levinson, J. (1996). *The seasons of a woman's life.* New York: Knopf.

Meleis, A. I. (1975). Role insufficiency and role supplementation: A conceptual framework. *Nursing Research, 24*(4), 264–271.

Mercer, R. T. (2004). Becoming a mother versus maternal role attachment. *Nursing Scholarship, 36*(3), 226–232.

Messias, D. K. H. (1997). *Narratives of transcultural migration, work, and health: The lived experience of Brazilian women in the United States.* Doctoral Dissertation, University of California, San Francisco.

Neugarten, B. L. (1976). Adaptation and the life cycle. *Counseling Psychologist, 6,* 16–20.

Neugarten, B. L., & Datan, N. (1974). The middle years. In S. Arieti (Ed.), *American handbook of psychiatry* (Vol. 1, pp. 592–608). New York: Basic Books.

Piaget, J. (1967). *The child's conception of the world.* Totowa, NJ: Littlefield, Adams.

Sawyer, L. M. (1999). Engaged mothering: The transition to motherhood for a group of African American women. *Journal of Transcultural Nursing, 1*(11), 14–21.

Schumacher, K. L. (1996). Reconceptualizing family caregiving: Family-based illness during illness care during chemotherapy. *Research in Nursing and Health, 19,* 261–271.

Schumacher, K. L., Jones, P. S., & Meleis, A. I. (1999). Helping elderly persons in transition: A framework for research and practice. In E. A. Swanson & T. Tripp-Reimer (Eds.), *Life transitions in the older adult: Issues for nurses and other health professionals* (pp. 1–26). New York: Springer Publishing Company.

Schumacher, K. L., & Meleis, A. I. (1994). Transitions: A central concept in nursing. *Image: Journal of Nursing Scholarship, 26*(2), 119–127.

Shanahan, M. J. (2000). Pathways to adulthood in changing societies: Variability and mechanisms in life course perspective. *Annual Review of Sociology, 26,* 667–692.

Shin, H., & White-Traut, R. (2007). The conceptual structure of transition to motherhood in the neonatal intensive care. *Journal of Advanced Nursing, 58*(1), 90–98.

Thoits, P. A. (1992). Identity structure and psychological well-being: Gender and marital status comparisons. *Social Psychology Quarterly, 55,* 236–256.

Wang, M. (2007). Profiling retirees in the retirement transition and adjustment process: Examining the longitudinal change patterns of retirees' psychological well-being, *Journal of Applied Psychology, 92*(2), 455–474.

Wheaton, B. (1990). Life transitions, role histories, and mental health. *American Sociological Review, 55,* 209–223.

3.2 BECOMING A MOTHER VERSUS MATERNAL ROLE ATTAINMENT

RAMONA T. MERCER

The transition to motherhood is a major developmental life event. Becoming a mother involves moving from a known, current reality to an unknown, new reality. A transition requires restructuring goals, behaviors, and responsibilities to achieve a new conception of self (Barba & Selder, 1995). Many strategies are used to adapt to a new reality while maintaining one's personal integrity. Strategies include recognizing the permanency of the required change, seeking information for construction of a new self-definition, seeking models for a new normalization, and competency testing of self in the new role (Deutsch, Ruble, Fleming, Brooks-Gunn, & Stangor, 1988; Mercer, 1995). Transitions may be facilitated or inhibited by the woman's personal conditions, cultural beliefs and attitudes, socioeconomic status (SES), preparation and knowledge, and community and societal conditions (Meleis, Sawyer, Im, Messias, & Schumacher, 2000).

Establishing a maternal identity in becoming a mother contributes to a woman's psychosocial development. In contrast to physical development, which is linear, some scholars have suggested that psychosocial development progresses as spiraling or widening, leading to an increase in a person's adaptive functioning (Kegan, 1982; Rubin, 1984).

Theory building is a continuous process as research findings provide evidence for clarification of concepts, additions, or deletions. In their review of research on women as mothers and grandmothers, McBride and Shore (2001) suggested retiring the phrase "maternal role attainment" (MRA) because it implies a static situation rather than a fluctuating process, and this implication discourages the study of motherhood from a life-span approach. The purpose of this chapter is to review the development of MRA theory and current research on the transition to motherhood, leading to the conclusion that the term MRA should be replaced with the term "becoming a mother" (BAM).

Background

Theory of Maternal Role Attainment

Rubin (1967) introduced MRA as a process leading to a woman's achievement of maternal role identity. Rubin described the progressive stages of the process that begins during pregnancy as mimicry, role-play, fantasy, introjection–projection–rejection, and identity. The woman moves from seeking information and mimicking observations, to seeking expert models, role-playing, and fantasizing about herself as a mother. She introjects observed behaviors of others, projects how those behaviors would be for her, and rejects behavior she judges as inappropriate for herself. An ideal image of self as mother is constructed from her extensive psychosocial work during pregnancy and postpartum, and through this image the maternal identity is incorporated into her self-system. Grief work accompanies the process as roles or parts of her life that are incompatible with motherhood are relinquished.

Selective perceptions of the woman's self-system (her ideal image, self-image, and body image) screen information that is taken in (Rubin, 1967). The ideal image reflects the qualities, traits, attitudes, and achievements the woman finds desirable for motherhood. The self-image is a representation of a consistent self in the present. The body image is reflected by body accommodations, functions, and capacity; maternal identity status is contingent on functional control of the body. Loss of functional control leads to lower self-esteem and risk of role failure. Rubin defined maternal identity as the end point in maternal role-taking, with a woman having a sense of being in her role, along with a sense of comfort about her past and future. This theory was based on nurses' field notes of their interactions with women during pregnancy and in the first month after birth.

In her 1984 book Rubin did not use the term MRA. She described maternal identity as an inseparable incorporation into the whole personality that is more than a role that can be stepped into and out of again (p. 38). Data for her book were drawn from nurses' field notes of their interactions with women during pregnancy and 6 weeks postpartum. Rubin reaffirmed the importance of tasks during pregnancy to establish the qualitative matrix of maternal behavior: ensuring safe passage for self and baby, seeking acceptance of and support for self and baby, "binding-in" to her infant, and giving of self (Rubin, 1975, 1984). She said that a woman's binding-in (a term Rubin thought more descriptive than "attachment") to her child and the formation of a maternal identity are interdependent coordinates of the same process.

Rubin (1984) also renamed two of the progressive stages in achieving maternal identity. She replaced the words "mimicry" and "role-play" with "replication"; the woman's mother was identified as her strongest model. Fantasy was retained. "Introjection-projection-rejection" was replaced by "dedifferentiation," which preceded the woman's establishment of a maternal identity as she shifted from models of expert-mothering persons to herself in relation to her child. In establishing maternal identity a mother's image of her child stabilizes, such that she anticipates her child's behavior, knowing "how, what, when, and why she does something for or with him as his mother, as her child" (p. 50). An operational location of the child as "you," the "I" in relation to "you," and the "you" in relation to "me" has occurred.

Rubin (1984) emphasized that maternal identity and behavior evolve as the age, condition, and situation of the child change, such that maternal identity, maternal behavior, and the quality of maternal and family life are anchored in the developmental age or stage, sex, physical condition, and behavior of the child. Furthermore, a new personality dimension is incorporated into a woman's self-system with the birth of each subsequent child, with no transference of maternal identity from one child to another. Each childbearing experience is different, just as the woman's life space and self-system are different. The uniqueness of each child, and of the mother at that particular point in her life, require systematic, extensive maternal work in getting to know and incorporate each child into her self and family systems.

Studies of Maternal Role Attainment

Rubin's work stimulated nurses to look beyond the physiological and pathological aspects of childbearing to the intricate process of becoming a mother, and to identify areas for providing help. For example, in Josten's (1982) research, primary clinic nurses' ratings of expectant mothers' behaviors on an instrument based on Rubin's (1975) tasks of pregnancy showed that women who prepared very little during pregnancy became inadequate mothers. These findings indicate the importance of assessing and fostering mothers' active preparation for motherhood.

Mercer (1980, 1981, 1985, 1986), a student of Rubin, began a series of studies focused on mothers' MRA in unique situations during the first 8 to 12 months of motherhood. Thornton and Nardi's (1975) four stages of role acquisition—anticipatory, formal, informal, and personal identity—were used to describe the process of MRA. The anticipatory stage, the period before incumbency (pregnancy), is a time of psychosocial preparation for the role. At birth, the mother moves to the formal stage of identifying her infant's uniqueness and begins caretaking tasks by copying experts' behaviors and following their advice. During the informal stage, the mother progresses from rigidly following directions of others to using her judgment about the best care for her infant. The stage of personal or maternal identity is characterized by the mother's sense of harmony, confidence, satisfaction in the maternal role, and attachment to her infant. She feels a congruence of self and motherhood as others accept her performance (Mercer, 1981, 1985).

Maternal variables identified as influencing MRA included maternal age, SES, perception of the birth experience, early mother–infant separation, social stress, social support, personality traits (temperament, empathy, and rigidity), self-concept, child-rearing attitudes, perception of the infant, role strain, and health status (Mercer, 1981, 1986). Infant variables identified as affecting MRA included temperament, appearance, responsiveness, and health status. Self-reported maternal behavior, observed maternal behavior, attachment to the infant, and gratification in the maternal role were constructs of MRA used to compare three age groups (15–19, 20–29, and 30–42 years) of women over their first year of motherhood. The majority (64%) achieved a maternal identity by 4 months; at 1 year 4% had not achieved it.

The patterns of self-reported maternal behaviors, feelings of attachment for the baby, and observed maternal competence did not differ by age group, although their levels of achievement differed (Mercer, 1985, 1986). These behaviors peaked at 4 months following birth. However, mothers reported feeling less competent and their observed maternal competence decreased significantly at 8 and 12 months. Feelings of attachment for their infants were significantly higher at 4 months than at any other test period. All mothers reported increased gratification in mothering at 4 months; teenagers reported a decrease at 8 and 12 months, but older mothers reported increased gratification.

Interview data at 8 months revealed a clash between the infant's evolving self in the form of greater demands on the mother, clinging behavior, willfully exploring and moving into hazardous situations, and the mother's need to regain a sense of herself as an organized, attractive woman and wife (Mercer, 1986). Mothers' difficulties in balancing wife, mother, and employment roles also contributed to their overall feelings of incompetence; role strain was a major predictor of observed competence.

Pridham, Schroeder, and Brown (1999) also reported a disruption in maternal behavior among mothers of term and preterm infants from 4 to 8 months after birth. Mothers' highest adaptiveness scores were at 4 months, and their lowest scores were at 8 months. In contrast, Elek, Hudson, and Bouffard (2003) observed that first-time mothers' infant care self-efficacy increased from 4 to 12 months; however, their satisfaction with parenting did not increase. Infant care self-efficacy was related to both parenting and marital satisfaction.

Women who were hospitalized for high-risk pregnancy during the third trimester, and women who experienced a low-risk pregnancy, were compared on two MRA constructs, attachment to the infant and perceived parental competence, at early postpartum, 1, 4, and 8 months following birth (Mercer & Ferketich, 1990). High-risk women (HRW) reported higher attachment to their infants than did low-risk women (LRW) during early postpartum, but their scores did not differ at 8 months following birth. Perceived parental competence was a constant predictor for both HRW and LRW. Additional predictors of HRW's attachment during early postpartum were fetal attachment, SES, and antepartal worry, and at 8 months pregnancy risk was a positive predictor. HRW's antepartal hospitalization and compliance to treatment indicated an early commitment to the health of their unborn infants and themselves. Additional predictors of LRW's attachment to their infants at early postpartum were anxiety, received support, fetal attachment, marital status, and relationships with their own mothers as children. Anxiety and marital status had negative effects. At 8 months more optimal family functioning, perceived support, and relationships with their mothers as children contributed to LRW's reported attachment to their infants. Anxiety and depression had negative effects on their attachment. An unexpected finding was that the latermothers held their infants following birth, the higher was their attachment.

No differences were found between LRW's and HRW's perceived parental competence at 1, 4, and 8 months following birth (Mercer & Ferketich, 1994). Both groups reported significant increases in parental competence at 4 and 8 months after a minimal decrease from birth to 1 month. Self-esteem and mastery (sense of control) were consistent predictors of competence for both HRW and LRW. HRW's prenatal attachment to their infants was a predictor of their feelings of competence at early postpartum, 1, and 8 months. Anxiety was a significant predictor of both groups' competence during postpartum hospitalization, and depression was a significant predictor at 1 month for both groups, and for HRW at 8 months. Significant correlations between the two constructs of MRA—perceived parental competence and feelings of attachment to the infant—among both HRW and LRW at all test periods indicated the interdependence of these two variables.

High-risk pregnancy did not seem to impede perceived maternal competence in parenting. However, the importance of prenatal attachment to HRW's parental competence shows that early commitment to their unborn infants might have helped offset the effects of obstetrical problems. Stainton, McNeil, and Harvey (1992) reported that HRW worked especially hard on maternal tasks of pregnancy while facing uncertain motherhood.

Sandelowski (1995) described infertile couples' extra work in reconstructing their thinking in pre-expectancy, expectancy, and parent phases, temporarily impeding their progress in the transition. Sandelowski and Barroso's (2003) meta-synthesis of qualitative findings on HIV-positive mothers showed consistent and profound negative effects of this illness on maternal behavior throughout the women's experience of motherhood.

Walker, Crain, and Thompson (1986a) delineated three constructs of MRA: maternal identity, and perceived and demonstrated role attainment. They proposed that maternal identity involves the cognitive and affective attributes of the reciprocal relationship between mothers and infants in which the mother establishes both linkages and boundaries between herself and her infant. Both primiparas' and multiparas' attitudes about themselves as mothers were correlated with attitudes toward their infants within and among the test periods at 1 to 3 days and at 4 to 6 weeks after birth. First-time mothers' formation of the relationship with their infants and their gaining self-confidence in the parenting role appeared to be interdependent; this finding is congruent with Mercer and Ferketich's (1994) and Rubin's (1984) findings. Multiparas' self-confidence in the parenting role was not reliably related to their relationship with their infants. Primiparas' self-confidence was moderately correlated with observed maternal behavior, maternal age, education, and SES at 4 to 6 weeks postpartum (Walker, Crain, & Thompson, 1986b). Multiparas' self-confidence during the first 3 days was related to observed maternal behavior at 4 to 6 weeks; however, their self-confidence at 4 to 6 weeks was related only to maternal age and infant size.

Koniak-Griffin (1993) also questioned the existence of discrete cognitive-affective and behavioral dimensions of MRA in her historical and empirical review of the theory. Zabielski (1994) reported that she did not find support for the separation of maternal identity from perceived role performance among mothers of preterm and term infants. Maternal identity was triggered by performance and cognitive-affective phenomena. Mothers reported from two to seven events that helped trigger their maternal identity recognition. These events included contact and interaction with the infant, assuming responsibilities of the maternal role, validation of their mothering by either an adult or their infant's recognition and response, feelings of love for the infant, and feelings of protectiveness and concern toward the infant. Although mothers of preterm infants were delayed in their early process of maternal identity achievement, by 4 months they did not differ from mothers of term infants. The more positive the mothers' perception of their infants, the earlier they recognized a maternal identity. Mothers' evaluation of their maternal competence and their satisfaction in the mother role were positively related. Mothers of exceptionally fussy infants and mothers who had problems attaching to their infants had difficulty in achieving maternal identity.

Observed maternal behavior may be inconsistent with a woman's perception of her confidence in mothering or how she feels as a mother. Variables such as her immaturity, definition of a good parent, or low self-esteem might affect her self-perception as a mother. However, observed mother-infant behavior has both clinical and research merit. Britton, Gronwaldt, and Britton (2001) reported that clearly observed and measured maternal behaviors with the infant (close contact, eye contact, loving touch, examination of infant, loving talk, positive comments, and appearance of happiness) shortly after delivery were related to the quality of the observed mother-infant relationship 6 and 12 months later, and to infant attachment behaviors at 12 months. These findings indicate that early-observed maternal behavior reflected the mother's emotional involvement with her child, and this early behavior was predictive of later mothering and infant behavior. However, only the mother can provide data about her perceptions of self as mother and of her infant for conclusions to be made about her cognitive assimilation of a maternal identity.

Questions raised by Walker, Crain, and Thompson (1986a) and Koniak-Griffin (1993) about MRA constructs, and McBride and Shore's (2001) suggestion about the timeliness of retiring the term, mandate reevaluation of MRA. Research findings about the transition to motherhood during the past 5 years provide a database for describing transition to a maternal identity in BAM, and for the argument to replace the term MRA with the term BAM.

BAM as Replacement for MRA

Several researchers have focused on the importance of mothers' work during pregnancy in preparation for becoming a mother and variables influencing this transition. Swedish mothers' prenatal attachment to their unborn babies predicted observed mother-infant relationships at 12 weeks postpartum (Siddiqui & Hagglof, 2000). Mothers who scored high on prenatal fantasy (thinking and daydreaming about the baby) were more involved when interacting with their infants. Mothers who scored high on prenatal interaction and affection stimulated their 12-week-old infants by using more proximal stimulation (touching and kissing). Mothers who scored high on differentiation of self with the unborn baby used more distal stimulation (maternal vocalizing).

Expectant mothers' representations of their own mothers mediated their internal working models of interpersonal relationships and their prenatal attachment to their babies (Priel & Besser, 2001). Mothers' current relationships with their own mothers tended to be recreated in their relationships with their infants (Kretchmar & Jacobvitz, 2002). Mothers who remembered being accepted by their mothers as children, and who were currently in balanced relationships with their mothers, were more sensitive and less intrusive with their 9-month-old infants.

Mothers' memories of maternal and paternal acceptance or rejection as children were also predictors of depressive symptoms and maternal sensitivity when their infants were 5 to 6 months old (Crockenberg & Leerkes, 2003). Self-esteem mediated these effects. Greater maternal sensitivity was associated with mothers' memories of parental acceptance. When memories of parental acceptance were high, depressive symptoms were unrelated to maternal sensitivity. Mothers who had memories of their parents as highly accepting of them as children reported fewer depressive symptoms during the third trimester of pregnancy and following birth. Mothers whose parents failed to let them know that they were loved and valued as children reported sadness and hopelessness throughout the transition to parenthood.

Women with postpartum depression had more negative perceptions of their infants, of themselves as mothers, and of their ability to provide appropriate care for their infants at 2 to 3 months following birth (Fowles, 1998). Women who reported higher levels of depression, anxiety, and marital ambivalence and conflict during pregnancy reported less efficacy in the parenting role (Porter & Hsu, 2003). More child care experience was associated with greater confidence in the mothering role during pregnancy, but it did not predict self-efficacy postpartum. Maternal efficacy increased at 1 month from the pregnancy measure; it was related to anxiety and marital love and maintenance, but it was no longer related to depression. By 3 months none of the psychosocial indicators of well-being were related to maternal efficacy, indicating that mothers' efficacy was becoming more differentiated and compartmentalized and less related to internal mood states or marital supports. Mothers' perceptions of infant temperament were associated with maternal efficacy at 3 months, indicating that mothers' parental competency was being shaped by the dynamic interplay between the infants' traits and the mothers' ongoing success in caregiving.

Clark, Kochanska, and Ready (2000) validated the bidirectionality of the early parent–child relationship. Maternal personality alone (power assertion and responsiveness) and in interaction with the infant's emotionality predicted future parenting behaviors.

A study of Finnish mothers' adjustment of their personal goals during pregnancy at 1 and 3 months postpartum showed that an increase in family-related goals predicted a decline in depressive symptoms (Salmela-Aro, Nurmi, Saisto, & Halmesmaki, 2001). Higher depressive symptoms during pregnancy predicted fewer birth-related goals. An increase in depressive symptoms at all stages predicted an increase in mothers' self-focused goals. Others reported that mothers who demonstrated higher levels of complexity of thinking during pregnancy about their future experiences as parents, and 6 months after birth about their experiences as mothers, were better adjusted than were mothers with simpler expectations (Pancer, Pratt, Hunsberger, & Gallant, 2000).

A comparison of maternal adaptation in Norway, Sweden, and the United States showed few differences (Kiehl & White, 2003). Mothers differed significantly in planned leave time from their employment, with Swedish mothers reporting the highest, Norwegian mothers the second highest, and U.S. mothers the lowest. Swedish mothers who had longer postpartum hospitalization had greater confidence in their ability to cope. Mothers with greater adaptation during pregnancy had greater adaptation postpartum. Prenatal identification with the mother role was related to mothers' satisfaction with motherhood.

Others reported that a positive experience of mothering was related to the husband's being a good father, the mother's warmth and interpersonal outgoingness, and a marriage low in conflict (Paris & Helson, 2002). First-time mothers described a "conspiracy of silence" about the realities of motherhood that they would not have been able to manage without the physical help and confidence building of their husbands (McVeigh, 1997).

Researchers using quantitative approaches have provided information about patterns of maternal behavior in the transition to motherhood and variables influencing the transition. Perceived confidence and competence in mothering and self-reported feelings about the infant were used consistently as constructs reflecting BAM in earlier and current research. Significant relationships between these variables were reported.

Qualitative research reports have included women's rich descriptors of their challenging experiences in the process of BAM. A core category, engaged mothering, was identified through interviews with middle-class African American mothers (Sawyer, 1999). Engaged mothering indicated an active, involved, and mutual process of preparation for motherhood through caring for themselves and their infants. The process began when the women either tried to get pregnant or became pregnant, the pregnancy was confirmed, and they decided to continue the pregnancy. Women's strategies in this process included getting ready, dealing with reality, settling in, and dreaming. The first three strategies were linear, but dreaming moved back and forth among past as context, present as experience, and future as vision. Dealing with reality began during pregnancy and extended into the postpartum period. Settling in began at birth and extended until the women were comfortable and confident in caring for, and making decisions about, their infants. Settling in was accomplished around 4 months following birth. Descriptions of settling in are congruent with Rubin's (1984) descriptions of establishment of maternal identity. The period of time for settling in is congruent with findings from quantitative studies. Dreams about the child in the future, their mothering, and world conditions, are congruent with Rubin's (1967, 1984) descriptions of fantasy.

Martell (2001) described first-time mothers' experiences as they began to orient themselves as mothers during their first 3 weeks following birth. The mothers' psychosocial development was a continuous process. The major theme was "heading toward a new normal" as mothers focused on appreciating their bodies, settling in, and becoming a new family. Mothers were deeply aware of bodily sensations and were appreciative of their bodies' capabilities in giving birth and slowly returning to a prepregnancy state. Mothers were also beginning to bond with their newborns, despite their inability to think clearly or to retain information. The settling-in process began as mothers began to feel competent and to develop confidence with their infants. They felt a need to leave the hospital so that they could test their ideas about integrating the newborn into their lives. In becoming a new family the women began realigning relationships, developing new routines, and delineating boundaries.

As the mothers began developing unique relationships with their infants during the first 2 weeks, the newborns became more real, and they realized the permanence of the relationship (Martell, 2001). Women described a warm, changing relationship with their partners and feelings of being more linked to their mothers, mothers-in-law, and other women.

In her synthesis of nine qualitative studies of mothers in North America and Australia, Nelson (2003) identified two often simultaneous processes in the transition to motherhood. The primary process is engagement, defined as making a commitment, striving and being engrossed in mothering through active involvement in the child's care, and experiencing the child's presence. At the same time, the woman's engagement or commitment in experiencing herself as a mother leads to the woman's growth and transformation as she becomes a mother. She has to deal with disruptions in commitments, relationships, daily life, self, and work outside the home. Mothers agonize over when to return to work, their decisions of timing, and their conflicts as they search for balance between motherhood and work roles (Nelson, 2003).

Selected phrases categorized as engagement included committing to new life circumstances, promoting the child's health and well-being, involvement in self-socialization, giving of self, experiencing love for the baby, settling in, coming to know, and learning to care for the baby (Nelson, 2003). These maternal activities do not differ from those described by other researchers, including Rubin (1975, 1984). Selected phrases that were categorized as women's growth and transformation included expansion of self, becoming, growth and development, widening scope of capabilities, redefining self and relationships, and incorporating motherhood into one's sense of self (Nelson, 2003).

Mothers of children aged 3 to 16 years reported that their work at self-definition was a continual process (Hartrick, 1997). Their process of self-definition involved a nonreflective doing (taking on roles and acting out a life modeled by parents and others), living in the shadows (a transitional period as their secure foundation crumbled), and reclaiming and rediscovering self. Reclaiming self led to a definition of their lives from a different perspective by reconnecting with, and learning to listen to, trust, and nurture, the self.

The qualitative research reaffirmed the transition to motherhood as an intensive commitment and active involvement that begins before or during pregnancy, with the woman beginning preparation by seeking information and caring for herself and baby. The woman's transformation and growth of self in becoming a mother is congruent with psychosocial developmental and transition theories. An enlargement of self occurs as a woman achieves a maternal identity in BAM. An expansion of her maternal identity continues as she rises to new challenges in motherhood by making new connections to regain confidence in the self.

Although the last stage in MRA is achievement of maternal identity, the dynamic transformation and evolution of the woman's persona are not captured by MRA. The theory of MRA does not include the continued expansion of the self as a mother.

New names for stages in the process of establishing a maternal identity in BAM were derived from the qualitative data: (a) commitment, attachment, and preparation (pregnancy); (b) acquaintance, learning, and physical restoration (first 2 to 6 weeks following birth); (c) moving toward a new normal (2 weeks to 4 months); and (d) achievement of the maternal identity (around 4 months). The times for achieving the last three stages are highly variable, and are influenced by maternal and infant variables and the social-environmental context. The stages also overlap; for example, physical restoration continues beyond the first few weeks, but it is predominant earlier. Moving toward a new normal may begin shortly after birth, but it becomes predominant when the mother learns the nuances of her baby's behavior.

The commitment, attachment, and preparation stage in which a woman's work in becoming a mother begins has long-range implications. The woman's active involvement in this stage has been consistently linked to a positive adaptation to motherhood.

The mother spends much time in the acquaintance, learning, and physical recovery stage learning about her newborn and looking for family resemblances, wholeness, and functioning of body parts. She studies her infant's responses to herself and others, and practices by trial and error as she learns how to comfort and care for her infant.

In moving toward a new normal stage the woman begins to structure her mothering to fit herself and her family according to her past experiences and future goals. She adjusts to the changing relationships with her partner, family, and friends. Much cognitive restructuring occurs as she learns her infant's cues and what is best for her infant, and adjusts to her new reality.

In the achievement of maternal identity, the mother has established intimate knowledge of her infant such that she feels competent and confident in her mothering activities and feels love for her infant; she has settled in. A new normal has been reached in her relationships and her family. The woman experiences a transformation of self in becoming a mother, as her self expands to incorporate a new identity and assume responsibility for her infant and her infant's future world.

The process of BAM should be studied in transitions such as becoming a mother of a school-age child, an adolescent, an adult, or becoming a grandmother. How does the process differ as a woman expands her maternal self? Identification of mothers' stressors and needed support as a child moves from dependence to becoming a peer as a parent should indicate areas for intervention in mothers' preparation, learning, moving to a new normal in family life, and achieving comfort with an expanded maternal identity. Are some variables more influential at different developmental milestones? How does a woman support her daughter in becoming a mother and a peer? The complexity of women's roles as wife, mother, and employee has increased much faster than has the health and social system in providing support. A life-span approach to the mothering role is needed, along with determining different ways to be happy and unhappy in the mother-child relationship in different situations such as whether one is a single mother, an adoptive mother, or a stepmother (McBride & Shore, 2001). These expanded investigations are needed to further develop and refine theories and practice related to maternal roles and transitions.

Conclusions

Women's descriptions of the life-transforming experience in becoming a mother with the concomitant growth, development, and new self-definition are not adequately encompassed in MRA terminology. The maternal persona continues to evolve as the child's developmental challenges and life's realities lead to disruptions in the mother's feelings of competence and self-confidence. The argument is made to replace "maternal role attainment" with "becoming a mother" to connote the initial transformation and continuing growth of the mother identity.

REFERENCES

Barba, E., & Selder, F. (1995). Life transitions theory. *Nursing Leadership Forum, 1,* 4–11.

Britton, H.L., Gronwaldt, V., & Britton, J.R. (2001). Maternal postpartum behaviors and mother–infant relationship during the first year of life. *Journal of Pediatrics, 138,* 905–909.

Clark, L. A., Kochanska, G., & Ready, R. (2000). Mothers' personality and its interaction with child temperament as predictors of parenting behavior. *Journal of Personality and Social Psychology, 79,* 274–285.

Crockenberg, S. C., & Leerkes, E. M. (2003). Parental acceptance, postpartum depression, and maternal sensitivity: Mediating and moderating processes. *Journal of Family Psychology, 17,* 80–93.

Deutsch, F. M., Ruble, D. N., Fleming, A., Brooks-Gunn, J., & Stangor, C. (1988). Information-seeking and maternal self-definition during the transition to motherhood. *Journal of Personality and Social Psychology, 55,* 420–431.

Elek, S. M., Hudson, D. B., & Bouffard, C. (2003). Marital and parenting satisfaction and infant care self-efficacy during the transition to parenthood: The effect of infant sex. *Issues in Comprehensive Pediatric Nursing, 26,* 45–57.

Fowles, E. R. (1998). The relationship between maternal role attainment and postpartum depression. *Health Care for Women International, 19,* 83–94.

Hartrick, G. A. (1997). Women who are mothers: The experience of defining self. *Health Care for Women International, 18,* 263–277.

Josten, L. (1982). Contrast in prenatal preparation for mothering. *Maternal–Child Nursing Journal, 11,* 65–73.

Kegan, R. (1982). *The evolving self.* Cambridge, MA: Harvard University Press.

Kiehl, E. M., & White, M. A. (2003). Maternal adaptation during childbearing in Norway, Sweden and the United States. *Scandinavian Journal of Caring Sciences, 17,* 96–103.

Koniak-Griffin, D. (1993). Maternal role attainment. *Image: Journal of Nursing Scholarship, 25,* 257–262.

Kretchmar, M. D., & Jacobvitz, D. B. (2002). Observing mother-child relationships across generations: Boundary patterns, attachment, and the transmission of caregiving. *Family Process, 41,* 351–374.

Martell, L. K. (2001). Heading toward the new normal: A contemporary postpartum experience. *Journal of Obstetric, Gynecologic, and Neonatal Nursing, 30,* 496–506.

McBride, A. B., & Shore, C. P. (2001). Women as mothers and grandmothers. *Annual Review of Nursing Research, 19,* 63–85.

McVeigh, C. (1997). Motherhood experiences from the perspective of the first-time mother. *Clinical Nursing Research, 6,* 335–348.

Meleis, A. I., Sawyer, L. M., Im, E., Messias, D. K. H., & Schumacher, K. (2000). Experiencing transitions: An emerging middle-range theory. *Advances in Nursing Science, 23,* 12–28.

Mercer, R. T. (1980). Teenage motherhood: The first year. *Journal of Obstetric, Gynecologic, and Neonatal Nursing, 9,* 16–27.

Mercer, R. T. (1981). A theoretical framework for studying factors that impact on the maternal role. *Nursing Research, 30,* 73–77.

Mercer, R. T. (1985). The process of maternal role attainment over the first year. *Nursing Research, 34,* 198–204.

Mercer, R. T. (1986). *First-time motherhood: Experiences from teens to forties.* New York: Springer.

Mercer, R .T. (1995). *Becoming a mother: Research on maternal identity from Rubin to the present.* New York: Springer.

Mercer, R. T., & Ferketich, S. L. (1990). Predictors of parental attachment during early parenthood. *Journal of Advanced Nursing, 15,* 268–280.

Mercer, R. T., & Ferketich, S. L. (1994). Predictors of maternal role competence by risk status. *Nursing Research, 43,* 38–43.

Nelson, A. M. (2003). Transition to motherhood. *Journal of Obstetric, Gynecologic, & Neonatal Nursing, 32,* 465–477.

Paris, R., & Helson, R. (2002). Early mothering and personality change. *Journal of Family Psychology, 16,* 172–185.

Pancer, S. M., Pratt, M., Hunsberger, B., & Gallant, M. (2000). Thinking ahead: Complexity of expectations and the transition to parenthood. *Journal of Personality, 68*(2), 253–278.

Porter, C. L., & Hsu, H. (2003). First-time mothers' perceptions of efficacy during the transition to motherhood: Links to infant temperament. *Journal of Family Psychology, 1,* 54–64.

Pridham, K. F., Schroeder, M., & Brown, R. (1999). The adaptiveness of mothers' working models of caregiving through the first year: Infant and mother contributions. *Research in Nursing & Health, 22,* 471–485.

Priel, B., & Besser, A. (2001). Bridging the gap between attachment and object relations theories: A study of the transition to motherhood. *British Journal of Medical Psychology, 74,* 85–100.

Rubin, R. (1967). Attainment of the maternal role. Part 1. Processes. *Nursing Research, 16,* 237–245.

Rubin, R. (1975). Maternal tasks in pregnancy. *Maternal–Child Nursing Journal, 4,* 143–153.

Rubin, R. (1984). *Maternal identity and the maternal experience.* New York: Springer.

Salmela-Aro, K., Nurmi, J. E., Saisto, T., & Halmesmaki, E. (2001). Goal reconstruction and depressive symptoms during the transition to motherhood: Evidence from two cross-lagged longitudinal studies. *Journal of Personality and Social Psychology, 81,* 1144–1159.

Sandelowski, M. (1995). A theory of the transition to parenthood of infertile couples. *Research in Nursing & Health, 18,* 123–132.

Sandelowski, M., & Barroso, J. (2003). Toward a meta-synthesis of qualitative findings on motherhood in HIV-positive women. *Research in Nursing & Health, 26,* 153–170.

Sawyer, L. M. (1999). Engaged mothering: The transition to motherhood for a group of African American women. *Journal of Transcultural Nursing, 10,* 14–21.

Siddiqui, A., & Hagglof, B. (2000). Does maternal prenatal attachment predict postnatal mother-infant interaction? *Early Human Development, 59,* 13–25.

Stainton, M., McNeil, D., & Harvey, S. (1992). Maternal tasks of uncertain motherhood. *Maternal–Child Nursing Journal, 20,* 113–123.

Thornton, R., & Nardi, P. M. (1975). The dynamics of role acquisition. *American Journal of Sociology, 80,* 870–885.

Walker, L. O., Crain, H., & Thompson, E. (1986a). Maternal role attainment and identity in the postpartum period: Stability and change. *Nursing Research*, 35, 68–71.

Walker, L. O., Crain, H., & Thompson, E. (1986b). Mothering behavior and maternal role attainment during the postpartum period. *Nursing Research*, 35, 352–355.

Zabielski, M. T. (1994). Recognition of maternal identity in preterm and full-term mothers. *Maternal–Child Nursing Journal*, 22, 2–35.

Reprinted with permission from: Mercer, R. T. (2004). Becoming a mother versus maternal role attainment. *Nursing Scholarship*, 36(3), 226–232.

3.3 THE CONCEPTUAL STRUCTURE OF TRANSITION TO MOTHERHOOD IN THE NEONATAL INTENSIVE CARE UNIT

HYUNJEONG SHIN
ROSEMARY WHITE-TRAUT

Abstract

Title: *The conceptual structure of transition to motherhood in the neonatal intensive care unit.* ***Aim:*** *This chapter is a report of a concept analysis of transition to motherhood for mothers with infants in a neonatal intensive care unit.* ***Background:*** *Mothers with infants in a neonatal intensive care unit have more difficulty in their transition to motherhood compared with mothers of healthy infants. The concept of transition to motherhood in the neonatal intensive care unit is not well-understood in nursing, often being confused with mothers' psychological responses in the neonatal intensive care unit.* ***Methods:*** *The concept analysis combined Rodgers' evolutionary method with Schwartz-Barcott and Kim's hybrid method. Thirty-eight studies were reviewed and a purposive sample of 10 Korean mothers with infants in a neonatal intensive care unit was interviewed.* ***Findings:*** *Three critical attributes of transition to motherhood in the neonatal intensive care unit were identified: (1) time-dependent process, (2) psycho-emotional swirling and (3) hovering around the edge of mothering. These are caused by the antecedents (1) unexpected outcome of pregnancy, (2) awareness of the situation and (3) mother–infant separation. The consequences were: (1) delayed motherhood and (2) developing a sense of meaning concerning family and life. Additionally, five influencing factors to be alleviated were identified: (1) negative meaning attribution, (2) uncertainty, (3) social prejudice, (4) lack of opportunities to make contact with the infant and (5) the neonatal intensive care unit environment.* ***Conclusions:*** *This concept analysis should help nurses to understand the process of becoming a mother in a neonatal intensive care unit and plan appropriate interventions for mothers with special needs.*

Introduction

Transition to motherhood has been described as a process of personal and interpersonal change, which occurs as a woman assumes maternal tasks and appraises herself as a mother (Pridham & Chang, 1992). For women, transition to motherhood is a universal developmental experience (Schumacher & Meleis, 1994; Meleis et al., 2000). The transition to motherhood in mothers with infants in neonatal intensive care units (NICUs), however, is different from mothers who have healthy infants. When compared with mothers of healthy infants, mothers with infants in a NICU may experience more difficulty in their transition to motherhood (Shin, 2003). Feelings of disappointment, fears about the infant's survival, and altered maternal experiences have been reported for these mothers (Affleck et al. 1990; Affonso et al. 1992). A mother's early experiences, when patterns of mothering and relating to the infant are being formed, are crucial (Walker et al. 1986) and a positive transition to motherhood has important consequences for the developing mother–infant relationship (Shin, 2003).

These experiences are deeply influenced by culture (Kurtz et al. 1992; Pinch & Spielman, 1996; Simkin, 1996). For example, many Koreans have negative impressions about infants in the NICU (for example, they will not be healthy) and they think that the mother is responsible for giving birth to an unhealthy infant (Shin, 2003). These negative social responses to mothers and infants in a NICU may inhibit mothers' healthy transitions (Shin, 2004).

Despite the importance of this transition and its cultural influences, the concept of transition to motherhood in the NICU is not well understood in nursing and has been confused with mothers' psychological responses in the NICU. There is not sufficient knowledge to describe or understand women's transition to motherhood in the NICU. Therefore, the purpose of this chapter is to analyse the concept of transition to motherhood for mothers whose infants are in a NICU.

Research Methods

Rodgers (2000) suggests that views of human beings and related nursing phenomena are constantly changing rather than static, and are context-dependent rather than universal or absolute. Rodgers' approach, therefore, seemed to be appropriate for clarifying the concept of transition to motherhood because the concept can change over time and be influenced by the context of the NICU (Shin, 2003). However, her model does not include the fieldwork that can provide important empirical data. For this reason, a combined framework was used (Hutchfield, 1999; Jacelon et al., 2004) and Rodgers' evolutionary method was used in conjunction with the Hybrid model of concept development (Schwartz-Barcott & Kim, 2000), which clearly identifies fieldwork as a part of the analytic process.

The combined framework consisted of three phases: the theoretical phase of the literature review; the fieldwork phase of collecting empirical data; and the analytic phase. Delineation of the working definition, which is the final step of the theoretical phase in the hybrid model, was replaced by the identification of attributes, antecedents, consequences, and additional organizing categories that emerged from the literature review and fieldwork. This resulted in a framework that seemed to be a more appropriate approach for clarifying the concept within the context using empirical data rather than seeking a universal definition based on the literature. The phases were conducted as follows.

Theoretical Phase

In order to have a better understanding of its use, an exploration of the application of the concept of transition to motherhood in NICUs across different cultures was undertaken through a review of English and Korean literature. The keywords mothering, motherhood, transition, high-risk infant, and NICU were used to search the CINAHL, Ovid, and MEDLINE databases. The same keywords were used for a search of Korean nursing journals. A manual search was conducted because there was no comprehensive electronic database of Korean nursing literature. However, only ten articles were found and most reported quantitative studies. Thus, unpublished master's theses and doctoral dissertations in Korea were added to the search. All the searches were limited to English or Korean language documents for the years 1990–2004. References were excluded if the focus of content was not relevant to becoming a mother in the NICU. The searches yielded 38 (21 English, 17 Korean) studies for review.

Fieldwork Phase

Participants for the interviews were recruited through purposive sampling, and data collection continued until interview content revealed repetitious data indicating common themes. Thus, 10 Korean mothers with infants in a NICU were recruited from a university hospital in Korea, and semi-structured interviews were conducted. Five were first-time mothers. Approval for the study was obtained from the hospitals, and participants gave oral consent to participate in the study according to usual practice in Korea. Based on the literature mentioning important periods for transition to motherhood (Rubin, 1961; Kitzinger, 1975; Park, 1991; Mun, 2000; Jackson et al., 2003), interviews were conducted three times during postpartum period: 3–10 days after the birth, near the day of infants' discharge, and 4–7 weeks following discharge. Interview data were collected between May 2002 and April 2003. Infants' health problems varied, e.g. prematurity, sepsis, pulmonary hypertension, low birth weight, pneumothorax, and cerebral hemorrhage. The length of infants' stays in the NICU was 20–65 days and their time at home after discharge varied between 4 and 7 weeks when third interviews were conducted. The primary interview questions concerned the definition, meanings, and impact of transition to motherhood. Interview data were analysed using content analysis.

Analytic Phase

In the third phase the data were analysed looking for common themes, and then Rodgers' analytic framework was applied to the data to identify critical attributes, antecedents, and consequences of the concept.

Findings

From the review of literature, common themes of becoming a mother in the NICU were found, namely time process, maternal psychological well-being, mother–infant attachment, and maternal role attainment. These themes will be addressed below, with supportive interview data and consideration of the time process.

Usually mothers of infants in NICUs pass through 'stages' in their adjustment, typically moving from shock, to denial, to anger and guilt, and finally to adjustment and acceptance (Affleck & Tennen, 1991). Transition to motherhood in mothers with high-risk infants has also been described as a process with four syntheses of experience: alienation, responsibility, confidence, and familiarity (Jackson et al., 2003). The process is distinct according to the meaning that mothers attribute to their situations (Shin, 2003). Those who attribute positive situational meanings move from a confusing phase to an accepting phase to a shaping phase; however, mothers who attribute negative situational meanings move from an avoiding phase to a conflicting phase to an accepting phase (Shin, 2003).

During the first few days after the birth, mothers face severe threats to their psychological well-being because of the new situation, which includes unexpected hospitalization of the infant and unfulfilled expectancy (Affleck & Tennen, 1991). Contrary to mothers with healthy newborns, they experience uncertainty, frustration, confusion, feelings of disappointment, and a sense of guilt and helplessness (Rapacki, 1991; Choi, 1999; Shin, 2003), which have an influence on mothers' negative neonatal perceptions (Kim & Jeong, 1995). Owens (2001) said of her NICU experience: "Waves of emotion pour over me, and it is often difficult to sort out the many conflicting feelings" (p. 68). These whirlwinds of emotion begin with sorrow, fear, and shock at the sight of the overwhelming NICU environment and the infant's appearance (Rapacki, 1991; Emily, 1999). After seeing their infants surrounded by many lines, devices, and monitors, for example, most mothers experienced fears that the infant would die, causing some to be afraid of visiting the infant until assured by their husbands that everything was fine (Shin, 2003). Other mothers experienced difficulty in leaving their infants because they were worried (Jackson et al., 2003; Shin, 2003). Despite these fears, mothers maintain a ray of hope for their infants' survival (Choi, 1999; Mun, 2000). They wish and hope for their infants' survival and health continuously, even 1 or 2 years after the birth (Choi, 1999; Mun, 2000).

Fears and feelings about the unfamiliar NICU environment, however, may cause difficulty in establishing mother–infant attachments (Moon & Koo, 1999). In NICUs a delayed or problematic process of attachment may occur, affecting mothers' perceptions of their own well-being (Bialoskurski et al., 1999). Uncertainty about the infants' survival also influences mother–infant attachment (Bialoskurski et al., 1999). Emily (1999) wrote of her NICU experience: "When the nurse asked if I would like to hold my daughter, I was tempted to answer, 'No.' I was frightened to bond with a baby who might not survive" (p. 22). One of our interview participants also said: "I think she is not my baby yet. Nobody knows her future. I think I cannot consider her as my baby until her discharge."

When an infant's health is poor and the outcome is uncertain, the mother may delay developing a relationship with them as a coping strategy to prevent excessive grief in case the infant dies (Bialoskurski et al., 1999). It is natural to use a self-protecting mechanism during the stressful time (Bialoskurski et al., 1999). However, mothers using this particular strategy may have more sense of shame and failure than those not using this strategy (Shin, 2003). One of our interview participants described her impression of becoming a mother in this way: "It's so shameful that I gave birth to this unhealthy, premature baby. Somehow I think, and I feel that I'm likely to have something lacking or a deficiency and so will my baby."

It appears that mothers' feelings of shame, guilt, and failure are related to social prejudice (Shin, 2003). It has been reported that Korean mothers perceived a strong social prejudice against the NICU infants (Lee, 1994; Lim, 1997; Choi, 1999; Mun, 2000; Shin, 2003). Mothers think that their infants in NICUs will have complications in growth and development, and that they are responsible for giving birth to an unhealthy infant (Choi, 1999; Mun, 2000). Nine of ten mothers interviewed in our study expressed these thoughts, one describing them thus: "I heard frequently that most of these babies will have problems somewhere in the body even when they grow up, and it may be difficult to be a normal person. Whenever I think of this, I want to give him up right now. I can be sure that people consider it as my fault. Anyway, I failed to give birth to a healthy baby. I have nothing to say."

An infant's admission to the NICU also may have serious effects on the attainment of the maternal role (Affleck & Tennen, 1991; McGrath & Meyer, 1992). Mothers often feel that they have relinquished primary caregiving for their own infants and feel that their maternal role is diminished while the infant is in the NICU, which leads to stress (Raines, 1999; Holditch-Davis & Miles, 2000; Kim, 2000). Sometimes, mothers feel ambivalent about their motherhood and maternal roles (Lee, 1994; Lim, 1997; Shin, 2003). They experience happiness about the infant on one hand, and grief about the infant's birth on the other (Rapacki, 1991; Jackson et al., 2003). They long to perform their maternal role themselves for their infants; however, they avoid this role and then are forced into engaging in mothering (Emily, 1999; Shin, 2003). This feeling of ambivalence at birth continues until the infant's discharge (Lim, 1997; Shin, 2003). Mothers' uncertainty also continues after infants' discharge, but may be changed in nature (Mun, 2000). One of our interview participants said: "I wanted to take my baby to my home. But, in a way, I was afraid of taking care of him. I was delighted when told about his discharge. But, I felt a somewhat heavy burden. I felt both good and depressed. I thought that all the problems would be solved with his discharge. But it was not. Still I cannot be sure whether he can grow up like other healthy babies." These comments suggest that uncertainty about the infant's survival changes to uncertainty about growth and development with the infant's discharge (Bialoskurski et al., 1999; Mun, 2000).

When discharged from an NICU, mothers experience a new sense of responsibility for care of the infant (Jackson et al., 2003), which gives rise to role strain as well as emotional strain (May, 1997; Singer et al., 1999). They feel unprepared for discharge from the hospital and for their new responsibilities (Jackson et al., 2003; Shin, 2003). They also feel insecure about caring for the infant (Shin, 2003). In our interviews, one of the mothers said: "I'm not ready to take care of him yet. So I asked a nurse whether I could delay his discharge for one week from now. Even though I learned how to bathe him, I'm afraid that he will be hurt when I bathe him by myself."

Mothers perceive that they are still not skillful at caring for their infants, and feel a lack of confidence (Shin, 2003). One mother in our study said: "I'm very nervous about my ability to take care of him. I have never slept well after his discharge. And still it's difficult to bathe him by myself. After bathing, I'm drenched in sweat. Always I think, 'What if he doesn't breathe? What if I don't notice something abnormal?' "

Even in the whirlwind of emotions and feelings, most mothers feel grateful towards their infants, families, and health care teams in the NICU, and they think that the birth of the infant has resulted in a developed sense of meaning about family, children, and life itself (Able-Boone & Stevens, 1994; Emily, 1999; Owens, 2001; Jackson et al., 2003). If infants thrive normally, mothers' lives at home become increasingly normal and routine (Choi, 1999; Mun, 2000; Jackson et al., 2003). This leads them to establish intimate knowledge of their infants so that they feel competent and confident in mothering activities and feel love for their infants (Jackson et al., 2003; Shin, 2003). However, some mothers, especially first-time mothers, experience difficulty viewing themselves as mothers or feeling competent as caretakers of their infants, even 3 months after the birth (Zabielski, 1994; Shin, 2003). For most mothers, their infants thrive and continue to develop normally, and these mothers see themselves as more mature as humans and as women after 1 or 2 years have passed since the birth (Choi, 1999; Emily, 1999; Rapacki, 1991; Mun, 2000). They have a new perspective on the world, which is different from the one they had before motherhood (Choi, 1999; Mun, 2000).

Critical Attributes of Transition to Motherhood in the NICU

Based on the literature review and interview data, three critical attributes were identified: time-dependent process, psycho-emotional swirling, and hovering around the edge of mothering.

Time-Dependent Process

Transition to motherhood in the NICU is not a static phenomenon, and there is a sense of flow, movement, and direction in it (Jackson et al., 2003; Shin, 2003). With the passage of time most mothers pass from unfamiliarity with the transition situation to acceptance and shaping motherhood in which they establish their own sense of motherhood (Jackson et al., 2003; Shin, 2003).

Psycho-Emotional Swirling

Whereas transition to motherhood in an NICU can be understood as a time-dependent process, this implies that psycho-emotional swirling is also a process. It has flow and direction with the passing of time. Contrary to mothers with healthy newborns, who begin the transition with many joys and congratulations, mothers with newborns in the NICU start their transition to motherhood in confusion, with mixed feelings such as sorrow and shock that progress to ambivalence and conflict near the time of their infants' discharge (Shin, 2003). Simultaneously with these mixed feelings, mothers continuously hope that their infants can survive and become healthy (Choi, 1999; Mun, 2000). After birth, mothers earnestly wish only that their infants can survive. These wishes change at the infants' discharge to wishes that the infants will grow up as normal and healthy (Mun, 2000). Whatever the circumstances, most mothers never discard their optimistic expectations (Mun, 2000).

Hovering Around the Edge of Mothering

In the NICU, the maternal role is diminished and distanced, either by mothers' own choosing or by the choice of others, resulting in diminished opportunity for mother–infant interaction (Kwon & Han, 1991; Raines, 1999; Holditch-Davis & Miles, 2000). The NICU environment and mothers' fears that infants will die inhibit establishing attachment (Bialoskurski et al., 1999). Thus, mothers are forced into engaging in mothering without enough time and preparation to becoming acquainted with their infants (Emily, 1999). All of these factors lead mothers not to engage actively in mothering, but to hover around the edge of it.

Antecedents of Transition to Motherhood in the NICU

Prior to the occurrence of a concept, certain events called antecedents must take place. The following are antecedents of transition to motherhood in the NICU:

- Unexpected outcome of pregnancy
- Awareness of the situation
- Mother–infant separation

First, an unexpected outcome of pregnancy resulting in the infant's admission to the NICU must exist. Most pregnant women desire to give birth safely to a healthy baby. However, if the outcome of pregnancy is different from what is expected, the transition to motherhood can also be different from what is expected (Affonso et al., 1992; Shin, 2003). Second, the mother has to be aware of the situation that she has to be a mother of a newborn in an NICU rather than a healthy newborn. In most cases, mothers' emotional swirling does not appear until they see and are aware of that situation (Shin, 2003). Third, there has to be mother–infant separation because of the infant's admission to the NICU. This period of separation leads a mother through a particular transition, which is different from that of a mother with a healthy baby (Cho, 1993).

Consequences of Transition to Motherhood in the NICU

The consequences correspond to events that may appear as a result of the presence of the concept and highlight the importance of the concept. The following are consequences of transition to motherhood in the NICU:

- Delayed motherhood
- Developing a sense of meaning concerning family and life

Delayed motherhood is an outcome of the transition to motherhood in the NICU (Kwon & Han, 1991; Zabielski, 1994). Usually, mothers with healthy infants are skillful in their maternal roles and are stable in motherhood by 2 or 3 months after the birth (Rubin, 1961; Kitzinger, 1975; Park, 1991). Compared with these mothers, mothers whose babies go through the NICU experience still have difficulty in performing maternal caretaking roles, establishing an attachment with their infants, and having an identity as a mother even after their infants' discharge or 3 months after birth (Kwon & Han, 1991; Zabielski, 1994; Shin, 2003). These mothers feel anxiety about their ability to care for their infants and feel guilty about ongoing follow-up care of the infants because of the complications (Choi, 1999; Mun, 2000; Shin, 2003). Although anxiety and a sense of guilt continue to exist, mothers reach a realization of the importance of the family and life in general, and of developing a sense of meaning about family and life itself (Able-Boone & Stevens, 1994; Emily, 1999; Owens, 2001; Shin, 2003). This realization is followed by personal growth and development, thus contributing to a healthy mother and a healthy baby (Emily, 1999; Rapacki, 1991; Mun, 2000).

In our interview data, however, none of the participants reached the final goal of healthy mother and healthy baby during the NICU period; more time was needed to reach that goal. In addition, the time required is different for each mother (Shin, 2003). Important turning points towards "personal growth and development" and "healthy mother and healthy baby" are (1) the time when the infant can be removed from the incubator (especially in the case of premature or low birth weight infants), (2) the time when the infant can be discharged from the NICU, and (3) the time when the infant looks normal compared with a healthy infant (Lim, 1997; Mun, 2000; Jackson et al., 2003; Shin, 2003).

Influencing Factors to Be Alleviated

Five influencing factors to be alleviated were identified in our combined data:

- Negative meaning attribution
- Uncertainty
- Social prejudice
- Lack of opportunity to make contact with the infant
- NICU environment

First, the meanings a mother attributes to a situation are cognitive representations and interpretations that are created by her and they symbolize her definition of reality (Wrbsky, 2000). Transition to motherhood in a NICU can be distinct according to the meaning a mother attributes to the situation, and negative meaning attributions to that situation can make this transition difficult (Shin, 2003). Second, uncertainty has to be alleviated to facilitate engagement in mothering. Mothers experience two kinds of uncertainty related to infants' survival in the NICU and growth and development up to 2 years, which can make it difficult for them to form attachment with their infants (Bialoskurski et al., 1999; Mun, 2000). Third, some social prejudices against the infant in an NICU have to be changed in order for healthy transition to motherhood to take place. The social prejudice that infants in NICUs will have some complications in the future or problems with growth and development, and that the mother has responsibility for giving birth to an unhealthy infant, can make the transition to motherhood difficult and cause mothers to feel a sense of shame, guilt, and failure (Lee, 1994; Lim, 1997; Choi, 1999; Mun, 2000; Shin, 2003). Fourth, lack of opportunities to make contact with the infant is a major factor leading to delayed transition to motherhood. Mothers' opportunities for interactions with their infants and caring them are reduced in NICUs (Raines, 1999; Holditch-Davis & Miles, 2000). Those who have less opportunity to make contact with their infants may have difficulty in establishing maternal attachment (Cho, 1993). Fifth, the NICU environment can be dehumanizing. Its overall sights and sounds, such as presence of unfamiliar equipment, sudden alarms, and large numbers of other sick infants, can lead mothers to feel uncomfortable and to distance themselves from the infant (Miles et al., 1993). Stressful and fearful feelings in terms of the NICU environment can be an obstacle for mothers in approaching their infants and establishing attachment with them (Moon & Koo, 1999).

What is already known about this topic:

Mothers with infants in a neonatal intensive care unit have more difficulty in their transition to motherhood when compared with mothers of healthy infants. The concept of transition to motherhood in neonatal intensive care units is not well understood in nursing, and is often confused with mothers' psychological responses in the neonatal intensive care unit.

What this chapter adds

A clearer understanding of the concept of transition to motherhood in the neonatal intensive care unit is based on a literature review and fieldwork. Factors influencing the transition to motherhood in the neonatal intensive care unit are negative-meaning attribution, uncertainty, social prejudice, lack of opportunity to make contact with the infant, and the unit environment.

Nurses need to encourage maximal maternal engagement in mothering while a baby is in a neonatal intensive care unit and provide opportunities to interact with the infant by supporting mothers to participate in infant care.

There may be interplay among these elements and they can influence each other. For example, a mother who has fewer opportunities to make contact with her infant in the NICU may give more negative-meaning attributions to that situation than a mother who has more opportunities, and a mother with more negative-meaning attributions may have fewer opportunities for making contact with her infant because she chooses to avoid such opportunities. A conceptual structure of transition to motherhood in the NICU, based on our findings, is shown in Figure 3.3.1.

Derived Definition

Based on the preceding analysis, our clarified definition is as follows: transition to motherhood in the NICU is a time-dependent process that leads mothers to develop a sense of meaning concerning family and life. However, without intervention, transition to motherhood presents as a hovering around the edge of mothering, with psycho-emotional swirling leading to a delayed motherhood. It

```
                                                    ┌──────────────┐
┌───────────────┐                                    │  Attributes  │ ──→  ┌──────────────┐
│  Antecedents  │ ──────────────────────────────→    └──────────────┘      │ Consequences │
└───────────────┘                                                          └──────────────┘
```

Antecedents	Influencing factors to be alleviated	Attributes	Consequences
- Unexpected outcome of pregnancy - Awareness of the situation - Mother-infant separation	- Negative meaning attribution - Uncertainty - Social Prejudice - Lack of opportunities to make contact with the infant - NICU environment	**Time-dependent process** - Sense of flow, movement and direction - Change through time **Psycho-emotional swirling** - Process - Mixed Feelings - Ongoing hopes and wishes **Hovering around the edge of mothering** - Distanced from maternal role - Diminished opportunity for interaction with the infant - Difficulty in establishing maternal attachment - Forced into engaging in mothering	- Delayed motherhood - Developing a sense of meaning concerning family and life itself **Turning points** - When the infant can be removed from the incubator (in case of premature or low birth weight infants) - When the infant can be discharged from the NICU - When the infant looks normal compared to healthy infant Personal growth and development Healthy mother and healthy baby

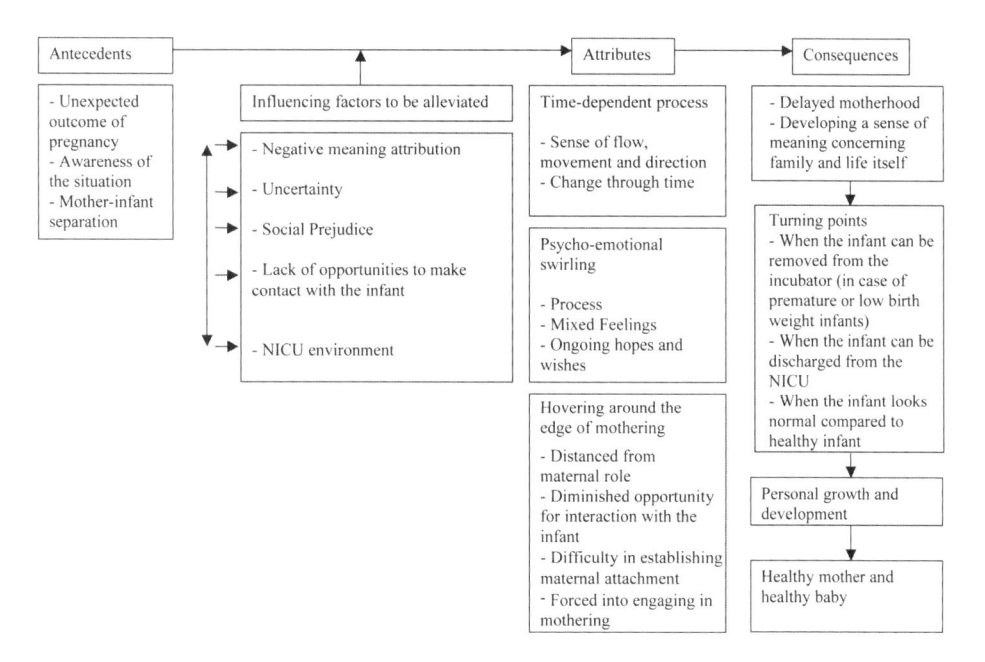

FIGURE 3.3.1 Conceptual structure of transition to motherhood in neonatal intensive care units (NICUs).

is preceded by the unexpected outcome of pregnancy, awareness of the situation, and mother-infant separation. Transition to motherhood in the NICU can be influenced by negative-meaning attributions, uncertainty, social prejudice, lack of opportunities to make contact with the infant, and the NICU environment.

Although these antecedents, attributes, and consequences were identified across cultures, an individual culture might influence the attributes and consequences of the transition to motherhood in the NICU in particular ways, making the transition to motherhood in the NICU more delayed by increasing difficulty in accessing mothering and psycho-emotional swirling.

Conclusions

It is well-documented that the birth and hospitalization of a newborn poses enormous challenges to mothers (Hurst, 2001). Mothers' experiences in NICUs, however, have only recently been the focus of nursing science (Shin, 2004). In this study we found that a consequence of transition to motherhood in the NICU is a delayed motherhood. Thus, nurses who care for mothers with newborns in the NICU need to support them to make an earlier transition to motherhood. To do this, nurses need to encourage maximal engagement in mothering during periods of forced separation such as NICU admission. For example, "kangaroo care" in the NICU is a strategy that promotes maternal engagement (Nelson, 2003). Nurses can provide more opportunities to make contact with and interact with infants by supporting mothers and encouraging them to participate in care. Frequent contact with their babies can also give mothers a sense of psychological stability and can initiate maternal attachment, which leads to calming down the psycho-emotional swirling. On the other hand, nurses may hinder attachment between mother and infant if they ask mothers of very ill or premature infants to touch them as little as possible (Bialoskurski et al., 1999). However, research shows that mothers' thoughts or emotions, such as feelings of distance from the infant or fear of developing a relationship with an infant who may not survive, are the main reasons for difficulty in establishing attachment (Shin, 2003). Therefore, feelings of maternal distance from infants should be diminished before encouraging early physical contact with them. Nurses can help mothers to reduce such feelings of distance by examining the environment of the NICU. The NICU should be a warm and welcoming place that facilitates mothers' getting to know their infants, as well as being a place for curing and caring (Owens, 2001).

Context and culture are also important elements for transition to motherhood in the NICU (Pinch & Spielman, 1996). While this may not be true worldwide, mothers interviewed in Korea perceived a strong social prejudice against infants in NICUs. Social norms, or mothers' perceptions of what others think right after the birth, are related to their outcome expectations and these influences may decrease over time (Kurtz et al., 1992). Thus, it is necessary for health care providers and family to show positive and consistent responses during the early NICU period in order to mitigate mothers' negative-meaning attributions.

This concept analysis has also verified Meleis and colleagues' (2000) transition theory as pertinent for explaining becoming a mother in the NICU, and has contributed to consolidating transition theory. Properties of transition experiences (e.g., awareness, engagement, change, time span) were identified as components of a theoretical framework for transition. In addition, influencing factors in a healthy transition for mothers with infants in NICUs were identified. Further endeavors should be directed towards developing and evaluating specific nursing therapeutics for these mothers.

REFERENCES

Able-Boone, H., & Stevens, E. (1994). After the intensive care nursery experience: families' perceptions of their well being. *Children's Health Care, 23*(2), 99–114.

Affleck, G., & Tennen, H. (1991). The effect of newborn intensive care on parents' psychological well-being. *Children's Health Care, 20*(1), 6–14.

Affleck, G., Tennen, H., Rowe, J., & Higgins, P. (1990). Mothers' remembrances of newborn intensive care: a predictive study. *Journal of Pediatric Psychology, 15*(1), 67–81.

Affonso, D. D., Hurst, I., Mayberry, L. S., Yost, K. & Lynch, M. E. (1992). Stressors reported by mothers of hospitalized premature infants. *Neonatal Network: Journal of Neonatal Nursing, 11*(6), 63–70.

Bialoskurski, M., Cox, C. L., & Hayes, J. A. (1999). The nature of attachment in a neonatal intensive care unit. *Journal of Perinatal and Neonatal Nursing, 13*(1), 66–77.

Cho, K. J. (1993). *A comparison of the mother–infant interaction in low birth weight infants and normal full-term infants.* Unpublished doctoral dissertation, Seoul National University, Seoul.

Choi, E. J. (1999). *A phenomenological study on mother's experience of premature infants.* Unpublished master's thesis, Pusan University, Pusan.

Emily, J. (1999). A mother's perspective: reflections on the NICU. *American Journal of Nursing, 99*(3), 22.

Holditch-Davis, D. H., & Miles, M. S. (2000). Mothers' stories about their experiences in the neonatal intensive care unit. *Neonatal Network: Journal of Neonatal Nursing, 19*(3), 13–21.

Hurst, I. (2001). Vigilant watching over: mothers' actions to safeguard their premature babies in the newborn intensive care nursery. *Journal of Perinatal and Neonatal Nursing, 15*(3), 39–57.

Hutchfield, K. (1999). Family-centered care: a concept analysis. *Journal of Advanced Nursing, 29*(5), 1178–1187.

Jacelon, C. S., Connelly, T. W., Brown, R., Proulx, K., & Vo, T. (2004). A concept analysis of dignity for older adults. *Journal of Advanced Nursing, 48*(1), 76–83.

Jackson, K., Ternestedt, B., & Schollin, J. (2003). From alienation to familiarity: experiences of mothers and fathers of preterm infants. *Journal of Advanced Nursing, 43*(2), 120–129.

Kim, S. J., & Jeong, K .H. (1995). Mothers' perception of their normal and high-risk newborn during the early postpartum period. *Journal of Korean Academy of Child Health Nursing, 1*(1), 5–15.

Kim, T. I. (2000). A study on the perceived stress level of mothers in the neonatal intensive care unit patients. *Journal of Korean Academy of Child Health Nursing, 6*(2), 224–239.

Kitzinger, S. (1975). Effects of induction on the mother–baby relationship. *The Practitioner, 21*(9), 263–269.

Kurtz, M. M., Perez-Woods, R. C., Tse, A .M., & Snyder, D.J. (1992). Antecedents of behavior: parents of high-risk newborns. *Children's Health Care, 21*(4), 213–223.

Kwon, M .K., & Han, K. J. (1991). A study on mother–infant interaction and maternal identity in mother–infant dyads of premature and full-term infants. *Journal of Korean Academy of Nursing, 21*(1), 79–87.

Lee, J. H. (1994). Perception and emotions of mothers of high-risk newborn infants. *Journal of Korean Academy of Nursing, 24*(4), 557–567.

Lim, J. Y. (1997). *Effect of supportive care and infant care information on the perceived stress level and health status of mothers of premature infants.* Unpublished doctoral dissertation, Yonsei University, Seoul.

May, K. M. (1997). Searching for normalcy: mothers' caregiving for low birth weight infants. *Pediatric Nursing, 23*, 17–20.

McGrath, M. M., & Meyer, E. C. (1992). Maternal self-esteem: From theory to clinical practice in a special care nursery. *Children's Health Care, 21*(4), 199–205.

Meleis, A. I., Sawyer, L. M., Im, E. O., Messias, D. K H., & Schumacher. K. L. (2000). Experiencing transitions: an emerging middle-range theory. *Advances in Nursing Science, 23*(1), 12–28.

Miles, M. S., Funk, S. G., & Carlson, J. (1993). Parental stressor scale: neonatal intensive care unit. *Nursing Research, 42*(3), 148–152.

Moon, Y. I., & Koo, H. Y. (1999). Parental role stress and perception of the newborn in mothers of preterm babies. *Journal of Korean Academy of Nursing, 29*(1), 174–182.

Mun, J. H. (2000). *The lived experience of mothers whose first baby is premature.* Unpublished doctoral dissertation, Yonsei University, Seoul.

Nelson, A. M. (2003). Transition to motherhood. *Journal of Obstetric, Gynecologic, and Neonatal Nursing, 32*(4), 465–477.

Owens, K. (2001). The NICU experience: a parent's perspective. *Neonatal Network: Journal of Neonatal Nursing, 20*(4), 67–69.

Park, Y. S. (1991). *Transition to motherhood of primipara in postpartum period.* Unpublished doctoral dissertation, Seoul National University, Seoul.

Pinch, W. J., & Spielman, M. L. (1996). Ethics in the neonatal intensive care unit: parental perceptions at four years postdischarge. *Advances in Nursing Science, 19*(1), 72–85.

Pridham, K.F., & Chang, A.S. (1992). Transition to being the mother of a new infant in the first 3 months: maternal problem solving and self-appraisals. *Journal of Advanced Nursing, 17*, 204–216.

Raines, D. A. (1999). Suspended mothering: women's experiences mothering an infant with a genetic anomaly identified at birth. *Neonatal Network: Journal of Neonatal Nursing, 18*(5), 35–39.

Rapacki, J. D. (1991). The neonatal intensive care experience. *Children's Health Care, 20*(1), 15–18.

Rodgers, B. L. (2000). Concept analysis: an evolutionary view. In *Concept development in nursing: Foundations, techniques, and applications,* 2nd edn (Rodgers, B.L. & Knafl, K.A., eds), W.B. Saunders, Philadelphia, pp. 77–102.

Rubin, R. (1961). Puerperal change. *Nursing Outlook, 9*(3), 743–755.

Schumacher, K.L., & Meleis, A.I. (1994). Transitions: A central concept in nursing. *Image: Journal of Nursing Scholarship, 26*(2), 119–127.

Schwartz-Barcott, D., & Kim, H.S. (2000). An expansion and elaboration of the hybrid model of concept development. In *Concept development in nursing: Foundations, techniques, and applications,* 2nd edn (Rodgers, B. L., & Knafl, K. A., Eds.), W.B. Saunders, Philadelphia, pp. 129–159.

Shin, H. J. (2003). *Maternal transition in mothers with high risk newborns.* Unpublished doctoral dissertation, Korea University, Seoul.

Shin, H. J. (2004). Situational meaning and maternal self-esteem in mothers with high-risk newborns. *Journal of Korean Academy of Nursing, 34*(1), 93–101.

Simkin, P. (1996). The experience of maternity in a woman's life. *Journal of Obstetric, Gynecologic, & Neonatal Nursing, 25*(3), 247–252.

Singer, L. T., Salvator, A., Shenyang, G., Lilien, L., & Baley, J. (1999), Maternal psychological distress and parenting stress after the birth of a very low-birth-weight infant. *Journal of American Medical Association, 281*, 799–805.

Walker, L. O., Crain, H., & Thomson, E. (1986). Mothering behavior and maternal role attainment during the postpartum period. *Nursing Research, 35*, 352–355.

Wrbsky, P. M. (2000). *Family Meaning Attribution in the Health-illness Transition to Preterm Birth.* Unpublished doctoral dissertation, University of Minnesota, Minneapolis, MN, USA.

Zabielski, M. T. (1994). Recognition of maternal identity in preterm and full-term mothers. *Maternal Child Nursing Journal, 22*(1), 22–35.

Reprinted with permission from: Shin, H., & White-Trout, R. (2007). The conceptual structure of transition to motherhood in the neonatal intensive care unit. *Journal of Advanced Nursing, 58*(1), 90–98.

3.4 NURSING PRACTICE MODEL FOR MATERNAL ROLE SUFFICIENCY

KATHLEEN FLYNN GAFFNEY

Abstract

In 1975 Meleis set forth a conceptual framework for nursing practice centered on the concepts of role insufficiency and role supplementation. Later, Millor introduced a parental role sufficiency model for nursing research in child abuse and neglect. Based on the works of both Meleis and Millor, a nursing practice model is proposed that focuses on maternal role sufficiency. It includes assessment of prenatal characteristics, measurement of developmental and health–illness outcomes, and preventive role supplementation intervention.

Nursing practice models serve as an organizing framework for clinical practice and research. The purpose of this chapter is to present a model for maternal–child nursing practice and research that addresses the need for primary prevention of special developmental and health problems of families with infants and children. Specifically, the model represents an expansion of earlier models developed by Meleis[1] and Millor.[2]

Background

In 1975 Meleis[1] set forth a theoretical basis for nursing practice based on the concept of role insufficiency. She explained that role insufficiency was a phenomenon individuals experienced during role transition and was accompanied by developmental and health–illness implications. She defined role insufficiency as "any difficulty in the cognizance and/or performance of a role or the sentiments and goals associated with the role behavior as perceived by self or by significant others"[1] (p. 266). Significant others included health care providers such as the community health nurse who made a nursing diagnosis and planned care for an expectant mother.

Central to the Meleis model were specific nursing actions designed to prevent or ameliorate role insufficiency, actions referred to as "role supplementation." The latter were described as a deliberate process that included conveying information or providing experiences for the role incumbent to become aware of anticipated role behaviors and goals, as well as the interrelationships between the new role and the roles of others.

Later, Millor[2] developed a nursing model for the complex phenomenon of parental role sufficiency. Specifically, Millor designed an organizing framework for nursing research in child abuse and neglect, the extreme manifestation of parental role insufficiency. Her model encompassed the transactional relationships among individual, family, and community characteristics, and parent role behaviors, as perceived by self and significant others. Millor's approach was an eclectic one that drew from symbolic interaction, stress, and temperament theories.[3–6] The core of her model was stress-appraised transactions between parent and child that, tempered by multifactoral individual and ecological components, led to a range of parental role behaviors, from normative nurturing (parental role sufficiency) to neglect and abuse (parental role insufficiency).

Rationale for the Expanded Model

Figure 3.4.1 depicts Millor's original nursing model for parental role sufficiency with the proposed expansion. The expanded model includes assessment of prenatal characteristics and measurement of developmental and health–illness outcomes, as well as direction for role supplementation intervention as described in the Meleis model.[1]

The primary reason for the proposed expansion of these models to the prenatal period is to provide nursing and related practice disciplines with a model for more fully examining the developmental and health–illness implications of role sufficiency throughout the period of transition to motherhood. To initiate examination of role sufficiency when the stress-appraised transactions between mother and child have already begun is to have missed the unique contribution of prenatal factors that occur early in the process of role transition. Examples of factors derived from the original model that may be assessed prenatally include the pregnant woman's perception of the mothering she received as a child with respect to nurturing and discipline (Parent's Own Childrearing History), her perception of current difficult life circumstances and her personal resources to cope with them (Parent Self-Characteristics), and her expectations of the maternal role and infant competencies (Parent Role Expectations).

In expanding the examination of role sufficiency, consideration is also given specifically to the impact of prenatal maternal role sufficiency on later role behavior. The term prenatal maternal role sufficiency is proposed to encompass the spectrum of prenatal behaviors that range from warm, affiliative nurturing to risky behaviors that may be deleterious to infant health.

Assessment Component of the Expanded Model

Parent's Own Childrearing History is one component of the original Millor model that may be expanded for prenatal assessment. Gaffney[7] compared prenatal plans for child discipline with pregnant women's own perceptions of having been disciplined as a child by their mothers and found a significant association. Further study is needed to determine the extent to which these prenatal plans predict later practices of childhood discipline.

However, the child abuse and neglect literature supports the notion that a woman's experience of having been maltreated as a child may put her at risk for continuing an intergenerational cycle of abuse and neglect. Based on their longitudinal, prospective study of the antecedents of child maltreatment, Egeland, Jacobvitz, and Papatola[8] concluded that the experience of being maltreated as a child may be a circumstance that leads mothers to lose control with their own children and neglect their physical or emotional needs. Their observation was that women who had been maltreated as children had suffered significant psychological trauma that impaired their capability for close interpersonal relationships. Sroufe and Fleeson[9] emphasized that women who were victimized as children often thought of themselves as victims and acted out the observed role of victimizer when caring for their own children.

However, studies[10,11] of maltreating parents also indicated that healthy parenting outcomes are possible despite earlier maltreatment, particularly when women have gained knowledge about relationships, relearned self–other concepts, and developed secure, emotional relationships that allowed them to deal with earlier traumas of childhood.

These findings support the notion that intervention to break the intergenerational cycle of abuse can be effective. It also argues favorably for early assessment and preventive intervention that supports the development of nurturing relationships *before* the mother is faced with stress-appraised transactions generated by an infant who may at times appear to be overly dependent and noncompliant.

A second concept from the nursing model for parental role sufficiency that may be assessed during pregnancy is Self-Characteristics. Specifically, a woman's perception of her chronic and current stressors, coupled with her perception of her own coping skills and supportive resources, may be considered within this concept.

The Children's Defense Fund[12] links dramatic rises in the incidence of child abuse and neglect with such stressors as poverty, homelessness, substance abuse, and domestic violence. Beckwith[13] cautions that most parents who experience high degrees of stressful circumstances do not abuse or neglect their children. In fact, a comparison of parents experiencing high stress found that those who did abuse or neglect their children were more likely to have also had a history of violence in their own childhood or current violent episodes with their partner and few satisfying social supports.

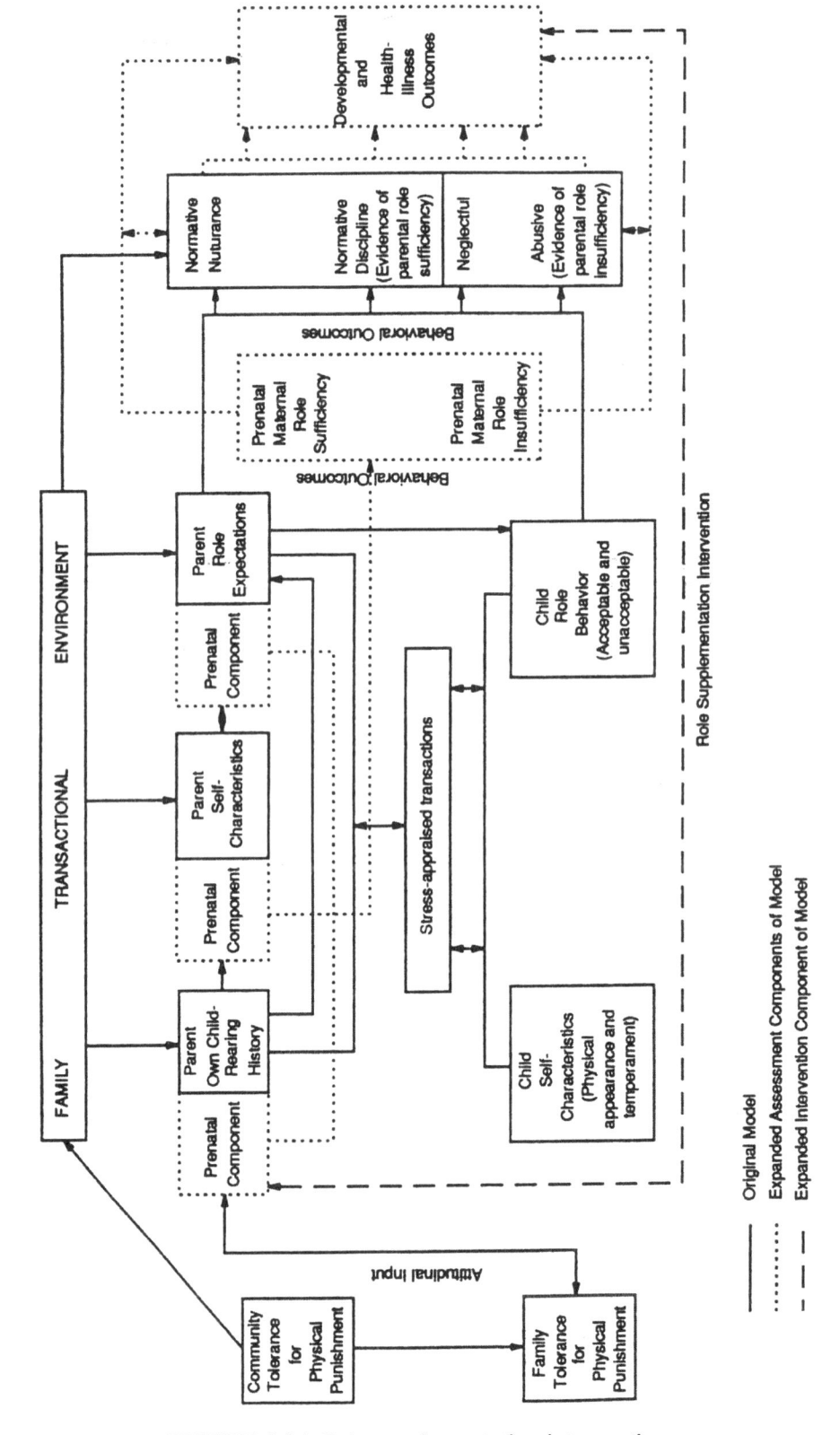

FIGURE 3.4.1 Role supplementation intervention.

The utility of prenatal assessments of perceptions women have of their own stressors and supportive resources has not been fully explored. However, Booth et al.[14] conducted a study of maternal competence that included prenatal assessment of both difficult life circumstances and perceived social support among women at social high risk. They found that women with low social skills who received individually planned, therapeutic home visits from nurses demonstrated improved competence in relation to both adult social skills and maternal–infant interactive skills. The researchers concluded that a connection may exist between these two outcomes. Specifically, they suggested that mothers who improved their own ability to communicate with adults were better able to reach out for the effective support needed to deal with difficult life circumstances and, in turn, became more emotionally available to respond to infant needs.

A third concept from the Millor model that may be extended for prenatal assessment when considering prevention of child maltreatment is Parent Role Expectations. According to Millor (personal communication, June 1992), this concept refers to the mother's expectations of herself in the maternal role and her expectations of her own infant's competencies.

By means of prenatal assessment of these factors, clinicians and researchers may be afforded a view of the distortions that contribute to a stressed relationship and heightened vulnerability to maternal role insufficiency. Snyder et al.,[15] for example, examined prenatal maternal expectations of infant capabilities with respect to early maternal–infant interaction. They found that inappropriate expectations by mothers during pregnancy were associated with lower scores on a measure of maternal provision of infant stimulation at 4, 8, and 12 months of age. The latter may be considered a measure of maternal role sufficiency. The Snyder et al. findings were confirmed in a later study by Gaffney,[7] using a larger sample at data collection points during pregnancy and 4 months infant age.[2]

Since the original Millor model identifies nurturing behaviors as evidence of parental role sufficiency and abusive and neglectful behaviors as evidence of parental role insufficiency, the concept of prenatal maternal role sufficiency is proposed to address entities, such as prenatal maternal attachment, that may be early indicators of later maternal role insufficiency.

Mercer and Ferketich[16] found that prenatal maternal attachment was a predictor of early maternal–infant attachment. Although studies are not available that link prenatal attachment levels with later parenting outcomes, it is increasingly clear that disorders of attachment lie at the root of abusive and neglectful parenting behaviors.[10,17,18] Consequently, early identification of normal and dysfunctional patterns of early attachment' are warranted.

Intervention Component of the Expanded Model

Beginning with the first prenatal assessment, role supplementation intervention may be initiated to prevent or ameliorate the incidence of maternal role insufficiency. As described by Meleis,[1] role supplementation intervention consists of two components. The first, role clarification, is defined as "the mastery of knowledge to perform the role." In order to efficiently target specific role clarification needs of new mothers, clinicians and researchers may use available indices including the Knowledge of Infant Development Inventory (MacPhee, D., 1982, unpublished data) and the Developmental Expectations Scale.[15]

The second component of role supplementation intervention, role taking, addresses the "empathetic abilities of self"[19] (p. 372) In the case of maternal role insufficiency, this component incorporates the woman's capacity to understand her role in relation to her infant's feelings and needs. The Maternal–Fetal Attachment Scale[20] addresses this phenomenon during pregnancy. The Nursing Child Assessment Feeding and Teaching Scales[21] with their Sensitivity to Cues subscales tap the role taking component.

In addition to the two components of role supplementation, three specific strategies for intervention have been described: role modeling, role rehearsal, and reference group interactions. All three were used in a study of couples expecting their first baby.[22] Role modeling consisted of teaching participants how to learn appropriate role behaviors from family, friends, and professionals who knew and utilized the behaviors and values of the expected role.

Role rehearsal was facilitated with the use of case studies. Couples were asked to think about and explain how they might handle a specific situation related to infant care. This intervention strategy helped the couples anticipate behaviors and sentiments associated with the parental role.

Reference group interactions were generated through weekly meetings with the couples and two nurse group leaders. The group forum allowed members to test ideas, receive reinforcements, and understand the normal range of feelings, fears, and experiences of others in a similar point of role transition.

Study findings supported the notion that role supplementation intervention had a positive effect on maternal role sufficiency.[2] Specifically, the mothers who received role supplementation intervention were less likely to show an attitude of ignoring infant cues and more likely to demonstrate an attitude of responding to infant needs than were mothers in two similar groups who did not receive the intervention.

More recent intervention studies provide some additional support for the use of role supplementation strategies to promote maternal role sufficiency. For instance, Unger and Wandersman[23] tested the effects of a resource mothers program for socially disadvantaged pregnant teenagers. The resource mothers were role models in that they were experienced mothers and paraprofessionals similar in race and socioeconomic status to the teenagers. The resource mothers visited the expectant mothers regularly during pregnancy and infancy and provided them with needed information about the anticipated maternal role. The researchers found that the visited mothers demonstrated greater knowledge of infant development, more satisfaction with the mothering role, and greater responsiveness to infant needs than did a control group. By using the expanded model as an organizing framework to conduct and evaluate nursing practice, a potential conclusion from these findings is that the role modeling strategy was effective in supporting maternal role sufficiency.

Olds[17] also conducted an intervention study of a prenatal home visit program for pregnant teenagers. His intervention involved the role rehearsal strategy. That is, nurses helped pregnant teenagers anticipate and recognize differences in infant temperament, especially crying behavior. The pregnant teenagers were helped to understand the meaning of crying from the child's point of view and not misinterpret it as an indication of the mother's failure in caregiving or a deliberate attempt by the baby to disrupt the mother's life. The teenagers in the home visit intervention program that experienced this role rehearsal strategy demonstrated fewer incidences of child abuse and neglect than did a similar control group. Olds concluded that subjects in the treatment group were able to interpret infant behavior more correctly and respond more appropriately, "thus forming the basis for secure attachments, which may protect the child from abuse and neglect"[17] (p. 752).

Although studies that demonstrate the effectiveness of the reference group interaction strategy in preventing or ameliorating maternal role sufficiency are limited, nursing has long used the group process as an intervention strategy.[24,25] Future nursing studies of the effectiveness of reference group interactions may consider injecting the focus group interview technique into this intervention strategy. The purpose of the focus group interview is to gather "information which, when performed in a permissive non-threatening group environment, allows the investigation of a multitude of perceptions on a defined area of interest"[26] (p. 1282). The purpose of the reference group is to provide members with a non-threatening situation for testing their ideas and for receiving positive reinforcements from others who are experiencing similar role transitions. By wedding the intervention strategy with the qualitative research technique, nursing is afforded the opportunity to meet the needs of clients in an immediate practice setting and to simultaneously generate data that leads to the ongoing evaluation and refinement of practice in a wider range of practice settings.

Scope of the Expanded Model

The proposed nursing practice model for maternal role sufficiency has potential application for clinical problems in addition to child abuse and neglect. Specifically, researchers may find it a useful framework for organizing studies of many health and developmental outcomes of infancy that have maternal precedents in the prenatal period. As an example, researchers who have studied causes and correlates of the incidence of low birth weight collectively present prenatal variables that fall within the umbrella of the expanded model. That is, just as the self-characteristics of prenatal perception of adverse life circumstances and prenatal perception of social support have been associated with later child maltreatment, these prenatal variables have been associated with the incidence of low birth weight (LBW). Bullock and McFarlane[27] examined the impact of one specific difficult life circumstance, battering during pregnancy, on later incidence of LBW and found a significantly greater incidence of LBW among women who had been battered compared with a control group. This finding concurs with the report of the Public Health Service Expert Panel on the Content of Prenatal Care[28] that indicated that living in abusive or other high-stress situations and experiencing inadequate personal support systems places a pregnant woman at risk for poor birth outcomes.

LBW researchers may find it useful to investigate prenatal behaviors such as abstention from smoking and alcohol, regular prenatal checkups, and healthy eating patterns within the expanded model concept of prenatal maternal role sufficiency. Each behavior fits within the definition of prenatal maternal role sufficiency and has been found to be a significant factor in reducing the incidence of LBW babies.[29-33]

Furthermore, the role modeling intervention strategy has been shown to have promising results in encouraging positive behaviors and preventing or reducing the incidence of LBW. Konafel[34] reported that, through the use of a resource mothers program with socially disadvantaged pregnant teenagers, the incidence of LBW dropped to 6%, compared with the prevailing rate of 9.6% in Virginia where the program was conducted.

By using the expanded model as an organizing framework, researchers are afforded an opportunity to examine multiple clinical outcomes with the same data set, thus yielding greater contributions to the current body of nursing knowledge. The intertwining nature of predictor variables and outcomes will yield information about interrelatedness that is unavailable with separate studies.

The proposed nursing practice model is directed specifically toward the prevention of health and developmental problems, such as child abuse and neglect, that may have underpinnings evident during pregnancy. Since the model includes a strong theoretical base, early prenatal assessment of maternal role sufficiency, simultaneous initiation of preventive role supplementation intervention, and an overall framework for ongoing empirical evaluation of health and developmental outcomes, it is considered to be a comprehensive model for maternal–child nursing practice.

REFERENCES

1. Meleis AI. Role insufficiency and role supplementation: a conceptual framework. *Nurs Res.* 1975; 24(4): 264–271.
2. Millor GK. A theoretical framework for nursing research in child abuse and neglect. *Nurs Res.* 1981; 30(2):78–83.
3. Mead GH. *Mind, Self, and Society, I.* Chicago, IL: University of Chicago Press; 1934.
4. Sarbin T. Role theory. In: Lindzey G, ed. *Handbook of Sociology.* Reading, MA: Addison-Wesley; 1954.
5. Lazarus R, Launier R. Stress-related transactions between person and environment. In: Pervin LA, Lewis L, eds. *Perspectives in Interactional Psychology.* New York, NY: Plenum; 1978.
6. Carey WB. A simplified method of measuring infant temperament. *J Pediatr.* 1970; 77:188–194.

7. Gaffney KF. *Prenatal Predictors of Maternal Role Sufficiency*. Final Report to the National Center for Nursing Research. Washington, DC: National Institutes of Health; 1991.
8. Egeland B, Jacobvitz D, Papatola K. *Intergenerational Continuity of Parental Abuse*. Proceedings from Conference on Biosocial Perspectives of Child Abuse and Neglect. York, ME: Social Science Research Council; May 20–23, 1984.
9. Sroufe LA, Fleeson J. Attachment and the construction of relationships. In: Hartum WW, Rubin Z, eds. *Relationships and Development*. New York, NY: Cambridge University Press; 1986.
10. Planta R, Egeland B, Erickson MF. The antecedents of maltreatment; results of the Mother-Child Interaction Research Project. In: Cicchetti D, Carlson V, eds. *Child Maltreatment*. New York, NY: Cambridge University Press; 1989.
11. Ricks M. The social transmission of parental behavior: attachment across generations. In: Bretherton I, Waters E, eds. *Growing Points of Attachment Theory and Research*. 50(1–2, Serial No. 209). *Monographs of the Society for Research in Child Development*. Chicago, IL: University of Chicago Press; 1985.
12. Children's Defense Fund. *The State of America's Children 1991*. Washington, DC: Children's Defense Fund; 1991.
13. Beckwith L. Adaptive and maladaptive parenting: implications for intervention. In: Meisels S, Shonkoff JP, eds. *Handbook of Early Childhood Intervention*. New York, NY: Cambridge University Press; 1990.
14. Booth CL, Mitchell SK, Barnard KE, Spieker SJ. Development of maternal social skills in multiproblem families: effects on the mother–child relationship. *Dev Psychol*. 1989; 25(3):403–412.
15. Snyder C, Eyres SJ, Barnard K. New findings about mothers' antenatal expectations and their relationship to infant development. *MCN*. 1979; 4:354–357.
16. Mercer RT, Ferketich SL. Predictors of parental attachment during early parenthood. *J Adv Nurs*. 1990; 15:268–280.
17. Olds DL, Henderson CR. The prevention of maltreatment. In: Cicchitti D, Carlson V, eds. *Child Maltreatment*. New York, NY: Cambridge University Press; 1989.
18. Main M, Goldwyn R. Predicting rejection of her infant from mother's representation of her own experience: implications for the abused–abusing intergenerational cycle. *Child Abuse Negl*. 1984; 8:203–217.
19. Meleis AI. The sick role. In: Hardy ME, Conway ME, eds. *Role Theory: Perspectives for Health Professionals*. Norwalk, CT: Appleton & Lange; 1988.
20. Cranley M. Development of a tool for the measurement of maternal attachment during pregnancy. *Nurs Res*. 1981; 30(5):281–284.
21. Barnard KE, Hammond MA, Booth CL, Bee HL, Mitchell SK, Spieker SJ. Measurement and meaning of parent–child interaction. In: Morrison F, Lord C, Keating D, eds. *Applied Developmental Psychology, III*. New York, NY: Academic Press; 1989.
22. Meleis AI, Swendsen LA. Role supplementation: an empirical test of a nursing intervention. *Nurs Res*. 1978; 27(1):11–18.
23. Unger DG, Wandersman LP. Social support and adolescent mothers: action research contributions to theory and application. *J Soc Iss*. 1985; 41:29–45.
24. Fullar SA, Lum B, Sprik MG, Cooper EM. A small group can go a long way. *MCN*. 1988; 13(6):414–418.
25. Snyder D. Peer group support for high-risk mothers. *MCN*. 1988; 13(2):114–117.
26. Nyamathi A, Schuler P. Focus group interview: a research technique for informed nursing practice. *J Adv Nurs*. 1990; 15:1281–1288.
27. Bullock L, McFarlane J. The birth weight/battering connection. *Am J Nurs*. 1989; 89(9):1153–1155.
28. *Caring for Our Future: The Content of Prenatal Care*. Report of the Public Health Service Expert Panel on the Content of Prenatal Care. Washington, DC: US Department of Health and Human Services; 1989.
29. Haglund B, Cratingius S. Cigarette smoking as a risk factor for sudden infant death syndrome: a population based study. *Am J Public Health*. 1990; 80(1):29–32.
30. Harwood HJ, Napolitano DM, Kristiansen PL. Economic costs to society of alcohol and drug abuse and mental illness: 1980. *Res Triangle Institute*. 1984; June.
31. Kleinman JC, Pierre MB, Madams JH, Land GH, Schramm WF. The effects of maternal smoking on fetal and infant mortality. *Am J Epidemiol*. 1988; 27:274–282.
32. Koop CE. *Memorandum from Surgeon General of Public Health Service*. Washington, DC: US Department of Health and Human Services; March, 1989.
33. National Commission to Prevent Infant Mortality. *Troubling Trends: The Health of America's*

Next Generation. Washington, DC: National Commission to Prevent Infant Mortality; 1990.
34. *Home Visiting: Opening Doors for America's Pregnant Women and Children.* Washington, DC: National Commission to Prevent Infant Mortality; 1989.

Reprinted with permission from: Gaffney, K. F. (1992). Nursing practice-model for maternal role sufficiency. *Advances in Nursing Sciences, 15*(2), 76–84.

3.5 A SITUATION-SPECIFIC THEORY OF KOREAN IMMIGRANT WOMEN'S MENOPAUSAL TRANSITION

EUN-OK IM
AFAF IBRAHIM MELEIS

Abstract

Purpose: *To extend the previous model of transitions by including the experiences of low-income Korean immigrant women in the United States during their menopausal transition. The extension results in a situation-specific theory of Korean immigrant women's menopausal transition.* ***Design:*** *Findings from a study of menopausal transition among Korean immigrant women were used as a main source for modification of the conceptual properties of transitions, conditions shaping the transitions, and indicators of healthy transitions. The study was cross-sectional with methodological triangulation. Quantitative analysis was based on data from 119 first-generation Korean immigrant women who engaged in low-status or low-income work outside their homes; qualitative study using theoretical sampling method included 21 women.* ***Methods:*** *Analyses included descriptive and inferential statistics and thematic analysis. Integrative conceptual analysis using deductive and inductive reasoning was conducted to determine modifications in theory based on the descriptions of menopausal transition of Korean immigrant women.* ***Findings:*** *Three main themes were identified: (a) the women gave their menopausal transition far less attention than they did their immigrant and work transition; (b) menopause was a hidden experience within the cultural background; and (c) the women "normalized," ignored, and endured symptoms. The findings indicated additions of the following concepts: (a) number, seriousness, and priority of transitions; (b) socioeconomic status; (c) gender; (d) context; (e) attitudes toward health and illness; (f) interrelationships among all conditions shaping transitions; and (g) symptom management.* ***Conclusions:*** *The proposed situation-specific model is limited in scope. However, it provides an understanding of the menopausal transition of Korean immigrant women in context, and is a guide for nursing interventions for immigrant women experiencing transition.*

Transition has been defined as a process that humans undergo when faced with changes in their lives or environments (Schumacher & Meleis, 1994). It is a human experience described as a constellation of responses over time and shaped by personal and environmental conditions such as the expectations and perceptions of individuals, the meanings they attribute to these experiences, their knowledge and skill in handling the changes, the experience at different points in the process, and their level of emotional and physical well-being (Chick & Meleis, 1986; Schumacher & Meleis, 1994).

Transition is a concept central to nursing practice. Meleis (1975, 1987, 1997; Chick & Meleis, 1986) reported that nurses spend much of their time and energy dealing with clients undergoing transitions precipitated by developmental, situational, or health and illness changes, and that these transitions have significant implications for well-being and health. Based on Meleis' early work, Chick and Meleis (1986) further developed the concept of transition using concept analysis. Schumacher and Meleis (1994) extended the effort by developing a model describing the types of transitions that nurses deal with, properties that characterize transitions, conditions that determine the nature of responses, indicators of healthy transitions, and nursing therapeutics most appropriate for people experiencing transitions.

We used the transition model by Schumacher and Meleis (1994) as a framework to describe how Korean immigrant women in the United States experienced menopausal transition i.e., the time beginning with perimenopause and ending a few years after menstruation has ceased (Li, Lanuza, Gulanick, Penckofer, & Holm, 1996). Based on our experiences with the population, we propose revision of the framework. Specifically, we propose modifications in the conceptual properties and conditions of the transition model and an additional indicator of healthy transition. The revisions produce a situation-specific theory of menopausal transition of Korean immigrant women. Situation-specific theories are "theories that focus on specific nursing phenomena that reflect clinical practice, are limited to specific populations or to a particular field of practice, and are developed to answer a set of coherent questions about situations that are limited in scope and focus" (Meleis, 1997, p. 18).

The basis for this integrative conceptual analysis was a study conducted to describe the perceived meanings of low-income Korean immigrant women about their menopause and menopausal symptoms with analysis of their responses in a context of immigration and work transitions (Im, 1997). This study was cross-sectional using methodological triangulation. A sample of 119 Korean women was recruited from one large Western city in the United States. Criteria for inclusion were self-defined first-generation Korean immigrant women, 40 to 60 years of age, who engaged in low-status or low-income work outside their homes. Only 21 peri- or post-menopausal women were included in the qualitative part of the study. Initially, the first 10 participants from the larger sample were invited to participate in the qualitative component of the study; subsequently the remaining 11 participants were recruited based on themes from the data collected from the first 10 women and using the theoretical sampling technique suggested by Strauss and Corbin (1990). The sociodemographic characteristics of the women are summarized in Table 3.5.1.

TABLE 3.5.1 Sociodemographic Profiles of Research Participants

Sociodemographic profiles	Quantitative part ($n = 119$) N (%)	Qualitative part ($n = 21$) N (%)
Age (years)		
Mean (SD)	47.94(5.77)	49.95(6.70)
Educational level		
No formal or elementary school	14(12)	2(9)
Middle school and high school	39(33)	9(43)
College and above	65(55)	10(48)
Family income (self-reported)		
Insufficient	36(31)	10(47)
Sufficient for essentials	57(48)	9(43)
More than sufficient	25(21)	2(10)
Marital status		
Married or partnered	107(90)	19(90)
Divorced or separated	3(3)	1(5)
Widowed	3(3)	1(5)
Single	4(4)	0(0)
Length of stay in the United States		
Less than 1 year	14(12)	0(0)
1 to 10 years	39(33)	19(90)
More than 10 years	65(55)	2(10)

Two interview protocols and a modified version of the Cornell Medical Index (Brodman, Erdman, & Wolff, 1949) were used. Women who agreed to participate were given a Korean version of the questionnaires. Interviews were scheduled at the convenience of participants. Locations included churches, homes, workplaces, and restaurants. Interviews lasted an average of 2 hours.

Quantitative data were analyzed using descriptive and inferential statistics. Qualitative data were analyzed using thematic analysis, including textual examination of interview transcripts, line-by-line coding of transcripts, categories, and descriptions of key relationships among the categories. Analysis was guided by the mode of qualitative analysis suggested by Strauss and Corbin (1990). Once codes were specified, data were sorted into categories based on the codes. Associations between categories were examined, and themes were constructed through analyses using both inductive and deductive reasoning (Denzin, 1978).

Women's Menopausal Transition

Several themes related to the menopausal transition of low-income Korean immigrant women were identified (Im, 1997). One theme was that the women gave their menopausal transition far less attention than they did their current immigration and work transitions. Given the lowest priority among the three transitions, menopause was "normalized" or ignored, i.e., they regarded menopause as a normal developmental process and considered symptoms experienced during menopause as normal and healthy. Demands because of multiple transitions—cultural, physio-psycho-social, and work (transition from housewife to employee)—may have influenced them to devote more of their energy, money, and time to meeting daily life demands. Some of these needs undoubtedly arose from additional hidden and in-between roles to maintain and nurture the values, expectations, and heritage of their country of origin while negotiating new skills required in the host country (Meleis, 1987).

Immigrant women are expected to negotiate complex educational and health-care systems, sometimes with limited language skills and capabilities. They are also expected to assume new roles in the host country's educational and health-care values and approaches. Self-care approaches to health care and parent partnerships in educating children are often in direct conflict with immigrants' value systems, skills, and customs. These demands and expectations in their multiple transitions may have led them to de-emphasize their menopausal transition and to normalize or ignore it. Two examples of participants' responses follow.

> Participant One: I didn't know it at that time. But, looking back...I was really busy in adapting to this new country and new work....My busy schedules and stress from work made me go through *pekyung* (menopause) easily. I did not have time to think about menopause. Maybe I had some symptoms due to *pekyung*. But I cannot remember anything. Compared with other stressful things, it was a very tiny part of my life.

> Participant Two: It just passed by. I had many difficult things. At the same time, everything happened. So I could not give attention to my *pekyung*. It just passed by....It's the same experience like being pregnant and having children....Later, I could remember it was difficult. What menopause meant to me, how I deal with the difficulties, I never thought about.

Another theme was that menopause was an experience hidden within the cultural background of patriarchy. Many feminists describe how reactions to menopause have been closeted and how women's experiences have been oppressed, neglected, and ignored. Talking about menopause has been taboo; menopause has been veiled in secrecy and dismissed as a biologic imperative not worth naming or discussing (Delaney, Lupton, & Toth, 1988; Dickson, 1990a, 1990b; MacPherson, 1981, 1985; Martin, 1987; Weideger, 1976). Women who participated in this study said they rarely talked about women-only experiences such as menstruation, pregnancy, and menopause directly in front of others. Such discussions were taboo even within families. One participant said, "No, I didn't do that" in response to a question about whether she talked about her menopause with her friends.

> I kept it to myself. I did not talk about it to my family [or] friends. Maybe I unconsciously talked about it. But I felt there were no problems due to menopause. It was shameful and embarrassing to talk about with my children.…Maybe if the relationships were good, then it would be easier to talk about [it]. But I did not want to talk about that to others, including my husband. It's shameful and it's not…something I could talk about in public.

Another participant said:

> It is shameful to talk about it. In fact, I did not have any problems regarding my daily activities due to *pekyung*. Indeed there were no difficulties due to physical symptoms. Rather, it was a conflict inside myself because I felt that I was not able to do anything. I went through my menopause very lonely because I considered it my own conflict.

Under the strong influences of their patriarchal cultural heritage, Korean immigrant women also made their menopausal transition "invisible" while putting family members' needs, especially male members' needs, ahead of their own. The need to pay children's school tuition or deal with financial crises often came ahead of seeking health care for themselves. Confucian patriarchal values might also have provided them with the rationale to behave, think, feel, and be like women, as biologically and socially ascribed, and to sacrifice themselves for their families (Cho, 1987; Kim & Hurh, 1987). These participants were socialized to sacrifice their own needs, including their health care needs, when their families had other needs, consequently making their menopausal transition invisible.

The following is what one woman said about Korean women and their responsibilities:

> [Women are] *ansaram*-person inside house. Men are *bakatyangban*-nobleman outside house. *Yeoja* [a woman] is *ansaram* and *namja* [a man] is *bakatyangban*. When introducing her husband, a woman says that this is my *bakatyangban*. And when a man introduces his wife, he says that this is my *ansaram*. I have been raised like that. *Yeoja* should take care of her responsibilities as an *ansaram* and men should take care of their responsibilities outside of the house. Then their families will be happy and peaceful.

Another said:

> It's useless to think that it is unfair for [Korean] women to do all the household tasks by themselves. Society and family do not accept it. Do you think Korean men who have been raised in Korean culture will accept it? Everyone thinks that women who fulfill their responsibilities as women are good women. Everyone thinks like that. Women's sin is the fact that they were born as women. Women should do their best to fulfill their responsibilities.

A third theme was that the women normalized, ignored, and endured symptoms experienced during menopausal transition. One of the reasons was that most women did not view the symptoms as serious because they usually connected their symptoms with life events (retirement, children leaving home, financial problems, spouse's death, children's independence, and interpersonal conflicts) or degenerative changes from aging instead of from pathologic etiologies. Consequently, they usually believed that their symptoms would disappear after they resolved the current conflicts and troubles. Or, they thought that they should live with these symptoms until they died because aging brought the symptoms. They also believed that these symptoms were inevitable and would continue regardless of any treatment because the symptoms were related to aging, which was perceived as normal. Another reason was the belief that the symptoms were temporary. This belief influenced meaning with an expectation that the symptoms would disappear after menopause. For example, when one of the women experienced "aches in the back of neck and skull," she did not seek help for the symptom because her friends informed her that the symptom was temporary and would disappear after menopause. A third explanation was that they regarded the symptoms as normal and appropriate changes for women's lives. Because menopause was regarded as natural, changes associated with it were not regarded as serious health problems. Only when the changes affected a woman's daily life so that she could not work as usual did she seek help from either a traditional or Western physician. A fourth explanation—the most important reason for normalizing, ignoring, and enduring symptoms—was that the women rarely have time for themselves or time to spend on being concerned about symptoms experienced during menopausal transition.

The following is what one participant said:

> I came here for my children. I want to provide better opportunities and a good education to them. So I work like an ant. Some people work for their pleasure. Some people work because others work. But I work for money. I need to eat and survive. I need to educate my children. I need to support their education. So I was indifferent to [menopausal symptoms]. I didn't care. Life as a working immigrant is very difficult and busy. Maybe women who are not busy would care. I didn't. So I think that my menopause passed by without any notice.

In summary, the women ignored but normalized their menopausal transition because of the demands of multiple roles and cultural heritage. Their cultural heritage, their immigration experience, and their gender made menopausal transition "invisible" and predisposed them to either ignore or normalize the symptoms that resulted from such a transition. Also the lack of connection between symptoms and menopause, the belief that the symptoms were temporary, the assumption that symptoms were normal and appropriate changes for women's lives, and lack of time for themselves made them normalize, ignore, and endure symptoms experienced during menopausal transition.

Modifications in the Transition Model

The findings support several modifications to the model described by Schumacher & Meleis (1994). The modifications are proposed to more fully explain low-income Korean immigrant women's responses to menopausal transition within the context of multiple transitions based on the study findings and our previous experiences with the population (Figure 3.5.1). Responses might also indicate transitions related to gender and sociocultural contexts.

Number, Seriousness, and Priority of Transitions

In multiple transitions, the number, seriousness, and perceived priority of each are as significant, if not more significant, than the type of transition. In the transition model by Schumacher and Meleis (1994), transitions are characterized only by the type of transition: developmental, situational, health and illness, and organizational. However, the type of transition did not fully explain the findings of the study. Research participants did not place much importance on their menopausal transition because of other transitions concurrently experienced. Because the demands of their daily lives as immigrants and workers were more serious and significant, menopause rarely meant much to them. To help explain the findings, we suggest that the number, seriousness, and priority of transitions be incorporated into explanatory models of transitions.

Additional Transition Conditions

Transition conditions (Schumacher & Meleis, 1994) include meanings, expectations, level of knowledge and skill, environment, level of planning, and emotional and physical well-being. The findings of this study indicate additional conditions that influenced the women's menopausal transition.

Socioeconomic Status

The findings indicated that symptoms experienced during the women's menopausal transition were influenced by their socioeconomic status rather than by their menopausal states. Indifference to their symptoms might have been because the women were immigrants with low socioeconomic status, had to generate income, and were preoccupied with daily life demands. Consequently, the women's menopausal transition was influenced by their socioeconomic status as low-income immigrant workers. Therefore, without considering socioeconomic factors, their menopausal transition cannot be described, explained, or understood adequately.

```
                                    ┌─────────────────────────────────┐
                                    │ Transition Conditions           │
                                    │ Meaning                         │
                                    │ Expectations                    │
                                    │ Level of knowledge/skill        │
                                    │ Environment                     │
                      ┌──────────┐  │ Level of planning               │
                      │ Universal│  │ Emotional & physical well-being │
┌──────────────┐      │ Properties│  │   - Socio-economic planning    │
│ Types of     │      │          │  │   - Gender                      │
│ Transitions  │◄────►│ Process  │  │   - Context                     │
│              │      │ Direction│  │   - Attitudes toward health    │
│ Developmental│      │ Change in│  │     & illness                   │
│ Situational  │      │ Identity │  │   - Interrelationships among   │
│ Health/illness│     │ Roles    │  │     transition conditions       │
│ Organizational│     │ Relationships└─────────────────────────────────┘
└──────────────┘      │ Abilities│
                      │ Patterns of  ┌─────────────────────────────────┐
┌──────────────┐      │ behavior │   │ Indicators of Healthy Transition│
│ Number,      │◄────►│ Structure│   │ Subjective well-being           │
│ Seriousness, │      │ Function │   │ Mastery                         │
│ and Priorities│     │ Dynamics │   │ Well-being of relationships     │
│ of Transitions│     └──────────┘   │ Effective management of symptoms│
└──────────────┘                     └─────────────────────────────────┘
        
                    ┌─────────────────────────────────────────┐
                    │         Nursing Therapeutics             │
                    └─────────────────────────────────────────┘
```

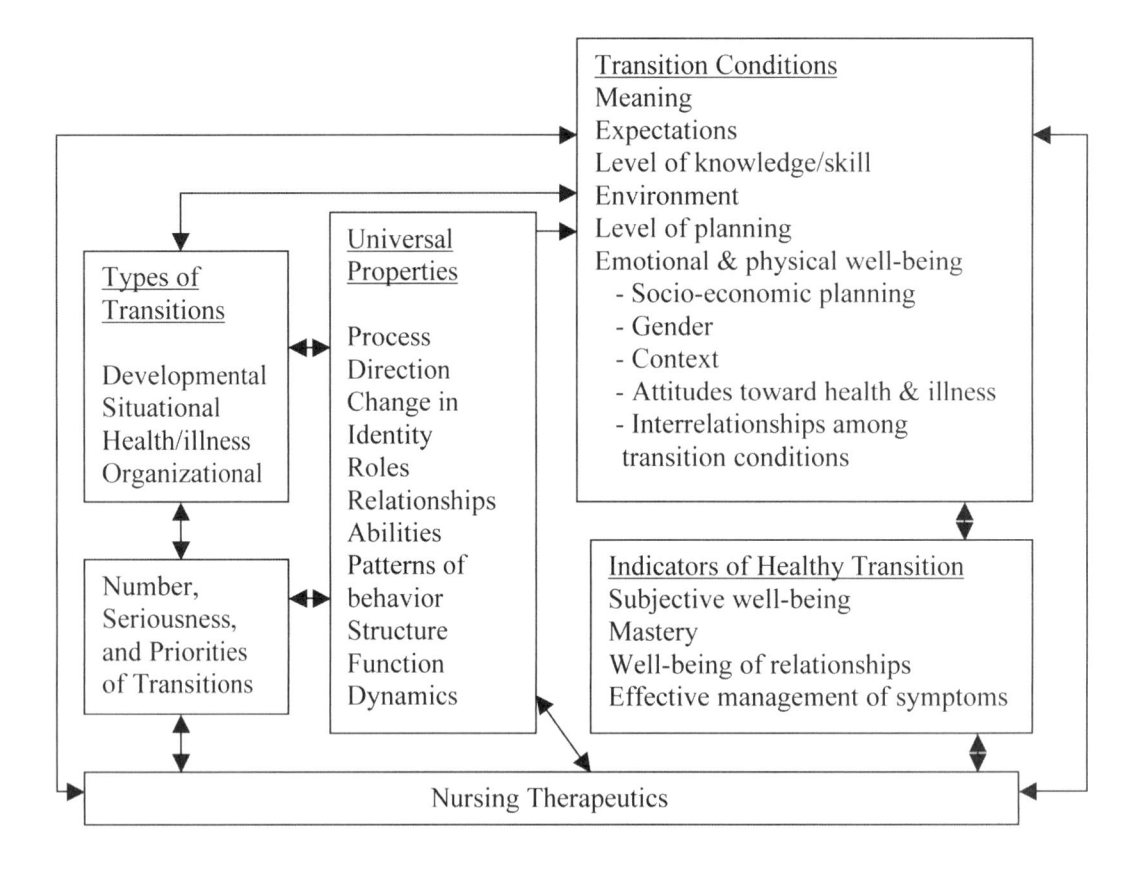

FIGURE 3.5.1 Model of a situation-specific theory: The menopausal transition experience of Korean immigrant women.

Gender

Menopausal transition cannot be adequately described and analyzed without careful attention to gender issues. Korean immigrant women's daily lives could be characterized by gender issues at the macroscopic societal level and microscopic family level (Cho, 1987; Kim & Hurh, 1987; Light & Bonacich, 1988). At the macroscopic societal level, many of the women worked in low-income jobs such as cleaners, seamstresses, waitresses, and family helpers. Even in their ethnic communities, the women occupied lower positions than did men. At the microscopic family level, the women often held lower positions than did their male partners, and were totally in charge of household responsibilities. In a patriarchal Korean culture, women's lower position in the family structure is relatively well known (Cho, 1987).

Context

Although the model includes environment as a transition condition, the concept of environment does not adequately address the dynamic interactions among cultural, social, political, historic, and psychological contexts. Context is more than the sum of the environments. Understanding the independent and interactive effects of the social, cultural, psychological, and biological changes within context is crucial for understanding women's unique menopausal experiences. As Ruzek, Olesen, and Clarke (1997) proposed, women's health cannot be fully understood without intertwining physical and psychological well-being as determined by the context in which the person operates. The results of this study are consistent with their position on context by showing that the women normalized or ignored their menopausal transitions under the strong influences of cultural attitude toward women's body experiences and the importance of family as a priority. Salient reasons for normalizing or ignoring health care needs during menopausal transitions existed for the women in this study.

Attitudes Toward Health and Illness

A fourth transition condition is the attitudes participants held toward health and illness. Although the model (Schumacher & Meleis, 1994) includes emotional and physical well-being as a transition condition, participants' attitudes toward emotional and physical well-being were not explicitly described. Women's menopausal transitions were influenced by their attitudes toward women's health problems. Because women in Korean culture tended to regard it as shameful behavior to talk about women's health problems in public (Im, 1994, 1997; Kim, 1993), their menopausal experience was lonely; they silently endured menopause alone.

Interrelationships Among the Transition Conditions

Interrelationships among the transition conditions should be incorporated in the model as a transition condition itself. While, in some cases, socioeconomic factors might be more important than other transition conditions in determining the nature of the menopausal transition, in other cases, the meanings of menopause were more important than was the socioeconomic variable. At other times, socioeconomic factors and the meanings of menopause were equally important.

Perceived Effective Management of Symptoms as an Indicator of Healthy Transitions

Within the transition framework (Schumacher & Meleis, 1994), subjective well-being, mastery, and well-being of relationships are included as indicators of healthy transition. Yet effective management of symptoms can be an additional indicator of successful menopausal transition. As the findings show, the women in this study ignored their symptoms for a variety of reasons. They thought that their symptoms would be temporary, were normal, and were caused by aging. Rarely did they have time to be concerned about their symptoms. When the symptoms were tolerable, they did not seek medical help. Only when the symptoms were so severe that they could not work adequately did they seek medical attention. Because their symptoms were tolerable, the symptoms did not have any special meanings, even though the symptoms could indicate potentially serious health problems such as cervical or ovarian cancer (Gorrie, McKinney, & Murray, 1994). To have healthy menopausal transitions, women are expected to promote their health through effective management of the perceived symptoms as well as to prevent other potential health problems through a program that might include taking supplemental calcium and getting exercise. In other words, a healthy menopausal transition can be indicated by effective management of actual and potential health problems. Therefore, effective management of symptoms is suggested as an indicator of healthy menopausal transition.

Implications for Theory Development

For further development of the theory of transitions, systematic research is an essential step. This chapter describes an integrative approach to theory development in which a study is used as a source of theory development along with the authors' previous experiences with the population. Using the theory-research-theory strategy, a theory of transition was modified and further developed through investigation of the menopausal transition of Korean immigrant women who were also experiencing other transitions. A situation-specific theory (Meleis, 1997) of the menopausal transition of low-income Korean immigrant women was proposed, with modification of the original model. The scope of application of the suggested situation-specific theory of menopausal transition of Korean immigrant women is limited. Yet the theory can be helpful for understanding the menopausal transition of Korean immigrant women. It might also be helpful in setting guidelines for the development of nursing therapeutics designed to support a healthy menopausal transition specifically for Korean immigrants. Some of the properties and concepts proposed could enhance understanding of the menopausal transitions of other immigrants.

The expansion and clarification of concepts through research using specific populations or particular fields of practice can provide more effective interpretation of transitions and guide nursing practice to be appropriate to the specific population. Theory-development efforts related to the responses and experiences of clients undergoing and experiencing transitions should consider diversities in transitions related to gender, socioeconomic status, culture, and other simultaneous transitions, and should be aimed at specific populations or particular fields of practice. Considering the results of the analysis and the modifications reported here, we propose that future theorists focus on situation-specific theories. This goal could be achieved through targeted research with diverse groups of clients who are experiencing transitions.

The findings of the study reported in this chapter support the notion that women's experiences are not one dimensional. For further theory development of transitions, the multidimensionality of women's experience during transitions should be incorporated by questioning the assumptions about concepts used in the theory, as well as the adequacy of the concepts in the theory. Assumptions about women's lives should be avoided, and uncovering properties, types, conditions, and interventions related to women's experiences should be among the strengths of the discipline of nursing.

REFERENCES

Brodman, K., Erdman, A. J., Jr., & Wolff, H. G. (1949). *Cornell Medical Index, health questionnaire: Manual*. New York: Cornell University Medical College.

Chick, N., & Meleis, A. I. (1986). Transitions: A nursing concern. In P.L. Chinn (Ed.), *Nursing research methodology: Issues and implementation* (237–257). Rockville, MD: Aspen.

Cho, O. (1987). Women in transition: The low income family. In E. Y. Yu & E. H. Phillips (Eds.), *Korean women in transition: At home and abroad* (71–84). Los Angeles: Center for Korean-American and Korean Studies, California State University.

Delany, J., Lupton, M. J., & Toth, E. (1988). *The curse: A cultural history of menstruation*. Chicago: University of Illinois.

Denzin, N. K. (1978). *Sociological methods: A source book* (2nd ed.). New York: McGraw-Hill.

Dickson, G. L. (1990a). The metalanguage of menopause research. *Image: Journal of Nursing Scholarship, 22*, 168–173.

Dickson, G. L. (1990b). A feminist poststructuralist analysis of the knowledge of menopause. *Advances in Nursing Science, 12*(3), 15–31.

Gorrie, T. M., McKinney, E. S., & Murray, S. S. (1994). *Foundations of maternal newborn nursing*. Philadelphia: W.B. Saunders.

Im, E. (1994). An analytical study of the relationship between menopausal symptoms and the stress of life events. *Journal of Korea Community Health Nursing Academic Society, 8*(2), 1–34.

Im, E. (1997). *Neglecting and ignoring menopause within a gendered multiple transitional context: Low-income Korean immigrant women*. Unpublished doctoral dissertation, University of California, San Francisco.

Kim, E. (1993). *The making of the modern female gender: The politics of gender in reproductive practices in Korea*. Unpublished doctoral dissertation, University of California, San Francisco.

Kim, K. C., & Hurh, W. M. (1987). Employment of Korean immigrant wives and the division of household tasks. In E.Y. Yu & E. Phillips (Eds.), *Korean women in tradition: At home and abroad* (199–218). Los Angeles, CA: California State University.

Li, S., Lanuza, D., Gulanick, M., Penckofer, S., & Holm, K. (1996). Perimenopause: The transition into menopause. *Health Care for Women International, 17*(4), 293–306.

Light, I., & Bonacich, E. (1988). *Immigrant entrepreneurs: Koreans in Los Angeles 1965–1982*. Berkeley, CA: University of California Press.

MacPherson, K. I. (1981). Menopause as disease: The social construction of a metaphor. *Advances in Nursing Science, 3*, 95–113.

MacPherson, K. I. (1985). Osteoporosis and menopause: A feminist analysis of the social construction of a syndrome. *Advances in Nursing Science, 7*, 11–22.

Martin, E. (1987). *The women in the body*. Boston: Beacon Press.
Meleis, A. I. (1975). Role insufficiency and role supplementation: A conceptual framework. *Nursing Research, 24*, 264–271.
Meleis, A. I. (1987). *Theoretical nursing: Development and progress*. Philadelphia: J.B. Lippincott.
Meleis, A. I. (1986). Theory development and domain concepts. In P. Moccia (Ed.), *New approaches to theory development* (3–21). New York: National League for Nursing.
Meleis, A. I. (1987). Women in transition: Being versus becoming or being and becoming. *Health Care for Women International, 8*, 199–217.
Meleis, A. I. (1997). *Theoretical nursing: Development and progress* (3rd. ed.). New York: J. B. Lippincott.
Ruzek, S. B., Olesen, V. L., & Clarke, A. E. (Ed.). (1997). *Women's health: Complexities and differences*. Columbus, OH: Ohio State University Press.
Schumacher, K. L., & Meleis, A. I. (1994). Transitions: A central concept in nursing. *Image: Journal of Nursing Scholarship, 26*, 119–127.
Strauss, A., & Corbin, J. (1990). *Basics of qualitative research: Grounded theory procedures and techniques*. Newbury Park, CA: Sage.
Weideger, P. (1976). *Menstruation and menopause*. New York: Alfred A. Knopf.

Reprinted with permission from: Im, E. O., & Meleis, A. I. (1999). A situation-specific theory of Korean immigrant women's menopausal transition. *Journal of Nursing Scholarship, 31*(4), 333–338.

3.6 HELPING ELDERLY PERSONS IN TRANSITION: A FRAMEWORK FOR RESEARCH AND PRACTICE

KAREN L. SCHUMACHER
PATRICIA S. JONES
AFAF IBRAHIM MELEIS

Abstract

Growing old is not an event. There is not a particular day or a certain birthday that marks a person as old. Growing old is a process of gains and losses that takes time. How this period of time is viewed by gerontological nurses shapes their work with elderly clients and their families. The nature of nursing assessment, the goals established with clients, and the interventions used are embedded in the nurse's perspective on aging. Similarly, the research questions posed by the gerontological nurse are embedded in a particular perspective. We propose that a transition framework provides a perspective on aging with significant potential for advancing gerontological nursing practice and research. Many transitions are experienced by elderly persons, and these transitions are inherently linked to the older person's health and need for nursing care. Indeed, it is often a transition that brings the older person into contact with professional nursing. The use of a transition framework recognizes the importance of transitions for the health of elderly persons. Thus, such a perspective leads to effective strategies for practice and productive lines of inquiry for research.

Introduction

The purpose of this chapter is to describe a transition framework for use in gerontological nursing practice and research and to demonstrate its use. We first provide an overview of transitions in elderly persons, briefly reviewing both conceptual work and nursing research on transitions. Next, we turn our attention to transitions and health, identifying characteristics and indicators of healthy transition processes. Finally, we describe several nursing therapeutics designed to facilitate smooth transitions for older clients. The use of this framework is demonstrated with a case example.

The Concept of Transition: Definition and Properties

A transition is a passage between two relatively stable periods of time. In this passage, the individual moves from one life phase, situation, or status, to another. Transitions are processes that occur over time and have a sense of flow and movement. They are ushered in by changes that trigger a period of disequilibrium and upheaval. During this period, the individual experiences profound changes in his or her external world, and in the manner in which that world is perceived. There often is a sense of loss or of alienation from what had been familiar and valued. During transitions, new skills, new relationships, and new coping strategies need to be developed (Chick & Meleis, 1986; Meleis, 1986; Meleis & Trangenstein, 1994).

Late life is a time of multiple transitions. Retirement, loss of spouse and friends, relocation to a new living situation, and the advent of chronic illness or frailty are just some of the transitions experienced by elderly persons. These transitions may be categorized as developmental, situational, or related to health and illness (Figure 3.6.1). Many of the transitions experienced by older persons involve loss and are undesired. However, some transitions are positive and are welcomed. For example, starting a new endeavor or developing new aspects of self are transitions that represent opportunities rather than losses.

What are the properties of a transition? First, a transition is precipitated by a significant marker event or turning point that requires new patterns of response. These markers prompt the recognition that business is not as usual and that new strategies are needed to handle even familiar, daily life experiences, such as managing one's finances, maintaining one's own health, or taking care of daily activities. Such strategies involve the development of new skills, new relationships, and new roles. Another characteristic of transitions is that they are processes that take time. Transitions span the whole period of time from the initial marker event until harmony and stability are again experienced. This time period is needed to experiment with different strategies and patterns of responses and to incorporate them into one's own repertoire. The time required for a transition is variable and depends on the nature of the change and the extent to which that change influences other aspects of a person's life. Another property of transition is that changes in identity, roles, and patterns of behavior occur. Transitions are not fleeting or superficial changes; rather, they involve fundamental changes in one's view of self and the world (Chick & Meleis, 1986; Meleis & Trangenstein, 1994; Schumacher & Meleis, 1994).

Transitions often are conceptualized in terms of stages to capture their movement, direction, and flow as they evolve over time. A classic description of the stages of transition is found in Bridges' study (1980). According to Bridges, the first stage of a transition is "a period of endings" in which there is disengagement from relationships or from ways of behaving as well as a change in the person's sense of self. The second stage, termed the "neutral zone," is an in-between period, a time when a person experiences disorientation caused by the losses in the first stage, followed by disintegration of systems that were in place. This is an uncomfortable but necessary period of time. Only by going through the neutral zone can persons become open to new possibilities. The final stage of a transition is that of "new beginnings," and is marked by finding meaning and experiencing some control. Persons must go through all three stages to deal effectively with the transition. However, the stages of a transition do not necessarily occur in a linear manner. Rather, they may be sequential, parallel, or overlapping.

Transitions also can be described in terms of patterns. Single or multiple transitions may occur within a given period of time, and they may be related or unrelated. Young (1990) alluded to the phenomenon of patterns of transition when she observed that relocation to a nursing home can occur in the context of other transitions and can catalyze further life changes. She also noted that relocation may include elements of situational, health/illness, and developmental transitions. Gerontological nurses often deal with such patterns of transition in clinical practice, but very little work has been done with theory development and research in this area. Fruitful directions for future scholarship would be to name and describe transition patterns and to explore the relationships between different patterns and client outcomes. In this chapter, we suggest three patterns of transition that we believe merit attention: (1) the sequential pattern, (2) the simultaneous/related pattern, and (3) the simultane-

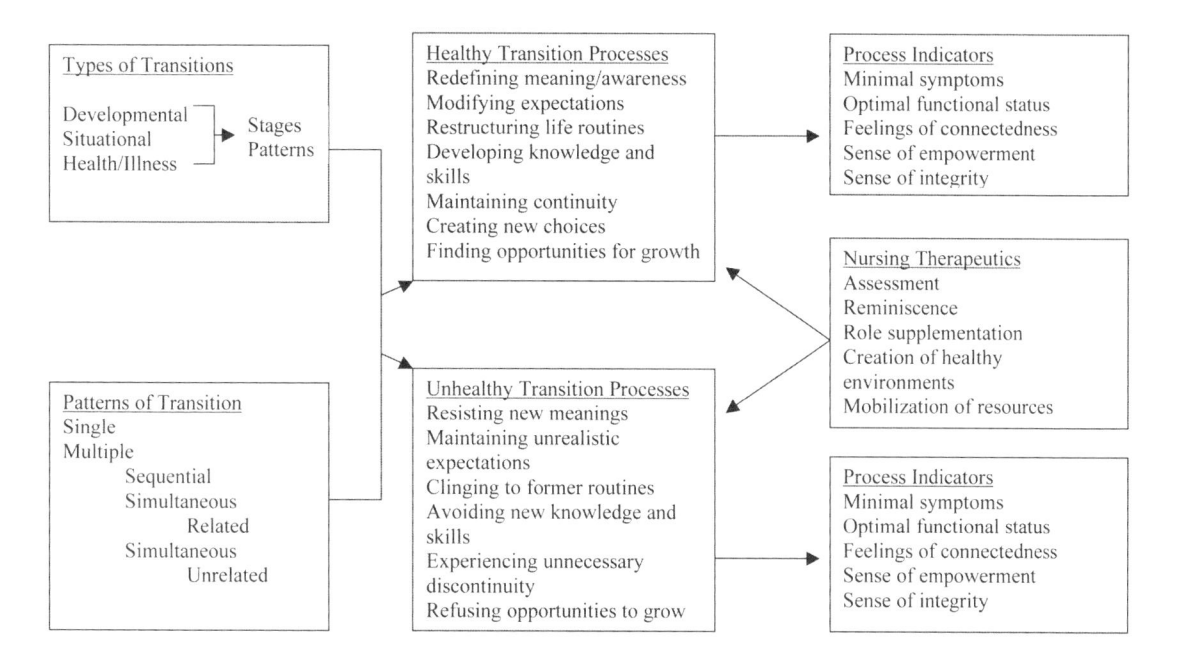

FIGURE 3.6.1 Transition and health: A framework for gerontological nursing.

Types of Transitions
- Developmental
- Situational
- Health/Illness

→ Stages, Patterns

Patterns of Transition
- Single
- Multiple
  - Sequential
  - Simultaneous Related
  - Simultaneous Unrelated

Healthy Transition Processes
- Redefining meaning/awareness
- Modifying expectations
- Restructuring life routines
- Developing knowledge and skills
- Maintaining continuity
- Creating new choices
- Finding opportunities for growth

Unhealthy Transition Processes
- Resisting new meanings
- Maintaining unrealistic expectations
- Clinging to former routines
- Avoiding new knowledge and skills
- Experiencing unnecessary discontinuity
- Refusing opportunities to grow

Process Indicators
- Minimal symptoms
- Optimal functional status
- Feelings of connectedness
- Sense of empowerment
- Sense of integrity

Nursing Therapeutics
- Assessment
- Reminiscence
- Role supplementation
- Creation of healthy environments
- Mobilization of resources

Process Indicators
- Minimal symptoms
- Optimal functional status
- Feelings of connectedness
- Sense of empowerment
- Sense of integrity

---

ous/unrelated pattern. Each pattern is described briefly.

In sequential transitions, there is a ripple effect in which one transition leads to another over time. For example, the death of one's spouse may lead to relocation to a nursing home, or retirement from paid employment may lead to the emergence of new dimensions of self. It is possible for this ripple effect to extend over a long period of time. The instance in which retirement leads to insufficient income, which in turn leads to a decline in health status, and eventually to chronic illness and loss of social interaction, is an example of a long-term, cumulative ripple effect.

Simultaneous transitions are clusters of related or unrelated transitions that occur together during a given period of time. In simultaneous, related transitions, a marker event precipitates numerous transitions. For example, the marker event of a stroke may usher in a cluster of transitions in functional abilities, identity, and living arrangements. The complexity of such transitions may be compounded by simultaneous transitions for the older adult's family members, who may take on the caregiving role and undergo changes in work and family roles. Ade-Ridder and Kaplan (1993) alluded to this pattern of transition when they noted that a transition for an older adult creates a variety of countertransitions for the family.

Simultaneous transitions also may occur without being initially related to one another. For example, an older adult may suffer a decline in health at the same time his or her adult child is experiencing the transition to an "empty nest." Such transitions in a given family happen concurrently and, although not directly related at first, may become intertwined over time.

Nursing Research on Transitions

What has nursing research shown about transitions? First, transitions may be accompanied by uncertainty, emotional distress, interpersonal conflict, and worry. Michels (1988) documented the uncertainty experienced by family caregivers of elderly persons during the transition from hospital to home. Johnson, Morton, and Knox (1992) found that nursing home admissions, too, are characterized by uncertainty. In this transition, uncertainty was related to lack of information and knowledge about the nature of nursing homes and the boundaries for family involvement there. Families also described feelings of sadness and anger, as well as a sense of failure when an older adult was admitted to a nursing home. Lack of communication with nursing home staff added to the emotional conflict. The transition to needing assistance with self-care activities also may bring about emotional distress. For example, Conn, Taylor, and Messina (1995) investigated the transition to needing medication assistance and found that some older adults were frustrated, depressed, or angry about requiring assistance. The researchers noted that nurses should expect some caregivers and care recipients to experience difficulties in their relationship as the caregiver begins assisting the older adult and that they should be encouraged to express their feelings about these transitions in role relationships.

Bull (1992) found that the transition from hospital to home was characterized by worry. In semistructured interviews, participants identified worries ranging from apprehension about learning new skills to distress about disruption in the family's usual activities of daily living. Bull also described the movement from worry to mastery as the transition evolved. By two months after discharge from the hospital, participants had established new routines and felt in control of the situation. The movement from worry to mastery found in the interviews was corroborated by quantitative data that showed a steady decline in anxiety and depression (Bull, Maruyama, & Luo, 1995).

The study by Bull and colleagues (Bull, 1992; Bull, Maruyama, & Luo, 1995) is noteworthy for the way in which the dimension of time was incorporated into the research design. In this study, change over time was documented by collecting data at two points in the transition. Such a design is congruent with the nature of the transition experience. Because transitions are processes, research designs need to be planned so that they capture the evolution of the transition experience.

There is some evidence that older persons and their family members do not always receive the professional support they need during a transition. In Michel's (1988) study, 73% of the older adults returned to their homes with a home-care regimen consisting of three or more components, such as prescription medications, dietary changes, assessment of signs and symptoms, and continuing care of an incision, tube, drain, or colostomy. Nearly two-thirds had been instructed on how to care for themselves and carry out their prescribed regimen, but only half acknowledged that someone had asked if they had questions or concerns about their care before the transition to home took place. Some family members had difficulties assuming caregiving responsibilities, and they did not always have the opportunity to participate in discharge planning to prepare them for the transition. Bull, Jervis, and Her (1995) also found that some family members of older patients were inadequately prepared for hospital discharge, did not have the opportunity for input into discharge decisions, and encountered problems with the coordination of services. Stewart, Archbold, Harvath, and Nkongho (1993) investigated a broad range of learning needs of family caregivers and found that health professionals were perceived as sources of information about taking care of the physical needs of the care receiver and setting up services in the home, but that caregivers reported learning very little from health professionals about taking care of the care receiver's emotional needs and handling the stress of caregiving.

Transitions and Health

We turn now to a consideration of transitions and health. What are the characteristics of a healthy transition? We approach this question by considering transition processes and process indicators (see Figure 3.6.1). Transition processes are the cognitive, behavioral, and interpersonal processes through which the transition unfolds. In other words, they are what happens during a transition. In healthy transitions, these processes move the individual in the direction of health, whereas in unhealthy transitions, they move the individual in the direction of vulnerability and risk.

Process indicators are measurable indices of how the transition is going at any point in time. A process indicator can be thought of as a stop-action snapshot of client well-being at a key point in the ongoing transition process. Assessed periodically, process indicators provide a way of tracking client progress through the transition. We use the term "process indicators" rather than "outcomes" because the process should be assessed periodically over the course of the transition, not just at its conclusion. When the older adult's experience is analyzed using a transition perspective, it is difficult to consider outcomes in the same way as when the older adult's experiences are viewed in isolation from time and significant others. From a transition perspective, "outcomes" evolve over the course of the transition and also are connected to life experiences prior to and after the transition. Process indicators could be used as client outcomes in research, but only with the caveat that they are part of the client's ongoing life experiences.

Healthy Transition Processes

Seven healthy transition processes and seven corresponding unhealthy processes have been identified (see Figure 3.6.1) and are described below. Over the course of the transition, there is a dynamic tension between healthy and unhealthy processes. Both the future toward which the transition is moving and the past that is being left behind exert a pull on the elderly client. These processes move the client through the "neutral zone" of the transition toward the next phase or situation in his or her life. The gerontological nurse should be alert to the presence of these processes in clients in transition and should monitor the direction in which they are proceeding.

1. Redefining meanings is one process that takes place during a healthy transition (Davis & Grant, 1994; Langner, 1995). The elderly client and his or her family actively engage in exploring the meaning of the transition and in finding new meanings. Previous meanings that do not apply to the new situation are recognized, and new meanings are discovered. The process of creating meaning is complex, and time is needed for the older person to work through it. When the transition is proceeding in a healthy direction, the general movement is toward rethinking and redefining meanings. In unhealthy transitions, there is resistance to redefining meanings. The older person and his or her family do not consider the meaning of the transition and attempt to apply old definitions to the new situation.

2. Modifying expectations is another process that characterizes healthy transitions. Long-standing expectations about self, others, and the future may be called into question during a transition (Dewar & Morse, 1995; King, Porter, & Rowe, 1994; Wilson & Billones, 1994), and the older person may be reluctant to give up these expectations. However, in healthy transitions, previous expectations are gradually modified and replaced with new expectations that are realistic for the new situation. In unhealthy transitions, the older adult and family maintain unrealistic expectations and anticipate a future that probably cannot happen.

3. Another characteristic of healthy transitions is the restructuring of life routines. Routines serve to order daily life and provide predictability, manageability, and even pleasure (Cartwright, Archbold, Stewart, & Limandri, 1994). In healthy transitions, routines are restructured in a way that is congruent with the new situation and allows the person to regain a sense that his or her life is predictable, manageable, and pleasurable (Daley, 1993). In unhealthy transitions, such restructuring does not take place. Instead, the older adult attempts to cling to former routines even though they no longer work in the new situation. If the person's abilities and the environment that sustained daily routines are no longer present, an unhealthy transition may lead to no routine at all. In such instances, daily life may become unpredictable, disordered, or empty, particularly for individuals who have a history of orderliness in their lives.

4. Healthy transitions are characterized further by developing new knowledge and skills (Brown,

1995; Edwardson, 1988). Specific needs for knowledge and skills are identified, and opportunities for their development are sought (Davis & Grant, 1994). Over time, the older adult's knowledge and skills closely fit the demands of the new situation. In unhealthy transitions, new knowledge and skills are avoided. Elderly persons and families try to manage the new situation with knowledge and skills that may have been sufficient in the past, but are no longer useful in the present situation. Opportunities for developing knowledge and skills are not taken, resulting in a gap between the demands of the situation and the knowledge and skills available to meet those demands.

5. Although transitions involve endings and disruptions, not everything in the life of the elderly client and his or her family changes. There are continuities, even as change occurs (Burgener, Shimer, & Murrell, 1992; Cartwright, et al., 1994). Healthy transitions are characterized by maintaining whatever continuity is possible in identity, relationships, and environment. Continuity facilitates coping with the changes brought about by the transition and fosters the elderly person's ability to integrate the transition experience into his or her life as a whole. In unhealthy transitions, there is discontinuity and disruption where it does not need to occur. There is lack of awareness of the possibilities for continuity, and change that could be avoided happens anyway. In such instances, transitions become more pervasive than they need to be and older adults sustain losses that could have been prevented.

6. The transitions experienced by elderly persons often are associated with losses, but it is possible that gains occur as well. One of the gains that may be experienced during a transition is the opportunity for new choices (Adlersberg & Thorne, 1990; Happ, Williams, Strumpf, & Burger, 1996). In healthy transitions, the elderly person is open to exploring new choices. He or she engages in seeking and creating new opportunities. Through the exercise of choice, the older adult actively shapes the transition process. Unhealthy transitions are characterized by limiting choices. Older adults themselves may limit the choices available, or choices may be limited by others in the environment (Nick, 1992). The process of limiting choices forecloses possibilities before they are explored. Choices that could be made are passed by, and the elderly person and family are passive with respect to determining the direction of the transition.

7. Finally, healthy transitions are characterized by finding opportunities for personal growth (Langner, 1995; McDougall, 1995; Young, 1990). New levels of self-awareness, new dimensions of identity and relationships, and new abilities can emerge during transitions. In healthy transitions, such opportunities for growth are embraced in a way that makes personal development and self-actualization possible. In unhealthy transitions, opportunities for growth are rejected. The developmental process is stalled or thwarted in a way that precludes the unfolding and emerging of self.

Process Indicators

As noted previously, process indicators are measurable indices of how a transition is proceeding. Many such process indicators can be used for assessment during a transition. In this chapter, we have identified five process indicators for consideration (see Figure 3.6.1), which are described below. We present them to exemplify an approach to evaluating the transition process and to stimulate others to identify additional indicators.

1. The elderly person's symptom experience is the first process indicator we consider. During a transition, the older person may experience new symptoms or exacerbation of previously existing symptoms (Ferrell & Schneider, 1988; Kozak, Campbell, & Hughes, 1996). Symptoms should be managed as much as possible so that the elderly person can attend to the transition process itself. If the beginning of the transition is marked by an increase in symptoms, there should be a measurable decline in their frequency and severity over the course of the transi-

tion. Although some physical and behavioral symptoms may be inevitable, they should be controlled as much as current symptom management strategies allow. The presence of symptoms that could be controlled suggests that the transition process is proceeding in an unhealthy direction. Patterns of symptoms and the management strategies used by the client should be noted carefully because they provide insight into how the transition is going.

2. Functional status is the next process indicator we propose. For the elderly person, changes in functional status may occur during a transition (Glass & Maddox, 1992; King, et al., 1994). However, when a healthy transition process is taking place, the highest possible level of physical and cognitive functioning is achieved over the course of the transition. The elderly person's self-care ability, independence, and mobility are enhanced to the furthest extent possible. A suboptimal level of functioning suggests an unhealthy transition process.

3. Another process indicator is the elderly person's sense of connectedness to a meaningful interpersonal network (Daley, 1993; Rickelman, Gallman, & Parra, 1994; Windriver, 1993). Although disruption in relationships may occur during a transition, there will be evidence of a regained sense of connectedness when the transition process is proceeding in a healthy direction. If the transition involved loss of one or more relationships, new or transformed relationships should be forged during the transition process to provide a stable source of connectedness by the completion of the transition process. Feelings of disconnectedness or isolation indicate unhealthy transition processes.

4. Another process indicator is a sense of empowerment (Jones & Meleis, 1993; Nyström & Segesten, 1994). The elderly person's sense of autonomy, self-determination, and personal agency may be threatened during the disruption brought about by the transition. However, a new sense of empowerment is found when the transition process is healthy. The older adult regains some control over his or her life. He or she is able to make decisions and put them into effect. For older adults with severe cognitive or physical limitations, there is an appropriate transfer of empowerment to a family member or significant other. Inappropriate disempowerment is indicative of an unhealthy transition process. Disempowerment may be manifested in loss of control, inability to make and carry out decisions, and inappropriate assumption of control by persons in the older adult's environment.

5. The final process indicator we propose is a sense of integrity (Erikson, Erikson, & Kivnick, 1986; Finfgeld, 1995; Mercer, Nichols, & Doyle, 1988). A sense of integrity includes a sense of wholeness and coherence. Personal growth and new insights about self are evidence of a healthy transition. There also is the sense that the transition fits into one's life story in a meaningful way. A loss of integrity indicates an unhealthy transition process. Loss of integrity may be manifested in a sense of fragmentation or meaninglessness in one's life course.

Nursing Therapeutics

The goals of nursing therapeutics from a transition perspective are to facilitate healthy transition processes, to decrease unhealthy transitions, and to support positive process indicators (Meleis & Trangenstein, 1994). Many nursing therapeutics could be used to facilitate transitions. We have selected five for discussion here that we believe have particular relevance for elderly clients (see Figure 3.6.1). These therapeutics take into account needs that are specific to this stage of the life cycle, such as the needs for life review and for integration into new living environments. They also take into account challenges often experienced by elderly persons, such as memory loss and changes in mobility.

Nursing Assessment

Nursing assessment is the basis for all nursing therapeutics. The use of a transition perspective suggests several principles for assessment. First, the nature of transitions as dynamic, ongoing processes suggests that nursing assessment must be continuous (McCracken, 1994; Moneyham & Scott, 1995). As the transition evolves, the nurse needs to address changes and developments in the client's situation. Because it is not possible to predict the course of a transition at its outset, assessment must be ongoing. A linear sequence of nursing actions beginning with assessment and moving in turn through planning, implementation, and evaluation is not congruent with a transition perspective. Rather, assessment must span the whole period of transition so that nursing care can evolve along with the movement of the transition process. Such ongoing assessment requires particular vigilance on the nurse's part, plus creation of a health-care context that supports frequent contact between the nurse and client.

Continuous assessment by the nurse takes into account patterns of transition. Knowing that multiple transitions often occur for elderly persons leads to the anticipation of simultaneous and sequential transitions. For example, knowing that the death of the spouse of a frail elderly person may mean that the elderly person must move from his or her home shapes the nurse's assessment of resources and options for the future. Knowing that a transition for an older adult often has a ripple effect through the family means that a thorough family assessment should be included in the assessment process.

Although assessment is a continuous process for the nurse practicing within a transition perspective, we suggest assessment of the process indicators identified previously at critical points during the transition. The use of process indicators provides the nurse with a way of tracking client progress and provides for early detection of difficulties at critical points in the transition.

The use of formal assessment instruments aids the nurse in making these periodic evaluations of the transition process. They provide an objective measure of the client's situation, allowing the nurse to identify deviations from population norms as well as deviations from the client's own norm. In Table 3.6.1, we provide examples of tools that could be used to measure process indicators. The use of process indicators is relevant with family members as well as with elderly persons. The timing and frequency of their use should be determined by the nature of the transition and the extent of the changes it precipitates.

TABLE 3.6.1 Tools for Measuring Process Indicators

Symptom Experience

State/Trait Anxiety Inventory (Spielberger, 1983)

Geriatric Depression Scale (Yesavage & Brink, 1983)

Mini-Mental State Questionnaire (Folstein, Folstein, & McHugh, 1975)

McGill Pain Questionnaire (Melzack, 1975)

Functional Status

Index of Activities of Daily Living (Katz, Ford, Moskowitz, Jackson, & Jaffe, 1963)

Multidimensional Functional Assessment (Duke University, 1978)

Connectedness

Mutuality Scale (Archbold, Stewart, Greenlick, & Harvath, 1992)

Adult Attachment Scale (Lipson-Parra, 1989)

Empowerment

Desired Control Scale (Reid & Ziegler, 1981)

Integrity

Fulfillment of Meaning Scale (Burbank, 1992)

Reminiscence

Reminiscence (Burnside, 1990; Burnside & Haight, 1992) is a nursing therapeutic that facilitates integration of the transition into the life course. Transitions must be viewed within the context of the elderly individual's whole life. Although they involve disruption and change, placing transitions within the context of the life course facilitates the processes of exploring meaning and discovering areas in which continuity with the past is still possible. The articulation of life themes through reminiscing supports the process of growth and development of identity. Reminiscence also can assist the older adult in reinterpreting the meanings of life situations, achieving resolution of ongoing issues, and transcending old pains. Thus reminiscence supports the process of new beginnings as the older adult proceeds through the transition.

Reminiscence is derived from "debriefing," an approach to therapy used with victims of disasters and with individuals who have encountered other crisis situations. Debriefing provides an opportunity to recount the difficult experience and to relive the reactions and emotions that were encountered. Reminiscence is like debriefing in that it provides an opportunity to reflect on important life experiences and to integrate the past into the present. For the person in transition, reminiscence provides an important bridge between the past and present as he or she ends one situation or stage in life and embarks on another.

For older adults with memory loss, the process of reminiscence must be tailored to individual needs. The memories that an older adult has depends on the type and extent of memory loss. Using reminiscence for older adults with memory loss may require innovative strategies (McDougall, 1994; Rentz, 1995). For example, finding a person who serves as a reservoir of memories for an elderly person with memory loss may facilitate reminiscing. The use of prompts, such as photographs or music (Cartwright et al., 1994) also may serve to stimulate memories.

Role Supplementation

Role supplementation is a nursing therapeutic that facilitates the process of developing new knowledge and skills. It is a nursing therapeutic that has been used for parental caregivers (Brackley, 1992), for new parents (Gaffney, 1992; Meleis & Swendsen, 1978; Swendsen, Meleis, & Jones, 1978), for Alzheimer's patients (Kelley & Lakin, 1987), and for cardiac rehabilitation (Dracup et al., 1984), and it has much potential for use with elderly persons. Role supplementation provides the support needed to revise skills and capabilities continuously as demands evolve in the new situation. It is defined as the process of bringing into awareness the behaviors, sentiments, sensations, and goals involved in a given role (Meleis, 1975), and it is particularly useful for persons taking on a new role or experiencing a transition in a long-standing role. In the process of role supplementation, information and experiences are conveyed to the role incumbent and his or her significant others so that the role transition can be made smoothly. It includes heightening awareness of one's own role and another's, and the dynamics of their interrelationships (Meleis, 1975).

Role supplementation has several components. One is role clarification or the identification of all aspects of a role. For example, role clarification may include a discussion of what is involved in being a nursing home resident. For a family member, it may be the identification of behaviors and feelings associated with the caregiving role. Another component of role supplementation is the process of role taking. Role taking is the empathetic ability to understand the position and point of view of another and to understand how one's role may affect other persons.

Several strategies are used in role supplementation. One is role modeling or the opportunity to observe someone in the role that is being taken on. Another is role rehearsal, the process of mentally or physically enacting the new role that the person is moving toward. Although there are multiple ways of enacting a given role, there are some aspects of roles that tend to be stable and consistent across individuals. For example, although there are some common features of nursing home roles, how they are enacted by a given individual is a dynamic and creative process. Providing clients and their significant others with opportunities to enact and rehearse both the common and creative features of a role leads to greater comfort with the role. Another strategy that facilitates transition for elderly persons and their families is the mobilization of a reference group that is responsive to the various situational and long-term needs of older adults. Reference groups may be for mobility and exercise, for eating, for recreation, and for dealing with chronic illness.

Creation of a Healthy Environment

Another nursing therapeutic for older persons in transition is creation of a healthy environment. We define "environment" broadly to include the older person's physical, social, political, and cultural surroundings. During a transition, the environment itself or the elderly person's interaction with a familiar environment may change. For example, in relocation or migration it is the environment itself that changes. It is the older person's interaction with the environment that changes when a decrease in mobility or cognition limits the ability to function in a familiar environment.

There are many facets to creating a healthy environment. One is to structure the environment so that it provides safety and security (McCracken, 1994; Taft, Delaney, Seman, & Stansell, 1993). Another is to facilitate access to what the elderly person needs and uses to accomplish daily routines (Daly & Berman, 1993). Honoring cultural traditions is another way of creating a healthy environment (Jones, 1995). Finally, freeing the environment of obstacles to dignity and personal integrity fosters a healthy environment (Magee, et al., 1993). The use of a transition perspective means that the goal of nursing is the creation of an environment that is dynamic and flexible enough to change in synchrony with the elderly person's evolving needs. It also means that the nurse maintains ongoing involvement with the older adult and family as they continuously modify, restructure, and reinvent the environment to meet the needs of the older family member.

Mobilization of Resources

Older adults in transition face new situations and demands for which previously developed resources may no longer be adequate. Therefore, mobilization of resources is an important aspect of nursing practice within a transition perspective. Enhancement of both personal and environmental resources appropriate to the individual's needs is necessary.

Resources include personal, family, and community resources. Specific resources in each category may be stable or changing, ongoing or newly developed. For example, personal resources may change during a transition, necessitating the mobilization of new personal resources. Similarly, the older adult may have long-standing family resources, but may need additional resources to meet the challenges of a transition. The community resources available to older adults differ according to geographic location and political policies, thus necessitating the ongoing mobilization of new community resources. In short, to mobilize resources, the nurse needs to consider not only the availability of resources, but whether or not they are stable or changing. Also, the nurse must consider whether existing resources are adequate or if new resources must be developed.

Mobilizing personal inner resources is one step toward facilitating healthy transitions in older adults. Scholars variously refer to personal resources as adaptability (Jones, 1991), coherence (Antonovsky, 1987), and hardiness (Kobasa, 1979). Magnani (1990) identified "hardiness" as antecedent to successful aging and recommended that nurses help older adults remain independent and optimize normal, healthy aging using three strategies: helping to strengthen the older adult's self-concept; helping the older adult to see his or her life events in perspective; and encouraging appropriate forms of activity.

Another personal resource is wellness (Alford & Futrell, 1992; U.S. Department of Health and Human Services [USDHHS] & American Association for Retired Persons [AARP], 1991; Walker, 1992). A healthy lifestyle should be promoted during a transition. The nurse can encourage regular exercise, a nutritious diet, control of alcohol intake, and abstinence from smoking. Regular primary health care services also are important during a transition.

A strong immune system is another resource that influences the transition process. Exposure to new environmental threats challenges the ability of the immune system to protect the body successfully and maintain physiological integrity. Therefore, promoting activities that strengthen the immune system is one way of mobilizing personal resources. Recent research has demonstrated a variety of behaviors that increase immune system competence, including laughter (Cousins, 1989), exercise (Nash, 1994), and a positive spirit (Kinion & Kolcaba, 1992). Regular immunizations against influenza and other infectious diseases provide extra immune protection. For some frail elderly persons, a compromised immune system may call for use of antibiotics to prevent as well as to treat infections.

Energy is another personal resource that facilitates smooth transitions. Energy is essential for developing new skills, for pursuing new opportunities for growth, and for maintaining functional status. The mobilization of energy must be a deliberate strategy if the older adult is to remain independent and empowered. Proper diet and regular exercise are key factors in energy mobilization. However, energy is holistic; thus psychological, social, and spiritual factors also are significant in its mobilization. These factors influence the older person's motivation to engage actively in life and to seek new opportunities for growth. In the Jones and Meleis (1993) Health Empowerment Model, mobilization of resources is an integral part of promoting energy for health and healthy transitions (see Figure 3.6.2).

Family resources also may need to be mobilized to assist an aging client in transition. Family resources can be described in terms of structural, economic, and cultural factors. The availability of family members to assist and support an aging person is a primary resource. However, it is possible that even in cultures where caring for aging family members is highly valued, the availability of family caregivers may be limited. In today's global society, potential family caregivers may be thousands of miles away from the person needing care. Furthermore, whole families may be in transition at the same time, as is the case with immigration. In such instances, the demands on each member are high. Thus, consideration of the needs of the whole family is necessary.

Community resources outside of the family may be needed to supplement what the family is able to provide. Some cultural groups tend to do more direct caregiving and to use community services less than others. For example, it has been shown that Blacks and Latinos enter nursing homes at lower rates than do European Americans and rely on informal, family-based support systems to a greater degree than European Americans (Angel, Angel, & Himes, 1992). This means that Black and Latino families caring for elderly family members may need more assistance in mobilizing and accessing community resources to support caregiving at home.

Throughout their lives, individuals participate as members of many different communities. Church and community service organizations are examples. In late adulthood, continued contact with members of these communities contributes to a sense of connectedness. The respect, common history, and affirmation that come with membership in these groups contribute to meaning, life satisfaction, and self-esteem.

Case Study

We demonstrate the use of a transition framework in practice by means of a case study. Mr. Adams is a 76-year-old widower whose wife died one month following the diagnosis of leukemia. With her illness and death, Mr. Adams entered a period of transition that lasted for over a year. This transition also involved his daughter, Gloria White. Mrs. White is a middle-aged woman who lives in another country with her husband and teenage children. Prior to her mother's death, Mrs. White visited her parents about once a year. Because of her family responsibilities and the expense of international travel, most of the communication between Mr. and Mrs. Adams and their daughter had been by telephone.

Mr. Adams had a long history of transient ischemic attacks that occasionally were accompanied by loss of consciousness. These episodes were followed by mental confusion and difficulty with activities of daily living. Prior to her death, Mrs. Adams had provided the assistance that he needed at these times.

After Mrs. Adams' death, family and friends encouraged Mr. Adams to move into a retirement center for increased assistance and social contact. However, he strongly resisted such a move. Throughout his home were pictures, paintings, furniture, and other items that represented significant memories, not only of his wife, but of his own

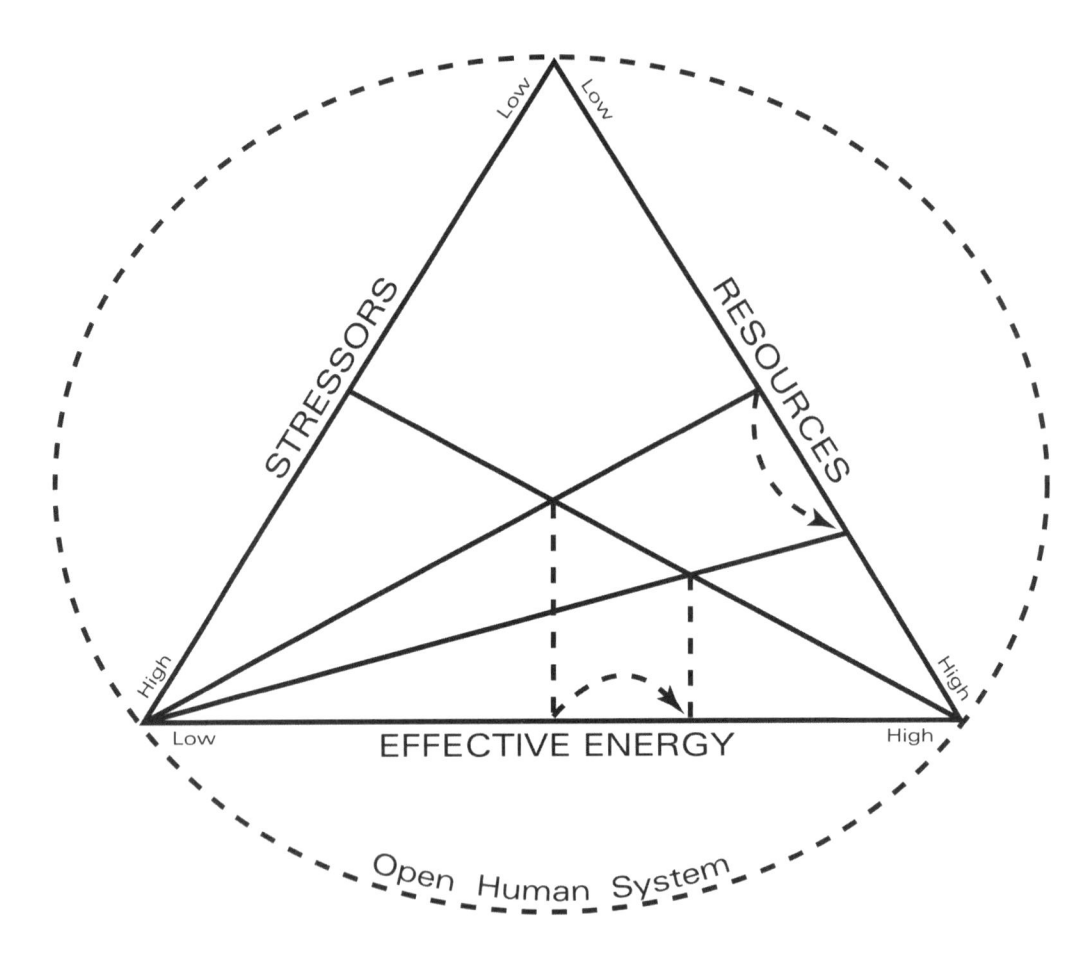

FIGURE 3.6.2 Mobilization of resources in the Jones and Meleis Health Empowerment Model (Jones & Meleis, 1993).

parents and childhood. On the property was a small workshop that housed an elaborate electric train, his lifelong hobby. In the garden were flowers and flowering shrubs that he and his wife had carefully chosen. Mr. Adams became angry and agitated when people encouraged him to move away from this familiar and meaningful environment.

Mr. Adams' health problems, compounded by his grief, emotional distress, and geographical distance from his daughter, worried his next-door neighbor. She contacted a gerontological clinical nurse specialist who worked with a local parish nursing program and asked for her advice. With Mr. Adams' permission, the nurse made a home visit and began providing nursing care using a transition perspective. Her initial assessment revealed the physical and emotional symptoms he was experiencing as well as his difficulties with activities of daily living. He felt isolated and alone. He also felt as if his autonomy and rights were being taken away and that he was going to be forced to leave his home. The initial nursing assessment included calls to Mrs. White and a complete assessment of her family responsibilities and resources. The nurse learned that Mrs. White was in the process of getting a divorce and thus was going through a simultaneous transition.

After the initial assessment, the nurse began to assist Mr. Adams with mobilizing community resources to enable him to remain in his home.

Obvious needs included assistance with activities of daily living, socialization, and supervision to prevent harm. Assessment of resources also included identifying his own strengths as well as what was necessary to supplement those strengths to continue living independently. Arrangements were made for home care attendants to assist with activities of daily living, domestic chores, grocery shopping, and transportation. "Meals on wheels" were arranged, medications were organized for easy administration, and an electronic personal alert system for use in an emergency was set up.

The nurse also helped Mrs. White negotiate the transition in her relationship with her father by assisting her to take on the caregiving role from a distance in the context of multiple family responsibilities and limited financial resources. Areas in which she could provide assistance and support to her father were identified. Also identified were realistic caregiving expectations for her. During this time, Mrs. White was a resource to her father, but at the same time was a family member needing support for her own transitions.

Because she realized that major transitions such as loss of one's spouse often are followed by further transitions, the nurse maintained ongoing assessment with Mr. Adams and Mrs. White. For about 6 months, the initial arrangements provided the support Mr. Adams needed and he continued to live at home. Then Mr. Adams' physical health began to decline. His episodes of transient ischemia increased, and he had several falls that caused injuries. It became clear that he could not continue to live alone, and Mrs. White came to help him make decisions and arrangements for a new living situation. He decided to enter a group living center where he could have his own two-bedroom duplex, but also would have all the assistance he needed.

In preparation for the move, extensive time was allowed for Mr. Adams to reminisce about the life he had enjoyed in his home. Possessions with special meaning were selected for relocation with him to the new environment. Role supplementation prepared him for his new role in the retirement center. Because the move was another major transition, arrangements were made for his daughter to be present to provide added support during this time.

The move to the assisted living center was difficult for Mr. Adams. He missed his home a great deal and initially had difficulty identifying the new environment as home. For a while his health problems continued with frequent fluctuations in his functional abilities and mental status. As the months passed, however, his health stabilized. His emotional well-being increased, and his cognitive status improved. He was able to engage in more self-care and began to participate in activities with other residents. Four months after his relocation, Mr. Adams felt at home in the retirement center. He had made friends there and found that he still had an acceptable degree of autonomy. Also, he had found meaning in assisting a blind resident who needed a companion to accompany him on outings. Mr. Adams expressed to his daughter and friends that the move had turned out to be the right decision after all.

Implications for Practice and Knowledge Development

The framework that we have proposed extends our previous work with the concept of transition (Chick & Meleis, 1986; Meleis, 1986; Meleis & Trangenstein, 1994; Schumacher & Meleis, 1994) by identifying specific transition processes, by suggesting indicators of client progress through transitions, and by identifying nursing therapeutics with particular relevance for older clients in transition. We have related transition processes to health by identifying processes that lead to well-being and those that lead to increasing vulnerability. This work is based on the premise that the mission of nursing is to facilitate healthy transitions and to prevent the risks to health that can arise during transitions (Meleis & Trangenstein, 1994).

How can this framework be used in clinical practice? Three possible answers are as follows:

1. It has implications for nursing assessment in that it identifies transition processes with enough specificity to guide observation and interview. The identification of healthy and unhealthy tran-

sition processes and indicators provides the nurse with greater ability to assess the direction of the transition and to identify clients at risk.
2. The nursing therapeutics included in the framework can be used to assist clients in many types of transition.
3. The framework can be used to advocate for an approach to practice that values continuity, family centeredness, and wellness.

These nursing values are threatened by a health-care climate in which cost cutting is leading to significant constraints on practice. This transition framework provides a way to articulate the complexity of transitions and the resulting need for nursing care that is holistic and continuous.

The framework also can be used to guide knowledge development through theory and research. Questions it suggests include: (1) How do different patterns of transition influence transition processes and process indicators? (2) What are the critical periods in the various patterns? (3) What are the relationships between patterns of transition and patterns of nursing intervention? To address these questions, preliminary work will be needed, including further description of transition patterns, processes, and process indicators; identification or development of additional tools for measurement; and continued specification and refinement of nursing therapeutics.

We conclude by emphasizing the importance of a transition perspective in gerontological nursing. Older adults experience multiple transitions related to their health and well-being. These transitions are not short-lived events. Rather, they are complex processes that evolve over a period of time and usually involve a number of individuals. To make nursing practice congruent with the experiences of older adults, the nurse must view their needs from a perspective that takes into account the complexity and temporal characteristics of the experience. We argue that a transition perspective provides the gerontological nurse with a powerful means of understanding and responding to the needs of older adults. We challenge gerontological nurses to use, refine, and extend the framework we have described.

REFERENCES

Ade-Ridder, L., & Kaplan, L. (1993). Marriage, spousal caregiving, and a husband's move to a nursing home: A changing role for the wife? *Journal of Gerontological Nursing, 19*(10), 13–23.

Adlersberg, M., & Thorne, S. (1990). Emerging from the chrysalis: Older widows in transition. *Journal of Gerontological Nursing, 16*(1), 4–8.

Alford, D. M., & Futrell, M. (1992). AAN working paper: Wellness and health promotion of the elderly. *Nursing Outlook, 5,* 221–226.

Angel, R. J., Angel, J. L., & Himes, C. L. (1992). Minority group status, health transitions, and community living arrangements among the elderly. *Research on Aging, 14,* 496–521.

Antonovsky, A. (1987). *Unraveling the mystery of health.* San Francisco: Jossey-Bass.

Archbold, P. G., Stewart, B. J., Greenlick, M. R., & Harvath, T. A. (1992). The clinical assessment of mutuality and preparedness in family caregivers to frail older people. In S. G. Funk, E. M. Tornquist, M. T. Champagne, & R. A. Wiese (Eds.), *Key aspects of elder care: Managing falls, incontinence, and cognitive impairment* (pp. 328–339). New York: Springer.

Brackley, M. H. (1992). A role supplementation group pilot study: A nursing therapy for potential parental caregivers. *Clinical Nurse Specialist, 6,* 14–19.

Bridges, W. (1980). *Transitions.* Reading, MA: Addison-Wesley.

Brown, D. S. (1995). Hospital discharge preparation for homeward bound elderly. *Clinical Nursing Research, 4,* 181–194.

Bull, M., Jervis, L. L., & Her, M. (1995). Hospitalized elders: The difficulties families encounter. *Journal of Gerontological Nursing, 21*(6), 19–23.

Bull, M. J. (1992). Managing the transition from hospital to home. *Qualitative Health Research, 2,* 27–41.

Bull, M. J., Maruyama, G., & Luo, D. (1995). Testing a model for posthospital transition of family caregivers for elderly persons. *Nursing Research, 44,* 132–138.

Burbank, P. (1992). Assessing the meaning of life among older adult clients. *Journal of Gerontological Nursing, 18*(9), 19–28.

Burgener, S. C., Shimer, R., & Murrell, L. (1992). Expressions of individuality in cognitively impaired elders: Need for individual assessment and care. *Journal of Gerontological Nursing, 19*(4), 13–22.

Burnside, I. (1990). Reminiscence: An independent nursing intervention for the elderly. *Issues in Mental Health Nursing, 11,* 33–48.

Burnside, I., & Haight, B. K. (1992). Reminiscence and life review: Analyzing each concept. *Journal of Advanced Nursing, 17,* 855–862.

Cartwright, J. C., Archbold, P. G., Stewart, B. J., & Limandri, B. (1994). Enrichment processes in family caregiving to frail elders. *Advances in Nursing Science, 17*(1), 31–43.

Chick, N., & Meleis, A. I. (1986). Transitions: A nursing concern. In P. L. Chinn (Ed.), *Nursing research methodology: Issues and implementation* (pp. 237–257). Rockville, MD: Aspen.

Conn, V. S., Taylor, S. G., & Messina, C. J. (1995). Older adults and their caregivers: The transition to medication assistance. *Journal of Gerontological Nursing, 21*(5), 33–38.

Cousins, N. (1989). *Headfirst: The biology of hope.* New York: E. P. Dutton.

Daley, O. E. (1993). Women's strategies for living in a nursing home. *Journal of Gerontological Nursing, 19*(9), 5–9.

Daly, M. P., & Berman, B. M. (1993). Rehabilitation in the elderly patient with arthritis. *Clinics in Geriatric Medicine, 9,* 783–801.

Davis, L. L., & Grant, J. S. (1994). Constructing the reality of recovery: Family home care management strategies. *Advances in Nursing Science, 17*(2), 66–76.

Dewar, A. L., & Morse, J. M. (1995). Unbearable incidents: Failure to endure the experience of illness. *Journal of Advanced Nursing, 22,* 957–964.

Dracup, K., Meleis, A. I., Clark, S., Clyburn, A., Shields, L., & Staley, M. (1984). Group counseling in cardiac rehabilitation: Effect on patient compliance. *Patient Education and Counseling, 6,* 169–177.

Duke University Center for the Study of Aging and Human Development. (1978). *Multidimensional functional assessment: The OARS methodology.* Durham, NC: Duke University.

Edwardson, S. R. (1988). Outcomes of coronary care in the acute care setting. *Research in Nursing & Health, 11,* 215–222.

Erikson, E. H., Erikson, J. M., & Kivnick, H. Q. (1986). *Vital involvement in old age.* New York: W. W. Norton.

Ferrell, B. R., & Schneider, C. (1988). Experience and management of cancer pain at home. *Cancer Nursing, 11,* 84–90.

Finfgeld, D. L. (1995). Becoming and being courageous in the chronically ill elderly. *Issues in Mental Health Nursing, 16,* 1–11.

Folstein, M. F., Folstein, S. E., & McHugh, P. R. (1975). Mini-Mental State: A practical method for grading the cognitive state of patients for the clinician. *Journal of Psychiatric Research, 12,* 189–198.

Gaffney, K. F. (1992). Nursing practice model for maternal role sufficiency. *Advances in Nursing Science, 15*(2), 76–84.

Glass, T. A., & Maddox, G. L. (1992). The quality and quantity of social support: Stroke recovery as psycho-social transition. *Social Science and Medicine, 34,* 1249–1261.

Happ, M. B., Williams, C. C., Strumpf, N. E., & Burger, S. G. (1996). Individualized care for frail elders: Theory and practice. *Journal of Gerontological Nursing, 22*(3), 6–14.

Johnson, M. A., Morton, M. K., & Knox, S. M. (1992). The transition to a nursing home: Meeting the family's needs. *Geriatric Nursing, 13,* 299–302.

Jones, P. S. (1991). Adaptability: A personal resource for health. *Scholarly Inquiry for Nursing Practice, 5,* 95–112.

Jones, P. S. (1995). Paying respect: Care of elderly parents by Chinese and Filipino American women. *Health Care for Women International, 16,* 385–398.

Jones, P. S., & Meleis, A. I. (1993). Health is empowerment. *Advances in Nursing Science, 15*(3), 1–14.

Katz, S., Ford, A. B., Moskowitz, R. W., Jackson, B. W., & Jaffe, M. (1963). Studies of illness in the aged: The index of ADL, a standardized measure of biological and psychosocial function. *Journal of the American Medical Association, 185,* 914–919.

Kelley, L. S., & Lakin, J. A. (1987). Role supplementation as a nursing intervention for Alzheimer's disease: A case study. *Public Health Nursing, 5,* 146–152.

King, K. B., Porter, L. A., & Rowe, M. A. (1994). Functional, social, and emotional outcomes in women and men in the first year following coronary artery bypass surgery. *Journal of Women's Health, 3,* 347–354.

Kinion, E. S., & Kolcaba, K. Y. (1992). Plato's model of the psyche: A holistic model for nursing interventions. *Journal of Holistic Nursing, 10,* 218–230.

Kobasa, S. C. (1979). Stressful life events, personality, and health: An inquiry into hardiness. *Journal of Personality and Social Psychology, 37,* 1–11.

Kozak, C. J., Campbell, C., & Hughes, A. M. (1996). The use of functional consequences theory in acutely confused hospitalized elderly. *Journal of Gerontological Nursing, 22*(1), 27–36.

Langner, S. R. (1995). Finding meaning in caring for elderly relatives: Loss and personal growth. *Holistic Nursing Practice, 9*(3), 75–84.

Lipson-Parra, H. (1989). Development and validation of the Adult Attachment Scale: Assessing attachment in elderly adults. *Issues in Mental Health Nursing, 11,* 79–92.

Magee, R., Hyatt, E. C., Hardin, S. B., Stratmann, D., Vinson, M. H., & Owen, M. (1993). Institutional policy: Use of restraints in extended care and nursing homes. *Journal of Gerontological Nursing, 19*(4), 31–39.

Magnani, L. E. (1990). Hardiness, self-perceived health, and activity among independently functioning older adults. *Scholarly Inquiry for Nursing Practice: An International Journal, 4,* 171–185.

McCracken, A. L. (1994). Special care units: Meeting the needs of cognitively impaired persons. *Journal of Gerontological Nursing, 20*(4), 41–46.

McDougall, G. (1994). Mental health and cognition. In P. Ebersole & P. Hess (Eds.), *Toward healthy aging: Human needs and nursing response* (4th ed., pp. 612–657). St. Louis: Mosby.

McDougall, G. J. (1995). Existential psychotherapy with older adults. *Journal of the American Psychiatric Nurses Association, 1,* 16–21.

Meleis, A. I. (1975). Role insufficiency and role supplementation: A conceptual framework. *Nursing Research, 24,* 264–271.

Meleis, A. I. (1986). Theory development and domain concepts. In P. Moccia (Ed.), *New approaches to theory development* (pp. 3–21). New York: National League for Nursing.

Meleis, A. I., & Swendsen, L. A. (1978). Role supplementation: An empirical test of a nursing intervention. *Nursing Research, 27,* 11–18.

Meleis, A. I., & Trangenstein, P. A. (1994). Facilitating transitions: Redefinition of the nursing mission. *Nursing Outlook, 42,* 255–259.

Melzack, R. (1975). The McGill Pain Questionnaire: Major properties and scoring. *Pain, 1,* 277–299.

Mercer, R. T., Nichols, E. G., & Doyle, G. C. (1988). Transitions over the life cycle: A comparison of mothers and nonmothers. *Nursing Research, 37,* 144–150.

Michels, N. (1988). The transition from hospital to home: An exploratory study. *Home Health Care Services Quarterly, 9*(1), 29–44.

Moneyham, L., & Scott, C. B. (1995). Anticipatory coping in the elderly. *Journal of Gerontological Nursing, 21*(7), 23–28.

Nash, M. S. (1994). Exercise and immunology. *Medicine & Science in Sports & Exercise, 26,* 125–127.

Nick, S. (1992). Long-term care: Choices for geriatric residents. *Journal of Gerontological Nursing, 18*(7), 11–28.

Nyström, A. E. M., & Segesten, K. M. (1994). On sources of powerlessness in nursing home life. *Journal of Advanced Nursing, 19,* 124–133.

Reid, D. W., & Ziegler, M. (1981). The desired control measure and adjustment among the elderly. In H. M. Lefcourt (Ed.), *Research with the locus of control construct: Vol. 1. Assessment methods* (pp. 127–157). New York: Academic Press.

Rentz, C. A. (1995). Reminiscence: A supportive intervention for the person with Alzheimer's disease. *Journal of Psychosocial Nursing and Mental Health Services, 33*(11), 15–20.

Rickelman, B. L., Gallman, L., & Parra, H. (1994). Attachment and quality of life in older, community-residing men. *Nursing Research, 43,* 68–72.

Schumacher, K. L., & Meleis, A. I. (1994). Transitions: A central concept in nursing. *Image: Journal of Nursing Scholarship, 26,* 119–127.

Spielberger, C. D. (1983). *Manual for the State-Trait Inventory (STAI) Form Y.* Palo Alto, CA: Consulting Psychologists Press.

Stewart, B. J., Archbold, P. G., Harvath, T. A., & Nkongho, N. O. (1993). Role acquisition in family caregivers for older people who have been discharged from the hospital. In S. G. Funk, E. M. Tornquist, M. T. Champagne, & R. A. Wiese (Eds.), *Key aspects of caring for the chronically ill: Hospital and home* (pp. 219–231). New York: Springer.

Swendsen, L. A., Meleis, A. I., & Jones, D. (1978). Role supplementation for new parents: A role mastery plan. *American Journal of Maternal Child Nursing, 3,* 84–91.

Taft, L. B., Delaney, K., Seman, D., & Stansell, J. (1993). Creating a therapeutic milieu in dementia care. *Journal of Gerontological Nursing, 19*(10), 30–39.

U.S. Department of Health and Human Services, & American Association for Retired Persons. (1991). *Healthy older adults 2000.* Washington, DC: AARP Health Advocacy Services.

Walker, S. N. (1992). Wellness for elders. *Holistic Nursing Practice, 7*(1), 38–45.

Wilson, S., & Billones, H. (1994). The Filipino elder: Implications for nursing practice. *Journal of Gerontological Nursing, 20*(8), 31–36.

Windriver, W. (1993). Social isolation: Unit-based activities for impaired elders. *Journal of Gerontological Nursing, 19*(3), 15–21.

Yesavage, J. A., & Brink, T. L. (1983). Development and validation of a geriatric depression screening scale. A preliminary report. *Journal of Psychiatric Research, 17,* 37–49.

Young, H. M. (1990). The transition of relocation to a nursing home. *Holistic Nursing Practice, 4*(3), 74–83.

Reprinted with permission from: Schumacher, K. L., Jones, P. S., & Meleis, A. I. (1999). Helping elderly persons in transition: A framework for research and practice. In E. A. Swanson & T. Tripp-Reimer (Eds.), *Life transitions in the older adult: Issues for nurses and other health professionals* (pp. 1–26). New York: Springer.

3.7 GERIATRIC SEXUAL CONFORMITY: ASSESSMENT AND INTERVENTION

MERRIE J. KAAS
G. KAY ROUSSEAU

Abstract

The interactional relationship between the elderly and society constitutes an important focus in health care. Negative cues of society toward the sexuality of the elderly render the aged susceptible to changes in sexual role behaviors and gender identity. Geriatric sexual conformity is an example of a socialized non-sexual role. Role theory provides a useful framework for explaining geriatric sexual conformity as a case of role insufficiency. Role theory, in conjunction with Annon's PLISSIT model for brief sexual therapy, offers a basis for specific sexual counseling interventions for the elderly and significant others.

The relationship between the elderly and the society, particularly changes in this relationship, constitutes an important focus in health care. The susceptibility of the elderly to the negative cues of society and the influence of this environment on the self-concept of the elderly has been well documented (Butler & Lewis, 1977; Kuypers & Bengston, 1973; Rosow, 1974). Rosow (1974) states that in the interaction between the elderly and society, dependency, deprivation, and indifference force the elderly to be "devalued, stereotyped, excluded from social opportunities, lose roles and confront role ambiguity, and struggle to preserve self-esteem through youthful self-images" (p. 12). It is through this interactive process between the aged and society that the elderly are socialized into an ambiguous and negative role. It is also through this same interactive process that the elderly are socialized into a non-sexual role.

Because one's sexuality is an integral aspect of self-concept, the societal, biological, and psychological forces that alter one's self-concept also affect one's sexuality. Many elderly conform to these forces by negating their sexuality and taking on a non-sexual role. This geriatric sexual conformity is an example of role insufficiency. Role theory provides a useful interactional framework in which to view the disparity between the sexual self-concept and behavior of the elderly and the sexual role expectations of society. Role theory also provides a basis for specific interventions in the sexual counseling of the elderly and their significant others.

The sexuality system is composed of four parts: biological sex, sexual identity, gender identity, and sexual role behavior (Sadock, Kaplan, & Freedman, 1976). Biological sex is the sex determined by chromosomes, hormones, and primary and secondary sex characteristics. It cannot be changed. Sexual identity is a person's sense of maleness and femaleness. The sexual identity can be in conflict with one's biological sex. An example would be the transsexual who has male chromosomes, hormones, etc., but whose sexual identity is female. Sexual identity cannot be changed, but physical appearance and behavior can be modified to match sexual identity. Gender identity is a person's sense of masculinity and femininity. Gender identity includes both feelings. A woman can feel "feminine" by the way she dresses and yet feel "masculine" in the way she relates to her co-workers. Gender identity can change frequently and be situationally determined. Sexual role behavior is both the behavior motivated by the desire for sexual pleasure (sex behavior) and the behavior with masculine and feminine connotations (gender behavior). Intercourse, masturbation, kissing, hugging, reading "sexy" books, and sexual fantasizing are all examples of sexual role behavior motivated by the desire for sexual behavior. Responding submissively, nurturing, initiating a date, being the "breadwinner" of the family, and assuming responsibility for housekeeping and cooking are examples of gender behavior. Sexual role behavior can be in constant flux depending on the situation. Geriatric sexual conformity assumes a change in gender identity and corresponding sexual role behaviors.

The symbolic interactional perspective of role theory is particularly useful as a theoretical framework for describing geriatric sexual conformity. This perspective considers the dynamic interactive process between culture, societal structure, and the individual (Cottrell, 1969). "Role" in this sense, then, is not "merely a set of behaviors or expected behaviors, but a sentiment or goal that provides unity to a set of potential actions" (Turner, 1962, p. 26). Roles develop interactively and are based in terms of other relevant roles. They are developed through a role-taking process in which the individual acts in reaction to his perceptions of significant others' views (Turner, 1978). Once a role is assumed by an individual, it is validated when others acknowledge acceptance of that role, and then it gives direction for role-appropriate behaviors (Meleis, 1975). These role behaviors are then continued or modified because of perceived positive benefits. In this sense, self-concept is a reflection of "how one relates to significant-other roles" (Meleis, 1975, p. 265).

Allport (1967) distinguishes four meanings of roles: role expectations, role conception, role acceptance, and role performance. Role expectations are what the culture prescribes; role conception is the individual's perception of his/her role; role acceptance or rejection is the affective response to that role; and role performance is the behavior the individual expresses relevant to that role.

Role Expectation

Role expectation is the set of expected behaviors that culture prescribes. Sexual role behavior at any age is dependent on several factors including prevailing mores concerning sexual behavior, actual physical capacities, the individual's past history of sexual behaviors, and available partners. For the elderly, "the 'symptoms' of being old are associated with the 'attitudes and actions' of those in one's society" (Kuypers & Bengston, 1973, p. 38). In the case of geriatric sexuality, our society prescribes sexlessness. The elderly are more susceptible to this prescription because of a number of factors. The first is the physiological changes in the sexual response cycle that occur with aging. Masters and Johnson (1966) found definite changes in sexual response in the geriatric population. According to their research there are four phases of the sexual response cycle: excitement, plateau, orgasmic, and resolution. Age changes occur in all phases for both men and women. Because of these age changes the elderly may feel as if they are losing their ability to be sexually expressive, i.e., the loss of specific sex behaviors that had been normal and satisfying. Other role losses that occur with age are losses related to family and friends, work, and social activities. These contribute to the changes in sexual role behaviors that have masculine and feminine connotations. All of these losses may induce diminished ego strength and self-identity, which make the elderly more susceptible to the acceptance of society's role expectation of sexlessness.

From where does this expected role of sexlessness originate? There is the myth that sexual expression is not characteristic of old people and that sex is wrong or sinful if continued into later life. Several explanations have been offered to account for these myths, including the notion that, traditionally, it has been felt that sexual activity should be engaged in primarily for procreative purposes, and only secondarily for recreative purposes. Because reproductive purposes in old age cannot be maintained, the myth of sexlessness continues. A second explanation is the extension of the Oedipal conflict. Observing or imagining parents engaging in sex created high levels of anxiety in some people. This anxiety may prevail because the elderly represent the parent generation (Pfeiffer, 1975). A third possible explanation for the continuation of these myths is the fear among the young that their own sexual abilities could be lost with age (Lobenz, 1975). One way to deal with this fear is to discount the importance of sex in later years. If sex is not important, then neither is the loss of sex. The young may also seek to eliminate the aged as competitors for sexual objects by fostering and generating the stereotype of the asexual elderly (Busse & Pfeiffer,

1969). Because of the physiological aging process and psychosocial factors, the elderly are predisposed to restricted sex role behaviors. The elderly depend on cues from the society to direct their sexual behavior. Society's sexual role expectation of sexlessness limits sexual activity in the elderly through restrictive cues based on myths and taboos.

Role Conception

Role conception is the individual's perception of his or her roles. How a person perceives a role is dependent on the role taking done with significant others in society. A change in one's own role mirrors a changed perception of the role of significant others, because roles exist in relation to their orientation toward other roles (Turner, 1962). This interactional approach to roles shifts the process of role conception from the idea of neat, prescribed behaviors to a dynamic, changing perception based on reflections of relationships with others.

Zusman (1966) states that "the person rendered susceptible, because of frames of reference derived from past experiences which are not available, becomes unusually dependent on current stimuli for cues regarding appropriate behavior, determining right and wrong, true and false, and judging what impulses to obey and which to inhibit" (p. 389). Society's current attitudes toward geriatric sexuality reflect sexlessness, so when the elderly role-take, the role they perceive as appropriate is NOT one of a sexually active and satisfied 75-year-old! Quite the contrary, the elderly are told they are incompetent, dangerous, and incapable of self control. Stereotypes such as "dirty old man" and "indecent old woman" are the negative messages that are conveyed. Based on the reflections from society, the elderly conceive of their sexual role as sexless, or non-sexual.

Role Acceptance or Rejection

This is the affective response to the role expectation, which, in this case, is the role of sexlessness in old age. Once this sexlessness (non-sexual role) has been identified by the elderly, they can accept it or reject it. If past sexual experiences of the elderly have been satisfying, and the importance of their sexuality cemented in their self-concept, this role will be rejected, and they will continue to express their sexuality in gratifying ways. In the case of sexual conformity, an elderly person involuntarily accepts the sexless role. Meleis (1975) describes this disparity between societal expectations and individual perception as role insufficiency. "Role insufficiency is any difficulty in the cognizance and/or performance of a role or of the sentiments and goals associated with the role behaviors as perceived by the self or by significant others" (p. 266). Role insufficiency may result from poor role definition, losses of roles with or without modifications of other roles, lack of knowledge of role behavior, or impaired or absent perceptions or interpretations of role behaviors.

Meleis (1975) also states that "once a role evolves, the need to reciprocate in role behaviors becomes actually a need for benefits received in order to continue receiving them" (p. 265). The costs incurred by remaining sexually active, namely, ridicule and scorn, may then lead older individuals who retain the physiological and psychological prerequisites for normal sex role behaviors into adopting what is essentially a "sick" role. Some behaviors inherent in the sick role, such as loneliness, sexlessness, or regression, are already perceived as characteristics of the elderly population, so they are already positively reinforced.

Role Performance

Role performance is what the individual actually does with the accepted role. It is the behavior in the social system. In this case, sexual role performance is the result of group pressure. Klein (1972) posited that older individuals, in comparison with younger individuals, would be more susceptible to external pressures and thereby conform more readily. His research results showed that, in general, older persons tend to be more conforming. The tendency toward conforming might be seen as a trait most characteristic of the elderly. His research indicated that this conforming nature may be due in part to elderly persons' perceptions of their own low competence. It follows, then, that if the elderly are more susceptible to conforming behavior because of their negative self-perceptions, that conforming sexual role behaviors and a change in gender identity may also ensue.

With the learning of new role appropriate behaviors comes the atrophy or extinction of other behaviors. Geriatric sexual conformity causes the elderly to lose their capacity to function sexually. Masters and Johnson (1966) state, however, that both aging males and females can continue to enjoy satisfying sexual relationships with continued, effective stimulation. Without this stimulation, emotional and physical, the ability to enjoy satisfying sexual relationships is diminished or lost. One forgets how to initiate and maintain a social conversation, or how to curl the hair or shave. When sexual role behaviors atrophy because of disuse, the elderly psychologically conform and see themselves as asexual or neuter. Hence, gender identity is also conformed. There is a real sense of change in feelings of masculinity and femininity.

The elderly learn to disavow any sexual feelings or desires as a result of guilt, fear, or shame. When asked about sexual feelings, one older woman told this author "Oh no, old people shouldn't have those anymore." The elderly also learn appropriate skills to hide their desires and activities to conform to the sexless role. Jokes about earlier sexual prowess mask the present sexual desires.

Finally, with the combination of sexual dysfunction, and learned behaviors to hide their sexuality, the elderly may consciously or unconsciously exhibit a change in gender identity. A well-dressed, stylish, pretty older lady may change to a drab, unkempt, old woman who isolates herself from interactions with others. The isolation serves to protect her from further negative reflections.

A Conceptual Scheme for Intervention

Geriatric sexual conformity results from an interactive process between social, biological, and psychological forces. It is the behavioral and affective outcome of the incongruence between the sexual self-concept and sexual behavior of the elderly, and the sexual role expectations of society or significant others. It is the difficulty in the understanding and/or performance of sexual role behavior as perceived by the elderly or their significant others. In role theory terms, it is an insufficiency in sexual role behavior.

Professional health-care providers can intervene to minimize this insufficiency in sexual role behavior. Meleis (1975) describes the process of role supplementation as a way to prevent and treat role insufficiency. *Role supplementation* is the process by which role insufficiency or potential role insufficiency is identified by the role incumbent and significant others, and the conditions and strategies of role clarification, role modeling, role rehearsal, and reference group, and are used to decrease or prevent role insufficiency (Swendson, Meleis, & Jones, 1978). In the case of geriatric sexual conformity, through role supplementation, the elderly and their significant others come to be cognizant of the sexual role expectations and behaviors, and educational strategies are developed to diminish the disparity between these expectations and behaviors.

Role clarification is the identification of the knowledge and behaviors associated with a role. Role modeling occurs when an individual is able to learn and emulate behaviors or attitudes through watching others enacting the same behaviors or attitudes. Role rehearsal occurs when an individual mentally enacts a situation or role, and anticipates or imagines the responses of significant others. *Reference groups* are a number of people gathered together with the same general interest for the purpose of supporting the development of different, adaptive behaviors, and discussing feelings and attitudes.

Just as role theory provides a framework for strategies for sexual role supplementation, Annon's (1976) PLISSIT model also provides a framework for behavioral treatment of sexual problems. This model designates four levels of approach for identifying and resolving sexual concerns. Inherent in this model is developments sequencing so that the least intrusive approach is used first, at the permission-giving level. The four levels are: (1) Permission, (2) Limited Information, (3) Specific Suggestions, and (4) Intensive Therapy.

Yoselle (1981) has used this model in conceptualizing nursing intervention with elderly clients. A synthesis of these two models offers a way of identifying specific interventions to reduce geriatric sexual conformity through sexual role supplementation in each of the four levels of approach to counseling. Because geriatric sexual conformity is an interactional process between the elderly and their significant others. The interventions suggested here may be useful for both elderly clients and their significant others, e.g., family, friends, partners, nursing staff, physicians, and so on.

Level I: Permission

At this first level of intervention, the elderly client (individual or group) is "permitted" to communicate about sexual issues. This level allows for the least intrusive discussion of various aspects of sexuality. Strategies of role clarification, role modeling, role rehearsal, and reference group facilitate the client's ability to discuss sexual attitudes and concerns. Role clarification at this level would involve letting the elderly know that it is normal to be sexual and to have sexual fantasies and dreams, and that the behavior they are engaging in is not perverted or abnormal. It is also important to discuss sexuality in broad terms, encompassing both sex and gender behavior. Frequently it is the job of the health-care professional to be a sounding board and to let the elderly know that many others share their concerns. It is also important at times to give the elderly permission not to engage in certain sexual behaviors, if they so choose. Role modeling is an important strategy at this first level. The healthcare professional can facilitate open communication by ensuring privacy and confidentiality, by not reinforcing defenses and anxiety by condoning jokes, testing, and distortions, by choosing appropriate but understandable vocabulary, by using open ended questions, and by not placing a value judgment on sexual role behavior. The way in which the health-care professional conducts the discussion of sexuality and the elderly will serve as a model for the elderly or others in discussing sexuality. Sensitive books such as Comfort's, *A Good Age,* or Butler and Lewis's, *Love and Sex After Sixty,* or films such as "Love Toads" or "A Rose by Any Other Name" may also serve as role models and stimulate discussion of various forms of sexual expression. The elderly may serve as role models and speakers at community groups interested in sexuality and the aged, as well as in seniors groups in the community and institutions. A problem with role modeling in geriatric sexuality is that there are not enough visible role models because the elderly are more isolated in society. Encouraging peer socialization and intergenerational socialization will facilitate the visibility of the elderly.

Role rehearsal, the mental enactment of a role can be used by both the elderly and significant others to imagine their own sexual development in the past or the future. This imagery will serve to facilitate discussion of attitude and value development and consequent sexual role behavior.

Reference groups also serve an important permission-giving function. It is through these groups that different attitudes, feelings, and concerns are shared. Both the elderly and their significant others can benefit by openly discussing general sexual issues and attitudes. Again, if the health care professional is facilitator of these groups, role modeling can take place and permission can be given to think about and talk about sexuality and the aged.

Level II: Limited Information

Providing limited information in conjunction with permission-giving can serve as a preventive and treatment intervention. In fact, it is difficult to give permission without limited information, and vice versa. Limited information gives key information that can minimize concerns and allow for attitudinal change.

Role clarification would include providing information about anatomy and physiology, normal age changes in the sexual response cycle, myths regarding attitudes toward geriatric sexuality, myths about appropriate sexual role behavior in the elderly, and the general effects of drugs, alcohol, medications, diet, and exercise on sexuality. Information about the effects of various illnesses on sexuality can also be included. Books on sexuality and aging can provide information, but, unfortunately, most literature about specific illnesses or medications do not include information on sexuality.

Role modeling can be facilitated by the use of books, magazines, and films that depict the normalcy of sexual expression in the elderly. One such film, "A Ripple in Time," can serve this purpose. Elderly role models can discuss personal experiences related to their sexuality with significant others.

Role rehearsal can be facilitated through role playing situations with the elderly or significant others in which aspects of geriatric sexual role behavior must be explained. For example, the health-care professional can role-play with other health-care providers a situation that would necessitate giving information about sexuality to elderly clients. Role-playing can also be used to try out responses of the elderly to those who disapprove of sexual expression in the elderly.

Reference groups also may be important in providing limited information about individual differences in normal age changes, responses to these changes, and experiences with various illnesses and treatments.

Level III: Specific Suggestions

At this level, specific suggestions are provided to help change sexual role behavior. Through role clarification health-care professionals can provide specific information about alternative sexual positions or techniques, use of self-stimulation, and use of lubricants and vibrators, various diets, or medications. These suggestions are specific to individual concerns, rather than discussed generally as might occur in Level I or II, and are intended for use in a brief therapy framework.

Role modeling can be useful when discussing various sexual techniques and positions. There are increasingly more films and literature depicting alternative techniques for clients with limitations of mobility, pain, or difficult respiration. Unfortunately, many of these resources aren't specifically oriented to a geriatric population as yet.

Role rehearsal can involve role-playing and fantasy. Role playing and/or fantasizing about initiating conversation with a friend, requesting a date, dressing up, carrying out the date, and responding to potential problems can all help the elderly and/or significant others anticipate new sexual role behaviors and prepare for possible problems. Fantasizing about previous sexual relationships and the positive feelings and satisfying behaviors can diminish anxiety and facilitate initiation of present-day action. Graduated dating sessions (Annon, 1976) can also help prepare for new sexual behaviors.

Reference groups can be supportive in times of trying out new behaviors. The threat of new behaviors can be diminished by discussing the fear and anxiety with others. The group is also a place where changes in attitudes and alternative plans can be discussed. The reference group may also become a place to meet new partners. Reference groups may be composed of couples, partners with special concerns, singles, heterosexuals, or gays/lesbians. These groups may also include families, friends, or other health-care providers who have specific concerns and want special information that will help them change their attitudes or behavior or help them to be supportive.

Level IV: Intensive Therapy

Intensive therapy constitutes treatment/counseling by a qualified sex therapist. As health-care professionals we need to give ourselves permission not to be an expert on all issues. When the sexual concerns of either the individual elderly person or significant others become too complex, referral to an appropriate sex therapist is necessary.

Geriatric sexual conformity is an interactive process between the elderly and their significant others resulting in a disparity in the understanding and/or performance of sexual role behavior as perceived by the elderly or the significant others. Health-care professionals can minimize this insufficiency through role supplementation. Utilizing strategies of role clarification, role modeling, role rehearsal, and reference groups with the elderly and significant others can change sexual role expectations and behaviors.

A Case Study for Role Supplementation

This case illustrates geriatric sexual conformity and interventions using the PLISSIT model and role supplementation. The health-care professional is a nurse practitioner in a senior citizens' drop-in clinic in a senior center.

The client, P.D., was a 65 year old male who was self-labeled as impotent. His personal history included an early retirement and a divorce in his early fifties. He had one daughter with whom had had minimal contact and there were no grandchildren. A medical history showed a seven year history of mild hypertension, which was being treated with a salt-restricted diet and diuretics. He had also had a mild myocardial infarction at age 60. In discussing his problem with achieving erections, he attributed the problem to age and antihypertensive medication. He had experienced major role losses without finding new meaningful ones and had accepted an asexual role for himself. There was also some deterioration in social skills and social distancing from others.

Interventions at Each Level

Level I: Permission

Permission to discuss sexual concerns was given by asking P.D. if he had any sexual concerns. Nonverbal permission was given by keeping a number of books on sexuality on the office bookshelves. Role modeling at the permission level occurred with an open attitude and with the use of appropriate vocabulary in discussions of sexuality.

This client responded quickly to the non-verbal message of the books by walking into the office on his first visit, picking up a book on sex and asking, "Why do you need this in a senior citizen's clinic?" Permission was extended by giving the response that people are sexual and that senior citizens are no exception. In the discussion that followed, P.D. labeled himself as impotent since starting blood pressure medication, but that it was all right because he was "too old for sex anyway." I pointed out that he engaged in other activities many people would say he was too old for. Why then was he too old for sex but still bicycled and jogged? At the end of his visit I invited him to return for discussion of his concerns and referred him to a group (reference group) on sexuality and aging that I was facilitating. Further individual counseling at the permission level included a discussion on sexual fantasies and dreams and the normalcy of fantasy.

The reference group consisted of four men and seven women who attended activities in the senior center. Reference group discussions at this level covered how family and societal attitudes can either inhibit or encourage sexual expression. The group identified family and societal messages indicating that it is not OK to be old and sexual and they explored their feelings about that message.

Level II: Limited Information

Role clarification at this level included giving information on the sexual response cycle and aging effects. He was also given information on his blood pressure medication, which did not have a direct physiological effect on the sexual response cycle. Fantasies were discussed as a pleasurable sexual activity and as a way to rehearse actual sexual role behaviors.

Reference group discussions at this level centered on personal values and beliefs and how they affected sexual behaviors. Where individuals expressed dissatisfaction with their sexual lives and held values that interfered with obtaining sexual satisfaction, we explored the option of modifying values.

Level III: Specific Suggestions

Role clarification included avoidance of alcohol prior to sexual activity and the need to use more direct genital stimulation. Since he had no partner, masturbation was suggested as a pleasurable sexual activity, as a way to learn about his own responses, and as an alternative to partner sex. It was also suggested that he incorporate some of the new information he gained from discussions and reading into his fantasies.

The group discussions at this level focused on topics such as stimulation techniques, positions, sex and illness, and alternatives to partner sex. Intensive therapy was not utilized with this client, although he was informed of the availability of those services through the group discussion.

During the 1-month period this client received individual counseling and participated in group discussions, he increased his social contacts and his self-pleasuring behaviors (fantasy, masturbation). He also reported having "wet dreams" again. Having achieved erections during sleep contributed to his ability to achieve erections during masturbation and renewed the possibility of partner sex.

While this man responded to a nonverbal invitation to discuss sexual concerns, other clients might need a more direct approach. They may also be less open in discussing concerns. Role supplementation and the PLISSIT model are flexible in tailoring counseling content and individual interventions.

REFERENCES

Allport, G. *Pattern and growth in personality.* New York: Holt, Rinehart and Winston. 1967.

Annon, J. *Behavioral treatment of sexual problems.* San Francisco: Harper & Row, 1976.

Butler, R., & Lewis, M. *Aging and mental health* (2nd ed.). St. Louis: C. V. Mosby Co., 1977.

Busse, E., & Pfeiffer, E. *Behavior and adaptation in later life.* Boston: Little, Brown and Co., 1969.

Cottrell, L. S. Jr. Interpersonal interaction and the development of self. In Goslin, D. A. (Ed.), *Handbook of socialization theory and research.* Chicago: Rand McNally, 1969.

Klein, R. L. Age, sex, and task difficulty as predictors of social conformity. *J. Gerontology, 27,* 1972.

Kuypers, J., & Bengston, V. Competence and social breakdown: A social psychological view of aging. *Human Development, 61,* 1973.

Lobenz, N. Sex after sixty-five. *Public Affairs Pamphlet No. 519.* Public Affairs Committee, Inc., 1965.

Masters, W., & Johnson, V. *Human sexual response.* Boston: Little, Brown and Co., 1966.

Meleis, A. Role insufficiency and role supplementation: A conceptual framework. *Nursing Research, 24,* 1975.

Meleis, A., & Swendson, L. Role supplementation: An empirical test of a nursing intervention. *Nursing Research, 27*(1), 1978.

Pfeiffer, E. Sexual behavior. In Howells, J. (Ed.), *Modern perspectives in the psychiatry of old age.* New York: Brunner/Mazel, 1975.

Rosow, I. *Socialization to old age.* Berkeley: University of California Press, 1974.

Sadock, B., Kaplan, H., & Freedman, A. *The sexual experience.* Baltimore: Williams and Wilkins Co., 1976.

Swendson, L., Meleis, A., & Jones, D. Role supplementation for new parents—A role mastery plan. *The American Journal of Material and Child Nursing,* 1978, 3(2).

Turner, J. *The structure of sociological theory.* Homewood, EL: The Dorsey Press, 1978.

Turner, R. Role taking: Process vs. conformity. In Rose, A. (Ed.), *Human behavior and social processes.* Boston: Houghton Mifflin Co., 1962.

Yoselle, H. Sexuality in later years. *Topics in Clinical Nursing.* 1981, 3(1).

Zusman, J. Some explanations of the changing appearance of psychotic patients: Antecedents of the social breakdown concept. *The Millbank Memorial Fund Quarterly, 64,* 1966.

Reprinted with permission from: Kaas, M. J., & Rousseau, G. K. (1983). Geriatric sexual conformity: Assessment and intervention. *Clinical Gerontologist, 2*(1), 31–44.

Chapter 4   Situational Transitions: Discharge and Relocation

4.1   PERCEIVED READINESS FOR HOSPITAL DISCHARGE IN ADULT MEDICAL-SURGICAL PATIENTS

MARIANNE E. WEISS
LINDA B. PIACENTINE
LISA LOKKEN
JANICE ANCONA
JOANNE ARCHER
SUSAN GRESSER
SUE BAIRD HOLMES
SALLY TOMAN
ANNE TOY
TERI VEGA-STROMBERG

Abstract

Purpose: The purpose of the study was to identify predictors and outcomes of adult medical-surgical patients' perceptions of their readiness for hospital discharge. **Design:** A correlational, prospective, longitudinal design with path analyses was used to explore relationships among transition theory-related variables. **Setting:** Midwestern tertiary medical center. **Sample:** 147 adult medical-surgical patients. **Methods:** Predictor variables included patient characteristics, hospitalization factors, and nursing practices that were measured prior to hospital discharge using a study enrollment form, the Quality of Discharge Teaching Scale, and the Care Coordination Scale. Discharge readiness was measured using the Readiness for Hospital Discharge Scale administered within 4 hours prior to discharge. Outcomes were measured 3 weeks postdischarge with the Post-Discharge Coping Difficulty Scale and self-reported utilization of health services. **Findings:** Living alone, discharge teaching (amount of content received and nurses' skill in teaching delivery), and care coordination explained 51% of readiness for discharge score variance. Patient age and discharge readiness explained 16% of variance in postdischarge coping difficulty. Greater readiness for discharge was predictive of fewer readmissions. **Conclusions:** Quality of the delivery of discharge teaching was the strongest predictor of discharge readiness. Study results provided support for Meleis' transitions theory as a useful model for conceptualizing and investigating the discharge transition. **Implications for Practice:** The study results have implications for the clinical nurse specialist role in patient and staff education, system building for the postdischarge transition, and measurement of clinical care outcomes.

With the contemporary focus on minimizing length of hospital stay, patients are discharged in an intermediate rather than complete stage of recovery.[1] Care needs extend beyond discharge into the home where the burden of managing the complexities of recovery falls on the patient and family members.[2-6] Readiness for discharge is typically a medical team decision based on achievement of clinical criteria. The patient's perception of readiness for discharge may be different than their care provider's evaluation.[7,8] In studies of hospital discharge and the transition to care at home, the patient's perception of readiness for discharge has rarely been included as a study variable. Assessment of readiness for discharge and the transition to home-based recovery and care has become increasingly important for patient safety, satisfaction, and outcomes. Identification of predictors of readiness or lack of readiness is essential for determining appropriate timing of discharge and subsequent postdischarge follow-up needs.

The purpose of this study was to identify patient characteristics, hospitalization factors, and hospital nursing practices that are predictive of adult medical-surgical patients' perceptions of their readiness to go home at the time of discharge and the relationship of perceptions of discharge readiness to posthospitalization coping and utilization outcomes. The study is of particular significance to Advanced Practice/Clinical Nurse Specialists, whose role responsibilities encompass outcome achievement for selected patient populations through patient and staff education, system building for continuity of care, optimization of outcomes during transitions between venues of care, and measurement and evaluation of clinical care processes and outcomes.[9]

Theoretical Framework

Going home following hospitalization has commonly been referred to as a transition for the patient and the family that begins prior to discharge and extends into the postdischarge period.[2,3,10-14] Meleis' middle-range theory of transitions[15] was selected as a guiding framework for conceptualizing the discharge transition and identifying relevant study variables because of the congruence between the concepts of this middle-range theory and the concepts of the specific transition situation of going home after hospitalization. Testing of transitions theory concepts and relationships in the specific situation of hospital discharge will not only develop knowledge to advance clinical practice but will also extend nursing knowledge about the phenomenon of transitions.[15,16] A transition is a process of passage from one life phase, condition, or status to another during which changes in health status, role relations, expectations, or abilities create a period of vulnerability.[15,17] Hospital discharge was viewed as a transitional process occurring in 3 sequential phases: (1) the hospitalization phase during which discharge preparation occurs; (2) the discharge when short-term outcomes of the preparatory process can be measured; and (3) the postdischarge period when patients' perceptions of their ability to cope with the demands of care at home and their needs for support and assistance from family and health services provide evidence of positive or adverse outcomes of the patient's transitional process. Four major dimensions of transitions theory were explored in this study: the nature of the transition (hospitalization factors including planned or prior admissions and length of hospital stay), transition conditions (patient characteristics including age, gender, race, socioeconomic status, payor, and living alone), nursing therapeutics (discharge teaching and care coordination), and patterns of response (readiness for hospital discharge, postdischarge coping difficulty, and postdischarge utilization of health services). Transitions theory proposes that the nature of the transition, transition conditions, and nursing therapeutic practices will affect patterns of response during a transition. Transitions theory concept definitions and specification of the related study variables and empirical indicators are presented in Table 4.1.1.

Background

Readiness for hospital discharge is a concept that is familiar to patients, families, and providers of hospital-based care. It has been described as an estimate of patients' and family members' ability to leave an acute care facility,[18] a perception of being prepared or not prepared for hospital discharge,[7,19] and as an indicator of sufficient recovery to allow safe discharge although the patient is in an intermediate rather than later stage of recovery.[1] Attributes of readiness for discharge include physical stability; functional ability, preparedness, and competence to manage self-care at home; psychosocial factors including coping skills; availability of social support; adequate education and information about what to expect; and access to healthcare system and community resources.[19-22]

A patient's readiness for discharge can be assessed from the perspectives of the care provider,

TABLE 4.1.1 Linkages Between Meleis Transitions Theory Concepts, Study Variables, and Study Measures

Transitions Theory Concept	Nature of the Transition	Transition Conditions	Nursing Therapeutics	Patterns of Response: a. Feeling confident and competent b. Feeling connected
Transitions Theory Definitions[15,17,30]	Descriptors of the type, pattern, and properties of a transition	Personal or environmental conditions that facilitate or hinder progress toward achieving a healthy transition	Focuses on the prevention of unhealthy transitions, promoting perceived well-being, and dealing with the experience of transitions A key nursing strategy is preparation for transition through education targeting assumption of new role responsibilities and implementation of new skills	Development of understanding of diagnosis, treatment, recovery, and living with limitations, and strategies for managing The need to feel and stay connected with, as examples, supportive persons and healthcare professionals
Study Variables	Hospitalization factors	Patient characteristics	Hospital nursing practices –Discharge teaching –Care coordination	Readiness for hospital discharge Postdischarge coping difficulty Utilization of postdischarge support and services
Study Measures	a. Planned admission b. First (no prior) hospitalization c. Previous admission for same condition d. Length of hospital stay	a. Age b. Gender c. Race d. Socioeconomic status e. Payor f. Lives alone	Quality of Discharge Teaching Scale Care Coordination Scale	Readiness for Hospital Discharge Scale–Adult Form Post-Discharge Coping Difficulty Scale a. Calls to friends and family b. Calls to provider c. Calls to hospital d. Office or clinic visits e. Urgent care/ER visits f. Readmission

patient, and family who may have different perceptions of the patient's readiness.[7,8] Most commonly, readiness for discharge is measured in the form of a criterion-based assessment using situation-specific criteria to guide clinical discharge decisions.[23] The need to include patient's perceptions of readiness for discharge has been identified as an important component of discharge assessment,[19,20] however, few studies have directly assessed readiness for discharge from the patient perspective. The method of assessment is often limited to a single-item question in yes/no response format on which more than 90% of patients report readiness for discharge.[20,24-26] Recently, Weiss et al.[22,27] have developed and tested a summated rating scale for measurement of patients' perceptions of readiness for discharge. Results indicated a general perception of readiness but not complete readiness at the time of discharge.

Despite the clinical relevance of the patient's perception of readiness for discharge, only a few studies have been conducted to determine the consequences of discharging a patient who is not ready from either the clinician's or the patient's own perspective. For example, failure to meet postsurgical discharge criteria has been associated with a higher incidence of symptoms at 24 hours postdischarge.[28] Adult patients who reported unmet needs for care after discharge had higher rates of posthospitalization complications and readmission than those who reported that their postdischarge needs were met.[29] Results of descriptive studies provide evidence of problems and concerns after hospital discharge that reflect lack of readiness for the transition from hospital to home, such as difficulties with activities of daily living, medication and pain management, health maintenance, emotional adjustment, family caregivers, and access to health and social services.[5,6,20,31]

Patient education in the form of discharge teaching and coordination of care through discharge planning activities are the primary hospital nursing strategies for preparing patients for discharge. Practice and research reports on these topics have focused on the needs and concerns for specific patient populations, essential content for the health condition, and evaluation of knowledge gained, satisfaction with programs and services, and postdischarge outcomes. Nurses and patients may have different priorities for discharge teaching,[32] but in general it includes activities of daily living, pain and wound management, treatments and medication, recognizing complications, and accessing follow-up services.[33] Extensive discharge teaching has become a standard of hospital care. However, anxieties related to the complexity of managing medical care needs at home, the amount and consistency of information, the timing of teaching, and the relevance of the content to personal needs and concerns are barriers to retention of discharge teaching.[34] Consequently, although most patients report receiving adequate information prior to discharge, they identify gaps in needed information when questioned after discharge.[33,35-37] In particular, patients report lack of anticipatory education to promote the knowledge, coping skills, confidence, and support needed for managing the stressful, complex, and changing realities of the posthospitalization experience.[6,38] When informational needs are not adequately addressed, patients experience difficulties in managing posthospitalization care[4] and increased postdischarge utilization of provider office visits.[35]

Care coordination activities have been successful in promoting positive perceptions of discharge readiness and ability to manage care at home.[39] Active patient communication, family participation, and interdisciplinary collaboration during discharge planning promotes congruent identification of learning needs and priorities by the patient, family, and clinician, leading to successful home transition and satisfaction with discharge planning services.[40,41]

Readiness for discharge is a transitional outcome in the continuum of care from hospital to home. Because the patient's perspective has only occasionally been included in studies of discharge readiness, little is known about adult medical-surgical patient characteristics, hospitalization factors, and nursing practices that promote feelings of readiness for discharge or the relationship of readiness for discharge to the patient's experience of coping with home management in the posthospitalization period.

CHAPTER 4 SITUATIONAL TRANSITIONS: DISCHARGE AND RELOCATION 157

Discharge   **Post-Discharge**

Transition Conditions
Patient Characteristics
- Age
- Gender
- Race
- Socioeconomic Status
- Payor
- Lives alone

Nature of the Transition
Hospitalization Factors
- Planned admission
- First hospitalization
- Previous admission for same diagnosis
- Length of Hospital Stay

Nursing Therapeutics
Hospital Nursing Practices
- Discharge teaching
- Care coordination

Readiness for hospital discharge

Coping difficulty

Utilization of post-discharge support and services
- Calls to friends and family
- Calls to providers
- Calls to hospitals
- Office/clinic visits
- Urgent care/emergency visit
- Readmission

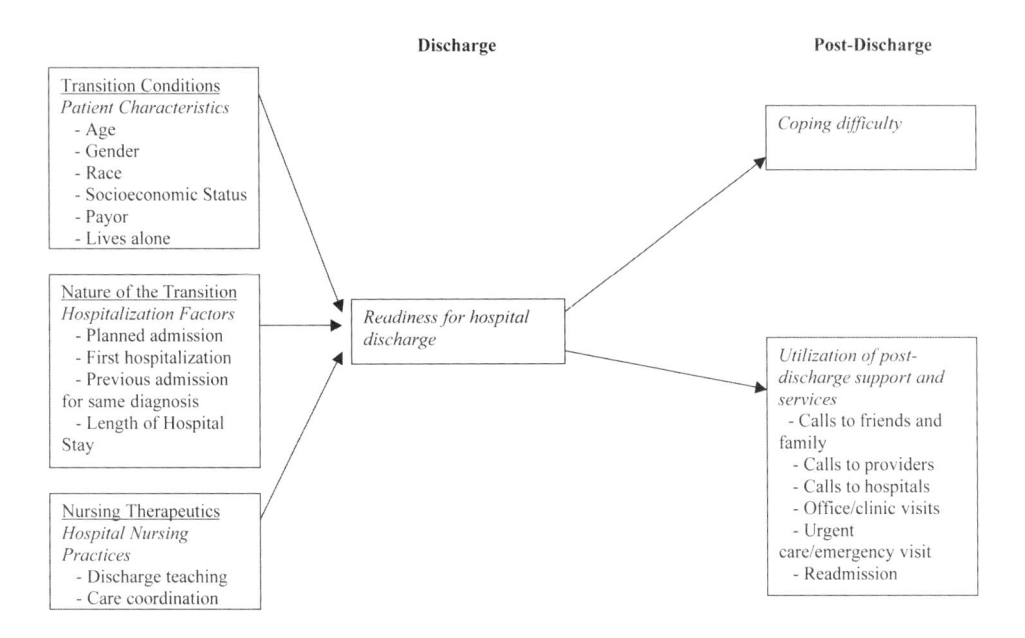

FIGURE 4.1.1 Proposed relationships between study variables.

Methods

The following research questions guided the selection of the correlational, longitudinal study design:

1. What patient characteristics, hospitalization factors, and hospital nursing practices are predictive of patients' perceptions of readiness for hospital discharge?
2. Do patients' perceptions of readiness for hospital discharge predict postdischarge coping difficulty and utilization of family support and health services?

The proposed relationships between the study concepts are presented in Figure 4.1.1.

This study was part of a larger study of predictors and outcomes of readiness for discharge among a broad sample of patients (adult medical-surgical patients, postpartum mothers, and parents of hospitalized children) discharged from acute care facilities.[42] The study reported here includes variables and results specific to the discharge transition of the adult medical-surgical portion of the larger study sample.

The sample consisted of adult medical-surgical patients at an urban tertiary-level medical center in the midwestern United States. Patients were recruited from general medical, surgical, and cardiac inpatient units. Patients met study inclusion criteria if they were at least 18 years old, were discharged directly home following hospitalization, had sufficient English language skills to read and respond to consent forms and study questions, and had telephone access for postdischarge data collection. Patients were excluded if they did not have sufficient cognitive skills to complete the consenting, questionnaire, and interview processes independently or they were discharged home with hospice care. A power analysis indicated that a sample of 120 would be sufficient to achieve a power of 80% in multiple regression analyses with up to 10 predictor variables at a moderate effect size.[43] A total of 147 patients enrolled in the study, 135 (92%) completed data collection at discharge, and 113 (77%) completed the 3-week postdischarge telephone interview. Loss to follow-up at the 3-week postdischarge period was due to inability to reach the patient using primary and alternate telephone contact information. There were more nonwhite ($\chi^2 = 3.98$, $df = 1$, $p = .046$) and public assistance patients ($\chi^2 = 5.60$, $df = 1$, $p = .02$) in the lost-to-follow-up group than among those who completed the follow-up interview. Two patients died during the 3-week interval after discharge.

Variables and Instruments

Patient Characteristics and Hospitalization Factors

During the inpatient hospitalization prior to the day of discharge, data on patient characteristics (age, gender, race, socioeconomic status, living alone) and hospitalization factors (planned admission [aware of admission date for at least 24 hours prior to admission], number of admissions to the hospital, previous admission for same condition) were collected from the patient during study enrollment. The Hollingshead 4-Factor Index of Social Status was used to calculate a family socioeconomic status score using education and occupation data from one or both parents depending on marital status.[44] Payor (a patient characteristic) and length of hospital stay (a hospitalization factor) data were abstracted from the medical record.

Four scales were developed and tested for the larger study:[22,42] The Readiness for Hospital Discharge Scale (RHDS) was a modification and extension of earlier work by Weiss and colleagues with postpartum patients.[27] The modified version of the RHDS and the Quality of Discharge Teaching Scale (QDTS), Care Coordination Scale (CCS), and Post-Discharge Coping Difficulty Scale (PDCDS) were developed for the specific purposes of measuring variables related to the discharge transition by 3 teams of nurse experts.

Readiness for Hospital Discharge

The adult patient version of the RHDS was used to capture patients' perceptions of readiness for discharge. The RHDS—Adult Form is a 22-item instrument that includes 21 items from a master version of the RHDS that can be used across patient populations[22] and 1 additional item specific to adult medical-surgical patients (knowledge about caring for personal needs). The items form 4 subscales: Personal Status, Knowledge, Coping Ability, and Expected Support. The RHDS is a self-reported summated rating scale with items scored on an 11-point scale (0–10) with anchor words (eg, not at all, totally) to cue the subject to the meaning of the numeric scale. Higher scores indicate greater readiness. The reading level of the instrument is grade level of 8.5 (Microsoft Word, 2003, Flesch-Kincaid Grade Level Score). Construct validity, using confirmatory factor analysis and contrasted group comparisons, and predictive validity have been established for the 21-item scale.[22] The Cronbach's alpha reliability estimate for the 22-item RHDS—Adult Form was .93.

Discharge Teaching

Educational preparation for discharge was measured using the QDTS. Discharge teaching was conceptualized as the composite of all teaching received by the patient (from the patient's perspective) during the hospitalization in preparation for discharge home and coping with the posthospitalization period. Principal components exploratory factor analysis of the QDTS data for the larger study sample identified a 2-factor structure (content and delivery) accounting for 54.2% of scale variance.[42] The QDTS consists of 18 items and uses a similar scaling format to the RHDS. The content subscale consists of 6 items representing the amount of "content received" during teaching in preparation for discharge. The 12-item "delivery" subscale reflects the skill of the nurses as educators in presenting discharge teaching and includes items about listening to and answering specific questions and concerns, expressing sensitivity to personal beliefs and values, teaching in a way that the patient could understand and at times that were good for patients and family members, providing consistent information, promoting confidence in ability to care for themselves and knowing what to do in an emergency, and decreasing anxiety about going home. The total scale score is calculated by adding the content received and the delivery subscale scores. For the adult sample, the Cronbach's alpha reliability coefficients for the total scale was .92 and for the content received and delivery subscales were .85 and .93, respectively.

Care Coordination

The CCS, with 5 items measuring care coordination during discharge preparations, used the same scaling format as the RHDS. With a small number of items, this scale did not perform adequately in reliability testing in the larger study and with the adult patient sample. Any results from its use should be viewed cautiously.

Postdischarge Coping Difficulty

The 10-item PDCDS used the same scaling format as the RHDS. Higher scores represented greater coping difficulty. Attributes of postdischarge coping that were included in PDCDS items were difficulties with stress, recovery, self-care, self-medical management, family difficulty, help and emotional support needed, confidence in self-care and medical management abilities, and adjustment. Exploratory factor analysis with the larger study sample indicated a single dominant factor accounting for 39% of scale variance. Reliability for the adult sample was 0.87.

Postdischarge Utilization of Support and Health Services

Utilization of support and health services was self-reported during a postdischarge telephone interview. The following occurrences were recorded in dichotomous format (yes/no): calls to friends and family for advice and/or support, calls to providers, office or clinic visits, calls to the hospital, urgent care/emergency room visits, and hospital readmission.

Procedures

Approval was obtained from university and hospital institutional review boards. The principal investigator trained the undergraduate nursing students who served as study research assistants in the study procedures for obtaining informed consent, data collection, and telephone interviewing. Before the day of discharge, the research assistants identified eligible patients from inpatient hospital records, described the study to potential participants, obtained informed consent, and abstracted medical records. Within 4 hours prior to discharge, patients completed the RHDS, the QDTS, and the CCS. The research assistant who enrolled the patient conducted a telephone interview at 3 weeks postdischarge to collect PDCDS and postdischarge utilization data.

SPSS 13.0[45] was used for the analyses. Incomplete responses on study questionnaires were replaced by substitution with item means if less than 20% of the responses on a scale were missing. Otherwise the respondent's scores were deleted from the affected analysis. This procedure resulted in different numbers of available respondents for each analysis. Descriptive statistics were used to describe the study sample and overall response pattern on study measures. Path analyses of relationships described in the proposed study model based on transitions theory (Figure 4.1.1) were conducted using multiple regression for examining outcome variables measured at the interval level (RHDS and PDCDS) and logistic regression for outcome variables measured at the nominal level (utilization variables). Preliminary analyses were conducted using variables associated with each of the transitions theory concepts (transition conditions [represented by patient characteristics], nature of the transition [represented by hospitalization factors], and nursing therapeutics [represented by hospital nursing practices]) in separate analyses for each of the 3 outcome variables (readiness for discharge, coping difficulty, and utilization of services). A final regression model was tested for each outcome variable using only the significant predictor variables from the preliminary analyses. This procedure assisted with retention of sufficient statistical power for the analyses and identification of additional relationships not originally specified in the research questions.

Results

Characteristics of the sample are presented in Table 4.1.2.

The 147 participants included 78 (53.1%) women and 69 (46.9%) men. The sample as a whole included a range of ages from 20 to 88 with a mean age of 53.4 (SD = 15.0). Half of the sample was married; 20% reported that they were living alone. The Hollingshead 4-Factor Index of Social Status score was greater than the scale's median value of 33, with 55% of the sample having post–high school education. The sample was predominantly white (63.2%) but included a substantial proportion of black patients (34.7%). Demographics for the geographic location (county/city) of the study sites[46] were 68.7%/53.7% non-Hispanic white, and 20.2%/31.4% black.

Overall, 93% of patients reported being ready to go home on a single-item yes/no format question. The sample as a whole reported that they felt reasonably ready for discharge (RHDS item mean = 8.0 [SD = 0.9], range of item means = 6.1 to 9.1), that they received good quality teaching (QDTS item mean = 7.6 [SD = 1.4], range of item means = 4.9 to 8.9), and that they had fairly low levels of difficulty coping in the postdischarge period (PDCDS item mean = 2.4 [SD = 1.0], range of item means = 0.9 to 4.0) [maximum item score on all scales = 10.0]. Postdischarge utilization of health services rates were calculated for all patients responding to the postdischarge interview and are presented in Table 4.1.3. Only 3 of the 113 respondents (2.7%) did not access any health service (call or visit to provider, emergency visit, or readmission) during the first 3 weeks following discharge.

TABLE 4.1.2 Patient Characteristics and Hospitalization Factors (n = 147*)

	Mean	SD
Age	53.4	(15.1)
Socioeconomic status†	38.0	(13.8)
Length of hospital stay (days)	5.0	(4.0)

	n	%
Gender		
Female	78	(53.1)
Male	69	(46.9)
Race		
White	91	(63.2)
Black	50	(34.7)
Hispanic	1	(0.7)
Asian	2	(1.4)
Marital status		
Married	75	(51.0)
Single	34	(23.1)
Widowed	19	(12.9)
Other (divorced, separated)	19	(12.9)
Lives alone	29	(19.9)
Payor		
Public	60	(41.1)
Private	80	(54.8)
Self	6	(4.1)
Education		
Less than high school	23	(15.9)
High school	42	(29.0)
Partial college	36	(24.8)
4-year college	28	(19.3)
Graduate education	16	(11.0)
Admission		
Planned admission >24 hours	73	(50.7)
First admission to hospital	14	(9.7)
Previous admission for same diagnosis	44	(30.8)

Values are presented as mean [SD] or n (%).
*The n in some categories is smaller due to missing data from incomplete responses. % indicates percent of actual respondents.
†Hollingshead 4-Factor Index of Social Status[44] scores range from 0 to 66.

TABLE 4.1.3 Utilization of Postdischarge Support and Services ($n = 113$)

Postdischarge Support and Services	n	%
Calls to friends and family	30	26.5
Calls to providers	34	30.1
Follow-up doctor visits		
Office/clinic visits	91	80.1
Unscheduled	12	10.6
Calls to hospital	12	10.6
Urgent care/ER visits	4	3.5
Readmission	8	7.1

Predictors of Readiness for Discharge

The results of multiple regression analyses of the RHDS are presented in Table 4.1.4. The first path to be analyzed was the relationship of patient characteristics and RHDS. The 6 predictor variables were entered simultaneously into the regression equation. The resultant model (Table 4.1.4, Model 1) explained 16% ($R^2 = 0.16$) of the variance in RHDS scores in this sample with a population estimate of 11% (Adj. $R^2 = 0.11$). The "lives alone" variable emerged as the only significant independent predictor. Next, the 4 hospitalization predictor variables were entered simultaneously into a regression equation for RHDS (Table 4.1.4, Model 2). The resultant model was not statistically significant.

The nursing practice variables of QDTS and CCS were then entered into a multiple regression analysis as predictors of RHDS. The QDTS total scale score and CCS accounted for 33% of the variance in RHDS (Table 4.1.4, Model 3a).

When QDTS subscale scores were entered in place of the total scale score with CCS (Table 4.1.4, Model 3b), these variables accounted for 44% of the variance in RHDS and all were significant predictors. As a final step, all significant predictors from the hospitalization phase were entered as predictors of RHDS (Table 4.1.4, Model 4). The resultant model accounted for 51% of the variance in RHDS. "Lives alone," QDTS content received and delivery of teaching, and CCS were significant predictors of patients' perceptions of readiness for discharge. The QDTS delivery of teaching subscale score was the strongest predictor. The direction on the relationships between QTDS—teaching delivery and CCS were in the expected direction, with more effective teaching delivery and greater care coordination associated with greater readiness for discharge. The direction of the relationship between amount of discharge teaching content received and readiness for discharge was inverse. In the regression analyses in Table 4.1.4 (Models 3b and 4), it appeared that less content received was associated with greater readiness for discharge, although both the amount of "content received" and "teaching delivery" were positively associated with RHDS ($r = 0.24$, $p = .01$ and $r = 0.62$, $p < .01$, respectively) and with each other ($r = 0.57$, $p < .01$) in bivariate correlations. This finding indicates that QDTS "content received" is a net suppression variable.[47] This effect indicates that when the stronger predictor variable (teaching delivery) was held constant, more content offered did not improve the readiness for discharge outcome, in fact, less may have been desirable in the presence of quality delivery of discharge teaching. To explore for the possibility of unanticipated differences in the amount of "content received" by patient characteristics or hospitalization factors, analysis of variance tests were performed with no significant differences found for any of the variables tested. For age, socioeconomic status, and number of days in hospital, the correlations with amount of content received were not statistically significant.

Outcomes of Readiness for Discharge

Two outcomes, postdischarge coping difficulty and utilization of support and healthcare services, were evaluated. The results of path analyses of predictors of PDCDS scores and utilization of services are presented in Tables 4.1.5 and 4.1.6, respectively. First, RHDS was entered as a predictor in a linear regression equation for PDCDS as the outcome variable. The results (Table 4.1.5, Model 1) indicated that RHDS scores explained 10% of the variance in PDCDS scores. To assess the contribution

TABLE 4.1.4 Predictors of Readiness for Discharge (RHDS)

| Predictor Variables | Model Statistics | Variable Statistics |||||
		B	SE B	Standardized β	t	p
Model 1: Patient Characteristics:	$F_{6,104} = 3.32$					
a. Age	$p = .01$	0.31	0.22	0.14	1.40	.17
b. Gender (0–male, 1–female)	$R^2 = 0.16$	3.56	6.27	0.05	0.57	.57
c. Race (0–white, 1–nonwhite)	Adjusted $R^2 = 0.11$	−5.51	7.34	−0.08	−0.75	.45
d. Socioeconomic status		0.40	0.26	0.16	1.56	.12
e. Payor (0–public, 1–private)		−5.15	11.09	−0.05	−0.47	.64
f. Live alone (0–no, 1–yes)		−30.66	8.16	−0.35	−3.76	<.01
Model 2: Hospitalization Factors:	$F_{4,106} = 0.18$					
a. Planned admission (0–no, 1–yes)	$P = .95$	3.50	6.65	0.05	0.53	.60
b. First hospitalization (0–no, 1–yes)	$R^2 = 0.01$	4.22	12.33	0.03	0.34	.73
c. Previous admission for same condition (0–no, 1–yes)	Adjusted $R^2 = -0.03$	−0.52	7.26	−0.00	−0.01	.99
d. Length of hospital stay		−0.47	0.97	−0.05	−0.49	.63
Model 3a: Hospital Nursing Practices	$F_{2,104} = 25.41$					
a. QDTS	$p < .01$	0.31	0.10	0.33	3.22	<.01
b. CCS	$R^2 = 0.33$ Adjusted $R^2 = 0.32$	1.03	0.33	0.32	3.12	<.01
Model 3b: Hospital Nursing Practices	$F_{3,103} = 27.46$					
a. QDTS—Content received	$p < .01$	−0.47	0.19	−0.23	−2.48	.02
b. QDTS—Delivery	$R^2 = 0.44$	0.83	0.14	0.58	5.83	<.01
c. CCS	Adjusted $R^2 = 0.43$	0.88	0.30	0.27	2.90	.01
Model 4: All significant predictors	$F_{4,103} = 26.50$					
a. Live alone (0–no, 1–yes)	$p < .01$	−21.09	5.73	−0.26	−3.68	<.01
b. QDTS—Content received	$R^2 = 0.51$	−0.40	0.18	−0.19	−2.25	.03
c. QDTS—Delivery	Adjusted $R^2 = 0.49$	0.77	0.14	0.54	5.61	<.01
d. CCS		1.93	0.29	0.29	3.26	<.01

QDTS indicates Quality of Discharge Teaching Scale; CCS, Care Coordination Scale.

Table 4.1.5 Predictors of Postdischarge Coping Difficulty (PDCDS)

Predictor Variables	Model Statistics	B	SE B	Standardized β	t	p
Model 1: RHDS	$F_{1,86} = 9.32$ $p < .01$ $R^2 = 0.10$ Adjusted $R^2 = 0.09$	−0.19	0.06	−0.31	−3.05	<.01
Model 2: Patient Characteristics	$F_{6,94} = 1.76$					
a. Age	$P = .12$	−0.29	0.13	−0.25	−2.24	.03
b. Gender (0–male, 1–female)	$R^2 = 0.10$	3.76	3.59	0.11	1.05	.30
c. Race (0–white, 1–nonwhite)	Adjusted $R^2 = 0.04$	3.94	4.13	0.11	0.95	.34
d. Socioeconomic status		−0.06	0.15	−0.04	−0.36	.72
e. Payor (0–public, 1–private)		7.39	7.09	0.12	1.04	.30
f. Live alone (0–no, 1–yes)		1.54	4.61	0.04	0.33	.74
Model 3: Hospitalization Factors	$F_{4,86} = 1.35$					
a. Planned admission (0–no, 1–yes)	$p = .26$	7.76	3.82	0.22	2.03	.05
b. First hospitalization (0–no, 1–yes)	$R^2 = 0.06$	4.33	6.58	0.07	0.66	.51
c. Previous admission for same condition (0–no, 1–yes)	Adjusted $R^2 = 0.02$	2.42	4.28	0.06	0.57	.57
d. Length of hospital stay		0.54	0.55	0.11	0.99	.33
Model 4a: Hospital Nursing Practices	$F_{2,79} = 0.36$					
a. QDTS	$p = .70$	−0.02	0.07	−0.05	−0.34	.74
b. CCS	$R^2 = 0.01$ Adjusted $R^2 = -0.02$	−0.11	0.25	−0.06	−0.46	0.65
Model 4b: Hospital Nursing Practices	$F_{3,78} = 1.93$					
a. QDTS—Content received	$p = .13$	0.31	0.17	0.28	1.89	.06
b. QDTS—Delivery	$R^2 = 0.07$	−0.25	0.12	−0.30	−2.04	.05
c. CCS	Adjusted $R^2 = 0.03$	−0.14	0.25	−0.08	−0.58	.57
Model 5: All Significant Predictors	$F_{3,81} = 5.22$					
a. RHDS	$P < .01$	−0.18	0.06	−0.30	−2.93	<.01
b. Age	$R^2 = 0.16$	−0.26	0.11	−0.24	−2.29	.02
c. Planned admission (0–no, 1–yes)	Adjusted $R^2 = 0.13$	4.26	3.50	0.12	1.22	.23

RHDS indicates Readiness for Hospital Discharge Scale; QDTS, Quality of Discharge Teaching Scale; CCS, Care Coordination Scale.

of all variables temporally antecedent to postdischarge coping, multiple regression analyses were computed for sets of predictor variables in their theory-based groupings: Model 2—transition conditions (patient characteristics); Model 3—nature of the transition (hospitalization factors); Model 4—nursing therapeutics (hospital nursing practices—QDTS and CCS). A final model (Model 5) was computed with all significant predictors from the preliminary models. The final model as a whole was statistically significant in predicting PDCDS, explaining 16% of its variance. Age and RHDS emerged as significant predictors in this final analysis. Younger adults and those who did not perceive themselves to be ready experienced greater coping difficulty.

To assess the predictors of postdischarge utilization, logistic regression analyses were conducted for each of the 6 utilization variables in the same manner as previous analyses, entering temporally antecedent variables and PDCDS (which was measured concurrently) in their theory-based groupings for preliminary analyses. The test statistics for the final models of all significant predictors are presented in Table 4.1.6. Readiness for Hospital Discharge Scale was predictive of readmission to the hospital but not of any other utilization variable. As expected, higher RHDS scores were associated with fewer readmissions, although only 8 study participants were readmitted. Living alone was the only patient characteristic variable associated with a utilization variable, with a more than 3-fold (OR = 3.53) increase in the number of patients calling family and friends for advice and/or support.

Higher PDCDS scores were also associated with a slightly greater use of family and friends (OR = 1.04). Patients reporting higher levels of care coordination made fewer calls to the hospital after discharge. Those with a longer length of stay made more office or clinic visits to providers. Of particular note, patients experiencing a first admission to the hospital were 7 times (OR = 7.76) more likely to have an unscheduled office visit than patients who had a prior hospitalization. Figure 4.1.2 displays the significant relationships identified in the regression analyses.

Discussion

Most patients feel ready for discharge but there was enough variability in the study data to suggest that those who are not ready have poorer postdischarge coping outcomes. The study's results also validate the importance of discharge teaching in preparing patients to feel ready to go home. The relationship of discharge teaching to postdischarge coping was indirect with readiness for discharge as an important intermediary. The findings suggest that discharge teaching places the patient in a state of readiness that sets the stage for successfully managing care and continuing recovery at home without substantial difficulty coping with the early postdischarge period. The significant relationships identified in the analyses indicate a trajectory of hospital-based nursing practices that impact patient readiness as an outcome of hospitalization, which then is reflected in postdischarge coping and utilization outcomes. This trajectory is consistent with the transitions theory propositions that generated the research questions for the study.

Higher quality discharge teaching was associated with more positive perceptions of discharge readiness. Both the amount of discharge teaching content and the skills of nurses in delivering the discharge teaching were associated with patients' perceptions of discharge readiness. The "delivery" of teaching was the strongest predictor of discharge readiness. This finding has important implications for development of nursing staff skills in discharge teaching and of programs and materials for patient education. Often, the focus of patient education is the content itself. The findings of this study suggest that the skills used in content delivery are associated with readiness as an outcome. In preparing nurses in discharge teaching, emphasis should be placed on the quality of the delivery of discharge teaching that results in the patient feeling prepared for the transition home. Specifically, delivery of teaching that included particular attention to listening and answering, sensitivity to personal beliefs and values, clarification, consistency, scheduling at times convenient for the family to attend, focusing on anxiety reduction, and confidence building improved patients' perceptions of their readiness to

TABLE 4.1.6 Significant Predictors of Postdischarge Utilization

Outcome Variables	Predictor Variables	Logistic Regression Statistics					
		B	SE	χ^2	Odds Ratio	95% CI	p
Calls to family and friends	Live alone (0–no, 1–yes)	1.26	0.61	4.28	3.53	1.07–11.66	.04
	PDCDS	0.04	0.01	7.99	1.04	1.01–1.06	.01
Calls to provider							NS
Calls to hospital	CCS	−0.15	0.06	6.25	0.86	0.77–0.97	.01
Office/clinic visits	Length of hospital stay	0.45	0.22	4.09	1.57	1.01–2.44	.04
Unscheduled office/clinic visits	First hospitalization (0–no, 1–yes)	2.05	0.85	5.88	7.76	1.48–40.66	.02
Urgent care/emergency visits							NS
Readmission	RHDS	−0.03	0.01	6.83	0.97	0.95–0.99	.01

RHDS indicates Readiness for Hospital Discharge Scale; CCS, Care Coordination Scale; PDCDS, Post-Discharge Coping Difficulty Scale; NS, nonsignificant.

go home. The combination of verbal and written modalities for presenting information for discharge has been recommended.[48] This study did not evaluate how the nurses used these modalities or how these modalities were customized to the patient's needs. What was evident from this study was that the skill of nurses as they provided for the patient's discharge learning needs was an important predictor of the patient's perception of readiness to go home.

The complexity of patient teaching was evident in the results of bivariate and multivariate analyses of the relationship between the quality of discharge teaching and readiness for discharge. As expected, in the bivariate correlations of the QDTS content received and delivery subscales with RHDS, both were positively correlated. When placed in the context of the totality of the teaching encounter (ie, both the content received and the way it is "delivered"), when both subscale scores were entered together into a model for predicting readiness for discharge as an outcome (Table 4.1.4, Model 3b and Model 4), the amount of content was negatively associated with RHDS, whereas delivery of teaching was still positively and more strongly related to RHDS. The complementary, synergistic, and complex nature of patient teaching is evident in these findings. Although providing information in preparation for discharge is, in general, beneficial, more may not always be better. In the presence of excellent teaching delivery skills, less content may be needed to produce the desired outcome. Overcompensation with excessive content may occur in the absence of high-quality teaching skills. Content in the absence of quality delivery skills is not as effective as when nurses with excellent teaching delivery skills provide the discharge preparation. Overloading the patient with all of the content the nurse perceives as beneficial may, in fact, interfere with retention. Anxiety, fatigue, and other illness responses; age-related memory; and medications can all potentially impact attention and retention of content presented in discharge teaching. Identification of information to meet individualized needs may reduce the amount of content but increase the accessibility of the information when needed. Several reports have indicated that patients

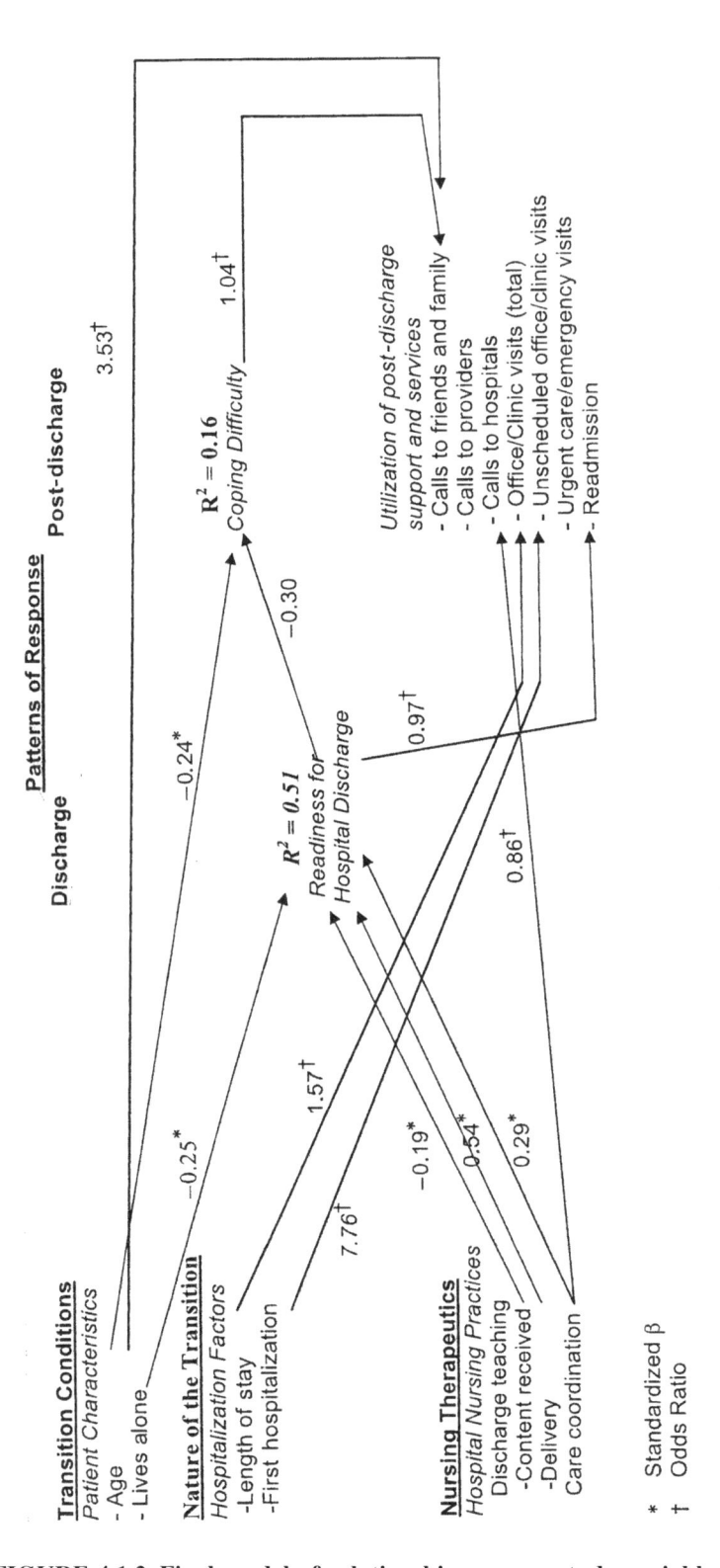

166 PART III THE EXPERIENCE OF AND RESPONSES TO TRANSITIONS

FIGURE 4.1.2 Final model of relationships among study variables.

report gaps in teaching once they are home, especially in the areas of expectations and realities of the postdischarge period and strategies for handling the complexities of postdischarge self-management.[4,6,31] Less but targeted content focused on expectations, realities, and problem-solving may be more effective than facts alone. Future research efforts should be directed to uncovering "best practices" for assessment of the desirable amount of content and the best methods of delivering discharge teaching.

Living alone and poor care coordination were associated with lower readiness for discharge scores. The importance of family support and continuity of care during the transition from acute to community-based care is well documented.[4,38,41]

Patients' perceptions of their discharge readiness were associated with difficulties with postdischarge coping and the occurrence of readmission in the first 3 weeks postdischarge. With only 8 patients readmitted, this finding should be viewed with caution. However, failure to institute anticipatory interventions for patients who do not perceive themselves to be ready for discharge may lead to unintended adverse clinical outcomes for the patient and cost outcomes for the health system. Readiness for discharge is a nurse-sensitive intermediate patient outcome in the transition from acute to community-based care. Patients with low readiness for discharge scores are not the only patients who need support and services following discharge. Perceived readiness for discharge explained a small portion of the variance in discharge coping difficulty and the likelihood of service utilization. Many patients with high perceived readiness for discharge also experienced difficulties and potentially preventable utilization of compensatory services in the postdischarge period. The need for continuing care and services beyond hospitalization is clear from the patterns of postdischarge utilization observed in this study.

Predictive pathways, in addition to those originally proposed, emerged from the analyses of the discharge transition model. Younger adults were more likely to experience coping difficulty, possibly related to the competing demands of family life, work responsibilities, and needs related to the illness and recovery. Likewise, older adults may have already developed successful coping behaviors during past health-related episodes that facilitate coping in subsequent health experiences. Patients who lived alone or who had difficulty coping, sought support and/or advice from friends and family. Nature of the transition variables, specifically a longer hospitalization and a first hospitalization, were associated with greater utilization of medical surveillance services in the postdischarge period.

Meleis' transitions theory was a useful model for conceptualizing and investigating the discharge transition. Many of the relationships identified using transitions theory as a guiding framework were supported by the study findings. Consistent with transitions theory, the findings indicate that transition conditions, the nature of the transition, transition conditions, and nursing therapeutics impact patterns of response across the posthospitalization transition.

Limitations

Patients' perceptions of their discharge transition, including their perceptions of the discharge teaching, their readiness for discharge, their postdischarge coping difficulty, and self-reports of service utilization were the data on which study findings were based.

These perceptions reflected the patient's reality but may not have accurately represented the clinical reality or the actual teaching that was provided. A legitimate question arising from this research is "Do patients accurately assess their readiness for discharge?" This question was not addressed in this study. Further exploration of the relationships between patient, family, and provider perspectives on discharge readiness is needed to determine the relative contribution of each to anticipating postdischarge outcomes.

Data for this study were collected in a single hospital and may not reflect the experience of patients in other facilities and geographic locations. The instruments for the study were developed for the specific purposes of this study and, for all but one scale (CCS), their reliability estimates were acceptable and validity was supported. These instruments will benefit from additional testing. Care coordination was positively associated with readiness for discharge, however, this finding should be considered with skepticism until the relationship between care coordination and readiness for discharge is tested with a better measure. The number of subjects was adequate for the number of variables entered into the multiple regression equations, providing sufficient power for analyses of readiness for discharge and postdischarge coping. However, more subjects are needed to confidently explore the relationship of predictor variables to utilization outcomes.

Conclusions and Implications for Advanced Practice Nursing

The results of this study are particularly relevant to the role of the clinical nurse specialist (CNS) across their 3 spheres of influence on patients/clients, nurses and nursing practices, and organizations/systems.[9] The results clearly point to the importance of nurses' patient education skills in promoting readiness for discharge and outcomes beyond discharge. Preparation of nursing staff to effectively deliver discharge teaching with emphasis on the appropriate amount of content and effective delivery methods is within the domain of the CNS. Readiness for discharge assessment should be part of discharge preparation for every patient and those who are less ready may benefit from rescue strategies to avert adverse outcomes. Readiness for discharge can be both a process measure to identify patients in need of additional interventions before and after discharge and a nurse-sensitive outcome measure of the hospitalization experience. Building systems of care that routinely assess progress toward readiness, outcome at the time of discharge, and implementation of strategies for addressing gaps in readiness that emerge after hospital discharge will promote optimal short-term and long-term outcomes of the hospitalization experience. This study also points to the value of using a nursing theory that incorporates the patient's experience and the role of the nurse, in this case, transitions theory, as a guiding framework for investigating and ultimately planning systems of care that address the important considerations of the discharge transition and other transitional processes.

Acknowledgments

The authors thank Marquette University College of Nursing undergraduate students Cheri Goepfert, Lindsay Gorectke, Meghan Jolly, Patrick McNally, Elizabeth Pricco, and graduate student Kim Nelson, who served as research assistants for the study. The nursing staff of Wheaton Franciscan Healthcare, St. Joseph, Milwaukee, WI, were active participants in the research process through their support of the study, involvement in study planning, and assistance with distribution of study questionnaires to their patients at the time of hospital discharge.

REFERENCES

1. Korttila K. Anaesthesia for ambulatory surgery: firm definitions of "Home Readiness" needed. *Ann Med.* 1991;23(6): 635-636.
2. Bull M, Maruyama G, Luo D. Testing a model of posthospital transition of family caregivers for elderly persons. *Nurs Res.* 1995;44(3):132-138.
3. Bull MJ. Managing the transition from hospital to home. *Qual Health Res.* 1992;2(1):27-41.
4. Bull MJ, Jervis LL. Strategies used by chronically ill older women and their caregiving daughters in managing posthospital care. *J Adv Nurs.* 1997;25(3):541-547.
5. Clark M, Steinberg M, Bischoff N. Patient readiness for return to home: discord between expectations and reality. *Aust Occup Ther J.* 1997;44:132-141.
6. LeClerc CM, Wells D, Craig D, Wilson JL. Falling short of the mark: tales of life after hospital discharge. *Clin Nurs Res.* 2002;11(3):242-263.
7. Congdon JG. Managing the incongruities: the hospital discharge experience for elderly patient, their families, and nurses. *Appl Nurs Res.* 1994;7(3):125-131.

8. Reiley P, Lezzoni LI, Phillips R, Davis RB, Tuchin LI, Calkins D. Discharge planning: comparison of patients' and nurses' perceptions of patients following hospital discharge. *IMAGE J Nurs Sch.* 1996;28(2):143-147.
9. National Association of Clinical Nurse Specialists. *Statement on Clinical Nurse Specialist Practices and Education.* 2nd ed. Harrisburg, Pa: National Association of Clinical Nurse Specialists; 2004.
10. Clark A, Nadash P. The effectiveness of a nurse-led transitional care model for patients with congestive heart failure. *Home Healthc Nurse.* 2004;22(3):160-162.
11. Coleman EA, Smith JD, Frank JC, Min S, Parry C, Kramer AM. Preparing patients and caregivers to participate in care delivered across settings: the care transitions intervention. *J Am Geriatr Soc.* 2004;52(11):1817-1825.
12. Esche CA, Tanner EK. Home health care. Resiliency: a factor to consider in facilitating the transition from hospital to home in older adults. *Geriatr Nurs.* 2005;26(4):218-222.
13. Shyu Y. Role tuning between caregiver and care receiver during discharge transition: an illumination of the role function mode of Roy's Adaptation Model. *Nurs Sci Q.* 2000; 13(4):323-331.
14. Woods LW, Craig JB, Dereng N. Transitioning to a hospice program. *J Hosp Palliat Nurs.* 2006;8(2):103-111.
15. Meleis AI, Sawyer LM, Im E-O, Messias DK, Schumacher K. Experiencing transitions: an emerging middle-range theory. *Adv Nurs Sci.* 2000;23(1):12-28.
16. Higgins PA, Moore SM. Levels of theoretical thinking in nursing. *Nurs Outl.* 2000;48(4):179-183.
17. Meleis AI, Trangenstein PA. Facilitating transitions: redefinition of the nursing mission. *Nurs Outl.* 1994;42:255-259.
18. Steele NF, Sterling YM. Application of the case study design: nursing interventions for discharge readiness. *Clin Nurse Spec.* 1992;6(2):79-84.
19. Fenwick AM. An interdisciplinary tool for assessing patients' readiness for discharge in the rehabilitation setting. *J Adv Nurs.* 1979;4:9-21.
20. Schaefer AL, Anderson JE, Simms LM. Are they ready? Discharge planning for older surgical patients. *J Gerontol Nurs.* 1990;16(10):16-19.
21. Titler MG, Pettit DM. Discharge readiness assessment. *J Cardiovasc Nurs.* 1995;9(4):64-74.
22. Weiss M, Piacentine LB. Psychometric properties of the Readiness for Hospital Discharge Scale. *J Nurs Meas.* 2006; 14(3):163-180.
23. Stephenson M. Discharge criteria in day surgery. *J Adv Nurs.* 1990;15:601-613.
24. Bernstein HH, Spino C, Baker A, Slora EJ, Touloukian CL, McCormick MC. Postpartum discharge: do varying perceptions of readiness impact health outcomes? *Ambul Pediatr.* 2002;2(5):388-395.
25. Greene M. *Adult Surgical Patients' Perceptions of Discharge Readiness and Postoperative Recovery* [Master's thesis]. Milwaukee, Wis: University of Wisconsin—Milwaukee; 1991.
26. Weiss M, Ryan P, Lokken L, Nelson M. Length of stay after vaginal birth: sociodemographic and readiness-for-discharge factors. *Birth.* 2004;31(2):93-101.
27. Weiss ME, Ryan P, Lokken L. Validity and reliability of the perceived readiness for discharge after birth scale. *J Obstet Gynecol Neonatal Nurs.* 2006;35(1):34-45.
28. Chung F. Recovery pattern and home-readiness after ambulatory surgery. *Anesth Analg.* 1995;80(5):896-902.
29. Mamon J, Steinwachs DM, Fahey M, Bone LR, Oktay J, Klein L. Impact of hospital discharge planning on meeting planning needs after returning home. *Health Serv Res.* 1992;27(2):155-175.
30. Schumacher KL, Meleis AI. Transitions: A central concept in nursing. *Image J Nurs Sch.* 1994;26(2):119-127.
31. Tierney AJ, Closs SJ, Hunter HC, MacMillan MS. Experiences of elderly patients concerning discharge from hospital. *J Clin Nurs.* 1993;2:179-185.
32. Ruchala PL. Teaching new mothers: priorities of nurses and postpartum women. *J Obstet Gynecol Neonatal Nurs.* 2000;29(3):265-273.
33. Jacobs V. Informational needs of surgical patients following discharge. *Appl Nurs Res.* 2000;13(1):12-18.
34. Paterson B, Kieloch B, Gmiterek J. "They never told us anything": postdischarge instruction for families of persons with brain injuries. *Rehabil Nurs.* 2001;26(2):48-53.
35. Henderson A, Zernike W. A study of the impact of discharge information for surgical patients. *J Adv Nurs.* 2001;35(3):435-441.
36. Lee NC, Wasson DR, Anderson MA, Stone S, Gittings JA. A survey of patient education postdischarge. *J Nurs Care Qual.* 1998;13(1):63-70.
37. Steele JM, Ruzicki D. An evaluation of the effectiveness of cardiac teaching during hospitalization. *Heart Lung.* 1987;16(3):306-311.
38. Berkman B, Millar S, Holmes W, Bonander E. Predicting elderly cardiac patients at risk for readmission. *Soc Work Health Care.* 1991;16(6):21-38.

39. Kleinpell R. Randomized trial of an intensive care unit-based early discharge intervention for critically ill elderly patients. *Am J Crit Care.* 2004;13:335-345.
40. Anthony MK, Hudson-Barr D. A patient-centered model of care for hospital discharge. *Clin Nurs Res.* 2004;13(2):117-136.
41. Bull MJ, Hansen HE, Gross CR. A professional-patient partnership model of discharge planning with elders hospitalized with heart failure. *Appl Nurs Res.* 2000;13(1):19-28.
42. Weiss ME, Piacentine LB, Johnson NL, Jerofke T. Readiness for hospital discharge: predictors and outcomes. In review.
43. Polit DF. *Data Analysis & Statistics for Nursing Research.* Upper Saddle River, NJ: Prentice Hall; 1996.
44. Hollingshead A. *Four Factor Index of Social Status.* New Haven, CT: Hollingshead; 1975. Working Paper.
45. *SPSS* [computer program]. Version 13.0. Chicago: SPSS, Inc.; 2004.
46. Census 2000. State and county quickfacts: U.S. Census Bureau. Available at: http://quickfacts.census.gov/qfd/states/55/55079.html. Accessed November 28, 2005.
47. Messick DM, van de Geer JP. A reversal paradox. *Psychol Bull.* 1981;90(3):582-593.
48. Johnson A, Sandford J, Tyndall J. Written and verbal information versus verbal information only for patients being discharged from acute hospital settings to home. In: *Cochrane Database Syst Rev.* The Cochrane Library; 2003.

Reprinted with permission from: Weiss, M. B., Piacentine, L. B., Lokken, L., Ancona, J., Archer, J., Gresser, S., et al. (2007). Perceived readiness for hospital discharge in adult medical-surgical patients. *Clinical Nurse Specialist, 21*(1), 31–42.

4.2 TRANSITION EXPERIENCES OF STROKE SURVIVORS FOLLOWING DISCHARGE HOME

MAUDE RITTMAN
CRAIG BOYLSTEIN
RAMON HINOJOSA
MELANIE SBERNA HINOJOSA
JOLIE HAUN

Abstract

Background: *Little is known about the transition experiences of stroke survivors after discharge home.* **Purpose:** *The purpose of this article is to describe three domains of psychosocial experiences of stroke survivors during the first month following discharge for acute stroke.* **Method:** *Data were collected from 125 stroke survivors interviewed at 1 month following discharge home.* **Results:** *Findings indicate that changes in sense of self, connectedness with others, and community integration presented the major challenges.*

Stroke is a leading cause of severe, long-term disability in the United States.[1,2] Approximately 80% of stroke survivors are discharged home to continue recovery, yet little is known about experiences of stroke survivors during the transition period after discharge home.[3-6] The purpose of this article is to describe three domains of psychosocial experiences of stroke survivors during the first month following discharge for acute stroke. Data were obtained from a multisite study to develop culturally sensitive models of stroke recovery across 2 years after discharge home.

Transition is a passage from one life phase, condition, or status to another and is embedded in the context of a particular situation.[7] A salient feature of a transition is that there is usually a triggering event that initiates a change in the way individuals look at themselves and their life situations.[8] The occurrence of a stroke is a triggering event that is accompanied by family members being focused initially on survival of the stroke victim during the acute phase of treatment. Once the family sees that the loved one will survive, they begin to anticipate changes needed after discharge and the stroke survivor begins coping with changes in functional abilities and body image.[9] These events usher in the onset of a transition. Two additional features of transitions are that the process occurs over time and involves changes in identities, roles, and behaviors.[10] The purpose of this article is to describe psychosocial experiences during the first month transition period.

Several studies using qualitative methods have reported on transition processes.[11-13] Findings indicate that the occurrence of a stroke affects the lives of other family members and the transition process is chaotic, resulting in changes in family relationships, caregivers coping with exhaustion, and survivors taking one day at a time and struggling to hang onto hope for recovery. The chaotic period is followed by reorganization during which life becomes a search gap by exploring the psychosocial transition experiences of stroke survivors during the first month after discharge home. Qualitative data from semi-structured interviews of 125 stroke survivors at 1-month postdischarge are used to answer the research question: What are the psychosocial domains of the transition experience following discharge home poststroke? The three domains include: changes in sense of self and bodily experiences, changes in connectedness, and changes in community integration. Quantitative data are used to describe the stroke survivor characteristics and functional changes between discharge and 1 month following discharge home.

Method

Data were derived from a longitudinal multisite study to develop culturally sensitive models of stroke recovery. For the longitudinal study, stroke survivors and their caregivers were invited to participate in the study while hospitalized for acute stroke. Informed consents were obtained prior to discharge. Data included in these analyses were collected during home visits at 1 month after discharge home at four Veterans Affairs Medical Centers (VAMCs) including Gainesville, Tampa, and Miami, Florida, and San Juan, Puerto Rico. The study was reviewed and approved by the institutional review boards and the VA Research and Development Committees at each of the VAMCs. Written informed consent was obtained from all participants prior to entering the study.

Sample

A total of 123 male veterans and 2 female veterans discharged home and their caregivers were included in this analysis. To be included in the study, the patient had to meet the following criteria: (1) ability to communicate as measured by a score of at least 6 on the communication subscale of the Cognitive Scale of the FIM™*; (2) mentally competent as measured by a score on the Mini-Mental Status Examination (MMSE) of 18 or above; and (3) presence of a caregiver who was willing to participate and signed an informed consent.

Data Collection

Qualitative data were obtained from in-depth, semi-structured interviews with stroke survivors and field observations made during home visits at 1-month postdischarge. Quantitative data were also collected and were used to describe the sample and examine changes in functional status (FIM™ motor scale) and mental status (MMSE) between discharge and 1 month. Depression (Geriatric Depression Scale [GDS]) and instrumental activities of daily living (Frenchay Activities Index [FAI]) were assessed at 1 month.

Data Analysis

Interviews were tape-recorded, transcribed verbatim, verified, and entered into N6 (QSR International Pty Ltd., Doncaster, Victoria, Australia), a computer program designed to assist with qualitative data analysis. The program allows researchers to code text data and retrieve data related to codes in specific themes or patterns of experiences. Four experienced qualitative researchers participated in coding the data using a coding tree developed from a preliminary analysis of 12 interviews. Each analyzed the data independently to identify aspects of recovery including transition from hospital to home, and consensus was achieved in team meetings. Three psychosocial domains were identified in the data. All data related to each of the psychosocial domains at 1 month after discharge were reexamined to identify characteristics of stroke survivors' experiences at 1 month following discharge home. The three psychosocial domains of the transition experience after discharge home include: changes in sense of self and bodily experiences, changes in connectedness, and changes in community integration.

Results

Description of Stroke Survivors

The sample included veterans from three racial and ethnic groups: African American (n = 33), Puerto Rican (n = 49), and non-Hispanic white (n = 43), with a total sample of 125 stroke survivors. Ninety-eight percent of the stroke survivors were male veterans with an average age of 66 (range, 40–93 years). Puerto Rican stroke survivors were the oldest (69 years), followed by whites (67 years) and African Americans (62 years), $F(2, 123) = 26.81$, $p < .001$. Type of stroke varied with 53% having ischemic stroke, 42% having cerebrovascular disease, and 4% having hemorrhagic strokes. Puerto Rican stroke survivors were more likely to suffer an ischemic stroke, $F(2, 123) = 6.35$, $p = .002$, and were less likely than whites or African Americans to suffer from cerebrovascular disease, $F(2, 123) = 5.38$, $p = .005$. Forty-seven percent of our sample had left body paresis (paralysis), 43% had right body paresis, 3% had both sides affected, and 7% had no paresis. The number of days spent in the hospital prior to discharge ranged from 0 days to 129 days with an average of 19.1 days. Puerto Rican stroke survivors spent significantly more time in the hospital (24 days) than did whites (17 days) or African Americans (15 days), $F(2, 123) = 4.92$, $p = .008$.

Changes during the transition in the first month included functional assessments that were taken at discharge and compared to assessments at the 1-month follow-up visit. Functional assessments (FIM™) at discharge indicated that most patients were in the high range of functional ability. The average of the total FIM™ score at discharge from the hospital was 106 out of a possible 126 score, and the average total FIM™ score at 1 month was 112. The average change from discharge to 1 month was an increase of 5.8 points. Though the average change was positive, 14 (11%) veterans had no change and 33 (26%) scored lower on the FIM™ during their 1-month interview.

The cognitive subscale of the FIM™ measures communication skills and social cognition and ranges from 5 to 35 points. The average cognitive subscale score at discharge was 31.2, and it was 32 at the 1-month interviews. Forty-six (37%) veterans had no change in their cognitive scores, 32 (25%) veterans showed lower cognitive functioning, and 48 (38%) had increases in their cognitive FIM™ scores. The second subscale we tested focused on the recovery of motor function. This subscale ranges from 13 to 91. The average FIM™ motor score at discharge was 74.8 and the average 1-month score was 79.9. Of all the veterans in our survey, 14 (11%) had no change in their motor function, 29 (23%) had a decrease in motor function, and 83 (66%) showed increases in motor functioning at the 1-month interviews.

The final measure of change during the transition is mental status as measured by the MMSE. This scale has 32 items, and scores range from 0 to 32 with higher numbers indicating better mental status. The average MMSE score at discharge was 26.5, and it was 26.7 at the 1-month interviews. Twenty-six veterans (21%) showed no change in their mental state, 46 (37%) had a reduction in mental state, and 54 (43%) had an improved mental state during the 1-month interviews. Overall these statistics demonstrate an average trajectory of recovery for the veterans in our study with the greatest gains in motor functioning.

The FAI was used to evaluate instrumental activities of daily living at 1 month following discharge. The mean score was 29.58 (range, 15–57). Puerto Rican stroke survivors had a score of 26.2, which is statistically similar to the 30.7 score for whites but is significantly different from the score of 33.1 for African Americans, $F(2, 123) = 4.8$, $p = .010$. The GDS was also collected at 1-month postdischarge to evaluate depressive symptoms. Higher scores on the GDS scale indicate more depressive symptoms, and a score of 10 or above is considered to be within the depressed range. The average GDS score for whites (8.98), Puerto Ricans (10.14), and African Americans (7.44) are statistically similar, $F(2, 123) = 1.63$, $p = .200$. The average GDS score for all stroke survivors is 9.04 (range, 0–29).

Changes in Sense of Self and Bodily Experiences

The most common experience following discharge is a disruption in a person's ability to construct self; more than two thirds of stroke survivors in this study experienced disruption or changes in sense of self. Interwoven throughout participants' discussions of their lives after discharge home were perceptions of how they now viewed their bodies and the impact of these changes on their self-image and self-esteem. Indicators of these changes were found in statements like "I'm not the same," "My life is different," "I feel worthless," "Life is meaningless," "I feel useless," "I'm stooped over shriveling," and "I'm handicapped." As one man commented, "My life's philosophy has changed because...I can't walk and I can't move my body freely." Participants also expressed feelings of social stigma. As one man said, "It's just self-degrading. I really hate the way I feel, feel about myself." Another participant stated, "When you are in this disgrace, you are apart (from others)."

The way people experience and talk about their body is one of many resources used in construction of sense of self.[14-18] When illness or injury interrupts the taken-for-granted functioning of the body, one's understanding of self can also change.[19] Changes in self-image and self-esteem are precursors to changes in overall self-perspective[20] or, more generally, sense of self. As an 80-year-old former Marine articulates changes in his sense of self at 1 month:

> You're supposed to be pretty straight and pretty macho...[but]...I am not that any more. I miss being that....Being in the Marine Corp and going from straight...with a cadence down to this is a long way and it does have some effect....I don't like to be stooped over shrivelin'.

Statements of disruption reflect the struggle that stroke survivors experience during the transition home as they attempt to make sense of the stroke in their daily lives. For many, the inability to use the body as before results in self-disruption and can make the return home bewildering as they attempt to reestablish a sense of normality in their daily lives. As one man tells us, "I see myself as different because of the way I walk and the way I act. I can't go anywhere like a normal person."

We found that depression, as measured by the GDS, and disruption in sense of self are linked. In the first month after discharge, 100% of Africans Americans, 83% of Puerto Ricans, and 81% of whites who experienced disruption of self also scored 10 or higher on the GDS indicating possible depression. Depression and consequently low self-esteem are common difficulties that occur after stroke.[21-24] As one stroke survivor commented when asked about how he sees his life now, "I wouldn't say frustrated, I would say sick, sick of life, once I even thought of killing myself to be clear, I thought of taking my life, I thought of a lot of things." Knowing the difficulties that can arise from changes in one's sense of self and related depression is important in preparing stroke survivors and their families to manage care at home.

It is important to note, however, that not all participants experienced disruption of sense of self. Participants who experienced continuity of self did not show signs of changes in their self-image, self-esteem, or overall self-perspective. These participants typically stated that they are "the same person" or feel that "nothing has really changed." "Life is about the same," says one participant. Another man states, "Basically nothing has changed for me, for me personally. My life really ain't changed that much." One participant told us that stroke was a "message for me to slow down," but he insists that he continues to "look at life the same way, you know."

We analyzed narratives of stroke survivors who did not experience disruption of sense of self to identify strategies used to maintain continuity. We found that bodily changes can be managed through the use of various symbolic resources that help to normalize them. Such resources include beliefs about age and God and spirituality. Berger[25] described symbolic resources as plausibility structures or conceptual frameworks for understanding and explaining the meaning of experiences.[25] Our findings that these resources can be useful strategies to normalize the situation after stroke are similar to other studies on stroke recovery and disruption, reflecting a growing body of literature on how people manage changes during an illness without experiencing disruption to sense of self.[26-29]

Interpreting the stroke as part of the aging process normalizes physical changes in the body. Part of the cultural understanding Americans have of illness is that it occurs with advanced years, making it part of the normal life trajectory.[26,27,30] One of the youngest participants of the study, aged 49, said "Well I'm getting older and I just don't have strength and energy that I used to have." Older participants framed it in the same way. One older man stated, "I guess it's just part of getting old. When you get eighty, why, things change." Attributing physical effects of the stroke to a function of age allows stroke survivors to normalize stroke-related physical changes, ameliorating or muting altogether the effects of bodily changes on one's sense of self.

Spiritual beliefs provide another strategy to normalize changes in bodily experiences and create continuity while coping with changes due to illness and disablement.[29] Many participants came to understand the stroke and its effects on their body as falling under the explanatory framework of spirituality or as part of God's plan. Though they remain unsure of God's purpose, they accept His role in the stroke. One man said, "I feel like the Lord put something on me that he wants me to have." This sentiment was echoed by another participant who said, "I think this is what God gave me." Another stated, "I've always been Catholic. I've always believed in God. So that's, I'm sure there's a reason for all this."

The belief that stroke onset was part of God's plan indicated that physical changes were sometimes viewed as consequences for personal behaviors, such as smoking and drinking. A number of men felt that God was punishing them and, consequently, they attributed physical changes to God's will. The stroke was a direct message from God conveying His displeasure. As one survivor commented:

> It'll make me appreciate the Lord more, things He do for me, and the way I hold it dear. That this stroke was, uh, supposed to happen 'cause when it happened, I know I didn't remember that I should a got my blood pressure checked good as I can remember, and so, this is supposed to happen to make me a better person.

Stroke reifies faith, as one man indicated: "With this stroke, it brought me closer to God, too." In this way, the stroke provides a clear sign that God's will is present in one's life.

In summary, stroke disrupts one's sense of self because it changes and alters the taken-for-granted body. Disruption creates a need to normalize the situation in an effort to create order from chaos.[19] Our study provides evidence that self-image, self-esteem, and overall self-perspective are often casualties of stroke. The transition period is fraught with confusion, anxiety, depression, and, for some, thoughts of suicide. For others, the transition from prestroke to poststroke is managed through symbolic resources that help normalize their experiences. The use of age and spirituality are ways to maintain continuity in one's sense of self. As people reconstruct the biography of self and tell the story of who they are, these symbolic resources serve to normalize their sense of self and represent the first steps on the road to stroke recovery.

Changes in Connectedness

Analyses of data from our study indicate that following discharge home poststroke, feelings of isolation were a major issue that stroke survivors faced. Participants reported a broad range of experiences reflecting their sense of connectedness or isolation based on their perceptions of social support and interactions with others at 1 month. These descriptions reflect their experiences during the transition following discharge. The model of a continuum of connectedness and isolation was developed from the data and consists of five domains that constitute the experience of being connected to others or feeling isolated: (1) availability of others, (2) support from others, (3) interaction with others and the community, (4) ability to contribute, and (5) the ability to engage in intimate relations. Stroke survivors' experiences in these five domains spanned the continuum from feeling connected to others to feeling isolated during the transition. Each domain is discussed below.

Availability of Others

At one end of the continuum, socially connected participants reported more social visits, adequate levels of support, and continued interaction with the community while managing their transition at 1 month poststroke. Their ability to maintain interaction with the community often involved support from others, as stated by one participant:

> Hell, if I didn't have her I'd be in a nursin' home. Let's face it. She does everything. Last night the youngest grandson had a concert...I was settin' there goin' to the left like that, kept slidin' to the left, cause the left side's gone...she pulls hers right up side of me, leans up there before so I can lean against her, instead of fallin' out of the chair.

At the other end of the continuum, stroke survivors who experienced isolation were more likely to be unmarried, and they reported having fewer social visits from family and friends, fewer people to confide in, and less psychological and instrumental support. For example, several isolated participants stated they spend much of their time isolated and alone. One participant commented, "I am always alone...I would like to have a companion...." Previous research has shown that social isolation may adversely affect those recovering from stroke. Small social networks are related to elevated risks of mortality among those with coronary disease, even when controlling for age and disease severity and adjusting for income, hostility, and smoking status.[31,32] Findings indicate that in a group of ethnically diverse participants, those who reported knowing fewer than three people well enough to visit in their homes were 1.4 times more likely to have an adverse outcome event than those with more social connections.[32]

Support From Others

Participants in our study experienced a range of support from others. Some participants enjoyed close ties with family and friends while others did not. Physical presence of others was not always related to feelings of support. Participants often talked about needing support and contact with others. Connected participants often talked about receiving support from others and the way it makes them feel. One participant stated:

> I feel good. My family loves me a lot and everybody and I don't have problems with anything...he [son in law] helps me, he...is very good. So I don't have reason to complain. My brothers are all great with me...life treats me well...they have more, more affection towards me.

This participant's perceptions of being loved and being treated well reflect his sense of connectedness with others while managing transition poststroke. Receiving support is critical for recovery and achieving an optimal quality of life.[6,32,33] Isolated participants did not have this level of support and often reported their families were not always able or willing to help them. As one participant who experienced isolation stated:

> I'm alone, no one takes care of me, if I need to do something difficult I have to grab myself from the wall just to walk....I have family but they all have their own things to do...except one of my sisters who comes from [mentions the city] to bring me something to eat, like a dog....

Inadequate emotional support diminishes a person's ability to manage transition at 1 month poststroke.[6] Furthermore, the experience of isolation diminishes the general well-being of the individual.[32] In addition to the physical presence of others, maintainence of an active social support system and social functioning has been reported to be critical for an optimal quality of life for individuals recovering from a stroke.[6,32-34]

Interaction With Others and the Community

Social and recreational interactions are also critical in maintaining a sense of connectedness with others poststroke.[35] In addition to the social support provided by a network of family and friends, church was identified as a major source of social interactions. One participant who maintained connections with the community spoke about his social life at length:

> Second Sunday every month, there's a Polish dance. And I belong to the Polish Church in Bellview. And ahh, there's a Polaski Club down there and they have Polish music and Polish food once a month. I'm very friendly down there. People are very friendly with me and the kind of people that I like to associate with...I might go to the store over there, I might go to the community center, I belong there. And just visit in general; a lot of friends over there...Friday nights I usually go to the VFW, fish fry, associate, have a couple of drinks...yeah, Elk's, Eagle's. I belong to both Eagle's and Elk's....

However, most participants, whether connected or not, were not able to maintain prestroke activity levels. The inability to interact with others was a common experience for isolated participants. As one isolated participant stated:

> I don't have public...I don't have neighbors...the one people that come here are my son and the lady that comes help me....I haven't gone out to buy anything...the lady and my son buy everything for me....I have little contact with other people...I spend my time at home and I don't go out unless it is to the hospital....

Social isolation not only inhibits the experience of connectedness with others but can also promote depression and physical illness for individuals managing transition at 1 month poststroke.[32]

Ability to Contribute

Survivors' ability to contribute to their home and their environment is important for sustaining a sense of connectedness with others poststroke.[35] Connected participants were more likely to talk about maintaining the ability to contribute to their environment. Connected participants reported contributing to their environment in different ways. One participant reported giving his family cooking lessons: "I'm teaching my son how to cook...him or my wife, cause neither one can cook. She can't cook but she'll try, so I go I go in there and I guide her." Another participant reported helping his son's neighbors:

> [A] neighbor of one of my sons cut his tree down and put all the logs over into his yard for his, my other son wanted to use it for burning for the fireplace and I told him, I said, I'll come out there and I'll load my little truck and I'll pull them over to your house...I hauled three or four truck loads over. Loaded them up myself. My wife helped me load some of 'em up. And I went over to my other house, other son's house, and unloaded and we stacked it up for him, and I was really exhausted, but it felt good.

In contrast, isolated participants were more likely to talk about their inability to contribute poststroke and being a burden to others as a result of their stroke, which often contributed to their experience of being isolated, One isolated participant stated:

> I don't wanna be a burden to anybody else....Now I can't seem to get out and do what I wanna do or get out and go, you know or get out and work or something....I mean I just seem to wanna just stay by myself more. It's been worse, get a little depressed....It's just that I've gotta feeling, like I'm just useless and you know, I can't do anything anymore you know, it's depressing....it's kinda depressing. All of a sudden you find out that you can't do much of anything, you gotta depend on people, you know.

The experience of being unable to contribute to one's environment has a negative influence on self-concept and thus the ability to feel connected to others.[35] Like the connected participants, isolated participants would benefit from the opportunity to contribute to their household and community during their first month of recovery poststroke.

Ability to Engage in Intimate Relations

Connected participants often spoke about intimate relationships with family and friends. One participant who enjoyed a strong connected family stated:

My boys have never had a day go by that they were with me that they never knew and heard me say that I love them. They say that to me a lot, and they hug me a lot....But I don't want to be just...just a hook, like a handshake. I want it to be something like I might not see you again Dad and this might be the last time. I want you to know that I love you...over the way that I used to think, that's...'it's a very much a positive thing.

This quote shows the role that love and intimacy with his sons has in sustaining this participant's daily life. The experience of intimacy with others has been described as a protective factor against isolation, and it promotes a sense of connectedness with others.[35]

However, at 1 month postdischarge, participants who experienced isolation seldom spoke about intimate relations. Rather, they talked about experiencing a lack of intimacy. One isolated participant talked about his choosing to remain alone and his difficulty with intimacy when he said:

I'd rather stay by myself, you know, this is even gonna make it worse you know....So I'll crawl a little bit more in my hole again, and I'll be more by myself....I dunno how the heck this is gonna work out, I'm gonna tell ya, because it's kinda depressing.

Our findings suggest that isolated participants' lack of intimacy and connectedness with others significantly contributed to a sense of isolation during their first month of transition poststroke.

Overall, findings suggest connected participants achieved feelings of intimacy and maintained social connections with others, whereas isolated participants experienced loneliness and a sense of disconnection from others, both physical and emotional. Reports from participants provided evidence for the range of experience of connectedness and isolation during the first month of stroke recovery, providing data to develop a model of a continuum of connectedness and isolation. Assessment of stroke survivors' experiences using the domains of the continuum of connectedness and isolation can provide valuable information for clinicians and informal caregivers. Understanding the stroke survivor's experiences of connectedness or isolation post-

stroke may contribute to individualized care and interventions to improve outcomes during the transition following discharge.

Changes in Community Integration

Community integration is defined as community activities that occur outside the home environment. Outside employment and education were also included in the definition of community integration. Interviews were examined to determine the level of community integration survivors described at 1 month following discharge home. In general, data indicate that at 1 month stroke survivors are in a period of adjustment, and participation in activities outside of the home is a major challenge for many. Our findings indicate that at 1 month following discharge most stroke survivors described low levels of community integration. However, community integration occurred on a continuum from low to moderate to high. We describe characteristics of these three levels and the impact this had on stroke survivors' lives.

Following discharge home, stroke survivors frequently reduce activities they enjoyed prior to the stroke. For example, activities such as walking and swimming are reduced or given up altogether, and, conversely, many participants increase the time spent in passive activities like daydreaming, sitting, and watching television. Survivors who experience low community integration express an outlook on life that consists of taking things easy, hoping they will improve physically as time goes by, eventually being able to return to important activities such as going out to see friends or resuming previous hobbies such as repairing automobiles. These survivors discuss adhering to their medication schedule, expecting that in time the medicine will help them physically improve enough that they are able to return to the activities they did before their stroke. The decline in participation in active, outside community and leisure activities is often attributed to physical and psychological barriers, including fear of falling, being afraid to leave the house, and transportation difficulties. Several participants with low community integration describe becoming emotionally over-whelmed by their limitations, saying that they are trying to stay out of other people's way until they get better. These findings are similar to a study by Holbrook and Skilbeck[36] who found that 75% of the 122 poststroke patients they surveyed reduced most of the community and leisure activities they had done before the stroke and never resumed them later in the recovery process.

Fatigue continued to be a problem that many stroke survivors discussed. Lacking the energy and strength to go out and participate in community activities, these participants remain indoors most of the time during their first month of recovery. Some tried to stay busy around the house, and others were trying to reestablish activites. One man, aged 57, said that he believes he could do the things he wants to do inside and outside of the house if he could only get the motivation to do it: "I can do the same things, it's just motivating myself to do them. I know they got to be done but I just don't get motivated to do it." A 73-year-old participant remarked, "I've never been a lazy man. I worked all my life, and there's things I want to do. I just let them go." Another participant, aged 52, summarized the experience that most of the participants with low community integration are facing 1 month poststroke when he says:

> I can't go out. I want to go places. It makes me you know, like I want to go places. I want to get dressed, put my nice clothes on and. I just feel lonesome. I feel trapped. I can't get out.

Feelings of living a more restricted life resulted in participants feeling "locked up," "in jail," and "incapacitated." Other survivors said they were okay with being homebound with minimal outside activities. They expressed pleasure in yard work or walking a little around their house, depending on other family members to do the shopping, banking, and other responsibilities the survivor had done before the stroke. Most survivors with low community integration are passive observers who witness life through television or radio. Without the support of their families, they would likely not be able to live at home. As another survivor commented, "My life has changed 100%. Before I used to exercise and play sports. And now nothing. Life is full of unhappiness." Those who can go out with the help of a family member and do some gardening or go out to eat express some hope and optimism for the future. For those who need constant assistance, their future is described as uncertain and bleak as seen in this statement:

> One is worthless, practically. You're alive, but you are worthless. Alive for what? They have to feed you, bathe you....What can you say that you are doing? Living a monotonous life, like a vegetable. Sometimes it is better that they give you something that leaves you dead and it is over.

The main variable in this shift from independence to dependence is walking ability. Many participants with low community integration report having fallen during their first month home. They realize that due to a loss of balance, stamina, and functional ability in one of their legs they are not able to walk the way they were used to doing prior to the stroke. One man commented on difficulties related to falling: "Yeah, fallin' is the worst. It's hard to describe 'cause it's like a sack of rocks, this side of my body." Another participant described the changes he has experienced since returning home from the hospital when he said:

> I wasn't very active but, I'd walk around and go different places. I've got a computer room out there. I'd go in the computer room and at Christmas time I used to like to put up the lights and stuff. This year I just can't do it. I know how to put up the lights but I used to fix our lights and we'd put them up together outside and stuff. This year I just can't do any of it. I can't walk.

Depression is linked with *low community integration*. Depressed participants typically see the future as bleak, uncertain, and filled with continued health problems, whereas others remain optimistic and hopeful for their recovery and make plans to travel and visit family and friends. Some survivors wait on time and medication to heal them; others exercise because they believe that pushing themselves physically will optimize their recovery. These veterans, however, remain uncertain about when and how much this exercise will "pay off" for them in terms of regaining the functioning and activity level they have lost since their most recent stroke. In other words, 1 month postdischarge marks a time of uncertainty during the transition for these stroke survivors as they continue to re-engage with meaningful activities.

At 1 month following discharge home, not all survivors experienced low community integration. Those with moderate community integration did get out into the community during their first month of recovery, albeit to a limited extent. A few of them stated they still worked part-time and were beginning to drive in a limited area around their home. These two activities were used by participants as major benchmarks for expecting future improvements. Fatigue and decreased physical strength were also major concerns for this group, and they adapted to these limitations when they went out into public places by using assistive devices. Survivors with moderate community integration described walking as an important exercise to improve their physical stamina and ensure they did not lose more functional ability. Walking for exercise was expressed as the major reason these survivors left their homes and entered community settings. These participants were actively engaged in continuing rehabilitation activities to strengthen their recovery.

Survivors with moderate community integration described engaging in casual public activities such as attending weekly bingo games, walking the dog, or going to a friend or neighbor's house to talk. Church attendance was regularly mentioned as an important part of many of these survivors' weekly routine. Some stated they were embarrassed in public due to hand impairments or other difficulties when eating out such as needing others to tell them they had food dangling from their mouth.

Survivors with high community integration described the stroke as having little or no impact on their community, social, and civic life. The ability to drive was an important difference between those with moderate and those with high community integration. Driving the car brought more independence and ability to go out into the community. Some continued to work full-time. Survivors with high community integration believed that remaining active in community life and doing the same community activities they did before the stroke was a very important aspect to their recovery. High community integration, however, did not always coincide with high levels of motor functioning. One person with high community integration described how others saw him as "handicapped" due to noticeable hand and leg impairments. Despite his handicaps, the survivor continued an active community life. He described attending up to three 12-step program meetings a day, biking daily, and continuing to go out with friends and socializing. Even with the same physical limitations as many persons with low and moderate community integration, this survivor participated in community and leisure activities daily and enjoyed rigorous physical activities.

Discussion and Conclusion

The experiences of stroke survivors during the first month after discharge home are characterized by a process of adapting to changes in their sense *of self, their connections with others, and their community participation*. Although participants scored high on the functional assessment, our findings indicate that, at *1 month postdischarge, they are managing multiple psychosocial changes and could benefit from interventions that prepare them for the transition back home and assist them during the transition*. Health care providers can use their knowledge about the experiences of stroke survivors as they learn to manage recovery *to promote* a better quality of life at home.

During the first month after discharge, stroke patients are often troubled by changes in their bodies, and consequently this changes the way in which they see themselves. Informal caregivers, family members, and friends play a significant role in helping stroke survivors manage these changes during the transition period. Our findings indicate that stroke survivors often experience isolation from others. Connectedness with others is a contributor to health and well-being following stroke. Positive health is defined as leading a life of purpose, having quality connections with others, possessing self regard, and experiencing mastery over the environment. Interventions are needed to help family members and friends maintain connections and strengthen relationships with stroke survivors during this recovery period.

Following discharge, participation in social, leisure, and physical activities in the community are often limited during the first month home. Community and leisure activities are positively related to higher levels of health, self-esteem, and quality of life.[37,38] Researchers have established links between quality of life, depression, and community and leisure activities.[39,40] For example, Holbrook and Skilbeck[36] found that some adults no longer experienced depression 6 months poststroke because they had adjusted psychologically to living with their impairments through reestablishing their daily, leisure, and community activities. The inability to regain full participation in leisure and community activities appears to be more closely linked to poor psychosocial outcomes such as depression and poor quality of life than do difficulties in performing basic activities of daily living.[41]

The transition period after discharge is a period of adjustment to psychosocial changes to reestablish a sense of normalcy in life. Interventions are needed that help stroke survivors and their caregivers understand the changes in the way they see themselves and their bodies. Stroke survivors may benefit from talking about these changes and developing some activities that could enhance positive self-image. Family members may need help to understand that visits and activities that promote connectedness with others not only reduces isolation but also communicates self-worth for the stroke survivor. Other implications for clinical practice include: assessing levels of support received in the home and matching the level of support with the needs of the stroke survivor; assessing the impact of disabilities on former social activities and making modifications or finding new social activities that foster connectedness and engagement with others; encouraging the stroke survivor and caregiver to find meaningful ways to contribute to the family and community; discussing alternative approaches to intimacy after stroke; and accessing transportation to promote community integration and increase social interactions and connectedness with others.

Acknowledgments

This study was funded by the VA Health Services Research and Development Program, Nursing Research Initiative, Culturally Sensitive Models of Stroke Recovery and Caregiving After Discharge Home.

REFERENCES

1. Fujiura GTP, Hye J, Rutkowski-Kmitta V. Disability statistics in the developing world: a reflection on the meanings in our numbers. *J Appl Res Intellect Disabilities.* 2005;18(4):295-304.
2. AHCPR. *Clinical Practice Guideline: Post-Stroke Rehabilitation.* US Department of Health and Human Services; Washington, DC: 1995.
3. Han B, Haley WE. Family caregiving for patients with stroke. Review and analysis. *Stroke.* 1999;30(7):1478-1485.
4. Michels N. The transition from hospital to home: an exploratory study. *Home Health Care Serv Q.* 1988;9(1):29-44.
5. Magilvy JK, Lakomy JM. Transitions of older adults to home care. *Home Health Care Serv Q.* 1991;12(4):59-70.
6. Glass TA, Maddox GL. The quality and quantity of social support: stroke recovery as psycho-social transition. *Soc Sci Med.* 1992;34(11):1249-1261.
7. Chick N, Meleis AI. Transitions: A nursing concern. In: Chinn PL, ed. *Nursing Research Methodology: Issues and Implementation.* Rockville, MD: Aspen Publishers; 1986:237-257.
8. Schlossberg NK. *Counseling Adults in Transition: Link Practice with Theory.* New York: Springer; 1984.
9. Farzan DT. Reintegration for stroke survivors. Home and community considerations. *Nurs Clin North Am.* 1991;26(4):1037-1048.

10. Schumacher KL, Meleis AI. Transitions: a central concept in nursing. *Image J Nurs Sch.* 1994;26(2):119-127.
11. Bull MJ. Managing the transition from hospital to home. *Q Health Res.* 1992;2(1):27-41.
12. Clarke-Steffen L. Waiting and not knowing: the diagnosis of cancer in a child. *J Pediatr Oncol Nurs.* 1993;10(4):146-153.
13. Fraser C. The experience of transition for a daughter caregiver of a stroke survivor. *J Neurosci Nurs.* 1999;31(1):9-16.
14. Bourdieu P. The social space and the genesis of groups. *Soc Sci Information.* 1985;24(2):195-220.
15. Freund PES. The expressive body: a common ground for the sociology of emotions and health and illness. *Sociol Health Illness.* 1990;12(4):452-477.
16. Goffman E. *Interactional Ritual: Essays on Face to Face Behaviors.* Garden City, NY: Anchor Brooks; 1967.
17. Hochschild A, Irwin N, Ptashne M. Repressor structure and the mechanism of positive control. *Cell.* 1983;32(2):319-325.
18. Mead GH. *Mind, Self, and Society.* Chicago: University of Chicago Press; 1934.
19. Becker G. *Disrupted Lives: How People Create Meaning in a Chaotic World.* Berkeley: University of California Press; 1997.
20. Cast AD, Burke PJ. A theory of self-esteem. *Social Forces.* 2002;80(3):1041-1068.
21. Doolittle ND. A clinical ethnography of stroke recovery. In: Benner P, ed. *Interpretive Phenomenology: Embodiment, Caring and Ethics in Health and Illness.* Thousand Oaks, CA: Sage; 1994:211-229.
22. Doolittle ND. The experience of recovery following lacunar stroke. *Rehabil Nurs.* 1992;17(3):122-125.
23. Hart E. Evaluating a pilot community stroke service using insights from medical anthropology. *J Adv Nurs.* 1998;27(6):1177-1183.
24. Chang AM, Mackenzie AE. State self-esteem following stroke. *Stroke.* 1998;29(11):2325-2328.
25. Berger FM. Control of the mind. *Am Sci.* 1967;55(1):67-71.
26. Faircloth C, Boylstein C, Rittman M, Young M, Gubrium J. Sudden illness and biographical flow in narratives of stroke recovery. *Social Health Illness.* 2004;26(2):242-261.
27. Sanders C, Donovan J, Dieppe P. The significance and consequences of having painful and disabled joints in older age: co-existing accounts of normal and disrupted biographies. *Social Health Illness.* 2002;24(2):227-253.
28. Idler E. Religion, health, and nonphysical sense of self. *Social Forces.* 1995;74:683-704.
29. Mansfield CJ, Mitchell J, King DE. The doctor as God's mechanic? Beliefs in the Southeastern United States. *Soc Sci Med.* 2002;54(3):399-409.
30. Pound P, Gompertz P, Ebrahim S. Illness in the context of older age: the case of stroke. *Sociol Health Illness.* 1998;20(4):489-506.
31. Brummett BH, Barefoot JC, Siegler IC, et al. Characteristics of socially isolated patients with coronary artery disease who are at elevated risk for mortality. *Psychosom Med.* 2001;63(2):267-272.
32. Boden-Albala B, Litwak E, Elkind MS, Rundek T, Sacco RL. Social isolation and outcomes post stroke. *Neurology.* 2005;64(11):1888-1892.
33. National Institute of Health. NIH Cognitive and Emotional Health Project: The Healthy Brain. US Department of Health and Human Services: 2001. Accessed February 2, 2007. Available at: http://nih.gov/cehp/.
34. Langford CP, Bowsher J, Maloney JP, Lillis PP. Social support: A conceptual analysis. *J Adv Nurs.* 1997;25(1):95-100.
35. Burkhardt MA, Nagai-Jacobson MG. *Spirituality: Living Our Connectedness.* Albany, NY: Delmar; 2002.
36. Holbrook MS, Skilbeck CE. An activities index for use with stroke patients. *Age Ageing.* 1983;12:166-170.
37. Niemi ML, Laaksonen R, Kotila M, Waltimo O. Quality of life 4 years after stroke. *Stroke.* 1988;19(9):1101-1107.
38. Ragheb MG, Griffith CA. The contribution of leisure participation and leisure satisfaction to life satisfaction of older persons. *J Leisure Res.* 1982;14:295-306.
39. Astrom M, Adolfsson R, Asplund K. Major depression in stroke patients. A 3-year longitudinal study. *Stroke.* 1993;24(7):976-982.
40. Bond MJ CM, Smith DS, Harris RD. Lifestyle activities of the elderly: composition and determinants. *Disabil Rehabil.* 1995;17(2):63-69.
41. Drummond AER, Walker MF. A randomized controlled trial of leisure rehabilitation after stroke. *Clin Rehabil.* 1995;9:282-290.

Reprinted with permission from: Rittman, M., Boylstein, C., Hinojosa, R., Hinojosa, M. S., & Haun, J. (2007). Transition experiences of stroke survivors following discharge home. *Topics in Stroke Rehabilitation, 14*(2), 21–31.

4.3 ASSESSING OLDER PERSONS' READINESS TO MOVE TO INDEPENDENT CONGREGATE LIVING

EILEEN K. ROSSEN

Abstract

Older adults are increasingly choosing to relocate to congregate-type independent living communities. Relocation to an independent living community is a late-life transition that is considered a stressful life event. Although relocation to an independent living community offers potential benefits, many older persons have difficulties during this transition, including poor adjustment, loneliness, and depression. All of these are associated with poorer health, higher healthcare costs, increased risk of institutionalization, and increased morbidity and mortality. This article provides guidelines for assessing the readiness of an older person to move to an independent living community and implications for advanced practice nurses whose role encompasses promoting the health and wellbeing of older adults. Using the assessment guidelines, the advanced practice nurse can identify older persons at risk for difficulty during relocation and intervene with guidance and strategies to promote positive relocation adjustment.

The U.S. population is aging rapidly, and by 2030, approximately 20% or 71 million people are expected to be 65 years or older.[1] With our aging society, an estimated 23% of persons 65 years or older experience relocation,[2] and increasingly, they are choosing relocation to independent congregate living communities (ILCs), where they can continue independent living in a "protected" setting with supportive services.[3-5] Independent congregate living communities are residential settings of multiunit independent living apartments adapted to meet the special needs of elderly persons with services such as meals, transportation, and housekeeping.

When older adults relocate to ILCs, they experience a disruption of their lives. The literature indicates, however, that those older adults who plan well for their move and use strategies to incorporate their new living arrangements into the structure of their daily lives are more satisfied with their move and experience better quality of life.[6,7] Older adults who plan poorly for the move and give little forethought to the effects of the move on their lives are less satisfied with their move and experience a poorer quality of life.[6,7] This article reviews the literature on factors that influence both positive and negative outcomes of relocation to ILCs. The article also provides 2 assessment tools for determining the readiness of an older person to move to independent congregate living and proposed areas for the older person to think about to promote readiness for the move. Older people's responses to the assessment tools can guide advanced practice nurses (APNs) to identify older persons at risk for difficulty during relocation process and identify the areas that put these older adults at risk. This knowledge will allow APNs to consider ways of intervening to promote positive relocation adjustment and quality of life in older adults.

Late-Life Relocation

Late-life relocation, a transitional process, comprises initiation of the move, the actual move, and subsequent adjustment to the new setting.[6] The reasons older adults give for relocating to ILCs vary, but they include concerns about health of self or spouse, need for help with cleaning and cooking chores, difficulty in maintaining their home and yard, the expenses of living and maintaining their home, safety, and social isolation.[4] Factors that older adults consider in choosing to move to an ILC reflect their reasons for moving and are related to (a) financial capability, (b) amenities provided, (c) relationships, (d) transportation, and (e) healthcare provision.[8] Krout and colleagues[8] report that the financial questions most asked are "Can I afford the ILC for my lifetime and how will the financial obligations at the ILC change my lifestyle?" The most often asked questions related to amenities of the ILC are "Does the ILC have an atmosphere I will like and fit into? Will I like the food served? Do they have activities I will enjoy?" Questions related to relationship concerns are "Will my relatives and friends visit me, or can I visit them after I move to the ILC? Will I make new friends and feel socially comfortable at the ILC?" Transportation concerns are reflected in the question, "Will I have transportation to places I will need or want to go to?" Finally, healthcare provision is reflected in the question, "Will my current and future health-needs be met when I move to an ILC?"

The literature suggests that older adults respond in varying ways to relocation transition: some are able to adapt effectively to the move with positive outcomes, whereas others have difficulty in adaptation, with subsequent negative outcomes. Positive relocation outcomes include improvements in health and social interactions[7] and psychological benefits such as experiencing unexpected gains,[6,9] finding meaning in the experience,[10,11] and experiencing feelings of safety and security.[12,13] Negative relocation outcomes include declining health, reduced functional independence, social isolation and loneliness, reduced quality of life, and dissatisfaction and depression.[4,6,7,12-16] These negative outcomes are associated with high healthcare costs, increased risk of institutionalization, and increased morbidity and mortality.[4,13,17]

Factors found to affect late-life relocation adjustment and physical, psychological, and social well-being include the person's perception about the choice to move, the predictability of the new environment, perceptions of self and others, preservation of relationships, presence of a confidant, maintenance of independence, and depression.[3,6,7,18] Perception of having a choice to move has been positively correlated with psychological adjustment, conceptualized as morale, congruence, and continuity and is a contributing factor to positive relocation adjustment.[3,6,19] Lack of choice or feeling forced to move has been associated with dissatisfaction with the new home,[6] poorer functional status and self-rated health, and higher levels of depression, loneliness and anxiety,[20] and this is a contributing factor to poor relocation outcomes.[6] Positive correlations have been found among perceptions of self and others and psychological adjustment to relocation.[9,19] Preserving relationships among family and friends and having a confidant were found to positively influence psychological adjustment to and satisfaction with a new home.[3,6,7] High self-esteem scores and low symptoms of depression were factors contributing to positive relocation adjustment, whereas low self-esteem and higher levels of depressive symptoms contributed to poor relocation adjustment.[7]

According to the nursing model of transitions, relocation is a situational transition.[21] Transitions are defined as complex person–environment interactions embedded in the context and the situation that consist of both the disruption of the person's life and the person's responses to the disruption. Transitions are process oriented. There are 3 major concepts in the transitions model: universal properties, transition conditions, and indicators of healthy transition. Universal properties include the characteristics of the process or movement from one state to another such as changes in identity, roles, relationships, abilities, and patterns of behavior. Transition conditions are personal and environmental factors that influence the transition, such as physical and emotional well-being as well as person–environment interactions. Indicators of healthy transition are factors that indicate the quality of the transition outcome, such as satisfaction with the new home and perceived quality of life. With the increasing numbers of older adults moving to ILCs, there is a need for healthcare professionals to assess the readiness of older adults to go through the situational transition of a move to an ILC, so that those who are at risk for negative outcomes and potentially costly healthcare use can be identified and interventions developed to prevent these negative outcomes. Implementing such interventions can contribute to meeting the *Healthy People 2010* objective of increasing older adults' quality and years of healthy life.[22]

Clinical nurse specialists and other APNs can play an essential role in meeting this need because they are in many settings where older adults seek healthcare and live.[23-27] For example, as healthcare delivery shifts from acute inpatient care to community-based settings,[27] APNs are moving into expanded community-based roles.[26] Many provide direct care to individuals, families, and communities (case management), and they may also be responsible for assessing the needs of populations such as older adults.[26] Thus, they are well positioned to assist elders who are relocating.

Assessment of Readiness to Move to an ILC

How does one know what an individual's risks are for negative relocation outcomes? Recent research[6,7,14,15] suggests that the parameters for assessing older persons' readiness to move to ILCs include (*a*) choice in relocation, (*b*) preparation for the move, (*c*) congruence between the ILC and the older person's expectations, (*d*) existence of a confidant, and (*e*) openness to forming new relationships. Two specific tools can be used to determine the readiness of older adults contemplating moving to an ILC. The first is a set of questions developed based on the review of literature that assess the above 5 factors. The questions in Table 4.3.1 can be used in an interview, and older adults' answers to the questions will help to assess the individual's readiness to move and provide potential indicators to develop strategies to promote the older person's positive adaptation to relocation to an ILC.

Question 1 explores the person's perception of having a choice to move and being an integral part of the decision. The literature points to better psychological adjustment following relocation when persons believe they have a choice about whether to move or not, whereas lack of choice or feeling forced to move has been associated with dissatisfaction with the new home, poorer functional status, and self-rated health as well as higher levels of depression, loneliness, and anxiety.[6,7,28] Therefore, it is important to determine the older person's desire to move. If the person wants to make the move, he or she should be supported; however, if the individual is resistant to the move or says that someone else strongly wants him or her to move, then the older adult should be encouraged to discuss feelings and desires about the move so that the individual can resolve those feelings and have a successful move, or choose not to move.

Questions 2, 3, 4, 5, and 6 explore the person's preparedness in many areas that will be affected by a move to an ILC. For example, in one study, women who adjusted well to their relocation to ILCs said that they had planned well for the move, knew what furniture and belongings to take with them, felt they had a good plan for disposing of unnecessary belongings (ie, what to give to children, sell, or throw out) and had planned in detail the progression of activities they needed to make to be ready to move (e.g., selling the home with closing date, shutting off utilities, etc), and knew who was going to help them pack, clean, and move.[6] Other women who adjusted well discussed how they had planned to eat dinner at different tables for the first month after they moved so they would meet as many new people as possible. One person planned to attend as many different functions as possible during her first few months at her new home, even those she was less interested in, so she could get better acquainted with her new neighbors.[6] Another person told how she had visited the ILC at different times of the day and evening and had eaten several meals at the ILC before moving to get "a feel" for the place.[6] The older person's answers to these questions reveal areas that have been thought of and planned for as well as areas that have not. To promote positive adjustment, support and encouragement can be given for those areas that have been well planned, whereas further discussion and problem solving can be used in areas that the older person has not thought of or planned for.

Positive psychological adjustment to and satisfaction with a relocation have also been shown to be influenced by preservation of positive relationships, continued social support from family and friends, and the presence of a confidant.[6,7,14,17] Older persons' answers to questions 7 and 8 in Table 4.3.1 will give a good indication of their thinking and planning in regard to their relationships. If they talk about maintaining ties with family and friends and discuss the ways they plan to do that (eg, have dinner with family every Sunday after church and continue to go shopping with a daughter at least once a week), then their continued relationships are likely to contribute to positive adaptation. If they do not discuss how they will continue relationships, then it may be useful to aid older persons to identify who they would like to remain in contact with and to problem solve ways they can do that (eg, weekly telephone calls, sending notes/letters, and inviting people to dinner). Older persons' answers to the questions in Table 4.3.1 can serve as the starting point for discussing and problem solving areas that are known to contribute to positive relocation adjustment.

A second tool to assess readiness for relocation to an ILC is the 32-item Self-Efficacy Relocation Scale.[28] Self-efficacy theory suggests that people are better able to meet challenges such as relocation when they believe that their thoughts, emotions, behaviors, and living situations are within their control and they have the confidence to carry out needed behaviors.[29,30] Beliefs in personal efficacy also contribute to ability to activate the motivation, cognitive resources, and actions necessary to accomplish specific tasks.[29] Therefore, older adults' self-efficacy or sense of control over their behavior, their environment, and their own thoughts and feelings can contribute to positive relocation adjustment. Nurses working with older adults in primary care and community health settings should assess clients planning relocation to determine their relocation self-efficacy.

The Self-Efficacy Relocation Scale consists of 3 subscales: transition management efficacy, daily living efficacy, and engagement efficacy. The transition management efficacy subscale is made up of 9 items that refer to the individual's confidence in planning and preparing the activities of moving (eg, hiring movers and unpacking boxes). The daily living efficacy subscale consists of 7 items that refer to the individual's confidence in meeting new and continuing demands of living at the ILC (eg,

TABLE 4.3.1 Questions Healthcare Providers Can Ask to Assess Readiness to Move

1. How was the decision to move made? Who participated in making the decision? How do you feel about the decision to move?
2. How do you plan to handle the actions necessary for relocating to an independent living community (ILC)?
3. What factors do you think will determine the fit between you and the ILC? For example:
    a. Is the ILC close to your current home, family, and friends?
    b. Have your visits to the ILC contributed to your decision to move there?
    c. What are your thoughts about the people who live there?
4. What kinds of things are you doing to prepare for the move? For example:
    a. How do you feel about giving up your current home?
    b. How did you determine what belongings/furniture to move?
    c. What kinds of plans do you have for the things that you are not taking with you?
    d. How do you plan to move your belongings? Who will help you?
5. How do you think the move will affect your life?
6. What kinds of things do you think will change? Remain the same?
7. How do you think the move will affect your relationships with family? Friends? Others?
8. Who do you have that you can talk about almost anything with?

learning the new address and telephone number and handling mail), and the engagement efficacy subscale is made up of 16 items that refer to the individual's confidence in engaging in social interactions and activities (eg, continue relationships with family and friends and make new friends).[28] The scale factors reflect relocation as process or phases of the move from the actual preparatory and completion actions (transition management efficacy) to consideration of new business and daily living arrangements (daily living efficacy) and to dealing with staying connected with friends and family as well as connecting with the new environment (engagement efficacy).[28] Items are rated on a 5-point scale indicating respondents' degree of confidence in their ability to carry out needed relocation behaviors (5 = extremely confident, 4 = very confident, 3 = moderately confident, 2 = a little bit confident, and 1 = not at all confident). Subscale and total scores are calculated by summing the responses, with higher scores indicating greater confidence in being able to carry out the behaviors necessary to move to an ILC. Answers on the tool can be used to guide development of interventions to support positive self-efficacy behaviors and encourage the development of behaviors that support relocation adjustment.

When older adults believe they have made the decision to move, have the confidence to make the move, feel there is a fit between themselves and their new home (ILC), sense that their plans to move are organized and pleasing to them, and know how they will continue relationships and develop new relationships with others, they experience a sense of control over their behavior and environment.[4,6,9,28] This sense of control contributes greatly to their well-being and successful relocation.

Thus, nurses who work with older adults need to recognize the role they can play in developing and implementing health promotion and illness prevention activities for those who are contemplating moving to an ILC. Assessment of readiness for this type of move with interventions for specific areas that put individuals at risk for poor relocation adjustment is essential. The problem is how do we get this assessment done? Advanced practice nurses need to identify a point of contact for the assessment. Readiness to move assessments may be made by APNs working in a retirement community during one of the initial visits made by a prospective "mover." Community health APNs can provide education and preventive consultations with older adults in senior centers, churches, and other organizations. Although it would be costly initially to insert this assessment in preliminary interviews or in community centers, in the long term, it would save costly hospitalizations prevent individuals from moving quickly across the continuum of care from independent living to assisted living and then to long-term care. Clinical nurse specialists and other providers of healthcare for older adults can help them meet the challenges of relocation and thus contribute to their quality and years of healthy life.

Acknowledgments

The author thanks Elizabeth Tornquist and Dr. Susan Letvak for their review and comments.

REFERENCES

1. Center for Disease Control and Prevention. U.S. Department of Health and Human Services (USDHHS), 2007. The state of aging and health in America 2007 report. http://www.cdc.gov/aging/saha.htm. Accessed May 10, 2007.
2. Administration on Aging. U.S. Department of Health and Human Services (USDHHS). A profile of older Americans. 2004. http://www.cdc.gov/aging/pdf/State_of_Aging_and_Health_in_America_2004.pdf. Accessed October 19, 2007.
3. Armer JM. Elderly relocation to a congregate setting: factors influencing adjustment. *Issues Men Health Nurs.* 1993;14:157-172.
4. Hays JC. Living arrangements and health: a review of recent literature. *Public Health Nurs.* 2002;19(2):136-151.
5. Lassey WR, Lassey ML. *The residential environment neighborhood, community, and home in quality of life for older people: an international perspective.* Upper Saddle River, NJ: Prentice Hall; 2001.
6. Rossen EK, Knafl KA. Older women's response to residential relocation: description of transition styles. *Qual Health Res.* 2003;13(1):20-36.
7. Rossen EK, Knafl KA. Women's well-being after relocation to independent living communities. *West J Nur Res.* 2007;29(2):183-199.
8. Krout JA, Moen P, Holmes HH, Oggins J, Bowen N. Reasons for relocation to a continuing care retirement community. *J Appl Gerontol.* 2002;21(2):236-256.
9. Smider NA, Essex JJ, Ryff CD. Adaptation to community relocation: the interactive influence of psychological resources and contextual factors. *Psychol Aging.* 1996;11:362-372.
10. Johnson RA. Helping older adults adjust to relocation: nursing interventions and issues. In: Swan-

son L, Tripp-Reimer T, eds. *Series on Advances in Gerontological Nursing.* New York, NY: Springer; 1999:52-72.
11. Tracy JP, DeYoung S. Moving to an assisted living facility: exploring the transitional experience of elderly individuals. *J Gerontol Nurs.* 2004; 30(10):26-33.
12. Choi NG. Older persons who move: reasons and health consequences. *J Appl Gerontol.* 1996; 15:325-344.
13. Danermark B, Ekstrom M. Relocation and health effects on the elderly: a commented research review. *J Sociol Soc Welfare.* 1990;17:25-49.
14. Heisler E, Evans GW, Moen P. Health and social outcomes of moving to a continuing care retirement community. *J Hous Elder.* 2004;18(1):5-23.
15. Lutgendorf SK, Tripp-Reimer T, Harvey JH, et al. Effects of housing relocation on immunocompetence and psychosocial functioning in older adults. *J Gerontol.* 2001;56A(2):M97-M105.
16. Castle NG. Relocation of the elderly. *Med Care Res Rev.* 2001;58(3):291-333.
17. Piven ML, Buckwalter KC. Depression. In: Maas ML, Buckwalter KC, Hardy MD, Tripp-Reimer T, Tiller MG, Specht JP, eds. *Nursing Care of Older Adults: Diagnoses, Outcomes, & Interventions.* St Louis, MO: Mosby; 2001.
18. Ryff CD, Essex MJ. The interpretation of life experience and well-being: the sample case of relocation. *Psychol Aging.* 1992;7:507-517.
19. Johnson RA. Relocation stress syndrome. In: Maas M, Buckwalter KC, Hardy MD, Tripp-Reimer T, Titler MG, Specht JP, eds. *Nursing Care of Older Adults: Diagnoses, Outcomes, & Interventions.* St Louis, MO: Mosby; 2001:619-630.
20. Rokach A, Brock H. Loneliness and the effects of life changes. *J Psychol.* 1997;131:284-298.
21. Schumacher KL, Meleis AI. Transitions: a central concept in nursing. *Image J Nur Scholarsh.* 1994;26:119-127.
22. US Department of Health and Human Services. Healthy People 2010. McLean, VA: International Medical Publishing; 2000.
23. DeJong SR, Veltman RH. The effectiveness of a CNS-led community-based COPD screening and intervention program. *CNS.* 2004;18(2):72-79.
24. Halm MA, Denker J. Primary prevention programs to reduce heart disease risk in women. *CNS.* 2003;17(2):101-111.
25. Lewis Y. Clinical nurse specialist practice: addressing population with HIV/AID. *CNS.* 2002;16(6):306-311.
26. Logan L. The practice of certified community health CNSs. *CNS.* 2005;19(1):43-48.
27. Mion LC, Palmer RM, Anetzberger GJ, Meldon SW. Establishing a case-finding and referral system for at-risk older individuals in the emerging department setting: the SIGNET model. *CNS.* 2001;49(10):1379-1386.
28. Rossen EK, Gruber KJ. Development and psychometric testing of the Relocation Self-Efficacy Scale. *Nurs Res.* 2007;56(4):244-251.
29. Bandura A. *Self-efficacy: The Exercise of Control.* New York: Freeman and Co; 1997.
30. Maddux JE, Lewis J. Self-efficacy and adjustment: basic principles and issues. In: Maddux JE, ed. *Self-efficacy, Adaptation, and Adjustment Theory, Research, and Application.* New York: Plenum; 1995:37-68.

Reprinted with permission from: Rossen, E. (2007). Assessing older persons' readiness to move to independent congregate living. *Clinical Nurse Specialist, 21*(6), 292–296.

4.4 WOMEN'S WELL-BEING AFTER RELOCATION TO INDEPENDENT LIVING COMMUNITIES

EILEEN K. ROSSEN

KATHLEEN A. KNAFL

Abstract

Late-life relocation to independent living communities is increasing, especially among women. This study described the impact of relocation on the health and well-being of 31 older women who moved from a private residence to an independent living community. Schumacher and Meleis' (1994) nursing model of transition guided the study. Health status, social activity, self-esteem, depression and quality of life were measured pre- and postmove. Postmove women reported a significant increase in engagement in social activities and higher quality of life. Participants' levels of self-esteem, depression, and quality of life were found to correspond with three relocation transition styles: full inte-

gration, partial integration and minimal integration. These preliminary findings suggest that nurses who identify older women with low self-esteem, high depressive symptoms and low quality of life premove may be at risk for poor relocation outcomes. Interventions to ease the transition process and improve relocation adjustment are needed.

The U.S. population older than age 65 years is increasing dramatically and expected to reach 71.5 million by 2030 (U.S. Department of Commerce, Economics and Statistics Administration [USDC-ESA], 2004). Older women are the fastest growing population segment in the rate of 1.4 times of men counterparts in 2003 (Department of Health and Human Services, Administration on Aging [DHHSAA], 2004). Approximately 23% of older persons age 65 years or older experienced relocation, a significant life transition and those older than age 85 years are moving at an even greater rate (DHHSAA, 2004). Although older adults prefer to continue living in their own home (DHHSAA, 2004), many are moving to an independent living community (ILC) where they can continue independent living in a "sheltered" environment with supportive services (Armer, 1993; Lassey & Lassey, 2001; Rossen & Knafl, 2003). ILCs are residential settings of multiunit independent living apartments adapted to meet the special needs of elderly persons.

Late-Life Relocation

Relocation is a transitional process that includes initiation of a move, the actual physical move and adjustment to the new environment (Remer & Buckwalter, 1990). Relocation sometimes has had negative outcomes, including declining health, reduced functional independence and quality of life, increased health care utilization, higher health care costs (Badger, 1998; Berkman, 1997; Castle, 2001; Choi, 1996; Johnson, 2001; Piven & Buckwalter, 2001), and increased risk for institutionalization, morbidity and mortality (Danermark & Ekstrom, 1990; Piven & Buckwalter, 2001). Research, however, has shown some psychological benefits of relocation, such as experiencing unexpected gains (Smider, Essex, & Ryff, 1996), finding meaning in the experience (Johnson, 1999; Tracy & DeYoung, 2004) and feeling secure (Choi, 1996). The impact of relocation is related to age, a person's perception about choice to move, predictability of the new environment and perceptions of self and others (Danermark & Ekstrom, 1990; Rossen & Knafl, 2003; Smider et al., 1996). Perception of having a choice to move has been positively correlated with psychological adjustment, conceptualized as morale, congruence and continuity (Armer, 1996; Johnson, 2001), whereas lack of choice or feeling forced to move has been associated with older women's dissatisfaction with the new home (Rossen & Knafl, 2003), poorer functional status and self-rated health and higher levels of depression, loneliness and anxiety (Rokach & Brock, 1997). Perceptions of self and others have been positively correlated with women's psychological adjustment to relocation (Johnson, 2001; Smider et al., 1996), and preserving relationships and social support were found to positively influence psychological adjustment to and satisfaction with a move (Armer, 1996).

The studies to date thus suggest that a person's perceptions about choice to move, preparation, psychological resources and relationships affect relocation adjustment and, in turn, physical, emotional and social well-being. The majority of relocation studies, however, have focused on relocation migration patterns (Duncombe, Robbins, & Wolf, 2003; Litwak & Longino, 1987; Longino, 1997), housing quality (Sweaney, Mimura, & Meeks, 2004) and relocation to nursing homes or assisted-living facilities (Kao, Travis, & Acton, 2004; D. T. F. Lee, Woo, & Mackenzie, 2002). Few studies have examined health-related effects and quality of life of women who relocated to ILC. Relocation has been identified as an important situational transition (Schumacher & Meleis, 1994). With the increasing numbers of older women moving to ILCs, there is a need to examine how relocation affects older women's health and quality of life to identify those at risk and to design nursing interventions to support women's transition to a new home, enhance health outcomes, prevent negative consequences and promote independent living (U.S. Department of Health and Human Services [USDHHS], 2000).

Purpose

This article reports a study designed to investigate the impact of moving from a private residence to an age-specific congregate ILC. Specifically, the current study describes: (a) pre- and postmove health-related characteristics (physical and emotional well-being); (b) person–environment interactions (perception of having a confidant and social activities); (c) subjective well-being (quality of life) of older women who moved to ILCs; and (d) the relationships between the measures of emotional well-being (self-esteem and depression) and quality of life and relocation transition styles (RTS; *RTS* refers to three distinct qualitatively derived late-life relocation types—full, partial and minimal integration; Rossen & Knafl, 2003).

Theoretical Framework

The nursing model of transitions (Schumacher & Meleis, 1994) that guided the current descriptive study is composed of three major concepts: universal properties, transition conditions and indicators of healthy transitions. Universal properties consist of the characteristics of process and movement from one state to another and involve changes in identity, roles, relationships, abilities and patterns of behavior. Transition conditions are personal and environmental factors that influence the transition. They include emotional and physical well-being and person–environment interactions. These conditions are conceptualized as facilitators or inhibitors to healthy transition (Schumacher & Meleis, 1994). The third major model concept, indicators of a healthy transition, are factors indicating the quality of the transition outcome, such as subjective well-being. The two model concepts used for the current study were transition conditions and indicators of a healthy transition. Transition conditions measured were physical well-being, emotional well-being and person–environment. Subjective well-being was considered the indicator of a healthy transition. Guided by Schumacher and Meleis' (1994) transition theory, Rossen and Knafl (2003) identified qualitatively three RTS—full integration, partial integration and minimal integration—to indicate the degree of success women experience in a move to an ILC. *Integration* was defined as the individual's adjustment or adaptation to the new living situation.

Method

Design, Setting, and Sample

The current study used a one-group pretest–posttest design to gain a more comprehensive understanding of women's late-life relocation to ILCs. The current study was a part of a large, mixed-methods study. Qualitative data from the current study have been reported elsewhere (Rossen & Knafl, 2003).

The target population was community-dwelling women age 61 years or older who could read, write and speak English and who had definitive plans to move (i.e., a scheduled move-in date) to an ILC. A convenience sample who met these criteria was recruited from 12 ILCs chosen from a roster of member ILCs in an association of independent housing communities for seniors in a large midwestern city and surrounding area. Women whose spouses had died within 13 months of the current study were excluded to reduce the possibility that the early stage of grieving, which itself is a transition (Scannell-Desch, 2003), would be a confounding factor. The ILCs provided similar programs and services for residents, including transportation, meals and social activities. A designated facility representative from each ILC identified potential study participants. Those who met the selection criteria were invited to participate, and informed consent was obtained.

Thirty-one community-dwelling English-speaking women completed the current study. Their ages ranged from 61 to 91 years with a mean age of 78 ($SD = \pm 6.34$); 23% were young-old (age

61–74 years), 61% old (age 75–84 years) and 16% old-old (age 85 years or older). Most (93%) were White, 6.5% were African American. The sample was diverse in marital status with 64.5% widowed, 19.4% married, 12.9% single and 3.2% divorced. The women were fairly well educated, with 45.2% reporting education beyond high school, 25.8% reporting a high school education and only 29% reporting less than high school education. Religious affiliations included Protestant (52%), Catholic (42%) and Jewish (6%); incomes varied, with 42% reporting less than U.S. $20,000 per year, 29% between $20,000 and $40,000 and 22% reporting incomes higher than $40,000. Although all of the women interviewed premove completed the move, one participant declined the postmove interview because her husband was ill.

Data Collection

The current study was approved by the human subjects' research committee at the first author's institution. Each ILC facility provided a letter of support for the current study. Data were collected in participants' homes via face-to-face interviews at two points approximately 4 months apart: within the month prior to the move and between the 3rd and 4th months after the move. After obtaining written informed consent from the participants, the authors collected demographic, health, self-esteem, depression, social and quality-of-life data.

Measures

Transition Conditions

Transition conditions measured in the study were physical well-being, emotional well-being and person–environment interactions (Schumacher & Meleis, 1994).

Physical Well-Being. Physical well-being was measured with six indicators; health, health satisfaction, health limitations, health habits, health service utilization and chronic medical conditions. Health was operationalized as self-report of health as excellent, good, fair, or poor. Health satisfaction was operationalized as self-report of satisfaction with health, as not at all satisfied, not very satisfied, very satisfied, or completely satisfied. Health limitations were operationalized as self-reported daily activity limitations related to health, from not at all limited, limited a little, somewhat, quite a bit or almost completely. Health habits were operationalized as a yes-or-no response to the questions: Do you smoke? Drink alcoholic beverages? Do physical exercise such as walking? Health service utilization was operationalized as number of physician visits, hospital nights and bed rest days due to illness in past 6 months. Chronic medical conditions were operationalized as self-reported number of chronic conditions in the past 12 months. These measures of physical well-being have been used in other studies of older adults (Adelmann, 1994; Ferraro & Kelley-Moore, 2001).

Emotional Well-Being. The second transition condition in the current study, emotional well-being, was measured with two indicators: self-esteem and depression (Table 4.4.1). Self-esteem was measured by the Rosenberg Self-Esteem Scale (RSE) that assesses global feelings of self-worth or self-acceptance (Rosenberg, 1965). Higher scores correspond to higher levels of self-esteem. For older adults, a score of 29 or less has been shown to indicate low self-esteem (Caserta & Lund, 1993). Depression was measured by the Geriatric Depression Scale (GDS; Yesavage et al., 1983), which assesses affective, cognitive and behavioral symptoms of depression. Scores of 0 to 10 indicate no depression, scores 11 to 20 indicate mild depression, and scores of 21 to 30 indicate moderate to major depression (Yesavage et al., 1983). Both measures have been widely used with reports of good reliability and validity in community elderly (Billipp, 2001; Cully et al., 2005; Gardner & Helmes, 2006; Stamatakis et al., 2004; Wang, 2004). For the current study, internal consistency reliabilities (Cronbach's alphas) for the RSE were

.86 premove and .88 postmove; the GDS Cronbach's alphas were .84 premove and .89 postmove.

Person–Environment Interactions. The third transition condition measured in the current study, person–environment interactions, refers to the relationship of the individual to the changing social environment (Schumacher & Meleis, 1994). It was measured in the current study by two indicators: perceived confidant and participation in social activities. Perceived confidant was operationalized as self-report of presence or absence of a confidant. Social activities were operationalized as the self-reported amount of participation in five areas of activity (Adelmann, 1994; Danermark & Ekstrom, 1990; Smider et al., 1996; see Table 4.4.1).

Subjective Well-Being

Quality of Life. Subjective well-being, a component of the concept indicators of healthy transition (Schumacher & Meleis, 1994) was measured as quality of life. Quality of life was chosen because the literature indicates that it is a component of subjective well-being (e.g., Ferrans & Powers, 1992) and it has been used by other researchers as a measure of subjective well-being (e.g., Lee & McCormick, 2004). The Quality of Life Index (QLI) quantifies an individual's appraisal of the importance and satisfaction or dissatisfaction with four areas of life: health and physical functioning, social and economic functioning, psychological and spiritual functioning, and family functioning (Ferrans & Powers, 1992). The range of possible scores is 0 to 30 for the total score and for each of the four subscales. Higher scores indicate better quality of life. The QLI has been used with older women (Ferrans & Powers, 1992), and reliability and validity have been established (Ferrans & Powers, 1992). For the current study sample, internal consistency reliability (Cronbach's alphas) for premove total scale, health and functioning, socioeconomic, psychological and/or spiritual, and family subscales were .94, .88, .87, .82 and .52, respectively; postmove they were .80, .72, .64, .89 and .65, respectively.

Data Analysis

All analyses were performed using SPSS (2004). Descriptive statistics were used to describe the magnitude of each variable, and nonparametric statistics (paired-samples sign test, McNemar test) were used to test differences between pre- and postrelocation variables. Statistical significance was based on a predetermined .05 level.

In the qualitative portion of the study (Rossen & Knafl, 2003), transition styles were developed from the iterative processes of reviewing categories of descriptive codes and subcodes, clustering codes, and identifying thematic patterns. Matrix display techniques described by Miles and Huberman (1994) facilitated categorizing participants into one of three RTS) based on 13 qualitative themes: full integration, partial integration and minimal integration. A *full integration RTS* was defined as voluntarily moving, being well-prepared for the move, having premove expectations fulfilled, having enduring confidant relationships and multiple other strong relationships, continuing premove daily patterns or centering life on routines of the new community, having a sense of competence in handling the demands of the new situation, and having a sense of belonging and satisfaction with the new community. A minimal integration RTS was defined as feeling forced to move and poorly prepared for the move, having only partially met premove expectations, discontinued confidant relationships, few or strained relationships and feeling essentially solitary and without friends, feeling a lack of belonging in the new setting, and being only somewhat satisfied or reluctantly accepting the new home. A *partial integration RTS* was defined as containing some of the characteristics of the full and minimal integration RTS. Each individual with a partial RTS had a unique combination of characteristics of the full and minimal integration RTS.

The current study looked at whether there was a correspondence between participants' self-esteem, depression and quality-of-life scores and their RTS. To describe the relationships between (a)

TABLE 4.4.1 Model Constructs and Measures: Emotional Well-Being, Person–Environment Interactions and Subjective Well-Being

Mode Construct	Measure	Description of Measures	Rating Scale
Transition conditions Emotional well-being	Self-esteem[a]	Affective judgments emerging from the individual's comparisons of what they are like to what they desire to be like (10 items)	1 = *strongly disagree*, 4 = *strongly agree*
	Depression[b]	Feelings of hopelessness, lack of control in response to events and or situations (30 items)	1 = no, 2 = yes
Person–environment interactions	Confidant	Self-report of a person they can confide in	1 = no, 2 = yes
	Social activities	Self-report # per week (a) visit family, (b) visit friends. (c) attend different groups, (d) total social activities attend. (e) total times attend social activities	
Indicators of healthy transition Subjective well-being	Quality of life[c]	Person's sense of well-being stems from satisfaction or dissatisfaction with areas of life that are important to the individual (64 items in two parts)	1 = *very dissatisfied*, 6 = *very satisfied*; 1 = *very unimportant*, 6 = *very important*

a. Rosenberg Self-Esteem Scale (Rosenberg, 1965).
b. Geriatric Depression Scale (Yesavage et al., 1983).
c. Quality of Life Index (Ferrans & Powers, 1992).

measures of self-esteem, depression and quality of life and (b) women's RTS, participants' levels of self-esteem, depression and quality of life were compared to their previous placement in one of the three RTS.

Findings

Transition Conditions

Physical Well-Being. Before the move, 77.4% of the women rated their health as "good or excellent," 87% said they were "somewhat to completely satisfied" with their health and 58% reported health-related limits on activities as "limited a little to not at all limited." Most (87%) of the women reported more than one medical condition. Arthritis was reported most frequently (65%), followed by high blood pressure (48%) and heart trouble (39%). Other medical problems included hearing loss, cataracts, macular degeneration, dizziness, headaches, high cholesterol and irritable bowel syndrome. Within the past 6 months, women had had an average of 3 days of bed rest, three physician visits and 3½ days in the hospital. Nearly all (90.3%) reported that they did not smoke, 67.7% did not drink alcoholic beverages, 48.4% did not walk for physical activity and 71% cleaned their own homes.

There were no significant changes in self-rated health after the move: 8 women rated their health higher postmove, 4 reported it lower and 19 reported no change. Nine women reported greater satisfaction with their health postmove, 4 reported less satisfaction and 18 reported the same satisfaction. As expected, there were no significant changes in the percentages of women reporting various health problems, for example, arthritis, heart trouble—with one exception. The percentage reporting high blood pressure decreased significantly, from 48.4% before the move to 29.0% after the move; the percentage of participants who walked for exercise increased from 51.6% before the move to 77.4% after the move, also a significant difference. There was no significant change in the total number of physical activities from premove ($M = 1.74$, $SD = 1.18$) to postmove ($M = 1.61$, $SD = .96$; paired sign test, $N = 31$, $p = .68$), or in the total number of times per week that participants engaged in physical activities (premove $M = 4.62$, $SD = 4.44$; postmove $M = 6.05$, $SD = 4.06$; paired sign test, $N = 31$, $p = .15$).

Emotional Well-Being. There were no significant changes in scores on the RSE after the move (see Table 4.4.2). For older adults, a score of 29 or less is indicative of low self-esteem (Caserta & Lund, 1993). In the current study, premove scores ranged from 21 to 40, with 25% scoring 29 or less. Two women who scored high on self-esteem premove scored low postmove, and two women who scored low on self-esteem premove scored high postmove.

As can be seen in Table 4.4.2, there were also no significant changes in depressive symptoms after the move. Premove GDS scores ranged from 0 to 19, with six women scoring in the mild depression range. Postmove scores ranged from 0 to 22, with three women scoring in the mild depression range and one in the moderate depression range. Four women who scored mildly depressed premove scored not depressed postmove.

Person–Environment Interactions. Pre- and postmove, 87% of the sample reported having a confidant with whom they could discuss almost everything. Two women reported having no confidant pre- or postmove, two reported gaining a confidant postmove and two who reported having a confidant premove reported no confidant postmove. At the time of the move, the women typically visited family twice a week, visited friends once a week, participated in three different kinds of social activities and attended four social activities per week. There were no significant changes postmove in the percentages that visited their families, visited friends, ate out with their husband and attended social activities. There was, however, a significant increase in the percentage who attended group social functions, from 41.9% ($n = 13$ premove) to 71.0% ($n = 22$ postmove); also, 42% ($n = 13$) reported an increase in social activities, and only 12% ($n = 4$) reported a decrease following the move. These differences were significant ($p = .049$) based on the McNemar test of dependent proportions. Although the total number of social activities did not change, the mean number of times per week that participants engaged in social activities increased significantly from 4.4 $SD = 3.5$ to 8.2 $SD = 5.0$ (paired sign test, $N = 31$, $p < .001$). Twenty-five participants reported an increase, five a decrease and one no change.

Subjective Well-Being

Quality of Life. The women showed a significant improvement in total scores on the QLI after their move (see Table 4.4.2) and on the Social and Economic and the Psychological and/or Spiritual QLI subscales, although not on the Health and Functioning and Family subscales. Postmove, 81% of the participants experienced greater overall life satisfaction, and 19% experienced less; 73% experienced greater satisfaction with their socioeconomic situation, 23% experienced less and 4% remained at the same level of satisfaction; and 63% experienced greater satisfaction with their psychological and/or spiritual life domain postmove, 19% experienced less satisfaction and 19% saw no change.

TABLE 4.4.2 Comparison of Premove and Postmove Self-Esteem, Geriatric Depression and Quality-of-Life Scores

	Premove			Postmove			
Measure	M	SD	n	M	SD	n	p
Self-esteem[a]	31.5	0.5	31	32.0	0.4	31	.664
Depression[b]	6.5	5.1	31	5.9	5.6	30	.690
Quality of life[c]							
Quality of Life Index total score	23.8	3.6	31	25.5	2.3	31	.001
Health and functioning	22.9	4.6	31	24.2	2.7	31	.151
Social and economic	23.4	4.7	31	26.4	2.3	31	.009
Psychological and/or spiritual	25.5	4.0	31	26.9	3.7	31	.015
Family	25.1	4.0	31	26.6	3.7	31	.523

Note: Differences between premove and postmove scores were found based on the paired sign test.
a. Rosenberg Self-Esteem Scale (Rosenberg, 1965).
b. Geriatric Depression Scale (Yesavage et al., 1983).
c. Quality of Life Index (Ferrans & Powers, 1992).

Integration. Table 4.4.3 presents participants' self-esteem, depression and quality-of-life levels by RTS. Low depression and high self-esteem and quality of life correspond with full integration RTS; high depression and low self-esteem and quality of life correspond with minimal integration RTS.

Discussion

Because nearly 25% of older adults change residence every 5 years (Sweaney et al., 2004), women's late-life relocation transition is important to understand (Rossen & Knafl, 2003: Schumacher & Meleis, 1994). The current study described older women's health, self-esteem and depression, presence of a confidant, social activities and quality of life before and after moving to an ILC. Postmove, the sample reported that they were healthier, engaging in healthier habits and enjoying a better quality of life. The women also tended to show improvements in most health measures after the move; they reported improved self-rated health and health satisfaction, an increase in walking, fewer bed rest days, hospital days, and number of physician visits; and significantly lower high blood pressure. Overall, 94% were somewhat, very, or completely satisfied with their health postmove. This finding is in contrast to previous reports that relocation negatively influences elders' mental and physical health (Choi, 1996; Dimond, McCance, & King, 1987: Ferraro, 1983; Johnson, 2001) and that women in particular report declines in self-rated health after relocation (Dimond et al., 1987).

The improvements in reported health may be explained by several factors, including provision of the main meal of the day, which offered good nutrition and social contact (McReynolds & Rossen, 2004), and accessible and varied physical, educational and social activities. Many of the women were walking more postmove than premove because their ILC provided walkable routes from their apartments to the common area for the evening meal, to get their mail, or to join in a social event.

Women who had a full integration RTS (45%) had high self-esteem, low depressive symptoms and high quality of life. Women who had a minimal integration RTS (13%) reported lower self-esteem, higher depressive symptoms and lower quality of life. Those with a partial integration (42%) had a

Table 4.4.3 Correspondence of Self-Esteem, Depression and Quality-of-Life Levels by Relocation Transition Styles (RTS)

	Relocation Transition Styles (RTS)		
	Full Integration RTS ($n = 14$)	Partial Integration RTS ($n = 13$)	Minimal Integration RTS ($n = 4$)
Self-esteem[a]			
Medium and/or high	11	10	2
Low	3	3	2
Depression[b]			
Not depressed (0 to 10)	13	11	2
Mild depression (11 to 20)	1	0	2
Moderate and/or major depression (21 to 30)	0	1	0
Quality of life[c]			
Highest 50%	14	7	0
Lowest 50%	0	6	4

Note: One case did not provide a Geriatric Depression Scale.
a. Rosenberg Self-Esteem Scale (Rosenberg, 1965).
b. Geriatric Depression Scale (Yesavage et al., 1983).
c. Quality of Life Index (Ferrans & Powers, 1992).

mix of high and low values for emotional and social functioning and quality of life. In spite of the positive postmove findings, more than one half (55%) of the study participants achieved only partial or minimal relocation integration, with the potential for lower self-esteem, higher depression and lower quality of life. Clearly it is important for health care professionals to understand the dynamics of relocation to an ILC and the ways in which this relocation affects the health and well-being of older women.

Pre- and postmove, the presence of a confidant appeared to contribute to a positive relocation transition. Others have also found that for older women, having a confidant acts as a buffer to the stress and anxiety associated with difficult life events such as relocation (Baltes & Silverberg, 1994; Crohan & Antonucci, 1989; Dimond et al., 1987; Hamilton, 1990; Huss, Buckwalter, & Stolley, 1988; Rossen & Knafl, 2003).

Women who were classified as achieving full or partial integration RTS had higher self-esteem scores and lower depression scores than women who were classified in the minimal integration RTS. Thus, low self-esteem premove should be considered a risk factor for an unhealthy response to relocation, as should high depressive symptoms either pre- or postmove.

After the move, there were significant improvements in QLI total scores, Social and Economic subscale scores, and Psychological and/or Spiritual subscale scores. Thus, relocation appeared to improve the women's satisfaction with quality of life and, contrary to much of the relocation literature, relocation proved to be beneficial.

This research demonstrates the applicability of transition theory in general and the nursing model of transition (Schumacher & Meleis, 1994) in particular to a community population of relocating women at risk for diminished emotional health and quality of life. The theory provides a framework by which a nurse can assess an individual's risk for poor relocation transition outcomes. In addition, the evidence of the usefulness of this model in guiding the study of relocation transition suggests its possible relevance for studying other situational, developmental and health and/or illness transitions.

The sample in the current study was small, participation was voluntary, and data were collected only at one follow-up point; therefore, the findings must be interpreted with caution (Cook & Campbell, 1979). Further research needs to be conducted with larger samples of men and women and samples that are heterogeneous in ethnicity, marital status (including newly widowed) and relocation type (i.e., independent, assisted living, long-distance relocation). A potential measurement limitation in the current study was the use of the Rosenberg's global self-esteem scale as a measure of emotional well-being; it may have lacked the sensitivity to change during the short period of follow-up. A more sensitive measure of state- or domain-specific self-esteem may be more useful than a global measure of self-esteem for measuring change in self-esteem (McCauley, Elavsky, Motl, & Konopack, 2005; McGannon & Spence, 2002). Studies with larger sample sizes and a more sensitive measure of self-esteem may help determine whether the relationships of self-esteem, depression and quality of life with RTS found here will hold for other samples and other relocation types.

Although the data from the current study are preliminary, nurses who identify older women with low self-esteem, high depressive symptoms and low quality-of-life indicators should be aware that these women may have difficulty in relocation adjustment and may need more support than other women in these areas. The correspondence found between emotional well-being, person–environment interactions, subjective well-being and RTS offer health care providers a basis for identifying those at risk for poor relocation outcomes and for planning and implementing programs for elders who are relocating.

REFERENCES

Adelmann, P. K. (1994). Multiple roles and physical health among older adults: Gender and ethnic comparisons. *Research on Aging, 16*(2), 144–166.

Armer, J. M. (1993). Elderly relocation to a congregate setting: Factors influencing adjustment. *Issues in Menial Health Nursing, 14,* 157–172.

Armer, J. M. (1996). Research brief: Degree of personalization as a cue in the assessment of adjustment to congregate housing by rural elders. *Geriatric Nursing, 17,* 79–80.

Badger, T. A. (1998). Depression, physical health impairment, and service use among older adults. *Public Health Nursing, 15,* 136–145.

Baltes, M. M., & Silverberg, S. B. (1994). The dynamics between dependency and autonomy. In D. L. Featherman, R. M. Lerner, & M. Perlmutter (Eds.), *Lifespan development and behavior* (pp. 52–90). Hillsdale, NJ: Lawrence Erlbaum.

Berkman, L. F. (1997). *Social relationships, connectedness, and health: The bonds that heal. A summary of a presentation.* Retrieved November 20, 2000, from www.obssr.od.nih.gov/Publications/SOCIAL.HTM

Billipp, S. H. (2001). The psychosocial impact of interactive computer use within a vulnerable elderly population: A report on a randomized prospective trial in a home health care setting. *Public Health Nursing, 18*(2), 138–145.

Caserta, M. S., & Lund, D. A. (1993). Interpersonal resources and the effectiveness of self-help groups for bereaved older adults. *The Gerontologist, 33,* 619–629.

Castle, N. G. (2001). Relocation of the elderly. *Medical Care Research and Review, 58*(3). 291–333.

Choi, N. G. (1996). Older persons who move: Reasons and health consequences. *Journal of Applied Gerontology, 15,* 325–344.

Cook, T. D., & Campbell, D. T. (1979). Quasi-experimentation: Design & analysis issues for field settings. Boston: Houghton Mifflin.

Crohan, S. E., & Antonucci, T. C. (1989). Friends as a source of social support in old age. In R. Adams & R. Blieszner (Eds.), *Older adult friendship: Structure and process* (pp. 129–145). Newbury Park, CA: Sage.

Cully, J. A., Gfeller, J. D., Heise, R. A., Ross, M. J., Teal, C. R., & Kunik, M. E. (2005). Geriatric depression, medical diagnosis, and functional recovery during acute rehabilitation. *Archives of Physical Medicine and Rehabilitation, 86,* 2256–2260.

Danermark, B., & Ekstrom, M. (1990). Relocation and health effects on the elderly: A commented research review. *Journal of Sociology and Social Welfare, 17,* 25–49.

Dimond, M., McCance, K., & King, K. (1987). Forced residential relocation: Its impact on the well-being of older adults. *Western Journal of Nursing Research, 9,* 445–464.

Duncombe, W., Robbins, M., & Wolf, D. A. (2003). Place characteristics and residential location choice among the retirement-age population. *Journals of Gerontology Series B, 58,* S244–S252.

Ferrans, C. E., & Powers, M. J. (1992). Psychometric assessment of the quality of life index. *Research in Nursing and Health, 15,* 29–38.

Ferraro, K. (1983). The health consequences of relocation among the aged in the community. *Journal of Gerontology, 38,* 90–96.

Ferraro, K., & Kelley-Moore, J. A. (2001). Self-rated health and mortality among black and white adults: Examining the dynamic evaluation thesis. *Journals of Gerontology Series B, 56,* S195–S205.

Gardner, D. K., & Helmes, E. (2006). Interpersonal dependency in older adults and the risks of developing mood and mobility problems when receiving care at home. *Aging and Mental Health, 10,* 63–68.

Hamilton, G. P. (1990). Promotion of mental health in older adults. In M. O. Hogstgel (Ed.). *Geropsychiatric nursing* (pp. 38–69). St. Louis, MO: C. V. Mosby.

Huss, M. J., Buckwalter, K. C., & Stolley, J. (1988). Nursing's impact on life satisfaction. *Journal of Gerontological Nursing, 14*(5). 31–36.

Johnson, R. A. (1999). Helping older adults adjust to relocation: Nursing interventions and issues. In L. Swanson & T. Tripp-Reimer (Eds.), *Series on advances in gerontological nursing* (pp. 52–72). New York: Springer.

Johnson, R. A. (2001). Relocation stress syndrome. In M. Maas, K. C. Buckwalter, M. D. Hardy, T. Tripp-Reimer, M. G. Titler, & J. P. Specht (Eds.). *Nursing care of older adults: Diagnoses, outcomes, & interventions* (pp. 619–630). St. Louis. MO: C. V. Mosby.

Kao, H. S., Travis, S. S., & Acton, G. J. (2004). Relocation to a long-term care facility: Working with patients and families before, during, and after. *Journal of Psychosocial Nursing and Mental Health Services, 42*(3), 10–16.

Lassey, W. R., & Lassey, M. L. (2001). The residential environment neighborhood, community, and home in quality of life for older people: An international perspective. Upper Saddle River, NJ: Prentice Hall.

Lee, Y., & McCormick, B. (2004). Subjective well-being of people with spinal cord injury: Does leisure contribute? *Journal of Rehabilitation, 70,* 5–12.

Lee, D. T. F., Woo, J., & Mackenzie, A. E. (2002). A review of older people's experiences with residential care placement. *Journal of Advanced Nursing, 37*(1), 19–27.

Litwak, E., & Longino. C. (1987). Migration patterns among the elderly: A developmental perspective. *The Gerontologist, 21,* 266–272.

Longino, C. F. (1997, Spring). On the move: The new migration patterns of older Americans. *Innovations in Aging, 26,* 23–26.

McCauley, E., Elavsky, S., Motl, R. W., & Konopack, J. F. (2005). Physical activity, self-efficacy, and self-esteem: Longitudinal relationships in older adults. *Journals of Gerontology Series B, 60B.* P268–P275.

McGannon, K. R., & Spence, J. C. (2002). The effect of exercise on self-esteem: Is it global or domain-specific? Research update. *Alberta Centre for Active Living, 9*(4). Retrieved December 6, 2005, from www.centre4activeliving.ca/Research/ResearchUpdate/2002/Active LivngSept.htm

McReynolds, J. L., & Rossen, E. K. (2004). Importance of physical activity, nutrition, and social support for optimal aging. *Clinical Nurse Specialist, 18,* 200–206.

Miles, M. B., & Huberman, A. M. (Eds.). (1994). *An expanded sourcehook: Qualitative data analysis* (2nd ed.). Thousand Oaks. CA: Sage.

Piven, M. L., & Buckwalter, K. C. (2001). Depression. In M. L. Maas, K. C. Buckwalter. M. D. Hardy, T. Tripp-Reimer. M. G. Titler. & J. P. Specht (Eds.), *Nursing care of older adults: Diagnoses, outcomes, & interventions,* (pp. 521–542). St. Louis, MO: C. V. Mosby.

Remer, D., & Buckwalter, K. (1990). Decreasing relocation stress for the elderly. *Continuing Care, 9,* 26–27, 42–50.

Rokach, A., & Brock, H. (1997). Loneliness and the effects of life changes. *Journal of Psychology, 131,* 284–298.

Rosenberg, M. (1965). *Society and the adolescent self-image.* Princeton, NJ: Princeton University Press.

Rossen. E. K., & Knafl, K. A. (2003). Older women's response to residential relocation: Description of transition styles. *Qualitative Health Research, 13,* 20–36.

Scannell-Desch, E. (2003). Women's adjustment to widowhood: Theory, research, and interventions. *Journal of Psychosocial Nursing and Mental Health Services, 41*(5), 28–36.

Schumacher, K. L., & Meleis, A. I. (1994). Transitions: A central concept in nursing. *Image: Journal of Nursing Scholarship, 26,* 119–127.

Smider, N. A., Essex, J. J., & Ryff, C. D. (1996). Adaptation to community relocation: The interactive influence of psychological resources and contextual factors. *Psychology and Aging, 11,* 362–372.

SPSS. (2004). *SPSS for Windows, rel. 13.0.1.* Chicago: Author.

Stamatakis, K. A., Lynch, J., Everson, S. A., Raghunathan, T., Salonen, J. T., & Kaplan, G. A. (2004). Self-esteem and mortality: Prospective evidence from a population-based study. *Annuals of Epidemiology, 14,* 58–65.

Sweaney, A. L., Mimura, Y., & Meeks. C. B. (2004). Changes in perceived housing quality among elderly movers: Does neighborhood and tenure matter? *Journal of Housing for the Elderly, 18*(2), 3–16.

Tracy, J. P., & DeYoung, S. (2004). Moving to an assisted living facility: Exploring the transitional experience of elderly individuals. *Journal of Gerontological Nursing, 30*(10), 26–33.

U.S. Department of Commerce, Economics and Statistics Administration. (2004). *We the people: Aging in the United States Census 2000 special reports.* Retrieved August 11, 2006, from www.census.gov/prod/2004pubs/censr-19.pdf

U.S. Department of Health and Human Services. (2000). *Healthy people 2010.* McLean, VA: International Medical Publishing.

U.S. Department of Health and Human Services, Administration on Aging. (2004). *A profile of older Americans: 2005.* Retrieved May 24, 2006, from www.aoa.gov/prof/statistics/profile/2004/2004profile.pdf

Wang, J. J. (2004). The comparative effectiveness among institutionalized and non-institutionalized elderly people in Taiwan of reminiscence therapy as a psychological measure. *Journal of Nursing Research, 12,* 237–245.

Yesavage, J., Brink. T., Rose, T., Lum, O., Huang, V., Adey, M., et al. (1983). Development and validation of a geriatric depression screening scale: A preliminary report. *Journal of Psychiatric Research, 17,* 37–49.

Reprinted with permission from: Rossen, E., & Knafl, K. (2007). Women's well-being after relocation to independent living communities. *Western Journal of Nursing Research, 29*(2), 183–199.

4.5 WOMEN IN TRANSITION: BEING VERSUS BECOMING OR BEING AND BECOMING

AFAF IBRAHIM MELEIS
IN ASSOCIATION WITH SANDRA ROGERS

Abstract

Women are at the center of all life transitions whether the transitions are within the family, such as maturation, or because of national modernization or a move to an urban center, or because of relocation to another nation. Ironically, women's roles in these transitions are ignored at best and misrepresented at worst. What we need is a raising of consciousness, an awareness of these women among us who are struggling with the being-versus-becoming dilemma of living in a new culture, and who would like to solve it by integrating being true to the values of their country of origin and becoming a valued citizen of the host country both for themselves and for their family.

I was recently sitting around a dinner table with a group of first-generation Middle Eastern immigrants to the United States. Among us were those who had immigrated 25 years ago and others only 5 years ago. Still others had recently come to the U.S. for a second time. They had returned to their home country or to another Middle Eastern country for a few years after deciding that they were not able to live for the rest of their lives with the so-called U.S. values toward marriage, children and aging. Though they were now back to live in the U.S. as immigrants, they were more determined than ever to preserve their *being* Middle Easterners and wanted to vehemently guard against *becoming* Americans.

Within this small group of diners, some had returned to their homeland to ensure that their teenage daughters maintained Middle Eastern values toward virginity, dating and the preference for a marriage initiated within their faith and culture. Others went back temporarily because their wives felt isolated and alienated in their neighborhoods and because they missed their extended families. Still others did the same because husbands were concerned about their changing role and image in the family. These husbands had become alarmed with sex-role changes in the family and sought to return to the home country in search of support for their discomfort with these changes. These were educated professional couples seated around that dinner table. None of them acknowledged or accepted the roles women played in the decisions for either the first or rotating immigration. Yet women were the center of all immigration decisions.

In analyzing immigration patterns and processes and in reflecting on that animated dinner conversation and the many interviews we have completed, I became aware of what the literature is beginning to support. Women are central in the immigration process. They are profoundly affected by it and they affect decisions about it. Even when they appear to have limited formal power in this process and even if the assumption that their informal power is limited is correct, the immigration transition exerts a significant influence on their roles in the family and society. That dinner conversation also represented a microcosm of the struggle that first-generation immigrants confront in *being* from a home country and maintaining all of the values and the sex-role behaviors of that home country and *becoming* an American and thus co-opting new sex-role behaviors. That struggle has been the center of many theoretical and methodological discussions on ethnic identity, assimilation and integration. The questions remain: Is it *being* versus *becoming or* being and becoming? More importantly, in what ways do *being* and *becoming* influence the health of women?

The purpose of this presentation is to discuss the roles of women in the immigration and postimmigration process and to identify some areas of neglect in knowledge development regarding women immigrants. Though I do not have many answers, I will make two points. First, we cannot really identify or understand the experiences, situation and health of immigrant women without paying special attention to women's situation in general and immigrant women's situation in their own country of origin. Therefore, there are equally compelling reasons for both international and cross-cultural research on women's roles and health. Second, feminism as it is conceptualized in the West may be an inappropriate and incongruent framework for understanding the situation of immigrant women. To develop these themes, I will offer some comments related to the following: a rationale for a focus on immigrant women, women's health in developing countries, immigrant women and their roles, women's health as immigrants in developed countries, and challenging questions that we continue to face in developing knowledge about immigrant women.

The framework for my analysis reflects of necessity my own areas of interest. As a nurse sociologist, my research reflects an interest in the roles that women enact in interactions with their significant others and reference groups, their transitions and their health status and behavior. My recent research further reflects a focus on Middle Eastern women in their home countries and as immigrants to California. The conceptual framework that I use for analysis considers identity, transition and health. The process by which women tend to develop identities is built upon the repertoire of roles that they enact and the health-care options that are available to them.

The numbers of immigrants and refugees are increasing in North America, and there is no reason to believe that their numbers will decrease (Reimers, 1985). As long as there is oppression in the world and as long as there are economic inequities, internal civil wars and conflicts between nations, populations will shift dramatically (Davis, 1974). The developed countries will continue military and economic interest in the troubled spots in the world and they will also continue to provide necessary aid. Some necessary assistance is the acceptance of refugees and immigrants. Therefore, most immigration movement is from low-income countries to high-income industrialized nations. Immigration trends indicate that there will be an increasing number of immigrants entering both the U.S. and Canada (Reimers, 1985). The problems of meeting the needs of these individuals become the responsibility of industrialized societies.

Census data indicate that of immigrants to the United States during this last decade, one-half of them were women. In Canada more than 30% of the total number of immigrants have been women. There have been many research studies addressing the immigration process, with a majority focusing on the adjustment of men during the immigration process, and the roles they play in the labor market.

Rationale

In spite of the number of women and their apparent centrality in the immigration process, I join the very respected Canadian authors Boyd, Lynam and Anderson in concluding that immigrant women are neglected as a group in studies of women at large, as well as in studies related to immigrants and migrants. We know very little about their experiences, their needs, their illnesses, their health status and their ways of coping with major transitions. This neglect is not confined to one country; the literature indicates a global neglect of measures regarding the movement of women across nations, as well as the migration of women from rural to urban areas within countries (Anderson, 1985; Boyd, 1975; Lynam, 1985).

Immigrant women may have been ignored in research studies because of the premise that has permeated immigration studies that women depend on males for their immigration (Boyd, 1984). Recent analysis of immigration patterns indicate that women are not simply following men in immigration nor is their immigration attached completely to kin immigration. There are some societal conditions such as the labor market of the developed world that attract the immigration of women. Some of these conditions are an increase in the availability of low-wage jobs that are particularly tailored for women. Examples are the electronics assembly lines and the sweatshops of the garment industry (Sassen-Kools, 1984). Women from the Southeast Asian countries (e.g., Indonesians, Sri Lankans, Taiwanese, Vietnamese and South Koreans) are preferred workers in electronic firms in California for several reasons. First, they were trained in their homes to perform manual work that is delicate in nature. Second, they are used to working under pressure, are cooperative and continue to show respect to those in authority. Third, they agree to work for relatively low wages (Taplin, 1986).

Therefore, it is apparent that immigrant women's labor and wage patterns and trajectories are simply different than immigrant men. Yet even reports of labor-force experiences of immigrants are largely based on male immigrants (Boyd, 1984; Kossoudji & Ranney, 1984). It is certainly possible that women's job market roles may lead to different health hazards than those facing men. Women's physical and mental health has been related to three central roles they play: marriage, employment and parenthood. Verbrugge and Madans (1985) analyzed data collected by the National Health Interview Survey (NHIS) for the periods 1964–65 and 1977–78 and concluded that, although employed women demonstrated the best health profile, nonemployed and nonmarried women have the worst. There is a definite trend toward a healthier women's population owing to participation in the labor market. The data and conclusions were focused mainly on white American women and black women. No such data exist on recent, first-generation immigrant women.

Considering that first-generation immigrants generally hold low-paying, dead-end jobs, they encounter other profound health hazards. In addition, their resources and support systems are somewhat limited and their access to health resources is severely hampered. All these conditions provide a strong rationale for making health care for immigrant women a global priority.

Women's Health in Developing Countries

A more effective approach to understanding the health-care needs of immigrant populations is one that takes into consideration the health of women in their own culture; their health being a product of the conditions in their country of origin.

I would like now to put immigrant women's health within the context of global issues in women's health. The United Nations' Decade on Women ended on July 26, 1985, with a summary of major health issues impinging on women. When global accomplishments related to improvement of the lot of women are looked at, several themes become apparent. In general, communicable, contagious and infectious diseases are declining; however, they continue to be responsible for high morbidity and mortality rates in some of the low-income countries. It is of note that in some countries such as India and Bangladesh, there are higher mortality rates for women and female children than for male children (Miller, 1981, 1984).

In addition to continuing to battle communicable diseases, many of the so-called stress diseases of the highly industrialized nations (such as cardiovascular diseases and accidents) are also finding their way to the less industrialized countries. Women are as much victims of a host of stress diseases as men are, but they are not equally considered when discussions are initiated about work and stress. There is also a universal myth that exists about women's work. The myth tends to classify women in larger proportion as nonworking women. Women's work is either hidden labor within a husband's business, or not classified because it is considered merely housework. Therefore, those who work as servants, prostitutes, or even those who are housewives are not considered to the same degree as men in health-care studies and analyses. In addition, although life expectancy for women in Egypt, for example, has increased from 49 years in 1965 to 59 years in 1983 (World Bank, 1985), there is still limited knowledge related to their aging process, caring roles for other elderly members in the family, and menopausal experience, to say nothing of the effect of osteoporosis on their lives.

When women's health is discussed, it tends to be circumscribed in terms of pregnancy and maternal roles and less in relation to the many other roles that women enact. Even at that, mortality rates attached to reproduction remain high (Stein & Maine, 1986). Some of the reasons for such high mortality rates remain related to limited access to health care, multiple pregnancies and nutritional problems. Even when it is very apparent that nutritional disorders play an important role in women's health and subsequently in children's health, women's nutritional problems are glossed over. These problems range from malnutrition owing to undernourishment or starvation in the developing world, to overnourishment that results in obesity and nutritional disorders such as bulimia and anorexia nervosa in the developed world (Maglacas, 1983; Ulin, 1982).

Environmental pollution plagues women whether they live in developing or developed countries. The developing countries experience pollution through inadequate sanitation, parasites and contagious diseases. The developed countries have created environmental pollution in the form of nuclear waste, chemical waste and noise; all of which influence the incidence of cardiovascular and neoplastic diseases (Ulin, 1982).

Limited access to health care is another global issue. A high percentage of the world population is medically underserved. Ulin (1982) asserts that "as many as 25% of the U.S. population live in medically underserved areas (that are) characterized by physician shortages, poverty, high infant mortality, and a high population of the aged" (p. 534). It is of concern to many that there remains a lack of research in other aspects of women's health that are of global interest such as hazards to health owing to female labor (Stein & Maine, 1986) and the mental-health consequences of various familial and societal roles.

Again, this may be due to a global myth that women are not involved in the labor force of the world or that they do not want to be involved in development. In fact, there are indications of the fallacy of this myth. I could cite historical examples of women in the Pharaonic era of Egypt or give the results of contemporary research, all of which point out that women like to be involved in development and that when they are not, they "feel left behind." For example, in a 1984 study of Nigerian women, the Nigerian scholar Tomilyo Adekanye concluded the following:

> Nigerian women are involved in all aspects of agriculture, production, processing, and trade. However, to enhance women's contributions and integrate them into rural development, it is necessary to increase the women's access to productive resources in agriculture. (p. 430)

It is society that may not be encouraging women's involvement. Nigerian women need access to cooperatives for purchasing power and for marketing of their products and access to the appropriate technologies that would support their products. They also need both formal and informal education to help them develop comfort and facility with technological innovations, ways by which they can have access to new jobs and ways by which they can communicate with the outside world (Adekanye, 1984, p. 430). They are not unlike women in any other developing nation.

That these third-world women are consistently a part of the economic support of their families is especially salient when we consider immigrant women. Although immigrant women may continue to value child-rearing and housekeeping roles, they also want to help achieve the North American dream for their extended family; a goal that mandates their participation in the labor force. Perez (1986) indicates that the economic success of Cuban immigrants in America can be traced to the labor-force participation of all family members, particularly mothers and daughters.

We have not been able to adequately and effectively use the fine resources of immigrant women. There are no adequate policies to open new options for them. They are deprived of demonstrating their highest potential and their host societies are deprived of making use of that highest potential. More importantly to this International Council on Women's Health Issues, their health may be profoundly influenced in the process.

Immigrant women from developing countries tend to suffer from triple negative status. They are women, they are immigrants and they are from developing countries. They are stigmatized with several social definitions. They are viewed as different with an emphasis on the negative aspects of their differences. They are considered a problem for society's agencies, such as educational and healthcare systems. They are considered to be dependent followers, qualities accorded negative meaning in the West. They are considered an economic problem because they are thought of as nonproductive as they prefer roles that are circumscribed by home and children. Finally, they have been viewed as barriers to family assimilation and integration.

At the heart of our misunderstanding of the roles of immigrant women is the misconception that arises from viewing them in terms of sex-role inequities. This negative conception pictures them as being oppressed and controlled by males in the family, with no options; totally dependent on their males and preoccupied by their roles as mothers and wives (Pontifical Commission of the Pastoral Care of Immigrants and Itinerant Peoples of the Holy See, 1981). To accept such roles is usually morally enraging to the North Americans who deal with these women. That vehement response coupled with a feminist approach tends to further alienate immigrant women who continuously feel that people in the host society simply do not understand their values, their commitments to family and their life goals. Moreover, such values, commitments and goals are devalued and discredited.

Unlike the individualism that is promoted in the West, immigrant women aspire to a better life for the family unit and not for the self alone. Feminism in third-world countries is defined not in terms of freedom from male oppression; rather, it is freedom from foreign oppression, from hunger, poverty, illness, malnutrition and from other forms of deprivation (Aguilar-San Juan, 1982). Navarro (1979), a Latin American social scientist, put it very well:

> In a continent where poverty, illiteracy, unemployment, extreme concentration of wealth, lack of civil liberties, and exploitation are major issues because they affect a large majority of the population, sex discrimination in all its aspects, as it is denounced by middle-class North American and European feminists, could easily be dismissed as secondary. (p. 114)

Immigrant women from developing countries come to interpret their experiences in terms of social inequities, not sex-role inequities. To them social inequalities are far more important than sex-role inequalities. Immigration heightens their sense of socioeconomic inequalities and makes it even more urgent for them to relegate sex-role inequities to a much lower priority than their sisters in the host society.

Immigrant Women and Their Roles

To understand the nature of the health needs of immigrant women, it is imperative to examine the unique roles they enact. Immigrant women participate in every aspect of the immigration process and, in some instances, have been the instigators of the movement from one locale to another. In these instances, the immigration process was initiated by a wife or a mother or even sponsored by one of her relatives:

> For every woman who was prompted by the male and followed willingly or regretfully, there were two who resisted and forced him to remain where he was; and there were five who had been the initiators of the idea: mother, sisters, wives, or daughters who worked at cajoling or pressuring males into taking the lead or forced them to make the move. (Smith, 1980, p. 79)

Although Smith was describing Portuguese immigrants specifically because Portugal is "supposedly a classic example of the male-dominated society," the same analysis could apply to the decision-making process of immigrants from any number of countries. Understanding the process of decision making related to immigration is significant in understanding the health and adjustment of immigrants in their new locale. Women who instigate and participate in decisions related to immigration may demonstrate a different adaptation pattern than those who have been coerced into immigrating.

All women in developing countries tend to have a negotiating or intermediary role in family interactions; perhaps more than is true in industrialized societies. By a negotiating, intermediary role, I mean a method of advocacy. It is advocacy for children in decisions that are made by the husband. It is also advocacy for males in the family to save face, to maintain their respect and protect them from direct confrontations with children and/or other members of the extended family. Although this negotiating role holds a great degree of informal power in influencing decisions, it is a burdensome role and has the potential to cause emotional distress and family polarization, thus draining energy and leading to emotional burnout.

A family negotiating role requires less confrontation, more tact, some evasiveness, a bit of indirectness in communication and some cover-ups. It is because of these properties that the negotiating role takes on significance for immigrant women. Although this role may have been expected, accepted and sanctioned in their home countries, it is fraught with ambivalence and mixed expectations in the industrialized host countries. Adult first-generation male immigrants continue to expect it, women may begin to want to relinquish it; but children have the most problems with it. Children learn new values in schools, values associated with openness and confrontation. They resist having to discuss matters of utmost importance to them with their fathers or other elderly male members of the family by going through their mothers. They resent their mothers' seeming evasiveness in communication and the mothers' attempts to perform the advocacy role between the father and other members of the family. This negotiating role is important but stressful for women. Immigrant women are given neither credit nor acknowledgment by the younger generation in the family or by the society at large for enacting this role.

Women are also expected to play an intermediary role in family negotiations with formal and informal agencies and other facilities in the new host country. Because of the nature of their commitment to the nuclear and extended family and to household responsibilities, immigrant women tend to be a key link between members of the family and educational, health and community sectors. They are the ones who tend to ease other family members into new roles (Pontifical Commission, 1981), In addition, women are the guardians of the family's ethnic identity, they are the ones who play an instrumental role in the maintenance of language, or in the development of a new language. They play an important role in how many and which of the values and norms of the host society are co-opted and integrated into the family's norms and roles and which traditional values are maintained (Seller, 1975). Women are also the ones who facilitate the necessary balance and harmony between the *being from* and the *becoming to*. In the process of playing this intermediary role, a woman may experience role stress.

The constraints and the forces inherent in the role of intermediary and the cost on the health of women in enacting such a role are not completely understood. Although women may have been, and most probably were, the negotiators and mediators in family, clan and community matters in their own countries, enacting an integrative role in the community of a new country may be more taxing and less rewarding. Stress may result because immigrant women in their new environment may have fewer resources to support these roles or they may have limited access to resources. The regular extended family that may have given them support in their homeland may have been replaced by a critical set of live-in in-laws, or nonunderstanding neighbors, or even an ethnic enclave consisting of individuals who adhere strictly to the values and beliefs of the country of origin.

It is indeed a marvel to watch these women play these two significant roles of decision maker and intermediary in spite of severe limitations imposed on them by their host country and its new values. We need to understand these roles and also the strategies that these women use on behalf of each family member. What are the constraints they encounter and ingeniously surmount; and how do they cope with the distress associated with these roles?

Similarly, women in general play a significant role in the health care of the family; immigrant women in particular play a more central role (Graham, 1985). They make many of the decisions about using health services and complying with ways to promote health and prevent illness. Knowing their beliefs and attitudes toward health, health care and health behavior will help health-care professionals provide necessary care to the immigrant family as a whole.

In the fifth seminar on adaptation and integration of permanent immigrants in Europe (1981), the Pontifical Commission proposed concentration on

the specific and important role that women migrants can play both in the process of group identity and in the dynamic relationship (of opposition or cooperation) which can be established within the receiving community taken as a whole (relations between the family–school–neighborhood and the community sector), that is, in the integration of the "knowledge" transmitted by the family, the "knowledge" transmitted by the school, and the "knowledge" that is acquired within the "framework of social life." (p. 4)

Another role of women is that of worker. Immigrant women's roles in the U.S. labor force are expanding, but their contributions have been neglected, misdefined and underestimated; as have been the consequences of their integration into the work force. Several aspects of their work role are important when we consider their health.

First, immigrant women tend to have different types of participation in the work force than other women in their countries of origin and other women workers in the host society. Although men predominate as laborers in industrialized countries (Taplin, 1986), Asian women are beginning to comprise a significant "number, if not the majority" of electronic industry workers in the U.S. They tend to be put in the low-income brackets. Immigrants' eagerness to acquire any job in the new land makes them vulnerable to accepting whatever low-paying, high-risk jobs are available. This allows the multinational companies that hire them to broaden their profit margins (Taplin, 1986, p. 191).

Second, immigrant women tend to develop lower occupational prestige than do male immigrants even from the same nationality. Their work experience in the U.S. does not help in enhancing this prestige. This has been due to their lack of knowledge of the world market, the necessity of obtaining training at their own expense, language problems and the nature of their foreign credentials, as well as family responsibilities that may require them to stay in nonprestigious jobs (Sullivan, 1984).

Third, immigrant women who are active in the labor force continue to carry the primary responsibilities of household activities, though it influences the balance of power in the family (Pessar, 1984). And even if there is a differential in their earning power that mandates more participatory household activities, role changes are bound to create tremendous stress reactions in the different members of the family (Kossoudji & Ranney, 1984). Therefore, a woman's integration in the work force makes her continue to be dependent on wages of men; increases her work load and her role responsibilities, and does not significantly improve her social status (Bloom, 1985; Griffith, 1985).

Difficulty in speaking the language of the host country increases the burden and energy expended in all these roles (Boyd, 1984). It is also a factor in the apparent lack of integration of these women in the communities in which they live. Though forced to act as links with these communities, they do not feel part of any of them. Questions related to balancing role demands and to job risks for these women remain untapped and unanswered.

There are other roles to consider. The longer the first-generation immigrants are in industrialized societies, the more roles will evolve. Immigrant women will follow the same universal trend in living longer than their male mates. In many of the countries from which the majority of women are currently immigrating, whether from the Middle East or Southeast Asia, women are cared for in their old age by daughters, daughters-in-law and sons. What are some of the potential aging problems that might happen to these women and what models of care will be useful for them? If cared for by their aging sons and daughters, what are some of the consequences of that care on the family members?

Consequences

The process of transition and the many competing roles that immigrant women enact and the limited supportive resources for those roles may act as stressors and increase the "potential of overuse" or the so-labeled abuse of the health-care system by women, as they may manifest a higher use of health-care services (Gallin, 1980). Immigrants may seek health care that is related to recent immigration in an attempt to receive support and assurance. They may turn to a spouse, which in turn increases stress in the family (Lynam, 1985). Immigrant women have turned to health-care systems for solutions to some unmanageable conditions that are not within the jurisdiction of attending physicians (Shuval, Antonovsky & Davies, 1970). Some of these conditions include spouse abuse and concerns about the school performance of their children (Ng & Ramirez, 1981). Gallin (1980) found that:

The poor, less educated, separated or divorced (women), were likely to (1) feel that their social resources were only nominally effective in mediating between them and the pressures of life strains, and (2) define the scope of physicians' roles and responsibilities broadly.

She also found that, when compared with women whose life situations were less burdened, these women visited the health-care system more frequently, reporting vague, disorganized and unrecognizable symptoms.

I am beginning to sense that some immigrant women are using the health-care system, as outpatients or as inpatients, as a cry for help, as a way for them to take "time out" from their truly burdensome roles. More accessible mechanisms for "time out" exist in their countries of origin and none exist in their new home country. What better and safer place to take "time out," a few days to bring back sanity and perspective, to maintain a sense of personal dignity and pride, than a bed in a health-care system? In the meantime, they are overtested and overmedicalized because a true understanding of their situation does not exist. I still do not have research data to support this hunch, but I have many clinical anecdotes.

Needs of Immigrant Women

As a result of their experiences, varied though these may be, immigrant women have similar needs. These include the need to receive credit for their roles, support during transition, knowledge of sources and resources and a more equitable deal in their new home.

Immigrant women need an approach that espouses the acceptance of differences and the reassurance that they are playing valuable roles that are important to group identity formation and to the integration of family members in society. They need to be credited for the different but significant roles they play in the family and in the host society. These women need an openness from health professionals who seek to truly understand the meaning of family identity that they hold. This includes understanding values promoted by various religions.

They need an approach from the receiving host society that indicates an interest in being and becoming. They need support during their transition through the period of relocation and training programs. It is important, though, to know that they tend to prefer to seek help through their relatives first or through those who are part of their private selves, rather than from outsiders (Lynam, 1985). Only when they have been here for a while do they seek help from outsiders.

Heller (1979) and Lynam (1985) propose the development of some ways to increase immigrant women's social competence and mastery in the new environment. Perhaps programs to assist in a successful relocation and for retraining modeled after Swedish programs could be explored. What these women do not need is a cursory list of resources; rather, they need a genuine interest in facilitating their participation in these resources. They need a sincere interest in helping them sort out some of their insurmountable hurdles and constraints that may be foreign to us, such as being home before their husband arrives or being home to prepare a lunch for male members of the family. Studies show that women tend to use the resource of personal contact if it is made by a person familiar to them. They will follow through only if persistence is present with personal contact (Lynam, 1985).

Immigrant women need resources (Nagata, 1969) to help them understand our North American, rather complex, systems. We need resources to help us understand their health-care needs. We need language and cultural interpreters and brokers, professionals who can interpret symbols for them and on their behalf. Presently we tend to depend on the women's family members for translations and, worse yet, for interpretations of meanings. The result is that we do not reach these clients.

An immigrant man related to me what he did when he was put in the position of translating and interpreting while his wife was in active labor. The obstetrician said to him, "Tell your wife not to push now." The man said to me, "How can I tell her not to push when she is screaming and when the head is about to pop out?" So I turned to her and said, "Push, push." The more he said, "Do not push," the more I urged her to push.

Finally, there are some critical points for provision of resources. One such critical point is always after the transition, whether it be the immigration transition, postpartum transition, or job transition (Lynam, 1985). We need resources to deal with illness transitions and resources to deal with marital distress (Chick and Meleis, 1986). Not all these resources have to be professional ones. Community resources are equally effective. Professionals can help by providing appropriate community contact and in matching needs and resources. In general, immigrant women need what a UNICEF study group called a fairer deal in society. They need to feel that they belong to, are not isolated from, the host society (Lynam, 1985).

Now the question is, What could the receiving society do to promote an understanding of immigrant women, without forcing them to abandon their being and their own country-of-origin identity and without forcing them to integrate totally by becoming a perceived American? What could be done to strike a balance between being and becoming?

Challenges and Questions

The challenge ahead of us in studying immigrant women and in focusing on identifying their roles in the immigration process and the relationship between roles and health-care options and outcomes, such as health status and health behavior, will ensure a healthy reproductive and productive national force. What is needed is an approach to the study of immigrant women that evolves from broader assumptions than the ones that have guided previous research. Two important components of that approach are that women must be active, not passive, participants in the process and that the focus must not be limited to the maternal role alone.

Recognizing women as valuable contributors to development in society may help in turning the government's attention to the social, physical and psychological needs of women (Ward, 1982). Therefore, women's roles, the ways by which women negotiate and mediate between different agencies and different cultures, need to be studied. In addition, studies of the strategies that immigrant women use on behalf of family members in helping them develop access to the new country's institutions, such as schools and health-care systems, will help to elucidate some of the constraints in their process of immigration.

We should also be attempting to answer questions related to understanding not only their cultural identity but our own as well. This understanding may decrease the racism and the potential of a ghetto-like existence. It could help in promoting a true integration of a mosaic of cultures. It could also increase the awareness of the expanding roles of women. Knowledge of the identity, values and norms of families in different sectors of community is essential to working with immigrant women. Such knowledge will promote collaboration between the different societal subsystems, "with a view to the protection of cultural identity and integration" (Pontifical Commission, 1981).

More studies are needed to understand the interior fabric of immigrant working and nonworking women. Such studies could help in deciphering their strategies for managing demands and the ways by which they maintain the family's ethnic being and enhance ethnic becoming. These studies would help us further to interpret how they plan and organize their lives to balance the multiple demands of work, family, community and extended family, all of which span at least two cultures (Bloom, 1985). There is a great deal to be gained from understanding the strategies that immigrant women have created to meet some of these competing demands and by comprehending the constraints and the forces on them in doing this.

Finally, because women as a whole are more receptive to making changes in their family and life situation and usually have more to gain by these changes (Nash, 1980), we need to collaborate in international research to find out whether immigration and/or development have benefited women in improving their status and expanding their roles. More significantly for us in the health field, we need to find out in what ways did the immigration and development process and resultant changes in women's experiences and situations influence health status, access to health care, and how these women maintain their health.

Conclusion

Women are at the center of all life transitions, whether the transitions are within the family, such as maturation, because of national modernization or a move to an urban center, or because of relocation to another nation. In each one of these transitions, women are profoundly influenced by change, particularly when they are not able to influence decisions regarding such change. Ironically, women's roles in these transitions are ignored at best and misrepresented at worst. That neglect is a two-edged sword. First, this neglect prevents the reflection of these experiences on policies related to women. Second, this neglect limits the wisdom that we are able to glean from their experiences that may then influence other women in the host society. This wisdom could come in the form of options and a range of positive coping styles that immigrant women may have used successfully in negotiating their new life experiences. What we need is a consciousness raising, an awareness of these women among us who are struggling with the being versus the becoming dilemma and who would like to solve it by integrating being and becoming.

In discussing gender inequities in food distribution internationally, Amartya Sen (1984) urges that "a low key and clinically academic discussion of the problem of intrafamily distribution is not quite adequate." She goes on to admonish us to add to those discussions "a bit more rage, a bit more passion, a bit more anger." Let us declare a focus on first-generation immigrant women to help us understand their experiences and provide them with adequate resources to meet their needs. We should approach this task as Sen urges, with anger for existing negligence, with embarrassment for lost time, and with a real passion and a sustained commitment to ensure that immigrant women, and all of us, can both *be* and *become*.

REFERENCES

Adekanye, T. O. (1984). Women in agriculture in Nigeria: Problems and policies for development. *Women's Studies International Forum, 7*(6), 423–431.

Aguilar-San Juan, D. (1982). Feminism and the national liberation struggle in the Philippines. *Women's Studies International Forum, 5*(34), 253–261.

Anderson, J. (1985). Perspectives on the health of immigrant women: A feminist analysis. *Advances in Nursing Science, 8*(1), 61–76.

Bloom, F. T. (1985). Struggling and surviving: The life style of European immigrant breadwinning mothers in American industrial cities 1900–1930. *Women Studies International Forum, 8*(6), 609–620.

Boyd, M. (1975). The status of immigrant women in Canada. *Canadian Review of Social Anthropology, 12*, 406–416.

Boyd, M. (1984). At a disadvantage: The occupational attainments of foreign born women in Canada. *International Migration Review, XVIII*(4), 1091–1119.

Chick, N., & Meleis, A. J. (1986). Transitions: A nursing concern. In P. L. Chinn (Ed.), *Nursing Research Methodology* (pp. 237–257). Rockville, MD: Aspen.

Davis, K. (1974). The migration of human populations. *Scientific American, 231*(3), 93–105.

Gallin, R. S. (1980). Life difficulties, coping and the use of medical services. *Culture Medicine and Psychiatry, 4*(3), 249–262.

Graham, H. (1985). Providers, regulators, and mediators: Women as the hidden careers. In E. Lewin & V. Olesen (Eds.), *Women, health and healing: Toward a new perspective.* New York: Tavistock.

Griffith, D. (1985). Women, remittances, and reproduction. *American Ethnologist, 12*(4), 676–690.

Heller, K. (1979). The effects of social support: Prevention and treatment implications. In A. P. Goldstein &: F. H. Kanfer (Eds.) *Maximizing treatment gains: Transfer enhancement in psychotherapy* (pp. 353–382). New York: Academic Press.

Kossoudji, S. A., & Ranney, S. I. (1984). The labor market experience of female migrants: The case of temporary Mexican migration to the U.S. *International Migration Review, XVIII*(4), 1120–1143.

Lynam, M. J. (1985). Support networks developed by immigrant women. *Social Science and Medicine, 21*(3), 327–333.

Maglacas, X. (1983). Health for all: A framework for action. In *Development of leadership strategies in the nursing change process in support for health for all through primary health care.* Tokyo: International Nursing Foundation of Japan.

Miller, B. D. (1981). *The endangered sex: Neglect of female children in rural North India.* Ithaca, NY: Cornell University.

Miller, B. D. (1984). Daughter neglect, women's work, and marriage: Pakistan and Bangladesh compared. *Medical Anthropology, 8*(2), 109–126.

Nagata, J. A. (1969). Adaptation and integration of Greek working class immigrants in the city of Toronto, Canada: A situational approach. *International Migration Review, 4*, 44–70.

Nash, J. (1980). A critique of social science roles in Latin America. In J. Nash & H. I. Safa (Eds.), *Sex and class in Latin America: Women's perspectives on politics, economics, and the family in the third world* (pp. 1–21). Brooklyn, NY: J. F. Bergin Publishers.

Navarro, M. (1979). Research on Latin American women. *Journal of Women in Culture and Society, 5*(1), 111–120.

Ng, R., & Ramirez, J. (1981). Immigrant housewives in Canada. Report available from the Immigrant Women's Centre, Toronto, Ontario, Canada.

Perez, L. (1986). Immigrant economic adjustment and family organization: The Cuban success story reexamined. *International Migration Review, 20*(1), 84–92.

Pessar, P. R. (1984). The linkage between the household and the workplace of Dominican women in the U.S. *International Migration Review, 18*(4), 1188–1211.

Pontifical Commission of the Pastoral Care of Migrants and Intinerant Peoples of the Holy See (1981). Fifth seminar on adaptation and integration of permanent immigrants: Situation and role of migrant women: Specific adaptation and integration problems. *Intergovernmental Committee on Migration,* Geneva. Information Paper No. 16.

Reimers, D. M. (1985). *Still the golden door. The Third World comes to America.* New York: Columbia University Press.

Sassen-Kools, S. (1984). Part IV, from household to workplace: Theories and survey research on migrant women in the labor market, notes on the incorporation of third world women into wage, labor through immigration and offshore production. *International Migration Review, XVIII*(4), 1144–1167.

Seller, M. S. (1975). Beyond the stereotype: A new look at the immigrant woman, 1880–1924. *Journal of Ethnic Studies, 3*(1), 59–70.

Sen, A. M. (1984). Food battles: Conflicts in the access to food. *Food and Nutrition, 10*(1).

Shuval, J. T., Antonovsky, A., & Davies, A. M. (1970). *Social functions of medical practice.* San Francisco: Jossey-Bass.

Smith, M. E. (1980). The Portuguese female immigrant: The marginal man. *International Migration Review, XIV*(1), 77–93.

Stein, Z., & Maine, D. (1984). The health of women. *International Journal of Epidemiology, 15*(3), 303–305.

Sullivan, T. (1984). The occupational prestige of women immigrants: A comparison of Cubans and Mexicans. *International Migration Review, XVIII*(4), 1188–1211.

Taplin, R. (1986). Women in world market: Factories, east and west. *Ethnic and Racial Studies, 9*(2), 169–195.

Ulin, P. R. (1982). International nursing challenge. *Nursing Outlook, 30,* 531–535.

Verbrugge, R. M., & Madans, J. H. (1985). *Milbank Memorial Fund Quarterly/Health and Society, 63*(4), 601–735.

Ward, C. (1982). Women and community development in Malaysia: The Kamila project. *Women's Studies International Forum, 5*(1), 99–101.

World Bank. (1985). *World development report 1985.* New York: Oxford University Press.

Reprinted with permission from: Meleis, A. I., & Rogers, S. (1987). Women in transition: Being versus becoming or being and becoming. *Healthcare for Women International, 8*(4), 199–217.

4.6 MELEIS'S THEORY OF NURSING TRANSITIONS AND RELATIVES' EXPERIENCES OF NURSING HOME ENTRY

SUE DAVIES

Abstract

Aim: This chapter explores the extent to which Meleis's mid-range theory of nursing transitions is supported by the findings of a study exploring relatives' experiences of the move to a nursing home. *Background:* Mid-range nursing theories are useful tools in helping to understand the scope of nursing practice in a range of contexts and situations. However, as yet, many formal mid-range theories have not been adequately tested. *Methods:* Findings from a constructivist study of relatives' experiences of nursing home entry were re-analysed in relation to the extent to which they reflected the domains of the theory of nursing transitions. Data for the original study were generated during 37 qualitative interviews involving 48 close family members of older people who had recently moved to a nursing home, and in observational case studies in three nursing homes. *Findings:* All domains of the theory of nursing transition were supported by the data generated within* the study. However, the model failed to represent adequately the interactive and dynamic nature of relationships between formal and informal caregivers in the nursing home context. ***Conclusions:*** The theory of nursing transitions has the potential to assist nurses in identifying appropriate strategies for supporting relatives throughout the period of an older person's relocation to a nursing home. However, to reflect fully the experiences of relatives at this time, the theory requires adjustment to recognize the contribution made by relatives themselves to positive outcomes. This therefore raises questions as to whether the relative absence of this reciprocal and interactive dimension is an element of Meleis's theory that requires further exploration in relation to other forms of transition.*

Introduction

With increasing levels of frailty among the ageing population, a growing number of family caregivers are finding themselves in the situation of needing to assist a relative to move into a nursing home. This frequently involves them in helping the older person to make the decision, find a suitable home, make the move and settle into their new environment. The move to a nursing home represents a major event in the life of the older person and can be a traumatic experience for all concerned (Reed & Payton 1996, Wright 1998). Temporal models of caregiving suggest that when family caregivers assist an older person to move into a nursing home, they enter a new but still involved stage and are likely to require support to achieve a smooth transition (Nolan et al. 1996a). However, there is little research evidence to suggest the type of support that will be most effective.

This chapter draws on evidence from an empirical study, the main aim of which was to develop a deeper understanding of the needs of relatives of older people who move into nursing homes (Davies 2001). Data derived from semistructured interviews with 48 family caregivers who had experience of such a move, together with observational case studies in three nursing homes enabled the development of a series of theoretical propositions. It was anticipated that these would suggest appropriate supportive interventions to enable a healthy transition. In comparing these insights with the existing literature, the relevance of Meleis's theory of nursing transitions (Meleis et al. 2000) as a potential framework for guiding practice in this area became apparent. In this chapter, the extent to which Meleis's theory was supported by data from the study is explored. Ways in which the theory of nursing transitions could be modified to reflect more fully family caregivers' experiences of assisting a relative to move into a nursing home are also outlined.

Background

Theoretical Perspectives on the Move to a Nursing Home

In the growing literature on experiences of long-term care, a number of conceptual and theoretical frameworks have been applied to the needs of older people living in nursing homes and their families. However, these are mostly derived from research carried out in settings other than nursing homes, and there is a need for more explicit empirical testing of a range of theoretical ideas in the nursing home context. Importantly, much of the literature on relatives' experiences of admission to a nursing home is devoid of references to theoretical or conceptual frameworks that might provide a basis for education, research and practice in this field. In terms of mid-range substantive theories, notable exceptions include Bowers' (1988) typology of family caregiving, Nolan et al.'s (1996a) temporal model of caregiving, and Nolan et al.'s (1996b) typology of admission types. A number of writers have attempted to apply mid-range theories developed in other contexts to the experiences of older people and their relatives in relation to nursing home entry. These are summarized in Table 4.6.1. However, with one exception, these theories are only useful in explaining certain aspects of the phenomenon of interest. An important exception is the formal mid-range theory of transitions described by Schumacher and Meleis (1994) and Meleis et al. (2000). This presents a comprehensive framework that recognizes the significance of transitions for health and attempts to encapsulate characteristics and indicators of healthy transition processes so as to suggest appropriate nursing interventions.

A Theory of Nursing Transitions

Meleis's theory of nursing transitions proposes that assisting people to manage life transitions is a key function of nursing (Schumacher & Meleis 1994, Meleis et al. 2000), with transition defined as: 'The passage or movement from one state, condition or place to another' (Chick & Meleis 1986, p. 237).

The rationale for considering this an important area for nursing and social care is that people undergoing transitions tend to be more vulnerable to risks that may affect their health and wellbeing. Transitions often require a person to incorporate new knowledge, to alter behaviour, and therefore to change the definition of self in the new social context (Wilson 1997, Meleis et al. 2000). The challenge for nurses and others involved in supporting those undergoing transition is to understand transition processes and to develop interventions which are effective in helping them to regain stability and a sense of well-being (Schumacher & Meleis 1994). Meleis and colleagues have conducted empirical work examining a range of transition experiences, including becoming a mother (Sawyer 1999), experiencing the menopause (Im & Meleis 1999), developing chronic illness (Messias 1997) and taking on a family caregiving role (Schumacher 1996). The findings of these studies have led them to develop a formal middle-range theory of transitions. The three domains of this theory—the nature of transitions, transition conditions and patterns of response—are illustrated in Figure 4.6.1.

This theory, in contrast to others described previously (e.g., Bowers 1988, Nolan et al. 1996b), is formal rather than substantive: that is, it is not concerned with a particular instance of a transition, i.e. nursing home entry, but rather focuses on transitions more generally.

TABLE 4.6.1 Application of Theoretical Frameworks Pertaining to Relatives' Experiences of Nursing Home Entry

Theoretical Framework	Examples	Definition/Description	Typical Application Within the Literature
Caregiving as a career	Cosbey (1994) Aneshensel et al. (1995) Murphy et al. (1997) Ross et al. (1997)	Career is defined as 'a series of statuses and clearly defined offices held throughout the life course, in which there are typical sequences of position, achievement and responsibility.'	The notion of the caregiving career can be used to explain the motivations of community-dwelling spouses at different stages in the care-giving career and their feelings associated with visiting.
Locus of control (LOC)	Morgan & Zimmerman (1990) Brown & Furstenberg (1992) Chen & Snyder (1996)	Locus-of-control (LOC) construct has three foci: internal control, external control and the influence of powerful others. Intervention of practitioners can result in changes in LOC orientation in client.	Shifting the LOC in decision making towards older people and family members will enhance satisfaction with care and ease adjustment.
Life crisis and transition	Oleson & Shadick (1993) Meleis and Trangenstein (1994) Schumacher & Meleis (1994)	Transition is defined as *the passage or movement from one state, condition or place to another.* Effective coping with transition/crisis requires understanding and effective management of the event.	Older people relocating to a nursing home and their families experience a life transition that they often perceive as a crisis. People experiencing transition are usually able to discern discrete phases in the process.
Continuity theory	Elliot (1995) Gladstone (1995) Reed & Payton (1995) Ghusn et al. (1996) Onega & Tripp Reimer (1997)	Continuity theory is concerned with *'maintaining a continuous sense of self in the face of the many internal and external disruptions accompanying old age.'*	Continuity is maintained not only by performing familiar activities, but also by engaging in a subjective process that brings about a feeling of order, consistency and a restoration of personal meaning in situations marked by physical, psychological or environmental change.
Social exchange theory	Clarke (1993) Nelson (2000)	Relationships are rooted in reciprocity.	Delayed reciprocity is an important concept for understanding why relatives continue to engage in seemingly unbalanced relationships with nursing home residents.
Family systems theory	Kaplan & Ade-Ridder (1991) Bogo (1987) Drysdale et al. (1993)	The family is perceived as a unitary group, with the consequence that change affecting one member will bring about change in the rest of the family unit. The implication is that the family as a whole will need additional support and information to re-establish equilibrium.	Family systems theory has been used to explain the impact of relocation on family caregivers and to suggest interventions that may assist families to preserve and enhance relationships following the move.

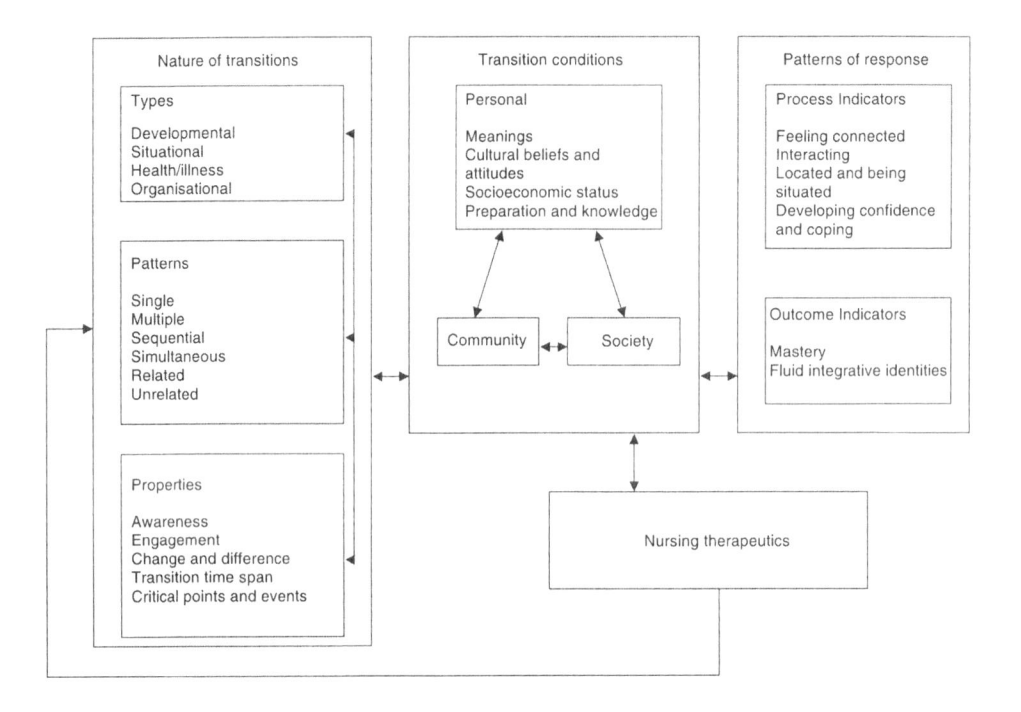

FIGURE 4.6.1 Model of nursing transitions (Meleis et al. 2000).

The Study

Aims

Given the dearth of literature exploring relatives' experiences of the move to a nursing home the aims of the study were:

- to describe and interpret the experiences of family caregivers in relation to helping a relative to move into a nursing home and continuing to support them in such a setting;
- to describe and interpret staff and family caregivers' perceptions of current practice within nursing homes in relation to supporting and involving family caregivers, particularly around the time of admission; and
- to generate understandings and insights to inform, assist and empower older people who experience admission to a nursing home in the future and their family caregivers.

Methods

discrete but related phases of data collection were undertaken within a broadly constructivist framework (Rodwell 1998) (Figure 4.6.2). The first phase comprised 37 semistructured interviews with 48 people who had experienced admission of a close relative to a nursing home. Participants were recruited using a range of strategies and essentially were a sample of convenience (Table 4.6.2). The most successful strategy involved contacting managers of local nursing homes and inviting them to distribute information packs about the project to relatives, who then contacted the researcher directly. Advertisements in local newspapers and carers' publications also produced some response.

Relationships between people who took part in the interviews and the nursing home resident are shown in Figure 4.6.2. For 16 of the main participants (11 spouses, four adult children and one niece), the older person had been co-resident

```
┌─────────────────────────────────────┐
│           Phase I                   │
│                                     │
│  Semi-structured interviews with    │
│  48 relatives of older people who   │
│  had moved to a nursing home        │
│                                     │
│  26 adult children and 9 spouses    │
│           11 spouses                │
│            2 nieces                 │
│            1 nephew                 │
└─────────────────────────────────────┘

┌───────────────────────────────────────────────────────────────────┐
│                          Phase II                                 │
│                                                                   │
│                 Case studies in three homes                       │
│                                                                   │
│           Observation (12-15 days in each home)                   │
│    Semi-structured interviews with residents, staff and relatives │
│                      Analysis of records                          │
├───────────────────┬───────────────────────┬───────────────────────┤
│  Nursing Home A   │   Nursing Home B      │   Nursing Home C      │
│                   │                       │                       │
│     88 beds       │      60 beds          │      24 beds          │
│ Registered for both│ Elderly frail residents│ Elderly mentally infirm│
│ personal care (20 beds)│ (personal care with │ residents (personal care│
│ and personal care with│     nursing)        │    with nursing)      │
│     nursing       │                       │                       │
└───────────────────┴───────────────────────┴───────────────────────┘
```

FIGURE 4.6.2 Overview of study methods.

prior to their admission to the nursing home. The interviews were conducted mostly in participants' own homes and focused on events leading up to the admission, the experience of relocation and involvement since admission.

The second phase of the study involved detailed case studies in three nursing homes. Here, the intention was to locate relatives' experiences in the context of everyday life within each home, using participant observation and field notes, interviews with staff, residents and relatives, analysis of documents and reflective accounts of the researcher's experiences within the setting. Homes were purposively selected from a list of those in the area to provide a range of size, type of ownership (private individual or large corporation) and location within the city. The nature of the research was discussed during an initial meeting with home managers, and all three approached agreed to take part. Participation was then negotiated with residents, staff and relatives on an individual basis. The principal data collection method was participant observation within the 'participant as observer role' (Junker 1960, Pearsall 1965). Between 12 and 15 days of observation were spent at each home over a 5- to 6-month period. Characteristics of the case study homes included in the second phase are shown in Figure 4.6.2.

Data for both phases of the study were gathered concurrently between 1999 and 2001.

TABLE 4.6.2 Number of Participants for Individual Interviews Recruited Using Each Strategy

Strategy	Participants (primary contact)
Contact with nursing home managers	20
Advertisement in local newspaper	6
Contacts made on visits to nursing homes	3
Advertisement in Carers' Newsletter	3
Sheffield Transitional Care Forum	3
Local branch of Relatives' Association	2
Total	37

Rigour

- Within both phases of the research the following features were designed to produce co-constructed narratives of each participant's experiences:
- Consent was negotiated over several days to ensure that the participant was aware of what their involvement would require.
- An outline interview schedule was handed or posted to each participant in advance.
- Throughout each interview the researcher attempted to check her understanding and interpretation of what was being said with the participant(s).
- The researcher fed in her own views and experiences to each interview when appropriate, including insights developed from earlier interviews and observations.
- A summary of each interview was posted to the participant(s) for comments.
- A summary of findings from each phase of the research was sent to participants for comments.

Ethical Considerations

An outline of the study was submitted to the Chairperson of the Local Research Ethics Committee, who decided that the research did not fall within the remit of the Committee at that time. This was because participants were not accessed via their use of health services. However, mindful of the ethical issues prompted by the study design, in particular the potentially distressing nature of some of the experiences that participants would be invited to recall, the researcher invited a small group of colleagues to discuss ways of minimizing risk to participants and a strategy was agreed, including the opportunity for referral to external agencies where indicated. The information provided by each participant was scrupulously protected as confidential, and data were coded and anonymized so that no notes or record of an interview could be associated with an individual.

Data Analysis

The approach to initial analysis of the data was inductive, and sought to develop theoretical propositions that would accurately reflect the participant's feelings, thoughts and actions (Maykut & Morehouse 1994). A similar approach was used to analyse the individual interview and case study data. Although detailed analysis of the data was undertaken in stages the process was essentially ongoing, with a written summary being prepared following each interview and on completion of each case study. This phased approach to data analysis is consistent with the constructivist method and comprised four steps:

- unitizing—locating units of meaning within the text,
- categorizing—taking all the units of data and sorting them into categories of ideas,
- filling in patterns—searching for convergent and divergent opinion and seeking explanation for these discrepancies and
- member checks—feeding back the categorization to participants (Lincoln & Guba 1985).

QSR NUD*IST (Qualitative Solutions and Research) was used to unitize and categorize the data. At the same time as data were extracted from each interview or set of field notes and aggregated in relation to categories, the integrity of each case was maintained by entering key categories on to a matrix for each participant so that linkages between themes could be examined. Examination of key themes was undertaken in parallel, comparing similar cases using the aggregation of data under the category headings and tracing the development of themes in relation to an individual participant's experiences. This process also facilitated the development of 'meta-themes' representing the range of experiences described.

Further details of the methods of data collection and analysis have been reported elsewhere (Davies 2001, Davies & Nolan 2003).

Findings

The main thematic framework that emerged from the findings is shown in Figure 4.6.3. Data analysis revealed three phases to the transition: 'Making the best of it'; 'Making the move' and 'Making it better,' with relatives' experiences across these phases being understood in terms of five continua, reflecting the extent to which they felt they were: feeling 'under pressure' or not; 'in the know' or 'working in the dark'; 'working together' or 'working apart; 'in control of events' or 'losing control,' and feeling 'supported' or 'unsupported' both practically and emotionally. These findings have the potential to inform health and social care practice in supporting family caregivers at this time and have been reported in detail elsewhere (Davies & Nolan 2003, 2004).

Following the initial analysis, the findings were re-examined in relation to the domains of the theory of nursing transitions. This involved a detailed consideration of each domain of the theory and its constituent parts, and mapping the empirical data on to these domains. This process was also facilitated by the use of QSR NUDIST, which creates a 'tree' structure, involving nodes and subnodes, to reflect the conceptual or theoretical framework emerging during the analytical process. It was a fairly straightforward process to create a new structure representing the domains and constituent elements of the theory of nursing transitions, and then to attach nodes resulting from the analysis of the relatives' data to this new tree. Components of the findings of the relatives' data that did not map on to the theory could then be easily identified. Once this process was complete the map was reviewed by an independent researcher, who confirmed the appropriateness of the allocation of data to each domain.

The extent to which the study findings were found to be consistent with the domains of the theory of nursing transitions is shown in Tables 4.6.3 to 4.6.5.

As can be seen clearly, there are numerous points of connection between the formal theory of Meleis et al. (2000) and findings of the current study, suggesting that the notion of transitions provides a broadly appropriate framework within which to locate these findings. The key question is whether it provides a complete framework or if the present theory could suggest ways in which that of Meleis et al. (2000) could be extended.

A significant limitation of Meleis's model for considering transitions to a nursing home setting (and thereby potentially other forms of transition) is the failure to acknowledge the reciprocal interrelationships between the key stakeholders. Analysis of data from both phases of the study revealed the sterility of attempting to understand and explain family caregivers' experiences of nursing home entry without also considering the experiences of older people and staff within nursing homes (see Davies 2003). The experiences of older people and family caregivers are shaped by the complexity of decision making in this context and are influenced by a range of perceived demands and responsibilities. The move to a nursing home creates a series of stressors and demands for older people and their caregivers. Staff within nursing homes also experience demands and stressors; yet the model of nursing transitions seems to underemphasize this interplay, and rather portrays professionals (nurses) as relatively detached 'experts' and the flow of support as 'one-way.' Thereby, the model fails fully to acknowledge the significance of 'emotional labour'—the emotional component of all nursing

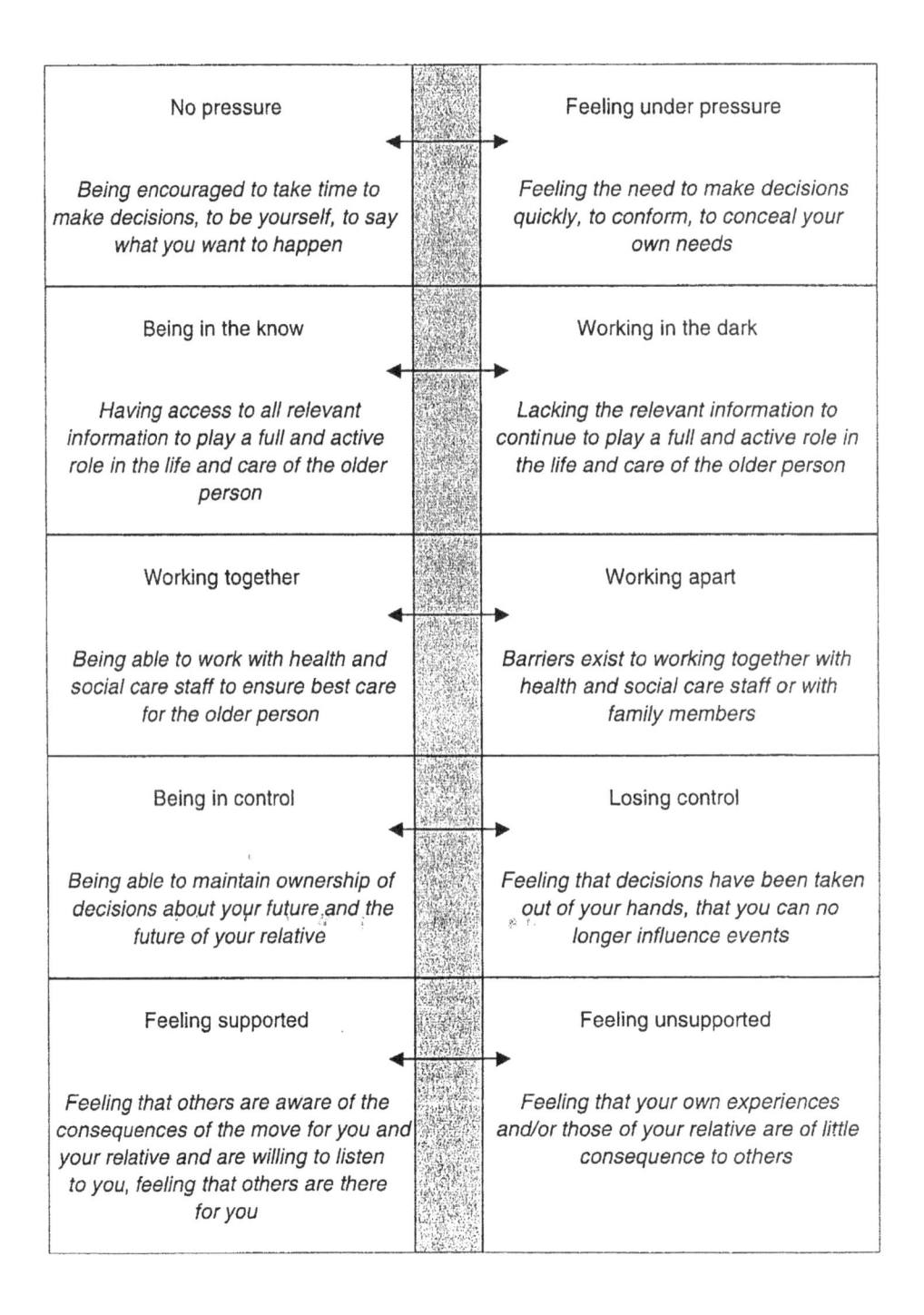

No pressure	Feeling under pressure
Being encouraged to take time to make decisions, to be yourself, to say what you want to happen	Feeling the need to make decisions quickly, to conform, to conceal your own needs
Being in the know	Working in the dark
Having access to all relevant information to play a full and active role in the life and care of the older person	Lacking the relevant information to continue to play a full and active role in the life and care of the older person
Working together	Working apart
Being able to work with health and social care staff to ensure best care for the older person	Barriers exist to working together with health and social care staff or with family members
Being in control	Losing control
Being able to maintain ownership of decisions about your future and the future of your relative	Feeling that decisions have been taken out of your hands, that you can no longer influence events
Feeling supported	Feeling unsupported
Feeling that others are aware of the consequences of the move for you and your relative and are willing to listen to you, feeling that others are there for you	Feeling that your own experiences and/or those of your relative are of little consequence to others

FIGURE 4.6.3 Relatives' experiences during phases of admission to a nursing home.

TABLE 4.6.3 The Nature of Transitions

Element	Description/Implications	Relevance to Current Study
Types Developmental Situational Health/Illness Organizational	Nurses regularly encounter four main types of transition in their work with individuals and families. *Interventions need to be tailored to the type of transition.*	All of these transition types may affect family caregivers involved in assisting an older person to relocate to a new long-term care environment.
Patterns Single Multiple Sequential Simultaneous Related Unrelated	Transitions are commonly patterns of complexity and multiplicity, with individuals experiencing more than one type of transition concurrently.	Many relatives were dealing with not only the situational transition of a change in the nature of the relationship with a close family member, but also with transition in their health status, often as a consequence of their own ageing or ill health. The result was that they were commonly dealing with a whole series of stressors and demands simultaneously, not all of which were necessarily related to the transition.
Properties	Meleis et al. (2000) describe a number of universal properties of transition or commonalities that are evident across the range of types of transition. *Consideration of these properties in relation to a particular transition is especially important in suggesting which nursing interventions are appropriate.*	
Awareness	Level of awareness is related to perception, knowledge and recognition of a transition experience.	Initially, most relatives were unaware of and therefore unprepared for the traumatic nature of the transition. Later, most experienced it as painful and emotional. However, few had been encouraged to consider or talk about their own experiences. There was a lack of acknowledgment that relatives were themselves undergoing a life transition.
Engagement	Engagement is the degree to which a person demonstrates involvement in the processes inherent within the transition. Indicators include seeking out information, using role models, actively preparing and proactively modifying activities.	Relatives varied in their degree of engagement in the process. Those who were proactive in seeking information tended to have more positive experiences.
Change and difference	Transitions result in changes in role, identity, relationships, abilities and patterns of behavior.	Relatives described changes in role, relationships and patterns of behaviour. Efforts to *maintain continuity* suggested attempts to retain their caregiving identity within the new context. New abilities related largely to strategies for negotiating care with staff to *ensure best care*.

(continued)

TABLE 4.6.3 *(continued)*

Element	Description/Implications	Relevance to Current Study
Transition time span and critical points and events	The process of transition takes place over time, commonly involves development, flow or movement from one state to another and can often be divided into a series of stages or phases. Critical points and events are associated with increasing awareness of change and more active engagement with the transition process.	Participants described their experiences in terms of three main stages: *making the best of it* (involving decisions about long-term care choices); *making the move* (involving the physical transfer and getting to know the individuals and routines within the new environment); and *making it better,* which involved them in identifying a new caring role, monitoring care, and maintaining their relationship with the older person. Critical events were most commonly associated with the decision to seek long-term care and with negative events within the new care environment that caused them to reflect upon whether they had made the right decisions.

work and specifically work in a nursing home. This component is clearly illustrated in the following data quote from our study:

> They're like my family. It's like I've got two homes. I worry about them when I'm not here and sometimes I ring up to find out how they are, if someone's been a bit poorly, for example. (Care assistant, case study home 3)

Furthermore, the model of nursing transitions tends to treat recipients of nursing interventions as passive and as if they have little potential to contribute to their environment or to influence their own destiny. On the contrary, relative participants in our study were very clear that they had an important contribution to make, and described three roles that they performed within the nursing home. These were: *maintaining continuity,* which involved helping the older person to maintain their sense of identity through the continuation of loving family relationships and through helping the staff to get to know them as an individual; *contributing to community* through interacting with other residents, relatives and staff, taking part in social events and generally providing a link with the outside world, and *keeping an eye,* by monitoring the care received, providing feedback to staff and filling any gaps. The following quotes are illustrative:

> We do try to help out when we visit. I've knitted about 12 blankets for them and we often take residents back to their rooms. Sometimes they say, 'Oh, we're glad to see you—you can give the teas out!' I don't mind this, and I enjoy being with them. You can have a laugh with some of them. (Elsie, Daughter, Interview no. 8)

> There's only one thing I've been a bit concerned with, and that is she doesn't seem to be awake at all at the moment. I'll have to talk to Steve about it. I think she needs to have the medication reduced. She's spending too much time asleep. Jim (manager) will see to that and the doctor or the nurse will sort that out. (Bill, Husband, Interview no. 15)

To perform these roles effectively, relatives must be prepared and encouraged to take the initiative and sometimes to challenge the status quo. This may require some adaptation on the part of staff who have been used to operating with a different mindset, one that sees relatives as potential adversaries or in some cases as 'customers'. The most positive experiences seem to result when relatives perceive that they too have a larger part to play in 'making it work' and this contribution is

TABLE 4.6.4 Transition Conditions

Element	Description/Implications	Relevance to the Current Study
Transition conditions	Wide variations occur among individuals, families or organizations in transition. *An appropriate framework for assessment needs to capture this variation to reflect transition experiences.*	
Personal meanings	These emerge from subjective appraisal of an anticipated or experienced transition and the evaluation of its likely effect on one's life.	Because of the overall lack of anticipation of placement as a life event, few relatives had given prior thought to its likely impact.
Cultural beliefs and attitudes	When stigma is attached to a transition experience, the expression of emotional states related to the transition may be inhibited.	Negative perceptions of nursing homes were held almost universally prior to the need to consider long-term care options. For most participants, these perceptions contributed to feelings of guilt and are likely to have inhibited relatives in expressing their own needs.
Socioeconomic status	Socioeconomic status has an important impact on transition experiences.	Older people and their relatives who were able to supplement social services fee levels, and those who were able to pay the full cost of nursing home care and therefore bypass the need for social services assessment, were able to choose from a wider range of accommodation. Low socioeconomic status often contributed to the experiences of being *out of control* of events.
Preparation and knowledge	People undergoing transition may or may not know what to expect and their expectations may or may not be realistic. As a transition proceeds, expectations may prove to be incongruent with unfolding reality. *Extensive planning helps to create a smooth and healthy transition*	Most relatives were *in the dark* as to what to expect in terms of levels of service and their own involvement following the move. Expectations of rehabilitation services within the home were usually unmet. Many participants were unaware of whether a detailed assessment of their relative's needs had taken place. Where relatives were involved in assessment, experiences were usually more positive.
Community conditions	The availability or lack of availability of community resources can facilitate or inhibit transitions. *Assessment of community conditions and adaptation and supplementation where possible can facilitate a smooth transition.*	Community resources include support from practitioners and from friends and other family members, and characteristics of the nursing home environment that support a smooth transition. Participants within the study derived support from a range of sources external to the nursing home. In particular, family members and friends frequently provided a listening ear and shared responsibility for continuing to support the older person living in the nursing home through regular visits. Health and social care professionals, particularly social workers, were identified as a source of valuable support. However, just as frequently, participants described a sense of isolation and a perception that they were *working apart*. The type of community model that was dominant within a nursing home had important implications for the experiences of relatives, residents and staff.

(continued)

TABLE 4.6.4 *(continued)*

Element	Description/Implications	Relevance to the Current Study
Society	The wider sociocultural environment shapes the transition experience. *Awareness of the sociocultural context of a transition can enable nurses to develop interventions at the group, community and societal level.*	Relatives felt *under pressure* from negative images of nursing homes portrayed in the media. *Relatives were aware of the poor working conditions and lack of training for staff working in nursing homes.* Staff within some homes often felt isolated, lacking in support and recognition.

TABLE 4.6.5 Indicators of Healthy Transitions

Element	Description/Implications	Relevance to the Current Study
Indicators of healthy transitions	These include both process and outcome indicators. Process indicators are helpful in identifying whether clients are moving in the direction of health or towards vulnerability and risk. *Ongoing assessment is therefore crucial in facilitating nursing interventions to promote healthy outcomes.*	Suggests the importance of ongoing and regular assessment and care planning in relation both to the needs of older people and those of their close relatives. This was absent for most of the relatives within the study, but, where it did take place, was associated with more positive experiences.
Process indicators Feeling connected	This is concerned with making new contacts and continuing old connections.	This was reflected in the importance attached by relatives in the current study to continuity in staffing and consistent allocation of individual staff members. Relationships with individual members of staff were important, both to residents and to relatives, enabling them to remain *in control* and to be *in the know*.
	Feeling connected to healthcare professionals who can answer questions and with whom they feel comfortable; also requires continuity in relationships between healthcare providers and patients/clients.	Maintenance of the relationship between the relative and the older person was an important element of *maintaining continuity*. Being able to continue the relationship in the same pattern as before or re-establishing a prior pattern was an important outcome for relatives within the current study; however, few had managed to achieve this.
Interacting	Through interaction, the meaning of the transition and the behaviours developed in response to the transition are uncovered, clarified and acknowledged.	The importance of effective communication at all stages of the transition was a key finding.

(continued)

TABLE 4.6.5 *(continued)*

Element	Description/Implications	Relevance to the Current Study
	Through interaction, a context is created in which self-care and caregiving can take place effectively and harmoniously.	The potential consequences when communication was less than effective were apparent in relatives' experiences of *working in the dark, feeling unsupported* and *working apart* from care staff. The effectiveness of communication had important implications for the type of relationship that developed between relatives and nursing home staff.
Location and being situated	Location involves understanding the new life by comparing it with the old; being situated involves finding justification for how or why they came, where they are and where they have been.	Participants within the current study varied in the extent to which they had reached an understanding and acceptance of how they came to be in their present situation. Those who felt they had been able to maintain control of decisions, had been able to take their time in planning the move and had been well supported appeared to adjust more easily
Process indicators Developing confidence and coping	The extent to which there is a pattern indicating that the individuals involved are experiencing an increase in their level of confidence; demonstrated by an understanding of the different processes inherent in diagnosis, treatment, recovery and living with limitations, in the level of resource utilization and in the development of strategies for managing. Involves a sense of wisdom resulting from lived experiences.	The current study provides evidence that the actions of health and social care staff are important influences on the extent to which relatives develop confidence and coping skills. Where relatives are provided with up-to-date and relevant information, are encouraged to recognize their own expertise and to contribute to an older person's care in the way that both they and the older person are comfortable with, then confidence in their ability to cope within the new environment developed rapidly. However, where such support was not forthcoming, and relatives lacked the inner resources to recognize their own abilities, then they frequently failed to reach this level of well-being.
Outcome indicators Role mastery	A sense of achievement of skilled role performance and comfort with the behaviour required in the new situation. May be represented by individuals starting to make their own decisions and by taking control of the situation.	The extent to which family members demonstrated 'mastery' was variable and to a degree dependent upon whether care staff facilitated or impeded their involvement in direct care-giving activities and in decision making. Many remained uncertain about their abilities to meet the needs of their relative within the new care environment. Others were more confident that skills developed over many years were transferable to the new setting and were able to resist staff efforts to 'take over'. Observations within the case study settings suggested limited attempts by staff to encourage relatives to recognize their own 'mastery' of the role of family caregiver within the nursing home.
Fluid integrative identities	Transition experiences have been characterized as resulting in identity reformulation. Perspectives become 'bicultural' rather than 'monocultural.'	Development of a bicultural perspective was reflected in participants' attempts to understand the pressures on nursing home staff, trying to see the situation from their point of view. A further application of this idea could lie in the relatives' ability or willingness to create a life outside of the home.

welcomed by staff. The importance of such a dynamic is missing from the theory of nursing transitions as currently described.

Discussion

The model of nursing transitions as first described by Schumacher and Meleis (1994) in 1994 and modified in later writings (Schumacher 1996, Meleis et al. 2000) provides a useful framework for considering the findings from a study of relatives' experiences of nursing home entry. In particular, the model's focus on transition types, conditions and outcomes is helpful in considering the factors that might facilitate or inhibit a successful transition to a new 'healthy' state. However, as with any developing mid-range theory, application to diverse situations is necessary to adjust and adapt the model to fit a range of circumstances. Comparing the model with the findings of a study of relatives' experiences of nursing home entry suggests a number of important omissions and insufficient emphasis within certain important dimensions of the framework. In particular, the failure of the model to represent the reciprocal nature of relationships within care homes and the suggestion that residents and family caregivers are passive recipients of care do not accord with these findings. The potential consequences of such a perception in the context of long-term care are tellingly summarized by Stanley and Reed (1999, p. 65):

> The vivid images that we have of recipients of charity, from frail older people to vulnerable children, do not include any notion that they might be giving something back to their benefactors—the traffic of kindness is entirely one way...This denial of reciprocity does a number of things. It diminishes the service user as an active agent and portrays him or her as entirely passive. This passivity is then taken as a rationale for privileging the expert's view, as this inability to act is taken as evidence of incompetence to act. A further idea is then brought into play, about the way in which the service user should be grateful to the practitioners for what they are providing as he or she would not be able to cope without this assistance. Any rejection of care is then viewed not just as a difference in opinion, but as a moral failing—service users are 'ungrateful' or 'awkward' or 'demanding.'

Data from both phases of this study and other work demonstrate that relatives can play an important role in enriching the lives not only of their own relative, but of other residents, their families and staff (McDerment et al. 1997, Ryan & Scullion 2000, Davies 2001). Such findings are consistent with emerging ideas about relationship-centred care (Tressolini & the Pew Fetzer Task Force on Advancing Psychosocial Health Education 1994, Nolan et al. 2004), which seek to redefine the provision of health and social care in ways that value and attest to the relationships that form the context in which care is provided.

According to its main proponents, relationship-centred care addresses the interdependences between care 'providers' and 'receivers' and 'captures the importance of the interactions amongst people as the foundations of any therapeutic or healing activity' (Tressolini & the Pew Fetzer Task Force on Advancing Psychosocial Health Education 1994, p. 11). There is, however, a need for further conceptual and empirical work to identify ways in which relationship-centred care can be elaborated upon and made a reality (Nolan et al. 2004).

The significance of organizational culture within nursing homes, in particular models of care, for the experiences of service users was an important finding of this study (Davies 2003) and finds support in the literature (McDerment et al. 1997, Stanley & Reed 1999). This aspect is also insufficiently emphasized within the model of nursing transitions for it adequately to represent key factors shaping relatives' experiences of nursing home entry. The culture of a particular home is influenced by the values held by staff, particularly those in senior positions, and by the model of care in operation. These factors in turn determine perceptions of roles and the nature of relationships within the home. Historical traditions, availability of resources, leadership style and expectations of service users are also likely to play a part (Stanley & Reed 1999). However, crucially, it would appear that staff, relatives and to a lesser extent residents also have the potential to influence the culture or 'type of community' that is created (Davies 2003).

Taken together, these findings raise questions, which at this point it is not possible to answer, about whether the relative absence of this reciprocal and interactive dimension is an element of Meleis et al.'s (2000) theory that requires further exploration in relation to other forms of transition.

Conclusion

Mid-range nursing theories require empirical testing in a range of care settings and environments if they are to develop as useful frameworks to guide nursing practice in all situations. Supporting people through times of transition is an important nursing function, and Meleis's theory of nursing transitions has been shown to have utility in understanding the impact of a wide range of life changes. Mapping the findings of a qualitative study of relatives' experiences of nursing home entry on to the model suggests that the three domains—the nature of transitions, transition conditions and patterns of response—may be helpful in considering the range of factors that shape each individual's journey through the transition, and in explaining the range of experiences that may be encountered. However, this process also suggests that the theory of nursing transitions may be incomplete, particularly within the domain of patterns of response, in its failure to consider the dynamic and reciprocal nature of the relationships between service users and service providers. Future applications of the theory of nursing transitions should take this into account. Furthermore, there is a need for further research to explore the impact of reciprocal relationships with care providers on experiences of life transitions in a range of settings and contexts.

Findings of the empirical study on which this paper is based confirm that the way in which the transition to nursing home care is managed exerts a significant effect on the quality of life for older people and their family caregivers, and suggest important developmental implications for practice within this field. In particular, the findings suggest that at each phase of the transition, practitioners should aim to:

- work in partnership with older people and their family caregivers,
- be aware of the range of pressures that family caregivers are experiencing and attempt to minimize these pressures wherever possible,
- ensure that older people and their family caregivers are well informed,
- enable older people and family caregivers to maintain control over events and decision making and
- ensure that older people and family caregivers are supported, both in practical and emotional terms.

Most of these interventions and strategies find support within Meleis's theory of nursing transitions. However, practitioners using this model to guide their practice are likely to miss opportunities to encourage family caregivers to recognize the important contribution that they themselves can make to ensuring a successful transition for all concerned.

Acknowledgments

The author would like to thank Mike Nolan for his supervision and comments on the original draft of this work.

REFERENCES

Aneshensel, C. S., Pearly, L. I., Mullan, J. T., Zarit, S. U., & Whitlach, C. J. (1995). *Profiles in caregiving: The unexpected career.* San Diego: Academic Press.

Bogo, M. (1987). Social work practice and family systems in adaptation to homes for the aged. *Journal of Gerontological Social Work, 1/2*(10), 5–20.

Bowers, B. J. (1988). Family perceptions of care in a nursing home. *The Gerontologist, 28*(3), 361–367.

Brown, J., & Furstenberg, A. (1992). Restoring control: Empowering older patients and their families during health crisis. *Social Work in Health Care, 17*(4), 81–101.

Chen, K. & Snyder, M. (1996). Perception of personal control and satisfaction with care among nursing home elders. *Perspectives, 20*(2), 16–19.

Chick, N. & Meleis, A. I. (1986). Transitions: A nursing concern. In P. L. Chinn (Ed.), *Nursing research methodology: Issues and implementation* (pp. 237–257). Rockville, MD: Aspen.

Clarke, E. (1993). *Family ties between nursing home residents and their relatives: A comparative perspective*. Unpublished doctoral dissertation, University of York, York, UK.

Cosbey, J. (1994). *Letting go: How caregivers make the decision for nursing home placement*. Unpublished doctoral dissertation, The University of Akron, Akron, Ohio.

Davies, S. (2001). *Relatives' experiences of nursing home entry: A constructivist inquiry*. Unpublished doctoral dissertation, University of Sheffield, Sheffield.

Davies, S. (2003). Creating community: The basis for caring partnerships in nursing homes. In M. Nolan, G. Grant, J. Keady, & U. Lundh (Eds.), *Partnerships in family care* (pp. 218–237). Maidenhead, UK: Open University Press.

Davies, S., & Nolan, M. (2003). 'Making the best of things': Relatives' experiences of decisions about nursing home entry. *Ageing and Society, 23*, 429–450.

Davies, S., & Nolan, M. R. (2004). Making the move: Relatives' experiences of the transition to a care home. *Health and Social Care in the Community, 12*(6), 517–526.

Drysdale, A. E., Nelson, C. F., & Wineman, N. M. (1993). Families need help too: Group treatment for families of nursing home residents. *Clinical Nurse Specialist, 7*(3), 130–134.

Elliot, K. (1995). Maintaining cultural and personal continuity in a Danish nursing home. *Journal of Women and Ageing, 71*(1/2), 169–185.

Ghusn, H. F., Hyde, D., Stevens, E. S., Hyde, M., & Teasdale, T. A. (1996). Enhancing satisfaction in later life: What makes a difference for nursing home residents. *Journal of Gerontological Social Work, 26*(1/2), 27–47.

Gladstone, J. W. (1995). The marital perceptions of elderly persons living or having a spouse living in a long-term care institution in Canada. *The Gerontologist, 35*(1), 52–60.

Im, E. O., & Meleis, A. I. (1999). A situation specific theory of menopausal transition of Korean immigrant women. *Image journal of Nursing Scholarship, 31*, 333–338.

Junker, B. (1960). *Fieldwork: An introduction to the social sciences*. Chicago: University of Chicago Press.

Kaplan, L., & Ade-Ridder, L. (1991). The impact on the marriage when one spouse moves to a nursing home. *Journal of Women and Ageing, 3*(3), 81–101.

Lincoln, Y. S., & Guba, E. G. (1985). *Naturalistic inquiry*. Beverly Hills, CA: Sage.

Maykut, P., & Morehouse, R. (1994). *Beginning qualitative research: A philosophical and practical guide*. London, UK: The Falmer Press.

McDerment, L., Ackroyd, J., Tealer, R., & Sutton, J. (1997). *As others see us: A study of relationships in homes for older people*. London, UK: Relatives Association.

Meleis, A. I., Sawyer, L. M., Im, E., Hilfinger Messias, D. K., & Schumacher, K. (2000). Experiencing transitions: An emerging middle-range theory. *Advances in Nursing Science, 23*(1), 12–28.

Meleis, A. I., & Trangenstein, P. A. (1994). Facilitating transitions: Redefinitions of the nursing mission. *Nursing Outlook, 42*(6), 255–259.

Messias, D. K. H. (1997). *Narratives of transnational migration, work and health: The lived experiences of Brazilian women in the United States*. Doctoral dissertation, University of California, San Francisco.

Morgan, M., & Zimmerman, M. (1990). Easing the transition to nursing homes: Identifying the needs of spousal caregivers at the time of institutionalisation. *Clinical Gerontologist, 9*, 1–7.

Murphy, K. P., Hanrahan, P., & Luchins, D. (1997). A survey of grief and bereavement in nursing homes: The importance of hospice grief and bereavement for the end-stage Alzheimer's disease patient and family. *Journal of the American Geriatrics Society, 45*(9), 1104–1107.

Nolan, M. R., Grant, G., & Keady, J. (1996a). *Understanding family care: A multidimensional model of caring and coping*. Buckingham, UK: Open University Press.

Nolan, M. R., Walker, G., Nolan, J., Williams, S., Poland, F., Curran, M., et al. (1996b). Entry to care: Positive choice or fait accompli? Developing a more proactive nursing response to the needs of older people and their carers. *Journal of Advanced Nursing, 24*(2), 265–274.

Nolan, M. R., Davies, S., Brown, J., Keady, J., & Nolan, J. (2004). Beyond 'person-centred' care: A new vision for gerontological nursing. *Journal of Clinical Nursing. International Journal of Older People Nursing, 13*(3a), 45–53.

Oleson, M., & Shadick, K. M. (1993). Application of Moos and Schaefer's (1986) model to nursing care of elderly persons relocating to a nursing home. *Journal of Advanced Nursing, 18*(3), 479–485.

Onega, L. L., & Tripp Reimer, T. (1997). Expanding the scope of continuity theory: Application to gerontological nursing. *Journal of Gerontological Nursing, 23*(6), 29–35.

Pearsall, M. (1965). Participant observation as role and method in behavioural research. *Nursing Research, 4*(1), 37–42.

Reed, J., & Payton, V. (1995). *Working to create continuity: Older people managing the move to the care home setting.* Newcastle-upon-Tyne, UK: Centre for Health Services Research, University of Northumbria.

Reed, J., & Payton, V. R. (1996). Constructing familiarity and managing the self: Ways of adapting to life in nursing and residential homes for older people. *Ageing and Society, 16*(5), 543–560.

Rodwell, M. (1998). *Social work constructivist research.* New York: Garland.

Ross, H. M., Rosenthal, C. J., & Dawson, P. (1997). Spousal caregiving in the residential setting—visiting. *Journal of Clinical Nursing, 6*(6), 473–483.

Ryan, A., & Scullion, H. F. (2000). Family and staff perceptions of the role of families in nursing homes. *Journal of Advanced Nursing, 32*(3), 623–634.

Sawyer, L. M. (1999). Engaged mothering: The transition to motherhood for a group of African American women. *Journal of Transcultural Nursing, 1*(11), 14–21.

Schumacher, K. L. & Meleis, A. I. (1994). Transitions: A central concept in nursing. *Image: Journal of Nursing Scholarship, 26*(2), 119–127.

Schumacher, K. L. (1996). Reconceptualising family caregiving: Family-based illness care during chemotherapy. *Research in Nursing and Health, 19,* 261–271.

Stanley, D., & Reed, J. (1999). *Opening up care: Achieving principled practice in health and social care institutions.* London, UK: Arnold.

Tressolini, C. P. & the Pew Fetzer Task Force on Advancing Psychosocial Health Education. (1994). *Health professions education and relationship-centered care.* San Francisco: Pew Health Professions Commission.

Wilson, S. A. (1997). The transition to nursing home life: A comparison of planned and unplanned admissions. *Journal of Advanced Nursing, 26*(5), 864–871.

Wright, F. (1998). *Continuing to care: The effect on spouses and children of an older person's admission to a nursing home.* York: York Publishing Services Ltd.

Reprinted with permission from: Davies, S. (2005). Meleis' theory of nursing transitions and relatives' experiences of nursing home entry. *Journal of Advanced Nursing, 52*(6), 658–671.

Chapter 5   Situational Transitions: Immigration

5.1   MIGRATION TRANSITIONS

DeAnne K. Hilfinger Messias

Transnational migration is a global phenomenon characterized by multidirectional flow and movement of persons, goods, and information across regional and national borders, resulting in new, fluid connections and social fields that cross host and home societies. A complex situational transition, migration may involve radical social, cultural, economic, and environmental changes, as well as potential disruption and difference in a wide range of human interactions and social networks (Jones, Zhang, & Meleis, 2003; Meleis, Sawyer, Im, Messias, & Schumacher, 2000). Migration experiences involve multidirectional, recurring movement across geographical places and social spaces, resulting in fluid and complex personal identities. Immigrants' experiences suggest that it is not the migratory movement or border crossing per se, but rather the accompanying passages between different life conditions, statuses, and phases and the resulting self-redefinitions over time, that characterize migration as a life transition (Messias, 1997, 2002).

Health is an integral component of migration transitions; health disparities among immigrant groups and between native-born and immigrant populations are of increasing concern to health practitioners and researchers. Critiques of existing theoretical models of immigration and health include ethnocentric bias, inadequate empirical support, and lack of applicability to diverse, heterogeneous immigrant populations (Hunt, Schneider, & Comer, 2004). The transitions framework is one of the more contemporary concepts and frameworks applied to migration (Meleis et al., 2000; Messias & Rubio, 2004). The three-fold aim of this chapter is to provide an overview of migration as a global transition phenomenon, briefly review other migration models, and examine migration through the lens of the transitions framework.

Migration: A Global Transition Phenomenon

Since the latter part of the 20th century, more people have moved faster and further across the globe than ever before, creating an expansive ecological migratory space (Carballo & Mboup, 2005). Pressures of population growth, environmental transformations, increasing wealth disparities and relative poverty, and natural and human-induced disasters all contribute to migratory streams from economically poor regions and countries to areas that are considered economically better off. More accessible international transportation and the rapid expansion of new technologies and global communication systems have facilitated this global phenomenon.

In- and out-migration, both internal (e.g., rural to urban) and cross-border, occurs across all regions and involves individuals across the spectra of gender, social and economic class, race/ethnicity, cultural groups, and health/illness status. Yet the social and cultural variability and heterogeneity among migrants is often masked by broad racial/ethnic categories used by the United States (U.S.) Census Bureau (e.g., Hispanic, Asian, and Pacific Islander) and in much public health research (Hoffman et al., 2008). Previously viewed primarily as a male-centered phenomenon in which women participated as dependents, migration has become increasingly feminized, with women making up about half of all international migrants (Carling, 2005; Fry, 2006). This trend is attributed to a wide range of factors, from changing gender norms and expectations to transformations in global agricultural practices, labor market dynamics, and increasing competition for goods and services (Fry, 2006). Women's independent participation in labor migration and an upswing in family and refugee migration, in which women usually outnumber men, have contributed to the feminization of global migration. An additional factor is the emergence of several female-specific forms of migration, including the commercialized migration of domestic workers, the migration and trafficking of women in the sex industry, and the organized migration of women for marriage (Carling, 2005).

Accelerated human migration is one of the hallmarks of globalization. According to the International Labour Organization (ILO, 2004), one in five Mexican workers currently lives abroad and increasing numbers of young, educated Argentineans are returning to the European countries from which their grandparents migrated. Participants in the globalization of higher education, students move across the globe for educational opportunities and some do not return home; Filipino women leave their own families behind to work as immigrant nannies and housekeepers in Taiwan, Saudia Arabia, and the United States; and transnational enterprises move managers around the world and "bodyshop" for skilled workers and professionals overseas. For lower-income countries, migration to industrialized countries has resulted in a significant brain drain of physicians, nurses, educators, engineers, and scientists, undermining efforts to build and sustain national economies (ILO, 2004). Within countries, similar economic, social, and environmental motives fuel domestic migration.

Migration Models and Frameworks

Scholars use various models to describe, explain, and predict the patterns and impacts of human migration. One such model identifies key interactive and dynamic components of population movement: The characteristics of the migratory population; the precipitants for mobility; and the movement process, composed of three phases: predeparture, transition, and postarrival (MacPherson & Gushulak, 2004). In the health sciences, there is a considerable body of scholarship on the relationships between immigration and health. One of the most common constructs is acculturation, referring to adaptive changes in behaviors, beliefs, and values of individuals or groups resulting from contact with another culture (Marin & Gamba, 1996). There is increasing recognition of the limitations of single-item proxy measures of acculturation (e.g., place of birth, duration of residency in the host society, or host-country language ability) in capturing complex acculturative processes (Barger & Gallo, 2008; Bathum & Bauman, 2007; Lutsey et al., 2008; Marmot & Syme, 1976; Messias & Rubio, 2004) and criticism of the inherent ethnocentricity and conceptual flaws of the construct itself (Hunt et al., 2004). In response, more sophisticated instruments that purport to measure multiple dimensions of acculturation have been developed (Abraido-Lanza, Armbrister, Florez, & Aguirre, 2006; de los Monteros, Gallo, Elder, & Talavera, 2008). However, much of the population-based immigrant health research has focused on the predictive power of specific factors (e.g., language, ethnicity, and acculturation) on health outcomes rather than on the complex underlying processes that may be contributing to immigrants' health status (Castro, 2008). Responding to these methodological and conceptual challenges, some immigrant health scholars have begun to move away from linear, ethnocentric models of acculturation to more fluid, dynamic explanations of immigration experiences, such as the transitions framework (Messias & Rubio, 2004; Portes & Zhou, 1993).

Application of the Transitions Framework to Migration

The transitions framework builds on interdisciplinary scholarship in immigration and health; incorporates the longitudinal aspects and multiple intersecting individual, population, and environmental factors of the migration phenomenon; and focuses on migrants' patterns of response and responsive nursing interventions, rather than static outcome measures. Use of the transitions framework allows for recognition of the complex, longitudinal, and iterative components and processes of migration. Its utility is further increased through its concurrent applicability to other health-related transition phenomena.

Nature of Migration Transitions: Types, Patterns, and Properties

Migration is a complex situational transition that rarely occurs in isolation (Meleis et al., 2000; Messias, 2002). For very recent immigrants or return-migrants, the migration transition may be the most visible or pressing. Given the longitudinal nature of a migration transition, it must be considered concomitantly when assessing or delivering interventions with immigrants undergoing developmental or family role (e.g., birth/parenthood, adolescence, aging, end-of-life), health–illness (e.g., chronic illness, post-hospitalization recovery), or situational (e.g., occupational, educational, professional) transitions. For example, international research indicates higher divorce rates among migrant populations and more deleterious emotional impact on the children of divorced migrants, when compared to nonmigrants (Carballo & Mboup, 2005). Factors that may mediate the multiple transitions within the migration experience include the contexts of the sending and receiving societies, age at migration, and gender (Birman & Trickett, 2001). In the United States, an example of an organizational transition embedded within the migration transition is the transition to the U.S. health care system, which requires sophisticated levels of knowledge and skills to understand, access, and navigate the complex and complicated system of insurers, services, and providers. Immigrant parents are at particularly high risk of alienation from systems of health care and support services available to low-income and other vulnerable populations in the United States (Yu, Huang, Schwalberg, & Kogan, 2005).

There is wide variability in individual and group patterns of relocation and settlement that may impact other characteristics and responses to the migration transition. Examples include planned, unplanned, forced, voluntary, temporary, permanent, cyclical, return, regular, legal, undocumented, and irregular migration. Patterns of migration may also be related to external precipitants or motives (e.g., economics, labor, political).

Recognized properties of transitions include awareness, engagement, change and difference, time span, and critical points and events (Meleis et al., 2000). Levels of awareness and engagement may vary with the patterns and conditions of the migration transition, as with migrants' characteristics (e.g., age at time of migration, current age, gender, social class, country of origin, educational level, marital status, employment and occupational history pre- and post-migration) and immigration status (e.g., legal immigrant, refugee, political asylum, migrant worker, undocumented). It is important to note that legal migration status may change over time. For example, individuals who enter the host country as tourists or business travelers may overstay their visas, becoming undocumented or out-of-status; or undocumented or irregular immigrants may eventually acquire legal temporary or permanent resident status.

The potential for change and difference associated with migration transitions is vast. It includes changes in social, political, economic, and environmental conditions; different modes of language, religious and cultural expression; and different or changing educational and employment opportunities and levels of individual, family, and community health, welfare, and security. Migrants may experience significant changes in climate, housing, living conditions, occupation, diet and physical activity patterns, health status, socioeconomic status, family and social networks, communication channels, and gender norms and relations. This is not to imply that immigrants live in a state of constant disconnectedness, flux, or change. However, such states may surface periodically, particularly in relation to health or illness concerns (Messias, 2002).

Migration tends to be an ongoing transition that has no set time span or universally applicable critical points or events. In most cases, identification of some key discrete migratory event may be possible. There may be critical events related to the decision to migrate, the migratory journey, entry, adaptation and settlement processes, or health/illness events. Detention and deportation are possible critical events among undocumented or irregular migrants. It is important to identify and explore other critical points within individual, family, and community migration experiences. Over time, although the migration transition may appear dormant, there is always the potential for reactivation by internal or external events or transitions, such as personal illness, death of a family member, or political turmoil in either host or home regions.

Conditions of Migration Transitions

Migration occurs within complex personal, community, and societal contexts. It is imbued with personal meanings, motives, expectations, and knowledge and impacted by levels of pre-migration preparation and postarrival support. The migration transition is also influenced by prevalent cultural beliefs and attitudes in both sending and host areas. These transition conditions may, in turn, facilitate or inhibit accompanying processes and patterns of response (Meleis et al., 2000). People relocate for a myriad of internal and external motives (e.g., political, social, economic, geographic, personal, educational, family). They may be subject to varying levels of influence, connections to, and support from earlier migrants, either in home or host society (Menjívar, 2000). Other migration conditions include the level of immigrant engagement in the social life and formal economic system of the host country (Nandi et al., 2008). Smuggled and trafficked migrants are particularly at risk for segregated living conditions and economic, labor, physical, psychological and sexual exploitation, and abuse and may live in constant fear of exposure or deportation (MacPherson & Gushulak, 2004).

At the level of community and society, migration transition conditions include the political and economic context of sending and receiving countries; existing structural support systems in receiving areas (e.g., housing, transportation, judicial, police) and access to culturally and linguistically appropriate health, education, social and legal services. An example of the challenging intersections of personal, community, and societal conditions is the knowledge, skills, and self-efficacy required of immigrants in order to successfully access and navigate complex social systems in the face of language, cultural, economic, social, and legal barriers. Carballo and Mboup (2005) reported that compared to U.S.-born citizens, noncitizens were at the highest risk of not being aware of health and community resources for most outcomes, followed by naturalized citizens. Noncitizens were least aware of services related to family discord, child care issues, and family violence.

The migration transition may be facilitated by the human capital that immigrants bring with them. Immigrants arrive with varying degrees of economic and social capital. Certain human resources, such as educational level, technical expertise, linguistic aptitude, social skills, and work ethic, may be valued and sought after by the host society. But across the globe, many immigrants arrive with little formal education, lacking proficiency in the host country language, possessing few marketable or technical skills, and locate in places with weak family and ethnic social networks (Castro, 2008). Common inhibitors of migration transitions include being subjected to xenophobia, discrimination, racism, and sexism. Such experiences may vary by immigrants' gender, race, and ethnic minority status (Carling, 2005). At the personal and family level, conditions that can inhibit a healthy migration transition include economic burdens related to debts incurred in the process of migrating and the commitment to send remittances to home and family; economic or employment insecurity; and family separation, disruption, and intergenerational conflicts. Many of these conditions also may contribute to poor or compromised health status among immigrant populations.

Immigration, health, and educational policies may facilitate or inhibit migration transitions. Directly or indirectly, policies may facilitate incorporation into host-country systems and institutions or increase psychosocial stress among immigrants, create barriers to social adjustment, and contribute to social deviance. Despite the fact that most receiving countries benefit from the labor of immigrants, there is increasing evidence that current policies and practices in these countries are "rendering migration and the life of migrants more insecure and risky from a health perspective" (Carballo & Mboup, 2005, p. 14). For example, policies restricting or denying family migration create disruptions in family and reproductive health, and may indirectly contribute to higher rates of sexually transmitted diseases. Similarly, policies that deny or restrict migrants' access to health care services contribute to the worsening health status of individual migrants as well as to the larger public health status within receiving countries.

Patterns of Response

In identifying and assessing patterns of response to migration transitions, it is important to take into account the potential multiplicity of immigrants' transition experiences and the possibilities of ensuing changes in identities, roles, relationships, and patterns of behavior (Meleis et al., 2000; Schumacher & Meleis, 1994). Individual-level process indicators of a healthy migration transition include a sense of satisfaction, competence, personal growth, and well-being (Messias, 2002). Examples of outcome indicators of a healthy migration transition include the development of language skills and cultural mastery that allows for meaningful interactions and communication with members of the host society; a fluid, integrated identity that incorporates and values components of both home and host societies; and sustained community connections and a sense of belonging. In contrast, social isolation, cultural conflicts, physical and psychosocial difficulties, anxiety, depression, and reliance on alcohol and other drugs are all potential indicators of a difficult or unhealthy migration transition.

Implications for Nursing and Health Interventions

In an increasingly interconnected world, transnational migrants tend to forge and sustain multistranded social, cultural, economic, and political relationships with their societies of origin and settlement (Glick Schiller, Basch, & Blanc-Szanton, 1992). Immigrants' health practices and decisions and actions related to seeking health care occur within transnational social fields; therefore, provision of care must take into consideration individual, family, community, and environmental patterns, properties, and conditions of migration transitions. The transitions concept and framework can guide the development of new initiatives and innovative health services to meet the needs of individuals and families as they move and settle, temporarily or permanently, in communities around the globe. Application of the transitions framework in nursing practice and research with international and domestic migrant populations broadens the possibilities of potential outcome variables beyond conventional concepts (e.g., acculturation). Through a transitions lens, the focus is on the complexities and richness of immigrant transitions, which may encourage nurses and researchers to envision and value the myriad ways in which fluid, integrative identities may be manifest. Future priorities include the assessment, development, and implementation of policies, programs, and nursing interventions designed to facilitate rather than inhibit migration transitions, improve mastery of requisite knowledge and skills needed to access (and provide) essential resources and services to emigrants and immigrants, and create and strengthen social connections and networks within and across sending and receiving communities and societies.

REFERENCES

Abraido-Lanza, A. F., Armbrister, A. N., Florez, K. R., & Aguirre, A. N. (2006). Toward a theory-driven model of acculturation in public health research. *American Journal of Public Health, 96*, 1342–1346.

Barger, S. D., & Gallo, L. C. (2008). Ability of ethnic self-identification to partition modifiable health risk among US residents of Mexican ancestry. *American Journal of Public Health, 98*(11), 1971–1978.

Bathum, M. E., & Bauman, L. C. (2007). A sense of community among immigrant Latinas. *Family and Community Health, 30*(3), 167–177.

Birman, D., & Trickett, E. J. (2001). Cultural transitions in first-generation immigrants: Acculturation of Soviet Jewish refugee adolescents and parents. *Journal of Cross-Cultural Psychology, 32,* 456–577.

Carballo, M., & Mboup, M. (2005). *International migration and health*. Geneva: Global Commission on International Migration. Retrieved December 28, 2008, from http://www.gcim.org/attachements/TP13.pdf

Carling, J. (2005). *Gender dimensions of international migration*. Geneva: Global Commission on International Migration. Retrieved January 3, 2009, from http://www.gcim.org/mm/File/GMP%20No%2035.pdf

Castro, F. G. (2008). Personal and ecological contexts for understanding the health of immigrants. *American Journal of Public Health, 98*(11), 1933.

de los Monteros, K. E., Gallo, L. C., Elder, J. P., & Talavera, G. A. (2008). Individual and area-based indicators of acculturation and the metabolic syndrome among low-income Mexican American women living in a border region. *American Journal of Public Health, 98*(11), 1979–1986.

Fry, R. (2006). *Gender and migration. Pew Hispanic Center Report*. Washington DC: Pew Hispanic Center. Retrieved December 28, 2008, from http://pewhispanic.org/files/reports/64.pdf

Glick Schiller, N., Basch, L., & Blanc-Szanton, C. (1992). Transnationalism: A new analytic framework for understanding migration. In N. Glick Schiller, L. Basch, & C. Blanc-Szanton (Eds.). *Towards a transnational perspective on migration: Race, class, ethnicity, and nationalism reconsidered* (pp. 1–24). New York: New York Academy of Sciences.

Hoffman, S., Beckford Jarrett, S. T., Kelvin, E. A., Wallace, S. A., Agenbraun, M., Hogben, M., et al. (2008). HIV and sexually transmitted infection risk behaviors and beliefs among Black West Indian immigrants and US-Born Blacks. *American Journal of Public Health, 98*(11), 2042–2050.

Hunt, L. M., Schneider, S., & Comer, B. (2004). Should "acculturation" be a variable in health research? A critical review of research on US Hispanics. *Social Science and Medicine, 59*(5), 973–986.

International Labour Organization. (2004). *Fair globalization: Creating opportunities for all*. Retrieved December 28, 2008 from http://www.ilo.org/public/english/wcsdg/docs/report.pdf

Jones, P. S., Zhang, X. E., & Meleis, A. I. (2003). Transforming vulnerability. *Western Journal of Nursing Research, 25*(7), 835–853.

Lutsey, P. L., Diez Roux, A. V., Jacobs, D. R., Burke, G. L., Harman, J., Shea, S., et al. (2008). Associations of acculturation and socioeconomic status with subclinical cardiovascular disease in the multi-ethnic study of atherosclerosis. *American Journal of Public Health, 98*(11), 1963–1970.

Marin, G., & Gamba, R. J. (1996). A new measurement of acculturation for Hispanics: The bidimensional acculturation scale for Hispanics (BAS). *Hispanic Journal of Behavioral Science, 18,* 297–316.

Marmot, M. G., & Syme, S. (1976). Acculturation and coronary heart disease in Japanese-Americans. *American Journal of Epidemiology, 104,* 225–247.

MacPherson, D. W., & Gushulak, B. D. (2004). *Irregular migration and health. Global Migration Perspectives No. 7*. Geneva: Global Commission on International Migration. Retrieved December 28, 2008, from http://www.gcim.org/gmp/Global%20Migration%20Perspectives%20No%20 7.pdf

Meleis, A. I., Sawyer, L. M., Im, E. O., Messias, D. K. H., & Schumacher, K. (2000). Experiencing transitions: An emerging middle-range theory. *Advances in Nursing Science, 23*(1), 12–28.

Menjívar, C. (2000). *Fragmented ties: Salvadoran immigrant networks in America*. Berkeley: University of California Press.

Messias, D. K. H. (1997). *Narratives of transnational migration, work and health: The lived experiences of Brazilian women in the United States*. Doctoral Dissertation, University of California, San Francisco.

Messias, D. K. H. (2002). Transnational health resources, practices, and perspectives: Brazilian immigrant women's narratives. *Journal of Immigrant Health, 4*(4), 183–200.

Messias, D. K. H., & Rubio, M. (2004). Immigration and health. *Annual Review of Nursing Research, 22,* 101–134.

Nandi, A., Galea, S., Lopez, G., Nandi, V., Strongarone, S., & Ompad, D. C. (2008). Access to and use of health services among undocumented Mexican immigrants in a US urban area. *American Journal of Public Health, 98*(11), 2011–2020.

Portes, A., & Zhou, M. (1993). The New School Generation: Segmented assimilation and its variants. *Annals of the American Academy of Political and Social Science, 430,* 4–96.

Schumacher, K. L., & Meleis, A. I. (1994). Transitions: A central concept in nursing. *IMAGE: Journal of Nursing Scholarship, 26,* 2, 119–127.

Yu, S. M., Huang, Z. J., Schwalberg, R. H., & Kogan, M. D. (2005). Parental awareness of health and community resources among immigrant families. *Maternal and Child Health Journal, 9*(1), 27–34.

5.2 A MODEL OF PSYCHOLOGICAL ADAPTATION TO MIGRATION AND RESETTLEMENT

KAREN J. AROIAN

Abstract

The purpose of this qualitative study was to investigate the implications of migration for emotional status over time. Analysis of interview data provided by 25 Polish immigrants, who resided in the United States ranging from 4 months to 39 years, allowed the construction of a model describing migrants' psychological adaptation. Loss and disruption, novelty, occupational adjustment, language accommodation, and subordination were described as predominant aspects of migration and resettlement. Psychological adaptation required the dual task of resolving grief over losses and disruption involved with leaving Poland and of mastering resettlement conditions associated with novelty, occupation, language, and subordination. The model provides assessment parameters and direction for intervening with migrants who are distressed. The model may also be generalized to other types of life change as well.

Nursing science is concerned with individual and group adaptations to environmental contexts in relation to health outcomes and populations at risk for illness (ANA Commission on Nursing Research, 1980; Stevens, 1984). Study of psychological adaptation to the experience of migration and resettlement is an exemplification of these nursing concerns. Migrants are confronted with major changes in lifestyle and environment, have many challenges for adaptation, and experience higher rates of emotional distress than their host populations (Brody, 1970; Hull, 1979; Rack, 1982).

Related Literature

Although the literature on migration and health has burgeoned with potential causes for migrants' high rates of emotional distress, there is still little understanding of the mechanisms by which stressors involved with migration and resettlement affect emotional health (Brody, 1970; Michalowski, 1987). For example, life change scales developed to tap typical life stressors have been commonly used to document both the magnitude and types of stressors involved with migration (Lin, Tazuma, & Masuda, 1979; Rahe, 1981). This "list approach" has major shortcomings: (a) it leaves the aspects of migration and resettlement that are most distressing and the reasons why to conjecture; (b) it does not explicate how generic stressors have components unique to migration and resettlement; and (c) it does not contribute to understanding migration and resettlement as a complex process that unfolds over time with cumulative interactions among multiple stressors.

A further limitation of extant research on the relationship between migration and emotional distress is that most studies have used static outcome measures such as rates of clinical morbidity or standardized outcome measures of psychological functioning that are unrelated to sources of distress. Using outcome indicators alone does not elucidate mechanisms of how life change affects health but merely documents a relationship between life change and health status. Thus, the mechanisms of how migration and resettlement influence emotional health remain ambiguous.

Scholars on migration and health also caution that viewing migration as risk is overly simplistic and criticize research on this topic as being conducted almost exclusively in a pessimistic fashion. They further note that less pessimistic approaches to the study of migration have found that migration and resettlement can present both opportunities and risks (Barger, 1977; Beiser, 1982; Graves & Graves, 1974; Kuo & Tsai, 1986). Consistent with refinements in the knowledge of life change and stress (McFarlane, Norman, Streiner, & Roy, 1983; Paykel, 1974), it can no longer be assumed that all life change has deleterious consequences for health. Therefore, the context of life changes and their meanings as well as those factors that are related to successful coping and adaptation must be considered.

Although understanding the reasons for migrants' high rates of distress is limited, even less is known about which conditions of migration and resettlement affect well-being or how people transform potentially stressful conditions into opportunities. Most likely, the meanings of phenomena change over time as individuals gain mastery over or transform conditions that initially pose challenges for adaptation. Since adaptation, by definition, is a process that unfolds over time (Cohen & Lazarus, 1983; Wild & Hanes, 1976), linking the sources of distress or well-being to changing conditions in the experience of migration and resettlement is crucial for explicating factors related to migrants' emotional status.

Rather than treating migration and resettlement as a unitary, static process, the purpose of this study was to explore the conditions under which migrants experienced psychological distress, and to explore the sources of their well-being. Resettlement was also investigated as a process unfolding over time and presenting changing demands as well as evolving opportunities in the host society. Specific aims of the study were to identify: (a) the type of migration and resettlement phenomena encountered; (b) the psychological meanings of and emotional reactions to these phenomena; and (c) how the experience of migration and resettlement and emotional reactions to it changed over time in response to adaptive strategies.

Method

Sample

A purposive sample of 25 Polish immigrants, who resided in the Seattle area and had been in the United States ranging from 4 months to 39 years, was obtained for this study. Purposive sampling involved stratifying study participants according to three historically distinct waves of Polish migration (Szulc, 1988), yielding three comparison groups or subsamples. Breakdown of the sample by wave of migration was as follows: Subsample 1 (post-World War II era) ($n = 6$), Subsample 2 (mid to late 1970s) ($n = 5$), and Subsample 3 (1980 to 1988) ($n = 14$). The mean length of time in the United States in years was: 30.83 (range: 23 to 29), 14.20 (range: 8 to 22), 3.86 (range: 4 to 7) for Subsamples 1, 2, and 3, respectively. The sample included 15 males and 10 females and the mean age was 43.92 (range: 26 to 77 years).

Grounded theory (Glaser, 1978; Glaser & Strauss, 1967) was the method used in this study. Study participants' initial and changing experiences of migration and resettlement were inductively explored and testable hypotheses regarding psychological adaptation to migration and resettlement were generated. Cross-sectional sampling and retrospective reports provided documentation of changes in the experience of migration and resettlement over time. Stratifying the sample according to three distinct waves of migration also fulfilled the criteria of maximum variation or "theoretical" sampling (Glaser, 1978) recommended for grounded theory methodology. This sampling allowed making case comparisons among the three wave subsamples with respect to differences in their experiences of and their adaptation to both migration and resettlement.

Sample recruitment as well as data collection, coding, and analysis were conducted by the same investigator. Sample recruitment and data collection occurred concurrently over an 8-month period as more people were invited to participate in the ongoing study. The sample was recruited by in-person and written advertisement in local Polish organizations and natural networks in the community. Recruitment ceased when attempts to obtain additional subjects yielded no new responses.

Instruments

Appointments were made with individuals who expressed interest in participating in the study. The appointments consisted of obtaining informed consent, conducting a semistructured interview, and administering a paper and pencil Demographic and Migration Questionnaire (DMQ) that was developed by the investigator for use in a larger study (Aroian, 1988). The DMQ elicited descriptive information about sex, marital status, religion, family income, education, prior and present employment status, length of time waiting for the first country of resettlement, number of external and internal migrations, citizenship, sponsoring agent, accompaniment, length of time in the United States, and availability and proximity of kin.

Procedure

The interviews were audiotaped and transcribed verbatim to ensure reliability of the data collection and analysis. During in-depth interviews, interviewees were asked to spontaneously introduce topics for discussion in response to the questions, "What prompted you to leave Poland?" "What is it like to be an immigrant?" and "How has the experience of being an immigrant changed over time?" Probes elicited emotional reactions to and psychological meanings of phenomena introduced by the interviewees. More specific questions about positive and negative aspects of migration and resettlement followed open-ended questions of the interviewees' overall perspective on the experience. This *funnel approach* (Chenitz & Swanson, 1986) was used to discover unanticipated responses and avoid imposing an a priori frame of reference on the respondents that the experience of migration and resettlement was necessarily stressful.

Preliminary data analysis occurred simultaneously with data collection. The process of interviewing and checking the accuracy of transcribed tapes provided the interviewer with initial global insights and tentative hypotheses regarding the emotional experience of migration and resettlement. This preliminary data analysis provided focus for the interviews conducted during later stages of data collection; in addition to the usual interview protocol, relevant themes and categories that emerged through analysis of earlier interviews were presented to subsequent interviewees as a way of validating impressions and verifying hypotheses that were generated from the earlier interviews.

Initial impressions of the data were solidified during a period of intensive data analysis discrete from data collection. During this period of data analysis, interview data were content analyzed by the constant comparative method (Glaser, 1978). This method was used to abstract the qualitative data into concepts and categories reflecting aspects of migration and resettlement that were reported as having implications for emotional status. An early level of coding involved isolating data that were sources of stress or well-being by linking the descriptions of migration and resettlement experiences to the accompanying meanings and emotions. A simple categorization, including positive experiences or gains and negative experiences or losses, was used to classify stimuli having implications for distress and well-being. Similarly, psychological affect was dichotomized as positive, such as happiness or comfort, and negative, such as distressing. A code book was developed simultaneously with the actual coding to increase intraanalyst reliability. The code book described the codes and defined characteristics of the data that would exclude or qualify the data segment as labeled by a particular code.

The next level of content analysis involved bringing the codes to higher levels of abstraction and identifying the central categories. Once the data were coded at this level of abstraction, a validity check involved discussion and verification of codes and categories with a research assistant who was familiar with the data. In addition, more specific questions from the interview schedule regarding the most positive and most stressful aspects of the immigration experience served as a second-order validity check for the centrality of interview data on different topics and coded categories. After major categories were developed, responses to these more specific questions were tallied and checked against the categories that emerged from the raw data. Once the categories were validated, case comparisons were made to examine variations of the categories among the three subsamples. Finally, preliminary hypotheses were developed and tested with respect to how the categories were linked to psychological adaptation.

Descriptive statistics were used to summarize the DMQ and these data were triangulated with factual data obtained during the interviews regarding the motivation for and conditions surrounding the migrations and resettlement. Data from the DMQ and factual data from the interviews were combined to provide a Demographic and Migration Profile for each of the three subsamples. These profiles provided the context for this study's findings on the emotional experience of migration and resettlement as well as document that the stratification scheme did achieve maximum variation sampling.

Findings

Demographic and Migration Profiles

Analysis of the DMQ revealed few demographic differences among the wave subsamples that were not a reflection of length of time in the United States. In addition, interview data suggested that the wave of migration subsamples were similar with respect to premigration social and economic status. Analysis of interview data, however, revealed marked differences among the three subsamples with regard to the motivation for and the conditions surrounding migration and resettlement. More specifically, every interviewee from Subsample 1 had sudden and involuntary migrations that were the direct result of Soviet or Nazi occupation of Poland during World War II, or a post-World War II agreement that consigned Poland and partitioned its eastern border to the Soviet Union. People in Subsample 1 also had the longest periods of temporary living while waiting for resettlement and the least formal or informal assistance with the resettlement process.

In sharp contrast, all interviewees who emigrated during the mid to late 1970s (Subsample 2) voluntarily chose and planned their emigration. Reasons given for emigrating by these interviewees were economic advancement or to join family members. These people had the shortest period of temporary resettlement, the highest percentage of family sponsors, and little formal assistance.

Subsample 3, interviewees who emigrated during 1981 to 1988, were a mixture of voluntary and involuntary immigrants; 9 of the 14 interviewees or their spouses were deported by the Polish government for their activities in the Solidarity movement in Poland. The remaining 5 interviewees left voluntarily for personal reasons such as wanting more freedom; 4 of these 5 defected and left Poland suddenly. In addition, people in Subsample 3 had the most formal assistance with resettlement (i.e., a period of public financial assistance and formal English lessons) and the highest percentage of non-family sponsorship.

The Experience of Migration and Resettlement

Although there were major group differences among the wave subsamples in the motivation for and the circumstances involved with leaving Poland, interview data from all three subsamples described remarkably similar experiences of migration and resettlement. Each interviewee characterized the experience as extremely stressful. Positive aspects of the experience included self-growth, financial opportunities, or having freedom. However, it was clear that leaving the homeland and the initial resettlement period posed many demands for adaptation and that monumental tasks and conditions had to be negotiated before the interviewees could begin to experience any opportunities afforded by migration. Content analysis of interview data yielded six central categories that summarize the universal process of migration and resettlement reported by the interviewees. The central categories include: Loss and disruption, novelty, occupation, language, subordination, and feeling at home.

Loss and Disruption

The frequency of and the intensity of affect associated with data reflecting the theme of loss led to the development of this central category. This category reflects how all 25 interviewees, even those who left voluntarily, felt that leaving Poland involved multiple, simultaneous losses that totally disrupted their lives and caused considerable distress. One man succinctly captured what it means to emigrate.

He stated, "Immigration has everything to do with intellectual and emotional attachment." Losses included valued possessions, careers, places of emotional significance, and, most important, the loss of family and friends. Descriptions such as "your whole life is gone" or "you have to divorce yourself from the past" were offered to explain what this experience was like.

Novelty

Immediately following the loss and disruption involved with leaving Poland, the interviewees described numerous distressing resettlement demands. Negotiating and limiting novelty was one major resettlement demand. Novelty reflects a theme common in much of the interview data that people had a great deal to learn about the host society. Knowledge deficits were described as having a variety of consequences; they jeopardized people's ability to live satisfactorily, both materially and psychologically in the host society. Lack of basic information made the simplest of tasks difficult. Not having basic information, although overwhelming, was a short-term problem for most interviewees. However, more complex information, such as cultural differences in styles of social interaction, took much effort and time to acquire.

Occupation

The theme of occupational hardship was readily apparent due to the frequency of interview data related to this topic and the intensity of the associated emotional responses. Occupational adjustment was described as most essential for successful resettlement; interviewees had to find means of financial support but had few resources to do so. Novelty either made it difficult to look for a job or created confusion during job interviews. Numerous additional occupational handicaps had to be overcome before gaining access to satisfactory jobs. As a result, most interviewees worked lengthy stints as menial laborers. For example, prior to emigrating, a professional man had been a guest researcher in the United States. He described his first work experience in the United States as a busboy: "I was one of those faceless people running around. This makes you feel even more like you're nothing. I was starting at the very bottom. I never was before that far down." Some people found status demotion the most distressing aspect of their entire migration and resettlement experience.

Language

Language, like occupation and loss, emerged as a central category due to the frequency of data and the intensity of affect associated with phenomena related to this category. Language accommodation was emphasized as the second priority for successful resettlement, partly because English was needed to secure satisfactory jobs. In addition, people needed English proficiency for nonwork-related tasks of daily living, gaining acceptance by the host society, and for psychological and social needs for communication. A woman explained, "When you don't know the language, you lose communication with people. This is like a handicap. To people who don't know me, I can't explain who I am and that depresses me."

Subordination

During content analysis of the interview data, what initially appeared as seemingly disparate data were recognized as reflecting the common theme of subordination. These data included descriptions that the interviewees had little choice or control over a variety of matters that were important to them, felt like second-class citizens, had suffered insults based on their ethnic identity, and had no choice but to accept American customs. The conclusion that these situations represent subordination is substantiated by literature on interethnic power relations that documents that immigrants have a lower status or rung in relation to native-born (van den Berghe, 1981; Lieberson, 1961). An example of data reflecting the theme of subordination includes an incident where one interviewee was chastised for going to nursing school. She was told, "you are an immigrant and you think you have all the same rights as people born here."

Feeling at Home

Together, data related to the central categories of novelty, occupation, language, and subordination represented major resettlement demands and characterized the resettlement environment as unfamiliar, distressing, and often hostile. The positive affective state of feeling at home was spontaneously introduced by many interviewees as the desired resolution for the distress experienced during resettlement. Feeling at home is defined as a positive affective state of psychological comfort derived from feeling at ease, familiar, and included in a social structure. In addition to interviewee statements regarding the desirability of this positive affective state, feeling at home is a logical indicator of no longer experiencing the resettlement environment as unfamiliar, distressing, and hostile. Thus, feeling at home represents the endpoint in psychological adaptation to the experience of migration and resettlement.

Content analysis of interview data revealed that mastery of resettlement tasks related to the central categories described above either directly or indirectly contributed to feeling at home. Interviewees stated that occupational adjustment, language accommodation, and overcoming subordination increased their sense of belonging, either by increasing host receptivity toward them, increasing their desire to mutually accept the host country, or by giving them a needed sense of purpose in the new environment. Language ability and working in nonmenial jobs also decreased novelty, and this familiarity was reported to make the United States feel more comfortable. Additionally, language ability and working in nonmenial jobs allowed interviewees to form satisfying social relationships with members of the host society and this level of social integration further contributed to feeling at home.

Grief Resolution and Return Visits

Despite interview data documenting a relationship between mastering resettlement tasks and feeling at home, the hypothesis that successful psychological adaptation required mastery of resettlement conditions was incomplete when checked against the interview data: Some interviewees from each of the three subsamples had achieved occupational adjustment and language accommodation and had limited novelty and subordination or had overcome them.

However, although they no longer experienced distress associated with these conditions, they reported not feeling at home. Instead, these people identified unresolved grief, such as missing their homeland and nostalgic illusion, as contributing to their feeling displaced or between two worlds. For example, one man who had successfully achieved all outward signs of material and social adaptation referred to the idealized memory of his homeland as a wound that interfered with his ability to enjoy his material gains. He stated, "I would like to eradicate this completely, forget my past and that would be OK. It's always coming back to me, after 47 years, the memories, this tremendous power that does not let you relax."

Analysis of interview data also revealed that return visits to the homeland were described as a powerful way of confronting the past and resolving nostalgic illusion. Furthermore, return visits were reported to cause a dramatic acceptance of the United States as home. Both the relationship between missing an idealized homeland and not feeling at home in the United States and the reported efficacy of return visits for facilitating acceptance of the United States as home, are consistent with theoretical perspectives on grief. More specifically, grief resolution requires emotionally experiencing and tolerating the pain of grief through confronting what was lost and relinquishing overidealized attachments to old bonds before reinvesting emotional energy in new ones (Benoliel, 1985; Parkes, 1972, 1983; Worden, 1982). Thus the tentative hypothesis that successful psychological adaptation requires mastery of resettlement conditions was revised with the qualifying statement that mastering resettlement conditions was necessary, but not sufficient. Instead, psychological adaptation to migration and resettlement requires the dual task of mastering resettlement demands and grieving and resolving the losses left in the homeland. (See Figure 5.2.1.)

Future Oriented Resettlement Tasks

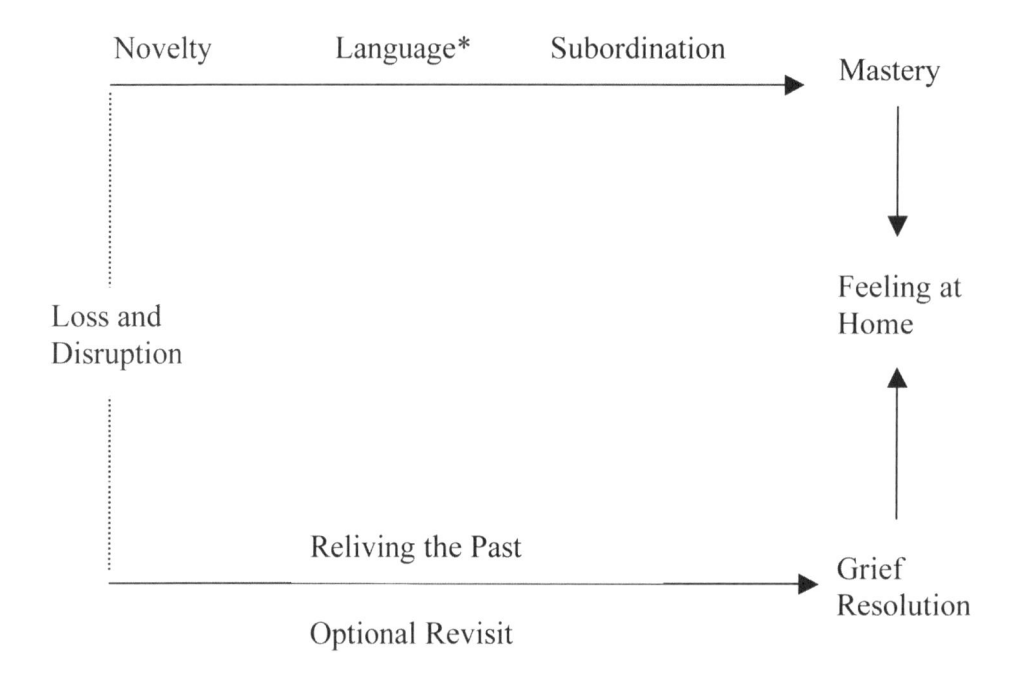

```
Novelty        Language*      Subordination      Mastery
                                                   |
                                                   ↓
Loss and                                        Feeling at
Disruption                                      Home
                                                   ↑
               Reliving the Past                Grief
                                                Resolution
               Optional Revisit
```

Past Oriented Strategies   *Priority tasks for resettlement

FIGURE 5.2.1 Psychological adaptation to migration and resettlement.

Despite how both grieving losses and mastering resettlement conditions were necessary for successful psychological adaptation, the dual effort of mastery and grieving was described by the interviewees as oppositional. For example, a woman stated, "If you started new life you must think about future and make many plans. Missing Poland comes later because you are too busy." The literature describing the magnitude of demands and the amount and timing of losses as key variables influencing adaptive outcomes supports interviewee accounts of the contrast between resolving loss and mastering resettlement tasks (Aquilera & Messick, 1986; Cohen & Lazarus, 1983; French, Rogers, & Cobb, 1981; Parkes, 1972; Worden, 1982). More specifically, the interviewees described experiencing multiple, simultaneously occurring losses and multiple resettlement demands that quickly followed losses and further required monumental coping efforts. The dual requirement of mastering major resettlement conditions and resolving losses may also be oppositional, not only because of the magnitude and timing of resettlement demands immediately following multiple simultaneous losses, but also because of the orientation needed for mastering resettlement conditions. For example, pressing resettlement tasks required pragmatic future-oriented adaptive strategies or involved putting all one's efforts into the present for the purpose of future gains. Grief resolution, on the other hand, represents an emotional goal and is a past-oriented strategy that requires energy to "remember and emotionally relive the past" in order to resolve past attachments (Benoliel, 1985; Parkes, 1972, 1983; Worden, 1982).

Future Considerations

The proposed model provides knowledge that can be used to guide valid assessment of psychological adaptation to migration and resettlement and to develop intervention protocols for migrants. More specifically, assessing migrants' psychological status should include how well they have accomplished crucial resettlement tasks, as well as investigating whether they have resolved grief over attachments left in the homeland. Interventions should assist migrants to find a balance between strategies aimed at mastery and those aimed at grief resolution.

The model on a more abstract level may also apply to psychosocial adaptation to various types of life change. Life change has been identified as always involving losses of some type, no matter how symbolic, and requiring some adaptive strategies (Holmes & Masuda, 1973; Parkes, 1971). More specifically, Parkes (1971) viewed losses and gains as two ways of classifying changes in state where final outcomes, positive or negative, actually represent a balance between the losses and gains inherent in all changes in life space. Parkes (1971) also discussed how life change requires a shift in assumptions about the world where old patterns of thought and activity must be given up and fresh ones developed. This conceptualization emphasizes both attachment to these prior ways of viewing the world and the need to adapt by developing a new set of assumptions that fit the new circumstances. Although some of the specific components of the migration and resettlement experience may not be applicable or be the most crucial elements of every type of life change, adapting to the new involves mastering the conditions associated with the new state. In addition, because of the nature of human attachment, grieving what was lost—even when the new state is a positive one—is most likely an essential requirement for accepting the change or feeling comfortable with the new.

However, few life changes may equal the magnitude of both the losses and demands and the sudden unanticipated nature of the losses people described here. In addition, some immigrant groups may have less traumatic departures and less demanding resettlements (Morrison, 1974). As previously discussed, the magnitude of demands and the unanticipated nature of the losses are most likely related to the contrast of simultaneously resolving losses while mastering the present. Since psychological adaptation is contingent upon these dual tasks of mastery and grief resolution, magnitude of losses and demands may be a crucial predictor of psychological risk for individuals confronted with life change.

Future research is needed to investigate the way both the magnitude of demands and losses and the unanticipated nature of the losses may make the pragmatic goal of mastering pressing resettlement conditions contrary to the more emotional goal of grief resolution. Even though interviewees from each wave subsample appeared to have equally demanding resettlement experiences, there were group differences in what the literature has identified as factors influencing grief resolution (Worden, 1982). For example, people from Subsample 1 had the most traumatic and sudden departures from Poland. It is unclear, however, whether a greater number of people from this subsample had the most difficult time resolving their losses and accepting the United States as their home.

The inability to investigate the consequences of these differences by subsample for both grief resolution and feeling at home resulted from the inductive design of this study where the initiative for introducing actual themes came totally from the interviewees. Because the importance of grief resolution and the concept of feeling at home as the core to psychological adaptation emerged from the data, and although many people offered information regarding grieving their losses and whether they felt at home in the United States, there were no data on these topics for every person. Furthermore, the large number of study participants in Subsample 3 and the recency of their arrival in the United States prevented investigation of the full trajectory of resolving losses and mastering resettlement conditions. Given the small sample and subsamples for this study, the consistent reports of the experience of migration and resettlement, and the fact that data on subjects from Subsample 3 were collected too soon after their arrival in the United States to predict resettlement outcomes, it was not possible to fully investigate all contingencies related to grief resolution and feeling at home.

Due to the limitations of this study, the proposed model presently lacks propositional statements regarding the relationship between magnitude of demands and losses and the ability to adapt to migration and resettlement. Developing such statements and testing how generalizable the model is for adaptation to other migrant groups and other life changes will increase the model's heuristic value for nursing assessment and intervention.

REFERENCES

Aquilera, O. C., & Messick, J. M. (1986). *Crisis intervention: Theory and methodology.* St. Louis: Mosby.

ANA Commission On Nursing Research. (1980). Generating a scientific basis for nursing practice: Research priorities for the 1980's. *Nursing Research, 29,* 219.

Aroian, K. J. (1988). *From leaving Poland to feeling at home: Psychological adaptation to migration and resettlement.* Unpublished doctoral dissertation. University of Washington, Seattle.

Barger, W. K. (1977). Culture change and psychosocial adjustment. *American Ethnologist, 4,* 471–495.

Beiser, M. (1982). Migration in a developing country: Risk and opportunity. In R. C. Nann (Ed.), *Uprooting and surviving: Adaptation and resettlement of migrant families and children* (pp. 119–146). Boston: Reidel.

Benoliel, J. Q. (1985). Loss and adaptation: Circumstances, contingencies, and consequences. *Death Studies, 9,* 217–233.

Brody, E. B. (1970). Migration and adaptation: The nature of the problem. In E. B. Brody (Ed.), *Behavior in new environments: Adaptation of migrant populations* (pp. 13–21). NJ: Prentice-Hall.

Chenitz, W. C., & Swanson, J. M. (1986). *From practice to grounded theory: Qualitative research in nursing.* Menlo Park, CA: Addison-Wesley.

Cohen, F., & Lazarus, R. S. (1983). Coping and adaptation in health and illness. In D. Mechanic (Ed.), *Handbook of health, health care, and the health professions* (pp. 608–635). New York: Free Press.

French, J., Rogers, W., & Cobb, S. (1981). A model of person-environment fit. In L. Levi (Ed.), *Society, stress, and disease, vol. 4* (pp. 39–44). New York: Oxford University Press.

Glaser, B. G. (1978). *Theoretical sensitivity.* San Francisco: University of California Press.

Glaser, B. G., & Strauss, A. L. (1967). *The discovery of grounded theory.* Chicago: Aldine.

Graves, N. B., & Graves, T. D. (1974). Adaptive strategies in urban migration. *Annual Review of Anthropology,* 117–151.

Holmes, T. H., & Masuda, M. (1973). Life change and illness susceptibility in separation and depression: Clinical research aspects. In J. P. Scott & G. Sengy (Eds.), *Proceedings of the American Association for Advancement of Science Symposium* (pp. 161–186). IL: AAAS.

Hull, D. (1979). Migration, adaptation, and illness: A review. *Social Science and Medicine, 13A,* 25–36.

Kuo, W. H., & Tsai, Y. M. (1986). Social networking, hardiness and immigrants mental health. *Journal of Health and Social Behaviour, 27,* 133–149.

Lieberson, S. L. (1961). A societal theory of race and ethnic relations. *American Sociological Review, 26,* 902–910.

Lin, K. M., Tazuma, L., & Masuda, M. (1979). Adaptational problems of Vietnamese refugees, part I. Health and mental health status. *Archives of General Psychiatry, 36,* 955–961.

McFarlane, A. H., Norman, G. R., Streiner, D. L., & Roy, R. G. (1983). The process of social stress: Stable, reciprocal, and mediating relationships. *Journal of Health and Social Behavior, 24,* 160–173.

Michalowski, M. (1987). Adjustment of immigrants in Canada: Methodological possibilities and its implications *International Migration Review, 25,* 21–39.

Morrison, S. D. (1974). Intermediate variables in the association between migration and mental illness. *International Journal of Social Psychiatry, 19,* 60–65.

Parkes, C. M. (1971). Psychosocial transitions: A study. *Social Science and Medicine, 5,* 101–115.

Parkes, C. M. (1972). *Bereavement: Studies of grief in adult life.* London: Tavistock.

Parkes, C. M. (1983). *Recovery from bereavement.* NY: Basic Books.

Paykel, E. S. (1974). Life stress and psychiatric disorder: Applications of the clinical approach. In B. S. Dohrenwend & B. P. Dohrenwend (Eds.), *Stressful life events: Their nature and effects* (pp. 135–150). New York: John Wiley & Sons.

Rack, P. H. (1982). Migration and mental illness: A review of recent research in Britain. *Transcultural Research Review, 19,* 151–172.

Rahe, R. H. (1981). Developments in life change measurement: Subjective life change unit scaling. In B. S. Dohrenwend & B. P. Dohrenwend (Eds.), *Stressful life events and their contexts* (pp. 63–84). Newark, NJ: Rutgers University Press.

Szulc, T. (1988). Poland: The hope that never dies. *National Geographic, 173*(1), 80–121.

Stevens, B. (1984). *Nursing theory: Analysis, application, and evaluation* (2nd ed.). Boston: Little, Brown.

van den Berghe, P. L. (1981). *The ethnic phenomenon.* Norwalk, CT: Elsevier.

Wild, B. S., & Hanes, C. (1976). A dynamic conceptual framework of generalized adaptation to stressful stimuli. *Psychological Reports, 38,* 319–334.

Worden, J. W. (1982). *Grief counseling and grief therapy.* New York: Springer Publishing Company.

Reprinted with permission from: Aroian, K. J. (1990). A model of psychological adaptation to migration and resettlement. *Nursing Research, 39*(1), 5–10.

5.3 IMMIGRANT TRANSITIONS AND HEALTH CARE: AN ACTION PLAN

AFAF I. MELEIS

Change should occur so that nursing is not compromised and the consumer is not placed at risk. This is another challenge for the profession to take on, and we need to lead the way. We are not willing to settle for less than the latest in technology; neither should we settle for less than the appropriate environment in which to practice or less than the presence of professional nurses to provide and direct the nursing care of patients. We must be willing to stand for quality and recognize that, although competition is forcing new boundaries, nursing excellence can continue to provide a competitive edge.

Immigrants and refugees have been part of the fabric of the United States since its inception, thanks to liberal immigration laws. However, today's immigrants and refugees are finding themselves in a more confusing social climate than did their predecessors, a climate characterized by ambivalence about whether they should be accepted and ambiguity about their status.

Two major trends characterize the current immigrant and refugee situation. First, because of a worldwide trend toward having pride in one's culture, immigrants often have an intense need to belong to a community that reflects the identity of their home country. Such communities provide support for newcomers and opportunities for cultural continuity through holiday celebrations, ethnic food, ethnic and religious schools, and community cooperatives. At the same time, belonging to such a community tends to set immigrants and refugees apart and isolate them from the larger community.

Second, newcomers are confronted by an environment that is both welcoming and hostile. On one hand, they find a tolerance of diversity, as manifested in acceptance of ethnic food and celebrations and sensitivity to employees of different backgrounds. On the other hand, a backlash exists that is manifested in policies to curb services for undocumented immigrants and to limit the potential of class action suits that challenge some practices of immigration and nationalization services *(San Francisco Chronicle,* Oct. 22, 1996, p. 1). Most recently, Californians voted to prevent undocumented immigrants from receiving educational, social, and health services. A backlash is also manifested in the hate crimes committed by confessed white supremacists. These crimes reflect fear of encroachment on otherwise homogenous communities.

Such backlash may be also a reflection of many myths that surround immigrants and refugees. One such myth is that newcomers take jobs that would otherwise be available for nonimmigrants. In reality, foreign-born workers tend to obtain jobs that are refused by those who are native-born. In northern California, immigrants and refugees work as housekeepers, manicurists, grocery store owners, seasonal farm workers, and janitors,—unwanted jobs that were quickly filled by first-generation immigrants who did not turn down demanding, low-status jobs for which they themselves are sometimes overqualified.

What does all this have to do with nursing? Everything! Nurses are concerned with the life experiences of people and how these life experiences may affect their health and responses to illness. Furthermore, to diagnose and treat immigrants who are ill, we must be able to put their responses within the context of their lives; otherwise, our understanding and interpretation of their responses to illness will be limited.

Immigrants and refugees experience a long and arduous transition. The transition from a homeland to a new home involves material and psychosocial losses. The manner in which immigrants and refugees experience these losses differs depending on whether they were forced out of their homes, whether their homes were devastated by war, and whether they were forced to get rid of their possessions to begin a new life. The degree to which attachment to objects and loss of such attachments may affect health and illness has not been considered or explored.

Much needs to be done to provide immigrants with culturally competent and transition-competent quality care. We must focus our scholarly efforts on uncovering transition experiences and examining the dynamic nature of the relationships between cultural explanatory frameworks, transition experiences, and the nature of health care actions. Research should focus on how these variables interact with responses to symptoms and symptom management and coping. These studies could be specific to the country of origin or specific to the transitional experience.

Equally important is the need to be vocal about policies designed to marginalize and disenfranchise immigrants and refugees that leave them at even higher risk of stress and illness. Although the issues surrounding undocumented immigrants are numerous, complex, and have no easy or quick solutions, I do not believe that denying health care to such persons solves the larger issues of documentation. Depriving families of preventive and primary care will only exacerbate health problems and lead to the need for more expensive emergency care; it also raises ethical and moral issues that must be addressed within our profession.

Reprinted with permission from: Meleis, A. I. (1997). Immigrant transitions and health care: An action plan. *Nursing Outlook,* 45(1), 42.

5.4 PRIMARY HEALTH CARE NURSES' CONCEPTIONS OF INVOLUNTARILY MIGRATED FAMILIES' HEALTH

KERSTIN SAMARASINGHE
BENGT FRIDLUND
BARBRO ARVIDSSON

Abstract

Background: Involuntary migration and adaptation to a new cultural environment is known to be a factor of psychological stress. Primary Health Care Nurses (PHCNs) frequently interact with refugee families as migrant health needs are mainly managed within Primary Health Care. ***Aim***: To describe the health of the involuntary migrated family in transition as conceptualized by Swedish PHCNs. ***Method***: Thirty-four PHCNs from two municipalities in Sweden were interviewed and phenomenographical contextual analysis was used in analyzing the data. ***Findings***: Four family profiles were created, each epitomizing the health characteristics of a migrated family in transition: (1) a mentally distressed family wedged in the asylum-seeking process, (2) an insecure family with immigrant status, (3) a family with internal instability and segregated from society, and (4) a stable and well-functioning family integrated in society. Contextual socioenvironmental stressors such as living in uncertainty awaiting asylum, having unprocessed traumas, change of family roles, attitudes of the host country and social segregation within society were found to be detrimental to the well-being of the family. ***Conclusion***: Acceptance and a clear place in society as well as clearly defined family roles are crucial in facilitating a healthy transition for refugee families. Primary Health Care Nursing can facilitate this by adopting a family system perspective in strengthening the identity of the families and reducing the effects of socioenvironmental stressors.

Introduction

Migration in general and involuntary migration in particular are known to be factors in psychological stress (Bhugra, 2004). The situational change of moving from one country to another leads into transition, defined as the transformation of identity because of the adjustments to various changes created by the new situation (Bridges, 2003). The transformation process consists of so-called acculturation—the adaptation to new cultural beliefs through social interactions (Berry, 1997). Transition occurs over time and is a three-phased process, first consisting of the letting go of the old identity, second, being caught in-between the old and the new identity, and finally the development of a new identity (Bridges, 2003). This process imposes the risk of acculturative stress (Berry, Kim, Minde, & Mok, 1987). For a family in cross-cultural transition, change in the family system is inevitable, and the full impact of the splitting of families because of migration and acculturation is shown most often after 3 to 5 years in the new host country (Sluzki, 1979). Changes are likely to occur related to family roles and obligations, memories and communication, relationships with other family members, and changes in family connections with the ethnic community and the host nation state (Weine et al., 2004). In addition, social degradation, marginality, racism, social passivity and loss of control increases the vulnerability to psychological distress and physical disease (Sundquist, Bayard-Burfield, Johansson, & Johansson, 2000; Westermeyer, Bouafuely, Neider, & Callies, 1989). Consequences of trauma as well as family members being resettled across different nations are additional stress factors for refugee families (Weine et al., 2004).

Studies in Sweden on involuntary migrated Chilean families show that loss of previous self-image caused an emotional threat (Nyberg, 1993). Living in uncertainty awaiting asylum, facing unemployment, changed roles within the family and perceived unfriendly attitudes of the host country were seen to influence the family causing, mental distress, physical disease and family conflicts (Samarasinghe & Arvidsson, 2002). Darvishpour (2003) found higher divorce rates of Iranian families compared with Swedes because of worse socio-economic circumstances, acculturative stress and a changed function of the traditional male role. Stress in the exiled family was one of the major determinants of poor mental health in refugee children during the first 18 months of exile (Hjern, Angel, & Jeppson, 1998). Both parents being refugees especially from non-European war zones were found to be an additional risk factor related to the psychological health of the child (Cederblad, Berg, & Höök, 2002).

The concept of transition is of interest to nursing because of its emotional and physiological impact on wellness (Schumacher & Meleis, 1994). According to Neuman & Fawcett (2002), health is equated with wellness, and is defined as the condition in which all parts and subparts are in harmony with the whole of the client where more energy is being generated than used. Neuman & Fawcett (2002) define a family as a group of two or more persons who create and maintain a common culture and whose central goal is one of continuance and to maintain system stability and integrity. The concept of family may have a wide range of definitions in a cross-cultural perspective but nevertheless always plays a central role in the various development processes of the individual, such as provision of social security and the preservation of cultural identity. Hence the whole of the family system should be taken into account when caring for refugees. However, there is little research performed on refugees in transition from this perspective (Weine et al., 2004). As Primary Health Care Nurses (PHCNs) play a vital role in the assessment and promotion of health (Allender & Spradley, 2001), it is essential to identify health issues of importance from a family perspective in order to facilitate a healthy transition for the refugee families. The aim of the study was to describe the health of the involuntary migrated family in transition as conceptualized by Swedish PHCNs.

THE STUDY

Design

A descriptive, explorative design, using phenomenography as a research method, was used. It is a way to describe how individuals think and understand the experienced world. Conceptions are central to phenomenography as they often represent implied meanings, which have not been subjected to reflection and made explicit (Marton, 1981). Individuals will conceptualize a phenomenon in qualitatively different ways, thus resulting in a spectrum of meanings. The outcome of this study will therefore describe qualitatively different meanings of the health of the involuntary migrated family in transition as conceptualized by Swedish PHCNs.

Participants and Setting

Thirty-four PHCNs were representatively chosen with regards to age, gender, ethnicity, civil status and family, number of years as registered nurse, specialist education, working sector within Primary Health Care (PHC) and number of years in PHC (Table 5.4.1). The study was carried out in 2003 within the PHC of two municipalities in southern Sweden with a refugee population of 2.7% and 3.4%, respectively (Statistics Sweden (SCB), 2004). From the mid-eighties there has been a great influx of asylum seekers and 2.6% of the Swedish population was considered refugees (SCB, 2004). The term refugee was defined as a person within the asylum-seeking process and the term immigrant was defined as a person with legal status holding a permanent residence visa. Involuntarily migrated family in this study is defined as a family originally holding a refugee status having obtained immigrant status. Each PHCN has worked with an average of 200 involuntarily migrated families.

Ethical Considerations

The Ethics Committee at Lund University approved the study and a written informed consent was obtained from all participants. In order to protect the anonymity of the participant and the refugee families concerned, the data were coded and kept personally unidentifiable.

Data Collection and Analysis

The first author conducted the tape-recorded interviews including two pilot interviews. The inter-

TABLE 5.4.1 Sociodemographic and Clinical Characteristics of the Participants ($n = 34$)

Age: mean (range)	49 (32–63)
Gender: Male/female	1/33
Marital status: Partner/no partner	32/2
Children: Child/none	31/3
Ethnicity: Swedish/non-Swedish	33/1
Registered Nurse in years: mean (range)	23 (4–37)
Specialist education: District nursing/midwifery/others	3/4/7
Sector within PHC	
Maternal health care/youth health care/school health care	2/3/7
Asylum health care/community health care	1/4
Clinic of district nursing in combination with	17
Asylum health care/telephone advisory service	2/3
Diabetes clinic/asthma clinic/child health care	3/3/6
Number of years in PHC: Mean (range)	7 (1–25)

PHC, Primary Health Care.

views lasted approximately 60 minutes each and were made at the workplace of the participants. The questions were: *What is your conception of the health of the involuntarily migrated family? How would the family obtain optimal health? How would the family be affected by returning to the country of origin?* All interviews were transcribed verbatim.

Contextual analysis was used in interpreting the data, which is a method characterized by an open and explorative approach through delimitation of wholes and parts within a given context, in order to give meaningful interpretation to the phenomenon being studied (Svensson, 1989). The first author carried out the analysis, while the two co-authors with specialized knowledge of methodology served as additional evaluators in the categorization procedure. The analysis was carried out in five steps: (1) the researchers read all data in order to obtain a feeling for the variation and limits of the study; (2) statements related to the aim were delimited and subjected to a structural analysis as to *What* and *How* the PHCNs expressed conceptions about the health of the families; (3) a short but comprehensive description was made of each interview on the basis of this analysis; (4) comparison was made in order that similarities and differences of the comprehensive descriptions could be recognized and grouped together; and (5) comparisons were also made of the entirety of the comprehensive descriptions so that similarities and differences could be recognized and subcategorized. The complete picture of the categorized data was compiled into a system of qualitatively different categories of description and subcategories characterizing the health of the families.

Findings

The analysis comprised of four qualitatively different categories of description and eight subcategories. Each category of description and subcategories illustrates a family profile epitomizing the health characteristics of a migrated family in transition, as conceptualized by the PHCNs. As transition is a process that occurs over time the profiles can be placed vertically beginning with the seeking of asylum, followed by having obtained the necessary permit in becoming legal settlers in the new home country, and finally either have become integrated or segregated in the Swedish society. The numbers within brackets (IP) refer to a particular PHCN's statements.

A Mentally Distressed Family Wedged in the Asylum-Seeking Process

The period of seeking asylum was conceived to be chaotic and stressful for all family members resulting in individual psychosomatic symptoms.

Living in Uncertainty. Parents' stress over the obtaining of a visa was conceived to be projected upon the children whose behavior reflected this stress. It was conceived that children either became withdrawn and stopped playing or took to self-harm such as biting themselves, or opposing their parents and becoming overactive and noisy. Psychosomatic symptoms such as chest or stomach pains were conceived to occur frequently in both adults and children and bedwetting occurred at times in older children. Parents were conceived as having lost all their energy because of the pressure of the uncertainty of being allowed to stay in Sweden or not, which in turn hindered them from functioning optimally as parents.

> The mental health has been badly affected…especially amongst the asylum seekers, they live in uncertainty too long, they do not have a future…they live in some kind of a vacuum and I believe this is extremely stressful to their sense of well-being. (IP3)

Living Without Any Rights. The asylum-seeking families were conceived as having no rights in Swedish society (e.g., as in cases such as where an asylum seeker having attempted suicide was discharged from hospital and sent back to the refugee camp without any 'follow-up' activity). Psychological trauma was conceived to be burdening refugees. The women especially felt lifelong suffering because of worry and guilt over those left behind in the home country as well as feelings of shame in cases of previous sexual assault. In these cases, the mother's depression was conceived to affect the children emotionally, which manifested itself by the child ceasing play activities or being afraid to leave the mother alone even for a short while.

> The asylum families are suffering and are not getting any help to relieve this. As long as they have no permit to stay in the country they have no right to get treatment or psychological counseling except for in an emergency situation. By then the problems have been magnified and take far longer to be resolved. (IP13)

An Insecure Family Having Immigrant Status

The condition of the family was conceived as improved on receipt of the permanent residence visa as the family was granted legal status although still vulnerable because of post-asylum reactions, unprocessed trauma, grief, and the lacking in understanding of the new culture. The absence of the extended family was conceived to create insecurity, causing family members to frequently visit the PHC clinics as well as seeking the company of fellow countrymen for security and comfort.

Living With Post-Asylum Reactions, Unprocessed Trauma and Grief. Depression and physical diseases; eczema, gastritis, and body pain were noted among family members and were conceived by the PHCNs as post-asylum stress reactions. Unprocessed traumas as well as grief resulting from loss of the home country were conceived to impact negatively on chronic diseases such as diabetes and asthma, and to be a hindrance for adaptation and learning ability. The women in particular were conceived to be isolated, in addition to having new and stressful demands to fulfill, thus suffering from tiredness, homesickness, and resultant somatic symptoms. The family was conceived as not communicating about the past within the family. Boys were conceived to be more closed and not wanting to speak about their refugee experiences, whereas girls were conceived to be more open to speaking about these experiences. The parents were conceived as worrying about their children having nightmares, but simultaneously being unaware of the mental strain their children were under in trying to cope in school in the new country.

> One does not talk about the recent past—one keeps within oneself this great sorrow that no psychiatric treatment can alleviate; as this type of help is neither found nor apparent in adults or children—this sorrow is something that lies as a lump of unresolved conflicts full of anguish, and which gives rise to physical and psychological symptoms. (IP1)

Being Misunderstood. Language problems and cultural differences were conceived as being commonplace, creating insecurity and frustration for the families. Differences were visible in the treatment forms preferred by the family, where immediate treatment by a doctor was expected whenever symptoms occurred, whereas, preventive forms of treatment and follow-up controls would be neglected. Other noted cultural differences were the breastfeeding period and food selection, which were conceived as making for irregular weight increases in infants causing pediatric investigations. Elders in turn were conceived as reluctant to meet with the PHC doctor, believing it would lead to hospitalization and death. The commonly occurring situation, where a male family member was speaking on behalf of the female, was conceived by the PHCNs as degrading to the woman.

> We don't understand them—they don't understand us—there can be so many mistakes. (IP4)

A Family With Internal Instability and Segregated From Society. An unstable family was conceived as a family who lives in disharmony because of not having clear-cut roles within the family, as well as a clear place within Swedish society, causing psychosocial distress and interpersonal conflicts.

Not Being Integrated. Negative attitudes of the host country toward immigrants were conceived to hinder the immigrant families from being accepted by society. Unemployment and inactivity accentuated the situation, which in turn was conceived to devastate self-esteem. Marginalized individuals were at risk of falling into criminal activity. Not all refugee families were conceived as wanting to accept Swedish society because of fear and prejudice about Sweden and its people, but also as a way of holding on to and idealizing the home culture for fear of forgetting what had been left behind.

> As long as they have not got a place in society it's very difficult for the children...as long as they are unemployed or not having a meaningful existence, we have lost both them and the children as well. (IP11)

Having Family Conflicts. Conflict situations were conceived to present themselves in the immigrant families because of several factors. The father being unemployed was conceived to create a poor role model situation for the sons of the family as well as being degrading in general for the family because of the resultant low income. The situation where the wife was employed, but the husband unemployed was conceived to aggravate the internal family conflicts because of the husband's lost role as the "bread-winner." This in turn could at times lead to violent behavior on the part of the husband. Teenagers were conceived as living a life in between the two cultural worlds in their efforts to adapt themselves. Girls especially were conceived to struggle with this situation, which caused them to turn to Swedish authorities for help thus leaving the parents in a further helpless situation. Language barriers forcing children to be used as an interpreter between the family and society was conceived to further destabilize the family, making parents and grandparents feel inferior.

> They come from a patriarchal society and when the father has no employment and when the daughters revolt—how are the families going to keep together? (IP17)

A Stable and Well-Functioning Family Integrated in Society

A stable and well-functioning family was conceived as one who has a clearly established position in society as well as well-defined roles within the family.

Living a Worthy Life. Family stability was conceived as being promoted when the family was treated with respect by society and valued as a resource, rather than a burden and discriminated against. Employment was conceived as an important factor in strengthening the parental role within the family as well as transferring positive attitudes about the new country to the children. The family's socioeconomic background was conceived to be a main reason for positive adaptation in the new country and well-educated parents were conceived to adjust themselves better than lesser-educated parents. This situation in turn was reflected in the adjustment success of the children.

> Families that have integrated...have started their own company or have some type of activity which brings them a reliable income—their children find it much easier to function harmoniously in society. (IP8)

Living in Togetherness. The families that maintained clearly defined roles in both the nuclear and extended family and who adjusted well in the new society were conceived as secure and possessing a sense of togetherness. This was conceived to manifest itself in respectfulness, as well as in aiding each other, resulting in the promotion of stability in the adjustment process.

> They stand together, really standing up for each other and are humble and respectful toward the elders. (IP30)

Discussion

Family Health Issues

The result of the study shows that according to Swedish PHCNs, transition is a stressful experience and a potential risk factor to the health of the involuntary migrated family as a whole. The study identifies several contextual socioenvironmental stressors such as living in uncertainty, having unprocessed traumas, change of family roles, attitudes of the host country and social segregation within Swedish society that threaten the wellness and the stability of the family in transition. These findings corroborate trauma with the findings of a study by Samarasinghe & Arvidsson (2002) that described the health of the involuntary migrated family living in transition from an inside perspective.

The long period of asylum was conceived by the PHCNs to have detrimental stress effects on the family's wellness as illustrated in the profile of *a mentally distressed family wedged in the asylum-seeking process.* Sourander (2003) demonstrated similar findings in that long periods awaiting asylum in Finland caused high levels of stress and psychiatric symptoms in asylum seekers. The obtaining of a residence visa improves this situation by allowing the family to relax to a degree. Nevertheless, there remains a risk of what is conceived as post-asylum stress reactions; a finding that needs to be addressed within Primary Health Care Nursing. The process of acculturation in turn, imposes the risk of acculturative stress as a result of changing family roles and functions. The transition of the father's role resulting from the loss of prestige in cases of being unemployed was conceived especially as a threat to family stability as illustrated in *a family with internal instability and segregated from society*. This finding is supported by Darvishpour (2003), who claimed that the high prevalence of divorces in Iranian families in Sweden was mainly due to the changed role of the male in the family. Furthermore and corroborating with De Montigny Korb (1996), the acculturation process can be additionally burdened by issues such as language barriers and cultural misunderstandings within healthcare services as demonstrated in *an insecure family having immigrant status*. In order to alleviate this difficulty, healthcare nurses need to be educated and aware of the issue at hand.

Additionally, PHCNs need to be sensitive to the reactions to the acculturation process such as refugee families rejecting the new culture, which hinders the creation of identity. As identity is fundamental to health, nurses need to support the identity creation process of the involuntary migrated family in order to promote self-esteem and subsequently the stability of the family. This is especially important during the family's first 3 to 5 years in the new country as the full impact of acculturation only then materializes (Sluzki, 1979). Moreover, the varying degrees of acculturation within a family need to be addressed in order to prevent the risk of imbalance. Such instances where children learn the new language and are required to attend regular schooling, while parents are lacking in interaction with the new society can be detrimental to the family identity. Hence, nurses need to be observant of these occurrences in order to prevent the deterioration of the issue.

Segregation, negative attitudes by the host country toward migrants, unemployment, and the resulting passivity were all conceived to have a negative impact on the migrant's self-esteem, family stability, and consequent health. Similarly, Wiking, Johansson, and Johansson (2004) showed that socioeconomic status, poor acculturation, and discrimination was found to explain the association between ethnicity and poor self-reported health. By contrast, the beneficial importance of integration for family wellness is illustrated in the profile *a stable and well-functioning family integrated in society*. Moreover, factors hindering stress for the migrated family are their own human resources, such as higher education and stronger socioeconomic backgrounds, which in turn allowed for an easier adaptation to the new culture. Additionally, being accepted by the host country proved beneficial to the adaptation process. Metha (1998) demonstrated the importance of a friendly and understanding attitude by the host country in emphasizing the feeling of acceptance and consequent better mental health. Similar findings of Nesdale, Rooney, and Smith (1997) indicated a relationship between ethnic identity and self-esteem, and the level of acceptance of the host country.

The findings express the necessity to promote health for involuntary migrated families from a system-orientated perspective. Several issues such as stress in parents, depression in mothers, change of the role of the father, as well as varying levels of acculturation within the family, all affect individuals within the family, and, in turn, affect the family as a whole as the family members constantly interact with each other. This is further supported by the findings of Hjern et al. (1998) who found parental stress being mirrored in their children. Furthermore, it was understood that trauma experiences and grief, because of loss of the former social network in the home country, were inadequately communicated within the families. Girls were conceived as needing to express these experiences to a larger extent compared with boys. According to Berman (2001), a common response to trauma is to deny and repress painful memories, rather than confront them, making it increasingly hard for PHCNs to deal with the family's trauma experiences. Especially as speaking about these experiences seemed to exacerbate any negative effects (Angel, Hjern, & Ingleby, 2001). There remains a need to develop new ways of nonstigmatizing treatment when clients are found to be suffering from psychological trauma (Yule, 2000).

Methodological Issues

The transferability of the study may be limited because of the study being carried out in Sweden. As Sweden is a smaller European country, the receiving and caring of refugees, non-European refugees in particular, is a relatively new experience. Another aspect that can be noted is that a more equitable gender and ethnic perspective would perhaps have surfaced if more male nurses and PHCNs with non-Swedish ethnicity had participated. However, the participants reflect a clear representation of Sweden's cadre of 7% male nurses and 5.5% non-Swedish ethnic nurses (SCB, 2004). As the research focused on the cognitive aspect of the PHCNs' experiences, phenomenography and its related contextual analysis in interpreting the empirical data with an holistic approach (Svensson, 1989) was found to be applicable. The credibility of the study was strengthened by strategically choosing the PHCNs, which is a norm in phenomenography, as well as two pilot interviews. In order to strengthen the confirmability of the research, the co-authors reevaluated the analysis of the data including the choice of cited quotations.

Conclusion

Transition is a stressful experience for the involuntary migrated family as conceptualized by Swedish PHCNs. Several contextual socioenvironmental stressors were found to affect the individuals of the family thus risking the wellness of the involuntary migrated family as a whole, as the family members constantly interact with each other. Acceptance and a clear place in society as well as clearly defined family roles are crucial for family wellness, as well as the family's own human resources, such as higher education and stronger socioeconomic backgrounds, which are factors hindering stress for the migrated family. The findings of this study therefore demand that PHCNs gain awareness of potential stressors and their impact on the individuals of involuntary migrated families by adopting a family system perspective and its consequent effect on health. Little attention has been paid to how these factors impact on the family as a whole in empirical literature, which motivates a more comprehensive model of the wellness of the involuntary migrated family in relation to transition experiences.

Implications for Practice and Research

Knowledge about acculturative stress should be made available to all categories of personnel who deal with refugee families. In turn, this will allow a stronger capability in nurses to assess stressors, cultural beliefs and values, past experiences, educational, and socioeconomic factors. Nursing interventions therefore need to focus on key issues in strengthening the identity of the families and reducing the effects of contextual socioenvironmental stressors. Factors that need to be addressed are the strengthening of family roles and the understanding of how these roles can be affected by the acculturation process. Additionally, supporting the parental role during the time of asylum is pivotal to the wellbeing of the children of the involuntary migrated family. Finally, unprocessed trauma needs to be resolved both from a gender perspective and in a non-stigmatizing way. Further research on the topic of health and involuntary migration families would benefit from emphasizing the essential nature of healthy transitions and ways in which these can be facilitated.

Acknowledgments

The authors wish to thank the PHCNs who participated in this study and Kristianstad University for financial support.

REFERENCES

Allender, J., & Spradley, B.W. (2001). *Community health nursing: Concepts and practice* (5th ed.). Philadelphia: Lippincott, Williams, & Wilkins.

Angel, B., Hjern, A., & Ingleby, D. (2001). Effects of war and organized violence on children: Study of Bosnian refugees in Sweden. *American Journal of Orthopsychiatry, 71*(1), 4–15.

Berman, H. (2001). Children and war: Current understandings and future directions. *Public Health Nursing, 18*(4), 243–252.

Berry, J. W. (1997). Immigration, acculturation, and adaptation. *Applied Psychology: International Review, 46*, 5–68.

Berry, J. W., Kim, U., Minde, T., & Mok, D. (1987). Comparative studies of acculturative stress. *International Migration Review, 21*(3), 491–511.

Bhugra, D. (2004). Migration and mental health. *Acta Psychiatrica Scandinavica, 109*, 243–258.

Bridges, W. (2003). *Managing transitions: Making the most of changes* (2nd ed.). London: Nicholas Brealey Publishing.

Cederblad, M., Berg, R., & Höök, B. (2002). *Regional study of children's psychological health.* FoU-report 36. The Council for health and health care research (in Swedish).

Darvishpour, M. (2003). *Immigrant women who break establishment patterns: How changing power relations within Iranian families in Sweden influence relationships* (Unpublished doctoral dissertation). Stockholm University: Sweden (in Swedish).

De Montigny Korb, M. (1996). Expectations in giving and receiving help among nurses and Russian refugees. *International Journal of Nursing Studies, 33*(5), 479–486.

Hjern, A., Angel, B., & Jeppson, O. (1998). Political violence, family stress and mental health of refugee children in exile. *Scandinavian Journal of Social Medicine, 26*(1), 18–25.

Marton, F. (1981). Phenomenography-describing conceptions of the world around us. *Instructional Science, 10*, 177–200.

Metha, S. (1998). Relationship between acculturation and mental health for Asian Indian immigrants in the United States. *Genetic, Social, and General Psychology Monographs, 124*(1), 61–78.

Nesdale, D., Rooney, R., & Smith, L. (1997). Migrant ethnic identity and psychological distress. *Journal of Cross-Cultural Psychology, 28*(5), 569–588.

Neuman, B., & Fawcett, J. (2002). *The Neuman Systems Model* (4th Ed.). Upper Saddle River, NJ: Pearson Education.

Nyberg, E. (1993). *Migration of families with children: Family relations in a changed life situation* (Unpublished doctoral dissertation). Department of Pedagogy, Stockholm University, Lange: Stockholm.

Samarasinghe, K., & Arvidsson, B. (2002). 'It is a different war to fight here in Sweden'—the impact of involuntary migration on the health of refugee families in transition. *Scandinavian Journal of Caring Sciences, 16*, 292–301.

Schumacher, K., & Meleis, A. (1994). Transitions: A central concept in nursing. *Journal of Nursing Scholarship, 26*(2), 119–127.

Sluzki, C. E. (1979). Migration and family conflict. *Family Process, 18*(4), 379–390.

Sourander, A. (2003). Refugee families during asylum seeking. *Nordic Journal of Psychiatry, 57*(3), 203–207.

Statistics Sweden (SCB). (2004). *Befolkningsstatistik och arbetskraftsunder-sökningen (Population Statistics and Employment Statistics).* Retrieved December 15, 2004, from http://www.scb.se

Sundquist, J., Bayard-Burfield, L., Johansson, L. M., & Johansson, S. E. (2000). Impact of ethnicity, violence and acculturation on displaced migrants: Psychological distress and psychosomatic complaints among refugees in Sweden. *Journal of Nervous and Mental Disease, 188*(6), 357–365.

Svensson, L. (1989). Phenomenography and contextual analysis. In R. Säljö (Ed.), *As we perceive it: Eleven contributions about learning and conceptions of reality* (pp. 33–52). Lund, Sweden: Studentlitteratur.

Weine, S. et al. (2004). Family consequences of refugee trauma. *Family Process, 43*(2), 147–158.

Westermeyer, J., Bouafuely, M., Neider, J., & Callies, A. (1989). Somatization among refugees: An epidemiologic study. *Psychosomatics, 30*(1), 34–43.

Wiking, E., Johansson, S. E., & Johansson, J. (2004). Ethnicity, acculturation and self reported health. A population based study among immigrants from Poland, Turkey, Iran, and Sweden. *Journal of Epidemiology and Community Health, 58*(7), 574–582.

Yule, W. (2000). Emanuel Miller Lecture. From pogroms to 'Ethnic Cleansing': Meeting the needs of war affected children. *Journal of Child Psychology and Psychiatry and Allied Disciplines, 41*(6), 695–702.

Reprinted with permission from: Samarasinghe, K., Fridlund, B., & Arvidsson, B. (2006). Primary health care nurses' conceptions of involuntarily migrated families' health. *International Nursing Review, 53*(4), 301–307.

5.5 TRANSNATIONAL HEALTH RESOURCES, PRACTICES, AND PERSPECTIVES: BRAZILIAN IMMIGRANT WOMEN'S NARRATIVES

DeAnne K. Hilfinger Messias

Introduction

Transnational lives, identities, and perspectives are created and maintained within the fluid migrant social fields that span geographic, cultural, and political borders. Transnational perspectives are formed in part by social relations and activities that take on meaning within the flow and fabric of daily life, as linkages between different societies are maintained, renewed, and reconstituted.[1–3] In recent years, advocates for feminist, postmodern, and transnational perspectives have argued for expanding and revisioning immigration frameworks to include gender, class, race, culture, ethnicity, nationalism, and transnationalism in migration research.[1, 2, 4–10] As a result, theorists and researchers have begun to include gender and transnational perspectives into conceptual frameworks and research when addressing the relationships of immigration and health. However, women tend to frame their stories in personal experiences rather than in theoretical frameworks. Women's own stories bring perspectives on their health practices and experiences that often are missing from the immigrant health literature.

Qualitative research, such as this feminist narrative interpretive study, in which immigrant women and researchers participate in the processes of telling, listening, and representing stories, can contribute to furthering health care professionals' understandings of immigrants' transnational health experiences. Through the lenses of individual women's experiences, such research can expand the knowledge and understanding of the diversity and multiplicity of immigrant women's lives and health practices.

The purpose of this chapter is to examine transnational health perspectives, practices, and resources through the presentation of Brazilian immigrant women's narratives. To date, there have been no published research studies related to the health of Brazilian immigrant women in the United States. This study is a contribution to the immigrant health research in that it focuses on the layered complexities of transnational health issues by exploring the experiences of Brazilian immigrant women through the lenses of transnationalism and gender.

Research Methodology

This chapter is derived from a broader qualitative study of the transnational migration, work, and health experiences of Brazilian women living in the United States.[3, 11, 12] An underlying assumption of the research is that women experience the world through the socially constructed phenomena of gender, class, race, ethnicity, and immigration status. The processes of feminist narrative inquiry and interpretation are based on the premise that the relationships between knower and what is to be known are subjective and interactive.[13–18] The resulting knowledge is a co-creation of the multiple voices of those who participate in research, narrators and interpreters alike. As a transnational–bicultural migrant, feminist, and advocate for the health of women and immigrants, the investigator brought personal identities, perspectives, and experiences to the research process. The researcher's perspectives and understanding of transmigrant health care practices initially informed the conceptualization of the research; in listening to and learning from other Brazilian women throughout the research process, these perspectives were expanded by the participants' stories and experiences.

A purposeful, convenience sample of diverse Brazilian women living and working in the United States was recruited for the study. Excluded were exchange students, visiting scholars, diplomats or employees of the Brazilian government, and women on guest worker visas. Participants were contacted through informal networking and snowball referrals within urban Brazilian immigrant communities on the east and west coasts. In-depth interviews were conducted in Portuguese with 26 Brazilian women; 4 of these women were interviewed more than once over the course of the study. The researcher's fluency in the Portuguese language and Brazilian culture were instrumental in creating a sense of rapport and mutual communication conducive for the women to tell their stories. The interviews, which lasted from 1 to 3 hours, were held at times and locations chosen by the participants. To accommodate participant preference and convenience, two of the interviews were collective, each involving three women who knew each other and arranged to be interviewed at the same time.

Institutional Review Board approval was obtained before initiating the study. A major concern regarding protection of the rights of the study participants was immigration status. Prior contacts and knowledge about potential participants strongly indicated that many could be undocumented immigrants. To minimize possible risks for those who might be undocumented immigrants, a waiver of a signed consent was granted by the institutional Committee on Human Research. However, written information regarding the study purpose and terms of voluntary participation was provided and reviewed with participants and verbal consent was obtained prior to initiating the interviews. To reduce the potential legal, social, political, or economic risks related to disclosure of immigration status, no direct or indirect inquiry regarding immigration status was made at any point in the research process. Specific measures taken to ensure confidentiality included not asking for or recording participants' full names. Because Brazilians commonly use only first names in social situations, this practice was not awkward or difficult. First names, telephone numbers, and addresses (when needed) were noted and kept separate from interview data.

Analysis of the transcribed interview data involved coding, identification of themes and story threads, locating stories within each interview text, and representing and interpreting the resulting narratives.[16] The final steps in the interpretive process involved translating the narrative representations into English and selecting the exemplars to present in reports of the completed research. In reporting the results, the participants are represented by pseudonyms. The direct quotations from the interview data have been translated from the original Portuguese. Editorial clarifications are included in square brackets and italicized text indicates verbal emphasis. The results are presented as both thematic categories[19] and as narrative co-representations and interpretations of individual women's stories.[16]

The Participants and Their Migration Contexts

The study sample consisted of 26 Brazilian immigrants living in the United States. The varying backgrounds and migration experiences of the women who participated in the study were an indication of the diversity among the recent wave of Brazilian immigrants.[20] The mean length of residency in the United States was 5.9 years, with a range of 2 months to 17 years. The women ranged in age from 22 to 60 years; the median age was 33. Age at the time of arrival in the United States varied from 17 to 56 years, with a median of 30.5. The diversity of the group was also evident in their Brazilian social class and geographic origins. The women came from low working class to upper middle class origins and from both urban and rural areas of the four major Brazilian regions. Eighteen were partnered or married, five were single, and three were separated or divorced. The majority of the participants had at least a high school education or above and nine women had completed a college degree. Six women reported having an eighth grade education or less. Occupation and employment prior to migration included a wide range of roles, including homemaker, domestic worker, student, and professional. Areas of formal sector employment in Brazil had included sales, business, clerical work, education, marketing, advertising, graphic arts, cosmetology, and nutrition and dietetics.

At the time of the interviews, all but two women reported being employed. The majority ($n = 17$) were employed as domestic workers (e.g., housecleaner, baby-sitter, home health aide, nanny, or housekeeper). Although most of the women were employed in some form of domestic labor, their employment conditions and characteristics varied greatly. Some women lived with their employers as full-time nannies. Others were autonomous jobworkers, engaged in baby-sitting or housecleaning for several different households. Two of the participants ran their own housecleaning businesses, in which they employed other Brazilian immigrants. Several were also engaged in other types of informal sector or temporary work, such as making and selling homemade food or catering Brazilian weddings and birthday parties. Two were artists who did freelance graphic work and also produced and sold their artwork; one woman ran an "informal" beauty salon in her living room; another was a teacher who also offered massage therapy at her home. Areas of current employment in the formal sector included food service, clerical work, mental health, and language education. Other temporary employment in the United States had included walking dogs, moving and packing services, and stuffing envelopes. Several women had been undergraduate or graduate students in the United States at some time point in time.

Some of the participants in this study fit the profile of economic or labor migrants who had come with the primary intent to work, earn and save up money, and then return to Brazil [20]. For others, migration was intimately connected to personal or family relationships. Some women had come to the United States expressly as immigrants. Others initially came as international tourists or to visit family or friends, and in the process of their travels became immigrant sojourner-settlers. Several were globetrotting adventurers who had lived and worked in other countries in addition to Brazil and the United States. The pursuit of new and different life experiences was the primary factor motivating their international migration. Although the participants were not asked about their immigration status, in the course of the research interviews a number of the women indicated that they were, or had been, undocumented immigrants.

Results

The presentation of the research results has been organized in two major sections. The first section focuses on the Brazilian immigrant women's *transnational resources, practices, and perspectives*. The second section, *crossing multiple borders and barriers*, presents the perspectives and meanings the women attached to their experiences and interactions with the U.S. health care system.

Transnational Resources, Practices, and Perspectives

These Brazilian women talked about their health in the context of their lives, work, families, and migration experiences. Prior to migrating, some women had engaged in specific *premigration health care practices*. In the United States they relied on a variety of *personal and communal transnational health resources and practices*, one of the most common being utilization of *transnational medications*. Migration not only expanded the borders of the world these Brazilian women inhabited; it also expanded and blurred the borders of their own *identities,* which became more *fluid and dynamic. Being Brazilian* was not only an identity, but also a *health resource.*

Premigration Health Care Practices and Concerns

One way women prepared themselves before coming to the United States was by taking steps to ensure their health. Premigration health practices, such as gynecological checkups, taking care of dental needs, and stocking up on medications, were commonly reported by women who had come to the United States with the express intention of settling, at least temporarily.

> I wanted to be well to come here, so I went to several doctors before coming…I was concerned about not bringing any disease with me, in coming here. (Flora)

> I had a gynecological exam and all the tests to see if everything was fine, if I needed anything. Dental treatment—I went for that so I wouldn't need to go here. Then I didn't go to the dentist again until I went back to Brazil again. My husband hasn't ever gone to the dentist here. He has good teeth, I don't. (Norma)

Underlying these premigration health practices was the need for assurance of a "clean bill of health," both a personal and public concern. Those who initially entered the United States on immigrant visas, or later adjusted their status, were required by federal law to have physical exams and other medical tests. For example, Ana Maria had come to the United States as an immigrant bride. She described in extensive detail the process involved in obtaining the medical clearance from U.S. immigration authorities in Rio de Janeiro and how, in the process, she was diagnosed with a thyroid disorder:

> I didn't have any health concerns at all, but the week that I came here I had a big scare. When I went to the immigration doctor in Rio, it turned out he was a thyroid specialist....He had to examine me first, before he requested the X-rays and the AIDS test. That's the function of this immigration doctor. So he started to examine me and he saw that my thyroid was either high or low. I still get confused with this business of the thyroid number. Anyway, I think it was almost zero, because I know that my leg didn't move the way it should....I had been walking my feet off and I thought it was just tiredness and I just didn't have the energy to walk ....So the doctor said he was going to ask for a thyroid test too....When I took him the results, he looked at them and said, "Go straight to the pharmacy and buy this medicine. You're going to take this medicine for the rest of your life." So I went and bought the medicine; I bought enough for a year ....He gave me a prescription written in English, to bring with me. I put it all in a little satchel and brought it with me.

For most of these Brazilian women, migration had been an excursion into the unknown. Many had very little, if any, knowledge of the U.S. health care system before they arrived. Premigration health care practices were in part an acknowledgment of this lack of information. Before venturing into uncharted territory, women often attempted to validate their perception of good health. In addition, they also were interested in preventing untoward medical expenses once they arrived in the United States. In contrast, women who had initially entered the country as visitors or tourists without the express intention of establishing residency did not report having engaged in specific premigration health preparations.

Personal and Communal Health Resources

On the whole, the women who participated in this study considered themselves to be in relative good health at the time they were interviewed. Responses ($n = 19$) to a tool rating perceived level of health on a ladder scale from 1 to 10 ranged from 4 to 10, with a mean of 8. In response to the question "What are your current health concerns?" women often reported not having any specific health concerns at the moment. However, in the course of the interviews, most identified or mentioned some type of personal and family health concerns. These included physical and mental health, specific illnesses and disorders, occupational health risks, health and nutrition practices, reproductive concerns, stress, overload, and emotional distress. Health care systems issues included access, language barriers, cost, and quality of care.

As immigrants, taking care of their health often depended on women's personal and communal resources. Responses to the question, "What do you do to take care of your health here in the United States?" included a variety of health maintenance and promotion practices. Nutrition and diet, exercise, risk reduction and avoidance behaviors, stress prevention, rest and sleep, and relaxation were the most common health maintenance practices mentioned. Avoidance of medications, caffeine, dietary fat, cholesterol, and smoking were also identified as health maintenance behaviors. Good nutrition was a frequently mentioned personal health practice, although some of the women related their nutrition and dietary practices more to weight loss concerns rather than health promotion per se.

Migration often upset the taken-for-grantedness of daily life. For example, among middle class women who had been accustomed to having live-in domestic help in Brazil, planning and preparing nutritious meals in the United States was identified as an added workload and stressor:

> I try to eat well, balanced nutrition, but other than that, no real preventive care. We try to eat at home, cook our own food, fresh food. The food isn't that much different from Brazil; the difference is that there's no maid to fix it! But here I had to take charge of the house; I have to worry about what it is that I'm going to eat. I always had everything done [by others]. For me, the situation here is horrible. I don't like it, and I find I still have to adapt. (Flora)

Lack of time was the most frequently mentioned barrier to personal health promotion practices:

I try to exercise, but usually when I'm going to school it's difficult, because I have classes twice a week at night, plus classes on Saturday morning, and I work from 8 to 3 during the week, and have to cook for myself and my husband, and do the laundry, and take care of the clothes—it gets difficult. (Sandra)

I'd like to be more active, do some exercise here, but I don't have time. I was taking some classes on Saturday, jazz, tap dance, and swimming, but now I don't have time. This weekend I'm working all day long, Saturday and Sunday. (Joana)

I have my own doctor now ....Every year I have my check-up. This year I haven't had it yet, but he's already sent me the notice. I urgently need to go, because I've got really bad pains in my back, down low. I don't know if it's stress, or kidney, or what. I've had them for about three months, really strong. And I go to work and in my mind I think, "I have to go to the doctor." Then I look at my schedule, it's full of things to do, and I never go. Always putting it off until tomorrow, putting it off until tomorrow. But he already sent me a little note, "time for your checkup." (Raquel)

The participants made frequent references to communal sharing of resources among family, friends, and other Brazilian immigrants. They exchanged information, advice, transportation, instructions for preparing home remedies, Brazilian medications, and prescription drugs obtained through American health care providers. Clara, a self-declared economic migrant who was both undocumented and uninsured, heard through the Brazilian immigrant "grapevine" that prescription medications were difficult to come by, even through physicians. When her husband became ill, rather than attempt to overcome the real and perceived barriers of the U.S. health care system, Clara relied on personal and communal resources such as folk remedies and Brazilian pharmaceuticals and the support of her Brazilian housemates:

My mother sends me Urobactrim® [an antibiotic]. She sends these medications from Brazil, because here, they say that they [health care providers] only know how to give you Tylenol® for pain. That they don't give you medication without knowing what it is. Here, I've only had a little kidney cramps, but it was only the beginning of kidney cramps; I didn't feel anything else. I used the medications from Brazil that my mother sent me. She always sends them, because now it's my husband who's got a kidney problem. These days he really was not feeling well and we thought we might even have to take him to the doctor. I'd given him the medication, and he got really sick, and when he got to work at the pizzeria he threw it all up...the pain hadn't gotten any better, so he even left work early and came home. So then Mariana and I made him some medicinal tea from nutmeg, because he thought it was gas ....Then Marcos said, "You guys go to bed and if he really doesn't get better, you can wake us up. There's a hospital here and we'll take him. And you don't need to be worried about the business of paying, you can parcel the payments and the bill comes later." But thank God he got better. I gave him 2 Buscopan® [pain medication] pills and 2 Urobactrim®, and he got better. But he's having to take the medication almost every other day, because he's feeling bloated.

Clara and others in this study were comfortable with an informal, family- and community-based approach to diagnosis and treatment, in which family members, friends, neighbors, and pharmacy clerks were considered to be trustworthy and reliable sources of information and medications.

Transnational Health and Medical Resources and Practices

Transnational medication practices, such as having a stock of Brazilian prescription drugs, practicing self-medication, and sharing medications with family and friends, were frequently noted. The women either brought medications with them from Brazil or sent for them as the need arose. Antibiotics and pain medications were among the most common "imported" Brazilian medications. Reasons given for having a personal source of Brazilian medications included convenience, familiarity, preference, and trust. Several other participants echoed the notion that U.S. physicians *only prescribe Tylenol®*, an attitude that also has been documented among Mexican immigrants [21]. Having their own medications was also one of the ways immigrants avoided having to seek professional health care in the United States, an important issue for those who were uninsured. But acquiring medications from Brazil also had its drawbacks, including the fact that these resources often went unused:

> We've got a mountain of stuff that's going to expire. Everything is going to go beyond the expiration date and we're never going to use it. There are pain medications and we've got things from Brazil for urinary infections. But I take very few medications. My husband has a back problem; he also has the medications he brings. He prefers to take medications from Brazil. (Flora)

Continued reliance on some type of Brazilian health resources and services was another common practice, although the degree and type of reliance varied widely. Some women's transnational migratory experiences involved multiple journeys between the United States and Brazil, allowing them to continue to rely on Brazilian medical coverage and providers:

> Well, I have very good health care coverage in São Paulo...and my gynecologist is very good. The first year I came here with a plan. I'd say it was a maintenance plan that the doctor gave me: the things that I should take, the precautions I should take. It was like a prescription for taking care of my health. And before I came I also had a checkup for all the necessary things, to check for osteoporosis, and blood and urine tests, thousands of things, heart, everything. And every time I've gone back to Brazil, I've gone to the doctor. Except for the last trip I made, because of extenuating circumstances I didn't go to the doctor when I was in Brazil. (Vera)

Luiza identified several transnational medical resources she called upon in times of need:

> When I came, my sister gave me a sack-full of medications. She also sent me some allergy medications, so whenever I have anything, I take one, but I don't take it a lot. I take vitamins, and I'm always very tuned in, like if I see that I'm going to come down with a cold, I take medications ....I asked my sister to send Buscopan® [pain medication]; when I have cramps I take that. So I have some of the medications that I used to take in Brazil, and I still take those. If I have something wrong, I'll go rummage through the sack, and if I find something interesting, I take it, I medicate myself ....Sometimes, I've done it a couple of times, I'll call my sister in Brazil and say, "I've got this and this and this." But I try not to do it very often, because otherwise they'll get worried about me ....I also call Vania [a friend who was a Brazilian physician living in the area]; I called another Brazilian doctor once, I don't know if he liked it or not, but I had called Vania and she wasn't home. I'm not really very close friends with him, but I was in really bad shape. I woke up in the morning vomiting and I couldn't even stand up, so I called to ask him about it, what he thought about it. I said, "A doctor's opinion, even from afar, is good."

Brazilian doctors, nurses, and dentists living in the area were a source of information and advice as well as formal and informal health care. Even when they provided care within the formal health care system, access had often been through informal contacts:

> I'm going to my first dentist appointment on Monday, at the university. There's a Brazilian dentist there, who's doing a residency there. My husband met him playing soccer. He plays soccer on my husband's team and he said, "I'm a dentist." Said and done. Now he's a friend of ours, so I'm going to have him do my dental work. (Norma)

Fluid Transnational Identities and Resources

One of the consequences of immigration was that these women's health practices become more dynamic and transnational. Similarly, in the transnational and transcultural contexts of their daily lives, homes, families, work, employment, and social milieu, these immigrant women's identities became more fluid. For example, Flora and her husband André were of middle-class origin in Brazil, but they did not have health insurance in the United States. As a result, in the process of identifying local health care services, Flora found she had to redefine her own transnational class identity:

> Then there was a time when my husband was sick and I ended up making a list of places where you could go, if you were low income. Because I *am* low income, maybe not the low income from here, but I *am* low income when it comes to health, because the money that we have is for education.

House, rent, food, these basic things, that's all guaranteed, but money for health, we don't have that. We'd have to pay for a health insurance...but we don't have coverage ....As a student, Andre used to have health insurance through his school, but he quit paying for it, since January. So ever since I arrived here we haven't had any insurance for either of us.

The stories the women told about transnational medication practices were as much about identity as they were about medicine. An example of how women framed their use of Brazilian medications both in terms of medicine and migration, Tereza considered use of American medications as an indication of her settlement mentality, a reflection of her desire to adapt and fit in:

In the beginning I used to bring a lot of medicine. In Brazil I had cystitis, and so I brought stuff for that kind of thing from Brazil. But later I said, "If we are going to live here, we have to adapt to things here." And getting the medication from Brazil was complicated. Every time I needed a medication I had to send for it, and it took three or four days to arrive. Finally I said "No, we are going to adapt here." So now everything is from here, [medications] for the children and for us, everything is from here.

For others, transnational health approaches and decisions reflected feelings of being a misunderstood outsider, an immigrant on the margin:

I used to use Microvular birth control pills. My mother would send me a batch every six months. I had my gynecologist in Brazil—but you don't need a prescription to buy birth control pills in Brazil. I could have gotten pills here—it wasn't that. I had my mother send me the pills because, you know the old adage "when you're winning the game, don't change the team." I never got pregnant using that pill, I didn't want to change pills, so send me that one. Initially I brought up my allergy medication too, but then I didn't bring them any more, partly because I know that here they don't use those medications. Then again, why am I asking my mother to bring medications, syringes, ampoules of Aerolin®, when it's so difficult to get through immigration with those kinds of things? Maybe security was a little bit of an issue, but I also think that there's the subconscious issue of "In Brazil, they are the only ones who understand me." You're never going to be *completely understood* in a place where you didn't spend your childhood, I think. Maybe—I think that today I don't have so much of a problem with being understood, being understood as a person, but when I'm fragile and vulnerable, of course, that's when I feel totally misunderstood. And I think that *only in Brazil* will I be understood. (Julia)

Although Julia reported she no longer actively sought to procure Brazilian medications, it did not necessarily mean she felt comfortable with U.S. resources and providers. Julia spoke fluent English and was married to an American; it was clear that her references to the phenomenon of *not being understood* by non-Brazilian health care providers were much deeper and more complex than the issue of language. What she was articulating was an immigrant's sense of the personal vulnerability and marginalization that comes with being *other*.

Depending on the situation or context, these women felt, acted, identified themselves, or were identified by others as being "Brazilian," "immigrant," "American," or somewhere inside, outside, or in-between. Their narratives illustrated how *being Brazilian* was more than an identity tied to national origin; it was also a way to situate oneself as an immigrant in America. Being Brazilian was a way of coping with difficulties, a way to make meaning out of the struggles and hurdles of life as an immigrant, and a personal resource to fall back on. The use of home remedies and herbal teas, the mainstays of Brazilian folk medicine, was a frequently cited response to illness concerns. Mariana's story about using herbal teas for a cold was also a story about transnational migration and identity transformation:

When I first got here, I had a very bad cold, and so I went to the drugstore to try to get some medicine, but because I didn't understand the inserts, I couldn't figure out what to buy. I didn't go to a doctor, even though I should have—because the colds here are so much worse than they are in Brazil. So I was drinking tea, lime tea, orange rind tea, chamomile tea, vitamin C, and honey. I didn't drink tea in Brazil, I hated it! No way! Because when I was a little girl I had the mumps and my aunt, who was very bothersome, would force tea down my throat. So after that, I came to hate tea. But here, what was I to do? I couldn't take medicine, I had to at least take tea that had a medicinal effect, you know. I told my mother, "I learned how to drink tea here." Not because I like it, mind you. I still don't like it.

Mariana had come to recognize a new, transnational perspective on her personal and cultural identity as a Brazilian. Rather than framing her approaches to health in terms of being or becoming Americanized or acculturated, Mariana provided an example of the "reverse" process. In one of those paradoxical twists resulting from migration, she became "Brazilian" in a way she had not been before, drawing on a cultural health practice she had previously rejected.

The complex, transnational nature of immigrant women's health care practices and decisions are illustrated in the following three personal narratives. These stories reflect the practices of *going back to my own ways, transnational syncretism, personal responsibility,* and *putting health on hold.*

Sandra: Going Back to My Own Ways. As a newly arrived immigrant, Sandra had been eager and willing to adopt what she perceived as "American" health care practices. However, as time went by, she began to question some of these practices and examine them from a transnational perspective.

> After I moved here, I found that in this country you gain a lot of weight, compared with Brazil. The tendency is to gain weight. There is a lot of food. In Brazil, we also eat a lot, but it's different. I think there's more sun [in Brazil] and it melts the calories away! [laughter] I also think that people in Brazil are more active. And the sun and the climate help. I'm not sure. Besides there's so much pizza here, so much hamburger, a lot of French-fries. So, recently I began to note that my body—like the problem with the [ovarian] cyst, and other little health problems start showing up, and I think that everything is related to diet, because my diet here is completely different than it was in Brazil. So I'm trying to go back to the diet that I had before. Not like eating rice and beans, which was the everyday diet, but in the sense of eating more vegetables. At home [in Brazil] everyday there was kale, a vegetable, a salad, and lots of fresh food. And I used to drink lots of carrot juice, beet juice, that kind of thing. So I'm trying to go back to a healthier diet. But I'm already feeling better, going back to my old ways, and I've already lost some weight, and as the time passes I'm feeling that my body is healthier.

Sandra's narrative contained constant comparisons of "American and Brazilian" practices, beliefs, and values and of her personal beliefs and practices "before and after" immigrating. Underlying these comparisons was a transnational experience of being very much connected to both worlds and moving back and forth between those worlds in very fluid ways.

> There's this other thing about medications. Here everybody takes medicine, aspirin and the like. There are advertisements for aspirin, for all kinds of aspirin on the television. And the way people just take aspirin here. Because in Brazil, people usually take something like chamomile tea for stomach ache, herbal tea when a child has colic, and even children in Brazil, they take tea with honey and more things like that for colds and the like, than here. In Brazil, it's more teas and that sort of thing. And I think that it's more healthy. And that's the sort of thing that I try to do now. But when I first got here, I'd go straight to Walgreen's, and I'd take aspirin. But now I'm trying to return to my former habits, that I think are more healthy....I don't know if it's diet, but there was another thing that I found very interesting. In Brazil, when you have a period, no one goes around talking about PMS [premenstrual syndrome]. No one goes around talking about stress, no one goes around saying "I'm depressed because I'm having my period." No one *ever* says that. After I came here, I heard so many women talking about that, that I caught it! In Brazil, sometimes people would say "Don't stay in the sun, don't drink a lot of coffee or Coca-Cola®," but in reality I don't think anybody paid much attention to that kind of thing—it really isn't that big of a thing. And even if I had a problem of depression, being sort of down or sad without a real reason, nobody would have related that with menstruation. Because nobody talked about it. But here, any little thing that happens at the time when you're menstruating, it's "Oh, it's [menstruation]." It's something that is automatic, like putting two and two together. So here women are conditioned, they are always thinking "Oh, I'm depressed, I'm

going to get my period." "Oh, I'm depressed, I just had my period." And here I was, already getting into this habit. But I think it's really very psychological. I really think it's an excuse for everything. So now that I've analyzed the fact that in Brazil people don't think like this, after that I stopped thinking like this myself—so much so that if I start having a thought [like that], now I stop and look, I say to myself, "Hold on." So now I try to put a question mark first, rather than automatically putting myself into everything.

Sandra was rather self-critical of certain "American" health attitudes and practices she had initially adopted. The perspectives reflected in her narrative of *going back to my own way* call into question the notion of transnational acculturation as a unidirectional phenomenon.

Sonia: Transnational Syncretism and Personal Responsibility. Sonia's *transnational and syncretic approach* to her own health and illness concerns illustrated a high degree of integration of allopathic, interpersonal, and spiritual health concepts and resources. As an immigrant, she attributed her strong sense of *personal responsibility* and need to be in control of her health to the feeling of being *alone*.

> I do a lot of yoga and stretching. I've always done exercise. Not that kind of thing they do here, to build muscles—no, I do it to maintain my health, to stay in shape, doing breathing exercises, going to the park, breathing deeply, that kind of thing. I used to do it in Brazil, but there I didn't need it as much as I do here. Here I do it more often, because I feel that I need it more here, the stress here is much greater. And here I'm alone, I have to take care of everything by myself.

Uninsured and unemployed at the time, she recognized the limits of her dependency on the formal health care system, but she also knew how to make her needs known.

> I don't have any health insurance, I don't have anything. I just have health. I already had a serious health problem when I lived in France. But I managed, I learned how to cope with it, to fight it, and to kill it. But it wasn't easy. I have, I had an ulcer, a duodenal ulcer. I already had it when I was in Brazil. In Brazil, before I came here, I went to the doctor about my ulcer. I suffered and I sought treatment, but the doctors in Brazil, they always prescribed that Zantac® stuff. And it never did much. I'd get a little better, the pain would be alleviated a little, but then if I stopped taking the medication because I wasn't going to take it forever, you're only supposed to take three bottles—the ulcer would come back. It never worked. I also tried to do what the doctors said—never let your stomach go empty, always try to fill your stomach, because if your stomach is empty, it creates that secretion that will cause the pain. I tried, but you know how it is, you can't always follow that rigid kind of thing, the occasions and circumstances don't allow for that, and working in other peoples' homes, and eating what they have. When I first arrived here I suffered a lot. I myself know that I was under a lot of stress, because of my live-in jobs, and I felt even more stress, and my ulcer hurt, and I'd be nauseated, and I had to go to the doctor several times. They'd give me antibiotics that also helped. I went to a doctor at a Free Clinic….I said to the doctor, I was quite sincere, "Look here Doc, I have this, and this, and this. Don't tell me to get tests done, because I know what I have. I have an ulcer." Because I'd already done that endoscopy. So I already knew what I had. I said "Look, I know that ulcers may be caused by bacteria, and that a combination of antibiotics can kill them." And he said, "That's great that you know." Because I had already done my homework, I already knew more or less what I needed.

Sonia had a strong sense of her personal responsibility for her own health. She had *done her own homework* and recognized the links between her own behaviors, work, environment, and health.

> Then I stopped smoking, I quit cigarettes. Because it was better to stop smoking than keep smoking and stay sick. So I decided that smoking was causing a good part of my illness, so I quit ….Then soon after that, about 3 or 5 months, I met my husband. And he brought me a 5-liter bottle of aloe vera juice, and said, "Look, this is a remedy for you." And I said, "Great!" So every day in the morning I'd have some, before eating anything, before even getting out of bed—it's there, at the bedside. But the ulcer is caused by cigarettes, and I smoked, I smoked a lot, and it's also a very emotional issue, because when you don't breath correctly, when you don't have good posture, these are things I'm learn-

ing about now—posture, breathing, a lot of meditation, a lot of yoga, and a lot of not worrying, not frying your brain over stuff. That's how I take care of my health now. My husband helps me a lot, also, because he works with crystals and with his hands; he cured my ulcer; he put my ulcer out. And he also cleansed me, using massage, and crystals, and giving me lots of love. It's love that cures, too. He'd kiss my tummy and say, "It's going to get better, it's going to go away, there won't be anything left," and he'd kiss me and care for me.

Sonia actively utilized the resources of both formal health care providers and traditional healing practices in addressing her health problems. In contrast to Sonia's *transnational syncretism*, Vera was very uncomfortable with a U.S. physician's advice to see an acupuncturist for treatment of the pain and swelling in her legs. She felt this put her in a position of having to make a choice between opposing systems of healing:

> See how bad this looks, how swollen my legs are? They've done blood tests twice, because it could be a serious disease, which I don't have ....This doctor thought that I should have gotten better, but I didn't get much better. So she sent me to another doctor [an acupuncturist]. I only had one acupuncture session. I don't know if I will go back or not. I've never had acupuncture in my life, and I don't think it goes well together, an oriental orientation with a western orientation. They sort of collide. I think I'd have to choose between them, so that they wouldn't collide.

Mariana: Putting Health on Hold. Limited time and resources, coupled with a transient mindset (even among long-term residents), contributed toward the attitude and practice of delaying or postponing the seeking of professional health care. Immigration status, economics, work and employment demands, and a multitude of access to care issues all factored into the practice of *putting health on hold*. This stance was particularly evident among women who indicated they were undocumented and those who had come specifically as economic sojourners with intentions of returning to Brazil. However, similar patterns of delayed care seeking behaviors also surfaced in the narratives of women with legal immigration status and even among the more long-term migrants.

Mariana's story of *putting health on hold* illustrated the complex, gendered negotiations that immigrants frequently engage in when making decisions about health and health care. In Mariana's case, the practice of putting her own health on hold resulted from both intentional and unintentional actions and decisions. She and her husband worked together in their own informal housecleaning business. In making decisions related to her own oral health needs, Mariana took into consideration financial concerns, premigration preventive practices, treatment options and costs, direct and indirect personal costs, and also weighed her personal health needs with those of her husband:

> I went to the dentist once. He examined my teeth and gave me an estimate of the treatment costs. Just for one tooth for which I need to replace the filling, it would have cost $800. But I am not going to have it done. I'm lucky that I have good teeth, and two years ago when I went to the dentist [in Brazil, before immigrating], I didn't have any cavities. Now this time when I went, I had one cavity. I'm only going to have that one cavity filled, so I won't have a problem later....We looked into the dental clinic at the university, but it's not that much cheaper...the difference in price isn't that much, and you have to have more time for the treatment at the university clinic. And for example, in our case, if we'd go to the university clinic, all of a sudden we'd lose a whole afternoon—that's a whole afternoon that we don't work. So I'm not going to take care of that now; I'm not going to have the dental treatment. I'll just wait and get my teeth fixed in Brazil. And if it were the case of having dental treatment, I'd prefer that my husband have his teeth taken care of, because his teeth are almost all gone.

Mariana noted that her intentions and actions related to delaying or seeking formal health care were not only related to cost, but also to a multitude of other factors, including information and knowledge barriers, her personal, culturally informed practices, and actual and perceived barriers to formal care:

> No, I haven't gone to a doctor here. Once when I had a lot of vaginal itching I needed to go to a doctor. It was very strong, really very strong. So I needed to go [to a doctor] and I just kept putting it off. You know? I don't know if it is so with Americans or not, but a Brazilian only goes to the doctor when there is no other way out. At least that's the way it is with me. So I was intending to go to a doctor, but how was I to do it? First you have to find someone who can give you a recommendation or a suggestion. Then you have to go, and then there is the issue of how much it's going to cost, and it just goes on and on. I finally did find out about a clinic in the [neighborhood], where you don't have to pay, you just help out with whatever you can. I even went to this clinic, but when I got there it was closed. And then I never went back, and the itching went away. I used a cream that is sold at Safeway. I used it and the itching stopped, but every once in a while it comes back. You know, I won't have it for four months, then it comes back, with discharge and with a strong odor, so I go and use the medicine. It stops for awhile then it comes back. I had the same thing in Brazil and I went to the doctor who gave me more or less the same thing. In Brazil I used it only once and I didn't need it anymore. I was lucky because I already knew the cream that you use. It has an applicator. After I came here [to the United Sates] it happens that it [the vaginal itching] comes back when I get tense. When I am very tense, very nervous and so forth, then it comes back.

In the end, Mariana resolved the vaginal itching by putting it temporarily on hold, relying on her own knowledge and resources constructed and accessed through her transnational experiences. Prior to immigrating, a Brazilian doctor had prescribed a vaginal cream, a treatment Mariana had deemed successful because the symptoms had subsided. In the face of multiple barriers to accessing a professional health care provider, Mariana drew on her premigration experiences, locating what she thought was a similar vaginal preparation (identified by the applicator) on the shelves of the local supermarket. What she probably did not realize is numerous vaginal preparations are sold with applicators, making the presence of an application an unreliable identification criterion. It is quite possible that the over-the-counter medication she had purchased was not appropriate or effective. Yet Mariana appeared confident that she had found an appropriate medication and interpreted the repeated flare-ups of vaginal symptoms to her state of nervous tension, which she in turn related to the level of stress in her life as an immigrant.

Mariana identified smoking as one of the ways she coped with the stress of her multiple responsibilities as a young immigrant domestic worker. Another example of *putting her own health on hold*, Mariana delayed further resolutions or attempts to stop smoking until some (idealized) time in the future, when she returned to Brazil:

> There are lots of worries and concerns, every day. Every day it's something different, something to do, a hurdle to get over. It's either the language, or the social aspect, or a problem that you have to call and take care of…everything that has to do with housekeeping, that's my own realm, and I'm on top of that. But if it's something outside that realm, I just don't feel as secure, and there are bigger communication problems. Yea. I think that's why I can't control it, why I can't quit smoking, because here [in the United States], for me, cigarettes are a form of relaxation, a tranquilizer. After I finish cleaning a house I get in my car and light up…I've already tried to quit smoking, but I turned into a nervous wreck. There's no way that I'm going to quit smoking here. In Brazil, when I'm tranquil and calm, yes. But here life is so worrisome and there is so much responsibility.

These individual women's stories illustrate different patterns and practices as well as diverse rationales for immigrants' practices of adopting, relying on, resorting to, or returning to home or host-based health approaches and resources.

Crossing Multiple Borders and Barriers

Life as an immigrant entails crossing multiple borders, of which national boundaries are only the first. In their efforts to cross the borders of the formal U.S. health care system, these Brazilian women confronted access and utilization issues related to language, culture, communication, information, transportation, cost, insurance coverage, satisfaction, and trust. In the process, they often relied on *informal social and employment networks*. The stories of women's experiences in *interfacing with the U.S. health care providers* in various contexts and settings revealed the diversity of their responses and interpretations, ranging from *satisfaction* and a sense of *being valued* to *disillusion, distrust, and resistance*. In telling their stories they represented views and perspectives from the margins that illustrated the economic, political, and cultural barriers that confront immigrants on the borders of the formal health care system. At the same time, they also highlighted the various transnational resources and practices immigrants create and use to gain information and access to health care.

Gaining Information

Information and access to the formal U.S. health care system were frequently gained through informal contacts and connections rather than directly through formal channels. In seeking and obtaining information about formal health care resources, women commonly relied on personal contacts, such as family members, friends, or acquaintances (either Brazilian or American).

> Asking, asking friends. I have a friend, he's an American ....He always oriented me, he'd show me things and say, "This is the Free Clinic," and he gave me addresses, and he'd give me a boost in that sense. He lives here in the neighborhood, and always talks with me, gives me strength and encouragement, you know. I ask him for information, and ask another friend too. (Sonia)

> My sister told me about the clinic. She'd been there. Because here they are more concerned about women's health than in Brazil. In Brazil, I had to do everything private pay, and it's very expensive, and the exams are very expensive. And here I haven't had any problems. I went to a clinic, and I'm taking birth control pills from the clinic. I went there, they gave me the medication, and I had an exam. It's not a private clinic. I have some friends who go to the clinic too. (Helena)

Although a commonly used resource, family and social networks were not always sources of useful or reliable information. When Raquel was going through the process to obtain her immigrant visa, she was diagnosed with tuberculosis and needed treatment. Her husband, a naturalized American citizen who had served in the U.S. military, did not know or understand the eligibility guidelines for his family members:

> At that time, I wasn't very well informed. I could have used my husband's military health service—because he was in the military...but he also wasn't very well informed, he didn't know what rights I could have as far as using the military health services.

In searching for information on affordable health care options, Flora combined her own resourcefulness with information she gathered from other Brazilian immigrants and health care professionals:

> Janaína had already told me about Planned Parenthood...and I have a cousin...and she has a friend, a Brazilian nurse who lives here, named Sibele. Anyway, my cousin came back to visit in January, and we went out to dinner with Sibele. So later, when André was sick, and agonizing over this thing about being sick, and agonizing even more just thinking about having to pay a hospital bill, I started looking around. I've been researching the materials from one health plan [a local Health Maintenance Organization] to see what we could do, what's most viable. I called Sibele and she told me some of the places that I could go, that had some kind of walk-in clinics, you know—places that would be some of the cheaper options. She told me about some places, and with the references she gave me I went out and did more research, and I ended up finding different places, such as a clinic here in the [neighborhood], near a church, some things like that. I made a list to have if one day we'd need it. Fortunately we haven't needed to use it yet. Sibele also told me about some things to do to take care of colds.

Informal Access to Professional Health Care Providers

Informal access to professional health care providers was a valuable resource because of the many barriers the women faced in accessing the formal health care system. Informal access to health care professionals was used to gain information, referrals, and even actual services. Several of the women had informal access to U.S. health care professionals through their employment as domestic workers.

> I go to the dental school. Because the first employer I had, he was a dental student, and he got me in at the dental school clinic and started my treatment. Then he passed me on to another student, and then another. (Sonia)

> [When] I was working for Dr. Janet, I had a gynecological exam with her, and a blood test—that sort of thing, and she didn't charge me anything. She told me to go to her office and she didn't charge me anything. (Adélia)

> Usually, if Judith [her employer, a physician] is around, I'll ask her, Like if I think that Rebecca has an ear infection, I'll ask her to check her ears, because Judith has all the instruments for checking ears and stuff. (Joana)

Joana's narrative illustrated how immigrants' own social networks intertwined with their health and employment networks, blurring the distinction between formal and informal systems. Several years after arriving in the United States to work as a nanny, Joana was diagnosed and treated for a gastric ulcer. As a result, she had developed a certain degree of expertise and understanding of the U.S. health care and insurance systems. Using her knowledge and connections, Joana provided an informal physician recommendation and referral service for other Brazilian immigrant domestic workers she knew. The physician, in turn, engaged her immigrant patients as domestic workers, creating an interactive, transnational network of women physicians, patients, domestic workers, and employers:

> After I got sick I decided to get health insurance .... I had this gynecologist, whom I'd gone to because of my [menstrual] cramps, and she recommended this general practitioner to me. Because, of course, [in this system] you always have to have a general practitioner. The gynecologist was a provider from my insurance plan. I looked in my little book. She was new, she had just gotten her credentials from my insurance plan. You have to go to a doctor on the insurance list, otherwise they won't pay. So I went to her, and then she recommended this other one [general practitioner] that I go to, this lady doctor. She's also Leonora's doctor; I'm the one who told her about this doctor, who speaks Spanish. Because Leonora doesn't speak English, and I'm the one who arranged for her to go to this doctor. The doctor lives and works around here and I also worked for her for some months; then I stopped, because she didn't need me any more. I babysat her two little kids. I met her at her office. Then she called me to see if I knew of someone [to do domestic work], and I gave her the names of a couple of people. One of them was Adélia.

Interfacing With U.S. Health Care Professionals

Most of the immigrant women reported some type of contact with the U.S. health care system, for reasons of either personal or family health care. In describing their experiences with U.S. health care providers, these Brazilian women voiced sentiments ranging from appreciation to frustration and even anger. Women made specific note of a variety of provider and setting characteristics, including cost, qualifications, efficiency, organization, personalized attention, and quality of care.

> A couple of weeks ago I went to the [Health Center], which is free. I found an excellent doctor, very socially conscious, good intellect. Of course, in order to work there in front of the [subsidized housing] projects, you have to be that way, not somebody old-fashioned. It was really great.... I also have a very good acupuncturist. But not very cheap. Nothing is cheap of course. And I had to pay out of my own pocket, because I didn't have insurance. So I didn't go there any more, but I liked him. (Julia)

> The other place I do go is to a women's clinic—it's another free clinic, where I can have a gynecological exam. They do everything, to check to see if everything is okay. And they treated me really super. It's very organized, they always send me letters, asking how I am, telling me it's time for another exam, and I go and have it. I give them a little dough to help out, when I go. I never get off for free, I always give 10 dollars, 15 dollars. It's super

efficient, and I like their work. They give out condoms and have all kind of assistance. (Sonia)

Personal receptivity and criteria for judging health care professionals obviously varied, but when U.S. health care providers attempted to reach across language and cultural borders and demonstrated personal interest and concern, their efforts usually met with acceptance and appreciation.

When I went [to the clinic] the first time I was received very well. They even tried to understand the language. There is a girl who speaks Spanish sort of mixed with Portuguese; she understands [Portuguese] well. They even do that, try to understand [me] better. That was the girl who called me [with the results of my Pap smear] and she sort of spoke Portuguese, and she said, "Don't worry, but your exam showed a change, so you need to redo it. But you have to wait to redo the test." But she said, "Don't worry, it doesn't mean you have cancer. But it's important that you come back in two months." (Helena)

The people at the [Public Health Clinic] pay attention to me ....Now I speak English with them, but in the beginning they didn't understand me, but they had people who spoke Spanish, and I'd go to the doctor and they'd send in a translator, a person who spoke Spanish to help me—it was great. They are great, too. (Ana Maria)

In contrast, impersonal treatment from health care providers was a source of frustration and disillusion for these immigrants. It might well be argued that on this point they did not differ from native-born users of the health care system. As illustrated in the following two personal narratives—immigrant women's personal experiences with the U.S. healthcare system, and their interpretations of these experiences, played out within dynamic and multilayered contexts of transnational migration, class, culture, gender, and personal and public health issues and concerns.

Julia: Personal and Political Resistance to Tuberculosis Prophylaxis. In the immigrant health literature on tuberculosis (TB), resistance usually refers to antibiotics, but Julia's story was about a different type of resistance. Julia worked as a waitress and also was enrolled as a graduate student at a local state university. In the process of seeking other employment, she was required to have a Purified Protein Derivative (PPD) tuberculin test. Her story presented an immigrant's personal and political perspective on a public health issue.

I had my TB test done at the university. I have the sense that people [health care providers] have to be very careful these days, because of all the suing and lawsuits, and they don't want to expose themselves, or sign on the dotted line. When I went there and the test came out positive, I told them, "Well, I've had BCG. I had three doses of BCG. In my day, in Brazil, you got BCG three times. I had it when I was 16, when I was 10, and before that, I don't remember exactly when." And at the time I was studying psychoneuroimmunology. That was like my biggest class last semester. And I was really into immunology. Then this woman turned to me and said, "You have to take this medicine, because you may have been exposed." She was a Registered Nurse. She was super nice, but very conservative. And I think that she has a certain degree of reason on her side, but I think that the greatest percentage is fear. There is a lot of fear. She is following what the American authorities are saying, because a lot of people come here, across the border, and don't do anything [about their own health], but it's not my case. Me, I don't want to take the medicine. Because you have to take it for six months, and I already have a hard time remembering to take my birth control pill every day, and I'm going to have to remember this other medication too? And I don't have insurance. And what if all of a sudden I get hepatitis, as a side effect? I understand that perhaps I'm not being totally correct, but I don't feel at all guilty, not even a little bit. Not at all. I got an X-ray, and it's clear.

In her narrative of personal resistance, Julia presented various perspectives and contexts from which her positive PPD results had been interpreted. She recognized immigration as both a political and public issue and also viewed the practices of U.S. health care providers within the context of a litigious society. Julia acknowledged that behaviors of individual health care providers are embedded within the broader context of public health concerns.

Again, I think that it's a political issue for the doctors. Everyone has a political posture, wherever ....The nurse has a political posture and the nurse can follow the politics or not. They [health care providers] are not very accommodating. My X-ray came out clear. But you know what they wrote? "Her TB skin test came out positive. Her X-ray is clear. *She is not contagious.*" Again, it's just a way of covering for themselves! "She is not contagious." But come on, am I gonna get a job when it says *"She is not contagious?"* I mean, it looks like I really have the bacteria, except that I'm not contagious, and I'm not contaminating anyone, but that I have it. They didn't say anything about the fact that I took BCG. But the other woman at [another medical center], she did write that down. But at the University Health Service, no. She *wanted* me to take the medicine. She said, "I want you to take this medicine" and she kept calling me, and I said, "Look, I understand the situation and I don't want to. It's my decision. If I want to in the future, I'll get in touch with you." So when I went to [the other medical center], I talked to a woman, and she said, "Look, I understand where you're coming from...I think that you take the medicine if you think it's important for you. You had your X-ray done, and it was clear, you took BCG, as far as I'm concerned, I think that you are 'eye-ball healthy.' She used that expression, you know, like you look at the person and say, "You're healthy." So now I don't worry about it. I turned in my papers, and I was accepted at the employment agency.

Underlying the individual nurse's behavior and the policies that guided it, Julia identified a common fear of immigrants. Julia branded the one nurse as *conservative* because she followed protocols and rules to the letter: Treat a positive PPD, no questions asked, no exceptions to the rule. From Julia's perspective, the nurse's recommendation for prophylactic treatment was based solely on protocol, without considering her individual variables or context. The nurse's insistence in *wanting me to take the medicine* smacked of authoritarian imposition and showed no consideration for her personal perspective or context. In contrast, the provider at the other facility acknowledged and understood her personal point of view, and considered other parameters (e.g., previous exposure to BCG) in interpreting the positive PPD result. Julia recognized the concern about tuberculosis as a public and immigrant health problem. But as an individual immigrant, she felt her personal perspectives and context had not been taken into consideration.

I think that when you are a child, your thymus, and the memory cells, they are more alert. And it's possible that I've been exposed; that's true. It's hard for me to be in this kind of situation in which I have to fight with the red tape and deal with the assumed situation that I might actually have the bacteria. But I think that perhaps because I'm very anti- whatever conservative, I interpreted that reality as a political situation much more than anything else. I have friends at the university who work in the Department of Immunology and they told me, "It's all because lots of Chinese came over here on boats, bringing TB. It's very logical that the immigration officials have to do something about it." So I thought, "Right on, that's true." But I felt discriminated against, I felt that I had been mistreated and abused by them, but at the same time, the first reaction that you have is an emotional reaction. I said, "Those SOB Chinese! Now I have to take this darn medicine [a merda deste remédio] because of these Chinese! Whoever told them to come over by boat?" Shoot [porra], I really don't have anything against the Chinese. But the health care providers aren't very understanding. Like that nurse that wants me to take the medicine and that's it.

Many, if not most, health care providers and public health officials would probably label Julia's resistance to prophylactic antibiotic treatment as "noncompliant" patient behavior. However, Julia's transnational interpretation of the situation reflected the intersection of personal, public, and political perspectives. Categorized as an immigrant, Julia felt marginalized, discriminated against, and stereotyped as a threat to the public health.

Fátima: A Disillusioned, Disheartened, and Distrustful Transnational Border Casualty. Fátima's interactions with the U.S. health care system had resulted in her feeling disillusioned, disheartened, and distrustful. In her case, neither her intentional premigration preparation and planning, nor the fact that she and her family had insurance provided through her husband's employment with a multinational corporation, made access to the U.S.

health care system easier or more satisfying. Many of the parameters she used to judge the U.S. health care system were based on her premigration experiences in Brazil. In particular, Fátima's relationship with her hometown homeopathic physician framed her perspectives on U.S. providers. In contrast to the health care she had received in Brazil, Fátima found the U.S. health care system unfamiliar, impersonal, alienating, and driven by an economic bottom line.

> Before we came here, in Brazil I only used homeopathic treatment. My children were brought up only with homeopathy. So I was accustomed to that kind of care and assistance, where you practically have a doctor at your disposition, even more so in a small town, where our doctor was more than a doctor, he was a friend. The minute I needed him, he found a way to see me. He talked with me, if I had a problem. He was just like family. He ended up becoming family. So there was a lot of trust, a lot of understanding. It was almost like I didn't even need to talk. Because he already knew what was going on in my life. So before coming here I loaded down with homeopathic medicine, and promised myself that I wouldn't change, no matter what. But when I got here I found everything so difficult. It's only when you get here that you see how difficult it is to find a person who is open, willing, and interested in taking care of you and in seeing you as a person. Everything is a question of money. Very practical. If it's worth it, yes, if it's not worth it, good-bye. This really shocked me. So when we moved here the company offered us a health plan. And since we didn't know where to go for assistance, we got this health plan which is the one I still have today, and I think it is *awful*. I have all the complaints about this health plan you could possibly imagine. But even today I still don't know how to get out of it, how to find something better, you know? Such as homeopathy, a more natural medicine, that's what I'd like to have for my family.

Initially Fátima was able to function as a self-sufficient family health practitioner, with an occasional long-distance consultation with her homeopathic physician in Brazil. However, migration disrupted her life in many ways. Although she came with the intention of maintaining her familiar health care practices, over time she discovered that she lacked the environmental and personal support and resources to do so.

> But before I came, I came prepared. I did everything I could to make sure that the children wouldn't need anything, and I was here for a good while without needing any attention here, taking care of everything myself, with the things that I knew, with the medications that I had. But, after about a year or so, it was over. I didn't have the medications, but besides not having the medications, I didn't have anyone with whom I could obtain the information I needed. There was a time when I'd call Brazil and ask for the doctor there to orient me, but then I didn't know where to buy the homeopathic medications here. And then I started having a lot of doubts. My husband started pressuring me a lot to have someone here as a backup, someone with knowledge, to look after the children. So I began to let it go, and I started going back to allopathy. I had to choose doctors by chance and luck, with my finger on the book. Whatever they gave me I had to take. My children never had one doctor, because I never liked any of them, so every time they'd go I'd take them to a different doctor. I don't like the care, because nobody looks you eye to eye, nobody treats you with interest and attention. I've found very few, if any, who do. So I go searching, and the minute I find one that fits, I'll stay, but so far I haven't found anyone. So when the children get sick, I take them, and when the people ask if I have a doctor, I reply, "No I don't have one. Give me anyone, whoever there is. I don't have a preference."

At the time of the interview, Fátima's adolescent daughter was undergoing treatment for a drug and alcohol problem. In her narrative, Fátima voiced stronger concerns and dissatisfaction for the "system" and the "treatment" than with her daughter's problem per se. She felt the culture and legalities of U.S. institutions tied her hands and found the professionals who were supposed to provide assistance and support to be disinterested and impersonal.

> I didn't mention that I have a family problem, my daughter has a drug and alcohol problem. And that's where I've seen the lack of support from the medical establishment, the lack of support from people in the community. Despite all the talk about it being a national concern, what you see here, anywhere, is that there is so little that is being done. What you hope would be done, and what there really is, it's very frustrating. But I haven't lost hope that

things will change, that things will get better ....We've been doing group treatment ever since February—in a group, and me alone, and her alone with a psychiatrist, and taking Prozac. But there was just this disinterest, how should I say it, it was so impersonal, the people who were there to assist you, it was like we were just one more case. There wasn't the concern that *this is a person, this is a being,* and *this is a family that is suffering* ....So I don't have any respect for the institution. I don't think that they are serious. They may want to be serious, but unfortunately the system doesn't function. That's how I see it ....Here, when the parents want to take a position, they can't because the children have rights that can't be infringed upon, so you end up not being able to do anything, not being able to help, not being able to take a position, because your hands are tied, whatever side you're on, it's wrong....So that's why I hope that by going to Chile, it will be different. There I'm going to be able to take a position that I think is best for her.

As Fátima was preparing for yet another transnational migration experience, she held on to the hope of being able to rely more on her own personal resources and feel more in control of her family's health, just as she had initially intended when she first came to the United States.

Discussion

Immigrant Transitions and Health

Transnational migration is a global phenomenon involving the constant flow and movement of persons and goods across national borders; it also involves fluid and complex fields of connections and ties to both host and home societies, of which health is an integral part. The results of this qualitative research support the conceptualization of health as a transnational phenomenon. The health experiences, attitudes, and behaviors reported in this study characterized the participants as transmigrants, persons who forge and sustain multistranded social relations linking their societies of origin and settlement [1, 2]. These immigrant women's health practices and health care seeking decisions and actions occurred within transnational social fields, at the intersections of Brazilian and U.S. personal, familial, social, cultural, economic, and political contexts.

Making comparisons and connections was one of the threads that ran through these Brazilian women's narratives. Making comparisons was a way of situating themselves and making sense of their host and home contexts. They compared their lives, work, and health pre- and post-migration; they compared Brazilian and American health care systems; and they compared their own health practices and beliefs to other Brazilian immigrants and to Americans. In the process, they identified a variety of health practices and resources rooted in their Brazilian culture or identity, and described the contacts and connections they forged in order to access resources in the United States.

From a nursing and health perspective, immigrants' experiences have been examined within a transitions framework.[11, 12] This research provided support for the concept of immigration as a transnational transition characterized by dynamic, multidirectional movement rather than a linear and unidirectional trajectory toward acculturation and assimilation. As Pessar [21] aptly noted in relation to migrants' transnational identities, practices, and institutions, "permanent settlement or permanent return are merely two of the possible outcomes; lives constructed across national boundaries is another" (p. 588). Even for those who settle permanently in the United States, it may be more appropriate to conceptualize transnational migration experiences as ongoing, recurring, or unending transitions. This does not necessarily mean that immigrants are constantly in a state of disconnectedness, flux, or change. However, such states may periodically surface, particularly related to health or illness concerns or crises.

Immigrants' Transnational Health Resources

Immigrant social networks are dynamic forces through which individuals and groups respond to forces in the larger environment.[23] Such networks have been shown to facilitate as well as constrain immigrants' access to health care.[24, 25] The women in this study created and benefited from their informal social networks to access information and formal U.S. health care resources. Transnational medication practices, similar to those that have been documented among the immigrant populations living in close proximity to the Mexican border, were clearly evident among these Brazilian immigrants.[21, 26, 27] The practice of combining multiple healing systems is certainly not unique to the immigrant women in this study; similar practices been documented among other immigrant groups in the United States.[25]

As demonstrated in the results of this study, cultural identity may serve as a health resource for immigrant women. The intertwining of cultural identity with women's household and community health production work has been noted in previous research. Kay[27] reported how some Mexican American women reclaimed their cultural identity by seeking older women kin to teach them traditional cultural health practices and birthing techniques. Clark[28] described how poor Mexican American women reaffirmed their cultural identity and reinforced their place in intergenerational and social networks through their household and community health production work. Immigrant women's roles and practices as family and community health care providers certainly warrant further attention by practitioners and researchers.

A wide range of factors may affect the ability or willingness of immigrants to access formal U.S. health care services.[25] As this study demonstrated, immigrants often intentionally avoid or delay seeking care from professionals in the formal health care sector. Difficulties and barriers to access also may increase the use of alternative or folk practices, or practitioners by immigrants.[30, 31] Such practices do not necessarily signify a rejection of formal biomedical practice, but may rather be an indication of parallel and simultaneous practices.[32-34] As immigrants move between folk and formal health care systems of both their home and host societies and cultures, they come in contact with different belief and normative systems, often selectively combining or eliminating elements from both systems.[35] In this study, there were examples of syncretism as well as selective adoption or elimination of strategies or approaches to personal health and illness care; whereas some women were receptive to new or different resources or practices, others actively resisted adaptation or change.

Implications for Research and Practice

On a national and international level, transnational migration has significant implications in terms of public health. For example, several women in this study related incidents with a focus on tuberculosis screening and prophylaxis programs and practices in the United States. On one level, their stories illustrated the trickle-down effects of public health practices on individual immigrant's lives; on another level, they highlighted the need for a transnational perspective in public health policy and practice. U.S. public health officials are rightly concerned about the spread of tuberculosis and immigrants have been identified as a high-risk population. However, the strategies for identifying and treating nonimmigrant Americans may not be the most appropriate strategies for diverse immigrant groups. The implications for public health go beyond the successful treatment of individual immigrants; designing and implementing public health approaches that are medically sound, accessible, and acceptable to immigrants would also prevent unnecessary waste of energy and resources.

Negative perceptions of relationships with U.S. health care providers, particularly feelings of being discounted, blamed, not understood, or acknowledged by health care personnel, as well as the expectations and satisfaction with providers who are patient, respectful, attentive, and friendly, have also been documented in research with Mexican Americans [36, 37]. The results of this research suggest the need for health care providers to recognize and acknowledge the adeptness and comfort level of their clients—immigrants and nonimmigrants as well—in crossing borders and moving between various health care systems and practices. Language, education, culture, migration history, employment, social support, expectations, health status, and transnational experiences all may contribute to the way immigrant women construct their identities, roles, expectations, and responses with regard to the U.S. health care system. Building trust and relationships with immigrant clients requires time as well as cultural, linguistic, and interpersonal skills on the part of health care providers. Despite the current trend in U.S. health care that equates time with higher costs, the benefits of spending time with immigrants and making the best use of that time must be considered and documented through practice and research. Incorporating "storytelling" approaches to medical history-taking may, at first, appear time-consuming, but the results of this research suggest it is an excellent way to explore immigrants' transnational perspectives and resources. One way for the clinician to gain entrée to immigrants' experiences is to incorporate questions about migration history and experiences, premigration health practices, and transnational sources of information, medications, and care into the health history interview.

The provision of quality health care for immigrants depends in part on the cultural competency of health care providers, institutions, and researchers.[38] Immigrant health care necessitates cultural competency on the part of health care providers and institutions. By offering nonjudgmental environments and contexts in which immigrants can explore and discuss their expectations and responses, practitioners and researchers can identify educational needs of immigrants in relation to the U.S. health care system and explore ways to improve the quality of health care. An equally important challenge is that of increasing the capacity and competency of immigrants in accessing health care services that meet their health needs and expectations. Community-based programs that incorporate immigrant social and employment networks are another resource that can be mobilized in the efforts to optimize immigrants' capacity to access the formal U.S. health care system more effectively and efficiently and to make better use of resources available to them. Because of women's roles as family and community health care providers, it is important to further identify and understand the gendered aspects of immigrant personal and communal health practices as well as care-seeking behaviors.

The results of this qualitative research highlighted the transnational nature of the health care perspectives, practices, and resources among a group of Brazilian immigrant women. Due to the methodological approach, the results are limited in the sense that they are informed by the specific social, cultural, class, occupational, health, and migration experiences of the women who participated in the study. However, the transnational perspectives, practices, and resources identified and described in this study may be used to inform future research on immigrant health. To date, studies of health seeking behaviors among very diverse groups of immigrants have used a variety of definitions and measures of acculturation, which have produced inconsistent findings.[27] Furthermore, the gendered nature of transnational migration has only recently been explored in more depth.[5, 22, 38] As a result, scholars and practitioners continue to face the challenge to pursue new frameworks for immigrant health research and practice. Longitudinal and comparative studies of other immigrant groups are necessary to expand the knowledge and understanding of the transnational nature of immigrant health. Researchers and practitioners also need to explore how the intersections of certain axes of inequality, such as gender, class, race, culture, ethnicity, sexuality, and immigration status affect transnational health practices, perspectives, and resources.

Acknowledgments

This research was funded by the National Institutes of Health (#NR07055, T32) and the University of California, San Francisco, School of Nursing Century Fund.

REFERENCES

1. Glick Schiller N, Basch L, Blanc-Szanton C: Towards a definition of transnationalism: Intro-

ductory remarks and research questions: In: Glick Schiller N, Basch L, Blanc-Szanton C, eds. Towards a Transnational Perspective on Migration: Race, Class, Ethnicity, and Nationalism Reconsidered. New York: New York Academy of Sciences; 1992: ix–xiv
2. Glick Schiller N, Basch L, Blanc-Szanton C: Transnationalism: A new analytic framework for understanding migration: In: Glick Schiller N, Basch L, Blanc-Szanton C, eds. Towards a Transnational Perspective on Migration: Race, Class, Ethnicity, and Nationalism Reconsidered. New York: New York Academy of Sciences; 1992:1–24
3. Messias DKH: Transnational perspectives on women's domestic work: Experiences of Brazilian immigrants in the United States. Women Health 2001; 33(1/2):1–20
4. Argülles L, Rivero AM: Gender/sexual orientation violence and transnational migration: Conversations with some Latinas we think we know. Urban Anthropol 1993; 22(3/4):259–275
5. Hondagneu-Sotelo P: Gendered Transitions: Mexican Experiences of Immigration. Berkeley, CA: University of California; 1994
6. Hondagneu-Sotelo P: Regulating the unregulated? Domestic workers' social networks. Soc Probl 1994; 41(1):50–64
7. Hondagneu-Sotelo P: Introduction: Gender and contemporary U.S. immigration. Am Behav Sci 1999; 42(4):565–576
8. Rogler L: International migrations: A framework for directing research. Am Psychol 1994; 49(8): 701–708
9. Rouse R: Mexican migration and the social space of postmodernism. Diaspora 1991; 1(1):8–23
10. Rouse R: Making sense of settlement: Class transformation, cultural struggle, and transnationalism among Mexican migrants in the United States: In: Glick Schiller N, Basch L, Blanc-Szanton C, eds. Towards a Transnational Perspective on Migration: Race, Class, Ethnicity, and Nationalism Reconsidered. New York: New York Academy of Sciences; 1992:25–52
11. Messias DKH: Narratives of Transnational Migration, Work, and Health: The Lived Experiences of Brazilian Women in the United States, Dissertation, University of California, San Francisco; 1997
12. Meleis AI, Sawyer LM, Im E, Messias DKH, Schumacher K: Experiencing transitions: An emerging middle-range theory. Adv Nurs Sci 2000; 23(1):12–28
13. Bell SE: Becoming a political woman: The reconstruction and interpretation of experience through stories: In: Todd AD, Fisher S, eds. Gender and Discourse: The Power of Talk. Norwood, NJ: Ablex; 1988:97–123
14. Devault ML: Talking and listening from women's standpoint: Feminist strategies for interviewing and analysis. Soc Probl 1990;37(1):96–116
15. Gorelick S: Contradictions of feminist methodology. Gender Soc 1991; 5:459–477
16. Messias DKH, DeJoseph JF: Feminist narrative interpretation: An approach to stories. In review.-Personal Narratives Group, ed.: Interpreting Women's Lives: Feminist Theory and Personal Narratives. Bloomington, IN: Indiana University Press; 1989
17. Riessman CK: Narrative Analysis. Newbury Park, CA: Sage; 1993
18. Strauss A, Corbin J: Basics of Qualitative Research: Grounded Theory Procedures and Techniques. Newbury Park, CA: Sage; 1990
19. Margolis MS: Little Brazil: An Ethnography of Brazilian Immigrants in New York City. Princeton, NJ: Princeton University Press; 1994
20. Pylpa J: Self-medication practices in two California Mexican communities. J Immigr Health 2001; 3(2):59–75
21. Pessar PR: Engendering migration studies: The case of new immigrants in the United States. Am Behav Sci 1999; 42(4):577–600
22. Salzinger L: A maid by any other name: In: Burawoy M, Burton A, Ferguson AA, Fox KJ, Gamson J, Gartrell N, Hurst L, Kurzman C, Salzinger L, Schiffman J, Ui S, eds. Ethnography Unbound: Power and Resistance in the Modern Metropolis. Berkeley, CA: University of California Press; 1991:139–160
23. Derose KP: Networks of care: How Latina immigrants find their way to and through a county hospital. J Immigr Health 2000; 2(2):79–87
24. Ell E, Castañeda I: Health care seeking behavior: In: Loue S, ed. Handbook of Immigrant Health. New York: Plenum; 1998:203–226
25. Lloyd LS: Border health: In: Loue S, ed. Handbook of Immigrant Health. New York: Plenum; 1998:243–260
26. Eisenstadt TA, Thorup CL: Caring Capacity Versus Carrying Capacity: Community Responses to Mexican Immigration in San Diego's North County (Mongraph Series 39). San Diego, CA: Center for U.S.–Mexican Studies, University of California; 1994
27. Kay MA: Mexican, Mexican American and Chicana child-birth: In: Melville M, ed. Twice a Minority: Mexican American Women. St Louis, MO: CV Mosby; 1980:52–65
28. Clark L: Gender and generation in poor women's household health production experiences. Med Anthropol Q 1993; 7(4):386–402

29. Bakx K: The "eclipse" of folk medicine in western society. Soc Health Illness 1991; 13(1):20–38
30. Laguerre MS: The Informal City. London: Macmillan; 1994
31. Cant SL, Calnan M: On the margins of the medical marketplace? An exploratory study of alternative practitioners' perceptions. Soc Health Illness 1991; 13(1):39–57
32. Murray J, Shepard S: Alternative or additional medicine? A new dilemma for the doctor? J R Coll Gen Pract 1988; 38:511–514
33. O'Brien ME: Pragmatic survivalism: Behavior patterns affecting low-level wellness among minority group members. Adv Nurs Sci 1982; 4(3):13–26
34. Kleinman A: Patients and Healers in the Context of Culture. Berkeley, CA: University of California Press; 1980
35. Warda MR: Mexican Americans' perceptions of culturally competent care. West J Nurs Res 2000; 22(2):203–224
36. Zoucha RD: The experiences of Mexican Americans receiving professional nursing care: An ethnonursing study. J Transcult Nurs 1998; 9(2):33–44
37. Meleis AI: Culturally competent scholarship: Substance and rigor. Adv Nurs Sci 1996; 19(2):1–16
38. Hondagneu Sotelo P, Avila E: "I'm here, but I'm there": The meanings of Latina transnational motherhood. Gender Soc 1997; 11(5):548–571

Reprinted with permission from: Messias, D. K. H. (2002). Transnational health resources, practices, and perspectives: Brazilian immigrant women's narratives. *Journal of Immigrant Health, 4*(4), 183–200.

5.6 EMPLOYED MEXICAN WOMEN AS MOTHERS AND PARTNERS: VALUED, EMPOWERED AND OVERLOADED

AFAF IBRAHIM MELEIS
MARILYN K. DOUGLAS
CARMEN ERIBES
FUJIN SHIH
DEANNE K. MESSIAS

Abstract

This study was designed to explore the daily lived experiences of a group of employed, low-income Mexican women in their maternal and spousal roles. The participants were 41 auxiliary nurses recruited from two large urban hospitals in Mexico. Data were collected through the Women's Roles Interview Protocol (WRIP) that solicited the participants' perceptions of the satisfactions and stresses they experienced in their roles as mothers and spouses, and their descriptions of the coping strategies and the resources they used to deal with stressful life experiences related to these roles. Data analysis consisted of a qualitative thematic analysis of the narrative responses to open-ended questions in the WRIP. Satisfying aspects of the maternal and spousal roles, as identified by the participants, included giving to and receiving from their children, and being valued and supported by their partners. Spousal approval of their work was also satisfying. These employed mothers, however, experienced many stressful aspects of functioning in multiple roles, including lack of resources, being absent from their children, self-doubt about their maternal role functioning, role overload, and spousal absences. The women coped by juggling priorities and utilizing family resources. From the data analysis, the investigators developed a conceptual framework for understanding these women's experiences with parenting and marriage. The centrality of the family, a sense of value and empowerment as women in maternal and spousal roles, and the reality of role overload are discussed within the Mexican cultural context of machismo, *its female counterpart* hembnsmo, *and family life. Implications for women's health are framed within a context of family and work.*

Introduction

Women in Mexico are entering the formal work force at an increasing rate, adding the role of worker and wage-earner to their traditional domestic roles of mother and wife. In 1930, only 4.6% of Mexican women were active in the workforce (Salazar, 1980), whereas 19.6% of Mexican females of 12 years of age and older were economically active in 1990 (Instituto Nacional de Estadística, Geografia a Informática, 1992). The harsh economic realities of urban lower-class life in Latin America have contributed to the expansion of women's roles as they move into the paid workforce in order to supplement household incomes. This situation challenges the traditional role conceptualization of male as the sole provider and female as the homemaker. The changes also challenge the levels and depth of involvement of women inside and outside the house. While contributing directly to the family income, taking on the role of wage earner also provides women with the opportunity to extend their social networks, develop new skills, and utilize personal and social resources (Neuhouser, 1989). However, as is the case with women worldwide, the fact that Mexican women are adding new roles to their repertoire does not imply that they have shed the responsibilities of their child-rearing role. Although there is evidence that changes are occurring in the traditional division of domestic tasks and conjugal decision-making styles, Mexican women continue to carry the bulk of domestic responsibilities (Elmendorf, 1977; Falicov, 1978; Zavella, 1987).

The questions of role occupancy, role quality, and sources of stress and satisfaction are of interest to social scientists and to health professionals. Previous research suggests that the quality of the role, not the occupancy of the role, is one of the predictors of distress among employed mothers, and provides increasing evidence that family role occupancy per se does not predict health outcomes. In their study of 403 women employed as licensed practical nurses and social workers, Barnett and Marshall (1992) examined the main effects of the quality of the employee and parent roles and the interaction effects between these variables. These investigators reported that psychological distress in mothers was not related to their parental status, but that employed mothers with positive mother-child relationships had lower levels of psychological distress than employed mothers with troubled mother-child relationships. They suggested that employed mothers reap mental health advantages from multiple roles, even when some of those roles are stressful. When women encounter difficulties in combining multiple roles, they frequently attribute these difficulties to a lack of time and to role overload. A study of Mexican nurses, school teachers, secretaries and housewives reported that women in all four categories were responsible for the same household tasks (Uríbe Vázquez, Ramirez Rodriquez, Romero Lima, & Gutierrez de la Torre, 1991). The work week was extended for those who were employed outside the home, and women in the four groups divided their time differently to accomplish all their tasks and responsibilities and deal with the many demands on their time. Work-related health problems were reported by women in all four categories, but the housewives had the highest reported morbidity rate. Similarly, in a landmark study Hochschild (1989) characterized employed women in the United States as working a *second shift* at home after completing their wage-earning work outside the home. In addition, Walker and Best (1991) cite various studies that show that employed mothers express concern about lack of time for their housework, family, friends, themselves, their own medical care, and opportunities for their children outside the home. Having children at home increases working women's total role responsibilities and has been cited as the most likely source of job-family conflicts (Barnett & Baruch, 1985). Investigating role stress in employed mothers of preschool children, Rankin (1993) reported lack of time, child-related problems and maternal guilt to be the major stressors identified by the women studied. Some studies have shown that even in the face of multiple role overload and consequential lack of time, working women have managed to maintain their health (Uríbe Vázquez et al., 1991; Barnett & Marshall, 1992).

Hall, Steven, and Meleis (1992) suggest that for health care providers to make comprehensive health assessment and intervention decisions, they need to understand how women integrate their multiple roles within a context of economic, social, political, and cultural forces and constraints. In light of existing research that suggests that understanding women's roles requires careful attention to the quality of their multiple roles and that a focus on women's lived experiences may uncover patterns of responses to health and illness (McBride & McBride, 1981), an investigation was completed of women's health and women's roles in Mexico, Colombia, Egypt, the United States, and Brazil. As part of the larger study, the analysis reported here sought to investigate the qualitative aspects of the daily lived experiences of a group of Mexican nursing auxiliaries. More specifically, we report here on the analysis of three aspects of working women's roles as mothers and spouses, their role satisfaction, role stressors, and coping strategies.

The Study

Participants

The women in this study were auxiliary nursing personnel recruited from hospital continuing education classes and acute care settings in two large urban areas in Mexico. Of the 41 auxiliary nurses in the convenience sample, 31 (76%) were nursing assistants and 10 (24%) were technical nurses. According to the Pan American Health Organization (1990), nursing assistants comprise 60% of Mexico's total nursing personnel. Nursing assistants in Mexico have had no formal nursing education other than on-the-job training, but have usually completed the 9 years of basic education offered in public schools. Technical nurses are the next largest group of auxiliary nursing personnel, comprising 26% of the total. They receive 3 years of hospital-based nursing training after having completed 9 years of general education.

All the participants were mothers and/or partners, 35 (85%) were mothers and 37 (90%) had partners. Of those with partners, 95% were married. The mothers had a mean of 2.17 children, ranging in age from 1 to 5 years The women ranged in age from 22 to 48 years, with a mean of 31.6 years. All the participants had at least 9 years of basic public education and the mean of educational level was 10.6 years. The mean household income for the sample was Mex $23.50 per day, equivalent to US $8.93 at the time of the study, with a range from less than Mex $10.00 (US $3.80) to greater than Mex $60.00 (US $22.81) per day. On the whole, the subjects described their household income as adequate, but reported that they did not have money available for anything other than basic necessities. Each respondent was paid the equivalent of US $4.00, as a modest reimbursement for the 2 hours required to complete the study questionnaires.

Data Collection

This investigation is part of a large international study examining stress, satisfaction, and coping strategies that are role specific for low-income women.

To obtain data related to women's roles as spouses and mothers for the present investigation, each participant was asked to complete a set of self-administered questionnaires. Two questionnaires were used for the analysis reported here, a demographic profile questionnaire, and the Women's Role Interview Protocol (WRIP). The demographic questionnaire contained questions related to participants' ages, education, and other socioeconomic variables not reported in the paper.

The WRIP was designed to be used as an interview protocol or as a self-administered questionnaire. It is a semistructured interview/questionnaire that focuses on obtaining data on the number of roles in women's lives, the degree of involvement in each of their roles, perceived satisfactions and stressors in each role, and the strategies that women use in dealing with the demands of stresses in each role. The open-ended questions used in the WRIP are grounded on the assumption that understanding the lives of people is based on uncovering their lived experiences in the central roles in their lives (Barnett & Baruch 1985; Turner, 1990) and on the centrality of uncovering the demands that women face in each role (Pearlin & Schooler, 1978; Pearlin, Lieberman, Menaghan, & Mullan, 1981). The WRIP as an interview protocol and as a self-administered questionnaire was used in other studies (Meleis, Norbeck, & Laffrey, 1989; Meleis, Laffrey, Solomon, & Miller, 1989; Meleis, Kulig, Arruda, & Beckman, 1990), linked with this one.

The WRIP was adapted for use in Spanish according to systematic translation protocols. First, it was translated by a bilingual translator. The translation was checked by Spanish-speaking judges and then a modified and refined version was piloted on a number of participants.

In the part of the study reported here, data from open-ended questions about maternal and spousal roles are analyzed. Narrative responses as perceived and articulated by participants were used as the texts for the analysis reported here.

Data Analysis

To analyze the narrative data from the WRIP, it was necessary that the written responses be translated from Spanish into English, since not all members of the research team were Spanish speakers. One of the researchers, who is a first-generation Mexican-American, served as the translator. The goal of the translation was to reflect an understanding of the participant's cultural context. The challenge of the interpretation was to get to know each respondent beyond the written word, and to form a conceptual picture of their thoughts rather than simply provide a literal translation. Each questionnaire was read and reread to search for similar word usages, and was then translated completely, without interruption, in order to capture that respondent's conceptual meaning and her personal expressive manner. Although a limitation of this strategy was translator fatigue caused by the length of the questionnaire and the intensity of the task, the process improved the overall trustworthiness of the translation.

The translated questionnaires were analyzed by the investigative team in search of response codes and categories (Strauss & Corbin, 1990) and a code map was devised. Subsequently, the entire data set was coded according to the code map, and the investigators re-analyzed, reviewed, collapsed, and refined the resulting categories as their properties were described within the framework of the research questions (Lofland & Lofland, 1984).

Results

For the purpose of this study, the unit of analysis was each individual response to the questions on the WRIP. A response was defined as a statement, a number of statements, a sentence, or a story that denotes an idea (Meleis & Stevens, 1992). In addition to the qualitative analysis of each category that emerged from the data, the authors deemed it useful to count the number of responses within each category in order to determine the relative strength of the type of response. In assigning percentage values to the responses, the authors do not intend to imply that the quantitative measure is more precise, accurate, or meaningful in understanding the phenomena at hand (Stern, 1991). Although the qualitative data analysis has attempted to uncover the meaning of the responses, the categories are intended to convey to the readers a sense of the type and range of the responses that were identified (Tables 5.6.1 and 5.6.2). Presentation of the results will include the analysis of the meaning as well as the quantitative value of the category (i.e., number of responses and percentage of the total responses in each category).

Maternal Role

In answer to questions related to their mothering role, participants described role satisfaction in terms of *giving to* and *receiving from their children*. Maternal role stressors described by these mothers were *sick child, lack of resources, absence, education, self-doubt, bad environment,* and *own health*. In order to deal with the stress of the mothering role, the coping strategies participants described included *juggling priorities, family resources, problem solving, outside help,* and *diversion*.

Maternal Role Satisfiers

As indicated in Table 5.6.1, of the 82 responses referring to maternal role satisfaction, 56 (68%) were categorized as *giving to child*. Participants described giving to, taking care of, feeding, loving, teaching, and being able to fulfill the needs of their children as intensely gratifying and rewarding expe-

TABLE 5.6.1 Maternal Role Experiences of 35 Employed Mexican Mothers

	% of Responses
Role satisfiers ($r = 82$)	
Giving to child	68
Receiving from child	32
Role stressors ($r = 124$)	
Sick child	26
Lack of resources	19
Absences	17
Child's education	10
Own health	10
Environmental dangers	9
Self-doubts	9
Coping strategies ($r = 173$)	
Juggling priorities	30
Family resources	27
Problem solving	15
Diversion	15
Outside help	13

r = number of response units

TABLE 5.6.2 Spousal Role Experiences of 37 Employed Mexican Partners

	% of Responses
Role satisfiers ($r = 91$)	
Being valued	57
Feeling supported	20
Approval of employment	18
Making husband happy	5
Role stressors ($r = 48$)	
Overload	50
His absences	23
Disapproval of employment	17
Inadequate income	10
Coping strategies ($r = 79$)	
Turning to spouse	42
Turning to family	32
Turning inward	20
Emotional release	6

r = number of response units

riences. These mothers reported satisfaction in the sheer involvement in attending to their children, meeting their needs, and *loving and educating them.*

Participants gave 26 responses (32% of the total) that were categorized as *receiving from child*. These responses described watching their children grow, receiving their affection, having pride in their development, and communicating with them as gratifying and a boost to their daily lives. Maternal satisfaction was "to know that there is something important in my life," stated one nursing assistant. Another was pleased with "being able to enjoy the companionship of my child and become interested in his play."

Maternal Role Stressors

In spite of the participants' feeling assured that their child care needs were well met and that they had resources to support their mothering role, 26% of the 124 responses related to maternal role stress revealed that they lived with a fear of the prospect of a *sick child* (Table 5.6.1). They worried about having their loved one ill, as well as the additional stress of working while their child was being cared for by someone else "When they are ill I have difficulty relating to the external work," was how one mother described her experience with having sick children.

These employed mothers cited *lack of resources* as the next most frequent source of stress in their maternal role (19% of the responses). They reported a lack of public resources such as transportation, parks, and youth centers, as well as inadequate personal financial resources to cover needed expenses. However, the resource identified as most lacking for their mothering role was an intangible one, *lack of time*. They lamented in particular, "not having enough time to spend with my children."

Responses indicated the constant struggle women have in their work and familial role, particularly in their mothering roles. Women described their daily stress related to *absence* with statements such as "having to go to work and leaving my children alone," and "having to leave them alone, healthy, or otherwise." Additional categories of maternal stress dealt with concerns about their children's *education* (both academic and parental guidance), worries about their *own health* and state of exhaustion, the *environmental dangers* inherent to living in a large urban area, and finally, their *self-doubts* about being a good mother.

Coping Strategies for the Maternal Role

The participants were creative in their use of coping strategies to deal with maternal role stressors. As seen in Table 5.6.1, *juggling priorities* was the most frequently used strategy (30%), and involved temporary shifting of maternal demands and priorities according to the pressing needs of the moment. When the demands of the mothering role became more prominent, the demands of other roles were temporarily ignored, submerged, or devalued. For example, a common solution proposed by these mothers for the problem of a child's illness was to "ask permission" from their nursing supervisor to stay home from work in order to care for the child. Another solution was to reduce the number of hours at work in order to spend more time with their children.

Participants also identified *family resources* (27%) and *outside help* (13%) as important strategies for coping with maternal stress. Family resources (i.e., mother, in-laws, sisters, daughters, and occasionally husbands) were solicited to help with child care and housework. Examples given of outside resources included individuals to help with child care and domestic chores. Interestingly, utilization of a day care center was cited only once from a total of 173 responses related to coping with maternal stress. Being well organized also helped reduce the stresses of motherhood.

In 26 responses, the participants identified *problem solving* as a maternal coping strategy. They described a process of turning the problem around and asking various questions before attempting to identify answers. A typical response was "I identify the problem and look for the best solution." Of the responses, 15% described how these women used *diversion* as a way to deal with stressful situations. A frequent response was *divertise* which means going out to have fun, but with no specific activity in mind. It is unplanned, spontaneous, and open-ended, like going for a ride with your friends and just seeing what will happen. Implicit in the concept, however, is the expectation that what happens will be pleasant and enjoyable. Other diversion strategies were singing, talking, and watching television.

Diversion was utilized as a coping strategy for the stresses of motherhood as well as for the pressures of work, however, when dealing with maternal stresses, they often took their children with them to partake in these diversionary activities.

Spousal Role

A total of 90% of the auxiliary nursing personnel in this sample were in a spousal relationship. They described the most satisfying aspects of being a partner as *being valued, feeling supported,* having spousal *approval of work* and *making husband happy.* They identified the most stressful aspects of their relationship as *overload and no help; his absences;* spousal *disapproval of employment;* and *inadequate income.* The strategies these employed wives used to cope with spousal stress were *turning to spouse, turning to family, turning inward,* and *emotional release.*

Spousal Role Satisfiers

Responses characterized as spousal role satisfiers are indicated in Table 5.6.2. *Being valued* was the most frequently cited spousal role satisfier (57% of the 91 responses), and is exemplified in the phrase *saber que tengo valor* (knowing that I have value). Feelings of affection, appreciation, companionship and love from their spouses were described as particularly gratifying. One woman wrote "he values me as a woman, wife, friend, companion, mother of the children, all beyond what is necessary." As partners, the participants expressed satisfaction in "our mutual relationship and the act of sharing our daily life experiences," "the understanding there is between us," and "in the way he behaves towards me." Another woman replied "he always respects me and gives me my place."

Another important source of spousal role satisfaction identified in 20% of the responses was the *support* and help that they receive from their spouses "Feeling the support all around me," and "I can count on his help all around me" were typical of such responses. One auxiliary nurse reported "while I am at the hospital, he helps me a lot because he works at night and he has time during the day to help me with the children and send them to school."

These Mexican women did not consider their employment as a personal decision or a guaranteed right. Participants in this study described how satisfied they were in their spousal relationship if and when their spouses demonstrated *approval of their employment* (18%). They felt that the quality of their spousal relationship was very much affected by their partners supporting their desire to work as nursing auxiliaries. Examples of responses were "my spouse thinks that work is a good therapy for me," "he says that I am self-sufficient," and "at first he did not like it, but now that I help him he doesn't say anything." The least cited category of spousal role satisfaction was *making husband happy* (5%).

Spousal Role Stressors

When asked to describe the stress they experience in their spousal role, the participants provided 48 responses, as compared to 91 responses describing satisfactions in being a wife. In other words, there were almost twice as many responses about spousal role satisfiers as there were about stressors. As indicated in Table 5.6.2, one-half of these responses indicated that the stress in their partner role stems from *overload*. The level of their responsibilities and the demands on their time, associated with the lack of help they received from their husbands in meeting these demands, contributed to this overload.

Another significant source of stress (23%) was a partner's lack of consideration in keeping his wife informed about his *absences* and whereabouts (e.g., when and why he will be late). Examples from the data were "he doesn't inform me when he will be late," and "it is stressful for me that my husband is late or works without taking the time to let me know." Others described feelings of jealousy about the absences and delays, and attributed the stress to this jealousy. These delays and absences magnified a lack of communication that these women sometimes experienced in their relationships. This lack of communication also contributed to disagreements about family decision making and about child-rearing practices.

How spouses felt about women's employment made a major contribution to how the women felt about their spousal relationship. Although some women described their husband's approval as a satisfying aspect of their relationship, others indicated by their responses that spousal *disapproval of their employment* could be equally stressful. Quotations reflecting disapproval were "he wants me to quit," "sometimes my work upsets him, but I know we need it," "he tells me the children need me and that I shouldn't be working," and "he asks me to stay home and I don't want to."

Although women frequently take jobs because of domestic economic needs, *inadequate income* still figured as a source of stress (10%) in their spousal role. Responses in this category of spousal role stress reflected not only a lack of sufficient income for meeting family needs, but also concern about how the available income was used (e.g., "for my husband's drinking"). However, inadequate income was cited least often by the respondents as causing stress in the spousal role.

Coping Strategies for the Spousal Role

Among the 79 responses regarding coping strategies for spousal role stress, 42% indicated using the approach of *turning to spouse* to talk about and try to resolve the issues that were creating stress in their lives (Table 5.6.2). In spite of recognizing that the spouse and the relationship were in and of themselves a source of stress, these women described how they were able to talk with their husbands, and how this dialogue helped resolve the underlying conflict and stress.

In responses characteristic of *turning to family* (32%), participants described how they reached out to other family members and utilized the help of parents, siblings, and children to provide them with support to cope with their marital stress. Of the responses, 20% described how *turning inward* helped them cope with spousal stress. Participants who coped by drawing on their own personal strength did so by reaffirming their own competence to deal with the situation. For example, "I am strong and self-sufficient," "I try to put things in perspective," is the way one woman described the process of reframing the meaning of the situation in order to get a sense of control over her life. Finally, only four responses (6%) described how an *emotional release*, such as crying or becoming angry, helped women cope with marital stress.

Discussion and Conclusions

Three main themes emerged from the data related to the daily lived experiences of this group of Mexican auxiliary nurses in their maternal and spousal roles: The central importance of the family in their lives, a sense of value and empowerment of the women themselves, and the reality of role overload with resulting implications for their health.

In analyzing the data, it became evident to the investigators that the cultural context of the Mexican family and the interplay of the concepts of *machismo* and *hembrismo* in spousal and maternal role expectations and behaviors were fundamental to understanding and interpreting the responses. *Machismo* is a Latin American, and particularly Mexican value concept that is generally understood from the stereotypical view of the unquestionable and absolute supremacy of the male and the inferiority of the female. The literature often refers to *machismo* without mention of the female counterpart, known as *hembrismo* or *marianismo*. *Hembrismo* is characterized primarily by a gender division of roles and labor that ascribes power and authority to women within the domestic sphere.

A conceptual framework has been developed to describe these themes and the relationships between them. Components of the framework are discussed in the following section.

Centrality of the Family

In Mexico, as in most of Latin America, the family still retains many of the traditional characteristics of the large, cohesive social network of the extended family (Keefe, Padilla, & Carlos, 1983). The extended family is a source of mutual psychological and economic support, and in those marriages where the spousal relationship is less supportive, it is the larger family network that provides women with affection and emotional support (Ross, Mirowsky, & Ulbrich, 1983). Children are an important part of the Latin American family, and appear to be less psychologically distressing for Mexicans, than for Americans. As they grow older, children also serve their mothers as a resource for the development and maintenance of social exchange networks (Neuhouser, 1989; Ross et al., 1983).

The results of this investigation support the explanation of the role and the centrality of the family in the lives of the participants. Family-centered role satisfactions included support and a sense of worth from their children, spouses, and extended family, as well as from society. Whereas childcare arrangements are generally considered a major issue in the life of working mothers, the majority of participants in this study did not consider childcare an issue because they were able to rely on the extended family as a childcare resource. Children were viewed by these working mothers as a personal resource, children provided women with their maternal role identity, but were also a source of support, as well as a source of joy and satisfaction.

The societal priority of women's role in the family is demonstrated by the support these workers had from their employers in order to fulfill their maternal role when necessary, even at the expense of their work role. When mothers needed to be home to take care of a sick child, flexible employee policies accommodated for this need, and supported maternal role priorities in times of increased family demands.

Valuation and Empowerment of Women

The second major theme in the findings is that in spite of the participants' involvement in multiple roles within the context of a perceived lack of economic and social resources, they described many satisfying aspects of their maternal and spousal roles and expressed feelings of being valued in these roles. In this study, a significant resource was the women's own sense of self-worth, evidenced by their utilization of inner resources (turning inward) and personal problem solving to cope with the many diverse stressors of being a mother, wife, and nursing auxiliary. The question that intrigued the researchers as the data were analyzed was related to the nature of women's power and value in their familial roles.

Traditional female roles may be stressful for women in modern industrial societies, but they are not necessarily as stressful for women in more traditional societies. This difference may be related to the value that societies attribute to the maternal role. More traditional societies place a higher value on the centrality of the family and the importance of women's roles in the home, with consequently less societal value on individual achievement. Several authors have proposed that married women in such societies experience relatively lower levels of psychological distress than women in more modern societies (Gove & Tudor, 1973; Ross et al., 1983).

For both males and females, the Mexican family is a very important source of social status and emotional support, in contrast to societies in which individuals derive more status from their jobs and tend to utilize family less than other resources for social and emotional support (Elmendorf, 1977; Ross et al., 1983). The Mexican female is the center of the family and is accorded honor and prestige not as readily available to her American counterpart (Ross et al., 1983). Mexican culture accords love and reverence to motherhood, and thus the great majority of women who bear children enjoy a higher status than non-mothers (Elmendorf, 1977).

The results of this study suggest a need to reevaluate the manner in which Mexican women have often been portrayed in the literature. A view, which has been held by some authors, is that the Mexican woman is confined to the home or to a repetitive, low-paying job; is unconditionally subordinated to men in general, her husband in particular; is passive and lacking initiative in making decisions; is self-abnegating and self-effacing before the interests of her husband and children, despite legal advances toward gender equality. This situation has been described as reducing "the majority of Mexican women to a situation of inferiority and material and psychological dependence on family and society" (Salazar, 1980).

Elmendorf (1977) and Stevens (1973) have refuted the myth of Mexican women as passive and submissive, arguing that women utilize and maximize the existing societal values to achieve their own ends. Ramirez and Arce (1981) cite several authors who take issue with the *machismo* myth of absolute male dominance as the basis for male-female roles in Mexican families. Within this framework the Mexican male (*el macho*) is dominant, whereas the female counterpart (*la hembra*) is passive and submissive. However, the Mexican interpretation of *machismo* also recognizes the male's inherent responsibility as the head of the household, which includes providing for the economic, social, emotional, and physical well-being of the family (Mirande, 1986). These prevailing cultural perspectives have not been adequately supported by research (Mirande, 1977).

Within the cultural context of *hembrismo*, women are responsible for providing the nurturing needs of the family, instilling the cultural belief system, and performing the domestic labor of the household (Mirande & Enriquez, 1979). Evidence of this in the present study is found in the participants' feelings of being valued, having the respect and support of spouse and family, and deriving joy, satisfaction, wonder and importance from their children. These findings also provide support for those aspects of *machismo* that emphasize the male's role in valuing and supporting their wives.

In general, spouses were described in this study as being supportive of their wives and families. Family figures as centrally in men's lives as it did in women's lives. On the other hand, nearly half the responses regarding spousal stress could be attributed to aspects of male dominance commonly associated with *machismo*. For example, women reported not knowing or not being informed of their husbands' whereabouts, being jealous of other women in their husbands' lives, and spousal disapproval of the woman's job, as causes for spousal role stress. These stressors reflect cultural values but are predominantly concerned with spousal role quality.

However, the verbal portraits these women paint of themselves in their maternal and spousal roles are evidence that they have resources that enable them to have a certain degree of active control in their lives. Their resources are their work, children, extended family, and own inner strength and resilience. Hall (1989) has proposed that having control over work outside the home is important because of the implications for the general social efficacy of women, and because working as a wage-earner is a major vehicle for adult socialization. This thesis may not be applicable to women in more traditional cultures that place a higher value on family and the maternal role. Therefore, in such societies, other sources of power for women should be considered.

Role Overload

Societal and personal valuing of the maternal role does not exempt women from role stress. In addition, the combination of domestic and work roles may result in role conflict or overload and consequently have an adverse effect on women's health (Barnett & Marshall, 1992; Froberg, Gjerdingen, & Preston, 1986; Houston, Cates, & Kelly, 1992; Uríbe Vázquez et al., 1991). The responses analyzed in this study included many descriptions of role overload, lack of redistribution of domestic tasks, lack of personal resources (particularly time and money), and limited social and health care resources. For the participants, perceiving family as a resource and having family support may, to some degree, have served as a buffer to the overall role stressors of overload and lack of resources that they experienced.

Over a period of years, research has found that the work of Mexican women outside the home has had a significant effect on traditional patriarchal roles and on conjugal decision making, leading to more egalitarianism and contributing to more shared decision-making (Hawkes & Taylor, 1975; Ybarra, 1975; Zavella, 1987). Although the participants in this study showed some signs of desire to change the traditional division of domestic labor in order to deal with their overload, they did not report having taken concrete steps to bring about such changes. The stricter traditional division of domestic labor in Mexican homes is encouraged by *hembrismo* and *machismo*, and the question thus arises of whether women would have to give up some of the benefits and resources derived from *hembrismo*, if they expect more profound changes in the division of domestic labor in order to cope with the strain of role and time overload.

Conclusion

This study was undertaken with the intention of describing role satisfactions, stressors, and coping strategies in a group of working women in Mexico. Although the study is limited by the small convenience sample and therefore results cannot be generalized to the larger population, the descriptions of these women's daily lived experiences hold potential implications for researchers and health care providers interested in the health care of women. Emphasis on the maternal and spousal roles may create a context of self-care neglect for women. For example, Mamede and colleagues (1991) reported that lower class Brazilian women relegated their own health to the last of their health care priorities, with the health concerns of their families achieving higher priority. Furthermore, the focus of health care delivery systems further supports women's self neglect. Women have been considered primarily in terms of reproductive capacity, or in terms of what they should do for the sake of their children, with little consideration for women's own growth and development issues (McBride, 1973; McBride & McBride, 1981). In other words, women become equated with their roles as mothers. More attention needs to be given to the family context in the lives of women and to women's multiple roles including their own self-care roles.

Future investigators could elucidate the health implications of other central roles in the lives of women in addition to the maternal and spousal roles, explore facilitators and barriers to women's ability to maintaining their own health, and compare and contrast the different strategies that women could use to enhance their own health within a multiple role context.

Acknowledgment

This study was made possible by the support of the Kellogg International Fellowship for the senior author.

REFERENCES

Barnett, R. C., & Baruch, G. K. (1985). Women's involvement in multiple roles and psychological distress. *Journal of Personality and Social Psychology, 49*, 133–143.

Barnett, R.C., & Marshall N. L. (1992). Worker and mother roles, spillover effects, and psychological distress. *Women and Health, 18*(2), 9–36.

Baruch, G. K., & Barnett R. C. (1986). Role quality, multiple role involvement and psychological well-being in midlife women. *Journal of Person, Society and Psychology, 51*, 578.

Elmendorf, M. (1977). Mexico: The many worlds of women. In J. Z. Giele & A. C. Smock (Eds.), *Women, roles, and status in eight countries* (pp. 3–31). New York: John Wiley.

Falicov, C. J. (1978). Mexican families. In W. D. Smith, A. K. Burlew, M. H. Mosley, & W. M. Whitney (Eds), *Minority issues in mental health.* Reading, MA: Addison Wesley.

Froberg, D., Gjerdingen, D., & Preston, M. (1986). Multiple roles and women's health: What have we learned? *Women and Health, 11*, 79–96.

Gove, W. R., & Tudor, J. (1973). Adult sex roles and mental illness. *American Journal of Society, 78*, 812–835.

Hall, E. M. (1989). Gender, work control, and stress a theoretical discussion and an empirical test. *International Journal of Health Services, 19*(4), 725–745.

Hall, J. M., Steven, P. E., & Meleis, A. I. (1992). Developing the construct of role integration: A narrative analysis of women clerical workers' daily lives. *Research in Nursing and Health, 15*, 447–457.

Hawkes, G. R., & Taylor, M. (1975). Power structure in Mexican and Mexican American farm labor families. *Journal of Marriage and the Family, 37*, 807–811.

Hochschild, A. (1989). *The second shift.* New York: Avon Books.

Houston, B. K., Cates, D. S., & Kelly, K. E. (1992). Job stress, psychological strain, and physical health problems in women employed full-time outside the home and homemakers. *Women and Health, 19*(1), 1–26.

Instituto Nacional de Estadística, Geografía a Informatíca. (1992). *La Mujer en México Una Visión Através de Estadísticas Nacionales [The Mexican Woman A Perspective From National Statistics]* Aguascalientes, Ags: Instituto National de Estadística, Geografía a Informatíca.

Keefe, S. E., Padilla, A. M., & Carlos, M. L. (1983). The Mexican American extended family as an emotional support system. *Human Organization, 38*(2), 144–152.

Lofland, J., & Lofland, H. (1984). *Analyzing social settings: A guide to qualitative observation and analysis.* Belmont, CA: Wadsworth.

Mamede, M. V., Messias, D. K. H., Shimo, A. K. K., Rodrigues, R. A. P., Nakano, A. M. S., Almeida, A. M. D., et al. (1991). Mulher e saúde suas preocupacções [Women and health their concerns]. *Revista Pauhsta de Enfermagem, 10*(3), 121–127.

Meleis, A. I., Kulig, J., Arruda, E. N., & Beckman, A. (1990). Maternal role of women in clerical jobs in southern Brazil: Stress and satisfaction. *Health Care for Women International, 11*, 369–382.

Meleis, A. I., Norbeck, J. S., & Laffrey, S. C. (1989). Role integration and health among female clerical workers. *Research in Nursing and Health, 12*, 355–364.

Meleis, A. I., Norbeck, J. S., Laffrey, S. C., Solomon, M., & Miller, L. (1989). Stress, satisfaction and coping: A study of women clerical workers. *Health Care for Women International, 10,* 319–334.

Meleis, A. I., & Stevens, P. E. (1992). Women in clerical jobs, spousal role satisfaction, stress and coping. *Women and Health, 18*(1), 23–40.

McBride, A. B. (1973). *The growth and development of mothers.* New York: Harper and Row.

McBride, A. B., & McBride, W. L. (1981). Theoretical underpinnings for women's health. *Women and Health, 6*(1–2), 37–55.

Mirande, A. (1986). Chicano fathers response and adaptation to emergent roles. *Stanford Center for Chicano Research, Working Paper Series, No 13.* Standford: CA: Stanford University.

Mirande, A. (1977). The Chicano family: A reanalysis of conflicting views. *Journal of Marriage and the Family, 39,* 747–756.

Mirande, A., & Enrigucz, E. (1979). *La Chicano: The Mexican American woman.* Chicago: University of Chicago.

Neuhouser, K. (1989). Sources of women's power and states among the urban poor in contemporary Brazil. *Journal of Women in Culture and Society, 14*(3), 683–702.

Pan American Health Organization. (1990). *Health conditions in the Americas 1985–1988.* Washington, DC: Pan American Health Organization.

Pearlin, L. I., & Schooler, C. (1978). The structure of coping. *Journal of Health and Social Behavior, 19,* 2–21.

Pearlin, L. I., Lieberman, M. A., Menaghan, E. G., & Mullan, J. T. (1981). The stress process. *Journal of Health and Social Behavior, 22,* 337–356.

Ramirez, O., & Arce, C. H. (1981). The contemporary Chicano family: An empirically based review. In A. Baron, Jr. (Ed.), *Explorations in Chicano psychology* (pp. 3–28). New York: Praeger.

Rankin, E. A. D. (1993). Stresses and rewards experienced by employed mothers. *Health Care for Women International, 14,* 527–537.

Ross, C. E., Mirowsky, J., & Ulbrich, P. (1983). Distress and traditional female role: A comparison of Mexicans and Anglos. *American Journal of Society, 89*(3), 670–682.

Salazar, G. G. (1980). Participation of women in Mexican labor force. In J. Nash & H. I. Safa (Eds.), *Sex and class in Latin America: Women's perspectives on politics, economics and family in the third world* (pp. 183–201). South Harley, MA: J F. Bergin.

Stern, P. N. (1991). Are counting and coding *a capella* appropriate in qualitative research? In J. M. Morse (Ed.), *Qualitative nursing research: A contemporary dialogue* (pp. 147–162). Newbury Park, CA: Sage.

Stevens, E. P. (1973). Marianismo: The other face of machismo in Latin America In A. Pescatello (Ed.), *Female and male in Latin America essays* (pp. 89–101). Pittsburgh: University of Pittsburgh Press.

Strauss, A., & Corbin, J. (1990). *Basics of qualitative research grounded theory procedures and technique.* Newbury Park, CA: Sage.

Turner, R. H. (1990). Role change. *Annual Review of Sociology, 16,* 87–110.

Uríbe Vázquez, G., Ramírez Rodríguez, J. C., Romero Lima, L. G., & Gutierrez de la Torre, N. C. (1991). El trabajo femenino y la salud de cuatro grupos de mujeres en Guadalajara, Mexico [Workers' health in four groups of women in Guadalajara, Mexico]. *Boletín de la Oficina Sarutária Panamencana 111*(2), 101–111.

Walker, L. O., & Best, M. A. (1991). Well-being of mothers with infant children: A preliminary comparison of employed women and homemakers. *Women and Health, 17*(1), 71–89.

Ybarra, L. (1982). When wives work: The impact on the Chicano family. *Journal of Marriage and the Family, 44,* 169–178.

Zavella, P. (1987). *Women's work and Chicano families.* Ithaca, NY: Cornell University Press.

Reprinted with permission from: Meleis, A. I., Douglas, M. K., Eribes, C., Shih, F., & Messias, D. K. (1996). Employed Mexican women as mothers and partners: Valued, empowered and overloaded. *Journal of Advanced Nursing, 23,* 82–90.

Chapter 6 Situational Transitions: Education

6.1 EXPLORING THE TRANSITION AND PROFESSIONAL SOCIALISATION FROM HEALTH CARE ASSISTANT TO STUDENT NURSE

GRAEME BRENNAN
ROB MCSHERRY

Summary

Background: Minimal research is available examining the socialisation process from the perspective of students with health care knowledge who prior to undertaking their training worked as a health care assistant (HCA). The transition and professional socialisation process undertaken by students is an important factor in contributing to the successful completion of a pre-registration nursing programme. Despite this, limited empirical research explores the impact prior health care knowledge plays in this process. ***Objective:*** The study's aim was to determine the transitional processes associated with moving from a HCA to Student Nurse. ***Design***: A descriptive qualitative study undertaken over an 8-month period at a university in the northeast of England. ***Population, sample, setting:*** A homogeneous sample of 14 students with previous experience as a HCA within the field of adult nursing was used. ***Methods:*** Data were collected through 4 focus group interviews and analysed using [Burnard, P., 1991. A method of analysing interview transcripts in qualitative research. Nurse Education Today 11, 461–466.] thematic content analysis. ***Findings:*** The main themes that emerged around culture shock and clinical issues identified both positive and negative perceptions on this process. Equally, a new concept is introduced from the findings identified as the comfort zone, which explores the intentional reversal into the HCA role by the participants of the study. From the findings a framework for the transition and professional socialisation from HCA to student nurse is provided. The findings will assist the university and others in identifying, addressing, and aiding the socialisation needs of these students into their new role as a student nurse.

Introduction

This qualitative study originated as a result of a senior nurse's comment that was made when visiting a student nurse on clinical placement who had had been a health care assistant (HCA) prior to commencement of her training. The senior nurse commented concerning the student nurse, "the problem is she is at the end of her first year, and she still thinks and acts like a health care assistant." This raised the question; "How do students who were HCAs stop thinking and acting like HCAs?" The study aimed to identify:

- The realities of the transitional and professional socialisation process undertaken by HCAs as they progress through their nurse training.
- What experiences alter a student's perception of thinking from a HCA to a student nurse?
- How this transition and its meaning affects the students' perspective upon their own prior level of knowledge?

This topic is important to fill a gap in existing research and literature. A HCA is a term used in the United Kingdom to describe a support worker for the qualified nurse. It is therefore timely at this juncture in nurse education to consider the impact of socialisation from HCA to student nurse. Current policy (Department of Health, 2000) is encouraging the increased recruitment of HCAs into nurse education. Understanding the realities and potential difficulties these students encounter will assist in raising the levels of awareness to their needs.

Literature Review

The socialisation and transitional process undertaken by nursing students is well documented (Du Toit, 1995; Fitzpatrick, While, & Roberts, 1996; Howkins & Ewens, 1999). Existing literature focuses on the student's experience and influencing factors such as culture and clinical areas. This literature review is important in understanding how student nurses develop, but fails to explore the influencing factor of prior health care knowledge.

A review of this literature identified that certain principals could be utilised in the exploration of the HCA's transition and socialisation process.

Defining Transition and Socialisation

In examining the transition and socialisation process it is necessary to define their meanings. The notion of transition is well documented, with Meleis (1986) cited in Hunter et al. (1996) being the most utilised. Meleis (1986) identifies that transition is never a singular event, but rather an individualised process, occurring over an undetermined period of time. During this transition, the individual's patterns of behaviour change in relation to abilities, identity, role, and relationships; and that the concept of transition demonstrates an acceptance of change.

Socialisation, according to Fitzpatrick et al. (1996) is the key aim of any pre-registration nursing programme, gradually socialising the student into their future professional role. Various definitions of socialisation exist. Howkins and Ewens (1999) cite Cohen (1981) as an appropriate definition relevant to nursing. Cohen views professional socialisation as:

The complex process by which a person acquires the knowledge, skills, and sense of occupational identity that are characteristic of a member of that profession. It involves the internalisation of the values and norms of the group into the person's own behaviour and self-conception. In the process a person gives up the societal and media stereotypes prevalent in our culture and adopts those held by members of that profession.

Cohen's (1981) definition recognises the importance of values as being a central concept within the socialisation process. Throughout training the student is attempting to acquire the values, knowledge and skills to enable him or her to be accepted into the established professional group of the registered nurse. Lacey (1977) emphasized that not only is an individual's personality and qualities important, but that past experience influences the socialisation process. This raises the question of how much impact prior health care knowledge has in this process and whether this knowledge leads to any confusion for the student as they clarify their future role and identity.

Role Identity, Role Confusion

If prior experience as highlighted by Cohen (1981) and Lacey (1977) affects the transition and socialisation process then it is important to find evidence within the literature. Holland's (1999) study challenges the importance health care experience plays in the transition from HCA to student nurse. Holland (1999) identified that role confusion exists in students who work as HCAs to supplement their income. This dual role and subsequent conflict raises questions about their socialisation. Holland (1999) suggests that a potential for confusion exists for the HCA turned student in identifying their new role. Therefore, when students enter nurse training—is being able to identify with the HCA role through past experience—a potential hindrance or advantage to their socialisation? In identifying what the role of the HCA is, the question arises whether they experience role confusion. Role identity is an important aspect of the transition and socialisation process, but how does the student cope with the demands of such a process?

Reality Shock

Kramer (1974) argues that transition and socialisation create a phenomenon known as *reality shock* that was used to describe conflicting emotions amongst newly qualified nurses in America. Kramer (1974) identified that nurses often found themselves unprepared for situations that they believed they were prepared to handle. Gerrish (2000), Maben and Clark (1998), and Kramer (1974)—identified that upon qualification, students experienced stress and felt unprepared for many situations.

In nurse training, Elkan and Robinson (1993), and Melia (1987) argue that socialisation occurs in both the practice and educational setting, with both settings regarded as interconnecting environments that the student becomes a part of in the socialisation process. Socialisation into the educational setting will be the same for all students, but is it the same for the practice setting? Students with no prior health experience have had no exposure to the nurse's role, and are instead left to draw upon their own set of values and preconceived ideas, which as Du Toit (1995) points out change over time. Gray and Smith (1999), as Du Toit (1995), identify the shock that students, with no prior nursing experience, feel when confronted with the realities of the clinical areas. Interestingly, Gray and Smith (1999) argue that students with prior nursing experience are protected by their prior knowledge and that this seems to reduce the reality shock in the clinical area. Gray and Smith (1999) raise the question that if HCAs are protected from this reality shock, what factors are at play in their protection?

Formal/Informal Exposure to the RGN Role

Socialisation occurs within any individual entering a professional role (Abbott, 1988), and it could be considered that HCAs also bring with them a degree of socialisation. The consideration for this perspective is the exposure the HCA has had to the qualified nurses role. Talotta (1990) argues that if qualified nurses are seen by students to be role models, then this group is unconsciously holding significant influence over the student in their socialisation process. This raises the question about how much influence staff and clinical areas have affected the HCAs' beliefs regarding their role, and how this has in turn affected them as students. Windsor (1987) demonstrated that students in the observation of other nurses drew upon these observations to inform, develop, and shape their practice and beliefs surrounding the nurse's role.

A Framework for Transition and Socialisation

Built from the existing literature review (Figure 6.1.1), this framework proposes that HCAs in their transition and socialisation have the potential to experience role identity confusion, reality shock, and a questioning of their preconceived beliefs about their future professional role, as a result of their exposure to the RGN role. This *journey* will be unique for each individual and is acknowledged by not putting any time limits on reaching the point at which they feel they have made the transition to a student nurse. What needs to be discovered, is how much of an impact the student's transition and socialisation process affects these themes.

Methodology

Qualitative research is concerned with the analysis and interpretation of the way in which people make sense of their lived experiences (Streubert & Carpenter, 1995). Since this study explores students in their transition to becoming a HCA, and seeks to understand their point of view, a qualitative approach was ideally suited.

Entry Issues and Ethical Considerations

Approval was obtained through the appropriate Local Research Ethics Committee along with management support to undertake the study. Furthermore, verbal and written consent was obtained from each of the studies participants.

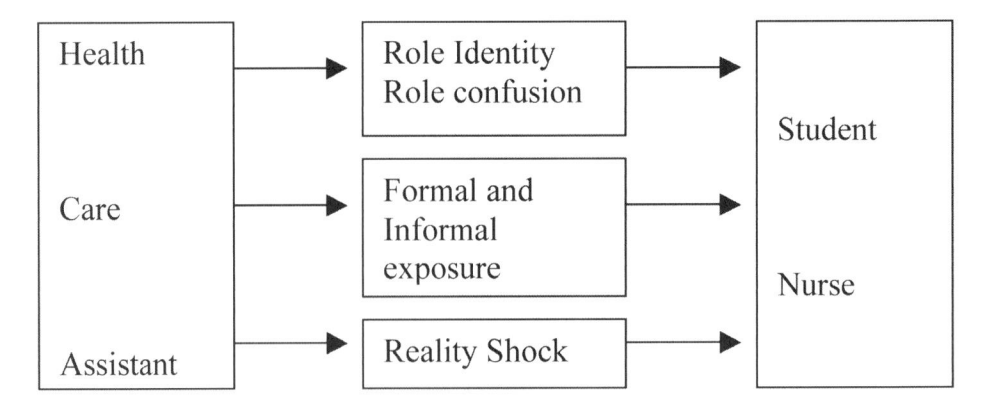

FIGURE 6.1.1 A framework for the transition and socialisation from HCA to student nurse.

The Sample and Setting

Based in a university in the North East of England, a homogeneous sampling was utilised, ensuring a good cross section of students' views and feelings, by randomly selecting student nurses undertaking a three-year adult nurse training programme. Participants for the study were identified in two ways. Potential participants, whose last employment positions were as HCAs, were identified from the university database. The researcher looked at the potential participants' file to confirm that they had at least 6-months experience in the adult field as HCAs. The rationale for this being that less than 6 months, would not ensure sufficient exposure to the HCA role to enable comparisons to be made when discussing the socialisation process. Any student with less than 6 months HCA experience or experience in other nursing disciplines was also excluded from the study since the student would have different cultural perspectives upon his or her transition and socialisation to that of adult nursing student.

Specific Techniques and Procedures for Data Collection

Four semi-structured focus group interviews were utilised. Focus group interviews are ideal methods for data collection in qualitative research providing a stimulus for ideas based on shared perceptions and experiences (Holloway & Wheeler, 2002). The interviews, lasting approximately 50 minutes, were performed with four groups of students at varying stages of their training (Figure 6.1.2). The participant numbers in each focus group were low, but were congruent with the perspective suggested by Greenbaum (1998) and Morgan (1998) who argue strongly that "mini focus groups" of 3–6 can be employed within qualitative research, particularly if the participants have a specific interest in the field of study.

In total, 14 participants were interviewed, of these 11 participants were women and 3 were men (Figure 6.1.2).

Results

Morse and Field (1996) argue that in qualitative research, researchers immerses themselves within the data. A key process in this immersion revolves around the method of data analysis. To this end, Burnard's (1991) thematic content analysis was utilised. All the focus group interviews were transcribed by the researcher verbatim, with participants given a unique code to maintain confidentiality.

Trustworthiness and Identification of Themes

To ensure trustworthiness of the research, a number of steps were followed. An impartial colleague in-

1 focus group midway through 1st year	4 participants
1 focus group at the beginning of 2nd year	4 participants
1 focus group at the beginning of 3rd year	3 participants
1 focus group at the end of their training	3 participants

FIGURE 6.1.2 Training position and participant numbers per focus group.

Themes	Sub Categories
Culture Shock	Professional role and accountability
	Private sector influences
	Skills
	University culture
Comfort Zone	Intentional reversal to HCA role
	Avoidance techniques
Clinical Issues	Forced reversal into HCA role with loss of learning opportunities
	Resource to others
	Confirmation of student role and gaining long term respect

FIGURE 6.1.3 Identified themes and subcategories.

dependently reviewed the transcripts identifying key categories and themes. Comparison between the researchers' and colleagues' categories identified that the original categories and themes were accurate and complete. One participant from each focus group was sent a copy of the group's interview transcripts and asked to identify what he or she believed were the key categories and themes. These themes were compared to the researchers' own, and adjustments were made as required—a process, that Holloway and Wheeler (2002) refer to as "member checking."

Burnard's (1991) thematic content analysis led to the identification of three main themes and nine subcategories (Figure 6.1.3).

Discussion

The findings are presented in themes with the use of direct quotes, a perspective supported by Sandelowski (1994) who views quotes as a means of giving a living meaning to the studies' participants.

Culture Shock

The socialisation process brought with it a significant culture shock from life as a student nurse on clinical placement. Many participants felt that upon entering nurse education, previously developed skills as a HCA would carry them through the initial stages of their training. This culture shock has many facets to it, one being accountability. The participants identified that their lack of understanding around the issue of accountability was due to their lack of appreciation of this issue whilst a HCA.

> I mean, you heard trained nurses talk about accountability, but you just didn't understand what they really meant did you? (3rd year student)

In line with accountability, the realisation of professional responsibility in the way regulations governed how they worked also came as a shock, yet this was not seen as a frightening issue as was the case with accountability, but rather as a positive means of helping them identify the differences between their role as a HCA and that of a student.

The realisation for some, that they were unprepared for the realities of their clinical placements caused a degree of anxiety, emphasising a clear link with their previous place of employment. The process of socialisation was more traumatic for those whose prior experience in health care originated from the independent sector. Here, the participants had a common belief that prior knowledge and skills would support them within the hospital setting.

> I realised that it was very different from what I was expecting, and I kept saying to myself, I thought I would be able to do this with working in the nursing home. I think that it is the shock factor of it being a totally different environment. (2nd year student)

Participants rationalised that the inability to apply their knowledge to the hospital environment was the belief that hospitals were more clinical in nature. Participants identified issues such as a faster pace of work and differing routines that affected their abilities to transfer their knowledge and adapt to new cultural pressures.

One area that united all participants was the belief in their abilities to perform practical skills developed whilst employed as a HCA, with some acknowledging the lack of theoretical understanding that went with these skills:

> I had done a lot of things like catheterisation, but it was not what I expected when we were taught it here (university). It was totally different. So I had come in here thinking, yeah, I've got knowledge, and I know what I am doing, when really, with my skills I didn't. (2nd year student)

Questioning perceived skills only served to increase the difficulties in the socialisation process. The realisation for some that what they had practiced gave them no *easy passage* into clinical practice and in some cases was clinically unsound, lead to questioning the knowledge they had developed as a HCA.

Whilst all participants identified that they redeveloped their skills as time progressed, some described the frustration of no longer being able to undertake tasks unsupervised, which they had previously performed as a HCA.

> I felt that my hands were tied behind my back. As a HCA, I use to do venepuncture, bladder scans, and other things. But in becoming a student it is all taken away from you and you have to start again, to learn as a professional person rather than as a HCA. (3rd year student)

It is evident that although participants go through a culture shock within their clinical placements, all were far less concerned with the cultural impact of the university setting, stressing the importance the university played in the development of their education. Equally, despite the culture shock, all were united in their view that any experience of health care prior to their training was seen as a distinct advantage. A finding supported by Gray and Smith (1999) who explored the socialisation of students, showing that students who had previous nursing experience obtained the advantage of insight into ward routines.

The Comfort Zone

Commencing clinical placements created the greatest degree of shock in the socialisation process. To off set this, participants developed strategies to aid this process. *The comfort zone* recognises that the participants viewed these strategies as a means of providing comfort and safety, while trying to socialise into the role of a student. The most common theme was the intentional act of reverting into the HCA role. This was utilised whenever participants felt unsure of their student role or wanted to demonstrate their abilities on a new placement to gain acceptance into the team. It was a process heavily utilised within the first year of training:

> Yeah, I think sometimes [during] your first week in placement you can sit back in the HCA role—you're comfortable with that, and you're team building, and you're getting to know the ward and staff. I mean if you've worked in medicine and you go to

surgery you could easily slip into the HCA role just to get a feel of the place. (3rd year student)

This approach to social acceptance demonstrates the need for a sense of professional incorporation. Cope, Cuthbertson, and Stoddart (2000) observed that to achieve professional incorporation there is a requirement to demonstrate confidence in one's abilities. In reverting to the HCA role, the participants were looking for professional acceptance as a means of defining their new identity. Equally, as they were prepared to adopt this strategy, the participants also realised and stressed the importance of being prepared to give it up.

The question arises as to whether the comfort zone was also being utilised as a shelter. The comfort zone was viewed by the participants to be a place to start their clinical placement and be secure in their known abilities as HCAs. However, this same zone could also be used as a shelter. In this context it could be seen as a place to escape from the pressures of being a student, through the reluctance to take on responsibility, or when lacking confidence. It can be seen that dropping into the comfort zone allows the opportunity to socialise with one particular group. In knowing that they were all HCAs before their training started, it was easier for the participants to socialise with the group to which they were once members, namely the HCAs. It was then a logical step to consider that socialising with a group that the participants were former members of, would help gain a quicker acceptance into the team. The comfort zone therefore serves a dual purpose, utilised at any stage of their training, it was particularly pertinent to the first year, when participants were still in the process of identifying their new roles. Between the two strategies, be it as a comfort zone or a shelter, the participants saw it as a vital means of protection, if not self-preservation.

Clinical Issues

Participants expressed concern regarding clinical placements use of them as HCAs, resulting in feelings of resentment at being utilised as HCAs, at

---

Intentional use of student as a HCA by placement
Short staffed on the ward
Lack of guidance from placement mentor
Lack of confidence to complain
Insufficient working time with placement mentor
Previous HCA role known by staff on ward
Busy clinical area

FIGURE 6.1.4 Participant's reasons for utilisation as a HCA.

the expense of their learning. A number of reasons were cited for this (Figure 6.1.4).

The participants recognised that staff shortages were a problem that everyone had to cope with, and were happy to work to meet the demands of the placement, but not at the expense of their learning. Their intentional use of them as HCAs was an occurrence cited by only a small number in the study, with participants exemplifying how their previous experience as a HCA was abused:

In my case the ward was very short staffed, and the charge nurse would come and say, "you are going to have to work as a team assistant today we don't have anyone who can mentor you." Even though my practice mentor would be there, and I found this nearly every shift I was on. So I was told to my face I was getting used as a team assistant. (3rd year student)

This overt method contrasted with the more covert approach used by other placements:

When I phoned up the nursing home and spoke to the matron she said, "I've already accepted one student and I don't want anymore," and then she said, "Can I just ask you something, do you have any experience as a HCA?" So I said, "I have actually, I have 15 years," then she said, "Oh well I think we will be able to fit you in, so you can come." So really, I knew before I started that I was going to be used as a HCA. (2nd year student)

Clinical placement's knowledge that the participants were former HCAs was cited by some as a reason that they were utilised as such. This disclosure of information was seen as a negative influence, since it encouraged staff to still view them as HCAs.

My first placement, when ever it was short of HCAs, I was always the one who would be sent to help the other HCA. The other student, because she had never done it before (nursing) was always doing the drug rounds or things like that. Because I had experience and they knew that, they thought, "She knows what she's doing. She will be able to do it quicker than the other student." (3rd student on completion of training)

To ensure that they did not miss out on learning opportunities, the participants resorted to varying methods to resolve the problem. For example, one method was not informing their clinical placement that they had HCA experience. Studies by Papp, Markkanen, and von Bonsdorff (2003); Jackson and Mannix (2001); and Nolan (1998) identified that student nurses view the attitudes of staff toward them as being important and that until the students felt accepted in their role, learning could not take place. A finding reinforced by the participants of this study.

Within the findings of this study lies a conundrum. On the one hand, the participants were happy to shelter in the *comfort zone* and revert back to the HCA role. But equally, they complained about being utilised as HCAs. This suggests that the participants saw a clear difference between the two in respect of this issue. Their utilisation as HCAs, along with the absence of learning opportunities lent itself to the overwhelming feeling of just continuing in their old HCA role. However, it is evident that they saw no problem in reverting back to the HCA role in moments of self-doubt. The participants viewed this as a coping strategy, and it is this independent ability to use the comfort zone as and when they saw fit that indicated to them when they were being seen and supported as students and not as HCAs.

A positive attribute of the socialisation process was the participants' willingness to share their knowledge. The participants found themselves being "looked up too" in the early stages of their training by students in their cohorts with no health care experience. As a result many saw this as a clear advantage, thus boosting their confidence and self-esteem in the clinical area.

A major concern for the participants was their long-term acceptance by others as qualified nurses. None of the participants, when asked, could give an exact point in their training when they felt as if they had fully socialised into the role of a student. But just as the socialisation to a student was a concern for them, many had their eyes fixed to the future and how they would be perceived as a qualified nurse. This was more acute for those who had been seconded from local trusts. Their main concern revolved around gaining respect and recognition in their new role as a qualified nurse. They highlighted occurrences of not being accepted as a student when on clinical placement, and of having doubts about being accepted back by staff who would forever perceive them as HCAs. Although acknowledging that ultimately respect is something they need to earn, some in identifying the difficulties of socialisation, realised they faced similar problems at the end of their training.

An Emerging Framework

The findings of this study offer a new framework for the transition and professional socialisation from HCA to student nurse. Initially based upon emerging themes from the literature, the findings of this study can now be extended, to demonstrate the transitional process undertaken by the HCA turned student (Figure 6.1.5).

Figure 6.1.5 identifies that issues around role identity, exposure to the RGN role, and reality shock, all play a part in the transition and socialisation process. Upon entering their nurse training these identified themes affect preconceived ideas and feelings around what participants expect their nurse training to be. The student now enters a new phase.

Here, what they know about their previous HCA role and how they perceived it would help them in their nurse training, is met by the reality of a culture shock. In order to progress, they work through this culture shock. This study highlights how professional and clinical issues affect the point at which students feel socialised into their student

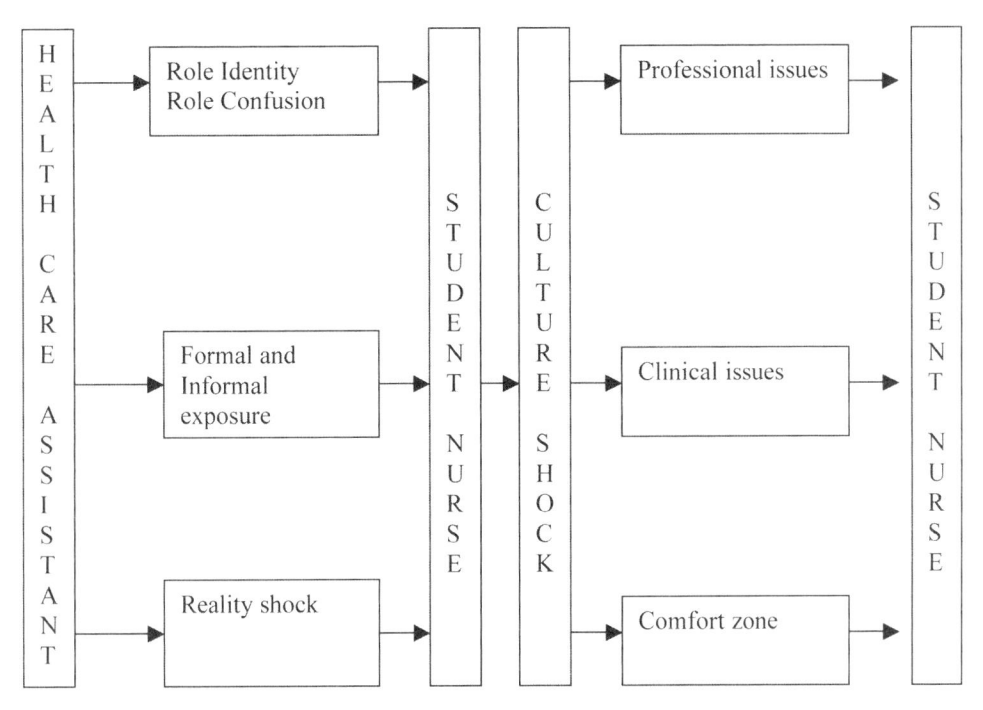

FIGURE 6.1.5 The transitional process undertaken by the HCA turned student.

role, and no longer see themselves as working or thinking like HCAs. To help this process, the student has the protection of the comfort zone. The comfort zone is in a constant fluid motion, which at any stage of his or her training, a student, based upon the findings of this study could drop back into. The ability to withdraw into the HCA role when feeling vulnerable is one that requires greater exploration. There is a need to understand what issues are at play and what drives students to retreat into their previous role.

Equally, there is a need to look at the role clinical areas play in this process. The agreement from all participants that they were utilised as HCAs should serve as a warning that the role students play in the clinical areas needs to be re-examined.

This new framework, through additional research, can be developed further. It takes the HCA turned student through a journey to the point of his or her socialisation. What is now open for exploration is: What happens to this student next?

Conclusion

Nursing students with a HCA background face different challenges in comparison to other nursing students. Although many would argue that these challenges are part of the realities of nursing, there comes a point when issues such as these need to be addressed. To ensure that the former HCA turned student nurse's transition and socialisation into the role of a student nurse is not detrimental to his or her education, but is in fact enjoyable.

REFERENCES

Abbott, A. A., 1988. Professional Choices: Values at work. National Association of Social Workers. In: Du Toit, D., 1995. A sociological analysis of the extent and influence of professional socialisation on the development of a nursing identity among nursing students at two universities in Brisbane, Australia. Journal of Advanced Nursing 21 (1), 164–171.

Burnard, P., 1991. A method of analysing interview transcripts in qualitative research. Nurse Education Today 11, 461–466.

Cohen, H.A., 1981. The nurses quest for a professional identity. In: Howkins, E.J., Ewens, A., 1999. How students experience professional socialisation. International Journal of Nursing Studies 36 (1), 41–49.

Cope, P., Cuthbertson, P., Stoddart, B., 2000. Situated learning in the practice placement. Journal of Advanced Nursing 31 (4), 850–856.

Department of Health, 2000. The NHS Plan: A plan for investment, a plan for reform. DoH, London.

Du Toit, D., 1995. A sociological analysis of the extent and influence of professional socialisation on the development of a nursing identity among nursing students at two universities in Brisbane, Australia. Journal of Advanced Nursing 21 (1), 164–171.

Elkan, R., Robinson, J., 1993. Project 2000: the gap between theory and practice. Nurse Education Today 13, 295–298.

Fitzpatrick, J.M., While, A.E., Roberts, J.D., 1996. Key influences on the professional socialisation and practice of students undertaking different pre-registration nurse education programmes in the United Kingdom. International Journal of Nursing Studies 33 (5), 506–518.

Gerrish, K., 2000. Still fumbling along? A comparative study of the newly qualified nurse's perception of the transition from student to qualified nurse. Journal of Advanced Nursing 32 (2), 473–480.

Gray, M., Smith, L., 1999. The professional socialisation of diploma of higher education in nursing students (Project 2000): a longitudinal qualitative study. Journal of Advanced Nursing 29 (3), 639–647.

Greenbaum, T.L., 1998. The Handbook for Focus Group Research, second ed. Sage Publications, London.

Holland, K., 1999. A journey to becoming: the student nurse in transition. Journal of Advanced Nursing 29 (1), 229–236.

Holloway, I., Wheeler, S., 2002. Qualitative Research in Nursing, second ed. Blackwell Science, London.

Howkins, E.J., Ewens, A., 1999. How students experience professional socialisation. International Journal of Nursing Studies 36 (1), 41–49.

Jackson, D., Mannix, J., 2001. Clinical nurses as teachers: insights from students of nursing in their first semester of study. Journal of Clinical Nursing 10 (2), 270–277.

Kramer, M., 1974. Reality Shock: Why Nurses Leave Nursing. Mosby, St Louis.

Lacey, C, 1977. The Socialisation of Teachers. Methuen, London.

Maben, J., Clark, J.M., 1998. Project 2000 diplomats perceptions of their experiences of transition from student to staff nurse. Journal of Clinical Nursing 7 (2), 145–153.

Meleis, A.I., 1986. Theory development and domain concepts. In: Hunter, L.P., Bormann, J.E., Lops, V.R. (Eds.), 1996. Student to nurse-midwife role transition process. Smoothing the way. Journal of Nurse-Midwifery 41 (4), 328–333.

Melia, K., 1987. Learning and Working. The Occupational Socialisation of Nurses. Tayistock, London.

Morgan, D.L., 1998. Planning Focus Groups. Focus Group Kit 2. Sage Publications, London.

Morse, J.M., Field, P.A., 1996. Nursing Research. The Application of Qualitative Approaches. Chapman and Hall, London.

Nolan, C., 1998. Learning on clinical placement: the experience of six Australian student nurses. Nurse Education Today 18, 622–629.

Papp, I., Markkanen, M., von Bonsdorff, M., 2003. Clinical environment as a learning environment: student nurses perceptions concerning clinical learning experiences. Nurse Education Today 23, 262–268.

Sandelowski, M., 1994. The use of quotes in qualitative research. Research in Nursing and Health 17 (6), 479–483.

Streubert, H.J., Carpenter, D.R., 1995. Qualitative Research in Nursing. Advancing the Humanistic Imperative, second ed. Lippincott, Philadelphia.

Talotta, D., 1990. Role conceptions and professional role discrepancy among baccalaureate nursing students employed as nurses aides. Journal of Nursing Scholarship 22 (2), 11–115.

Windsor, A., 1987. Nursing students perspectives of clinical experience. Journal of Nursing Education 26 (4), 150–154.

Reprinted with permission from: Brennan, G., & McSherry, R. (2007). Exploring the transition and professional socialization from health care assistant to student nurse. *Nurse Education in Practice, 7*(4), 206–214.

6.2 CLINICAL TRANSITION OF BACCALAUREATE NURSING STUDENTS DURING PRECEPTORED, PREGRADUATION PRACTICUMS

Diane M. Wieland
Geralyn M. Altmiller
Mary T. Dorr
Zane Robinson Wolf

Abstract

Transition into the role of registered nurse after graduation from nursing education programs results in new nurses feeling overwhelmed and unprepared for the challenges of the workplace. The purpose of this triangulated, descriptive study was to describe the clinical transition experience of senior baccalaureate nursing students during pregraduation preceptored practicums, which took place three times per week for three weeks. Data were collected from student journal entries, liaison faculty, and clinical preceptors. Thematic analysis was performed on responses students recorded on the Daily Feedback Sheet on Transition to the Graduate Nurse Role and on preceptor- and liaison faculty-documented journals. According to students, preceptors, and liaison faculty, students' knowledge and skills increased during the preceptorship, and many students became integral members of hospital unit teams. Strategies to modify the preceptorship included maintaining consistency with liaison faculty and increasing communication between preceptors and liaison faculty.

Following graduation, during their initial employment, new nurses often feel overwhelmed and unprepared for the challenges of the workplace [1]. Preceptored, senior-year practicums can ease the stress of adaptation and socialization intrinsic to independent nursing practice and serve as a transition for nursing students to the role of registered nurse.[2-4] Successful preceptor programs support nurses and help ensure their retention in nursing.

The literature describes experiences of new nurse graduates who are assigned preceptors in orientation programs [5-10]. However, there is a dearth of research literature on the transition of students to the graduate nurse role through preceptored experiences that take place during the final year of a baccalaureate nursing program. This chapter reports on a triangulated, descriptive study designed to describe the clinical transition experience of seniors during a pregraduation, preceptored clinical experience. Two research questions were posed:

1. From the perspectives of students, liaison faculty, and clinical preceptors, what is the clinical transitional experience for BSN students who participate in an intensive preceptorship, three days per week for three weeks, during the senior year?
2. What patterns in the clinical transitional experience reveal issues for continuous improvement of the BSN program?

Consistent with VanGennep, the clinical transitional experience was defined as a social and physical passage in which students progress to the graduate nurse role during preceptorship prior to graduation [11]. Issues for continuous quality improvement were defined as matters for discussion by faculty to improve the preceptored experience, and the preceptorship program was defined as a pregraduation "intensive, reality-based clinical experience to facilitate transition into the real world of nursing."[12, p. 26]

Review of Literature

The clinical transition from the nursing student role to the graduate nurse role can be viewed as a rite of passage that encompasses three major phases: Separation, transition, and incorporation [11]. As a transition, the preceptored practicum in the senior year might include the separation of students from dependence on faculty, their feelings of increasing competence, and their incorporation into the new role of professional nurse.

The clinical competence of baccalaureate nursing students participating in a summer preceptorship was compared to that of a similar group who worked as nursing assistants in a non-instructional clinical setting [13]. Clinical competence was rated by head nurses. Students in the summer preceptor groups demonstrated greater gain in clinical competence, problem solving, application of theory to practice, and performance of psychomotor skills. Similarly, Yonge and Trojan [14] compared the nursing performance of nonpreceptored and preceptored students in their final clinical course of a BSN program. Nonpreceptored students were assigned to a small clinical group with one clinical faculty member; preceptored students were assigned to individual preceptors. Students in the preceptored group had statistically significantly higher postclinical scores compared to the nonpreceptored group.

Following a 12-week preceptorship that took place during the last term of the BSN program, students rated their perceptions of the demands of nursing practice, environments, and their learning competencies.[12] They rated themselves higher on all competencies and skill levels, including testing theories and experimenting with new ideas.

White[15] reported on how students, enrolled in a management clinical rotation in their final semester, described their clinical decision making. Students described their decisions and nursing actions as consistent with patients' immediate needs. A model of clinical decision making emerged that included gaining confidence in skills, building relationships with staff, connecting with patients, achieving comfort with self as a nurse, and understanding the clinical picture. The support and participation by staff nurses fostered the development of self-confidence in students.

An integrative clinical preceptor model was implemented as a collaborative partnership between a school of nursing and nurses in community health settings [16]. Students underwent an intensive orientation period, adopting a service-learning approach. Faculty, who served as resources for students and preceptors, participated in students' projects, made site visits, and assessed the achievement of service-learning goals and objectives related to population-focused care. They also evaluated the outcomes of the experience and student performance. Preceptors attended a course on the characteristics of a good preceptor, role expectations and responsibilities, conflict resolution, and an overview of teaching/learning principles for effective clinical teaching. They developed relationships with faculty members, functioned as clinical teachers and role models, and participated in planning and implementing clinical experiences.

Rogers described the preceptor role as essential to a preceptorship program, whether it takes place before or after graduation [17]. In helping neophytes transition to the role of professional nurse, preceptors serve as coaches, role models, socializers, and evaluators. They ease new nurses through the honeymoon, shock, and recovery phases into the resolution phase and help them identify with positive professional behaviors and develop a balanced perspective on health care settings. Preceptors validate interpersonal competencies, critical thinking, and decision-making skills; their evaluations are beneficial if they are timely and factual, include criticism and praise, promote professional growth, and affirm respect for new nurses.

Hrobsky and Kersbergen [18] reported on clinical preceptors' perceptions of associate degree nursing students whose clinical performance during a practicum was deemed unsatisfactory. Identified themes were: Hallmarks of poor clinical performance, preceptors' feelings, and the role of liaison faculty. Poor performance consisted of unenthusiastic behavior toward nursing, not asking questions, and unsatisfactory skill performance. Although concerned about patient safety, preceptors were fearful, anxious, and self-doubting, especially when they knew that students would fail based on their negative evaluations. Liaison faculty provided support for the preceptors, listening to them and following up at the end of the practicum.

Yonge, Ferguson, Myrick, and Haase examined preparation for the preceptorship experience.[19] Faculty liaisons noted that the preparation of preceptors was inconsistent and the frequency of faculty visitation with students and preceptors varied. Liaisons saw their role as one of supporting students and preceptors, communicating curriculum trends, and fostering students' application of knowledge to clinical situations.

Method

This triangulated, descriptive study used journal entries [20,21] to foster students' critical thinking and reflection [22] about their practice. A form titled "Daily Feedback Sheet on Transition to the Graduate Nurse Role" (DFSTGNR) was the chief data source.

Triangulation was achieved by analysis of textual data from three sources: The DFSTGNR, liaison faculty, and clinical preceptor journals. Two themes were identified using the narratives recorded by participants: The transitional experience and process improvement issues.

Thirty-two senior nursing students attending a full-time undergraduate nursing program and enrolled in an adult, acute care, senior-level course at the end of the program were invited to participate.[23–25] Fourteen students completed journals. Three clinical or liaison faculty employed by the university and nine clinical preceptors employed by health care agencies also participated.

Students ranged in age from 21 to 42 years old. Two of the 14 students were male and two were married. Most, 11 students, were white; two were African American; and the ethnic background of one student was not identified. All but one student spoke English as their primary language.

The institutional review board of the university approved the study; participants' anonymity was maintained. Each participant signed a consent form and complied with Health Insurance Portability and Accountability Act (HIPAA) regulations regarding patient assignments.

Students recorded handwritten comments on the DFSTGNR. This journal, constructed to document the transition to the graduate nurse role during the preceptorship, asked students to record as follows: Describe your patient assignment (comply with HIPAA guidelines and do not include identifying information); number of patients assigned; gender; diagnosis; comments on changes you are experiencing; your goals and additional comments.

A Preceptor Form was created for preceptors to comment on changes they saw in students. Similarly, clinical or liaison faculty completed a Nursing Faculty Form, which elicited comments on the performance of individual students as well as group changes. The forms were also used to provide individual feedback to students throughout the preceptorship, by both the preceptor assigned to the student and the faculty member responsible for the student.

Students worked at clinical sites for a total of nine eight-hour shifts (each Tuesday, Wednesday, and Thursday for three weeks). This schedule was selected following a focus group with employers that took place at the university and centered on the logistics of when, and in which units, the preceptorships would be provided. Employers attending the focus group preferred that a nine-day experience be provided to allow for greater exposure to the nursing role. Faculty adopted their recommendation. Previously, the school had offered a six-day experience.

Students were given a packet of three DFSTGNRs that they completed on the third, sixth, and ninth days of the practicum. On the same days, faculty and clinical preceptors also recorded their responses. Often, preceptors were not paired with the same students from day to day, depending on the nurse preceptor's work schedule.

Data were analyzed using the constant-comparative methods of Glaser and Strauss as adapted by Lincoln and Guba [23–25]. Checks were performed at the completion of data analysis; students, faculty, and preceptors confirmed the findings. Trustworthiness was established with peer review and an audit trail. Transferability was achieved by two current students and a liaison faculty member participant who read the study and confirmed that it described many aspects of pregraduation, preceptored practicums.

Results

Student Observations

Students selected their own units of preference and were assigned to patients with many different diagnoses. Four students were in the medical–surgical unit; three selected oncology; and the others were in the emergency unit, maternity, the operating room, a cardiac catheterization laboratory, the intermediate neuro-intensive care unit, the acute psychiatric unit, and a short procedure unit.

Among the patients cared for were a 68-year-old woman with breast cancer who had nausea, vomiting, and diarrhea; an 80-year-old woman with diverticulitis and pseudomonas colitis; a 69-year-old woman with anemia pancytopenia; a 98-year-old with dehydration, urinary tract infection, and dementia; and a 59-year-old with metastatic lung cancer with rule-out spinal cord compression. The number of patients assigned increased gradually over the 9-day period.

Students wrote of enjoying nursing care and relishing patients' appreciation of their care: "My patients were very receptive to my presence; I enjoyed their company." They were thankful that their knowledge was demonstrated: "I felt really good when I was able to answer their questions." One student, however, was exhausted by the preceptorship and the demands of her courses: "It was very difficult for me to come home and attempt to study or do homework." Financial stress was a concern as some students who were employed on a part-time basis as patient care associates while attending the university found that they were unable to work during the three weeks of the preceptorship.

The preceptorship enabled students to expand their knowledge base and skill performance. Stimulated by the challenge, students became increasingly comfortable with, and proud of, their developing skills: "I feel very comfortable giving meds, assessments, trache care, suctioning, and using pumps." They appreciated seeing procedures, such as a paracentesis and a central line flush, learning about more medications and IVs, learning how to administer different medications, and gaining information regarding medical conditions as well as nursing care specific to abnormal laboratory values. One wrote, "I have gotten much better at reading fetal heart monitoring which was one of my goals." Students' capacity to access information from computers and understand staff assignment strategies increased, along with their assessment documentation and charting abilities.

The comfort of students corresponded to their increased independence and competence. One wrote, "I felt much more involved with patient care, talking to doctors and other care providers." Another wrote, "I now feel comfortable dealing with vented patients. Throughout the week (three days) the nursing staff on the unit has placed me with a vented patient....I feel more comfortable now, when I graduate, to handle a patient in this condition. One patient had a PEG tube, so I did a lot of work with putting meds down the tube, checking residual, and flushing."

During the second week, as nursing care progressed more smoothly, most students became increasingly independent and communicated more easily with staff when they needed assistance. Students were challenged by how much there was to learn about caring for patients, but their self-confidence increased: "I feel like I can do anything," and "I feel proud because I am competent and learning." Students were also proud that they managed an increased number of patients and felt part of the culture and functioning of units. One wrote, "I have come to know the staff members here very well and I feel like I am part of the team."

Students had specific as well as general goals. Some focused on such areas as knowing how to set up patient-controlled analgesia equipment, knowing when to call physicians, using better time management, teaching patients about medications, and learning more about the actions and side effects of medications: "[I want to] become comfortable using pumps and other hospital technology."

During the final week, students persisted in setting their agendas for learning. One shared her plan: "I hope to have a general understanding of psychiatric meds, multidisciplinary approaches to psychiatric management, the role of the psychiatric nurse, and effective communication techniques for patient/nurse interaction." They began to see a broader scope of learning possibilities. One student was determined to become more knowledgeable in the area of oncology and to take care of an "entire nurse's assignment," another was interested in understanding cardiac drugs and principles of triaging emergency unit patients. Students learned how to practice in specialized settings such as cardiac catheterization ("I am better able to identify what I see as the heart as viewed with dye and x-ray"); the operating room ("I am learning how to set up sterile fields for the procedure"); and to care for difficult patients ("I had a couple of noncompliant patients so I have had a firsthand account in the nursing position dealing with these patients").

Although improvements in time management were noted over the nine days, more skill was desired. Students became aware of competing and sometimes unequal needs and priorities of patients: "I realize how difficult it is to care for four patients, especially when one of them requires more care than others."

Students were very comfortable with their preceptors, who answered their questions and positioned them to "see new things." Some thought that their preceptors trusted them: "My RN lets me take on the entire workload and helps me with problems such as PD (peritoneal dialysis) and urinary irrigations." Some regretted that they had more than one preceptor, but tried to make the best of the situation. A few had a more difficult time meeting the expectations of preceptors. "Everybody is possessive over what they feel we should be doing" and "It was difficult to assess what changes/improvements I was making since I had a different preceptor every day."

Students gained confidence in interacting and working with the nursing staff. They felt free to ask questions and appreciated receiving "excellent" explanations. One felt privileged when working with the team of nurses and physicians: "I have come to know the staff members here very well and I feel like I am part of the team."

Students valued the preceptorship most of the time. Many realized immediately that they needed to reach out to the staff by asking questions and becoming accustomed to the independence associated with the preceptorship. "The nurses were very helpful, but in order to learn I had to ask questions or else they thought you knew what you were doing." Later they recognized the preceptorship as "integral in my development from nursing student to graduate nurse." Their adaptation to the units was facilitated by preceptors and enhanced by their commitment to learning.

For some students, who were concerned about their performance in class, the nine-day preceptorship was too long. One student wrote: "Although the preceptorship was a little too long for me in my setting, I am proud I have finished my clinical experience well. I feel the three days a week is a lot to handle, perhaps two days a week for an extended period would be more beneficial. I found by the third day [the preceptorship], along with studying, was very tiring."

A few students criticized the role of liaison faculty. They did not appreciate the brief time spent with them and the fact that faculty completed a clinical evaluation form on student performance. They noted also that the first phase of the preceptored experience was disorganized: "[We] were made to go to the units themselves, even if [we] were unsure of how to get there." In some cases, students were "hostile to the clinical (liaison) instructor" and hoped for better communication among the administrator, liaison faculty, students, and classroom teacher. They also were annoyed about competition among nursing programs for clinical sites and limited assignments due to low patient census. They appreciated the opportunity to select the clinical sites that most interested them.

Liaison Faculty Observations

As the practicum began, liaison faculty saw students as apprehensive about the immersion experience and, at the same time, excited about its challenges. Although some students seemed detached, it was understood that they might have been concentrating on the challenges ahead. Initially, students did not seem to trust faculty members and gave the impression that they were confused about their role as preceptee. Some complained that the preceptored experience was extended from six to nine days and that the goals of the immersion experience had not been discussed with them. They were frustrated since fewer patients were assigned during the preceptorship compared to the clinical experience during the previous semester when they were expected to care for up to four patients per day. In addition, a few patient units accommodated students from different nursing programs, which led to competition for patients.

On the whole, students settled in comfortably as they took care of patients with different diagnoses. They worked somewhat autonomously and seemed confident. One faculty member mentioned that they might have been too confident. Although on some specialty units, students seemed to be helping nursing staff rather than caring for patients independently, they were involved with patient assignments and asked for increasing independence.

As the days went by, students tested the limits of their role as they tried to perform as much nursing care as allowable, and most seemed comfortable with greater responsibility. Some called physicians to follow up on patient problems. They modeled nursing staff behavior and acted more like staff, for example, giving a change-of-shift report. Some stood out as particularly confident, competent individuals. In general, students' documentation abilities improved and they progressed in organizational skills and time management.

By the last day of the preceptorship, students were more accountable for their actions and demanded challenges to improve their critical thinking. They followed through in discussions of patient problems with physicians and pharmacists, and some students were too busy to pay attention to the liaison faculty when they were observed on the last day. Although a few students had "bad" attitudes about the experience, most were very positive about the preceptorship, interacted well with the nursing staff, and were respected by them. As they gained the trust of staff, they were assigned more patients and given greater independence.

Preceptor Observations

Preceptors were conscious that students looked to them as role models. As the days of the practicum progressed, preceptors were eager to hire some students as coworkers and singled certain students out for praise. In general, they saw students becoming more aware of patients' needs, taking initiative, organizing patient care, prioritizing the needs of patients, and understanding the workflow and needs of the unit. Students were alert to physicians' orders, progress notes, and patient regimens, and were also very willing to help the members of the team.

Although some students needed to improve their skill base, organizational skills, and knowledge of patient chart information, most were motivated to learn and actively sought additional learning opportunities. They were efficient and organized, friendly and outgoing with nursing staff, and attentive to the subtleties of the role differences among the nurses working in different settings. Gradually, students gained independence and confidence, began to ask more questions, adjusted to unit environments, and managed time more efficiently as they administered medications. Several adjusted to having more than one preceptor, and all became more comfortable with the increased number of patients assigned.

Students handled stressful situations, asked questions, were eager to learn, and worked well with preceptors and nursing staff. They knew their limits and continued to sharpen documentation, organization, knowledge recall, and prioritization skills. They looked more competent and confident and completed assignments in a timely fashion.

Discussion

Students made many gains during the preceptored experience. Their time management abilities and documentation skills increased, and they became comfortable with more assignments and expanded responsibilities. They emulated the practice of nursing staff and began to act like staff members. By the final day of the preceptorship, they requested challenges to improve their critical thinking, were more accountable for their actions, and collaborated more often with other health care providers. They were more efficient, organized, and performed clinical skills more competently, and they began to adjust to unit environments, handle stress, and manage medication administration proficiently. Most students felt supported by preceptors and clinical liaison faculty and believed that they had achieved goals identified at the beginning of the preceptorship.

Students' confidence in their performance, the relationships they built with staff, their connections with patients, and their comfort as nurses were consistent with findings from White's[15] study.

Planning, evaluation, interpersonal relationships, and communication also corresponded with performance changes reported by Yonge and Trojan.[14]

The investigation provided a voice for students, liaison faculty, and preceptors to contribute to continuous quality improvement of the preceptored experience. Issues for continuous improvement include facilitating connections between students and preceptors; having one preceptor, if possible, throughout the preceptorship; having clinical liaison faculty conduct clinical rounds at least twice daily; enhancing the orientation for preceptors and preceptees; clarifying guidelines concerning final student clinical evaluations; reviewing with students reality-based expectations of the preceptored experience; and maintaining consistency among liaison faculty by retaining those who had taught the students earlier that semester.

Other recommended strategies include liaison faculty escorting students to assigned units or settings; encouraging the development of positive student-preceptor relationships; contacting students at least twice during a shift and more often if assignments increase in complexity due to workload or unforeseen events; and developing an evaluation form specific to the preceptorship. It may also be beneficial to clear students' schedules of all other class demands and allow them to follow preceptors' schedules, regardless of the day of the shift. This might eliminate the stress that comes with having multiple preceptors with varying styles.

Future research on the perceptions of clinical liaison faculty about the preceptorship experience via a focus group might yield insights for continuous program improvement. Pretest/posttest design studies measuring differences in student competencies and skills before and after the preceptorship are also recommended. A possible tool would be Yonge and Trojan's Six Dimensional Scale of Nursing Performance (measuring leadership, critical care, teaching/collaboration, planning/evaluation, professional development, communication, and interpersonal relationships)[14]. Another area for study might involve comparing traditional and nontraditional students in a preceptorship in order to tailor preceptorships specifically to each group.

Finally, a national survey is recommended. Such a survey should ask how preceptorships are structured, where in the curriculum they are implemented, the length of time for preceptored experiences, and procedures used in the implementation of preceptorships. The results could provide guidance for evaluation, managing increased student enrollment, and obtaining clinical sites.

REFERENCES

1. Brasler, M. E. (1993). Predictors of clinical performance of new graduate nurses participating in preceptor orientation programs. *Journal of Continuing Education in Nursing, 24*(4), 158–165.
2. Dobbs, K. K. (1988). The senior preceptorship as a method for anticipatory socialization of baccalaureate nursing students. *Journal of Nursing Education, 27*(4), 167–171.
3. Ellerton, M. L. (2003). Preceptorship: The changing face of clinical teaching. *Nurse Educator, 28*(5), 200–201.
4. Ridley, M. J., Laschinger, H. K., & Goldenberg, D. (1995). The effect of a senior preceptorship on the adaptive competencies of community college nursing students, *Journal of Advanced Nursing, 22,* 58–65.
5. Baltimore, J. J. (2004). The hospital clinical preceptor: Essential preparation for success. *Journal of Continuing Education in Nursing, 35*(3), 133–140.
6. Casey K., Fink R., Krugman, M., & Propst, J. (2004). The graduate nurse experience. *Journal of Nursing Administration, 34*(6), 303–311.
7. Delaney, C. (2003). Walking a fine line: Graduate nurses' transition experiences during orientation. *Journal of Nursing Education, 42*(10), 437–443.
8. Godinez, G., Schweiger, J., Gruver, J., & Ryan, P. (1999). Role transition from graduate to staff nurse: A qualitative analysis. *Journal for Nurses in Staff Development, 15*(3), 97–110.
9. Kilstoff, K., & Rochester, S. F. (2004). Hitting the floor running: Transitional experiences of graduates previously trained as enrolled nurses. *Australian Journal of Advanced Nursing, 22*(1), 13–17.
10. McKenna, B. G., Smith, N. A., Poole, S. J., & Coverdale, J. H. (2003). Horizontal violence: Experiences of registered nurses in their first year of

practice. *Journal of Advanced Nursing, 42*(1), 90–96.
11. VanGennep, A. (1960). *The rites of passage.* Chicago: University of Chicago Press.
12. Laschinger, H. K., & MacMaster, E. (1992). Effects of pregraduate preceptorship experience on development of adaptive competencies of baccalaureate nursing students. *Journal of Nursing Education, 31*(6) 258–264.
13. Sheetz, L. J. (1989). Baccalaureate nursing student preceptorship programs and the development of clinical competence. *Journal of Nursing Education, 28*(1), 29–35.
14. Yonge, O., & Trojan, L. (1992). The nursing performance of preceptored and non-preceptored baccalaureate nursing students. *Canadian Journal of Nursing Research, 24*(4), 61–75.
15. White, A. (2003). Clinical decision making among fourth-year nursing students: An interpretive study. *Journal of Nursing Education, 42*(3), 113–120.
16. Mallette, S., Loury, S., Engelke, M. K., & Andrews, A. (2005). The integrative clinical preceptor model: A new method for teaching undergraduate community health nursing. *Nurse Educator, 30*(1), 21–26.
17. Rogers, B. (2003). *The effective nurse preceptor handbook.* Marblehead, MA: HCPro.
18. Hrobsky, P., & Kersbergen, A. (2002). Preceptors' perceptions of clinical failure. *Journal of Nursing Education, 41*(12), 550–553.
19. Yonge, O., Ferguson, L., Myrick, F., & Haase, M. (2003). Faculty preparation for the preceptorship experience: The forgotten link. *Nurse Educator, 28*(5), 210–211.
20. Brown, H., & Sorrell, J. (1993). Use of clinical journals to enhance critical thinking. *Nurse Educator, 18*(5), 16–19.
21. Callister, M. (1993). The use of student journals in nursing education: Making meaning out of clinical experiences. *Journal of Nursing Education, 32*(4), 185–186.
22. Boud, D. (2001). Using journal writing to enhance reflective practice. *New Directions in Adult Continuing Education, 90,* 9–17.
23. Glaser, B., & Strauss, A. (1967). *The discovery of grounded theory: Strategies for qualitative research.* Chicago: Aldine.
24. Lincoln, Y. S., & Guba, E. G. (1985). *Naturalistic inquiry.* Beverly Hills, CA: Sage.
25. Morse, J. (1994). Designing funded qualitative research. In N. K. Denzin, & Y. S. Lincoln (Eds.), *Handbook of qualitative research* (pp. 220–235). Thousand Oaks, CA: Sage.

Reprinted with permission from: Wieland, D., Altmiller, G. M., Dorr, M. T., & Wolf, Z. R. (2007). Clinical transition of baccalaureate nursing students: During preceptored, pregraduation practicums. *Nursing Education Perspectives, 28*(6), 315–321.

6.3 THERE REALLY IS A DIFFERENCE: NURSES' EXPERIENCES WITH TRANSITIONING FROM RNs TO BSNs

COLLEEN DELANEY
BARBARA PISCOPO

Abstract

The purpose of this phenomenological study was to explore and describe the experience that associate degree and diploma nursing graduates have when transitioning from RN to BSN. Twelve nurses with a variety of clinical backgrounds and completion of different RN–BSN programs were interviewed to elicit the lived experience of transitioning from RN to BSN. Eight theme clusters emerged when the formulated meanings were organized into categories: (1) Varied Expectations, (2) Tentative Beginnings, (3) Cornerstone Courses, (4) Translating Knowledge into Empowerment, (5) Becoming Assertive Leader and Advocate, (6) Confronting and Conquering Challenges, (7) Envisioning the Whole, and (8) Recreating Everyday Practice. Findings indicate that both the quality of patient care and nurses' practice were enhanced as a result of BSN completion programs.

A *transition* is a pause between what was and what will be that is typically characterized by changes in identities, roles, relationships, abilities, and patterns of behavior (Schumacher & Meleis, 1994). For a small but increasing number of nurses, a significant but often overlooked transition is that from being RNs (registered nurses) to becoming BSNs (bachelor of science nurses). An RN–BSN program graduate, summarizing her perceptions at the beginning and at the end of her BSN completion program, captured the overall sentiments of the study participants:

> When I returned to school, I felt I was already a quality nurse. In the beginning, I did not think education would change my practice. But as I got deeper into nursing and the BSN [program], I began to pull the whole picture together just as if I was reading the whole story...and, I never thought I'd say this, but there really is a difference.

Baccalaureate preparation in nursing, as an important requisite to the advancement of the profession and optimal patient outcomes, is supported by national nursing organizations as well as accreditation bodies and validated in nursing research. A national objective for the profession of nursing collectively stated by nursing leaders is to reverse the current statistic of one third of the nursing force holding a BSN degree to two thirds by 2010 (National Council on Nurse Education and Practice. 2001). Referred to as the new nursing shortage, the lack of BSN program-prepared nurses is resulting in a deficiency of nurses adequately prepared to meet certain areas of patient needs in a changing health care environment (National League for Nursing, 2002). In addition, for hospitals to achieve a magnet status, the highest award given by the American Nurses Credentialing Center (2005) to organized nursing services, there must be among other criteria a high percentage of BSNs.

Although nursing organizations and accreditation bodies support the importance of increasing the number of BSN program-prepared nurses, empirical evidence linking nursing education to improved outcomes provides an even stronger rationale. Recent research suggested that there is a correlation between BSN program-prepared nurses and reduced mortality among surgical patients (Aiken, Sean, Cheung, Sloane, & Silber, 2003) as well as professional behaviors important to patient care, such as critical thinking (Brown, Alverson, & Pepa, 2001), professionalism (Phillips, Palmer, Zimmerman, & Mayfield, 2002), and creativity (Ku, Lo, Wang, Hsieh, & Chen, 2002).

The RN–BSN population has come into center stage as one of the key venues through which to achieve the national nursing objective. Further research is needed to better understand the unique needs of RN–BSN program students and facilitate school reentry. The aim of this study was to explore and describe nurses' experiences with transitioning from being RNs to becoming BSNs. A phenomenological approach provided the conceptual framework for researching the complexity of the study participants' lived experience and the methodology to uncover the essential structure of this phenomenon that changed the nurses, in their own way, from the nurses they were to the nurses they became.

Background

The changing health care system is demanding that health care workers be more knowledgeable, that care be linked to identified patient outcomes, that practice be evidence based, and that providers be accountable for the care provided. Registered nurses, accounting for the largest number of health care providers, must be knowledgeable workers delivering care based on best practice standards. There is a need for RNs, but, more importantly, there is also a need for RNs prepared at the baccalaureate and advanced levels of practice. Since the inception of articulation agreements in the 1980s, numerous strategies to facilitate BSN completion have been developed. However, in spite of diverse program formats, accelerated curricula, and tuition reimbursements, over the past 10 years, only approximately 16% of ADNs (associate degree nurses) and 24% of diploma nurses return to school to complete their baccalaureate degree (Spratley, Johnson, Sochalski, Fritz, & Spencer, 2000). In the past 2 years, the number of ADNs and that of diploma nurses returning to school have shown a modest increase across the country (North Atlantic = 3.8; Midwest = 0.8; South = 3.0; West = (18.5), but continue to lag behind other nursing enrollment statistics (American Association of Colleges of Nursing, 2005). Although ADNs and diploma nurses recognize the personal development and professional growth that accompany furthering their education, lack of support and recognition from employers and the difficulties of finding time, financial resources, and flexible class schedules are perceived as major barriers to returning to school (Delaney & Piscopo, 2004).

A review of the literature over the past decade revealed that several researchers have studied the RN–BSN population using quantitative methods most frequently and qualitative methods to a lesser extent. During this time, no phenomenological study concerning RN–BSN transitions had been published.

Brown et al. (2001) examined the influence of baccalaureate education on the critical thinking abilities of traditional, RN–BSN program, and accelerated students. Students completed the Watson–Glaser Critical Thinking Appraisal at the beginning and at the end of their nursing course sequence, Findings revealed a significant difference in pretest and posttest scores for traditional ($p = .007$) and RN–BSN program ($p = .029$) students, but not for accelerated students. Brown et al. concluded that further research was needed to determine the best course mix to facilitate critical thinking. These findings are inconsistent with those of a similar study conducted by White and Gomez (2002), who found no significant difference on two measures of critical thinking with 19 RNs at the beginning and at the end of a baccalaureate degree completion program.

Phillips et al. (2002) examined professional development as RNs progressed through their program. Students completed the Professional Development Self-Assessment Matrix (Beeler, Young, & Dull, 1990; Sovie, 1983), which addresses the four levels of professional development and competencies within each of these four levels at the beginning and at the end of the program. An analysis of 223 entering and 168 graduating students showed that the scores of graduating students were significantly higher ($p = .001$) on all five professional development dimensions than the pretest scores. Clark (2004), also interested in the concept of professionalism, asked whether RNs who graduated from a degree completion program have the same professional socialization as do graduates of a generic nursing program. Both groups had similar mean scores in the "higher level of professional autonomy" on the Nursing Activity Scale developed by Schutzenhofer (1987). Clark concluded that the socialization of generic baccalaureate students and the resocialization of RNs into the professional role were effective in the participating programs.

During the past few years, several researchers explored nurses' transition from being RNs to becoming BSNs from a qualitative perspective. Trainor (2000) examined the work environment as a factor in the persistence or nonpersistence of RNs in completing their baccalaureate degree. Findings revealed that many students did not continue because of family, work, and financial factors. The study also showed that the students did not continue when work was novel and fresh, but remained when work was stressful.

Zuzelo (2001) examined the concerns and priorities of RNs seeking a baccalaureate degree as well as the impact that this education had on their nursing practice patterns. Eighteen themes with additional subthemes were identified. Study findings demonstrated that the nurses believed they were more holistic and aware of cultural diversity as well as the influence of research on practice and described themselves as better communicators. They did not see the changes in their direct relationship with patients.

Lillibridge and Fox (2005) examined the impact that degree completion had on the personal and professional lives of RNs enrolled in a baccalaureate program. The researchers identified six themes: Having an edge for career advancement; not fitting in with basic students; need for support especially from peers; looking at things differently or seeing the bigger picture; developing new thinking skills; and becoming a change agent. In addition, the growth of knowledge for the RNs, gaining a more global perspective, and, finally, having a feeling of personal accomplishment were identified.

The current literature, albeit limited, provides evidence of the effectiveness of baccalaureate education in improving critical thinking and professionalism, as well as facilitating personal and professional growth, speaks to the importance of developing programs that meet the unique needs of this population, and indicates the need for further research.

Methods

Research Design

Descriptive phenomenology was used to explore and describe nurses' experiences with their transition as RNs to BSNs from the participants' perspectives. The phenomenological method is grounded on the belief that truth can be found in the lived experience and that human experience (the transition from being RNs to becoming BSNs in this study) is composed of essential structures despite individual differences (Spiegelberg, 1965). A central objective in phenomenology is to enter into the investigation with an a priori knowledge—to authentically listen rather than impose preconceived beliefs or the researcher's interpretive lens on a phenomenon. As Husserl (1960), the father of phenomenology, stated, to use phenomenology is "to return to the things themselves." Bracketing is used as a reflective process to temporarily suspend opinions as well as biases and facilitate focus on what is essential in the phenomenon. In this study, we engaged in active dialogue and private contemplation to uncover the participants' assumptions related to their transition as RNs to BSNs and continued the process throughout the study. Examples of the presuppositions included the following:

- Transitions, by their very nature, tend to be stressful;
- RN–BSN program education benefits nurses personally and professionally;
- the value of RN–BSN program education is often not recognized, valued, or rewarded; and
- RN–BSN program graduates provide a higher level of nursing care.

Procedure

The research protocol was submitted to the university institutional review board, and approval to conduct the study was obtained before data collection. The inclusion criteria for this study required that the participants (1) be English-speaking nurses older than 21 years, (2) have an RN–BSN status, and (3) have the ability and willingness to articulate their experience. All participants were assured of confidentiality and informed of the purpose and benefits of the study as well as their right to withdraw at any time. Participants were asked to sign an informed consent form acknowledging that they have read and understood the research and were willing to participate. Data collection occurred over a 12-month period. Each nurse was asked to describe his or her experience with transitioning as an RN to a BSN in as much detail as possible. The interviews were conducted at the place and time of the participants' choice to increase their comfort level and facilitate free expression. Interviews were audiotaped and later transcribed by a professional transcriptionist.

Sample

The purposive sample of 12 nurses consisted of 11 women and 1 man who graduated from all types of RN–BSN program formats (i.e., conventional, accelerated, and online). The participants' ages ranged from 32 to 52 years (mean = 44.6 years). Most of them were Caucasian (91.6%), married (66.6%), and working full time (58.3%). The sample included both ADNs and diploma nurses, and the length of time since the participants' RN–BSN completion ranged from 4 months to 5 years.

Data Analysis

The nurses' stories of their experiences with transitioning as RNs to BSNs were analyzed using the method of phenomenological analysis as proposed by Colaizzi (1978). We began data analysis by independently reading and rereading the transcripts to obtain an overall feel of the participants' experience. We then came together to extract the significant statements, which totaled 220. Significant statements were then jointly transposed into formulated meanings and later collapsed into theme clus-

304   PART III   THE EXPERIENCE OF AND RESPONSES TO TRANSITIONS

TABLE 6.3.1 Selected Examples of Significant Statements With Corresponding Formulated Meanings

Significant Statement	Formulated Meaning
"I thought returning to school is going to be beneficial in the future…it was something I always wanted to do."	Nurses saw future professional and personal benefits in obtaining a BSN degree
"My classmates were great. It was really good to hear from other people that worked in other hospitals…it was almost like a different culture."	Classmates shared information with each other, which broadened learning
"My school experience told me that if you want something, you could achieve it. Just overcoming the challenge of school gave me inner peace."	Nurses felt increased confidence in their ability to achieve goals
"I felt more secure in myself. I am better able to question things and present my ideas."	Nurses were better able to communicate

ters. The results were integrated into an exhaustive description that was subsequently validated by a subgroup of study participants as prescribed by Colaizzi's method. Tables 6.3.1 and 6.3.2 show partial audit trails of these steps.

Results

Analysis of the 12 stories describing the participants' transition as RNs to BSNs resulted in eight themes that illustrate the essence of their experience.

Theme I: Varied Expectations

The nurses decided to return to school to complete their BSN program under different circumstances and with varied hopes and expectations. For some, incentives and pressures in the workplace motivated their decision. One nurse stated, "A job came up in the family birth center but it required a degree, so I applied for the RN–BSN program and the job on the same day." Another nurse described feeling pressured to complete her BSN program: "I was told [that], in order to keep my position as a charge nurse, I would need a BSN [degree] within 5 years."

For other nurses, school reentry was viewed as a springboard to an advanced degree and an investment for the future. One participant explained, "I was interested in getting my BSN [de-

TABLE 6.3.2 Examples of Theme Clusters with Corresponding Significant Statements

Theme Cluster	Significant Statement
Cornerstone courses	"The research class was challenging, but it made me think more critically and look at evidence-based practice."
	"There is more depth in my practice now. I see the nursing theory behind everything I do."
	"Being in the leadership class gave me more confidence to venture into different committees."
	"Before I took community health, I just discharged people and life goes on…now I make sure things are set up for them at home."
Envisioning the whole	"I think of the whole picture now instead of just half the picture."
	"I look at things more holistically now." "Your thinking is just broader. You don't think of one thing, you think of the whole person."
	"I am more aware of how families and culture impact health."

gree] just because I wanted to continue on after that. I wanted to go for some kind of advanced degree because, although I liked what I was doing, I wanted to do more." Another nurse commented:

> I see my BSN degree as a self-preservation tool because I am getting older and I do not know how long I will actually be able to do bedside nursing with the 12-hour shifts and nights; it is a heavy job, most people do not understand how physical it actually is.

For whatever reason, all the nurses mentioned that a primary motivation was their love of learning and that pursuing a baccalaureate education was something they wanted to do for themselves. As one nurse put it: "Returning to school was a gift to myself."

Theme 2: Tentative Beginnings

Most of the nurses began their RN–BSN program tentatively, both in the number of courses they took and in their perceptions of what they would take away from the experience. In addition, most of them started with one or two courses; as one nurse described, "I started slowly, with one course, and once I felt like I could do it, I started taking more classes." Initially, many nurses were unsure of what to expect from the program. One nurse described her feelings at the beginning of the program as follows:

> I started on the road. I found myself in the first class, and we were told that a BSN [program] nurse was at a different level than an associate or diploma [nurse]. I found myself, as did other students, feeling a little defensive. We felt as though we were already fine nurses, we had been doing this as a career all our lives.

It was apparent that the classroom environment was significant in facilitating the early phases of the participants' transition. When the class cohort consisted of mainly younger students, the transition was more challenging; one nurse described:

> I was 38 when I went back to school, and I remember looking around the classroom thinking, 'Oh my God, I am old.' It was hard because we RN–BSN [program] students were such a minority compared to the majority of people in the classroom.

Conversely, when their classmates were of a similar age, the participants' transition was smoother; as expressed by another nurse: "Coming back and starting in a class where everyone was older too was comforting. I liked the RN–BSN [program] students, they had a little bit more maturity…we had a connection."

Theme 3: Cornerstone Courses

As nurses got further into the RN–BSN program curriculum, their knowledge base expanded. Repeatedly, nurses mentioned the same courses that formed the cornerstones of this new knowledge foundation; research, theory, leadership, and community health were the courses most frequently mentioned.

Research was mentioned by most nurses as an important component of their education. Nurses began to see research as one of the keys to change and the core of the profession. One nurse described her increased awareness of the relationship between research and change:

> There is a lot more focus on nursing research these days than there used to be, so it makes you think about best practice. I realize now that if I want to change a policy or do something differently, I need to do some research first.

Another nurse related research to nursing in general: "Research made me realize I love nursing for the science of it more than anything else. I don't take things at face value anymore, I think more critically."

Nursing theory provided meaning for the nurses and fostered a new way of thinking about their profession. One of the nurses recounted a class experience that led her to look at nursing in a new way:

> We had a discussion in class as to whether nursing was a job or profession. We had to really define it, and then I realized that we are a profession

and [that], though I had always [seen] myself as a professional, I didn't know why before.

Leadership classes provided nurses with an expanded viewpoint of their work and gave them a skill set that they were able to apply to numerous situations. One nurse commented on the effect of her leadership course:

> I gained a lot of leadership skills from the RN–BSN program, which were what I was looking for. We talked about how you might handle certain situations like conflict with peers, visitors, or families. It also raised my awareness as far as what the budget is, what the bottom line is, and how much things cost and trying to keep the costs down so that we can still do our job, do it well, and protect our patients at the same time.

For nurses already in management, leadership courses changed the way they approached the nursing staff; as one nurse who is an assistant head nurse said, "It made me more thoughtful, in my speech and how I respond to people."

Community health classes broadened nurses' perspectives and led them to look beyond the present. One nurse described how it changed her hospital nursing practice:

> The community health course was completely different from anything we do in the hospital. To see how people function on the outside really blew my mind, but I think it also opened my mind to other things. I'm more conscious of their home situation now.

Interweaved in nurses recounts of important educational content was the crucial importance of computer skills to succeed academically. Over and over again, nurses described computer skills as "absolutely essential and one of the greatest challenges."

Theme 4: Translating Knowledge Into Empowerment

The knowledge gained from the cornerstone courses caused an internal change in all the nurses and allowed them to formulate a new worldview. Their perspectives began to shift as they saw themselves and others—as many described—in a new light. One nurse recalled how the RN–BSN coursework changed her thought process:

> In course after course, we learned about history [and] research, and we learned where we came from. It was more than a knowledge base, it is a feeling. I could see a transition. Even everyday practice I saw in a different light.

She went on to explain how this knowledge affected her self-perception and translated into empowerment: "It was as if I was fed Miracle-Grow. I am stronger and see more direction personally and professionally."

As nurses' perspectives shifted, they saw others differently. One nurse expressed how her perception of her manager changed:

> We have one of those managers who always says, 'If you don't like it, you can leave.' Most of the staff [are] threatened by her, but I am seeing her in a different perspective. She is most likely stressed and doesn't have the answers. I don't take it personally anymore.

Another nurse echoed similar thoughts: "I used to be hard on my coworkers. I now see myself and others in a different light. I am more tolerant and forgiving."

Theme 5: Becoming Assertive Leaders and Advocates

As nurses changed internally, they interacted with others differently. For most nurses, the external expression of their empowerment was manifested in becoming a stronger leader and advocate. One nurse's story exemplifies this theme:

> I recently had a patient whose baby had an abnormal head ultrasound, so the physician was going to go to the family and tell them that there was a possibility that the baby would be mentally retarded or have seizures but that he was not sure yet and needed a CAT scan. I stopped him and I said this family is Muslim and the baby is a girl and the wife is already being treated differently. I said I was concerned how the child would be treated and

asked him to wait until there were conclusive results and I don't think I would have brought up anything to the physician culturally before this.

As nurses increased their knowledge and their perspectives broadened, their communication skills improved. One nurse described the feeling:

> I am able to present how I view things to physicians better. I am not afraid to speak up and say what I think because I feel I have more knowledge to present to them in a proper way. I know now that I have to do a little research and be prepared not only to say what I think is wrong but to offer solutions.

Theme 6: Confronting And Conquering Challenges

Like all transitions, there were challenges to confront as nurses completed their BSN program. For some, the greatest challenge was in the beginning of the BSN completion program; as recounted by one nurse: "I was frustrated with the initial registration when I found out I would have to repeat some courses." For others, the main challenge was trying to balance the responsibilities of home, work, and school; as illustrated by one nurse's comment: "It was tough to juggle it all, especially when papers were due. Sometimes I would ask myself, why am I doing this?"

Nurses did not always find support from their work colleagues. One nurse elaborated: "The most common reaction I got from my coworkers was, 'Why are you doing this, you won't get any more money.'" Another nurse added: "My coworkers were threatened and asked me if I was planning to leave."

Classmates provided a major source of support and encouragement to the nurses in this study. Most of the study participants mentioned their classmates as playing a major role in their transition. One nurse's comment illustrates the importance of classmate relationships: "There was a group of us working on our BSN [degree] together, and one of us was quitting every week. We kept each other going." Even in virtual settings, the classmate connection was invaluable. A nurse who graduated from an online program expressed the importance of her classmates: "Most of us had some problems with the computers, especially in the beginning. We would talk over the computer and sometimes over the phone to help each other. I still keep in touch with some of them."

Theme 7: Envisioning the Whole

Almost all the nurses stated that being able to see the bigger picture was the most significant result of their education experience. Although articulated differently, the nurses became conscious of a larger context surrounding their nursing practice. As if a curtain was lifted, the nurses saw the whole picture. One nurse described the transformation in her clinical practice:

> I am able to see the bigger picture now. Instead of just seeing the person and this is what I'm doing for them, I see a lot more. I can see where we are going and where we came from. I think about their disease process, what I am doing to help them now, and what I need to anticipate in the future.

The larger picture that nurses described went beyond the patient; one nurse explained: "I am looking at the family now, how they interact, and what their disease is doing to the family." Another nurse extended this thought: "You start putting things together on a different level when you go through the program. You see their families and their culture."

Theme 8: Recreating Everyday Practice

With the bigger picture in focus, the nurses began to recreate their everyday practice. By the end of the RN–BSN program, the nurses were aware of a difference in the way they approached patient care. One nurse reflected on how the program affected her nursing practice:

> I used to be very task oriented. I would think we need to get this and that done, wait 2 hours, and do it again. The interaction with patients was missing. Now, when I look at my patients. I say, 'Ok, there are some chores to do,' but I take a look at how they are feeling and I take more time to communicate with them to actually find out what they need.

Most of the nurses believed that the program had a direct benefit for their patients. One nurse explained how: "The whole experience has inspired me, and that is good for me and my patients. I think I am in a good mental place because I see that I am growing and I'm sure that benefits my patients." Another nurse's simple statement summarized: "I feel more like a nurse now than I did before."

Exhaustive Description

Nurses embarked upon the common road to BSN completion with varied expectations. Career advancement, role changes, job security, and love of learning were the primary motivators and the desired destinations in their return to school. Most of the nurses began the program slowly and tentatively, with one or two courses and feeling unsure of what they would gain. As the curriculum progressed, the nurses were exposed to key courses, such as research, theory, leadership, and community health, which formed the cornerstones of their new knowledge base. This newly acquired knowledge allowed the nurses to develop an expanded worldview and changed the way they perceived themselves and related to others. Knowledge was translated internally into empowerment and expressed externally as the nurses became assertive advocates and leaders.

Throughout the BSN completion program, it was apparent, that the nurses' classmates played an important role in their transition process. Their classmates, particularly those of a similar age, provided support, encouragement, and the determination to confront and conquer challenges. However, their classmates' being younger or unengaged caused a delay in the nurses' transition. On the other hand, coworkers often presented another challenge for the nurses and tended to question their decision and agenda for continuing their education.

The ability to see the bigger picture was the most powerful common experience for the nurses. They were able to move beyond old patterns of thinking and behavior to envision the whole person, critically analyzing the complexity of the human experience. The biggest change occurred in their thought process, although skill levels also advanced for many. By the end of the program, the nurses saw their work in a different light and began recreating their everyday practice. The nurses had successfully transitioned as RNs to BSNs and emerged with a renewed commitment to their profession, forever changed by the experience.

Discussion

This phenomenological study contributes to the understanding of the transition from being RNs to becoming BSNs with its identification of the essential structure of this phenomenon and focus on the nurses' experiences with achieving their BSN completion. The findings validate and extend those of previous quantitative and qualitative studies. Nurses in this study believed that they had better critical thinking skills, consistent with the findings by Brown et al. (2001), and enhanced professionalism, as found in the studies by Phillips, Zimmerman, and Mayfield (2002) and Clark (2004). The themes in this study are similar to and extend the six themes identified by Lillibridge and Fox (2005). In addition, although our findings are consistent with those of Zuzelo (2001), unlike the participants in that study, the participants in this study saw a direct relationship between their education and their approach to patient care.

This study uniquely contributes to this body of knowledge by providing a rich description of the lived experience, particularly by identifying the courses that made the greatest impact on the nurses and how this knowledge transformed their perspective and, subsequently, their approach to everyday practice.

Several implications for nurse educators in academia and work environments, as well as current and potential students, can be drawn from this study. Implications for nurse educators in academia include the importance of facilitating the early transition phase by creating caring environments, focusing on what nurses bring to the classroom, and avoiding inferences related to the knowledge deficit among non-BSNs. Nurses will discover the difference on their own. This implication is congruent with the finding of Cangelosi (2004) that faculty who acknowledge students' experiences, provide a caring environment, and empower students were most helpful to RN–BSN program students. In addition, developing curricula with an emphasis, as most BSN programs have, on research, theory, leadership, and community health that include group work to build classmate connections can foster persistence and motivation throughout the program. The findings also suggest that RN–BSN program students have the best experiences when they are in a cohort rather than integrated with traditional students.

Implications for nurse educators and managers in work environments include the need to encourage RN–BSN program graduates to become involved in committees, leadership roles, and other activities that allow RN–BSN program graduates to develop their full potential. Finally, current and potential RN–BSN program students can benefit from this study by gaining a greater insight into the positive effect of furthering their education, which may lead to an increase in reentry into BSN completion programs.

REFERENCES

Aiken, L. H., Sean, S. P., Cheung. R. B., Sloane, D. M., & Silber, J. F. (2003). Educational levels of hospital nurses and surgical patient mortality. *Journal of The American Medical Association, 290,* 1617–1623.

American Association of Colleges of Nursing. (2005). *Enrollment and graduations in baccalaureate, and graduate programs in nursing.* Washington, DC: American Association of Colleges of Nursing.

American Nurses Credentialing Center. (2005). *The magnet 2005/2006 instructions and application process manual.* Silver Spring, MD: American Nurses Credentialing Center.

Beeler J. L., Young, P. A, & Dull, S. M. (1990). Professional development framework: Pathway to future. *Journal of Nursing Staff Development, 6,* 296–301.

Brown, J. M., Alverson, E. M., & Pepa, C. A. (2001). The influence of a baccalaureate program on traditional, RN–BSN, and accelerated students' critical thinking abilities. *Holistic Nursing Practice, 15,* 1–4.

Cangelosi, P. R. (2004). The tact of teaching RN–BSN students. *Journal of Professional Nursing, 20,* 167–173.

Clark, C. L. (2004). The professional socialization of graduating students in generic and two-plus-two baccalaureate completion nursing programs. *Journal of Nursing Education, 43,* 346–351.

Colaizzi, P. (1978). Psychological research as the phenomenologist views it. In R. Vale, & M. King (Eds.). *Existential phenomenological alternative for psychology* (pp. 48–71). New York: Oxford University Press.

Delaney, C., & Piscopo, B. (2004). RN–BSN programs: Associate degree and diploma nurses' perceptions of the benefits and barriers to returning to school. *Journal for Nurses in Staff Development, 20,* 157–161.

Husserl, E. (1960). *Cartesian meditations* (D. Carins, trans.). The Hague, Netherlands: Martineus Nijhoff.

Ku, Y., Lo, C. K., Wang, J., Hsieh, J. L., & Chen, K. (2002). The effectiveness of teaching strategies for creativity in a nursing concepts teaching protocol of the creative thinking of two-year RN–BSN students. *Journal of Nursing Research, 10,* 105–112.

Lillibridge, J., & Fox. S. D. (2005). RN–BSN education: What do RNs think? *Nurse Educator, 30,* 12–16.

National Council on Nurse Education and Practice. (2001). *Nursing: A strategic asset for the health of the nation policy on the nursing workforce shortage.* 102nd meeting Silver Spring, Maryland.

National League for Nursing Tri-Council for Nursing Policy Statement. (2002). Strategies to reverse the new nursing shortage. Retrieved May 3, 2006, from http://www.nln.org/aboutnln/news_tricouncil2.htm

Phillips, C. Y., Palmer, V., Zimmerman, B. J., & Mayfield, M. A. (2002). Professional development: Assuring growth of RN–BSN students. *Journal of Nursing Education, 41,* 282–284.

Schumacher. K. L., & Meleis. A. I. (1994). Transitions: A central concept in nursing. *Image: Journal of Nursing Scholarship, 26,* 119–127.

Schutzenhofer, K. K. (1987). The measurement of professional autonomy. *Journal of Professional Nursing, 3,* 278–283.

Sovie, M. (1983). The role of staff development: Part II. *Journal of Nursing Administration, 12,* 30–33.

Spiegelberg, H. (1965). *The phenomenological movement: A historical introduction.* The Hague, Netherlands: Martineus Nijhoff.

Spratley, E., Johnson, A., Sochalski, J., Fritz, M., & Spencer, W. (2000). *The registered nurse population: Findings from the national sample survey of registered nurses.* Rockville, MD: U.S. Department of Health and Human Services, Health Resources and Service Administration Bureau of Health Professions Division of Nursing.

Trainor, J. M. (2000). *A study of the work environment as a factor in persistence or non-persistence of RN students in a baccalaureate nursing program.* Unpublished doctoral dissertation. Pennsylvania State University.

White, M. J., & Gomez, G. A. (2002). Outcomes of critical thinking and professional attitudes in RN–BSN completion programs. *Nurse Educator, 27,* 71–72.

Zuzelo, P. R. (2001). Describing the RN–BSN learner perspective: Concerns, priorities, and practice influences. *Journal of Professional Nursing, 17,* 55–64.

Reprinted with permission from: Delaney, C., & Piscopo, B. (2007). There really is a difference: Nurses' experiences with transitioning from RNs to BSNs. *Journal of Professional Nursing, 23*(3), 167–173.

6.4 A QUALITATIVE STUDY OF HOW EXPERIENCED CERTIFIED HOLISTIC NURSES LEARN TO BECOME COMPETENT PRACTITIONERS

LEIGHSA SHAROFF

Abstract

Purpose: Artistry of holistic nursing requires practitioners to be equipped with the ability to integrate and assimilate knowledge and experience. This integrated wisdom is woven into proficiency and expertise, thus allowing for the transition to an experienced competent health care provider who can meet the complex melange of practice. This qualitative naturalistic study was designed to explore how 10 experienced certified holistic nurses (HNCs) learned to become competent holistic nurses. ***Method***: In-depth interviews of 10 HNCs, critical incident reports, and a summative focus group. ***Findings***: (a) Disjuncture existed between the structure of traditional nursing and the need of nurses for continued personal and professional growth and development; (b) need for credibility was key to nurses becoming competent holistic nurses; (c) use of informal learning strategies to help them achieve competency; and (d) overcoming challenges emanating from the traditional system as they transitioned to becoming holistic nurses.

Experienced certified holistic nurses (HNCs) are continually influenced by factors in their internal and external environments that lead to a more competent and confident holistic nurse. Some of these factors include more personal and professional growth and development; increased awareness of health care trends; mentors; attending conferences and educational seminars; and increased knowledge, skills, and attitudes learned outside of the formal educational setting. Yet we know too little about how experienced holistic nurses learn to become competent HNCs. The essence of this study asked: How do experienced HNCs know what needs to be learned in order to become competent and successful holistic nurses?

Separation from mainstream nursing occurs when a nurse acknowledges that the old model (of healing) is no longer fulfilling, or that the same philosophy of nursing with colleagues is not shared (Slater, Maloney, Krau, & Eckert, 1999). This is the time when traditional nurses, whose epistemology is influenced more by traditional science models, begin to question their assumptions (*epistemology* is the theory of what counts as valid knowledge and valid ways of knowing; Yorks & Sharoff, 2001). As the literature states, some of the reasons nurses transition to holistic nursing may be because of feeling burnout from traditional nursing, personal reasons (i.e., an illness), or for professional/personal growth, development, and personal ethics (AHNA, 2000; Dossey, 1997; Dossey & Guzzetta, 2000).

The knowing that emerges from various forms of learning has a significant effect on the HNC's ability to participate in the healing process of others and self. This knowing contributes to HNCs' expertise, thus affecting their ability to participate in the healing process. By gaining the knowledge of how nurses learn to become competent providers, nurse educators will be potentially better able to assist HNCs in becoming professional healers who can meet the complex, ill-defined mélange of problems in the workplace and, therefore, become competent and successful practitioners.

The inquiry for this study was driven by four central questions: (a) What motivates a professional registered nurse to become an HNC? (b) What knowledge, skills, and attitudes did experienced HNCs perceive they needed to become competent as holistic nurse practitioners? (c) How did those practitioners acquire the knowledge, skills, and attitudes they perceived they needed? and (d) What factors facilitated and/or impeded their ability to become competent practitioners?

Literature Review

To ground the nurse in the concepts of holistic nursing, of being one with self and others, the American Holistic Nurses Association (AHNA) developed the Standards of Holistic Nursing Practice, which defined and established the scope of holistic nursing and the expected level of care from a holistic nurse (Dossey, Frisch, Forker, & Lavin, 1998; Dossey & Guzzetta, 2000). The Standards of Holistic Nursing Practice were revised in 2000 following the results of the Inventory of Professional Activities and Knowledge of a Holistic Nurse (IPAKHN) survey.

Studies on holistic nursing (Bishop & Scudder, 1997) and client-nurse interactions (Schubert & Lionberger, 1995) have added to the understanding of holistic nursing and holistic nursing theory. Cary's (2001) study explored the benefits and drawbacks of nursing certification. The consensus that certification is an important component for validation of a practitioner's knowledge and skills depicts the 21st-century citizens' demand for expertise and competency in their health care providers.

Transition is a process of movement. Becoming-to-being a HNC requires a transitional experience that culminates with the legitimization by the certifying body. This study focused on situational transitions (Schumacher & Meleis, 1994) exploring the experienced HNC at the proficient and expert levels of competency. The researcher used the concept of proficient and expert to assist in the purposeful sampling of HNCs. Proficient practitioners perceived situations as wholes and performance is guided by a deep understanding of the situation (Dreyfus & Dreyfus, 1996). Expert practitioners have an enormous background of experience and have an intuitive grasp of each situation (Dreyfus & Dreyfus, 1996).

Studies on transition (Holland, 1999; Slater et al., 1999; Ventre & Bowland, 1995) explored the transitional process and motivation for change. Daley's (1999) study explored the different learning processes of the novice and expert nurse. This researcher's intention was to complement Daley's study by furthering the understanding of how experienced HNCs learned to become competent practitioners, thus gaining the higher level of knowledge and skills needed to meet challenges of practice.

The journey of becoming an expert and professional competent practitioner requires nurses to incorporate various stores of knowledge and skills, beyond the practical level, into their personhood and professional practice. One can conclude that the epistemological center of professional expertise is made up of tacit knowing, incidental knowing, practical knowledge, informal knowing, explicit knowledge, reflection in action, critical rationality, reflection-on-action, and reflection-in-action (Jarvis, 1992a, 1992b, 1999; Patel, Arocha, & Kaufman, 1999; Schön, 1987, 1991; Sullivan, 1995).

The transition from a novice to experienced practitioner culminates with expert practitioners embodying the practical knowledge and the extant understandings of how to integrate practical and theoretical knowledge (Benner, Tanner, & Chelsea, 1996). Experts can arrive at a solution to complex situations without conducting extensive research (Glaser & Chi, 1988) because they develop a "feeling-sense of the problem" (Boreham, 1992). Competent practitioners must not only solve technical problems by selecting the means appropriate to clear and self-consistent ends but also reconcile, integrate, or choose among conflicting appreciations of a situation so as to construct a coherent problem worth solving (Schön, 1987). Competency in one's practice is an interactive process of acquiring skills, knowledge, and experience. A conceptual framework of professional competency is built on the triple foundations of the practitioner's knowledge, skill, and attitude (Jarvis, 1995).

The technical training of HNCs occurs in formal classrooms and formal programs; however, these programs only go so far with regard to the dissemination of knowledge and skills. Yet the core of the HNCs' ability to transition to competent health care providers does not occur with the completion of this formal training. It requires the acknowledgment of the "spectrum of learning opportunities available to adults, from the highly structured to the more informal ways adults go about learning" (Merriam & Caffarella, 1999, p. 24).

The researcher has explored several learning opportunities, including informal learning, experiential learning, learning from experience, reflection, reflection-in-action, critical reflection, transformative learning, and mentoring (Boud, Cohen, & Walker, 1993; Boud, Keogh, & Walker, 1985; Cohen & Galbraith, 1995; Merriam & Caffarella, 1999; Vance, 2001).

For HNCs to be able to learn, they must be able to make that experience meaningful. Numerous adult educational theorists have explored this basic ideology, such as Mezirow (1990a, 1990b), Schön (1987, 1991), and Dewey (1938). To learn and make that experience meaningful, the HNC must reflect on it to gain a deeper understanding of the event. Mezirow (1990a, 1990b), as well as Jarvis (1992, 1999), Schön (1987), and Brookfield (1990), agree that two types of change can occur as a result of the learning process:

> Learners may be changed and they may act to change the situation within which they function. (Jarvis, Holford, & Griffin, 1998, p. 64)

It is through learning from one's experiences, from reflecting on what those experiences have to offer, that new skills and knowledge are constructed. To reflect on one's action is to be an autoresearcher in one's practice.

Method

Design

The purpose of this naturalistic qualitative study was to explore how experienced HNCs learn to become competent practitioners. Institutional Review Board (IRB) approval for the protection of human participants' rights was obtained from Columbia University.

Participants

The study focused on a sample of 10 HNCs who have been practicing as holistic nurses for more than 3 years and have incorporated the philosophy of holistic nursing into their lives and practice. The initial criteria for inclusion in this study were being an HNC and the time frame of the practicing HNC. All participants were initially contacted via e-mail with a general description of the purpose of this study, participant eligibility, and participant involvement. Purposeful sampling occurred when the researcher contacted the AHNA and requested a list of all current HNCs. In addition, the researcher reviewed the AHNA's Member Directory, which was available to all members. E-mail addresses were obtained through the AHNA's Member Directory. Once a participant agreed to be in this study and his or her eligibility was confirmed, an introduction letter, critical incident, and demographic inventory were sent via e-mail attachment (see Table 6.4.1).

Data Collection Methods

Demographics were collected to provide basic information about the HNC participant population, including age, gender, racial/ethnic background, highest level of nursing degree held, area of nursing practice, location of practice, incorporation of holis-

TABLE 6.4.1 Description of Participants

Demographic Inventory Data	Demographic Inventory
Summary	
Gender	Female, 100%
Age	44–67 years, mean 51.6 years
Ethnicity	90% Caucasian, 10% Asian
Highest degree	BS 20%, BSN 20%, BA 10%, MSN 30%, EdD 10%, PhD 10%
Years of experience in nursing	9–27 years, mean 26.7 years
Year obtained HNC certification	1996 10%, 1998 50%, 1999 10%, 2000 30%
HNC certification process	Portfolio, 100%
Area works in	East Coast 40%, Midwest 40%, West Coast 20%
Practice setting	Parish nursing 10%, education 30%, home health care 10%, consulting 10%, private 20%, hospital 10%, mental health 10%
Position	Retired 10%, career specialist 10%, client-centered 30%, professor 10%, case manager 20%, consultant 20%
Incorporate HNC philosophy	Yes, 100%
AHNA member	Yes, 100%

HNC = certified holistic nurse.

tic nursing philosophy, and the year credentials were received. A critical incident was used to obtain a real-life experience that pertained to the research question.

> "The critical incident technique consists of a set of procedures for collecting direct observations of human behavior" (Flanagan, 1954, p. 327) and to enter another's "frame of reference" to "highlight particular, concrete, and contextually specific aspects of people's experiences" (Brookfield, 1990, p. 180).

The critical incident was an instrument designed to obtain additional data, and the analyses of those findings were used to further refine the interview questions as well as provide data. After 8 of the 10 participants completed the original critical incident and analyses of those 8 critical incidents were completed, a more precise and brief critical incident was developed. The revised instrument asked the participant to think of an important event in his or her career and briefly describe how that experience affected his or her practice as an HNC.

A semistructured, open-ended-question interview guide was developed to glean the stories of the participants. All interviews were audiotaped and conducted via telephone. A summative focus group was also used for triangulation to validate conclusions. The researcher recruited 11 different HNCs to participate in a 2-hour focus group. The volunteer participants were HNCs with at least 3 years of experience, thus forming a focus group comparable to those participants who were interviewed.

Data Analysis

To confirm the researcher's perception of theme and category coding, review of the data was confirmed through interrater reliability checks, summative focus group, and discussions with three consultants (all doctoral professors at Columbia University). In addition, participants were asked to review the interview for accuracy. The coding scheme was developed for each of the four central research questions. Descriptors were formulated from the critical literature review with additional descriptors constructed after analyzing the interviews. Triangulation between the critical incident, interview, and summative focus group provided for reliability of the research findings with confirmation of replication ability.

Limitation

The researcher, an experienced HNC, brought her own assumptions and experiences to this research study, which may have influenced the analysis. Another limiting factor was the small sample size of all female participants; henceforth, findings of this study are not widely generalizable to the universe of HNCs. However, this study's participants were comparable to that of the larger studies (Cary, 2001; Dossey et al., 1998).

Findings

Research Question 1: "What motivated a professional registered nurse to become an HNC?" Was it the disjuncture between the structure of traditional nursing and the HNCs' own personal and professional growth and development?

Research participants were asked to describe what led them to move into holistic nursing, and all 10 participants described feelings of disillusionment between the reality of traditional nursing and the ideal of what they would like nursing to be. Some disillusionments discussed included the following: A lack of and need for professional and personal growth and development; a loss of connection with people; living with one philosophy and working in another philosophy (concept of causality/duality); and personal events/burnout from traditional nursing.

One of the primary findings in this study was that all participants were highly motivated to become an HNC. One of the reasons for this motivation appears to be a limitation in traditional nursing. Traditional nursing, the style of nursing that was taught in the academic setting, although a vital aspect to health care, no longer satisfied these participants. The participants were fiercely committed to finding a nursing paradigm where they could practice the type of nursing that they wanted to. Thus, to become competent, the experienced HNC must first be committed to working in a medical paradigm that is congruent with their personal and professional beliefs.

One participant, who presently works in home health care, was motivated to become an HNC because she found traditional nursing unrewarding. She stated:

> My relationship to nursing...felt was very unrewarding...very task oriented...not what I had in mind in going into nursing...looking for a meaning behind being a nurse other than...task-master...learn how to do a lot of tasks...don't approach the fundamental essence of nursing.

Another participant, with more than 30 years of experience as a nurse and 7 years as an HNC, related her own need for self-healing. She said,

> I do not think I had a good self care model...my body was giving me a message that I would likely become ill if I did not shift and change. And I heard that loud and clear...fall into...path of disease if I did not really improve my own habits...get my life into a better pattern. It was a self healing thing...let go of agreeing with traditional medicine...wanted my personal and professional life to be in congruency.

Research Question 2: "What knowledge, skills, and attitudes did experienced HNCs perceive they needed to become competent as holistic nurse practitioners?" Was it the need for credibility?

The participants were asked to discuss what they thought they needed to know as they made the transition to becoming an HNC. They were asked to discuss the early stages of this transition and if they felt they were prepared or unprepared for the challenges that they faced. There were differences in their explanations for needing credibility, yet all commented on the effect of how having others judging them fueled their desire for credibility. There were also similarities in how they felt negatively judged by others, particularly by nursing colleagues, the medical community, fellow academicians, and family members. Several participants discussed needing credibility for a personal sense of confidence and competency.

One of the primary findings of this study was that experienced HNCs felt that needing credibility was a key feature in being perceived as competent. The philosophy of holistic health care has been well received by most consumers, but health care professionals have been slower to embrace the concepts. Thus, legitimacy and credibility were perceived as necessities by experienced HNCs. Nurses who practiced within the domain of holistic nursing had to overcome the stigma of being perceived differently by their colleagues. Obtaining the credential of an HNC brought about a certain level of credibility for these nurses, which then elevated their confidence and competency levels. Thus, a key issue is the experienced HNCs' perception of competence because of the validation provided by the certification process.

One participant stated that she needed credibility because other health care professionals perceived holistic nursing as a form of voodoo. She said,

> Always ridiculed…by peers, physicians, therapists, nurses…people of higher education…frustrating…felt my hands were tied…they felt I had no credibility…was considered Satanism…occult …looked upon as very evil. Voodoo is the nickname that it was for a long time, "How's your voodoo work going?…How's that waving your hands and scaring people?" Holistic nurses…compared to voodooism…was…a religion…not of God, not of Christ…wasn't ready for that…didn't see it coming. I think that was the hardest thing that I had to deal with.

As one participant shared, she felt frustrated by her workplace environment. She said,

> Almost a perennial effort to remind…faculty about holistic nursing philosophy and practice. What is frustrating and even painful is how fear will cause us to sabotage each other for being different…how that contaminates the work environment.

Research Question 3: "How did those practitioners acquire the knowledge, skills, and attitudes they perceived they needed to know?" Was it through the inclusion of informal learning strategies to help them achieve competency?

Participants were asked to discuss what strategies they used to get to know what to do and how to do it in order to become competent. In addition, participants were asked to discuss key lessons they learned in becoming competent health care providers. Finally, they were asked what and who may have helped them as they made their journey as holistic nurses. The participants discussed variations in the learning strategies, such as increased awareness; learning with and through others (mentors, role models); finding like-minded individuals; reading and attending conferences and workshops; learning through experiences; and an increased sense of confidence. All 10 participants referred to an increased awareness as they journeyed through the process. This ranged from an awareness of how to attend to feelings and emotions, to self-care, to learning to tolerate ambiguity and be nonjudgmental, and the learning strategies used that assisted in gaining this awareness.

One of the primary findings in this study was that experienced HNCs described using informal learning strategies, yet there were variations in the learning strategies. For experienced HNCs to learn to become competent as holistic nurses, they must be open and willing to foster that knowing via a variety of learning opportunities. The majority of learning opportunities that the HNCs in this study described were interpreted as either informal learning or incidental learning.

One participant, a nurse with 33 years of experience and 7 years as an HNC, commented that the tool needed was increasing awareness of self and others. She stated,

> Needed tools…if I needed tools, other people needed…tools…knowledge, I mean awareness…it is really about awareness…increasing awareness. Honor who we are as we are but to also honor the process that continues to allow us to evolve.

One participant, who has 24 years of experience as a nurse and 3 years as an HNC, described how her awareness resonated with her own self-caring. She said,

> Started to align my accidents…incidents…when I was out of control without, nurturing…when would my back go out…get pneumonia again…wasn't listening to my body to rest…listening to myself…took 2 years but I got it…a very hard lesson…have to constantly relearn it though.

All 10 participants also described how the process of learning with and through others assisted in their becoming competent health care providers.

There were variations in the learning process and all participants described using more than one form of learning.

Seven of the participants described how a mentor was an important figure in their journey. One participant, who practices as a family nurse practitioner in the New York region, described how important her mentor was to her. She stated,

> Mentorship...really the thing that saved me...had a mentor...somebody that took me through...my personal mentor...mentoring was a big part....-Mentor...already had awareness...experience with skills I was seeking to develop in myself.

Five of the 10 participants discussed how learning through networking and finding people who were like-minded was another strategy used in becoming competent practitioners.

One participant, who has been a nurse for 9 years and an HNC for 5 years, commented on how she received support from like-minded people. She said,

> Networking...support from like-minded people...different networking groups...really helpful...get support emotionally for how hard it is sometimes just to be a nurse.

Research Question 4: "What factors facilitated and/or impeded their ability to become competent HNCs?" What were the challenges that they had to overcome as they transitioned from traditional nursing and in their practice as HNCs?

Participants were asked to discuss what obstacles may have stood in their way that they wished weren't there. They were also asked to reflect on what they might have done differently in their journey.

Four of the 10 participants commented that they would have done nothing differently as they made their journey into holistic nursing, yet all did experience some obstacles as a source of growth, such as educational choices; the need for more time and money; self-imposed beliefs and fears; and lack of support in the work environment.

One participant, a nurse for 9 years who presently works in community service, stated that obstacles eventually became catalysts for growth. She said,

> Made the decision, to walk the path...more I did ...able to facilitate a healthier environment, for myself...learned about my self care...more empowered I became to change whatever needed to be changed...do not think...allowed obstacles...if they were there they became catalysts.

Six of the participants commented that they would have done things differently; however, there was no consensus on what they would have done differently. Three of the six commented on making different educational choices.

One participant, a diploma RN who has a BA degree, stated that she would have worked toward different educational degrees but also feels she has not made any wrong choices. She stated,

> Never really wanted my BSN...always had a negative attitude about it...if there was one possibility...would have a BSN and then a master's in holistic nursing. I do not know if...actually made any wrong choices or could wish it to be different...guess it has to play itself out...think what I have is wonderful...it has served me well.

A nurse with 38 years of experience who has her doctorate commented that the only obstacle might have been time and money. She stated,

> Only obstacle might have been time and money...had more time...might have gotten places.

Five of the participants shared how their self-imposed beliefs and fears were obstacles. An example of this is provided by one participant, a master's-prepared family nurse practitioner, who described how she self-imposed obstacles. She stated,

> Obstacles were my own...any obstacle...ever had ...always self-imposed obstacles...really resistance to change...an unwillingness to really thoroughly commit to a new direction.

However difficult the obstacles have been, the participants in this study all expressed that the process of learning to become competent practitioners has led them down a wonderful and exciting road.

The journey to becoming an HNC has been a process of love, growth, and being true to oneself. There has been an acceptance of the obstacles and of the people who were unable to understand or accept the process. In other words, to learn to become competent practitioners, experienced HNCs learned to view all obstacles and experiences as part of the learning process, thus the obstacles became facilitators of growth. One participant, a nurse with 24 years of experience, stated,

> Everything was for a purpose…truly believe that it helped me grow…helped me learn…more about me…as frustrating as it was…I learned things that I couldn't learn in the classroom…the process taught me to be gentle with walking quietly…teaching…persistence…it is a passion…and the passion will drive you.

One participant who works in a hospital critical care setting stated,

> [I] feel blessed from all my experiences…which have been enhanced because of my acquired HNC…[I] believe by furthering my knowledge by pursuing my HNC…I opened pathways from within myself.

Discussion

The first step in the process of learning to become competent health care providers is awareness of the need to work in a nursing paradigm that is congruent with one's own personal and professional beliefs and values. The commitment to foster personal and professional growth and development and the need for self-care and to reconnect with others is the driving force that propels this need. The next step is the awareness of what knowledge, skills, and attitudes are needed to make such a change. The awareness that credibility and legitimacy are necessary for acceptance and respect by others continues to foster personal and professional growth and development. Openness and willingness to use a variety of learning opportunities to acquire the necessary knowledge, skills, and attitudes complements this journey. By becoming reflective practitioners and establishing healthy interpersonal relationships, one continues to foster the process of learning. Finally, being aware of and accepting the challenges and obstacles that one faces on the journey of learning is an integral part of the entire process.

Conclusions and Recommendations

The researcher has drawn six conclusions based on the findings of this interpretative qualitative study. One of the conclusions is that people who learn to be competent HNCs have awareness of what they need to foster their own growth and development. In addition, people who learn to become successful competent HNCs are dedicated to their own personal growth and development. They understand that caring for oneself is an important prerequisite to helping others.

A third conclusion is a commitment to maintaining equilibrium between satisfying personal needs and professional goals and aspirations. There is no separation between the personal and the professional. A fourth conclusion is the necessity to being open and willing to use a variety of learning strategies to achieve their goals. By being conscious of how to incorporate the learning gained from different situations into their practice, by being reflective practitioners and exploring alternative perspectives to beliefs and assumptions, successful competent health care providers are able to problem solve and meet workplace challenges.

Furthermore, having a good support system is vital to learning to become a competent HNC. Successful practitioners surround themselves with individuals who can provide guidance, support, and learning opportunities. Finally, viewing challenges and obstacles as learning opportunities is integral to the process. Competent holistic nurses have the ability to reconstruct assumptions and to revise and refine their beliefs and values, thus improving their vision of what is and what can be.

The principal recommendation is that there should be a continued dialogue between the leaders of the holistic nursing community and traditional nursing programs to discuss the incorporation of holistic nursing principles into nursing curricula. In addition, there needs to be a demystification of what holistic nursing is.

In sum, experienced HNCs learned to become competent by being committed and motivated to continue to foster their personal and professional growth and development. There was disillusionment with the traditional nursing paradigm and awareness that change was needed. The most influential perceived need that the HNCs credited with influencing their learning was the awareness of the need for additional knowledge and skills and the need for credibility and legitimacy by others. With experience and knowledge, HNCs gained more confidence in their skills and capabilities.

Formal learning provided the foundation for the HNCs' knowledge base, but it was through informal and incidental learning where the HNCs learned how to become competent. For experienced HNCs to learn to become competent health care providers, they needed to acquire the knowledge and skills via a variety of learning opportunities, become reflective practitioners, continue to develop their self-awareness and self-care, and establish interpersonal relationships. Finally, the transition from a novice to an experienced HNC was fraught with a multitude of challenges, yet all of the challenges eventually brought HNCs to where they are today. In other words, difficult times are sometimes necessary to allow for growth to occur. Thus, experienced HNCs learned to become competent by being aware of the challenges and obstacles that they faced and to view these obstacles as part of their learning process.

REFERENCES

American Holistic Nurses' Association. (2000). *Standards of holistic nursing practice* (rev. ed.). Flagstaff, AZ: Author.

Benner. P., Tanner, C., & Chelsea, C. (1996). *Expertise in nursing practice.* New York: Springer Publishing Company.

Bishop, A., & Scudder, J. (1997). A phenomenological interpretation of holistic nursing. *Journal of Holistic Nursing, 15*(2), 103–111.

Boreham, N. (1992). Harnessing implicit knowing to improve medical practice. In H. Baskett & V. Marsick (Eds.), *Professionals' ways of knowing: New findings on how to improve professional education* (pp. 71–78). San Francisco: Jossey-Bass.

Boud, D., Cohen, R., & Walker, D. (1993). Understanding learning from experience. In D. Boud, R. Cohen, & D. Walker (Eds.), *Using experience for learning* (pp. 1–17). Buckingham, UK: Open University Press.

Boud, D., Keogh, R., & Walker, D. (1985). Promoting reflection in learning: A model. In D. Boud, R. Keogh, & D. Walker (Eds.). *Reflection: Turning experience into learning* (pp. 18–40). London: Kogan Page.

Brookfield, S. (1990). Using critical incidents to explore learners' assumptions. In J. Mezirow & Associates (Eds.), *Fostering critical reflection in adulthood: A guide to transformative and emancipatory learning* (pp. 177–193). San Francisco: Jossey-Bass.

Cary, A. (2001). Certified registered nurses: Results of the study of the certified workplace. *American Journal of Nursing. 101,* 44–52.

Cohen, H., & Galbraith, M. (1995). Mentoring in the learning society. In M. Galbraith & N. Cohen (Eds.), *Mentoring: New strategies and challenges* (pp. 5–14). San Francisco: Jossey-Bass.

Daley, B. (1999). Novice to expert: An exploration of how professionals learn. *Adult Education Quarterly, 49*(4), 133–147.

Dewey, J. (1938). *Experience and education.* New York: Touchstone.

Dossey, B. (1997). *Core curriculum for holistic nursing.* Gaithersburg. MD: Aspen.

Dossey, B., Frisch, N., Forker, J., & Lavin, J. (1998). Evolving a blueprint for certification: Inventory of professional activities and knowledge of a holistic nurse (IPAKHN). *Journal of Holistic Nursing, 16*(1), 33–56.

Dossey, B., & Guzzetta, C. (2000). Holistic nursing practice. In B. Dossey, L. Keegan, & C. Guzzetta (Eds.), *Holistic nursing: A handbook for practice* (pp. 5–38). Gaithersburg, MD: Aspen.

Dreyfus, H., & Dreyfus, S. (1996). The relationship of theory and practice in the acquisition of skill. In P. Benner, C. Tanner, & C. Chelsea (Eds.), *Expertise in nursing practice* (pp. 258–372). New York: Springer Publishing Company.

Flanagan, J. (1954). The critical incident technique. *Psychological Bulletin, 51*(4), 327–358.

Glaser, R., & Chi, M. (1988). Overview. In M. Chi, R. Glaser, & M. Farr (Eds.). *The nature of expertise* (pp. xv–xxviii). Hillsdale, NJ: Lawrence Erlbaum.

Holland, K. (1999). A journey to becoming: The student nurse in transition. *Journal of Advanced Nursing, 29*(1), 229–236.

Jarvis, P. (1992a). Learning practical knowledge. In H. Baskett & V. Marsick (Eds.), *Professionals' ways of knowing: New findings on how to improve professional education* (pp. 89–96). San Francisco: Jossey-Bass.

Jarvis, P. (1992b). *Paradoxes of learning.* San Francisco: Jossey-Bass.

Jarvis, P. (1995). *Adult and continuing education: Theory and practice* (2nd ed.). New York: Routledge.

Jarvis, P. (1999). *The practitioner-researcher: Developing theory from practice.* San Francisco: Jossey-Bass.

Jarvis, P., Holford, J., & Griffin, C. (1998). *The theory and practice of learning.* London: Kogan Page.

Merriam, S., & Caffarella, R. (1999). *Learning in adulthood: A comprehensive guide* (2nd ed.). San Francisco: Jossey-Bass.

Mezirow, J. (1990a). How critical reflection triggers transformative learning. In J. Mezirow & Associates (Eds.), *Fostering critical reflection in adulthood: A guide to transformative and emancipatory learning* (pp. 1–20). San Francisco: Jossey-Bass.

Mezirow, J. (1990b). Toward transformative learning and emancipatory education. In J. Mezirow & Associates (Eds.), *Fostering critical reflection in adulthood: A guide to transformative and emancipatory learning* (pp. 354–376). San Francisco: Jossey-Bass.

Patel, V., Arocha, J., & Kaufman, D. (1999). Expertise and tacit knowledge in medicine. In R. Sternberg & J. Horvath (Eds.), *Tacit knowledge in professional practice* (pp. 75–99). Mahwah, NJ: Lawrence Erlbaum.

Schön, D. (1987). *Educating the reflective practitioner.* San Francisco: Jossey-Bass.

Schön, D. (1991). *The reflective practitioner.* New York: Basic Books.

Schubert, P., & Lionberger, H. (1995). Mutual connectedness: A study of client-nurse interaction using the grounded theory method. *Journal of Holistic Nursing, 13*(2), 102–116.

Schumacher, K., & Meleis, A. (1994). Transitions: A central concept in nursing. *Image: Journal of Nursing Scholarship, 26*(2), 119–127.

Slater, V., Maloney, J., Krau, S., & Eckert, C. (1999). Journey to holism. *Journal of Holistic Nursing, 17*(4), 365–383.

Sullivan, W. (1995). *Work and integrity: The crisis and promise of professionalism in America.* New York: HarperCollins.

Vance, C. (2001, February/March). The value of mentoring. *National Student Nurses' Association, Imprint,* pp. 38–40.

Ventre, F., & Bowland. K. (1995). The transition from lay midwife to certified nurse-midwife in the United States. *Journal of Nurse-Midwifery, 40*(5), 428–437.

Yorks, L., & Sharoff. L. (2001). An extended epistemology for fostering transformative learning in holistic nursing education and practice. *Holistic Nursing Practice, 16*(1), 21–29.

Reprinted with permission from: Sharoff, L. (2006). A qualitative study of how experienced certified holistic nurses learn to become competent practitioners. *Journal of Holistic Nursing, 24*(2), 116–124.

Chapter 7   Health and Illness Transitions

7.1 SELF-CARE OF HEART FAILURE: A SITUATION-SPECIFIC THEORY OF HEALTH TRANSITION

BARBARA RIEGEL
VICTORIA VAUGHAN DICKSON

Heart failure is the most common and expensive chronic illness among older adults in developed countries. In the United States alone, the prevalence of heart failure is 5,300,000, with one in eight deaths attributable to heart failure (American Heart Association, 2008). In persons with chronic heart failure, transitional care involves coordination and continuity of care as patients transfer from hospital to home and cycle between phases of relative physiologic stability to acute decompensation. The cost associated with heart failure has risen exponentially over time as well due to frequent and repeated exacerbations and hospitalizations. In the United States, the estimated direct and indirect cost of heart failure for 2008 was $34.8 billion (American Heart Association, 2008).

Over the past 15 years, heart failure disease management has become an exemplar model of transitional care. However, only about 20% of persons with heart failure are referred to heart failure specialty teams able to provide full-service disease management (Fonarow, 2006). Even fewer investigators have used continuity of care models in this patient population (Naylor et al., 2004). For these reasons and others explored in the text that follows, my program of research has focused on improving the ability of heart failure patients and their families to engage in self-care as an adjunct or an alternative to disease management.

Self-Care Defined

We defined self-care as a naturalistic decision-making process that patients use in the choice of behaviors that maintain physiologic stability—symptom monitoring and treatment adherence—and the decision-making response to changes in signs and symptoms (Riegel et al., 2004). Patients who engage in routine and consistent self-care have better outcomes; several studies have demonstrated that poor treatment adherence, a component of self-care, is common among patients who are admitted to the hospital with worsening heart failure (Bennett et al., 1998; Ghali, Kadakia, Cooper, & Ferlinz, 1988; Opasich et al., 2001; Tsuyuki et al., 2001; Vinson, Rich, Sperry, Shah, & McNamara, 1990). We have demonstrated that event-free survival is significantly better in symptomatic heart failure patients who engage in above average self-care management compared with those who are poor in self-care management (Lee, Moser, Lennie, & Riegel, 2008).

A Situation-Specific Theory of Heart Failure Self-Care

My program of research in self-care as a means of facilitating transitions in heart failure began during my tenure as a Clinical Researcher at Sharp HealthCare in San Diego, California. In the mid-1990s, administrators focused on heart failure as one of the top 10 causes of hospitalization. As the Clinical Researcher responsible for the cardiovascular service line, I began a series of studies testing disease management approaches to decrease the need for rehospitalization in persons with heart failure (Riegel & Carlson, 2004; Riegel, Carlson, Glaser, & Hoagland, 2000; Riegel, Carlson, Glaser, & Romero, 2006; Riegel et al., 2002).

Very early in that process I began to focus on self-care as the mechanism responsible for the outcomes we achieved. We developed a model of self-care that evolved in later years into a situation-specific theory of heart failure self-care (Riegel & Dickson, 2008). Compared with grand and middle-range theories, situation-specific theories are more concrete, less abstract, and address a specific clinical phenomenon seen in practice (Im & Meleis, 1999). Consistent with the definition of situation-specific theory, we limited our theory to adults with heart failure. We used the integrative approach to the development proposed by Im and Meleis (1999) and included the crucial elements of a nursing perspective, a clear link between the theory, research, and clinical practice, and a conceptual scheme based on abstract thinking, memo or journal writing, and dialogue with colleagues, students, and research participants.

Theory Link

The theory and research by prior investigators greatly enhanced our understanding of self-care as a process performed by patients with the support of clinicians (Becker, Gates, & Newsom, 2004; Dodd, 1997; Leenerts, Teel, & Pendleton, 2002; Orem & Vardiman, 1995). That is, although self-care is ultimately an individual patient responsibility, self-care is performed most effectively with the support of clinicians who coach and support patients (Becker et al., 2004). It would be extremely unusual for a person with a chronic illness as complex as heart failure to master self-care without the guidance of a nurse. Embedding our theory in clinical practice, we had observed that nurses help patients learn how to monitor and interpret symptoms, set priorities, and make decisions about their care. Others have used terms such as self-observation, symptom perception and labeling, judgment of severity, treatment consultation, choice of assessment and treatments, and symptom outcome to capture this process of self-care (Dodd, 1984; Levin, Katz, & Holst, 1979; Sorofman, Tripp-Reimer, Lauer, & Martin, 1990).

The situation-specific theory described here evolved from our early conceptual model, which was codified for the purposes of instrument development (Riegel, Carlson, & Glaser, 2000). Key concepts in the conceptual model were self-care maintenance and self-care management to comprise the behaviors of symptom monitoring, treatment adherence, and decision making, as described previously. The selective attention that occurs with symptom monitoring is crucial for recognizing and interpreting symptoms. Treatment adherence, a component of self-care (Lorig & Holman, 2003), involves following the advice of providers to follow the treatment plan and attend to taking care of oneself with behaviors such as exercise and smoking cessation.

Decision making in response to symptoms is the quintessential element of self-care management, which is defined as an active, deliberate process. Self-care management is essential in heart failure if patients are going to control the precarious balance between relative health and symptomatic heart failure. Five stages of management were described: recognizing a change in health status (e.g., new swelling), evaluating the change in status, deciding to take action, implementing a treatment strategy (e.g., taking an extra diuretic dose), and evaluating the treatment implemented (Figure 7.1.1). This definition of management is consistent with the definition from Wilde and Garvin (2007) who define self-monitoring as encompassing bodily awareness, a concept similar to recognizing a change in status. It is also consistent with the work of Wilson et al. (1993) who note that in self-management, patients undertake tasks that are the traditional province of professionals such as prescribing drug dosages. Once changes in signs and/or symptoms are recognized, a response must be decisive and timely. An assumption of the self-care management process is that patients able to recognize their symptoms will be better at subsequent steps in the process.

Figure 7.1.1 illustrates the conceptual model of heart failure self-care. Stage 1 reflects self-care maintenance, a process focused on symptom monitoring and treatment adherence. Stages 2–5 reflect

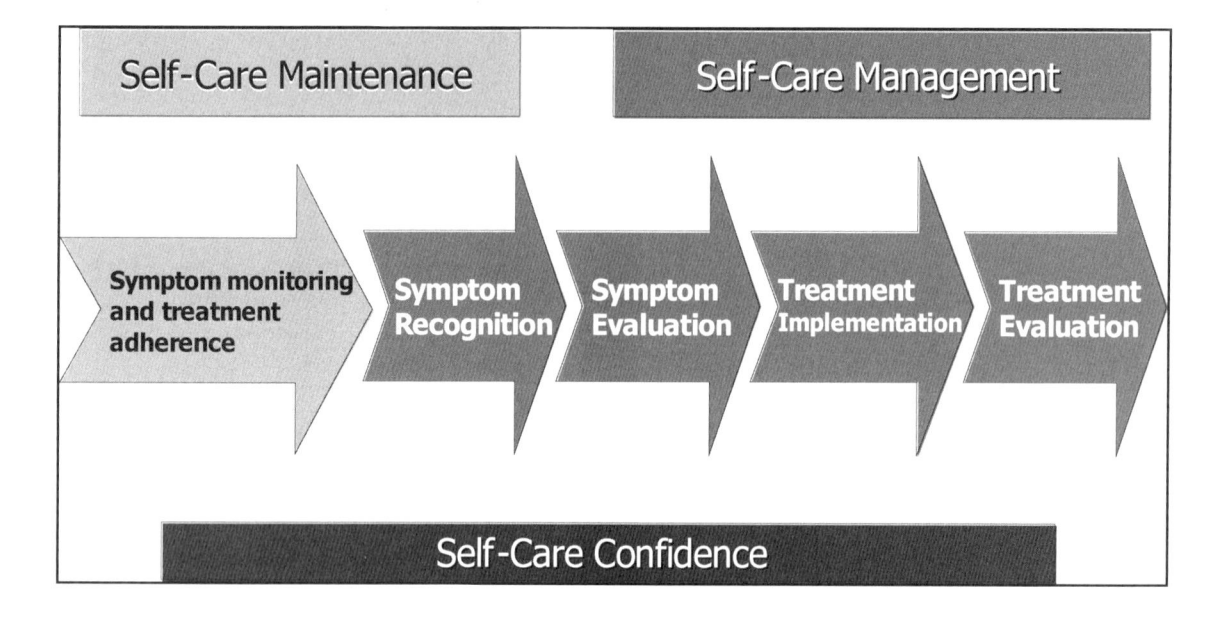

FIGURE 7.1.1 Self-care of heart failure model.
Reprinted from the *Journal of Cardiovascular Nursing* with permission of Lippincott Williams & Wilkins (Riegel & Dickson, 2008).

self-care management, a process in which patients recognize and respond to their symptoms. Confidence is thought to influence the self-care process in important ways.

Since that early work, two major advances occurred in our thinking. First, in our early work, self-care was defined as a rational process, involving purposeful choices and behaviors, reflecting knowledge and thought. Later we questioned the rationality and critical thinking abilities of patients making decisions about symptoms. Naturalistic decision making (Lipshitz, Klein, Orasanu, & Salas, 2001) was thought to better reflect the process by which people make decisions in real-world settings. Four characteristics exemplify naturalistic decision making: (a) focusing on process rather than outcome, (b) using decision rules that match the situation and the action, (c) letting context influence decision making, and (d) basing practical decisions on the empirical information available at the moment. Naturalistic decision makers rely on developed expertise to mentally simulate an action and anticipate how it will play out and less on normative models of rational behavior. The factors most influential in developing that expertise are knowledge, experience, skill, and compatibility with values (Figure 7.1.2).

Figure 7.1.2 illustrates the naturalistic decision-making process underlying the situation-specific theory of heart failure self-care. In order to make a decision in a particular situation or context, four criteria are needed: experience with and knowledge about the situation and the decision, skill to act on the decision, and the decision and action must be compatible with values.

The second major advance in our thinking is related to the concept of confidence. Initially, confidence was conceptualized as a component of self-care based on early pilot work interviewing heart failure patients about their self-care. In later discussions with colleagues, we came to see confidence as a mediator and/or a moderator of the relationship between self-care and outcomes rather than a core component of self-care itself.

Research Link

In a recently published description of our situation-specific theory of heart failure self-care (Riegel &

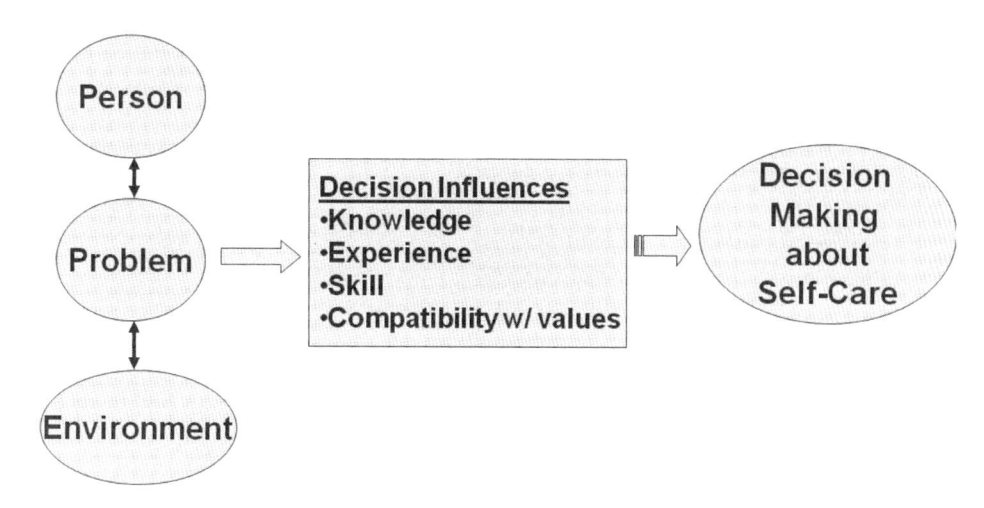

FIGURE 7.1.2 Decision-making model of heart failure self-care.

Dickson, 2008), we proposed and tested a series of propositions using existing data sets from our prior research. The theoretical propositions tested were: (a) symptom recognition is the key to successful self-care management; (b) self-care is influenced by knowledge, experience, skill, and compatibility with values; and (c) self-care confidence mediates and/or moderates the influence of self-care.

For the first proposition, we hypothesized that the patients who were unable to recognize their symptoms would be unsuccessful in subsequent steps in self-care management. This hypothesis was supported when treatment initiation scores were higher in persons who recognized their symptoms quickly versus those who did not. Treatment evaluation ability also was higher, although the difference between the groups in this analysis did not reach statistical significance.

In testing the second proposition, we hypothesized first that self-care would be higher in patients with more knowledge about their heart failure, but interestingly, that hypothesis was only partially supported. Self-care maintenance was lower in patients with higher knowledge, contrary to our prediction, but self-care management was higher in those high in knowledge, albeit not significantly so. Self-care maintenance and management were higher in patients with more self-care skill, as hypothesized. Self-care management was better in patients experienced with heart failure compared with those who were inexperienced. Persons with positive values regarding self-care had higher self-care maintenance than those with predominately negative values. A similar picture was seen in self-care management.

Then we tested the proposition that confidence moderates the relationship between self-care and outcomes, hypothesizing that higher levels of heart failure self-care would be associated with better economic outcomes, but only when confidence is high. This hypothesis was supported (Lee, Carlson, & Riegel, 2007). Specifically, self-care predicted the likelihood of readmission for heart failure. Level of self-care also explained a significant amount of the variance in heart failure direct and total inpatient cost.

Finally, we hypothesized that self-care confidence would mediate the relationship between social support and self-care in patients with heart failure. The proposed mechanism was that social support would improve self-care confidence and thereby improve patients' abilities to perform self-care. In testing, support was a significant predictor of self-care confidence and a significant predictor of self-care management. When support and confidence were entered into the equation simultaneously, there was evidence of a mediator effect (Riegel & Dickson, 2008). Based on this analysis, we believe that social support improves self-care management by improving patients' confidence in their abilities to perform heart failure self-care.

Practice Link

Knowledge and skill are conditions known to be extremely important in influencing transitions (Schumacher & Meleis, 1994). Both knowledge and skill are believed to be essential for successful heart failure self-care. Nurses have a long history of promoting knowledge acquisition (Saarmann, Daugherty, & Riegel, 2000), but skill acquisition is virtually ignored in heart failure patients. We have used our situation-specific theory of heart failure self-care to guide the development of interventions focusing on skill development. Little attention has been given to identifying how to improve skill in HF self-care. We used qualitative descriptive meta-analysis techniques to assess what self-care skills heart failure patients perceive needing and how they developed the skills needed to perform self-care. Themes identified in data from 85 adults with chronic heart failure enrolled in three prior studies were re-examined using within-study and across-study analysis and translated to create a broader and more complete understanding of the development of skill in heart failure self-care (Dickson & Riegel, 2009).

In that analysis, we identified that both tactical (e.g., "how to") and situational skills or "what to do when" are needed to perform adequate self-care. Tactical self-care skill involves the performance of routine behaviors (e.g., meal preparation, ordering low-salt food in a restaurant). Situation skill involves making decisions about signs and symptoms. In prior research, we demonstrated that skill in self-care maintenance is needed before persons with heart failure can successfully master self-care management (Riegel, Vaughan Dickson, Goldberg, & Deatrick, 2007). So, we think there is a hierarchy in the development of these processes. These skills evolve over time and with practice, as patients learn how to make self-care practices fit into their daily lives and as they gain experience in successfully managing heart failure symptoms.

Assisting patients in the development of self-care skill requires a shift in the patient education paradigm from a traditional model characterized by authoritarian, prescriptive, and generalized information to a patient-centered, collaborative approach in which patients learn the tactical and situational skills necessary for true self-care. A skill-building paradigm needs to begin with assessment of the level of tactical skills needed for self-care and any unique circumstances that need to be considered in teaching these skills. Skill-building exercises focus on skill deficits and managing unique situations.

Assessing what situations pose the greatest challenge to the patient (e.g., vacation, family situations, workplace) will help identify circumstances that place the individual at risk for lapses in self-care. Assisting in planning through these special situations may be facilitated by role-playing scenarios and think-aloud exercises. Identifying the trusted resources most likely to influence the patient's self-care practices and including them whenever possible in educational sessions may reinforce behaviors and correct misconceptions held by those trusted others.

A skill-building paradigm also must include the critical element of coherence—linking the individual's unique symptoms, the heart failure mechanism, the cause of symptoms, and specific action needed to avert an exacerbation of heart failure. In prior research, we identified coherence as the construct that ties it all together for patients (Dickson, Deatrick, & Riegel, 2008). Thus, coherence needs to be a constant theme during any skill-based intervention. Without that link, patients will continue to tell us that they know they need to follow a low-salt diet, but they do not know how to do it or what to do when faced with a difficult situation like a family holiday gathering.

To maximize the ability of heart failure patients to successfully transition from hospital to home and to avoid future hospitalization because of an acute exacerbation, skill acquisition needs to be developed in these patients. True skill in self-care evolves over time and with practice, as patients learn how to make self-care practices fit into their daily lives. We found in prior research that proficiency in skill acquisition was attained primarily through input from family and friends (Dickson et al., 2008). Health care professionals rarely made significant contributions to the learning of essential skills, so including family and friends in teaching sessions is essential.

Traditional patient education does not support development of skill in self-care in persons with heart failure. New patient teaching strategies are needed that support the development of tactical and situational skill, foster coherence, and use trusted resources. Research testing coaching interventions that target skill-building tactics such as counseling, role-playing, and practice is ongoing. This new skill-building paradigm is a unique opportunity for nurses in home health settings to contribute to skill development, because self-care skills are typically mastered at home (Dickson & Riegel, 2009). Assessing self-care skills, reinforcing positive skill development and correcting inadequate behaviors should be part of the continuum of care for all HF patients as they transition from hospital to home.

Conclusion

In this chapter we have described our situation-specific theory of heart failure self-care, summarized some of the testing done to support the theory, and summarized the practice implications that guide our future directions. An important limitation of this situation-specific theory is that it is a biomedically derived approach to health that focuses on a specific illness. As such, important cultural, gender, and psychosocial influences on self-care are ignored (Becker et al., 2004). It is also essential to recognize that the decision making discussed in relation to the self-care of heart failure is greatly influenced by the broader context in which patients live.

The major strength of this approach is the clinical relevance of the topic. For nurses, self-care is a particularly important construct, as it captures the essence of our philosophy and a key dimension of our practice in transitional care. Im and Meleis (1999) note that there are probably several reasons for the seeming disconnect among theory, research, and practice, but one likely reason is the tension between theoretical vision and clinical wisdom. Situation-specific theories such as the self-care of heart failure theory described here may be one way of linking theory, research, and clinical practice. The theory described here directly reflects the experiences of clinicians in their daily practice.

REFERENCES

American Heart Association. (2008). *Heart and stroke statistical update: 2008.* Retrieved April 23, 2008, from www.americanheart.org

Becker, G., Gates, R. J., & Newsom, E. (2004). Self-care among chronically ill African Americans: culture, health disparities, and health insurance status. *American Journal of Public Health, 94*(12), 2066–2073.

Bennett, S., Huster, G., Baker, S., Milgrom, L., Kirchgassner, A., Birt, J., et al. (1998). Characterization of the precipitants of hospitalization for heart failure decompensation. *American Journal of Critical Care, 7*(3), 168–174.

Dickson, V., & Riegel, B. (2009). Are we teaching what patients need to know? Building skills in heart failure self-care. *Heart Lung, 38*(3), 253–261.

Dickson, V. V., Deatrick, J. A., & Riegel, B. (2008). A typology of heart failure self-care management in non-elders. *European Journal of Cardiovascular Nursing, 7*(3), 171–181.

Dodd, M. J. (1984). Measuring informational intervention for chemotherapy knowledge and self-care behavior. *Research in Nursing and Health, 7,* 43–50.

Dodd, M. J. (1997). Self-care: Ready or not! *Oncology Nursing Forum, 24*(6), 983–990.

Fonarow, G. C. (2006). How well are chronic heart failure patients being managed? *Reviews in Cardiovascular Medicine, 7* (Suppl.) 1, S3–11.

Ghali, J. K., Kadakia, S., Cooper, R., & Ferlinz, J. (1988). Precipitating factors leading to decompensation of heart failure. Traits among urban blacks. *Archives of Internal Medicine, 148*(9), 2013–2016.

Im, E. O., & Meleis, A. I. (1999). Situation-specific theories: philosophical roots, properties, and approach. *Advances in Nursing Science, 22*(2), 11–24.

Lee, C., Carlson, B., & Riegel, B. (2007). Heart failure self-care improves economic outcomes but only when self-care confidence is high (abstract). *Journal of Cardiac Failure, 13*(6) (Suppl. 2), S75.

Lee, C., Moser, D., Lennie, T. A., & Riegel, B. (2008). Event-free survival in adults with heart failure who engage in self-care management. Lee: Heart failure self-care event-free survival. [abstract]. *Circulation, 118*(18), (Suppl.).

Leenerts, M. H., Teel, C. S., & Pendleton, M. K. (2002). Building a model of self-care for health promotion in aging. *Journal of Nursing Scholarship, 34*(4), 355–361.

Levin, L., Katz, A., & Holst, E. (1979). *Self-care: Lay initiatives in health*. New York: Predist.

Lipshitz, R., Klein, G., Orasanu, J., & Salas, E. (2001). Taking stock of naturalistic decision making. *Journal of Behavioral Decision Making, 14*, 331–352.

Lorig, K. R., & Holman, H. R. (2003). Self-management education: History, definition, outcomes, and mechanisms. *Annals of Behavioral Medicine, 26*(1), 1–7.

Naylor, M. D., Brooten, D. A., Campbell, R. L., Maislin, G., McCauley, K. M., & Schwartz, J. S. (2004). Transitional care of older adults hospitalized with heart failure: a randomized, controlled trial. *Journal of the American Geriatrics Society, 52*(5), 675–684.

Opasich, C., Rapezzi, C., Lucci, D., Gorini, M., Pozzar, F., Zanelli, E., et al. (2001). Precipitating factors and decision-making processes of short-term worsening heart failure despite "optimal" treatment (from the IN-CHF Registry). *American Journal of Cardiology, 88*(4), 382–387.

Orem, D. E., & Vardiman, E. M. (1995). Orem's nursing theory and positive mental health: practical considerations. *Nursing Science Quarterly, 8*(4), 165–173.

Riegel, B., & Carlson, B. (2004). Is individual peer support a promising intervention for persons with heart failure? *Journal of Cardiovascular Nursing, 19*(3), 174–183.

Riegel, B., Carlson, B., & Glaser, D. (2000). Development and testing of a clinical tool measuring self-management of heart failure. *Heart & Lung, 29*(1), 4–12.

Riegel, B., Carlson, B., Glaser, D., & Hoagland, P. (2000). Which patients with heart failure respond best to multidisciplinary disease management? *Journal of Cardiac Failure, 6*(4), 290–299.

Riegel, B., Carlson, B., Glaser, D., & Romero, T. (2006). Randomized controlled trial of telephone case management in Hispanics of Mexican origin with heart failure. *Journal of Cardiac Failure, 12*(3), 211–219.

Riegel, B., Carlson, B., Kopp, Z., LePetri, B., Glaser, D., & Unger, A. (2002). Effect of a standardized nurse case-management telephone intervention on resource use in patients with chronic heart failure. *Archives of Internal Medicine, 162*, 705–712.

Riegel, B., Carlson, B., Moser, D. K., Sebern, M., Hicks, F. D., & Roland, V. (2004). Psychometric testing of the self-care of heart failure index. *Journal of Cardiac Failure, 10*(4), 350–360.

Riegel, B., & Dickson, V. V. (2008). A situation-specific theory of heart failure self-care. *Journal of Cardiovascular Nursing, 23*(3), 190–196.

Riegel, B., Vaughan Dickson, V., Goldberg, L. R., & Deatrick, J. A. (2007). Factors associated with the development of expertise in heart failure self-care. *Nursing Research, 56*(4), 235–243.

Saarmann, L., Daugherty, J., & Riegel, B. (2000). Patient teaching to promote behavioral change. *Nursing Outlook, 48*, 281–287.

Schumacher, K. L., & Meleis, A. I. (1994). Transitions: a central concept in nursing. *Image: Journal of Nursing Scholarship, 26*(2), 119–127.

Sorofman, B., Tripp-Reimer, T., Lauer, G. M., & Martin, M. E. (1990). Symptom self-care. *Holistic Nursing Practice, 4*(2), 45–55.

Tsuyuki, R. T., McKelvie, R. S., Arnold, J. M., Avezum, A., Jr., Barretto, A. C., Carvalho, A. C., et al. (2001). Acute precipitants of congestive heart failure exacerbations. *Archives of Internal Medicine, 161*(19), 2337–2342.

Vinson, J. M., Rich, M. W., Sperry, J. C., Shah, A. S., & McNamara, T. (1990). Early readmission of elderly patients with congestive heart failure. *Journal of the American Geriatrics Society, 38*(12), 1290–1295.

Wilde, M. H., & Garvin, S. (2007). A concept analysis of self-monitoring. *Journal of Advanced Nursing, 57*(3), 339–350.

Wilson, S. R., German, D. F., Lulla, S., Chardon, L., Starr-Schneidkraut, N., & Arsham, G. M. (1993). A controlled trial of two forms of self-management education for adults with asthma. *American Journal of Medicine, 94*, 564–576.

7.2 HEALTH-ILLNESS TRANSITION EXPERIENCES AMONG MEXICAN IMMIGRANT WOMEN WITH DIABETES

MARYLYN MORRIS MCEWEN
MARTHA BAIRD
ALICE PASVOGEL
GWEN GALLEGOS

Abstract

Multiple and complex health-illness transitions are required for successful diabetes self-management. Diabetes health-illness transitions influence the daily lives and interactions of Mexican immigrant women with diabetes. This chapter reports the findings from an intervention study designed to facilitate the health-illness transition in Mexican immigrant women with type 2 diabetes who reside in the Arizona-Sonora region of the U.S.–Mexico border. There was a significant (p < 0.001) increase from preintervention to postintervention in diabetes knowledge and diabetes self-efficacy, and a significant decrease (p = 0.001) in psychosocial and health-related behavior problems. Immigrants are confronted with multiple and complex social, cultural, and situational transitions that may adversely affect their health.[1-3] The nature, conditions, meanings, and processes of health–illness transitions associated with diabetes influence the daily lives and interactions of Mexican immigrant women residing in the U.S.–Mexico border region. This article reports the findings of a pilot intervention study designed to facilitate the health-illness transition of Mexican immigrant women diagnosed with type 2 dibetes who live in the Arizona–Sonora region of the U.S.–Mexico border.

Hispanic Immigration Trends

Persons of Hispanic origin (hereafter referred to as Hispanics) are the largest and fastest growing minority group in the United States, and are projected to represent 25% of the U.S. population by 2050.[4] Although the majority (59.8%) of Hispanics in 2005 were U.S. citizens at birth, 40.2% were foreign born or immigrants,[5] primarily from Mexico.[6] The majority of Mexican immigrants are concentrated in the western part of the United States.[7] The state of Arizona, the site for this study, reported in 2000 that 66.4% of the state's foreign-born population was born in Mexico.[6] Arizona has the sixth-largest proportion of Hispanic households in the nation (28.9%), and experienced a 32.4% increase from 2000 to 2005.[5]

Diabetes in the Hispanic Population

Diabetes disproportionately affects Hispanic Americans. The majority of data that describe the prevalence of diabetes in the Hispanic population were generated from 4 large studies that established a 2 to 3 times greater prevalence of noninsulin diabetes in persons of Mexican origin than in non-Hispanic Whites.[8] Findings from a random household survey conducted along the Arizona-Sonora region of the U.S.–Mexico border demonstrated that the prevalence of diabetes in Hispanics (primarily of Mexican origin) aged 40 years or more was 20%, or 2 to 2.5 times greater than in non-Hispanic Whites.[9] Contributing to the rapidly increasing prevalence of type 2 diabetes in Hispanics is a family history of diabetes, an elevated body mass index, an increase in sedentary lifestyle, and an underlying genetic susceptibility.[10] Compared with diabetic non-Hispanic Whites, Mexican Americans with diabetes have a greater incidence of macrovascular and microvascular complications, including end-stage renal disease.[11]

Culturally Situating Diabetes Self-Management

Diabetes self-management necessitates daily engagement in a complex set of behaviors that include (a) healthy eating, (b) physical activity, (c) blood glucose monitoring, (d) taking medications, (e) problem solving, (f) healthy coping, and (g) reducing risks.[12] Successful management of behavioral changes needed to attain glycemic control is often challenging for Hispanics with diabetes.[13] Many researchers attribute this to the fact that most traditional diabetes self-management models are culturally insensitive, culturally inappropriate, acontextual, and ineffective for this population.[14,15]

Oomen and colleagues[15] suggested a shift from viewing self-management as personal beliefs and values, self-efficacy, and lifestyle modifications to incorporating the constructs of social support, interpersonal behavior, group interaction, language, community, and cultural values.

Culturally relevant interventions intended to increase diabetes self-management skills for achieving glycemic control in persons of Mexican origin who reside in the U.S.–Mexico border region have been tested.[16-19] Although the majority of the participants in these studies successfully achieved short-term glycemic control, they were unable to adapt diabetes self-management behaviors for a long term. Inadequate intervention dose[14] and culturally inappropriate models have been suggested as contributing factors for failure to sustain diabetes self-management.[15] The development of culturally congruent Hispanic diabetes interventions requires research aimed at developing culturally appropriate outcome measures and exploring motivating factors and strategies for diabetes self-management within a cultural context.[14,15]

The Diabetes Health-Illness Transition Among Hispanics

The middle range nursing theory of transitions[1] provided the theoretical framework for this study. Transition theory is an effective way to understand complex adaptations that immigrant women make as they manage the health-illness transitions associated with a chronic illness such as diabetes. Health-illness transitions are complicated because immigrants are at risk for discrimination, lower socioeconomic status, and language and cultural barriers, which may prevent access to necessary resources.[20]

Transitions have been defined as "a passage from one life phase, condition, or status to another."[21(p. 256)] Individuals and families experiencing developmental, situational, and health-illness transitions come in contact with nurses and the health care system. Nursing practice is concerned with how people respond to transitions, as well as those factors that assist them during transition periods.[22] Health-illness transitions may involve the processes of getting ill, being diagnosed, recovery, adapting to a chronic illness, accessing health care services and support, as well as seeking and using traditional healing practices. Transitions seldom occur alone and frequently precipitate other transitions.[1] Mexican immigrant women who have type 2 diabetes experience multiple and complex transitions simultaneously[23,24]; this chapter focuses on their health-illness transition experiences associated with diabetes.

Transitions are fluid because they involve ongoing processes and outcomes over time (Figure 7.2.1).[22] Factors affecting transition processes and outcomes include the nature and meaning ascribed to the transition and critical events occurring throughout the process, as well as individual, family, and community facilitators and inhibitors. Five properties have been associated with transition experiences: (a) awareness, (b) engagement, (c) change and difference, (d) time span, and (e) critical events. Awareness and engagement are evidenced by the women's recognition of the chronic illness and their involvement in diabetes self-management behaviors. Change, difference, and time span are reflected in their personal accounts of the ways in which the illness has affected their daily lives. An example of a critical event is the day of diagnosis[1] or hospitalization for a diabetes-related complication.

Healthy transitions are facilitated and inhibited by personal, community, and/or societal factors.[1] Personal factors that could facilitate or inhibit the diabetes health-illness transition include meanings, knowledge, cultural beliefs, and practices surrounding diabetes. Early assessment of process indicators that facilitate health or increase vulnerability is essential for developing interventions that facilitate healthy outcomes. Examples of process indicators that characterize healthy transitions are feeling connected and interacting with others, being situated, and developing confidence and coping strategies.

Outcome indicators that characterize healthy transitions involve "mastery of new skills needed to manage a transition and the development of a fluid yet integrative identity."[1(p. 25)] Belief in one's ability and actual daily engagement in healthy eating, physical activity, blood glucose monitoring, and medication management represents mastery of skills for a healthy diabetes transition.[12] Nursing interventions in the community can promote a healthy transition at many points during the health-illness transition process by facilitating or diminishing inhibitors affecting the transition outcome. In this study, we implemented a culturally tailored community-based nursing and *promotora*[25,26] (community health worker) intervention within the con-

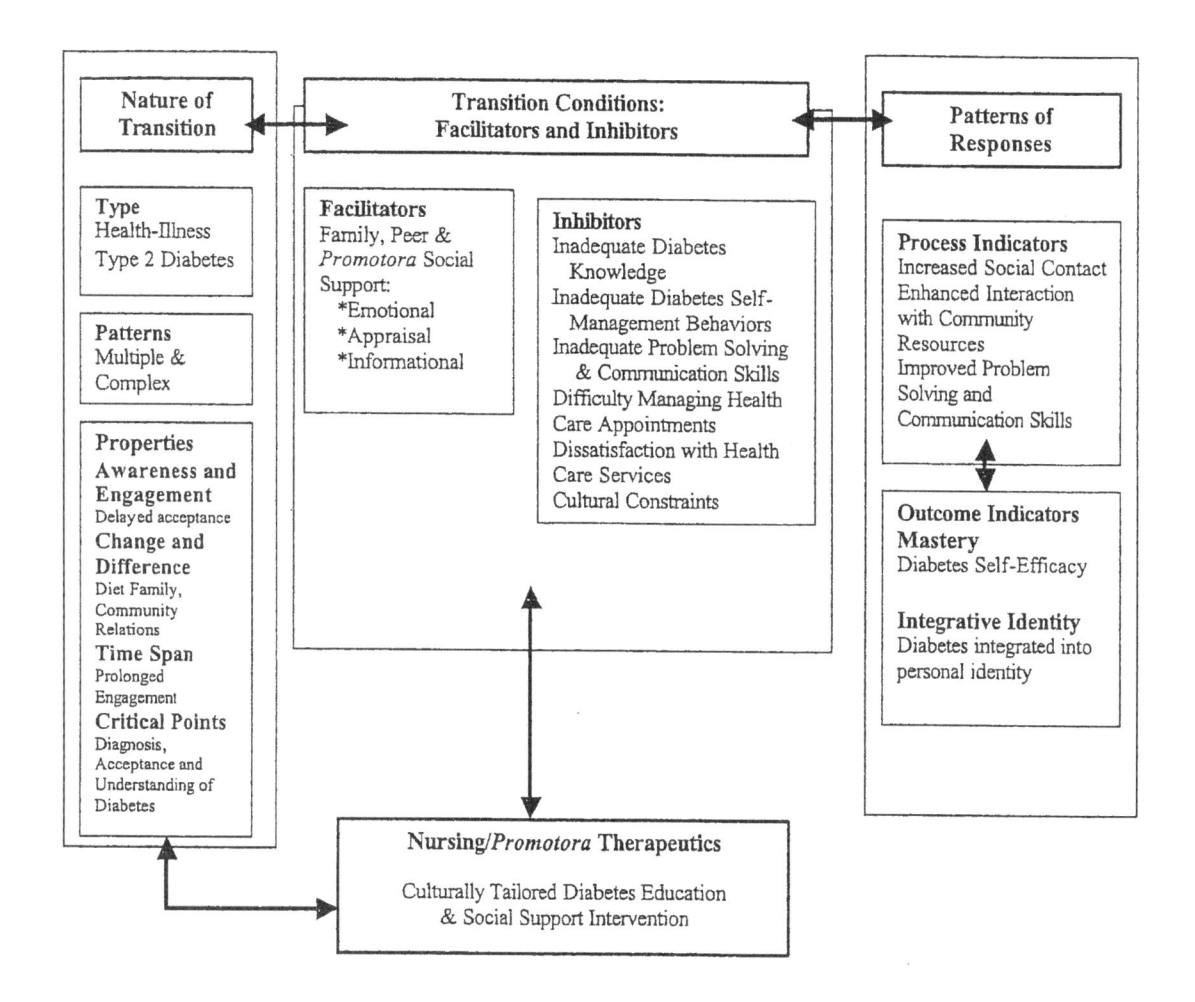

FIGURE 7.2.1 Health-illness transition experiences among Mexican immigrant women with diabetes.

Adapted with permission from Meleis et al. (p. 17).

text of the health-illness transition in a group of Mexican immigrant women with type 2 diabetes.

Methods

The purpose of the study was to explore the potential effect of the intervention on the health-illness transition of Mexican immigrant women with type 2 diabetes. The research design was an equivalent status mixed-method design[27] using both quantitative and qualitative approaches. The design for this exploratory investigation uses the advantages of both the quantitative and qualitative paradigms, and reflects the research process of working back and forth between deductive and inductive models of thinking in a research study.[28(p. 178)]

Intervention

A team consisting of a nurse researcher and a bilingual nurse/certified diabetes educator (CDE) developed the *Promotora*-Diabetes Education and Social Support Intervention (P-DESSI). The goal of the P-DESSI was to facilitate Mexican immigrant women's diabetes health-illness transition by increasing diabetes knowledge and social support, decreasing psychosocial and health-related behavior problems, and increasing diabetes self-efficacy. We recruited and trained 2 bilingual *promotoras* employed by the local community health center, who were knowledgeable about diabetes and experienced in conducting home visits, to deliver the 6-month community-based intervention. Because the participants did not speak English, the entire intervention was delivered in Spanish.

The intervention consisted of a group component delivered once a month at the local community health center, and an individual component delivered in the participants' homes. The group component was organized around a 30-minute class, followed by a 1-hour focused discussion session, and ended with 10 minutes of physical activity. The research team and invited professionals conducted the classes. Over the 6-month period, 5 of the 7 recommended diabetes self-management behaviors[12]—healthy eating, physical activity, problem solving, healthy coping, and reducing risks—were addressed in the classes. During 3 of the 6 group sessions, the *promotoras* facilitated a focused discussion session that was audiotaped. The topic of the focused discussion session was consistent with the class content. For example, when a bilingual, bicultural nutritionist presented on healthy eating, the focused discussion session also addressed healthy eating. The *promotoras* used 2 questions developed by the researcher to facilitate the focused discussion sessions. During the final 10 minutes of the monthly group meetings, the *promotoras* facilitated a physical activity session (e.g., dancing, stretching, or walking).

The *promotoras* delivered the individual component of the intervention at each participant's home, in four 60–90-minute sessions. The purpose of the first home visit was to establish rapport and identify psychosocial and health-related behavior problems (transition inhibitors) using the Omaha System.[29] During the other 3 home visits, the *promotoras* provided individually tailored diabetes education and social support. The home visit curriculum consisted of 3 modules: healthy eating, managing stress, and physical activity. The *promotoras* delivered each module within 3 weeks following the corresponding group session. The intervention was individually tailored to the context of needs of each participant. For example, during the nutrition module, the *promotora* and the participant sat at the kitchen table and read food labels on the packaging of breakfast foods the woman usually ate.

Sample and Recruitment

Prior to recruiting participants, the institutional review board (IRB) of The University of Arizona and the local community health center IRB reviewed and approved the research. We selected a convenience sample of 15 participants from attendance logs of diabetes education programs conducted in the community. Inclusion criteria included the following: (a) being of Mexican origin, (b) aged 18–65, (c) diagnosed with type 2 diabetes (confirmed by medical record), (d) patients of the local community health center, (e) able to speak Spanish, (f) able to walk at least 1 mile (self-report), and (g) had previously attended a diabetes education program. Health center staff contacted potential participants by telephone and used a recruitment script to review the study and seek their permission to be contacted by the nurse researcher and/or the CDE. Once enrolled, *promotoras* mailed monthly postcard reminders about the group sessions and made telephone calls to schedule the 4 home visits.

Design and Measures

The quantitative approach used established instruments to compare differences between (a) diabetes knowledge, (b) social support, (c) psychosocial problems, (d) health-related behavior problems, and (e) diabetes self-efficacy in participants both before and after the intervention. Quantitative data collection consisted of completion of a set of self-reported questionnaires collected during the first and last group sessions. In addition, a demographic questionnaire was administered during preintervention data collection. The *promotoras* and/or the bilingual CDE read in Spanish the questionnaires for those participants who had visual impairments, were illiterate, or had low health literacy levels.

The qualitative approach was used to obtain different and/or complementary data on the same phenomena. Qualitative data collection consisted of 2 semistructured questions that were presented to participants during the focused discussion sessions: (a) What are the strategies that you use that allow you to be successful in managing your diabetes? (b) What are the challenges or barriers that get in the way of successfully managing your diabetes? The focused discussion sessions were audiotaped and transcribed.

Quantitative Measures

The 10-item demographic questionnaire was administered at the preintervention session and included country of origin, number of years in the United States, language first learned, years of formal education, years with diabetes, and number of diabetes classes previously attended. Instruments used to collect data in the preintervention and postintervention sessions included the 24-item Diabetes Knowledge Questionnaire (DKQ)[30] and the 19-item Medical Outcomes Study (MOS) Social Support Inventory.[31] The DKQ is a reliable and valid measure of diabetes-related knowledge.[30] The MOS Social Support Inventory measures the availability of social support in 4 functional domains: informational/emotional, tangible, affectionate, and positive social interaction. Internal consistency for the overall scale is 0.97, and subscale values range from 0.91 to 0.96.[31] Psychosocial and health-related behavior problems were identified by the *promotoras* during the first and last home visits using 2 domains of the Omaha System.[29] The psychosocial domain includes 12 potential problems, and is defined as patterns of behavior, emotion, communication, relationships, and development. The health-related behavior domain has 9 potential problems, and is defined as patterns of activities that maintain or promote wellness, promote recovery, and decrease risk of disease. Finally, diabetes self-efficacy served as a process indicator of a healthy diabetes transition. The 8-item Self-Efficacy for Diabetes Scale[18] was administered in the postintervention data collection session. The Self-Efficacy for Diabetes Scale was administered first as a posttest and then readministered as a retrospective pretest. A retrospective pretest assumes that the participant's pretest and posttest response is made with respect to the same internal standard. The expectation is that the comparison of posttest scores with retrospective pretest scores would eliminate treatment-produced response shifts and give an unconfounded indication of the treatment effect.[32] Reliability and validity of the scale has been established in Spanish- and English-speaking individuals.[33,34]

Data Analyses

Data analysis consisted of both quantitative and qualitative methods to study the same phenomenon—the health-illness transition of Mexican immigrant women with diabetes. Quantitative data analysis was conducted using SPSS for Windows version 14. Descriptive statistics were used to identify trends and characteristics of the sample. Paired t tests were produced for comparison of preintervention and postintervention questionnaire data. The significance level was set at $p < 0.05$. The qualitative data from the tape-recorded 1-hour focused discussion sessions were transcribed by a bilingual graduate assistant and subsequently translated into English; cultural equivalency was ensured through backtranslation.[35] The researcher and the graduate assistant analyzed the translated qualitative data from the focused discussion sessions using thematic analysis.[36] Ongoing consultation and reference to the original Spanish-language transcripts provided further assurance of semantic and cultural equivalence of the findings.

Results

Sample

A total of 15 Mexican immigrant women were recruited and enrolled into the 6-month intervention pilot study of the P-DESSI. Word of mouth and telephone calls were the most effective recruitment strategies used by the *promotoras*. All of the participants received the individual component of the intervention (4 home visits). However, only 20% of the women participated in all 6 of the group sessions; 80% participated in at least 3 of the group sessions. Reasons for missing group sessions were primarily related to sick children, school activities, and other competing family events.

Fifteen ($N = 15$) women with a mean age of 53 years ($SD = 11.05$, range 36–72) participated in this study conducted in an Arizona community adjacent to the Mexico border. All of the women were Mexican citizens at birth who immigrated to the United States. The mean number of years they had lived in the Arizona community was 21 years ($SD = 12.35$, range 5–46). Despite the fact that they were long-time U.S. residents, the immigrant women spoke only Spanish. The mean number of years of formal education—primarily from Mexico—was 8.33 years ($SD = 3.54$, range 0–14). The majority ($n = 8$) were married, 2 were widowed, 1 was divorced, and the other 4 were single. The mean number of years diagnosed with type-2 diabetes was 3.0 ($SD = 2.58$, range 6 months–10 years). The average number of previous American Diabetes Association diabetes education classes attended by the women was 5.6 ($SD = 1.3$, range 1–6). The women were not outsiders to the formal U.S. health care system; they had health care providers at the local community health center, but were challenged by the multiple and complex factors that inhibited and facilitated the diabetes health-illness transition.

Quantitative Results

Results from the quantitative measures suggest that the intervention had a statistically significant effect on diabetes knowledge, psychosocial problems, health-related behavior problems, and self-efficacy. Table 7.2.1 presents the preintervention and postintervention scores.

The mean diabetes knowledge scores increased significantly from 16.27 to 18.93 ($p < 0.001$). There were no significant changes between preintervention and postintervention scores related to social support (Table 7.2.1). Because the items in the informational and emotional subscale of the social support instrument were the most likely to be influenced by the intervention, they were analyzed separately from the other items; there were no significant changes between preintervention and postintervention in those scores. The potential influence of a dose effect on social support was assessed by selecting those participants who attended at least 2 of the 3 focused discussion sessions ($n = 12$). There were no differences between preintervention and postintervention for the informational and emotional social support subscale in this subgroup ($t_{11} = -0.72, p = 0.49$). The diabetes self-efficacy questionnaire was administered during the postintervention data collection period as a posttest and retrospective pretest, and was also significant ($p < 0.001$).

There were significant changes between preintervention and postintervention in the numbers of problems identified in the 2 domains of the Omaha System: psychosocial ($p = 0.001$) and health-related behaviors ($p < 0.001$) (Table 7.2.1). Problems with interpersonal relationships were reported by the majority (93.3%) of the women and were most frequently attributed to minimal shared activities (80%), difficulty problem solving (47%), prolonged tension (40%), and inadequate communication skills (33%). The second most frequently reported psychosocial problem was difficulty with communicating with community resources (86.7%). An inability to communicate their concerns (60%), dissatisfaction with services (47%), transportation (33%), and language barriers (27%) contributed to problems with interacting with community resources. Mental health problems experienced by 80% of the women were manifested by sadness, hopelessness, and low self-esteem (53.3%) and difficulty managing stress (40%). The women reported a reduction in psychosocial problems between preintervention and postintervention; problems related to mental health and role change decreased by 33.3%, communication with community resources and social contact decreased 20%, and problems

TABLE 7.2.1 Changes From Preintervention to Postintervention ($N = 15$)*

Measures	Preintervention Mean	SD	Postintervention Mean	SD	T value
Diabetes knowledge	16.27	3.71	18.93	3.31	−6.01†
Social support	80.17	16.32	82.00	15.12	−0.38
Diabetes self-efficacy	48.33	17.84	76.73	3.95	−5.82†
Omaha System					
Psychosocial	3.80	1.15	2.67	1.35	4.43†
Health-related behaviors	4.07	1.10	2.07	1.10	6.48†

*Paired samples t test.
†$p \leq 0.001$.

related to interpersonal relationship decreased by 6.6%.

Health-related behavior problems included nutrition, physical activity, health care supervision, medication regimen, and sleep and rest. Problems with nutrition were reported by the majority of the women (93.3%), and the most frequently reported contributing factor was hyperglycemia (73.3%). Physical activity (80%) was the second most frequently reported health-related behavior problem due to sedentary lifestyle (40%). Problems with health care supervision (80%) were related to lack of follow-up appointments (60%) and inability to coordinate appointments (40%).

Problems with managing medications were reported by 80% of the women; contributing factors included not following the recommended protocol (66.7%) and an inadequate system for taking medications (66.7%). The women reported a reduction in health-related behavior problems between preintervention and postintervention; problems related to physical activity decreased by 66.7%, medication management problems reduced by 53.3%, health care supervision problems reduced by 33.3%, sleep and rest problems reduced by 26.6%, and nutrition problems reduced by 20%.

Qualitative Results

Thematic analysis[36] of the qualitative data from the transcripts of the focused discussion sessions resulted in 3 themes: (1) *Difficulty in Acknowledging Diabetes As Part of My Life*, (2) *Still Adjusting to Change and Difference*, and (3) *Putting Family First*. Three major themes that address the properties in the Transitions Model[1] (Figure 7.2.1) will be discussed.

In the first theme, *Difficulty in Acknowledging Diabetes As Part of My Life*, the transition properties of awareness, identity, engagement, and time span are evident. Several women addressed the difficulty of admitting to themselves that they had diabetes. Examples that illustrated the difficulty women had in accepting diabetes as part of their personal identity included the following:

> It took a lot for me to say this problem, but it is the truth.
> Well, for me it was very difficult to accept that I have diabetes.

It is important to note that the relationship between time span and awareness of the reality of the illness was a common theme among these participants. Many of these women were still trying to come to terms with their diagnosis and the implications diabetes had on their daily life and their long-term health:

> When I was told I had diabetes, it was hard to admit until after a year. I think that is when I started to take it more serious.
> It was difficult to recognize this as an illness and I am going to have it for the rest of my life and I am learning how to eat.

I am conscious about 80% of the time that I have diabetes and if I do not take care of my diabetes, it is not going to lead me to nothing good.

Inadequate and inaccurate diabetes knowledge that precluded active engagement in diabetes self-management activities was revealed by the women during the focused discussion sessions. Questions asked by the women during the classes included the following:

How is the sugar [level] supposed to be in the morning before you eat?
Do pain and other illnesses cause the sugar levels to rise?

These women were *Still Adjusting to Change and Difference*. This theme illustrated the transition property of change and difference and was best reflected in the women's narratives about the dietary and physical activity changes they experienced during the intervention. In the first focused discussion session, the women were asked, "What has been the most difficult in controlling your diabetes?" The unanimous response was, "the food!" They clearly had changed their dietary habits and recognized the difference it made in their life:

I feel sad because I can't eat what I like, but when I see my sugar it makes me happy and eager to keep going.
I have stopped eating many things, salt, sodas, flour, fat, and cereals. The doctor recommended the 12-grain bread and that is what I eat.

These changes were not easy. Making food selections during the Thanksgiving holiday was particularly difficult for one woman:

I cried because I could not eat. I am not one of those people that can [just] taste it, so I avoid it. I cannot eat small portions.

In the case of physical activity, several women noted the benefits of their changes in activity levels:

I wasn't used to walking and now I walk 30–40 minutes.
I used to feel very bad. I couldn't bend over because I felt like I was suffocating due to the love handles, it used to bother me. Now it doesn't, not the same. I have more flexibility in the sense that I can bend over and tie my shoes without a problem and that is a benefit.

Others described critical turning points in the diabetes transition—those events associated with increased awareness of change, difference, or more active engagement. One participant described such a turning point as being the link between her awareness of the severity of her diabetes and the importance of self-management:

When we learn we are sick and all that [high blood sugar] is harmful, that is when we begin to become conscious [of the need to engage in diabetes self-management].

Another woman described how her mother's diabetes complications increased her own awareness and engagement in self-management of her own diabetes:

My mother never took care of herself and her sugar didn't get lower than 400 or 500. She got really sick, all of her body is numb, she gets burns, horrible things happen to her and she does not feel it. I see her and I do not want to end up like her. That is why I am taking care of myself and doing everything I can so I do not get to that point.

For these Mexican immigrants, *Putting Family First* was one of the ways they engaged in diabetes self-management and still took care of their families. Several women described the changes they made in cooking for themselves and their family:

I love tortillas and I have to make them, my children love them. But I will restrain myself and will not eat them.
My children are already older and it is difficult too because they take care of me a lot. And I know it is difficult for them because I don't make the foods they like, I used to put fresh cheese in the beans and now they are eating like me.

Taking care of personal physical and mental health was important not only for the women themselves but for the well-being of their families as well:

It is not good to be depressed because you transmit those feelings to those around you. For example, the kids get annoyed and uncontrollable and instead of trying to relax them you get desperate and things get out of hand and you feel like going crazy.

Discussion

This pilot intervention study extends the application of the theory of transitions to a specific type of transition—the health-illness transition related to diabetes in Mexican immigrant women. The quantitative and qualitative data from this intervention pilot study offer overlapping and divergent facets of the health-illness transition related to diabetes as experienced among a group of Mexican immigrant women. We presented the study findings in Figure 7.2.1, an adaptation of the Transitions model[1] that represents the complex and multidimensional process of these Mexican American women's health–illness transition experiences.

Figure 7.2.1 captures the critical dimensions of the process that moved the women toward a healthy transition outcome, facilitated and mediated by a diabetes education and social support intervention with professional and *promotora* components. These results suggest that redefining self as a person with diabetes and engaging in diabetes self-management activities may be delayed for as long as 1 year after diagnosis. In fact, findings demonstrate that the interrelated and essential properties of the diabetes health-illness transition are complex and unfold in an undulating and protracted fashion. Consequently, formal diabetes education programs that are traditionally offered following the initial diagnosis may not be the most optimal timing for this population. A more appropriate model might be one in which an individual could enroll in the program when they have achieved sufficient awareness and are prepared to engage in diabetes self-management behaviors.

A healthy transition is characterized by process and outcome indicators.[1(p. 22)] Therefore, we used multiple measures to assess the indicators of Mexican immigrant women's diabetes health-illness transition. Whereas there was convergence between the quantitative and qualitative data related to diabetes knowledge (outcome indicator) and diabetes self-efficacy (process indicator), there was divergence between the findings related to social support (process indicator). The difference between preintervention and postintervention scores in the MOS social support instrument was not statistically significant. However, there were statistically significant differences between preintervention and postintervention scores for Omaha psychosocial problems that tapped dimensions of social support. For example, problems related to emotional support—such as social isolation or not having someone to confide in, talk about problems and share worries and fears with, and help with problem solving—decreased between preintervention and postintervention measures. An explanation for the divergent findings between the 2 quantitative measures may be related to the Likert scales and potential lack of semantic equivalence[37] with the MOS social support instrument. An alternative perspective for interpreting the divergent findings related to social support is the way in which the Omaha data were collected. The *promotoras* collected the data in the women's homes and in the context of discussion and reflection over a 60–90-minute time period. This method of data collection represents a more culturally congruent approach when compared with the method used to collect the other quantitative measures.

This study supports earlier findings,[25,26,38–40] about the significant contributions of *promotoras* to community-based interventions, and suggests that *promotoras* can be effective interventionists in facilitating healthy transitions among Mexican American women with diabetes. The *promotoras* brought multiple strengths to this intervention study. They had an insider's perspective of the community and environmental conditions that facilitate or inhibit progress toward achieving a healthy diabetes transition. For example, *promotoras* understood the meanings, beliefs, and attitudes attributed to diabetes. Finally, the *promotoras* were knowledgeable about the community diabetes education program, familiar with the health care providers and policies of the local community health center, and life in the Arizona-Sonora region of the U.S.–Mexico border.

Limitations

Several study limitations need to be acknowledged. The small sample size ($N = 15$) and sample demographics limit the generalizability of the findings to other populations. The intervention was constructed to facilitate the health–illness transition related to diabetes for Mexican immigrant women residing in a rural U.S.–Mexico border community. The intervention may not be as effective for Mexican immigrants in other border communities or for those living in urban communities. Because both *promotoras* and participants were female, it is possible that findings may differ with male participants and/or with male *promotores*. Furthermore, the single group did not allow for empirically testing the effectiveness of the intervention. A future study that uses a 2-group experimental design would provide an opportunity for empirically testing the effectiveness of the intervention. In addition, a future study that includes biomarkers would allow for an objective evaluation of outcome criteria specific for diabetes self-management. Lastly, there is a need for more community-based studies that investigate community-level facilitators and inhibitors of healthy transitions among immigrant women with diabetes.

Conclusions

This study demonstrates the value of transition theory for providing an understanding of the nature, conditions, and processes of the health–illness transition associated with diabetes as experienced by a group of Mexican immigrant women. The findings from this pilot study suggest that the 6-month diabetes education and social support intervention successfully facilitated the outcomes that characterize a healthy transition for immigrant women with diabetes who reside within the U.S.–Mexico border region. Future research that clarifies the complexity and dimensionality of the health-illness transition associated with diabetes can be used to inform culturally congruent nursing therapeutics that aim to reduce the disproportionate burden of diabetes in Mexican immigrants.

REFERENCES

1. Meleis, A. I., Sawyer, L. M., Im, E. O., Messias, D. K. H., & Schumacher, K. (2000). Experiencing transitions: An emerging middle-range theory. *Advances in Nursing Science, 23*(1), 12–28.
2. Meleis, A. I. (1997). Immigrant transitions and health care: An action plan. *Nursing Outlook. 45,* 1–42.
3. Jones, P. S., Zhang, X. E., & Meleis, A. I. (2003). Transforming vulnerability. *Western Journal of Nursing Research, 25*(7), 835–853.
4. U.S. Census Bureau. *Census bureau projects tripling of Hispanic and Asian populations in 50 years; non-Hispanics may drop to half of total population.* Retrieved September 28, 2006, from http://www.census.gov/Press-Release/www/releases/archives/population/001720.html
5. PEW Hispanic Health Center. *A statistical portrait of Hispanics at mid decade. Reports and factsheets.* Retrieved September 15, 2006, from http://pewhispanic.org/reports/middecade/
6. Malone, N., Baluja, K. F., Costanzo, J. M., & Davis, C. J. (2003). *The foreign-born population: 2000. Census 2000 brief C2KBR-34.* Retrieved September 13, 2006, from www.census.og/prod2003pubs/c2kbr-34.pdf
7. Larsen, L. J. (2004). *The foreign-born population in the United States: 2003. Current population reports, P20-551, U.S. Census Bureau, Washington, DC.* Retrieved September 12, 2006, from http://www.census.gov/prod/2004pubs/p20-551.pdf
8. Stern, M. P., & Mitchell, B. D. (1995). Diabetes in Hispanic Americans. In M. I. Harris, C. C. Cowie, M. P. Stern, E. J. Boyko, G. E. Reiber, & P. H. Bennett (Eds.), *Diabetes in America* (2nd ed., pp. 631–659). Washington, DC: U.S. Department of Health and Human Services, National Institutes of Health; DHHS Publication No. (NIH) 95-1468.
9. West, S. K., Klein, R., Rodriguez, J., et al. (2001). Diabetes and diabetic retinopathy in a Mexican-American population: Proyecto VER. *Diabetes Care, 24,* 1204–1209.
10. Mitchell, B. D., Almasy, L. A., Rainwater, D. L., et al. (1999). Diabetes and hypertension in Mexican American families: Relation to cardiovascular risk. *American Journal of Epidemiology, 149*(11), 1047–1056.
11. National Diabetes Information Clearinghouse. (2002). *Diabetes in Hispanic Americans.* Retrieved September 15, 2006, from http://diabetes.niddk.nih.gov/dm/pubs/hispanicamerican. NIH Publication No. 02-3265.
12. American Association of Diabetes Educators. (2005). *Setting the standards for behavioral measurement in diabetes self-management training.* Retrieved September 14, 2006, from http://www.diabeteseducator.org/AADE7/index.shtml

13. Portillo, C. J., Villaruel, A., de Leon Siantz, M. L., Perigallo, N., Calvillo, E. R., & Eribes, C. M. (2001). Research agenda for Hispanics in the U.S.: A nursing perspective. *Nursing Outlook, 49*(6), 263–269.
14. Brown, S. A., Garcia, A. A., Kouzekanani, K., & Hanis, C. L. (2002). Culturally competent diabetes self-management education for Mexican-Americans. *Diabetes Care, 25*(2), 259–268.
15. Oomen, J. S., Owen, L. J., & Suggs, L. S. (1999). Culture counts: Why current treatment models fail Hispanic women with type 2 diabetes. *Diabetes Educator, 25*(2), 220–225.
16. Brown, S. A., & Hanis, C. L. (1995). A community-based, culturally sensitive education and group-support intervention for Mexican Americans with NIDDM: A pilot study of efficacy. *Diabetes Educator, 21*(3), 203–210.
17. Brown, S. A., Blozis, S. A., Kouzekanani, K., Garcia, A. A., Winchell, M., & Hanis, C. L. (2005). Dosage effects of diabetes self-management education for Mexican Americans: The Starr County Border Health Initiative. *Diabetes Care, 28*(3), 527–532.
18. Lorig, K., Ritter, P., & Gonzales, V. M. (2003). Hispanic chronic disease self-management: A randomized community-based trial. *Nursing Research, 52*(6), 361–369.
19. Vincent, D., Pasvogel, A., & Barrera, L. (in press) A feasibility study of a culturally tailored diabetes intervention for Mexican-Americans. *Biological Research for Nursing*.
20. Aday, L. A. (2001). *At Risk in America* (2nd ed.). San Francisco: Jossey-Bass.
21. Meleis, A. I., & Trangenstein, P. A. (1994). Facilitating transitions: Redefinition of the nursing mission. *Nursing Outlook, 42*, 255–259.
22. Schumacher, K. L., & Meleis, A. I. (1994). Transitions: A central concept in nursing. *Image: Journal of Nursing Scholarship, 26*(2), 119–127.
23. McEwen, M. M., & Slack, M. K. (2005). Factors associated with Latino health behaviors. *Hispanic Health Care International, 3*(3), 143–152.
24. Messias, D. K. H. (2006, February). *Border crossing and health: Concepts and frameworks for nursing research*. Paper presented at the U.S.–Mexico Border Health Symposium, University of Arizona, Tucson.
25. Nemcek, M. A., & Sabatier, R. (2003). State of evaluation: Community health workers. *Public Health Nursing, 20*(4), 260–270.
26. Swider, S. M. (2002). Outcome effectiveness of community health workers: An integrative literature review. *Public Health Nursing, 19*(1), 11–20.
27. Tashakkori, A., & Teddiie, C. (1998). *Mixed methodology: Combining qualitative and quantitative approaches*. Thousand Oaks, CA: Sage.
28. Creswell, J. W. (1995). *Research design: Qualitative and quantitative approaches*. Thousand Oaks, CA: Sage.
29. Martin, K. S. (2005). *The Omaha System: A key to practice, documentation, and information management*. St Louis, MO: Elsevier Saunders.
30. Brown, S. A., Harrist, R. B., Villagomez, E. T., Segura, M., Barton, S. A., & Hanis, C. (2000). Gender and treatment difference in knowledge, health beliefs, and metabolic control in Mexican Americans with type 2 diabetes. *Diabetes Educator, 26*(3), 425–438.
31. Sherbourne, D. C., & Steward, A. L. (1991). The MOS social support survey. *Social Science and Medicine, 32*, 705–714.
32. Sprangers, M., & Hoogstraten, M. (1989). Pretesting effects in retrospective pretest-posttest designs. *Journal of Applied Psychology, 74*(2), 265–272.
33. Lorig, K., & Gonzales, V. M. (2000). Community-based diabetes self-management education: Definition and case study. *Diabetes Spectrum, 13*(4), 234–240.
34. Lorig, K., Ritter, P., & Jacquez, A. Outcomes of border health Spanish/English chronic disease self-management programs. *Diabetes Educator, 31*(3), 401–409.
35. Brislin, R. W. (1970). Back-translation for cross-cultural research. *Journal of Cross-Cultural Psychology, 1*, 185–216.
36. DeSantis, L., & Ugarriza, N. D. (2000). The concept of theme as used in qualitative nursing research. *Western Journal of Nursing Research, 22*(3), 351–372.
37. Flaskerud, J. H. (1988). Is the Likert scale format culturally biased? *Nursing Research, 37*(3), 185–186.
38. Gary, T. L., Bone, L. R., Hill, M. N., et al. (2003). Randomized controlled trial of the effects of nurse case manager and community health nworker interventions on risk factors for diabetes-related complications in urban African-Americans. *Preventive Medicine, 37*(1), 23–32.
39. Kim, S., Koniak-Griffin, D., Flaskerud, J. H., & Guarnero, P. A. (2004). *Journal of Cardiovascular Nursing, 19*(3), 192–199.
40. American Association of Diabetes Educators. (2003). Position statement: Diabetes community health workers. *Diabetes Educator, 29*(5), 818–824.

Reprinted with permission from: McEwen, M. M., Baird, M., Pasvogel, A., & Gallegos, G. (2007). Health-illness transition experiences among Mexican immigrant women with diabetes. *Family and Community Health, 30*(3), 201–212.

7.3 TRANSITIONS IN CHRONIC ILLNESS: RHEUMATOID ARTHRITIS IN WOMEN

Muriel P. Shaul

Abstract

This article describes transition theory as it relates to a qualitative study of women with rheumatoid arthritis (RA) and the importance of this theory in nursing practice. Rheumatoid arthritis is prototypical of many chronic illnesses because it has a profound impact on activities of daily living. It frequently occurs during a person's most productive years and continues throughout life. Because a person with RA typically experiences a number of exacerbations and remissions over the course of many years, transition theory was chosen as a framework for this study. The study sample consisted of 30 women with RA, who were interviewed about their experiences of living with this chronic illness. The women described four distinct phases in learning to live with RA, which began with awareness and proceeded to mastery. These findings are consistent with the stages of transition described by other investigators.

Nurses work with people experiencing developmental, situational, and health and illness transitions. Understanding what precipitates the transition process from health to illness and the stages experienced with specific illnesses could facilitate the planning and implementation of appropriate nursing interventions.

Living with a chronic illness often requires management of symptoms and treatment modalities on a daily basis, as well as coping with the demands of daily life. Rheumatoid arthritis (RA) is a systemic disease that is thought to be the result of an autoimmune response (American Academy of Family Physicians, 1990; McCance & Huether, 1995). It poses many challenges due to its characteristic pattern of exacerbation and remission, as do many other chronic illnesses. RA typically affects the joints, causing pain, inflammation, swelling, and deformity. Fatigue, weakness, and general malaise, along with joint and muscle symptoms, also occur.

The experience of living with RA can be described as an ongoing transition process or as one in which the individual uses many intuitive and intentional strategies to balance resources and demands, including those that are intrapersonal, interpersonal, and environmental (Thorne, 1993). It is a process of living with the unexpected—of not knowing from one day to the next how one might feel or what one can do. For people with chronic illness, particularly RA, there is not one identifiable end point at which the health and illness transition is complete (Anderson, Blue, & Lau, 1991).

The study on which this chapter is based used transition theory as an organizing framework to explore the experience of learning to live with RA over time. The study and findings have been published previously (Shaul, 1995), and are summarized here to provide the context for a discussion of transition theory and the implications these findings have for nurses who provide care for people with RA and other chronic conditions.

Background

The word *transition* stems from the Latin preposition *trans*, which can mean across, over, beyond, or through (*American Heritage Dictionary*, 1969) and a root word conveying the meaning of movement and change. *Transition* has been defined as, "the process or an instance of changing from one form, state, activity, or place to another." (p. 1364) One of the earliest applications of transition theory was by van Gennep in 1906 (1906/1960), who described the three stages of transition used by agrarian societies to commemorate the developmental passage from childhood to adulthood (Chiriboga, 1979). Called "rites of passage," these stages were marked by primitive societies with a public ceremony. The stages were labeled (a) segregation, (b) liminal, or transition, and (c) incorporation (van Gennep). Segregation refers to the actual separation of an individual from the rest of the society in preparation for the transition phase. The segregation stage is followed by the liminal, or transition, stage, during which the individual is neither what he or she was nor what he or she will become. The transition phase ends with the onset of the incorporation stage, which is the point at which the individual has embraced a new identity (van Gennep).

Transitions can be initiated by developmental stages, as described by van Gannep (1960) and others (Dixon, Dixon, Spinner, Sexton, & Perry, 1991; Mercer, Nichols, & Doyle, 1989) as well as by situations (Aroian, 1990; Dimond, McCance, & King, 1987; Murphy, 1990) and health and illness events (Catanzaro, 1990; Chick & Meleis, 1986). Developmental transitions are those that occur predictably as part of maturation (Baltes, 1987). Situational transitions are those that involve changes in one's living, work, or family situation (Schlossberg, 1984; Silverman, 1982) and can include relocation, immigration, divorce, and job loss. Health and illness transitions involve a change from one state of health to another (Chick & Meleis, 1986; Corbin & Strauss, 1991; George, 1982).

Thus, transitions can occur at predictable developmental milestones, can be precipitated by an unexpected crisis, or can be a more gradual process from one state of being to another. The consistent thread in all transition experiences is change—change to or within an individual, the environment, or both. Meleis and Trangenstein (1994) further explain that although transitions include change, the transition process is complex, occurs over time, and incorporates flow and movement.

The model of transition described by Chick and Meleis (1986) provided the organizing framework for the study of the women described in this chapter and of how they learned to live with RA.

Transitions—A Nursing Model

Chick and Meleis (1986) describe a health and illness model of transition that is applicable to nursing practice. The major components of this model are process, awareness, perception, disconnectedness, patterns of response, and health outcomes.

Process

The word *process* refers to the dynamic nature of a transition experience. It has a beginning and an end, yet the characteristics identifiable at one end of the continuum may not resemble those at the other. Furthermore, the process is ongoing, and more than one type of transition can occur simultaneously.

Awareness and Perception

A transition process is precipitated by a change-inducing event that is perceived by an individual as important (Chick & Meleis, 1986). A person's awareness of the change and the perceived importance of the event, which can occur separately or simultaneously, depend upon the person's individual interpretation. For example, a person may be aware of pain and stiffness but may perceive both as tolerable. However, fatigue, which is typical in many chronic illnesses, may be perceived as intolerable. This individual perception is grounded in the interpretation of sensations and events and in the meaning these have to a person at a particular time.

Disconnectedness

A period of disconnectedness, characterized by uncertainty and ambiguity, follows as the individual attempts to adapt to changing circumstances or situations. Disconnectedness produces a disruption in the stability and predictability in daily life. Theoretically, the transition concludes with a return to a stable state. The individual has changed during the process by incorporating changes in physical, psychological, social, economic dimensions, or in all of these dimensions, into a new self-identity.

Patterns of Response

Responses to the transition process, which are individual and dynamic, are influenced by contextual, situational, and biological factors. These factors, referred to as antecedent and mediating factors by Chick and Meleis (1986), include life stage, other health problems, genetic and cultural inheritance, and inadequate housing or income. Individual mediating factors include both physiologic and psychological responses (Chick & Meleis, 1986). Physiologic factors include the body's ability to tolerate or respond to certain medications and physical symptoms, decreased mobility and strength, and the severity of comorbid conditions. Psychological factors include personality traits such as hardiness, locus of control, or learned responses such as problem-solving capabilities, tolerance for uncertainty, and the ability to find meaning in experiences. Some individual mediating factors may be therapeutic, such as the ability to assess the need for rest and to act on that need, or they may be nontherapeutic, such as continuing activities that produce stress on the joints or avoiding exercise, thereby increasing the likelihood of developing joint contractures and increased weakness.

Environmental mediating factors are those that occur external to the individual and include access to appropriate care, medications, or assistance; support from significant others and care providers; adequate or inadequate housing; and the presence or absence of appropriate work opportunities (Chick & Meleis, 1986).

Health Outcomes

According to Chick and Meleis (1986), there are four possible health-related outcomes in transition processes: restoration, maintenance, protection, and promotion. Health restoration refers to the return to a state of health that is equal to or better than what the individual experienced prior to the transition. Health maintenance refers to a stable state in which the individual may have a chronic illness but is able to maintain a level of wellness necessary for role function. Health protection indicates that a person requires the care of others to prevent further deterioration or disability. Health promotion indicates that a person has the ability to engage in activities that increase overall health and well-being.

Schumacher and Meleis (1994) expanded on the conceptualization of transitions by identifying defining characteristics such as emerging life patterns and new identities. These concepts reflect the change that occurs during the period from the initiation to the completion of a transition experience and the development of revised patterns of living and self-concept.

Method

Sample

This qualitative study was part of a larger study that examined the changes experienced by women with RA over a 3-year period (Shaul, 1994). Study participants were drawn from a panel of people with RA involved in a longitudinal study, maintained by the Arthritis Research Group of the Rosalind Russell Multipurpose Arthritis Center at the University of California, San Francisco. Panel recruitment procedures have been reported previously (Katz & Yelin, 1993; Shaul, 1995). The panel was composed of approximately 745 people, 75% of whom were women. Participants in the panel were interviewed every year by telephone regarding their physical, psychological, social, and economic function, medication usage, use of health care services, and RA symptoms.

This secondary data analysis examined indicators of physical, psychological, social, and economic function among all women in the panel during the preceding 3-year period ($N = 422$) to identify a subset who experienced significant change in two or more areas of function ($n = 119$). Participants meeting the following criteria were eligible for an interview in their home: (a) experienced two or more changes in function indicative of transitions in health status during the preceding 3-year period,

(b) had an RA duration of 15 years or less, (c) lived within prescribed geographic boundaries, and (d) were between 30 and 75 years old (Shaul, 1995). The inclusion criteria identified 45 eligible women, 30 of whom were interviewed in their homes.

Participants were contacted by telephone to explain the purpose of the study and to request a personal interview. Of the 45 women who were eligible, 9 refused to participate and 6 were not contacted because theoretical saturation was reached after 30 interviews. (Theoretical saturation occurs when no new data emerge, all possible categories are evident, and the relationships among them are clear.) The 9 who refused gave the following reasons: They were too busy (2), they don't like to dwell on it (1), they were too sick (3), or they would be away from home during the data collection period (3). Those who refused to participate did not differ significantly from the entire group as to either functional level or demographics.

Demographics

The mean age for the interview sample was 54 years; mean duration of disease was 9 years. Of the 30 interviewees, 19 (63%) were married; and 22 (73%) were Caucasian. All of the women had had at least two negative changes in physical, psychological, social, or economic function during the 3 years preceding the interview.

Procedures

The University of California, San Francisco, Institutional Review Board approved the larger study, of which this qualitative study was a part. Informed consent was obtained from participants before the interviews in their homes.

Two assumptions were central to the study: The first was that learning to live with RA is a transition process, and the second was that women experience changes in various dimensions of life that can be measured and can serve as indicators of this transition process. This led to the development of research questions aimed at expanding what is known about living with chronic illness and the specific challenges faced by women.

The interview guide consisted of open-ended questions aimed at facilitating the descriptions of the women's experience of living with RA, beginning with the first symptom to the time of the interview. Also, questions were included to identify the types of health care providers involved with the diagnosis and treatment of the illness and maintenance of routine health, the sources of social and emotional support, and the strategies for meeting role expectations. Each interview was audiotaped and transcribed.

Prior to the study, the interview guide was evaluated for face and content validity. Two women who had RA but were not part of the sample critiqued the questions for appropriateness and credibility. The guide was also critiqued by one registered nurse who had extensive experience working with people with RA and by a rheumatologist. The reviewers agreed that the questions and format of the guide would facilitate learning about how women experience RA from the time of the earliest signs and symptoms to the time of the interview. Suggested revisions in the wording of the questions were made before data collection began.

As the interviewer, I kept a journal to record my impressions and experiences during data collection and analysis. The use of a journal facilitated the reflection that was necessary for objectivity and insight.

Analysis

I verified demographic and functional data with the participants, and tabulated the data by using frequencies, means, and standard deviations. During the fieldwork, I used a process of constant comparative analysis to identify categories and themes that appeared with regularity in the qualitative data. I read each transcribed interview while listening to the audiotape to verify the accuracy of the transcription. I then coded the interviews and entered the codes into Ethnograph, a computer software program that helps to organize and retrieve data (Seidel, Kjolseth, & Seymour, 1988). I reread the transcripts, code sets, and exemplars to refine the codes and categories, search for contrast cases, give alternative explanations of the phenomena, and verify emerging themes (Shaul, 1994). I also gave transcriptions of three randomly selected interviews to two nurse researchers for coding. This was done to assess consistency in analytic decisions and interpretations (Sandelowski, 1986). I compared the codes that I had assigned to those assigned by the nurse researchers; there was consistency 95% of the time in the codes that the three of us had assigned.

Results

I found exemplars of the transition process in the women's descriptions of how they recognized and learned to live with RA (Shaul, 1994). The stages of the transition process have been reported elsewhere, but are provided here to structure the discussion of the transition theory as described by Chick and Meleis (1986) and the relationship of the theory to nursing interventions.

The Transition Process

The women in the sample described the experience of living with RA in overlapping and recurring stages. These stages were labeled "becoming aware," "getting care," "learning to live with it," and "mastery" (Shaul, 1994).

Becoming Aware. The women described symptoms that occurred at this stage as "early twinges" and said that they often discounted them or attributed them to the aftereffects of recent physical activity. These twinges signaled an awareness that something was happening physically, and when the twinges became constant, severe, or disabling, they sought a diagnosis and medical treatment. For example, when a woman could not tend to her infant or had difficulty meeting work-related expectations, she labeled her symptoms as a problem. It was at this stage that the women noted that they began to feel isolated because the symptoms were less apt to be taken seriously by others. Once the symptoms were labeled as a problem, however, the women began the challenge of getting care. For some, the stages of "becoming aware" and "getting care" overlapped because the symptoms were often vague or transitory. For others, there was a clear demarcation between becoming aware that there was a problem and the process of finding appropriate care. These women experienced a sudden and profound onset of symptoms that usually precipitated an early diagnosis, but not always the appropriate treatment. Generally, women at the "becoming aware" stage responded with denial and disbelief that anything serious was occurring and hoped that the symptoms would be transitory and that their strength and agility would be restored.

Getting Care. This period was not a distinct stage; it emerged first during the "becoming aware" stage and then reemerged during the "learning to live with it" stage. However, it is treated separately here to add clarity to the experiences reported by the women.

For example, one woman, who first experienced symptoms in her hands right after her son was born, had difficulty changing his diapers. Her doctor decided it was the result of a postpartum hormonal imbalance and told her to go home and take some aspirin. It took several months and several more trips to the doctor for her to be diagnosed with RA. Another woman complained to her doctor about fatigue, morning stiffness, and swollen knees. Her doctor tested her for a thyroid problem and gave her leg exercises to do. Her thyroid turned out to be normal, and her knees got worse. Sometime later, she was tested for RA and was found to be positive. She was then referred to a rheumatologist.

The initial serious flares (or flare-ups) were times of new learning, because the women did not know what to expect, what was normal, or how to best cope with the experience. The women described being overwhelmed by their symptoms of pain, stiffness, joint swelling, fatigue, and depression. "Shopping" for a doctor and trial-and-error treatment were common experiences. Many women also experienced the frustration of getting care later in the process due to changes in their health care coverage, relocation, dissatisfaction with their physician, or their physician's retirement.

Learning to Live With It. This was a distinct stage that began once the diagnosis was made. The phrase, "You'll just have to learn to live with it" was a repeated prescription from physicians, but it did nothing to relieve the suffering or diminish the sense of anguish about the diagnosis. The "learning to live with it" stage varied in length from months to years and included periods of remission. This period was characterized by a sense of isolation, of being out of touch with others, and of having symptoms taken lightly by physicians, family members, and friends. Typically, the next flare could not be predicted, so the women continued to feel out of touch or isolated even when in remission. The disease and its symptoms assumed a dominant place in their daily lives as the women attempted to attend to self-care needs, role responsibilities, and relationships. Many withdrew from activities, social relationships, and work due to the limitations imposed by the disease, further reinforcing a sense of being disconnected from their lives before RA.

As the women described how they lived with RA, four general patterns of responses emerged as part of the process of "learning to live with it." These were labeled "listening to the body," "keeping a positive attitude," "asking for help," and "pretending." By "listening to the body," the women learned to recognize cues of oncoming flares, learned how to titrate medications to obtain the best effect, and learned when to exercise and when to stop, as well as when to rest and when to keep moving.

A second response pattern involved maintaining a positive attitude. This included the following strategies: setting realistic goals, using humor, being with family and friends, doing things they enjoyed, helping others as much as possible, helping others to understand what they were going through, praying, and refusing to "give in" to the condition. The key to successfully maintaining a positive attitude was recognizing the negative feelings and immediately pursuing strategies that counteracted them.

A third response pattern involved asking others for help with everyday tasks. This was one of the most difficult things the women learned to do because of the inevitable feelings of guilt that accompanied this response pattern. Several women spoke of asking others for help only when they absolutely could not perform a certain activity and it was necessary to do so for their family's or their own well-being. Other women said they were comfortable asking for help when they were involved in a reciprocal relationship.

A fourth response pattern that emerged was pretending. Pretending served as a means of responding to others who tended to disbelieve or minimize the physical symptoms and limitations the women experienced. Several women noted that at times they pretended to be all right in front of others, even family members. Younger working women acknowledged that admitting to physical limitations at work could preclude them from being considered for advancement.

The experience of invisible symptoms was a problem for many of these women and precipitated the need to pretend they were all right. More than half of the women I interviewed looked healthy and had no outward, visible signs of the disease. During a flare, joints would swell and be inflamed, but during remission the illness was invisible. Also invisible were the fatigue and decrease in stamina and strength that often continued beyond the flare. The women noted that it was very difficult for others to comprehend the extent of their pain, weakness, and fatigue, which were with them daily even when they were in remission. Pretending and minimizing the pain created frustration because the symptoms were real and were often severe, and yet they were not taken seriously or understood by others. The women expressed frustration about not having anyone who would understand to talk to about their experiences.

Mastery. The final stage in the transition process was mastery, when women were able to incorporate the disease and its symptoms into everyday life and recognize the cues that signal the onset of a flare, overwork, or the need to change a pattern of activity (Shaul, 1995). Through the acquisition of knowledge about the disease, its treatment, and the experience of living with it, they developed a level of expert insight. They learned as much as possible about the treatment of RA and also employed their own learned strategies to cope with the symptoms and maintain life roles. Of the 30 women interviewed, only 2 said that they felt helpless about taking care of themselves and managing their illness.

Health Outcomes

Chick and Meleis (1986) describe outcomes related to health restoration, maintenance, protection, and promotion. Although health may be restored, it may be at a different level than the one prior to the flare. Most of the women in the sample experienced what one described as a gradual loss in ability. She said, "Every time it flares, I lose a little bit more strength. There are a few more things I can either no longer do or have to do differently."

Maintenance of health depended on a woman's economic status and her ability to purchase health care insurance. All of the women in this study were covered by some form of medical insurance, and the majority sought routine health care within the limits of their coverage. The third outcome—health protection—was necessary when a woman either required the care of others to prevent further deterioration or disability or when her activities were limited to prevent further deterioration. Most of the women required assistance and care only during a flare; however, 2 women required daily assistance with all activities of daily living. The fourth outcome was health promotion. Most of the women expressed an understanding of the importance of health-promoting activities such as exercise, nutrition, and rest. However, less than one-third actively engaged in specific health-promoting exercise, whereas the majority said they had a nutritionally sound diet and obtained adequate rest.

Markers of the Transition Process

Another major finding was the identification of significant life events as markers of the transition process. Living with RA was punctuated by life events that were unpredictable and beyond a person's control. These events included significant personal loss, relocation, changes in lifestyle, or physical and psychological trauma. These events created stress and elicited a variety of coping strategies. What was interesting was not that these events happened or that they produced stress, but that there was a perceived relationship between these events and the onset or exacerbation of the illness.

Of the 30 women interviewed, 28 attributed the cause of RA to stressful life events or situations. From the early twinges that piqued their awareness of physical symptoms, to the women's acknowledgment that something was wrong and needed attention, life events served as markers and, often, explanations for the onset of an illness that was to last a lifetime.

Nursing Support

A somewhat surprising finding was that nurses were rarely identified as care providers who helped these women learn to live with their illness. Unless a woman experienced an acute exacerbation, requiring surgery and hospitalization, there was little or no nursing involvement in helping her learn to live with the illness. The only consistent reference to health care providers was to physicians, and those experiences were described as having been more negative than positive.

Discussion

This study provides a preliminary understanding of the transition process that occurs with a chronic illness or disability. The transition process for these 30 women began with an awareness that a change was occurring. A woman who actively denied the severity of a symptom or attributed the pain or unrelenting fatigue to some other cause had not yet become aware of the transition. Chick and Meleis (1986) describe this as a pretransition phase. The period of becoming aware was characterized by denial that alternated with fear of the unknown when the women acknowledged that something was wrong and sought medical attention. During this stage, women were not apt to encounter nurses unless it was for another problem or through an informal relationship. Nurses must be alert to subtle, even vague, complaints or symptoms, explore these fully, and encourage patients to seek and pursue medical care. This stage was consistent with the stages of awareness and perception described by Chick and Meleis.

Getting care was for some a subphase of the "becoming aware" stage and for several women recurred in the "learning to live with it" stage. It began when they first sought help, and it often continued beyond the diagnosis. For several women, being given a diagnosis did not solve the need for appropriate medical management. "Shopping" for a doctor was common, as was trial-and-error treatment.

"Learning to live with it" was synonymous with the period of disconnectedness. The women tended to withdraw from activities, social relationships, and work due to limitations imposed by the disease. The transition continued in an uneven and sometimes unpredictable manner, much like the course of RA. This was a time of uncertainty, of learning, and a time for establishing new patterns that eventually provided a sense of control or mastery over their lives (Shaul, 1995). As the women progressed through this stage of the transition process, they regained a sense of connectedness and stability. This stability, which lasted for weeks or even years, was not a final state in most instances. A few women became quite disabled during this time, but most were able to live with their symptoms and achieve mastery in managing their lives despite their limitations.

Health outcomes, as defined by Chick and Meleis (1986), were not clearly evident in these findings. Rather, they serve as descriptors of a woman's status in relation to the restoration, maintenance, protection, and promotion of health at a particular point in time. The primary outcome in this study was the achievement of mastery that included knowledge and awareness of the illness and how to manage it.

Illness-precipitated transitions occur simultaneously with other transition experiences, such as loss of a loved one, relocation, or a change in or loss of a job (Corbin & Strauss, 1988). Thus, the ability to cope with an illness-precipitated transition is influenced by events that are unrelated to the illness experience. The study of human responses to illness must address factors that are not illness-related to fully understand the process of coping with a chronic illness (George, 1982). The women in this study related numerous traumatic life events that they believed to be implicated in the disease process. The impact of life events cannot be discounted when nurses and other health care providers provide support and guidance related to living with a chronic illness. Rather, support must extend beyond the diagnosis and facilitate coping through various simultaneous transitions.

Nurses are particularly interested in how people live with a disease, situation, or problem, and seek ways by which they can help people live more fully despite a chronic illness or disability (Christman et al., 1988; Corbin & Strauss, 1991; Dimond et al., 1987). Although appropriate medical management is essential, the process of living with a disease requires far more than medication regimes and treatments. To continue to live independently and care for oneself, a person must make frequent adaptations and accommodations to symptoms that characteristically come and go, change in frequency and severity, and pose the constant threat of increasing disability (Thorne, 1993). It is from the experience of living with a disease such as RA that people learn new ways to accommodate and adapt to the changing demands and capabilities of their bodies. By increasing their knowledge about the process of living with the disease and its impact on quality of life, nurses and other care providers will be better able to support and guide people through health and illness transitions (Meleis & Trangenstein, 1994).

Summary

The transition experience is also influenced by individual interpretations of events, individual and environmental mediating factors, physiological and psychological responses, and available resources.

A transitions framework is dynamic, incorporating the concepts of individuality with regard to awareness and perceptions of an illness and the development of patterns of response that are unique to individuals with similar problems. Many life transitions are clearly identifiable by a beginning and an ending, by the achievement of a new role or a new set of behaviors; yet some people with a chronic illness do not clearly complete a health-related transition.

Studies of transitions present methodological challenges in that longitudinal studies are expensive and difficult to sustain. Retrospective reports may be the result of the accumulation of experiences and may not reflect reality. Further, the use of existing data sets or medical records provides only one view of this complex human experience. Time is an essential element in transitions. Variables must be measured over a specified period to capture the initial interpretation, the midcourse experience, and the outcome of the transition experience.

This study was limited to predominantly Caucasian married women with RA, who were insured. Although there are similarities between RA and other chronic illnesses in terms of the impact of the symptoms on daily life, generalizing these findings to other ethnic or racial groups, single women, men, or people with other chronic illnesses must be done with caution. The small sample size also was a limitation. Future study should focus on women of color, men, and people with other chronic illnesses to identify commonalities and differences in health and illness transitions.

Nurses are best suited to support and guide people with chronic illness through transitions, but they need to know how and when to intervene. Future study should be directed toward learning more about the key points in a transition process when intervention would be most effective and about how to intervene to promote positive health outcomes, mastery, and improved well-being. Additionally, research aimed at exploring and describing the connection between stress and illness will answer questions related to the impact of life events and transitions on health and wellness.

Acknowledgment

This study was funded in part by an Institutional Predoctoral National Research Service Award, Afaf Meleis, Ph.D., R.N., FAAN, Project Director, PHS Grant #l-T-NRO7055-01. The author gratefully acknowledges Dr. Meleis' comments on an earlier draft of this chapter.

REFERENCES

American Academy of Family Physicians. (1990). *Current concepts in managing rheumatoid arthritis* [Videotape]. Kansas City: Author.

American Heritage Dictionary. (1969). Boston: Houghton Mifflin.

Anderson, J. M., Blue, C., & Lau, C. (1991). Women's perspectives on chronic illness: Ethnicity, ideology and restructuring of life. *Social Science Medicine, 33,* 101–113.

Aroian, D. J. (1990). A model of psychological adaptation to migration and resettlement. *Nursing Research, 39*(1), 5–10.

Baltes, P. B. (1987). Theoretical propositions of life-span developmental psychology: On the dynamics between growth and decline. *Developmental Psychology, 23,* 611–626.

Catanzaro, M. (1990). Transitions in midlife adults with long-term illness. *Holistic Nursing Practice, 4*(3), 65–73.

Chick, N., & Meleis, A. I. (1986). Transitions: A nursing concern. In P. L. Chinn (Ed.), *Nursing research methodology* (pp. 237–257). Rockville, MD: Aspen.

Chiriboga, D. A. (1979). Conceptualizing adult transitions: A new look at an old subject. *Generations, 4*(3), 4–6.

Christman, N. J., McConnell, E. A., Pfeiffer, C., Webster, K. K., Schmitt, M., & Ries, J. (1988). Uncertainty, coping, and distress following myocardial infarction: Transition from hospital to home. *Research in Nursing & Health, 119*(2), 71–82.

Corbin, J. M., & Strauss, A. (1988). *Unending work and care: Managing chronic illness at home.* San Francisco: Jossey-Bass.

Corbin, J. M., & Strauss, A. (1991). A nursing model for chronic illness management based on the trajectory framework. *Scholarly Inquiry for Nursing Practice, 5,* 155–174.

Dimond, M., McCance, K., & King, K. (1987). Forced residential relocation: Its impact on the well-being of older adults. *Western Journal of Nursing Research, 9,* 445–464.

Dixon, J., Dixon, J., Spinner, J., Sexton, D., & Perry, C. (1991). Psychometric and descriptive perspectives of illness impact over the life span. *Nursing Research, 40*(1), 51–56.

George, L. K. (1982, November). Models of transitions in middle and later life. *Annals of the American Academy of Political and Social Science, 464,* 22–37.

Katz, P., & Yelin, E. (1993). Prevalence and correlates of depressive symptoms among persons with rheumatoid arthritis. *Journal of Rheumatology, 20,* 790–796.

McCance, K. L., & Huether, S. E. (1995). *Pathophysiology: The biologic basis for disease in adults and children.* St. Louis, MO: C. V. Mosby.

Meleis, A. I., & Trangenstein, P. A. (1994). Facilitating transitions: Redefinition of the nursing mission. *Nursing Outlook, 42*(6), 255–259.

Mercer, R. T., Nichols, E. G., & Doyle, G. C. (1989). *Transition in a woman's life: Major life events in developmental context.* New York: Springer.

Murphy, S. A. (1990). Human responses to transitions: A holistic nursing perspective. *Holistic Nursing Practice, 4*(3), 1–7.

Sandelowski, M. (1986). The problem of rigor in qualitative research. *Advances in Nursing Science, 8*(3), 27–37.

Schlossberg, N. K. (1984). *Counseling adults in transition.* New York: Springer-Verlag.

Schumacher, K. L., & Meleis, A. I. (1994). Transitions: A central concept in nursing. *Image: Journal of Nursing Scholarship, 26,* 119–127.

Seidel, J. V., Kjolseth, R., & Seymour, E. (1988). *The Ethnograph: A program for the computer assisted analysis of text based data.* Corvallis, OR: Qualis Research Associates.

Shaul, M. P. (1994). From early twinges to mastery: The transition experience of women learning to live with rheumatoid arthritis. (Doctoral dissertation, University of California, San Francisco, 1994). *Dissertation Abstracts International, 55*(9B), DAO-72699.

Shaul, M. P. (1995). From early twinges to mastery: The process of adjustment in living with rheumatoid arthritis. *Arthritis Care and Research, 8,* 290–297.

Silverman, P. R. (1982, November). Transitions and models of intervention. *Annals of the American Academy of Political and Social Science, 464,* 174–187.

Thorne, S. E. (1993). *Negotiating health care.* Thousand Oaks, CA: Sage Publications.

van Gennep, A. (1960). *The rites of passage* (translated). Chicago: University of Chicago Press. (Original work published 1906.)

Reprinted with permission from: Shaul, M. P. (1997). Transitions in chronic illness: Rheumatoid arthritis in women. *Rehabilitation Nursing, 22*(4), 199–205.

7.4 RECURRENCE OF OVARIAN CANCER—LIVING IN LIMBO

EWA EKWALL
BRITT-MARIE TERNESTEDT
BENGT SORBE

Abstract

Few studies have shed light on women's life situations after being informed of having recurrent ovarian cancer. The present study aimed to elucidate women's experiences of living with this knowledge. Interviews were conducted with 12 women who were undergoing or had just completed chemotherapy, 5 to 10 months after learning of the recurrence. Data were collected and analyzed based on a life world perspective using a descriptive phenomenological method. The women's experiences are described via three key constituents; being denied one's future and simultaneously hoping to be able to delay the cancer's advancement, feeling alienated from both oneself and one's surroundings, and being responsible. The key constituents were integrated into the structure "living in limbo." The women lived on the threshold to the unknown. They were preparing themselves both for a continued life and for death. "Living in limbo" can be described as a phase of a health-illness transition characterized by loneliness. The vulnerable position and existential struggle of these women should be focused upon in nursing. The sensitive dialogue is essential in these cases.

It is known that certain cancer diagnoses carry a more intense charge than others do. Gynecologic cancer can be considered one of these.[1] Women with gynecologic cancer experience their diagnosis as less socially and emotionally accepted than do women with breast cancer.[2] One of many possible reasons for this could be that gynecologic cancer affects organs considered private and taboo.[3] The diagnosis can also cause a woman to lose her fertility,[4] a reality that can be difficult to live with. It is known that primary gynecologic cancer changes women's relationships and roles, regarding both family and friends. Life undergoes changes, compared with how it was before the diagnosis.[5] This can affect the woman's self-image.

Few studies illuminate women's experiences of living with gynecologic cancer during the disease's various stages, for example, how a recurrence of cancer affects a woman's life situation.[6] As regards other diagnosis groups, studies have shown that many who have been informed that they have been cured of their cancer are afraid—and are aware—of the risk of a recurrence.[7,8] This awareness, however, does not seem to reduce the shock that news of a recurrence brings.[9] Being informed of a recurrence is experienced differently than is being informed of primary cancer.[9] Previous experience of living with cancer and undergoing treatment can contribute to the recurrence being experienced as extra frightening.[10] For those who have a recurrence, it becomes clear that the treatment that was considered to give the best chance for a cure has failed.[11] They must once again undergo a treatment that they know will have side effects. Existential issues take on a specific significance in the case of recurrence,[10] which changes how an individual looks at the world[12] and her relationship to the surrounding world.[13] Even if most of the studies mentioned previously do not focus particularly on how women having recurrence of gynecologic cancer have experienced the situation, it is reasonable to assume that the experiences are similar. There is a need for studies elucidating this from a nursing perspective, and the present study is a step in this direction.

In 2002 in Sweden, approximately 800 women received the news that they had ovarian cancer.[14] Of these women, half are expected to experience a recurrence within 5 years of completed treatment.[15]

The purpose of this study was to deepen the understanding of how women having a recurrence of ovarian cancer experience live with this knowledge, and what it means in their daily lives. This knowledge is expected to form a basis for how support from nurses can be developed for this group of women.

Method

To deepen the understanding of how the recurrence of ovarian cancer was experienced and lived through by the women, a phenomenological method has been chosen.[16,17] The method has its starting point in phenomenological philosophy. Edmund Husserl, the founder of the modern phenomenology, considered the everyday life, or the life world, as the base of the human science. The life world can be described as the world we live in daily and that we constantly, if unconsciously, take for granted.[16] A life world perspective applied in research is characterized by openness and flexibility regarding the phenomenon being studied, usually referred to as a "return to things themselves." It also requires that prior experiences and knowledge be set aside and "bracketed." According to Giorgi and Giorgi,[16(p.32)] this, "does not mean to be unconscious of these other sources, but rather to engage them so that there can be no influence from them on the instance being considered." The phenomenological method aims to illuminate the invariant aspects or the structure/essence of the phenomenon.[17]

Sample and Settings

The study was conducted at a university hospital in central Sweden. Inclusion criteria were that women must have been clinically "free" from cancer for at least 1 year after completion of primary treatment, that they did not have any other malignant disease, and that they understood and spoke Swedish. The hospital maintained a clinic register of women who had been treated for gynecologic cancer. Women who had been treated for recurrence of ovarian cancer were consecutively selected from this register during a period of 1 year. The women were informed on numerous occasions regarding participation in the study, as well as of the fact that the care they were receiving would not be affected if they declined to participate. Twelve women (50–74 years old) agreed to participate, whereas 8 declined. Ten women lived with someone, and 2 lived alone. Ten had children, and of these, one had small children. Primary diagnosis was ovarian cancer, stages 1C to 3C.

Ethical Considerations

There was a risk that the interview discussion forced the women to be confronted with a reality they would rather repress. However, respect for the women's integrity, autonomy, and private life formed the foundation of the interview and was exercised through the interviewer being sensitive to what the particular woman did or did not want to discuss. The women were offered the opportunity for discussion after the interview; however, none of them requested such a dialogue. The study was approved by the research ethics committee, D-nr 1177/99.

Data Collection

The interviewer (E.E.) asked the women to narrate, as concretely as possible, their experiences of being informed of recurrence and how the time since learning of the recurrence had been. Open-ended follow-up questions were requested, to obtain as rich and varied a description of the women's experience of the phenomenon as possible. Questions such as, "How did you feel then?," "What were you thinking?," "How did you act?," and "Would you like to tell more?" were asked. The entire interview lasted between 1 and 2 hours and, in 10 cases, was conducted in the woman's home. The remaining 2 interviews were conducted at the hospital, according to the women's wishes. All interviews were audio recorded and have been transcribed verbatim.

Data Analysis

After completion of all interviews, the transcribed interviews were analyzed in the following 4 steps[17(pp. 251–253)]:

- Reading for a sense of the whole: every interview was read and listened to numerous times, to obtain a feeling for the entire interview;
- Determination of parts: the text was reread, and meaning units were established and marked with slashes where there was a shift in meaning;
- Transformation to nursing perspective: meaning units were transformed into nursing-sensitive expressions, with respect to the phenomenon under study. This step is described as the heart of the method and entails that the meanings of the women's statements were made explicit and transformed into a language considered relevant from a nursing perspective; during this process, we struggled to avoid using theory-laden terms;
- Determination of the structure; to see what was truly essential in the nursing-sensitive expressions, we practiced imaginative variation. The invariant meaning emerged through 3 key constituents—(a) being denied one's future and simultaneously hoping to be able to delay the cancer's advancement, (b) feeling alienated from both oneself and one's surroundings, and (c) being responsible (Table 7.4.1). The key constituents were then integrated into the structure "living in limbo."

Findings

At the time of the interview, 5 to 10 months (mean = 7 months) had passed since the women had learned of the recurrence. Even if they had been conscious of the risk on a certain level, the discov-

TABLE 7.4.1 Examples of Statements Contributing to the Structure/Essence of Living in Limbo

Patient Statement	Meaning Units From a Nursing Perspective	Key Constituents	Structure
1. Days when I've felt that I won't get better; this is totally meaningless, why should I be tortured when I'm not going to get better anyway. Then a couple days go by, and I've started thinking, "Well, of course I'm going to get better."	There are days when S. has doubts, when nothing has meaning or hope of becoming cancer-free. Then come days when she feels the opposite and is optimistic.	Being denied one's future and simultaneously hoping to be able to delay the cancer's advancement	
2. I don't know which role I have. I'm not where I was last fall before I became ill. Then, I worked and had someone to share my life with. Just now I feel like I'm in some kind of vacuum state (upset). I don't know whether I'm healthy or ill. I do know that they've said that they don't feel anything anymore, that it's the lump and what I felt before I started the treatments, they've called it complete remission, but I've come to understand that that's not completely reliable. They haven't opened me up and gone in and looked. It could be hiding somewhere. Today, I know it can be there anyway, even if you can't see it, and sit there and smolder like it's presumably done.	S. is confused and insecure in her identity. She is living in a vacuum that is reinforced by the fact that neither she nor her doctor can reliably conclude that she is healthy. The tumor that was there before the treatment (that she hadn't felt) is gone according to the medical assessment, but she has learned not to trust such assessments; cancer is an elusive disease that, in her case, was present without her taking notice.	Feeling alienated from both oneself and one's surroundings	**Living in Limbo**
3. I reason a little with myself, that I have to bring out this mental strength I have...so I don't break down if they say "sorry, we've found new lumps" or...I thought...I have to, like, have the mental readiness so I can get started on a new kind of treatment.	S. is working with and preparing herself to come to grips with possible negative news about the cancer. She thereby assumes responsibility for maintaining a mental preparedness.	Being responsible	

ery was often unexpected. It had been between 1 and 5.7 years (mean = 2.8 years) since the women had completed treatment for the primary cancer. Their life situations when they received diagnosis varied greatly, with some experiencing a serious illness in their immediate surroundings or having recently experienced the death of someone close to them. One woman had small children, which strengthened her will to fight for survival at any cost. She could not imagine being forced to abandon the children who needed her so. At the time of the interview, the women were undergoing or had just completed a treatment series of chemotherapy. The treatment's effect was not yet known to the women, who were living in uncertainty. Some had sought help to manage living with the death threat that a recurrence is said to have initiated.

Despite differences regarding the women's life situations, there were similarities in the way they related their experiences of having a recurrence and living with this knowledge for a number of months. The 3 key constituents will be introduced initially, followed by the description of the structure.

Being Denied One's Future and Simultaneously Hoping to Be Able to Delay the Cancer's Advancement

Learning of a recurrence was experienced as an obvious death threat and a confrontation with death in a different way than learning of the primary cancer was. The women described how they had previously avoided thinking about death. Now, the atmosphere they lived in was characterized by sorrow over possibly not being able to experience the future they had taken for granted. The women related to this realization in different ways; some discussed it, whereas others preferred to avoid thinking and talking about the future, although, as can be seen in the following quote, the thought was there nonetheless.

"I don't think too far into the future. I think it's kind of sad that you (sighs)…even these retirement information letters that come in the mail (upset)…I don't want to look at it. I think I won't even exist then (crying); honestly, I'm not sure if I will. What if I'm not alive in 6 months; it's no use buying a new dress…but then I think that you can't think that way! You can just have it as long as you can (upset). We [husband and wife] never reasoned like this the first time I was ill, because then I was more convinced that I'd beat this."

Despite deep despair, the women had hope, at least at times, that they would somehow be able to restrain the disease. They seldom imagined a completely healthy existence, but instead one in which they were able to live a while longer despite the disease. The will to live was often very strong, and they hovered between hope and despair.

"I'm secure and hopeful and insecure and not hopeful, all at the same time. It goes up and down-…then I think more that it's the healthy part of me that makes it go up and down, but even so, it's…(sighs deeply)…the hope…that it's at least a little bigger than hopelessness."

The feeling of uncertainty was reinforced by the doctor's inability to give a prognosis. They understood that it was beyond doctor's ability to declare whether a particular woman would survive, and at the same time, this medical uncertainty strengthened the women's fear of an approaching death.

Feeling Alienated From Both Oneself and One's Surroundings

The obvious physical changes caused primarily by chemotherapy had a negative effect on the women's view of themselves. Their bodies were altered by both the treatment and the disease, and as a consequence, they often felt that they had lost their female attractiveness. When they saw their own reflection, it was not the same as the image they had of themselves, and they therefore avoided mirrors. Some also described a negative effect on their sex life. They described an alienation from themselves, a feeling that seemed to be reinforced by the fact that they had seen themselves as healthy when they were notified of the recurrence, or they had only diffuse symptoms, which they seldom associated with the cancer. One woman expressed this as follows.

"The last time, I went to see a doctor for my upset stomach. When I found out that it was something, that I was ill, that they could do something about it, it felt like a relief in some way. Now [with the recurrence], it doesn't feel like a relief, it only feels like 'No, God, this isn't how I want it to be.' I'm healthy now, and I'm going to be healthy. I didn't even have pain anywhere; I felt great."

The situation was even more confusing for the women when the recurrence was discovered only through positive tumor marker (CA-125) or cancer cells in abdominal fluid. Many of the women thus had an unclear picture of both the cancer's localization, the rationale for the treatment, and the prognosis. One woman expressed her dissatisfaction at not having received understandable and optimal medical information as follows.

"Where is it right now? Yeah, they don't know; maybe it's on my abdominal wall, and that's not something that can be seen so they can't...but it's so unclear. Is it just in this liquid? Where does it come from? That's what I want to know. Those thoughts were easier last time."

When the disease showed symptoms, or when the women experienced a certain, if faint, feeling of being ill, it appeared to be easier for them to understand what was happening. Women experiencing symptoms were also more emotionally motivated to undergo treatment, because they wanted to be free from the symptoms. However, side effects from the treatment intensified the feeling of illness, and in certain cases, the women described the situation as nearly unbearable. This limited the women in their daily life.

After completion of the treatment for the primary cancer, the women were seen by their surroundings and themselves as "strong survivors." Being a strong survivor was integrated into the women's self-concept and strengthened their view of themselves. They had managed a difficult event well. When they then learned that they had had a recurrence, they saw themselves as failures. One woman narrated:

I shocked everybody who had been so happy...like the children, who had let go of the thought of Mom having cancer and feeling bad and who were now happy that life had turned out all right. I felt like I let them down...because everybody had believed in this thing, that...Mom had proven that you can beat cancer. My coworkers, who've stuck with me through this all these years since 1993, through all the phases...who time after time have said 'Just think, it's unbelievable, you're bubbly, you're alive, you're living proof that you don't have to die of cancer, you can beat it. It's just fantastic.' Everybody around me, including myself, was completely convinced that I'd beaten this and was going to be healthy. I had made it through the first time so well and looked healthy and had been so lively; that had helped them get over their fear of the cancer.

Like many others, this woman was disappointed in both herself and life, because she had not succeeded in staying healthy. In various ways, they sought explanations for why they had gotten cancer again. They thought a great deal about their lifestyle and wondered whether stress and worry had contributed to their having a recurrence. Some women expressed a personal guilt, whereas others had a more fatalistic attitude and asserted that disease strikes unfairly. However, they did express in other ways a feeling that the diagnosis of a recurrence was a great disappointment and contributed to feelings of alienation.

"(Sighs) I don't know what I thought, but I was disappointed. I was disappointed in myself, in life...yeah, sort of in everything. I felt sad and thought that everything was just shit. It was a huge disappointment to get sick again."

The women's self-image changed and contributed to the women at times avoiding interaction with people, mainly outside the family. The changes to their appearance were described as a great hindrance to socializing. The women felt that, by simply showing themselves, they were telling everyone else that they had something terrible in their body, and they were doing all they could to hide it. The women's stories even contain a fear of being rejected or abandoned by those who were closest to them. One woman was worried about how her partner would react to the changes she was now going through.

Is he going to put up with me when I'm going to look like a monster again? You're quick to cry and get angry...your identity disappears in a way...it's not me. I mean, when you get out of the shower, you don't have your wig on...so you're forced to see yourself, but I hate...I hate this misery! That's almost the worst thing, not having hair. I can't show myself. He wakes up early in the morning, and I'm so afraid he's going to wake up before I have a chance to put my wig on. I think that's the worst, actually.

The women also related that people around them treated them differently, now that they were ill. Close relatives and friends withdrew, and few talked with the women about the disease and the situation they were experiencing. They felt that now that they could no longer be the positive example they had been for those around them; they would do all they could to avoid being a burden.

Being Responsible

As is clear in the prior key constituent, "feeling alienated from both oneself and one's surroundings," that the women assumed responsibility—partly for having had a recurrence and partly for having made those around them uncomfortable because of this. They assumed responsibility for their immediate health and fought to regain the best possible health and were confident that by "living right," they could affect the cancer's advancement and avoid any further recurrences. They also believed that a positive attitude would bring about a successful result. One of the women expressed this as follows.

Being active, happy, and positive in various ways is a way to take your part of the responsibility. If it doesn't work out (laughs), it's because you're not being positive. Believe in this, and it'll be fine. It's like a requirement that you have to be so positive that you're lifting yourself up by the hair.

A healthy diet, exercise, and positive activities helped the women recover between chemotherapy treatments.

I've had a whole week to myself, and it's been so nice; I've rested and recovered, I've done something fun during the third week every time. Built myself up. You have to be active yourself; that's more clear when you have a recurrence.

The women strove, actively and goal oriented, to regain their former selves. Through caring for and looking after themselves, as well as seeking information on the disease, they hoped to contribute to a successful treatment and to delay the cancer's advancement. To be able to take responsibility, the women wanted to become knowledgeable. One woman expressed that, with the first diagnosis, it had been enough to simply know she had cancer. She did not have a need for more information, but now she wanted to know more.

If you have more knowledge, then you also get strong in your disease.

When they have not received enough information, they have created their own explanation models to be able to face the new and unknown that was waiting. In the women's minds, keeping the cancer away depended a great deal on themselves.

The new awareness of life's fickleness had helped them, according to themselves, appreciate togetherness—especially with their family and also with significant friends—more strongly than they previously had. The women saw this as the disease's positive side effect. Something that was clear, however, was that the women assumed great responsibility, often protecting those close to them, and were afraid of being seen as a burden. This was expressed, for instance, in the women crying alone. Another way the women protected and spared those close to them was to visit their doctor alone and later "give doses" of the information to those around them. The women found it difficult to ask for help and felt that although they had people around them, they were nevertheless alone in their struggle. Women without a partner seemed to have extra difficulty, because they did not want to burden their children.

When you don't have a partner to live with, it's a huge difference. It's just that, as a mother, you want to perhaps spare your children from some of it and not burden...not call and cry as soon as it feels ...you just don't do it.

Some of the women felt, in light of this, that during certain periods, it was easier to talk to friends than to their immediate family.

Structure—Living in Limbo

By integrating the 3 constituents (that have strong contact points) into an indivisible whole, a structure describing the women's experiences of the phenomenon "living with recurrence" has been created. The constituents "being denied one's future and simultaneously hoping to be able to delay the cancer's advancement," "feeling alienated from both oneself and one's surroundings," and "being responsible" have been synthesized into the structure "living in limbo." Living in limbo means that the women found themselves on the threshold to something unknown. This situation was characterized by an existential loneliness. Even if many of the women had a social network, they were, for the most part, alone with their thoughts. The threat of death contributed to the women valuing relationships with others in a new way. They wanted to feel that they belonged and were afraid of being rejected. They assumed great responsibility for their own health and for the well-being of those around them. The latter meant that they protected those closest to them by, for example, not spreading their worry. Because of this, they were very isolated and vulnerable, and at the same time, their accounts also showed courage, strength, and a desire to care for others.

Discussion

The aim of this study was to deepen the understanding of the phenomenon living with a recurrence of ovarian cancer during the first 5 to 10 months after learning of a recurrence. The findings showed that the women's daily life had changed markedly. The women described feelings of alienation from both themselves and others. They were living in a limbo, on the threshold to the unknown. Death became a stronger threat than it had been in the past. It can be said that they simultaneously prepared themselves for death as well as continued life while trying to live in the present. The threat of death contributed to a change in meaning and charge for the women's close relationships. A sense of belonging was important to the women; however, they described how the recurrence and the treatment brought them suffering and how the changes to the body had a negative effect on their experiences of both themselves and their relations to others. Their complete existence and, with it, their identity were threatened. According to Merleau-Ponty,[18(p. 206)] not only does a person have a body, but *is* also her body. Although a person is more than just a body, it is through that body she meets the world. Without a body, she can neither perceive nor act. This means that when the body changes, access to the surrounding world is also described as changing. Applied to our study, this means that women's identities have been formed by how they have experienced themselves and their interplay with their surroundings.

The concept of transition is central in nursing.[19,20] From a nursing perspective, the significance of the phenomenon "living in limbo" is deepened by being described as a health-illness transition. The women in our study described living on the threshold to the unknown, a significant turning point in life and, as such, a phase of a health-illness transition. The transition process starts with separation, followed by a phase of liminality, and ends with a phase of incorporation. For the women in our study, the transition was initiated at the time of the diagnosis of recurrence. The phase of liminality is described as state of being in between, encompassing loss of control, uncertainty, and ambivalence.[21] Being between two worlds can be likened to finding oneself in between the world of the healthy and the ill[22,23]—a condition marked by alienation. Sontag[24] has stated that all individuals, even if we do not acknowledge it, have double citizenship—one in the realm of the healthy and one in that of the ill. According to Schumacher and

Meleis,[25] a healthy transition is characterized by connectedness, confidence, subjective well-being, mastery, and successful coping.

The significance of finding oneself in limbo is close to the concept described as existential homelessness,[26] a condition in which the world is no longer experienced as familiar. This can be said to apply to the women in this study. In our study, the women described themselves as alienated and alone. Both the woman herself and the society had contributed to placing her in what we have described as limbo. They were strangers to themselves and to others and felt that those around them treated them differently. It is likely that all of this worked interactively. The women strove to be treated like "normal people," and they had a strong desire to belong to "the healthy." Similarly, cancer patients in the study of Halldorsdottir and Hamrin[27] described a desire to be taken back to "the land of the well."

The experienced isolation can also be linked to feelings of guilt. It is known that women who have cancer recurrence have feelings of guilt, and that these are more common in cases of recurrence than with primary cancer.[6] The feelings of guilt are described as increasing with the disease's advance.[28] For those having recurrence, these guilt feelings can bring unnecessary suffering. In such a situation, those who live alone can be especially vulnerable,[29] something that should be given attention in nursing. Patients are often left alone with their thoughts and questions of vital importance. This is found in a study by Strang et al.,[30] which shows that patients with brain tumors and their spouses need to discuss existential matters. However, the nurses in their study did not feel that they had the competence or time to address these needs. This might reinforce the feeling of existential loneliness. It is important to stress that even existential loneliness cannot merely be discussed away—it is part of life—it can be alleviated if it is respected and if patients were offered opportunities to talk about it. In our study, we have the impression that the interviews that served as the basis of the study filled this need to a degree. The women have been able to talk about their experiences with a person who was motivated to listen. Many of the women also expressed this opinion.

In addition to the questions already mentioned, this study raises other thoughts. For this study's subjects, recurrence was discovered relatively early, thanks to the regular checkups performed on women with ovarian cancer. This early discovery is likely the reason that many of the women had not yet felt any symptoms. This raises an ethical question, as research has not shown any difference in survival for women with gynecologic cancer, depending on whether they showed symptoms at the time of diagnosis. If this result is rigorously substantiated, the question can be posed as to whether an early discovery of recurrent ovarian cancer benefits a woman or instead causes harm. This question must be both discussed and studied.

We have not found any other studies in which this behavior of assuming responsibility for health is as clear. In their struggle to belong to life, the women felt responsible for having the best health possible. In our earlier study of how women with primary cancer experienced health care, we found that they wanted to take an active part in their own care. At the same time, they placed themselves in the hands of the health care professionals, convinced that the tumor would be removed as soon as possible and that everything would return to normal.[3] This result is in agreement with results from other studies.[31,32] However, the women in the current study asserted that, by assuming responsibility, they contributed to a good result. For the women to be able to take responsibility, they depended on receiving the information they needed. Knowledge is a condition of participation and autonomy (cf. Andershed and Ternestedt[33]) and involvement in care (cf. Sahlberg Blom et al.[34]).

The driving force behind this substantial assumption of responsibility can be interpreted in various ways. A reasonable interpretation, based on the women's accounts, is that they have tried to manage on their own as long as possible for fear of being rejected or being a burden to their families. They exerted themselves in various ways to let life go on as usual as much as this was possible; they avoided showing their own tiredness and sadness as much as they could. The women's accounts of isolation can thus have been supported; in certain cases, they may have refused help with the intention of, for example, protecting those around them who did not need to be confronted with death and the fears it awakens. This attitude is in accordance with other studies.[10,35-37] Previous studies have shown that women with cancer see themselves as alone despite the fact that they have close relatives and friends.[2,38] Studies have also shown that recurrence of cancer can have a negative effect on close relationships, regardless of sites.[39,40] Both partners in a relationship can avoid showing their feelings to the other, who they believe to be weaker.[41] Consequently, this can mean that those close to a sick individual are not active participants in their situation. Such a pattern emerged in our study as well. How the women felt about this is not evident; however, it is reasonable to assume that they had their reasons for acting as they did, even if it may have contributed to their being unnecessarily isolated. It therefore seems important that nurses be aware of women's experienced isolation and give them the support they need.

The study also brings up the question of why the women assumed such great responsibility for others and whether there might be feelings of guilt, anger, and/or fear of abandonment behind this behavior, and whether the withholding of information, for example, may have been a way to maintain mastery over their everyday life in a highly vulnerable situation. Alternatively, caring for others may have become more central than it had been previously, in the light of the women's realization that life could soon be over. From an ethical caring perspective, the latter appraisal can be seen as most likely. According to Gilligan and Wiking,[42] women often define themselves through their relationships to others. In our study, it is reasonable to regard the women's behavior as both an expression of care and a way to preserve as much of their identity as possible in a situation in which their existence is threatened. It has been described earlier that close relationships take on a particular meaning when death is at hand[9,43] and that relationships promote identity. A number of other factors likely contribute to the women's behavior and should be considered at this point, in the short time that has passed after they have learned of the recurrence.

In the previously mentioned study of how women with primary cancer experience health care, we found that it could be important to provide certain information to a woman's partner as well, at the same time that the woman is informed, given that the woman desires this.[3] It is reasonable to assume that such support would also help to lessen a woman's fear of abandonment, which emerged in this study. However, it is doubtful that the women in this study would have accepted this type of support if it had been offered. They showed signs, in some cases, of refusing help from those close to them, taking an apparently conscious responsibility for their disease. On the other hand, we cannot rule out the possibility that it could have served as a support during a very difficult time if the women had been offered support sessions with a person of their choice. More knowledge is needed in this area.

Trustworthiness

In judging this study's trustworthiness, it should be considered that it was conducted 5 to 10 months after the women had learned of a recurrence, a period in the course of the disease described as difficult for the patient. This can have been complicated by the fact that many women had been completing a treatment series, which is described as extra difficult in the case of recurrent cancer.[44] The study's aim was, however, to try to capture the women's experience in the midst of this vulnerable situation and describe what is truly essential about the phenomenon of living with recurrence. According to Giorgi and Giorgi,[17] the structure is meant to be typical for this phenomenon and not universal. This means that none of the 3 key constituents comprising the structure can be removed without markedly changing the phenomenon. Another important trustworthiness criterion is giving the reader as much information as allows him or her to follow certain basic steps, and thus test the results' trustworthiness himself or herself. An endeavor in this study has been to be as open and accurate as possible regarding the women's accounts, and to be conscious of our own assumptions and knowledge (clinical and theoretical) and place these in parentheses.

The transferability of the findings is limited by the sparse amount of research in this area. However, it is reasonable that the findings can be applied to women with recurrent cancer. More research on recurrent female cancer is needed.

Implications for Practice

In the care of women living with a recurrence, it is a central theme to focus on the phenomenon "living in limbo" and the transition women undergo, as well as how their life world changes. The women's isolation, especially, should receive attention, as well as the fact that they may need to talk with someone outside their situation. Of main importance when promoting a healthy transition is an individual support from the perspective of the unique woman. The goal is to support the woman's own strength and will, so she can achieve the highest possible level of well-being. Dialogue, counseling, information, and education may help the process. In certain cases, it should even be helpful to the woman if her husband or another close relative or friend is invited along with her to a dialogue on what the recurrence can imply, if the woman wants this. There is a need for studies evaluating various interventions with the aim of supporting this group of women.

REFERENCES

1. Fitch MI. Psychosocial management of patients with recurrent ovarian cancer: treating the whole patient to improve quality of life. *Semin Oncol Nurs.* 2003;19(3 suppl 1):40–53.
2. Auchincloss SS. After treatment. Psychosocial issues in gynecologic cancer survivorship. *Cancer.* 1995;76(10 suppl):2117–2124.
3. Ekwall E, Ternestedt B, Sorbe B. Important aspects of health care for women with gynecologic cancer. *Oncol Nurs Forum.* 2003;30(2 part 1): 313–319.
4. Maughan K, Clarke C. The effect of a clinical nurse specialist in gynaecological oncology on quality of life and sexuality. *J Clin Nurs.* 2001;10(2): 221–229.
5. Howell D, Fitch MI, Deane KA. Impact of ovarian cancer perceived by women. *Cancer Nurs.* 2003;26(1):1–9.
6. Howell D, Fitch MI, Deane KA. Women's experiences with recurrent ovarian cancer. *Cancer Nurs.* 2003;26(1):10–17.
7. Fitch M. Supportive care for cancer patients. *Hosp Q.* 2000;3(4):39–46.
8. Ferrell B, Ervin K, Smith S, Marek T, Melancon C. Family perspectives of ovarian cancer. *Cancer Pract.* 2002;10(6):269–276.
9. Mahon SM, Casperson DM. Exploring the psychosocial meaning of recurrent cancer: a descriptive study. *Cancer Nurs.* 1997;20(3):178–186.
10. Mahon SM, Casperson DS, Psychosocial concerns associated with recurrent cancer. *Cancer Pract.* 1995;3(6):372–380.
11. Holland JC. Clinical course of cancer. In: Holland JC, Rowland JH, eds. *Handbook of Psychooncology: Psychological Care of the Patient With Cancer.* New York: Oxford University Press; 1989:75–100.
12. Duesund L, Thorell J. *Kropp, Kunskap och Självuppfattning [in Swedish].* Stockholm: Liber utbildning; 1996.
13. Burnet K, Robinson L. Psychosocial impact of recurrent cancer. *Eur J Oncol Nurs.* 2000;4(1): 29–38.
14. Socialstyrelsen, National Board of Health and Welfare. Cancer incidence in Sweden 2002. Available at: http://www.sos.se/FULLTEXT/42/2003-42-11/2003-42-11.pdf. Accessed December 2003.
15. Heintz AP, Odicino F, Maisonneuve P, et al. Carcinoma of the ovary. *Int J Gynaecol Obstet.* 2003;83(suppl 1):135–166.
16. Giorgi A, Giorgi B. Phenomenology. In: Smith JA, ed. *Qualitative Psychology: A Practical Guide to Research Methods.* London: Sage; 2003:25–50.
17. Giorgi AP, Giorgi BM. The descriptive phenomenological psychological method. In: Camic PM, Rhodes JE, Yardley L, eds. *Qualitative Research in Psychology: Expanding Perspectives in Methodology and Design.* Washington, DC: American Psychological Association; 2003: 243–273.
18. Merleau-Ponty M. *Phenomenology of Perception.* Repr. ed. London: Routledge & Kegan Paul; 1962.

19. Olsson K, Ek A. Transition; how a concept has been used in nursing science. *Theoria J Nurs Theory.* 2002;11(4):4–12.
20. Meleis AI. *Theoretical Nursing: Development and Progress.* 3rd ed. Philadelphia: Lippincort-Raven; 2005.
21. Little M, Jordens CF, Paul K, Montgomery K, Philipson B. Liminality: a major category of the experience of cancer illness. *Soc Sci Med.* 1998;47(10):1485–1494.
22. van Gennep A. *The Rites of Passage.* Chicago: University of Chicago Press; 1960.
23. Turner VW. *The Ritual Process: Structure and Anti-Structure.* London: Routledge & Kegan Paul; 1969.
24. Sontag S. *Sjukdom som Metafor [in Swedish].* Stockholm: Bromberg; 1981.
25. Schumacher KL, Meleis AI. Transitions: a central concept in nursing. *Image J Nurs Scholarsh.* 1994;26(2):119–127.
26. Svenaeus F. The phenomenology of health and illness. In: Toombs SK, ed. *Handbook of Phenomenology and Medicine.* Boston: Kluwer Academic; 2001:87–108.
27. Halldorsdottir S, Hamrin E. Experiencing existential changes: the lived experience of having cancer. *Cancer Nurs.* 1996;19(1):29–36.
28. Gotay CC. Why me? Attributions and adjustment by cancer patients and their mates at two stages in the disease process. *Soc Sci Med.* 1985;20(8):825–831.
29. Houldin AD, Jacobsen B, Lowery BJ. Self-blame and adjustment to breast cancer. *Oncol Nurs Forum.* 1996;23(1):75–79.
30. Strang S, Strang P, Ternestedr BM. Existential support in brain tumour patients and their spouses. *Support Care Cancer.* 2001;9(8):625–633.
31. Jefferies H. Ovarian cancer patients: are their informational and emotional needs being met? *J Clin Nurs.* 2002;11(1):41–47.
32. Ekman I, Bergbom I, Ekman T, Berthold H, Mahsneh SM. Maintaining normality and support are central issues when receiving chemotherapy for ovarian cancer. *Cancer Nurs.* 2004;27(3):177–182.
33. Andershed B, Ternestedt BM. Involvement of relatives in the care of the dying in different care cultures: involvement in the dark or in the light? *Cancer Nurs.* 1998;21(2):106–116.
34. Sahlberg-Blom E, Ternestedt B, Johansson J. Patient participation in decision making at the end of life as seen by a close relative. *Nurs Ethics.* 2000;7(4):296–313.
35. Znajda TL, Wunder JS, Bell RS, Davis AM. Gender issues in patients with extremity soft-tissue sarcoma: a pilot study. *Cancer Nurs.* 1999;22(2):111–118.
36. Maughan K, Heyman B, Matthews M. In the shadow of risk. How men cope with a partner's gynaecological cancer. *Int J Nurs Stud.* 2002;39(1):27–34.
37. Kirsch SED, Brandt PA, Lewis FM. Making the most of the moment: when a child's mother has breast cancer. *Cancer Nurs.* 2003;26(1):47–54.
38. Thome B, Haliberg IR. Quality of life in older people with cancer—a gender perspective. *Eur J Cancer Care (Engl).* 2004;13(5):454–463.
39. Halliburton P, Larson PJ, Dibble S, Dodd MJ. The recurrence experience: family concerns during cancer chemotherapy. *J Clin Nurs.* 1992;1(5):275–281.
40. Northouse L. Sharing the cancer experience: husbands of women with initial and recurrent breast cancer. In: Baider L, Cooper CL, De-Nour AK, eds. *Cancer and the Family.* New York: John Wiley & Sons Ltd; 1996:305–317.
41. Glaser BG, Strauss AL. *Awareness of Dying.* 10th pr. ed. New York: Aldine; 1980.
42. Gilligan C, Wiking P. *Med kvinnors röst: Psykologisk teori och kvinnors utveckling [in Swedish].* Stockholm: Prisma; 2001.
43. Anderson B. Quality of life in progressive ovarian cancer. *Gynecol Oncol.* 1994;55(3 pt 2):S151–S155.
44. Jenkins PL, May VE, Hughes LE. Psychological morbidity associated with local recurrence of breast cancer. *Int J Psychiatry Med.* 199

Reprinted with permission from: Ekwall, E., Ternestedt, B. M., & Sorbe, B. (2007). Recurrence of ovarian cancer—Living in limbo. *Cancer Nursing, 30*(4), 270–277.

7.5 ADMITTED WITH A HIP FRACTURE: PATIENT PERCEPTIONS OF REHABILITATION

LARS-ERIC OLSSON
ANNE E. M. NYSTRÖM
JÒN KARLSSON
INGER EKMAN

Abstract

Aims and Objectives: The aim of this study was to describe the hip fracture patients' own *perceptions of their situation and views of their responsibility in the rehabilitation process.* **Background:** *Although much research has been conducted on various aspects of the rehabilitation process in patients with a hip fracture, no attention has been given to the patients' own views of their situation at the start of this transitional process.* **Method:** *Thirteen informants with a hip fracture, aged 71–93 years, were interviewed postoperatively at a Swedish hospital. Phenomenographic analysis of the interview transcripts was performed.* **Results:** *The informants varied greatly in their engagement in the rehabilitation process, in their conceptions of who was responsible for their recovery, and in their views on the need for information pertinent to their condition. Three categories of description were formulated: the* Autonomous, *i.e., patients who were self-sufficient and used to taking care of themselves and who searched for relevant information; the* Modest, *i.e., frail patients in need of more support who wanted information, but did not ask for it; and the* Heedless, *i.e., patients who were already dependent, who were not aware of their own responsibility and not interested in information. The informants also shared some traits: they all needed more information, although not all were aware of it, they all worried about their future ability to walk again, and they all had a strong zest for life.* **Relevance to Clinical Practice:** *Our results suggest that differences in patients' perspectives on the rehabilitation process need to be taken into account to enhance outcomes. Inadequate knowledge and engagement on the part of patients with a hip fracture probably have an impact on their rehabilitation outcome, but the degree of impact is uncertain.*

Background

Hip fractures represent a large and increasing health problem today. The incidence of hip fractures increases exponentially with age (Hedlund, 1985), and the annual number in Sweden has increased from 18,000 in the late 1980s (Thorngren, 1996) to around 28,000 in 1998 (The National Board of Health and Welfare, 1998). Patients with a hip fracture are in a vulnerable position, and the fracture poses a potential and fundamental threat to their life situation. Postoperative rehabilitation aims to help the patient regain the same functional status as before the fracture, however, only 25–50% ever achieve this goal (Egan et al., 1992; Marottoli et al., 1992; Hall et al., 2000). With the increase in average age of patients with a hip fracture, the group has become more heterogeneous and the difference in care requirements between patients needing the least versus most care is considerable. The reason for this difference is related to the patient's physical, mental, and social condition before the fracture (Ceder et al., 1980; Zetterberg et al., 1990; Ensberg et al., 1993; Sonn et al., 1994; Koval et al., 1996, 1998; Cree & Nade, 1999; Overend et al., 2000; Zuckerman et al., 2000a, b). Hence, the requirement for nurses to work effectively within the multiprofessional team is increasingly important, and their contribution within rehabilitation is the ability to maximize patients' choice to enhance independent living (Long et al., 2002).

A hip fracture constitutes a sudden traumatic event threatening all aspects of the older person's functional status. The rehabilitation of patients with a hip fracture is a transition from initial complete dependency to recovery of optimal functional status (Robinson, 1999). The initial period of the rehabilitation is particularly stressful for the patients, involving uncertainty, fatigue, and postoperative pain. Whereas attempting to cope with these changes, the older person must also diligently participate in the rehabilitation process. Many people experience transitions, and for older people, such transitions may be linked to their health and need for nursing care. Transitions are conceptualized as complex multidimensional processes that both cause and affect changes in life, health, relationships, and environment. They include five different properties: awareness, engagement, change and difference, time span, and critical points and events

(Meleis et al., 2000). These properties are probably interrelated in the transition process. Although much research has been conducted on various aspects of the rehabilitation process in patients with a hip fracture, no attention has been given to the patients' own views of their situation at the start of this transitional process.

Knowledge is empowering to those who develop it, to those who use it, and to those who benefit from it. Understanding the properties and conditions inherent in the process for patients with a hip fracture would help nurses to assess and/or promote the individual patient's possibilities for a healthy transition. Hence, the aim of this study was to describe the patients' own perceptions of their situation and views of their responsibility in the rehabilitation process.

Methods and Informants

Qualitative methods are particularly appropriate for gaining a fuller understanding of what constitutes reality for patients in a special situation. Phenomenography, developed at the Department of Education and Educational Research at Göteborg University, Sweden (Marton 1981), is a method for describing the way people understand their experiences. A distinction is generally made between the first-order perspective, which basically comprises facts that can be observed from without, and the second-order perspective, which is the informant's experience or perspective of a phenomenon (Larsson, 1986). Phenomenography focuses on issues relating to the second-order perspective. Knowledge of the way in which a certain group of people conceives phenomena in the world around them will facilitate teaching (Uljens, 1989). We can assume that there is a relationship between the effects of health care measures, patients' recovery and the way patients view themselves as patients, how they view their illness or injury, and the kind of knowledge they have about the treatment that is offered. Accordingly, a central issue for the health sciences is to investigate patients' conceptions of the phenomena they encounter (Wenestam, 2000). Thus, to describe different conceptions among patients with a hip fracture, we used a phenomenographic approach, as described by Marton (1981) and Booth (1992).

Informants

Informants were recruited from a geriatric/orthopedic ward at a Swedish hospital. Inclusion criteria were: age 70 years or more, noninstitutional residence, and acutely operated on for a hip fracture. Exclusion criteria were: severe illness, cognitive impairment or dementia, or pathological fracture. Thirteen patients strategically selected, and 2 men and 11 women, aged 71–93 years (median 81 years) met inclusion criteria and were invited by the patient's primary nurse to participate in the study. They were provided with both oral and written explanations of the study, and assured that participation was voluntary and that the data would be treated confidentially. Informed consent was obtained and all 13 patients agreed to participate. The study was approved by the hospital administration and the Human Ethics Committee, Göteborg University, Sweden.

Interview

The interviews were conducted in the informants' room or in a secluded area of the ward as soon after the operation as the informants felt strong enough, to obtain the patients' personal conceptions. Each interview lasted 30–45 minutes, and was recorded and later transcribed verbatim by the first author. The interviews took the form of a dialogue and were semistructured such that the main questions, related to the informants' perception of the transitional properties, were included in all interviews. During the interviews, deliberate efforts were made to encourage informants to reveal and comment freely on their personal experiences of and reflections on their situation, without imposing the interviewer's own values on what was being said (Kvale, 1996). The interviewees talked freely, and all appeared to be grateful for the attention and for having someone to listen to their reflections.

Data Analysis

Transcripts were first perused several times to become familiar with the data and to form an impression of the material as a whole. They were then analyzed to determine the patients' perceptions of the five transitional properties, and meaning-units relevant to the study were identified and pooled. A total of 542 meaning-units could be identified, and a saturation of conceptions was observed when nine interviews had been analyzed. These meaning-units were then read and compared with each other. In the next step, meaning-units describing qualitatively similar conceptions were grouped together and the nature of this similarity was articulated. This grouping resulted in a limited number of categories of description. These categories were labeled in accordance with their characteristics and exemplified with representative quotations from the interviews. An example of a meaning-unit that led to a category is, "If there is something I do not understand I will ask, I think I am entitled to do so," a statement exemplifying the "Autonomous" category. To test the reliability of the categories, the second author evaluated the categories in relation to the interviews.

Results

The main findings in this study concern variation in the informants' conceptions, which were possible to group into three distinct categories. However, analyses also revealed similarity in informants' conceptions. These common traits appeared in various forms and degrees in all interviews.

Different Conceptions

Informants differed in their conceptions regarding their need for information and views of their own responsibility in the rehabilitation process. Informants could be classified into three distinct categories of description: the Autonomous, the Modest, and the Heedless.

The Autonomous

The Autonomous appeared to be confident and accustomed to managing for themselves and being in control of their lives. They were willing to listen to the staff, but made their own decisions. One patient described how she acted in conjunction with an earlier fracture:

> This leg was in plaster for nearly a year, and then I was supposed to have physical therapy at the hospital, but I found it just too much trouble, so after a while I didn't bother. I exercised the leg myself.

The Autonomous knew what they wanted after discharge from hospital. One woman was determined to obtain community aftercare, even though she knew it was very difficult to get:

> I have been thinking and I know that I shall have to stay there for some time, a few weeks or so, since I can't manage to go home straight away, definitely not.

Even if the Autonomous appeared to be strong, they felt just as vulnerable as the other groups. However, they were aware of the importance of information, personal support, and their own responsibility. One informant pointed out that more information given preoperatively could have made a great difference:

> Of course, if someone had come and sat down for a little while and talked. If they had said something like, this is what it will be like, and so on, and after a while you will be able to walk and maybe manage on your own again. That would have been reassuring, it really would. Because, I really must say, at moments like that, you get a feeling of being small and insignificant.

It was apparent that they understood the importance of taking responsibility for their rehabilitation. They realized that the most important immediate information they needed was how to exercise the leg without disturbing the fracture, and that many other questions would arise later.

The Modest

The Modest gave the impression of being vulnerable and dependent on others, and they expressed themselves cautiously. They wanted to be restored to their previous functional status, but appeared hesitant about saying so. Instead of demanding community aftercare like the Autonomous, they were willing to go along and accept what was offered:

> I've asked to be sent to a community facility after discharge, to get some more rehabilitation. But the doctor said that it wasn't possible, this is the rehabilitation. I had been hoping I could stay a little longer, but then I figured, there is nothing to do about it, maybe I can get some help at home, my children will come, and then I have my older sister.

These informants appreciated and were grateful for the information offered to them, but for some reason they did not request more, even though they seemed to want to. Asked whether she had been given all the information she needed, one woman said

> No, I can't say that I have, but I guess I haven't asked enough either.

The Modest worried more about their future ability to walk and to maintain their former lifestyle than did the others. They feared being discharged, saw only problems, and appeared unaware of the progress they had made. They were reluctant to talk about their hopes and wishes for the future and did not see their own responsibility as clearly as the Autonomous.

The Heedless

The Heedless differed dramatically from the other two groups in terms of how they regarded their situation. They appeared to view their situation with some detachment, almost as if it did not really concern them. The Heedless did not doubt that they would recover, and they were confident that people around them would care for them. In some ways, their position was enviable in not having to worry about the future. When asked who was responsible for their rehabilitation, one 84-year-old woman said:

> I don't know, it must be the physiotherapist who is involved in the treatment I think, hope. I don't care. It is not for me to say, but they usually come to help me.

The Heedless were characterized predominantly by a reluctance to reflect on their situation, by a refusal to accept responsibility, and by their need for information. They did not accept any responsibility for their rehabilitation and relied entirely on their physicians, nurses, and significant others. They were not interested in receiving or discussing information that might be useful to them. Their strategy was to simply follow instructions and let the staff help them through the transition. They did not appear to have reached a stage where planning for the future was relevant.

Common Traits

Awareness

Informants lacked adequate knowledge about their condition, what to do and how to act, and needed more information. Only one informant knew someone who had undergone rehabilitation for a hip fracture. On the second day after surgery, one woman was unaware of which joint had been operated on or what she could do with her leg:

> I sat here thinking that I have bent my leg, so obviously it is possible to bend it.

Shocking Event

Many older people live alone, so in the event of an accident, it may take some time before they can get help. One of the informants spent the whole night waiting:

It was ten o'clock in the evening, I was in my bedroom, and fell to the floor. I was in terrible pain. The balcony door was open, I wanted to shut it, but I could not move and I could not get up into bed. I spent the whole night on the floor, and at seven in the morning I could finally call my sister.

Although several suspected they had sustained a fracture, all of the informants were very distressed by the diagnosis and felt as if they had received an ominous verdict. One informant described how he lost his sense of reality:

I just could not believe it, was this really happening to me? My thoughts went back and forth. Was my leg broken or was it a bad dream? After a while, I came to my senses and realized that my leg really was broken.

The period before surgery was described as mostly blurred and filled with fear and the pain. They worried about how they would function postoperatively and characterized the experience both before and after the operation as alarming. One female informant repeated several times the thoughts she had both before and after the operation, "It's not at all sure that I shall ever be able to walk again, maybe I will have to spend the rest of my life in a wheelchair."

Zest for Life

All patients, regardless of age, health status, or abilities, expressed a strong desire to recuperate. Although they were still confined to bed, they were very worried, remembering the pain and inability to move their leg. All the suffering they had experienced in anticipation and preparation for the operation led them to believe they might not be able to walk with their leg again. One informant said that she had been convinced that she would not be able to walk again, but that it all changed when the physiotherapists got her up for the first time:

They came in with the walker and helped me up on my feet, and then I told them I do not think I can walk, but they said, come on, we know you can do it, and I did. After that I thought, damn it, I can do it and so it is, it may work. One can not give up, you see, one needs to keep at it to the final breath.

A 93-year-old woman, admitted for a third fracture that year, said she was not going to give up:

You have to give it all you've got—if you're stubborn enough.

Discussion

Results from the present study indicate that patients with a hip fracture, in general, lack adequate knowledge about their fracture and their rehabilitation. More importantly, our findings pointed to a significant difference in patients' engagement in the rehabilitation process. This difference indicates that patients cannot be considered a homogeneous group who do, or do not, participate in their transitional process. Variation in patient participation in rehabilitation has previously been described in different ways in studies of patients actually undergoing rehabilitation (Jewell, 1996; Larsson-Lund et al., 2001). Furthermore, Carlsson et al. (1991) found that older people develop different behavioral patterns during the course of their lives, which correspond to the different strategies found in our study. These findings may also shed some light upon the communication gap revealed in studies on patient satisfaction with information and discharge planning. For example, Dahlberg and Herlitz (1997) and Zidén and Wenestam (1991) found that their patients were dissatisfied with information, and Jewell (1993) and Smith et al. (1997) found that their patients were equally dissatisfied with discharge planning. Both Jewell (1996) and Bull et al. (2000) reported that older people want to be involved in planning, and that patient participation in planning yields better health outcomes from the perspective of both the patient and family carer after discharge. These results indicate that although patients wish to participate, they may not feel that they are afforded those opportunities.

In all the interviews, the informants conveyed a sense of distress. They viewed their situation as threatening, and worries of permanent dependency and impaired walking ability were prominent. Little research interest has focused on patient worries and concerns, and we found only one study in which patients described their condition as alarming (Bowman, 1997). Clearly, such worries and concerns represent yet another hurdle to successful rehabilitation. However, it has been shown that these feelings can be reduced by brief supportive nursing interventions, including improved information (Houldin & Hogan-Quigley, 1995). For older people, a hip fracture is a devastating transitional process spanning from an initial state of complete dependency to a restoration of former functional status, a goal reached by few (Cooper, 1997; Robinson, 1999; Hall et al., 2000; Norton et al., 2000; van Balen et al., 2001). The fears and worries expressed by our informants clearly suggest that they needed more attention and emotional support to ensure a healthy start in the transition.

Some transitions are associated with identifiable marker events, critical points and events. These could be associated with an increasing awareness of change or difference, or more active involvement in dealing with the transition experience (Meleis et al., 2000). Some critical points were salient for our informants. Two negative critical points were noted: the fall itself, because some informants were alone and helpless for hours; and the diagnosis, which the informants experienced as distressing and threatening. One positive critical point was identified: when the informants were first able to put weight on the fractured leg, and thus, realized they might be able to walk again. Even though trying to walk involved both discomfort and pain, it also seemed to trigger a strong zest for life, and none of the informants was ready to give up. All transitions are characterized by flow and movement over time, but it is debated whether or not transitions are also characterized by an identifiable endpoint (Meleis et al., 2000). For patients with a hip fracture, the endpoint is probably not identifiable because so many of them never regain their previous level of physical function. Stability and acceptance of the situation are probably more appropriate endpoints. Patients with a hip fracture are a very heterogeneous group, and some of them are already in one or several transitions. Coordination of these transitions is essential for achieving stability.

Study Limitations

In spite of the small number of informants, different categories of description were easily formulated from the interviews. The phenomenographic method is regarded as highly applicable when this goal has been reached and the results have led to categories that describe different conceptions. A saturation of the conceptions was reached before all the interviews had been completed, which attests to the validity of the results (Taylor & Bogdan, 1984). A larger study might further refine the categories and possibly add additional ones; however, with more data, there is a risk that the analysis will become superficial, and thereby undermine the aim of the work (Larsson, 1986).

Relevance to Clinical Practice

Our results suggest that differences in patients' perspectives on the rehabilitation process need to be taken into account to enhance outcomes. The willingness of patients to participate in rehabilitation documented in earlier studies, combined with the zest for life found in our patients, underscore the importance of nurses carefully assessing each individual's resources and barriers for rehabilitation. Understanding the patients and encouraging their willingness to participate are important tasks for nurses, and will potentially enhance the patients' chances for recovery. Our results suggest that we need to develop different ways to inform and educate these patients that better take into account the patients' ability to absorb and digest the information. They all need the information to be provided both in writing and orally as early as possible, not all at once, but rather step by step and repeated as necessary. The Autonomous group only needs better information, and the Modest group also needs enhanced emotional support, especially during the initial period. The Heedless are more difficult to know how to handle. They do not only need better information, but they also need to be made aware of their own role during their rehabilitation. The first postoperative ambulation should start as soon as possible to abate their worry and stimulate their zest for life.

Suggestion for Future Research

The care of patients with a hip fracture is very complex, and requires the involvement of many staff members. Our result suggests the need for more individualized care based on the patient's prerequisites. To achieve this, a structured quality care may be used, where the contribution of all the members of the multiprofessional team is specified and further developed. Further research is needed to develop methods to more efficiently identify and classify patients according to the categories identified here. Moreover, efforts need to be made to better manage the Heedless and to encourage them to take greater responsibility for their rehabilitation.

REFERENCES

van Balen, R., Steyerberg, E. W., Polder, J. J., Ribbers, T. L. M., Habbema, J. D. F., & Cools, H. J. M. H. (2001). Hip fracture in elderly patients. *Clinical Orthopaedics and Related Research, 390*, 232–243.

Booth, S. (1992). *Learning to program. A phenomenographic perspective*. Unpublished doctoral dissertation, Göteborg University, Göteborg, Sweden.

Bowman, A.-M. (1997). Sleep satisfaction, perceived pain and acute confusion in elderly clients undergoing orthopaedic procedures. *Journal of Advanced Nursing, 26*, 550–564.

Bull, M. J., Hansen, H. E., & Gross, C. R. (2000). A professional-patient partnership model of discharge planning with elders. *Applied Nursing Research, 13*, 18–28.

Carlsson, M., Berg, S., & Wenestam, C.-G. (1991). The oldest old: Patterns of adjustment and dependence. *Scandinavian Journal of Caring Sciences, 5*, 93–100.

Ceder, L., Thorngren, K. G., & Wallden, B. (1980). Prognostic indicators and early home rehabilitation in elderly patients with hip fractures. *Clin Orthop, 152*, 173–184.

Cooper, C. (1997). The crippling consequences of fractures and their impact on quality of life. *American Journal of Medicine, 103*, 12s–19s.

Cree, A. K., & Nade, S. (1999). How to predict return to the community after fractured proximal femur in the elderly. *Australian & New Zealand Journal of Surgery, 69*, 723–725.

Dahlberg, L., & Herlitz, C. (1997). *Vägen från sjukhuset: Om äldre människors återhämtning efter ortopediska skador* (in Swedish). Dalamas forskningsråd;. Report no. 1997:2. Falun.

Egan, M., Wairen, S. A., Hessel, P. A., & Gilewish, G. (1992). Activities of daily living after hip fracture: Pre- and post discharge. *Occupational Therapy Journal of Research, 12*, 342–356.

Ensberg, M. D., Paletta, M. J., Galecki, A. T., Dacko, C. L., & Fries, B. E. (1993). Identifying elderly patients for early discharge after hospitalization for hip fracture. *Journal of Gerontology Medical Sciences, 5*, 187–195.

Hall, S. E., Williams, J. A., Senior, J. A., Goldswain, P. R. T., & Criddle, R. A. (2000). Hip fracture outcomes: Quality in older adults living in the community. *Australian New Zealand Medical Journal, 30*, 327–332.

Hedlund, R. (1985). *Incidence of femur fractures*. Unpublished doctoral dissertation, Karolinska Institutet, Stockholm, Sweden.

Houldin, A. D., & Hogan-Quigley, B. (1995). Psychological intervention for older hip fracture patients. *Journal of Gerontological Nursing, 21*, 20–26.

Jewell, S. E. (1993). Discovery of the discharge process: A study of patient discharge from a care unit for elderly people. *Journal of Advanced Nursing, 18*, 1288–1296.

Jewell, S. E. (1996). Elderly patients' participation in discharge decision-making. *British Journal of Nursing, 2*, 1065–1071.

Koval, K. J., Skovron, M. L., Polatsch, D., Aharonoff, G. B., & Zuckerman, J. D. (1996). Dependency after hip fracture in geriatric patients: A study of predictive factors. *Journal of Othopaedic Trauma, 8*, 531–535.

Koval, K. J., Skovron, M. L., Polatsch, D., Aharonoff, G. B., & Zuckerman, J. D. (1998). Predictors of functional recovery after hip fracture in the elderly. *Clinical Orthopaedics, 348*, 22–28.

Kvale, S. (1996). *Interviews. An introduction to qualitative research interviewing*. Newcastle Upon Tyne, UK: Sage.

Larsson, S. (1986). *Kvalitativ analys av exemplet fenomenografi* (in Swedish). Lund, Sweden: Studentlitteratur.

Larsson-Lund, M., Tamm, M., & Bränholm, I.-B. (2001). Patients' perception of their participation in rehabilitation planning and professionals' view of their strategies to encourage it. *Occupational Therapy International, 8*, 151–167.

Long, A. F., Kneafsey, R., Ryan, J., & Berry, J. (2002). The role of the nurse within the multi-professional rehabilitation team. *Journal of Advanced Nursing, 37*, 70–78.

Marottoli, R. A., Berkman, L. R., & Cooney, L. M. (1992). Decline in physical function following hip fracture. *Journal of the American Geriatrics Society, 40*, 861–866.

Marton, F. (1981). Phenomenography: Describing conceptions of the world around us. *Instructional Science, 10*, 177–200.

Meleis, A. I., Sawyer, L. M., Im, E.-O., Messias, D. K. H., & Schumacher, K. (2000). Experiencing transitions: An emerging middle-range theory. *Advances in Nursing Science, 23*, 12–28.

Norton, R., Butler, M., Robinson, E., Lee-Joe, T., & Campbell, A. J. (2000). Declines in physical functioning attributable to hip fracture among older people: A follow-up study of case-control participants. *Disability and Rehabilitation, 22*, 345–351.

Overend, T. J., Mackenzie Chesworth, B., Sandrin, M., Stroud, S., Petrella, R. J., & McCalden, R. (2000). Determination of prefracture physical function in community-dwelling people who fracture their hip. *Journal of Gerontology Medical Sciences, 11*, 698–702.

Robinson, S. B. (1999). Transitions in the lives of elderly women who have sustained hip fractures. *Journal of Advanced Nursing, 30*, 1341–1348.

Smith, M., Rosseau, N., Lecouturier, J., Gregson, B., Bond, J., & Rodgers, H. (1997). Are older people satisfied with discharge information? *Nursing Times, 93*, 52–53.

Sonn, U., åsberg Hulter, K., Hultin, G., Mellström, D., & Zetterberg, C. (1994). ADL-förmågan förutsäger vaoårdtiden (in Swedish). *Läkartidningen, 91*, 2962–2963.

Taylor, S. J., & Bogdan, R. (1984). *Introduction to qualitative research methods: The research for meanings* (2nd ed.). New York: Wiley-Interscience.

The National Board of Health and Welfare. (1998). *Yearbook of health and medical care* (in Swedish). Stockholm, Sweden: Norsteds tryckeri AB.

Thorngren, K. G. (1996). *State of the art: Höftfraktur. [State of the art: Hip fracture]*. Stockholm, Sweden: Socialstyrelsen.

Uljens, M. (1989). *Fenomenografi –forskning om uppfattningar* (in Swedish). Lund, Sweden: Studentlitteratur.

Wenestam, C.-G. (2000). The phenomenographic method in health research. In B. Fridlund, & C. Hilding (Eds.), *Qualitative methods in service of health* (pp. 97–111). Lund, Sweden: Studentlitteratur.

Zetterberg, C., Gneib, C., Mellström, D., Sundh, V., Zidén, L. (1990). Rikshöft –utvärdering av fysisk funktion och vårdkonsumtion efter höftfraktur. *Läkartidningen, 23*, 2040–2045.

Zidén, L., & Wenestam, C.-G. (1991). The band aid is the evidence. Eight women's knowledge and understanding of their hip fractures, the care and the surgical treatment. In B. Fridlund, & C. Hilding (Eds.), *Qualitative methods in service of health* (pp. 111–113). Lund, Sweden: Studentlitteratur.

Zuckerman, J. D., Koval, K. J., Aharonoff, G. B., Hiebert, R., & Skovron, M. L. (2000a). A functional recovery score for elderly hip fracture patients: I: Development. *Journal of Othopaedic Trauma, 14*, 20–25.

Zuckerman, J. D., Koval, K. J., Aharonoff, G. B., Hiebert, R., & Skovron, M. L. (2000b). A functional recovery score for elderly hip fracture patients: II: Validity and reliability. *Journal of Othopaedic Trauma, 14*, 26–30.

Reprinted with permission from: Olsson, L. E., Nyström, A., Karlsson, J., & Ekman, I. (2007). Admitted with a hip fracture: Patient perceptions of rehabilitation. *Journal of Clinical Nursing, 16*(5), 853–859.

7.6 TAIWANESE PATIENTS' CONCERNS AND COPING STRATEGIES: TRANSITION TO CARDIAC SURGERY

FU-JIN SHIH
AFAF IBRAHIM MELEIS
PO-JUI YU
WEN-YU HU
MEEI-FANG LOU
GUEY-SHIUN HUANG

Cardiovascular disease was reported as the second leading cause of death in Taiwan.[1,2] Despite the fact that the overall heart disease mortality rate has declined by 40% over the past 20 years, the prevalence of cardiac disease is reported to increase continuously in Western, as well as Eastern, society.[3,4] Studies on recovery from cardiac surgery are of interest to both Eastern and Western health care professionals. Recovery is often thought to be a process that begins from the moment a disease diagnosis is made and a treatment starts, and continues until the person subjectively perceives himself or herself to be fully functional, or has completed his or her rehabilitation program.[5–10]

The consequences of heart disease usually affect an individual's total performance, and create many physiologic and psychologic hardships, such as chest pain, depression, altered body image, and increased dependency.[5,6,9–15] This frequently leads to the fear of an uncertain future and a decreased sense of well-being.[7,10,11,16,17] Although the success of surgical treatment of cardiac disease has been well established, there are still many risks for postoperative complications of cardiac surgery: wound infection, coagulopathies, thromboembolisms, neurologic impairments, renal failure, dysrhythmia, valve degeneration, endocarditis, heart failure, and death.[10,18–22] Because of the highly threatening nature of cardiac surgery and the psychologic ties to the heart itself, cardiac surgery and the physiologic and psychosocial responses related to it have been the foci for researchers.

Some of the preoperative concerns of patients that relate to cardiac surgery have been identified and grouped into five types: (a) the waiting itself; (b) physical responses, such as postoperative pain; (c) psychologic responses, including mourning the loss of good health and control, disappointment, anger, and fear of the appearance of wounds, impairment, seriousness of surgery, and death; (d) cognitive responses, including helplessness and guilt, and knowledge deficit of additional tests, procedures, and medication; and (e) sociologic issues, such as extended hospital stay and increased cost.[4,11,12,15,23]

However, few investigators have researched further to include the patients' concerns regarding cardiac surgery, and the strategies patients have used to deal with these concerns during the preoperative hospitalization stage that extends from diagnosis until the date of surgery. The purpose of our study was to explore Taiwanese patients' concerns and their coping strategies during their admission transition for cardiac surgery, as well as the background context that has framed this phenomenon.

For the purpose of our study, the patient's concerns were tentatively defined as "a single or multiple event(s) that bothers one's mind" and the coping strategies were tentatively defined as "one's efforts in managing the aforementioned concerns." The admission transition for cardiac surgery conceptualized in our study is the stage extending from the day the patient is hospitalized until the moment she or he is sent into the operating room. The admission period is not only part of the preoperative period, but is also a component of the overall recovery transition of patients.

Method

An exploratory research design was used to reveal the nature of patients' concerns at the beginning of their recovery transition.

Sample

Because coronary artery bypass grafting (CABG), valvular replacement surgery (VRS), and atrial or ventricular septal defect (ASD or VSD) repair are three major types of cardiac surgeries in Taiwan, a purposive sample of subjects who met the following criteria was obtained: (a) more than 18 years old; (b) able to understand and speak Mandarin, Taiwanese, or Hakka, or having family members willing to interpret for them; and (c) planning to have surgery for CABG, VRS, ASD, or VSD repair. Excluded were subjects who were intubated with nasal, oral, or tracheostomal tubes; those who were not fully conscious (Glasgow Coma Scale < 15); and those who had a degree of mental illness (confirmed by at least one psychiatric physician) before conducting interviews by the principal investigator (FJS).

Procedures

Our study protocol was reviewed and approved by the Committee for Research on Human Subjects at the University of California–San Francisco and the four study sites. Permission to conduct the study also was obtained from the directors of the surgical and nursing departments of one national and three general hospitals in northern Taiwan—each institution having a reputation for successful cardiac surgery. The list of all patients scheduled to receive cardiac surgery was obtained through daily contact with the clerk or head nurse of the surgical cardiovascular floor units at four hospitals. All patients who met the inclusion criteria, and who expressed an interest in participating in our study before surgery, were considered as potential candidates. They were then individually approached by us and informed of the purpose of our study, the extent of participation expected, and the potential risks involved. A consent form was read to them before they were asked to participate. All patients were given time to read the consent form and ask questions. A signed consent form was obtained from each patient who chose to participate, and each patient was offered a copy of his or her consent form.

Instruments

Two types of data collection tools were used: a semistructured interview guide and the patient profile. The semistructured interview guide, entitled "Suggested Interview Questions and Probes for the Patient," was developed on the basis of literature reviewed pertaining to surgical cardiac recovery, as well as on Chinese health and culture. In addition, the principal investigator's empiric knowledge, based on more than 16 years of surgical cardiovascular nursing work in Taiwan, and periodic (once or twice per week) consultation with her four internationally respected interdisciplinary experts—a surgical cardiac nursing scientist, a nursing theorist, and two sociologists familiar with the use of multiple qualitative methods—also constituted valuable sources of input in devising this guide. The final modification of the interview guide was made after interviewing four male and three female Taiwanese patients 1 day before their cardiac surgery in Taiwan (before our study protocol was approved). The interviews were conducted in the patients' rooms on the surgical cardiovascular floor unit 1 day before cardiac surgery. The exact time of the interview was scheduled by consulting with the patient's primary nurse and obtaining the patient's agreement. Following the semistructured interview format, patients were asked questions with the aim of constructing a patient profile. The patient profile consisted of the patient's demographic information, such as age, language, marital status, socioeconomic status, living arrangements, and religious affiliation. After finishing the interview, the principal investigator went to the nursing station to review the patient's chart and to record the patient's health status, medical history, and medications.

Sixty patients were approached by us, but only 40 (20 men and 20 women) actually met the requirements and completed the interview. Sixteen patients were too weak to participate or finish the interview as a result of various preoperative signs and symptoms, such as fatigue, shortness of breath, severe coughing, pain, and gastrointestinal discomforts. Four patients' family members insisted that patients should talk as little as possible to save their energy for the cardiac surgery, although the patients themselves agreed to participate in the study.

Twenty-five percent of the participants ($n = 10$) came from one medical center, 30% ($n = 12$) from one military hospital, and 25% ($n = 10$) and 20% ($n = 8$) from two private hospitals. The participants' ages ranged from 20 to 70 years ($M = 50.10$; $SD = 17.24$). Most of the participants were married. Most had received more than seven years of schooling. Eighty-seven percent were employed. Seventy-three percent ($n = 29$) of the subjects' annual family income was between $3703 (U.S.) and $22,222 (U.S.). Because five of the subjects did not have steady incomes, the mean income of the other 35 subjects ($26,121 [U.S.]) was used for purpose of analysis. Eighty percent of subjects ($n = 32$) perceived their annual family income as adequate. The severity of cardiac disease ranged from NYHA functional class 1 (38%) to IV (5%). Thirty percent of subjects ($n = 12$) planned to have CABG; others planned to have septal replacement, or VRS,

TABLE 7.6.1 Sample Demographics ($n = 40$)

Demographic	M (SD)	Range	n	%
Age (yr)	50.10	20–30	7	18
	(17.24)	31–40	7	18
		41–50	6	14
		51–60	10	25
		61–70	10	25
Education			2	5
Graduate school				
College			8	20
Senior high school		7	17	
Junior high school		7	17	
Elementary school		11	28	
None		5	13	
Religious affiliations			32	80
Buddhism				
Protestantism		3	7	
Confucianism			5	13
Occupation			4	10
Not working				
Housewife			7	18
Self-employed			6	14
Laborer			16	40
Administrator			4	10
Teacher			2	5
Student			1	3
Family Income/yr	512,989	NT 40,000–99,999	4	10
(27.0 NT = $1 US)	(492,867)	NT 100,000–199,999	7	17
		NT 200,000-299,999	5	13
		NT 300,000-399,999	5	13
		NT 400,000-499,999	5	13
		NT 500,000-599,999	7	17
		= NT 600,000	7	17
Perceived adequacy of income				
Very satisfied			4	10
Satisfied			9	23
Okay			19	47
Unsatisfied			5	13
Very unsatisfied			3	7
Number of caregivers	1.95			
1			14	35
2	(0.85)		14	35
3			7	17
4			5	13
NYHA Functional Class			15	38
I				
II			13	32
III			10	25
IV			2	5
Type of surgery			12	30
CABG				
VR			9	23
SR			8	20
Redo VR			6	14
CABG and VR			3	7
SR and annuloplasty			1	3
Annuloplasty			1	3
No. of preoperative	5.12	1–7	30	75
hospitalization days	(3.14)	8–14	7	18
		15–18	3	7

NT, New Taiwan dollar.

or both CABG and VRS, or other surgeries. The duration of the subjects' stay in the floor unit before the surgery ranged from 1 to 18 days ($M = 5.12$, $SD = 3.14$) (Table 7.6.1).

Analytical Methods

The data were first transcribed from audio tape in the patient's native language (Mandarin, Taiwanese, or Hakka) in written Chinese, and later translated into English by Chinese, and later translated into English by the principal investigator and three individuals, who are each proficient in both Chinese and English, have a good knowledge of Eastern and Western culture, and were well trained by the principal investigator.

The accuracy of the data translation was checked by translating the English version back into Chinese, and then having it reviewed by other investigators. Data analysis took a total of 21 months, starting with the first interview and continuing to the end of the research period. To keep the emerging codes, categories, themes, and concepts firmly grounded in the subjects' actual experiences, a unique mode of qualitative content analysis was used.[24,25]

The various analytic codes, categories, and themes related to the concept of patients' concerns about cardiac surgery were developed by means of seven different levels of analysis. We developed this analytical approach by periodically (once or twice per week) discussing the data with the aforementioned consultation group during the data analysis process. The seven levels included: (a) accurate transcribing and translating, (b) obtaining a holistic understanding of the subjects' responses, (c) codifying emerging patterns in each interview in the field notes, (d) creating an action/interaction strategy–examining work sheet, (e) carrying out action/interaction strategy–examining work with use of the action/interaction strategy–examining work sheet, (f) creating themes with use of data linkage and constant comparison, and (g) generating categories and subcategories.

For example, the categories in this study are concerns, coping strategies, and contexts of the phenomenon. The subcategories of the participants' concerns revealed in this study were the presence and the absence of concerns. The subcategories of the participants' coping strategies identified in this study were the presence or absence of coping strategies. The themes of the subjects' concerns were the different levels (consisting of various components) of the subjects' concerns. Likewise, the themes of the subjects' coping strategies were the three types (consisting of various methods) of the subjects' coping strategies.

Trustworthiness

Some strategies were used to enhance the rigor of the findings. Informant-checking was agreed to by all respondents.[24–28] Negative cases were investigated and analyzed.[26,29–31] All patients' charts were reviewed.[26,28,29,31] Additionally, each subject's primary nurse or caregiver was asked to confirm specific events.[25,26,29,32] For example, when the subjects addressed concerns related to their hospital experiences, or other medical or nursing issues, the principal investigator would contact the subjects' primary nurse as well as their caregivers to clarify the related information. In addition, if the subjects' concerns were related to their family members or to socioeconomic issues, the principal investigator would contact the subjects' caregivers to get more background information to better understand the subjects' concerns.

Results

Participants' Concerns at Admission

When asked about their impending surgery, 90% of the participants ($n = 36$) expressed and described their feelings, whereas the rest indicated that they had no particular concerns, questions, or fears related to the surgery. This 10% of the participants ($n = 4$) felt concerned about the surgery, but were unable to describe their concerns in more specific terms.

Analysis of the responses to questions about concerns revealed three levels of concerns, questions, and feelings of participants related to their surgery. Each level was differentiated by the intensity, severity, and sentiment associated with the responses. The, "caring or thinking about concerns" in this project means, "the lowest level of concerns that consume one's least cognitive efforts, and cause the least intensive and significant impact on one's well-being." The, "worrying about or being afraid of concerns" is, "the middle level of concerns that consume one's more cognitive efforts, and cause an intensive and significant impact on one's well-being." The, "experiencing a mortal fear of concerns" indicate, "the strongest level of concerns that consume one's most cognitive efforts, and cause the most intensive and significant impact on one's well-being."

Fifty-two percent of the subjects ($n = 21$) described concerns that have caused the least intensive and significant impact on their cognitive or emotional responses. The participants labeled these concerns as the level of "caring or thinking about" concerns (Table 7.6.2). Forty-three percent of the subjects ($n = 17$) described another set of concerns about which they expressed a stronger level of intensity and emotion. They named these concerns as the level of "worrying about or being afraid of" concerns (Table 7.6.3). Participants emphasized the second level of concerns more through language, facial expressions, and tension in their bodies. Thirty percent of the participants ($n = 12$) had "experiencing a mortal fear of" concerns (Table 7.6.4) that were described to have made the participants be truly "afraid of" and intensely worried about each of the concerns related to the recovery process.

"Caring About" Type of Concerns

Fifty-two percent of the participants ($n = 21$) reported experiencing the first level of concerns, such as process of recovery, the unfinished responsibilities and life goals, significant others and places, hospital experiences, and death.

Process of Recovery

Fifty-two percent of subjects ($n = 21$) described their concerns about lack of knowledge of what to expect during their recovery, such as the optimal degree of recovery and its course. The process of recovery and what to expect through it gave them pause, and having the interview at this time provided them an opportunity to reflect on their thoughts. They were able then to express such statements as, "I didn't have the experience of surgery, so I don't know what will happen after surgery. I really care about it."

Unfinished Responsibilities and Life Goals; Significant Persons and Places

Half of the participants ($n = 20$) cared about how the surgery and the recovery period might interfere with their daily lives, their life goals, and the lives of their significant others. They were concerned that the recovery transition would deprive them of carrying out their familial obligations, impede their life goals, and interfere with their job continuity. For this group of participants, a sense of unfinished responsibilities was of concern to them. Their concerns were about unfinished responsibilities including extended families, such as parents and parents-in-law, in addition to their immediate nuclear families.

The concerns about leaving their responsibilities suspended included those related to raising children, providing them with a quality education, helping them get married, and helping them set up their own business. Among the reasons why they perceived responsibilities toward their children as being unfinished were that their children were still young, or had not finished college yet, were still single, did not have the ability to buy their own house, or were still dependent on their parents because of lack of income or unemployment, even though they are adults. Participants also felt that they were leaving their children without a resource person to help them with school work.

Participants expressed many reflective concerns about their parents, as well. They cared about

TABLE 7.6.2 What Taiwanese Patients Cared About During the Admission Transition (n = 40)

Things Cared About	n*	%
Process of recovery	21	52
The unfinished responsibilities and life goals, and significant people and places	20	50
Hospital experiences (including maintaining daily living activities, pain at admission, and expectant discomforts and disability in the ICU)	14	35
Death	13	33

*Each participant may have more than one response.

TABLE 7.6.3 What Taiwanese Patients Worried About During the Admission Transition (n = 40)

Things Worried About	n*	%
The unfinished responsibilities	16	40
Hospital experiences (expectant discomforts and disability in the ICU)	12	30
Death	10	25
Financial needs	9	23
Process of recovery	7	18
Poor quality of care	4	10

*Each participant may have more than one response.

TABLE 7.6.4 What Taiwanese Patients Feared During the Admission Transition (n = 40)

Things Feared	n*	%
Death	11	28
Hospital experiences (expectant discomforts and disability in the ICU)	10	25
Process of recovery	8	10

*Each participant may have more than one response.

their parents deeply and were concerned about who might be their caregivers while they were going through the entire surgical and recovery transition. Obligations towards parents and parents-in-law included *Faan-Buu* (Mandarin, meaning giving parents financial and emotional support in the future, thus showing filial piety) ("I have done little in rewarding my mom" "I want to repay them after getting a job"), and not letting parents or parents-in-law worry about them ("My responsibility is to live well, not to let parents worry about me"). In addition, the participants described *Faan-Buu* to include protecting their parents from worrying about them, and how their "lack of health," as reflected in the diagnosis, the planned surgery, and the recovery period, will inflict worry and pain on their parents. Their responses included such statements as "I should not let my mother endure so much stress; she has been so tired in caring for me, and she is worried about the surgery so much."

Factors that influence *Faan-Buu* are the number of male siblings ("I'm the only son in my family"), the birth order of the participant ("I'm the eldest son"), the sex of the participant ("How can

I avoid this kind of responsibilities as a son?"), the marital status of the participant ("I'm still single"), and the participant's parents' health status ("In case something happens to them, I need to help.").

Thirty-five percent of the participants (*n* = 14) were also concerned about their spouses, such as the spouses' quality of life. Women were particularly concerned about their spouses' need for their companionship as they attempted to fall asleep ("My husband can't fall asleep without seeing me"). The sense of interruption in responsibilities for some female elderly participants extended also to their grandchildren ("Who will tutor my grandchildren?"; "I miss my grandchild; I care about his homework since I used to tutor his homework every day"), and neighbors and places that were significant to them ("All the neighbors in Hsin-Chu are old friends; it's hard for me to leave").

Forty percent of the participants (*n* = 16) cared about their unfinished work-related responsibilities. Executives were concerned about the daily management of their companies, and one stated, "Working with the employees is a great responsibility" that he would miss. Others worried about unfinished office projects they had been supervising before they were admitted to the hospital: "I hope my colleagues can handle the project, which I really care about." Two career soldiers (5%) were concerned about leadership responsibilities to their country ("to fight for our country in case of war"), which required their presence and health—both of which were missing at the time of the interview.

Finally, 20% percent of the participants (*n* = 8) described their concerns about the anticipated interruptions in their life goals, including pursuing higher education ("I wish I can [sic] finish my graduate study after I recover"), getting a job, doing social services, such as helping in an orphanage, and pursuing their global life plan ("I have a lot of things that I want to do in the future").

Hospital Experiences

Thirty-five percent of the subjects (*n* = 14) described their concerns about their hospital experiences, including how it will interrupt their daily activities, the extent of their discomforts, and their pain at admission and subsequently. Most in this group cared about how to maintain their daily activities, including getting enough sleep and rest, nutrition, taking showers, buying personal items, and doing laundry in the hospital. These concerns may have been highlighted because the participants experienced disruptions in their daily activities as a result of the hospitalization. The wake–sleep changes caused by institutional demands and the level of noise in hospital settings are inevitable. For instance, "It's too noisy here; it's like going to a supermarket" and "The people who have difficulty in falling asleep usually fell asleep late, and early morning was the time they slept most soundly." These experiences may have contributed to why the participants expressed some concerns about their hospital experiences. Their concerns included whether the food was adequate and healthy, should and could they take showers, and whether they would be able to replenish their personal items. For example, "I do not know how much food is needed for [someone like] me, who has diabetes," "The facilities [rest rooms] here are good, but I'm not used to taking a bath here" and "I don't like the public bathroom."

Twenty-three percent of the participants (*n* = 9) cared about discomforts and temporary disabilities they expected in the intensive care unit (ICU) while they were in pain and intubated. The expected discomfort during ICU recovery included cold and feeling pain; the expected kinds of pains were overall pain, pain specific to a location, such as wound pain, and pain caused by the insertion of tubes.

Thirteen percent of the participants (*n* = 5) were concerned about whether their current pain would be managed adequately and whether they would be able to achieve some level of comfort ("I felt very painful [sic] yesterday," and "I have felt very *Tong-Kou*" [Mandarin and Taiwanese, meaning physiologically, psychologically, and/or spiritually painful.]).

Death

Finally, 33% of the subjects (*n* = 13) had concerns about such security issues as the survival rate ("I don't know if the surgery will be 'peaceful' [safe] or not"), waiting for surgery alone in the operating room (OR), and the hospital environment ("I am hypersensitive to any, even little changes, in the environment, particularly in the hospital; any changes will make me nervous, [and] then my heart will speed up, and I will start to sweat a lot").

"Worry About" Type of Concerns

The second level of concerns were those that were described with more intensity than the previous concerns. These concerns were described by 43% of the participants ($n = 17$) and included unfinished business, hospital experiences, death, financial matters, process of recovery, and quality of care.

Unfinished Responsibilities

Forty percent ($n = 16$) of the participants who described concerns in this category expressed moderate concerns about unfinished business in their lives with more feelings, emotions, and intensity than the participants' responses that were discussed under the previous category of "caring about." These responses included worrying about the future raising of children, their children's education, and responsibilities regarding, "marrying and settling" their children. Examples are, "I worry about my children. If my surgery failed, I would pity my children since they will have no mother to take care of them," and, "No one can take care of my children."

Hospital Experiences

Thirty percent of the participants ($n = 12$) worried about specific discomforts, such as catching cold or flu, being unable to talk ("I worry that I cannot speak out to express myself"), having their body harmed or violated by tube insertion ("I'm afraid that they will insert tubes into my body"), suctioning ("I worry about suctioning sputum; it will be painful according to my experience"), having their hands tied up, pain ("I'm afraid of pain"), and being unable to handle their excreta ("I'm afraid that it will be inconvenient for me to handle my stool and urine by myself").

Death

Participants' third worry was concerning their death. Twenty-five percent of the participants ($n = 10$) worried about death ("I'm afraid that the surgery will not go smoothly," "I'm afraid that I'll be one of the few people who will not survive after the surgery."), and the unconscious state during surgery ("I worry about surgery; I mean I feel insecure since I will be unconscious at that time.").

Financial Needs

Twenty-three percent of the participants ($n = 9$) worried about their financial problems. These participants, all men, were concerned about the financial demands for family, which included family routine expenses ("After I got married, I had to support my family"), children's expenses, whether the savings left for the wife and the children would be enough, and children's tuition fees. The source of this worry was that, for some, their income had ceased on admission to the hospital, and it would be terminated altogether if they were unable to return to work as soon as possible after discharge ("I do not have any income now since I'm a self-employed taxi driver"). Some of the financial worries included payment for medical expenses, such as whether the percutaneous transluminal cardiac angiography would be covered by insurance.

Process of Recovery

Eighteen percent of participants ($n = 7$) worried about specific postsurgical matters, such as the appearance of wounds or scars ("I'm worrying about my wounds" "I wonder how my wounds will look like after recovery"), the condition of their hearts after surgery ("I'm worrying whether my heart will be overloaded in the ICU or not"), and the impact of preoperative and postoperative complications on their recovery. Other participants' worries were more general, encompassing the entire process of recovery, because they had other health problems:

"I'm worrying about my recovery since I've had diabetes for so many years."

Poor Quality of Care

Finally, 10% of the participants (*n* = 4) worried about the potential of receiving a poor quality of care from ICU nurses, either by being treated as "abnormal individuals," or because they anticipate that they themselves by their "bad mood" may trigger nurses' "bad temper." They pleaded, "Please do not treat me as an abnormal person when my mood is not good; I might behave like a person out of her mind."

"Experiencing a Mortal Fear" Type of Concerns

Thirty percent of the participants (*n* = 12) expressed the strongest degree of concern, "experiencing a mortal fear of" about dying, hospital experiences, and process of recovery during their admission transition. This determination is based on subjective and objective observations of the subjects throughout the interviews. These observations include terminology as well as visual and auditory signs of distress, such as tone of voice, facial expressions, tremors or shaking, sweating, and crying.

Death

Twenty-eight percent of the participants (*n* = 11) had a fear of death. For some, it was because they were having cardiac surgery for a second time. The intensity of their fear was evident in remarks such as, "I don't know what will happen this time; it is so frightening" and "I'm scared to death to have surgery again." The underlying cause of some participants' concern was the nature of cardiac surgery: "I'm very scared since this is open heart surgery. I don't want to know anything about the surgery and other things." For others, it was lack of knowledge about the surgery and the recovery process: "I'm scared to death since I don't know whether the surgery will be a success or not, and what would happen after the surgery. I know little about that. I wish I can [sic] learn more about that."

Hospital Experiences

The anticipated experiences in ICU provided a fertile field of concerns for 25% of the participants (*n* = 10). Some of them feared discomforts specific to the surgery, such as catching cold; having their hands tied up, later to become numb and painful; being unable to do anything; lying all day, unable to move; having tube insertions ("I feel it would be terrible to have so many tubes in my body"); being unable to talk; suctioning and having physical pain ("I have a great fear of pain"), or even feeling *Tong-Kou* ("If I feel very *Tong-Kou*, I would rather jump into a volcanic crater").

Some participants' fear was general, encompassing their overall discomfort in the ICU: "I'm so scared that I will have discomfort in the ICU" and "I'm very scared of *Jer-Mwo*" (Mandarin, meaning submitting to an ordeal; undergoing trials and afflictions). Participants' fear of expectant discomforts in the ICU appeared to be the result of reading the informational booklets ("I think it's terrible when I see the pictures that there would be tubes in my nose and mouth") and previous experiences ("I don't know if I can tolerate those pains in the ICU again this time.").

Process of Recovery

Eight participants (20%) had fears about their condition after surgery, such as the appearance of the scar or wound and complications. They feared that their wounds might be unsightly and that significant others, such as spouses or boyfriends, would be offended, which might adversely affect their relationships in the future. For example, one said, "He (her husband) doesn't say anything about this (the appearance of the wounds) now, but I fear that he might not like it in the future, and this concern really bothers me."

Uncertain Concerns

Finally, 10% of the participants (*n* = 4) described having concerns, but they could not be certain what specifically concerned them during the admission component of their recovery transition. Their responses were categorized as having a vague apprehension without specificity about what concerned them. Examples are "I don't know what I'm concerned about," "I don't know what I'm worrying about," and "I'm not sure what I'm scared of."

Coping Strategies Used to Manage Concerns

Participants were asked throughout their interview how they had managed to cope with their concerns or how they were planning to do so. Three strategies for coping emerged: person-focused efforts (50%), seeking help from others (30%), and turning to metaphysical resources (10%).

Coping by Use of Person-Focused Effort

The most frequently cited coping strategy was use of intrapersonal efforts, both cognitive and psychomotor. Fifty percent of the participants (n = 20) coped with concerns of security, such as death, the expectant discomfort, and the uncertainty about their condition on recovery through several cognitive efforts. These efforts included maintaining maximal preoperative health status, not thinking, thinking less, avoiding negative thinking, positive thinking, stoically tolerating pain, planning to grimace while in pain and being intubated, and letting go ("If the surgery failed, you [family members] should not feel upset; instead, I could go [leave the world] happily and *Huen-Huen-Duen-Duen* [Mandarin, meaning properly and securely; safely and soundly] without feeling any pain.").

Some participants reported that they made up their mind not to worry about the survival rate because they had no alternative to surgery. Others coped with their concerns of unfinished office responsibilities by anticipatory care and arranging their office work before their surgery. Some also said that they tried to use psychomotor behaviors to cope; they did simple exercises, such as daily walking and constant body movements, to enhance their physical strength for surgery.

Coping by Seeking Help From Others

Thirty percent of the participants (n = 12) sought help from others, such as family members, health professionals, and other patients. They coped by coaching their family members in taking care of unfinished business, such as teaching one's husband or sibling to "Cook the rice at home" and "Buy lunch and dinner from the cafeteria."

Others coped with the worries about the ICU experience, death, and condition on recovery by getting psychological support from their children (daughters), who talked to them in an encouraging and positive way, and from their parents (fathers), who gave them *Hong-Bou* (Mandarin, meaning red envelope containing money as a gift; red envelope of "good-luck money"). However, two female subjects (5%) addressed coping with the expectant pain in the ICU by asking their spouses to help terminate their lives if their condition became hopeless: "I asked my husband to turn the oxygen off if I were hopeless in the ICU."

Some participants' work roles and responsibilities were assumed by family members (siblings), who had the same occupation. Others received sick leave from their companies.

Another coping method was to ask for help from health care professionals, including nurses and doctors. Some participants coped with their concerns about maintaining daily activities, such as obtaining enough sleep, by suggesting that the nurses change their routines: postpone their daily visit from 5:00 a.m. to 6:00 a.m. Other participants coped with such concerns as awaiting surgery alone in the OR by asking the nurses on the floor unit to convey this concern to the OR head nurse to get permission to have their family members' company.

Still other participants informed the ICU nurses who visited them on the day before the surgery of their concerns regarding their worries about the ICU experience. They described their needs for protection from catching a cold, getting psychological support through a friendly attitude on the nurses' part, and asking for their toleration of the mood changes that they expect they may have. Some asked the doctors to prescribe pain medication for them when they needed it. Getting support from other patients, such as their roommates, was a useful strategy to cope with the concerns of some participants. An example of one patient's response is, "I chatted with my roommates, so I feel less fearful, and don't feel so lonely. They are very helpful."

Coping by Turning to Metaphysical Resources

Ten percent of subjects ($n = 4$) who particularly feared death described how they coped by turning to metaphysical resources, including gods and *Miah* (Taiwanese, meaning fate or destiny). They faced the uncertain future by trusting in gods, such as Jesus Christ or Buddha, or making a deal with their gods ("If my gods keep me in this world after the surgery, I will serve them in the future."). Some of them attributed the surgery's failure to another metaphysical factor, such as *Miah*, or God's will: "If the surgeon didn't perform a good surgery, it would be my *Miah*. Otherwise, what could I do?" and "If you [god] want to forgive me this time, you will save me by the doctors' hands. Otherwise, it will be the time for me to go and I will not have any regret about my life."

Absence of Concern

Four participants (10%) indicated that they did not have any concern on admission. Several reasons were offered for their lack of concern. First, for some subjects, their responsibilities had been fulfilled or covered with help from family members, relatives, and colleagues. The need to attend children was covered by help from family members and, with use of the bedside telephone in the hospital, participants were able to communicate with their children daily. Some had no children, whereas others had children who were grown and independent (children had finished college education, had jobs, or were married): "I no longer have family responsibilities since all three children (sons) are all independent," and "I have done my duties for them." Some participants' housekeeping role was also assumed by family members, as was the role as cook, which was temporarily taken over by relatives or was dealt with by family members cooking for themselves, buying meals, and eating out. Regarding office work, colleagues were a resource of support for other participants; the colleagues were willing to take over participants' office responsibilities.

Second, the needs of participants related to surgery have been met by various support resources. These needs include security, understanding surgery and the recovery process, how the medical instruments will be used on them, maintaining daily activities, maintaining optimal physical condition for surgery, and receiving quality treatment. Two Buddhists and one Christian valued their friends' help in providing spiritual support.

A third explanation for the lack of concern was subjects' confidence in the survival rate for the surgery. These participants had confidence in modern medical science. They also had confidence in their cardiac surgeon, because he had professional knowledge and good medical skills: "I trust in the cardiac surgeon's capabilities." Other participants' confidence in the survival rate was based on the available information as to the high survival rate for atrial septal defect surgery in Taiwan and for CABG in America, on the testimony of patients in other successful cases, and on the simplicity of surgery. As one participant said, "I think this is just a minor surgery. It won't affect my body."

The last reason was their expectation of optimal recovery from cardiac surgery. They expected to recover faster because they were young, or their preoperative physical strength was good. They also expected that their symptoms of cardiac disease would be improved or even totally disappear, and that they would be cured.

Discussion

Ninety percent of Taiwanese patients ($n = 36$) experienced certain concerns during the admission transition to cardiac surgery. From the least to the strongest, 52%, 43%, and 30% of the participants, respectively, reported experiencing three levels of

TABLE 7.6.5 What Taiwanese Patients Are Concerned About During the Admission Transition (n = 40)

	Cared about		Worried about		Feared		Total	
	n*	%	n*	%	n*	%	n*	%
Things concerned about	21	52	17	43	12	30	36	90
Process of recovery	21	52	7	18	8	20	36	90
Hospital experiences (including maintaining daily lives, expectant discomforts and disability in the ICU, and pain at admission)	14	35	12	30	10	25		
Death	13	33	10	25	11	28	34	86
The unfinished responsibilities and life goals, and significant people and places	20	50	16	40	0	0	0	90
Financial needs	0	0	9	23	0	0	9	23
Poor quality of care	0	0	8	20	0	0	8	20

* Each participant may have more than one response.

concerns. The components of their concerns identified in this study were process of recovery, hospital experiences, death, the unfinished responsibilities and life goals, significant persons and places, financial needs, and poor quality of care. The comparison of three levels of concerns shows that the most prevalent concerns, experienced by 90% of the participants and constantly appearing at all three levels of concerns, were process of recovery and hospital experiences (including maintaining daily activities, pain at admission, and expectant discomfort and disability in the ICU). The concern about death was also highly cited by the participants (86%) across three levels of concerns. The participants' unfinished business was the only kind of concern that appeared in the first two levels of concerns. Last, financial needs and poor quality of care were found to fall in the intermediate level (the second level) of concerns (Table 7.6.5). In addition, the aforementioned concerns were found to be commonly experienced by the subjects undergoing different types of cardiac surgeries including CABG, VRS, or ASD/VSD, although the risks for different types of cardiac surgeries would be different.

Although the components and the detailed issues of the patients' concerns revealed in this study were not identical to the Western data, the dimensions of the Taiwanese patients' concerns in this study were similar to those of the Western patients, except for the waiting itself.[23] The components and dimensions of the patients' concerns shared by both Western and Taiwanese patients were physical responses, such as postoperative discomforts; psychological responses, such as death; cognitive responses, such as knowledge deficit; and sociologic issues, such as financial needs.[4,11,12,15,23] However, the levels of Western patients' concerns, or the comparison across different levels of concerns (if they exist in the Western society), as well as the type of strategies that Western patients used to cope with their concerns during the admission transition to cardiac surgery, all seem not to have been well documented yet.

On the other hand, patients' concerns that were unique to Taiwanese patients seem to depend more on their daily basic functional activities, social roles such as the unfinished business, and their interactions with the critical care nurses. The three themes that emerged from the data help in understanding the context and the living experiences of Taiwanese patients' concerns and coping strategies during their admission transition to cardiac surgery. These three themes are being a person, resuming normality, and empowerment of self. We describe and discuss each of these.

Being a Person

Several Western patients' preoperative concerns about cardiac surgery have been identified, which include the waiting itself; the patient's physiologic, psychological, and cognitive responses; the treatment; and the cost-related sociologic issues.[4,11,12,15,23] It appears as though Western patients' preoperative concerns about cardiac surgery centered around the individual person and the surgery-related treatment or outcomes, rather than around a person's social roles and his or her interpersonal relationships.

Some scholars believe that the primary task of personhood for Chinese people is learning to be a person,[33-36] and most Taiwanese people are deeply influenced by the traditional Chinese culture.[9,10,34-38] Central to the concept of being a person are doctrines of role identification in the person himself or herself, family, and community (neighborhood), national, and universal levels, as well as the social relationships required to perform these roles. That is why some participants in this study addressed their concerns about the unfinished obligations to family members, friends, significant persons and places, and then job obligations to the company and country. However, because the family, rather than the individual, was identified by Taiwanese people as the basic unit of society, their primary task is to maintain the centrality of the family.[9,10,33-36] This value is evidenced by the fact that several Taiwanese subjects repeatedly expressed their concerns about unfinished responsibilities toward their nuclear and extended family members and relatives. Several male participants—valued in traditional Chinese culture as the ones responsible for family incomes—worried about their parents and children because their obligation to their families were interrupted, and their family income became inadequate as a result of the expenses for cardiac surgery and recovery. In addition, married female subjects, identified in traditional Chinese culture as the ones responsible for managing events within the family, cared for or worried about the maintenance of their daily lives and prospects for their spouse, children, and even grandchildren, although they themselves were facing an impending stressful event. However, although family makeup, birth order, sex, marital status, and parental health status were reported as factors that influence subjects' burdens, the relationship among these factors and the patient's perceived levels of concern needs further investigation.

The impact of cultural norms on Taiwanese patients' concerns about interpersonal relationship also can be seen in the patients' worry that possible conflicts with the critical care nurses may undermine the quality of their care. Because Chinese culture values interpersonal relationships,[9,10,36,38] most Taiwanese patients are sensitive to their relationships with health care providers, particularly when one expects his or her health condition to be more critical in the ICU ("My temper is bad, but I can control myself while things go smoothly; I mean when I'm not under stress. I need people to treat me good, but I worry that I may lose control if the critical care nurses' attitudes are not friendly, while I'm suffering discomforts in the ICU…although I know I need to be very careful about my relationship with the doctors and nurses there.").

Resuming Normality

Although waiting for cardiac surgery was in itself a major cause of stress,[7,35] most of the participants in this study expressed concerns across three levels about the management of their experiences or anticipated hospital experiences, such as pain at admission and various discomforts and disability in the ICU. In addition, 35% of the subjects cared about how to maintain their daily activities during hospitalization, including getting enough sleep and rest, nutrition, taking showers, buying personal items, and doing laundry in the hospital. Resuming normality is itself probably one of the realistic expectations for the people who are undergoing major stress from such an impending surgery.[7-9,14]

On the other hand, the expectation for resuming normality also provided plausible context for 63% of the participants who worried about their unfinished business or financial needs. This was because, without the benefit of resumption or improvement of their health condition, patients' expectations for resuming their unfinished business or having a better quality of life after cardiac surgery would be impossible.[8,9,14]

In addition, resuming normality was also probably one of the realistic strategies useful for some patients who were undergoing cardiac surgery,[7,8] although subjects did not name it as one of their coping strategies. Participants in this study came from areas throughout Taiwan, and most lived in an urban area. For most, this was the first time they stayed in such a complex metropolitan city as Taipei for a cardiac surgery, which was perceived as a life-threatening event by the majority of the participants across three levels of concerns. Resuming as many daily routine activities as possible could help subjects and their family members settle themselves down to concentrate on preparing for the impending surgery, and even further help in preparing subjects for recovery when they reentered the same floor unit from the ICU after surgery.

Empowerment of Self

In spite of experiencing multiple levels of preoperative concerns within the context of being a person and resuming normality, the participants empowered themselves by using human efforts, such as getting help from self and others and turning to metaphysical resources to cope with their concerns. The resources that Taiwanese participants used to empower themselves involved intra-, inter-, and extrapersonal (metaphysical) dimensions. Intrapersonal strategies include use of person-focused efforts, both cognitive and psychomotor. Taiwanese subjects empowered themselves by practicing not thinking, thinking less, avoiding negative thinking, thinking positively, stoically tolerating pain, and letting go. Some also said that they tried to use psychomotor behaviors to cope. For instance, they planned to grimace while in pain and while being intubated, and to make up their minds not to worry about the survival rate—because they had no alternative to surgery. Furthermore, they did simple exercises such as daily walks and constant body movements, to enhance or maintain their physical strength for surgery.

An interpersonal strategy that participants used to empower themselves was getting help from others. Participants reported seeking help from family members, friends, health care professionals, and other patients to manage their concerns about maintaining daily activities, unfinished family and job responsibilities, security, preoperative signs and symptoms, and condition on recovery.

Extrapersonal strategies that participants used to empower themselves to cope with the concern of security involved metaphysical resources, including culture, god or gods, and fate. Ten percent of the subjects conceived metaphysical power as another alternative to social support to help them cope with their concerns about death. Confucianism teaches that humans need to maintain a harmonic relationship with heaven. They are predestined by metaphysical factors, such as *Ten* (Mandarin, meaning heaven), to fulfill their mission on earth.[34] This is similar to some Western Christian beliefs. Confucians allow *Ten* or *Miah* to guide their lives, and believe that one who does not follow the guidance of fate will get lost on earth, and bad luck or disease may follow him or her.

The Taoist view of nature follows cyclic changes: birth and death, the onset of the seasons, the rhythm of night and day, and the waxing and waning of the moon. On a more esoteric level, the Taoist philosophy advocates *Wu-Wei* (meaning nonaction), detachment from the world, and allowing things to be. In other words, it is the philosophy of let it be.[34,36] Both Confucianism and Taoism regard heaven as the highest authority and proclaim the human being's total obedience to it. These beliefs provide a basis for understanding Taiwanese patients' needs for spiritual support during their admission transition to cardiac surgery.

The findings in this study also support these beliefs. What the Taiwanese participants feared the most during the admission transition was death, followed by the expected discomforts and disabilities in the ICU, and their condition on recovery, in that order. In managing the intense uncertainty of life or death, 10% of the participants turned to metaphysical powers, such as heaven and their gods, including Jesus Christ and Buddha and their ancestors, as their major coping mechanism to meet their security needs. They asked these metaphysical powers to protect them from bad luck, such as failed surgery and postsurgical complications, and to promote their recovery. They believed that human beings have no control over heaven's (God's) will. Nor should human beings question the result of surgery—to prevent bad luck caused by disobedience. That is why a female subject made a will to ask her family members to help terminate her life support if her health condition became hopeless after surgery. She believed that it would be useless to struggle for her fresh life if her gods do not intend to save her life through the surgeon's hands.

Another example is that, in addition to providing psychological support, the subjects' parents (who are acknowledged as the person's lifelong protector in Taiwanese society) planned to bring good luck to the subjects by giving the latter a symbolic blessing—*Hong-Bou*. The subjects' parents, and particularly elderly people, believe that by doing this, the subjects would be empowered, and the possibility of death, the expectant uncomfortable ICU experiences, and other negative conditions on recovery would, therefore, be decreased. This finding was also supported by White,[39] who proposed that the purpose and function of culture is to make life secured and enduring to people, which can be a valuable factor in providing physical, emotional, mental, social, and spiritual health to a cultural group. Most Taiwanese Buddhists believe that heaven can be touched by their sincerity, which they show by increasing intensity and frequency of worship and the numbers of gods worshiped.

In addition, some Buddhist participants also valued a person's will to suffer. They believed that if they can endure the physical or psychological *Tong-Kou*, they will be rewarded in the afterlife.[38] The significance of this kind of reward is proportional to the intensity of the *Tong-Kou* they had tolerated. Consistent with this belief, several participants still decided to undergo cardiac surgery, although they expected to suffer from a lot of physiologic and psychological *Tong-Kou*, particularly in the ICU stage, because most surgeons would not allow them to use pain medications for fear that the subjects' neurologic and pulmonary functions would be influenced by the pain medications. Therefore, the data from this study seem to support the impact of Taiwanese patients' belief in the presence of a sense of personhood, rooted in their cultural values and religion, on their concerns and coping strategies during their transition to cardiac surgery.

Conceptual Definitions of Patients' Concerns About Cardiac Surgery

Little research has discussed the definition of patients' concerns during their admission transition to cardiac surgery. The conceptual definitions of patients' concerns may now be tentatively modified as, "a single or multiple event(s) that usually consumes one's cognitive efforts, causes one's emotional responses, and may further interfere with one's biophysiological, psychological, cognitive, social, spiritual, or global functional well-being." One may experience it in the forms of, "caring or thinking about," "worrying about or being afraid of," or "experiencing a mortal fear of." The, "caring or thinking about" type of concerns disclosed in this project may be modified as, "the lowest level of concerns that consumes one's least cognitive efforts, and causes the least intense and significant impact on one's well-being." Likewise, the "worrying about or being afraid of" type of concerns may be modified as, "the middle level of concerns that consumes one's more cognitive efforts, and causes a stronger, intense, and significant impact on one's well-being." Last, the "experiencing a mortal fear of" type of concerns may be modified to tentatively indicate, "the strongest level of concerns that

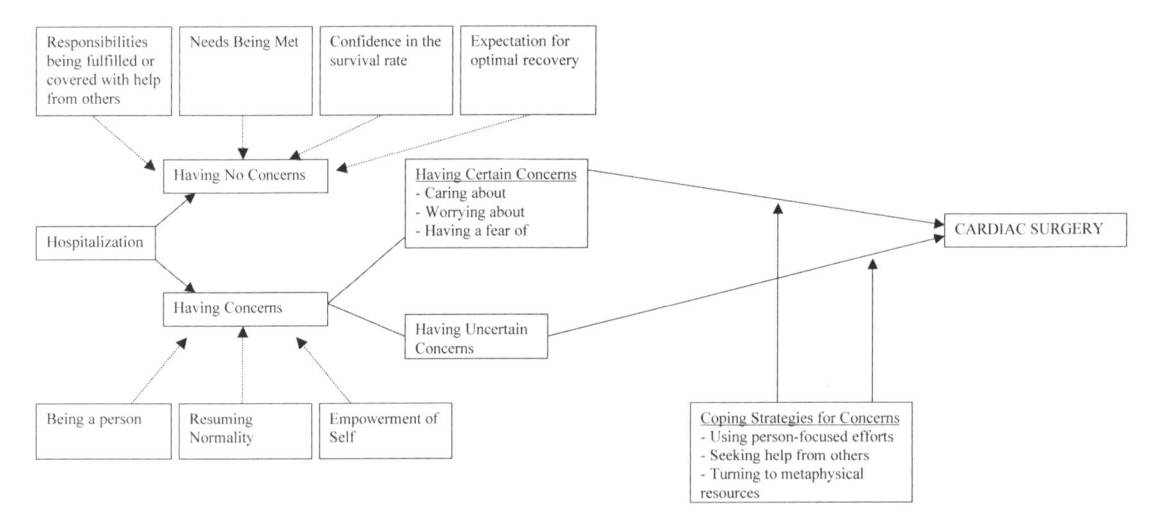

FIGURE 7.6.1 Conceptual framework of Taiwanese patients' perceptions of concerns during admission transition to cardiac surgery.

consumes one's cognitive efforts the most, and causes the most intense and significant impact on one's well-being." Finally, a conceptual framework (Figure 7.6.1) also has been drawn from the data to describe and depict this phenomenon.

Limitations and Implications

There are several limitations inherent in this study. First, the time for the interview data was not standardized. The subjects' perceptions of concerns about cardiac surgery were investigated based on a period of hospitalization ranging from 7 to 24 hours, depending on their readiness for the interview. In addition, the patients' preoperative hospitalization days fell into a range of 1 to 18 days, with a mean of 5.12 days. The patients' concerns may be different between those who were admitted to the hospital for 1 day, and those who had been hospitalized for a longer period.

Second, the representativeness of the sample was limited. This is because a purposive sample was used, and most of the subjects were from the middle or upper socioeconomic class, who had family caregivers with elective cardiac surgery and NYHA functional class less than IV. In addition, 20 patients failed to participate in the interview as a result of various preoperative signs and symptoms, or because of their family members' concerns about them losing energy during the interview process. Therefore, the findings in this study may be only directly applicable to the patients with the aforementioned characteristics, rather than being valid for all patients undergoing cardiac surgery; patients' preoperative concerns about cardiac surgery may differ for patients who are to undergo nonelective cardiac surgery, have poor ventricular function, come from a lower socioeconomic class, or lack a primary caregiver.

Third, because the data were collected and analyzed with the patients' perspective in mind, the difficulties in confirming the validity and totality of the data need to be addressed.

Because some participants may not report the whole story, or the background rationale for their concerns or lack of concerns, we have tried to lessen this drawback by confirming the patients' concerns with their primary nurses and caregivers. For example, 10% of the subjects reported having no concerns during the admission transition. This may be due to their conscious or unconscious use of a coping strategy such as denial or other considerations, in addition to the four rationales provided by them.

Fourth, the process of transcription, followed by translation from Chinese into English, and conducting data analysis based on the English version, may have resulted in some loss of meaning and accuracy.

Last, because the study was limited to one culture, valid cross-cultural comparisons cannot be made until the study is replicated in another culture. Nevertheless, because most Taiwanese people are deeply influenced by Chinese traditional culture, the findings in this study may be valuable for Western cardiovascular health care providers who have opportunities of caring for patients with Chinese beliefs of health.

Several suggestions for nursing clinicians and educators can be made based on the results of this study. First, nursing educators may incorporate the findings of this study into surgical cardiovascular nursing education programs for both nursing clinicians and students to help them better understand Chinese patients' subjective concerns during the admission transition to cardiac surgery. Nursing diagnosis, nursing care plans, and different strategies aimed at exploring patients' concerns, helping them to address and cope with their concerns while waiting for an impending major surgery, such as cardiac surgery, may also be developed further.

Second, nurses on the floor unit should be aware of the components, levels, and background context of their Chinese patients' concerns about cardiac surgery. If the patients report being under a lot of stress awaiting surgery alone in the OR, the nurses on the floor unit may help convey their clients' concerns to the OR nurses. It is suggested that Taiwanese patients, particularly the elderly, should not be left alone. Instead, the OR nurses may take the initiative to comfort the patients, or encourage the patients' family members or friends, if present, to provide verbal, as well as nonverbal, support for the patients during this critical transition.

Third, for the patients who are concerned about maintaining daily activities, such as being unable to follow hospital routines and having difficulties in overnight sleep, particularly in the first few days after hospitalization, the nurses on the floor unit may postpone their first daily visit to 6:00 a.m., or help arrange daily activities to allow their Chinese patients to take a nap during the daytime, and instruct them to do so.

Fourth, because concerns about condition on recovery are pervasive in three levels of concerns, Taiwanese subjects in this project seemed to lack knowledge of the whole picture of their health status. Nurses may do preoperative teaching based on the knowledge of patients' concerns about recovery from cardiac surgery. Subjects in this study seemed to want more information about the influence of preoperative signs or symptoms on their recovery process, survival, normality of the recovery process, the expectant discomforts and disability while in the ICU, and the resumption of their social roles. By having this information, patients will better understand their recovery process and be prepared for cardiac surgery. The related intensity or frequency of their preoperative concerns may, therefore, be lessened.

Fifth, findings of this study may sensitize the nurses on the floor unit and ICU to more precisely evaluate their Chinese clients' concerns about cardiac surgery and recovery process, and provide more effective nursing interventions to manage events or conditions that might have a negative impact on patient's concerns during the admission transition. For example, for subjects who are concerned about the postoperative ICU experience or worried about possible conflicts with critical care nurses, it is suggested that nurses on the floor unit take the initiative to convey the patients' concerns to the critical care nurses or arrange for the patients to have a preoperative ICU visit. By doing this, patients may have a clearer picture of the physical environment and the rationale of the nursing interventions in the ICU. This visit may also provide the patients with opportunities for direct verbal communication with the ICU nurses. During that time, patients have not been intubated or sedated yet, and are possibly better able to address their concerns more precisely to the critical care nurses. Both Chinese patients and critical care nurses may clarify their mutual concerns through direct communication before the surgery. As a result, not only is unnecessary misunderstanding between them avoided, but also the unpleasant sense of an inhuman physical environment and unfamiliarity with the hectic pace of critical care nursing may be decreased.

Nurses need to be aware that most Chinese patients, particularly the elderly, value the psychological support that a friendly attitude on the nurses' part conveys; they ask for the nurses' toleration of the mood changes that they expect to have as a result of their condition. If trusting and respectful relationships with health care providers are established, Taiwanese patients would possibly be encouraged to express their thoughts, feelings, and needs during the recovery process. Therefore, not only would their actual concerns and needs be more accurately assessed, but also their concerns about conflicts with nurses may possibly be prevented or managed.

Sixth, nurses on the floor unit or critical care nurses may take the initiative to discuss with Chinese patients the options of pain control. If the pain medication is legitimate for the patients after surgery, nurses may acknowledge this to their Chinese clients in advance, and teach them how to express their concerns about pain and needs for pain control with some easily learned hand motions.

Last, because some subjects cited getting support from family members and other patients as a useful strategy for coping with the concerns of death, nurses on the floor unit and ICU should allow companionship from the patients' significant others, and encourage other patients who have successfully undergone cardiac surgery to visit the patients who have a mortal fear for their security before the surgery or in the ICU.

Future researchers are encouraged to explore further the level, components, and nature of certain and uncertain concerns across various recovery transitions; the impact of patients' age, sex, family makeup, birth order, marital status, parental health status, religious affiliations, preoperative hospitalization days, and type of surgery on the severity of their concerns or the options and effectiveness of their coping strategies; the comparison of the severity of patients' concerns across various recovery transitions; the impact of patients' subjective concerns and coping strategies on their postoperative outcomes, such as degree of recovery, activity levels, and use of pain medication; the comparison of the effectiveness of the nursing interventions in managing different levels of patients' concerns across recovery transition, the background context for Western patients' concerns and coping strategies; and the comparison of background context for both Western and Chinese patients' concerns and coping strategies during various recovery transitions. The proposed conceptual definitions and framework also requires further validation. Finally, determining reliable indicators and carefully recording patients' concerns and related effective nursing interventions during different recovery stages also deserve attention.

REFERENCES

1. Department of Health. The table of the twenty leading causes of mortality in Taiwan (in Chinese). Taipei (Taiwan): Department of Health; 1994.
2. Hu, YH. The exploration of variation in health related to gender in Taiwan [in Chinese]. Proceedings of the Conference on Women and Health. Taipei (Taiwan): Population Studies Center, National Taiwan University and Department of Health Ministry of Education; 1990 June 1-3.
3. American Heart Association. Heart and stroke facts. Dallas (TX): American Heart Association; 1991.
4. Bresser, PJ, Sexton, DL, Foell, DW. Patients' responses to postponement of coronary artery bypass graft surgery. Image J Nurs Sch 1993;25:5-10.
5. Gortner, SR, Gilliss, CL, Moran, L, Sparacino, P, Kenneth, H. Expected and realized benefits of coronary bypass in relation to severity of illness. J Cardiovasc Nurs 1985;21:13-18.
6. Gortner, SR, Jaeger, AA, Harr, J, Miller, T. Elders' expected and realized benefits from cardiac surgery, J Cardiovasc Nurs 1994;30:9-15.
7. Shih, FJ. Taiwanese patients' expectations for recovery from cardiac surgery during admission transition. NAROC Nurs Res 1995:3:309-322.
8. Shih, FJ. Patients' needs and their coping strategies: transition to cardiac surgery. Kaohsiung J Med Sci 1996;12:114-127.

9. Shih, FJ. The experiences of Taiwanese patients during recovery transitions from cardiac surgery [dissertation]. Ann Arbor: University of Michigan; 1995.
10. Shih, FJ. Perception of self in the intensive care unit after cardiac surgery. Int J Nurs Stud 1997;34:17-26.
11. Bradley, KM, Williams, DM. A comparison of the preoperative concerns of open heart surgery patients and their significant others. J Cardiovasc Nurs 1990;5:43-53.
12. Carr, JA, Powers, MJ. Stressors associated with coronary bypass surgery. Nurs Res 1986:35:243-246.
13. Cozac, J. The spouse's response to coronary artery bypass graft surgery. Crit Care Nurs 1988;8:65-71.
14. Hwang, SL, Lin, BG, Liou, MG, Chang, E, Hwang, SF. Stressors associated with heart surgery—a follow up and comparison study of patients' and nurses' perceptions of pre- and post-heart surgery stressors [in Chinese]. NAROC Nurs Res 1994;2:17-27.
15. King, KB. Measurement of coping strategies, concerns and emotional response in patients undergoing coronary artery bypass grafting. Heart Lung 1985;14:145-150.
16. Quinless, R, Cassese, M, Atherton, N. The effects of selected preoperative, intraoperative, and postoperative variables on the development of postcardiotomy psychosis on patients undergoing open heart surgery. Heart Lung 1985; 14:324-341.
17. Rahimtoola, SH, Grunkemeier, GL, Starr, A. Ten year survival after coronary bypass surgery for angina in patients aged 65 years and older. Circulation 1986;74:509-517.
18. Gregersen, RA, McGregor, MS. Cardiac surgery. In: Underhill, SL, Woods, SL, Froelicher, ESS, Halpenny, CJ, editors. Cardiac nursing. Philadelphia: JB Lippincott; 1989. 537-560.
19. Hole, J., Forfang, K. Arrhythmias and conduction disturbances following aortic valve implantation. Scand J Thorac Cardiovasc Surg 1980;14:177-183.
20. Kern, LS. Advances in the surgical treatment of coronary artery disease. J Cardiovasc Nurs 1986:1:1-14.
21. Kern, LS, Norris, SO, Constancia, P. Coronary bypass grafting. In: Riegel B, Ehrenreich D, editors. Psychological aspects of critical care. Rockville (MD): Aspen; 1989. 150-170.
22. Kirklin, JW, Kouchoukos, NT, Blackstone, EH, Oberman, A. Research related to surgical treatment of coronary artery disease. Circulation 1979: 60:1613-1618.
23. Rakoczy, M. The thoughts and feelings of patients in the waiting period prior to cardiac surgery: a descriptive study. Heart Lung 1977;6:280-286.
24. Patton, MQ. Qualitative evaluation method. Newbury Park (CA): Sage; 1980. 44-45,306-329.
25. Emerson, R, Pollner, M. On the use of members' respondents to researchers' accounts. Human Organization 1983:47:189-198.
26. Lincoln, YS, Guba, EG. Naturalistic inquiry. Beverly Hills (CA): Sage; 1985. 281-331.
27. Sandelowski, M. The problem of rigor in qualitative research. ANS 1986;8:27-37.
28. Hammersley, M, Atkinson, P. Ethnography principles in practice. New York: Routledge; 1990. 195-200.
29. Woods, NF, Catanzaro, M. Nursing research theory and practice. St. Louis (MO): CV Mosby; 1988.
30. Katz, J. A theory of qualitative methodology: the social system of analytic framework. In: Emerson, RM, editor. Contemporary field research—a collection of readings. Prospect Heights (IL): Waveland; 1983. 127-148.
31. Strauss, A, Corbin, J. Basics of qualitative research—grounded theory procedures and techniques. Newbury Park (CA): Sage; 1990.
32. Fielding, NG, Fielding, JL. Linking data: the articulation of qualitative and quantitative methods in social research. Beverly Hills (CA): Sage; 1986. 41-53.
33. Chen-Louie, T. Nursing care of Chinese American patients. In: Orque MS, Bloch B, Monrroy LSA, editors. Ethics in nursing care: a multicultural approach. St. Louis (MO): CV Mosby; 1983. 183-218.
34. Redfield, R. The primitive world and its transformation. Ithaca (NY): Cornell University Press; 1953.
35. Yang, LS. The concept of Pao as a basis for social relations in China. In: Fairbank, JK, editor. Chinese thought and institutions. Chicago (IL): University of Chicago Press; 1967. 290-309.
36. Shih, FJ. Concepts related to Chinese patients' perceptions of health, illness and person: issues of conceptual clarity. Accid Emerg Nurs 1996:4:208-215.
37. Teng, JE. Religion as a source of oppression of creativity for Chinese women [in Chinese]. I Women Gender Stud 1990:1:165-194.
38. Kleinman, A, Lin, TY. Normal and abnormal behavior in Chinese culture. Boston: Reidel; 1981
39. White, LA. The evolution of culture. New York: McGraw-Hill; 1958.

Reprinted with permission from: Shih, F. J., Meleis, A. I., Yu, P. J., Hu, W. Y., Lou, M. F., & Huang, G. S. (1998). Taiwanese patients' concerns and coping strategies: Transitions to cardiac surgery. *Heart and Lung, 27*(2), 82–98.

7.7 SUFFERING IN SILENCE: THE EXPERIENCE OF EARLY MEMORY LOSS

PETRA ROBINSON
SIRKKA-LIISA EKMAN
AFAF IBRAHIM MELEIS
BENGT WINBLAD
LARS-OLOF WAHLUND

Abstract

This chapter presents the early experience of memory loss among eight individuals who were assessed clinically by a comprehensive memory evaluation because of a perceived gradual loss of memory. A qualitative approach was used, based on interview data, in order to understand and describe the situation from the sufferer's perspective. The findings demonstrate how a patterned sequence of unfolding stages was identified in the interview data, through which the participants moved before seeking professional help, revealing the overall concept of "suffering in silence." These stages included experiencing forgetfulness, a recognition that "something is wrong," and a search for meaning. During the process of seeking help, strategies were used to compensate for the memory loss, to maintain a sense of competence, and to prevent others from recognizing their difficulties. Because stages of memory loss in patients with a dementia disease have mainly been described from a medicopathological perspective, the focus of this study was shifted toward understanding the subjective experiences of persons confronting early memory loss.

Introduction

It has often been described how persons with a dementia disease are aware of their cognitive decline, and complain of symptoms clearly related to cognitive impairment early in the course of their illness (McCormick et al., 1994; Jonker et al., 1996). Subjective memory complaints should therefore not be neglected, but should rather be considered a promising indicator of memory impairment that signals the need for further evaluation of cognitive function. Taking into consideration the fact that tests for subtle memory impairment may be insensitive in identifying any objective decline early in the course of a dementia disease (Kurz et al., 1990), it may be suspected that persons with memory complaints who do not meet rigorous criteria for dementia have what has been referred to as a "subclinicar dementing" illness (Morris & Fulling, 1988) or a "preclinical phase" of dementia, sometimes extending over several years before it is diagnosed (Linn et al., 1995).

Because most current research on early-stage dementia has taken place primarily from a biological and pathological perspective, focusing on identifying diagnostic markers, the subjective experiences of those persons have until now been largely overlooked (Cotrell & Lein, 1993; Cotrell & Schulz, 1993; Bahro et al., 1995). The disease process in persons with early-onset dementia has, therefore, rarely been described, and the literature on the needs of these sufferers and their carers is equally sparse (Williams et al., 1995). Recognizing that there is an absence of information from the patients themselves, especially the younger ones, epidemiological studies need to be accompanied by research that aims specifically at highlighting the experiences of persons suffering from early-onset dementia and includes persons who may be in a preclinical phase of a dementia disease.

To learn more about the life situations of our clients and how they perceive their increasing memory loss, the focus of research on dementia has to be shifted toward the lived situations of those persons, and be grounded in the first-hand experiences of the person afflicted.

Furthermore, this form of understanding may come to play a crucial part in future dementia care, as it is most likely to provide information and assist health care professionals in the development of meaningful interventions that correspond to the specific needs of our clients during the early phase of memory loss.

Memory Loss as a Transition

When a disease process occurs over time with a movement toward greater complexity in the disease and the illness experience, and with changes that create more disruptions in the person's life, it may be more useful to consider it within a transition framework (Meleis & Tangenstein, 1994). By shifting the focus from the disease as an event to the experiences of the person who has the disease over time and the responses of people during these transitions, there is a greater potential for a better understanding of the nature of the experience as a whole. Considering each phase as part of a larger transition experience may be the key for interpreting the progressive impact of the illness experience on the life of the client.

The transition is a familiar concept in developmental and adaptation theories. It accommodates both the continuities and the discontinuities in the life processes of human beings (Chick & Meleis, 1986). A transition is defined as the passage from one life phase, condition, or status to another, involving elements of process, disconnectedness, perception, and patterns of response (Golan, 1981). It denotes a process of changes in health status, in role relations, in expectations, or in abilities (Meleis, 1991). In some transitions, there is an identifiable event associated with the process, such as the diagnosis of an illness or the loss of a job, whereas in other transitions such as gradual memory loss, specific marker events may not be as evident (Bridges, 1980, 1991). Considering the transition as a process suggests phases and sequence, and involves both the disruptions that the transition creates and the person's responses to this experience.

For the purpose of this study, the transition has been used as a framework for a better understanding of the experiences of participants who are confronted with early memory loss. Using a transitional framework makes it possible to describe the situation of participants as they begin to experience memory loss more specifically, even though a new state of stability may not be reached. The aim of this chapter is then to describe the experience of early memory loss and the transition toward seeking professional help among patients who requested treatment because of a perceived gradual loss of memory.

Methodology

This study is the first part of a larger ongoing longitudinal study in which eight persons with early symptoms of memory loss have been assessed clinically and followed up by interviews over a period of two years. The study is designed to capture the early experience of memory loss from the perspective of the person afflicted, and is being conducted in Sweden at a major university medical center in the Greater Stockholm area.

Description of Clinical Assessment

The memory clinic is a unit for examining inpatients for memory impairment and suspected dementia, in which the purpose of the examination is to make a reliable diagnosis. A workup consisting of a detailed physical examination, including medical history, Mini Mental State Examination (MMSE) (Folstein et al., 1975), neurological examination, routine blood and lumbar puncture tests, computed tomographic scan, single photon-emission computed tomographic scan, electroencephalography, and electrocardiography, is conducted over a two-week period. The examination also includes a comprehensive neuropsychological diagnostic test battery and an occupational, physiotherapeutic, and verbal assessment. Following the *DSM-III-R* diagnostic criteria (American Psychiatric Association, 1987) and the guidelines outlined by NINCDS–ADRDA (National Institute of Neurological and Communicative Disorders and Stroke, and the Alzheimer's Disease and Related Disorders Association) (McKhann et al., 1984), a consensus diagnosis is reached between the members of the interdisciplinary team.

Permission to carry out the study was received from the Committee for Ethical Research, Karolinska Institute, and from the Swedish Computer Inspection Board.

Participants

The first eight individuals who entered the clinic for their initial medical consultation were identified by a geriatric specialist and assessed clinically by a comprehensive memory evaluation for suspected dementia. The criteria for the inclusion of participants in the study were being under 65 years of age and reporting symptoms of early memory loss that had interfered with daily functioning for more than six months, but not having a diagnosis of dementia (see Table 7.7.1 for patient characteristics). All the participants were responsible for initiating their referral to the clinic, although their decisions were mostly supported by their spouses. One of the authors (P.R.) approached the participants on the first day of their designated memory examination. She introduced the study, invited them to participate, and gave them consent information. As informed consent was obtained verbally from all participants, an appointment was made for the interview at a convenient time for each person.

Method of Data Collection

During the time of data collection, none of the participants had yet been diagnosed as having a dementia disease. A semistructured interview guide was used, which centered on certain themes, although it allowed the participants freedom to speak about their situations and experiences. The guide was designed to capture the experiences of participants as far back as they could remember. During the interview, they were encouraged to describe their own experiences, feelings, and thoughts, as well as their reactions and responses. Interviews were carried out without any distractions or time pressure, in a separate room apart from the ward. All the interviews took place during the first few days of their memory investigation. They were audiotaped, lasted for an average of 2 hours, and yielded 400 pages of transcribed computer text. All the interviews were completed and transcribed by the same person (P.R.).

Method of Data Analysis

The interviews were analyzed using a phenomenological hermeneutic approach inspired by Ricoeur's philosophy (1971, 1976; cf. Ekman et al., 1993; Jansson et al., 1993). Data analyses were performed in a series of steps. First, all the interviews were read "naively," in order to acquire a sense of the whole. Then, an open structural analysis was performed to identify the themes in each interview, searching for words or phrases that captured the meaning in each transcript relating to their experiences of memory loss. This meant that sequences of the interviews not related to their memory loss were left out of the analyses in this study. The themes were contrasted for similarities and differences between the eight persons, in order to allow overall themes to emerge. The relationship between the themes began to emerge from the data, showing the process of experiencing memory loss. These themes were then again confirmed within the context of each interview. The main themes emerging from the open structural analyses were: (a) an awareness that there was something wrong, with a strong perception of subtle changes over time, which were affecting their personality, work, and daily activities; and (b) patterns of responses with the underlying themes of reactions and responses, efforts made to prevent others from recognizing their situation, and the decision to seek professional help.

Because the emerging themes showed a movement over time, from a state of stability toward a more disrupted reality through different phases, the concept of transition was chosen as the framework

TABLE 7.7.1 Clinical Data on Participants

Patient no.	Age (years)	Sex	MMSE	Diagnosis 1	Diagnosis 2
1	56	M	29/30	S	S
2	63	F	30/30	S	S
3	53	F	27/30	S	S
4	55	M	24/30	AD	AD
5	64	F	26/30	O	AD
6	49	M	27/30	S	S
7	59	F	26/30	O	O
8	61	F	28/30	O	O

MMSE (Folstein et al., 1975) is a widely used screening scale of mental function in patients with dementia, with scores ranging from 0 to 30. A score below 24 is considered to indicate a possible mild dementia, scores below 18 a moderate dementia, and scores below 10 a severe dementia.

Diagnosis 1 is the diagnosis made from the first clinical examination and diagnosis 2 is made at a follow-up examination 6–12 months later, following the *DSM-III-R* and NINCDS-ADRDA criteria. No other confounding diseases were found during the time of examination.

S = Subjective memory disturbances: the person reports experiences of subjective memory disturbances; however, no objective evidence that confirms any cognitive decline could be found through neuropsychological testing.

AD = Alzheimer's disease: presence of objectively verified signs that meet criteria for diagnosis.

O = Objective memory disturbances: presence of objective signs that confirm cognitive decline but do not fulfill diagnostic criteria for dementia.

for continuing analyses. To understand better the relationship between the themes, a second structural analysis was performed within the concept of transition. Finally, all the data were brought together, looked at as a whole again, and reflected upon with the account of the naive reading and the structural analyses within the context of early memory loss.

Results and Comments

"Suffering in silence" was identified as the overall organizing theme. The participants' suffering was characterized by subthemes that were understood as a three-stage process of forgetfulness, a recognition that "something is wrong" and a search for meaning (see Figure 7.7.1). These provided a structure for their movement through three stages before they decided to seek professional help. As they moved through these stages, it became clear that the participants developed and used different strategies to deal with the consequences of their memory loss. These strategies were labeled normalizing, watching and analyzing, and avoiding and vigilance.

Similar patterns of unfolding stages were uncovered in all interviews. They are not distinct or mutually exclusive, unfolding in a passage from one stage to another over time, although it is not claimed that this sequence is invariable. It does, however, provide a framework for understanding the experiences and responses of our clients. These stages involve in-between periods, serving as specific milestones for entering the next stage. These in-between periods were characterized by a spill-over from two stages as a sense of lack of ability to manage their situation emerged, followed by attempts to develop new strategies for achieving a sense of stability.

The time span ranged from one to five years of subtle but increasing changes, reflecting the progress of their difficulties. The stages, in-between periods, and strategies developed are, in context, an overall feeling of agonized suffering, which, in general, they kept to themselves, accompanied by feelings of uncertainty and unsettlement. They also perceived themselves as constantly making efforts to maintain their self-competence in managing their lives and to prevent others from becoming aware of their situation. Each stage includes the participants' experiences and the challenges they encountered during that stage. The stages will be presented sequentially, in order to capture the process of movement from one phase to another over time, re-

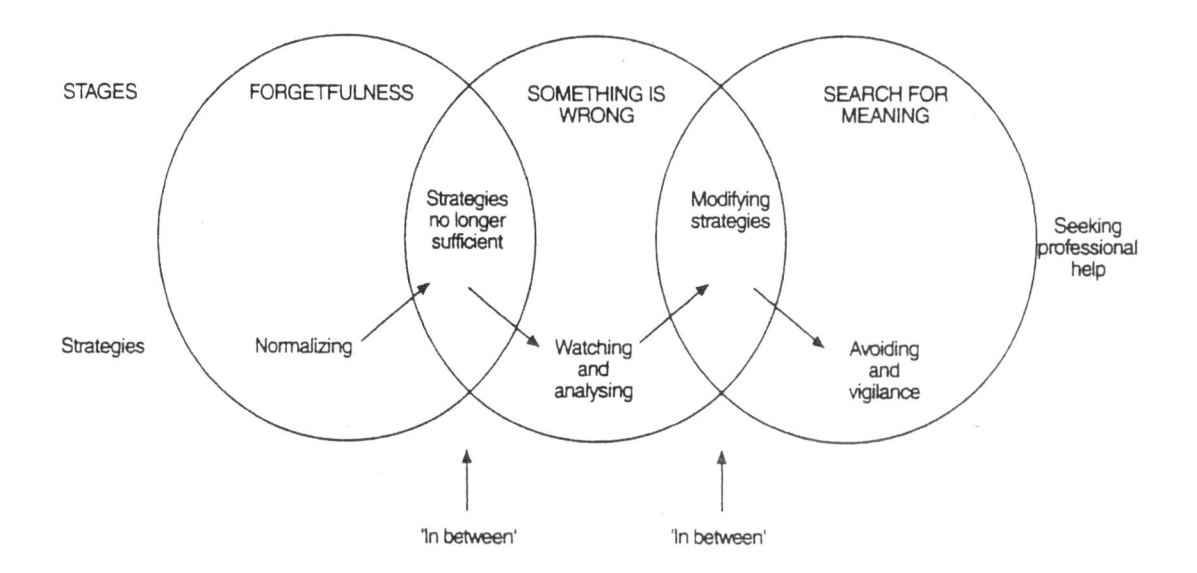

FIGURE 7.7.1 The transition of persons with early memory loss toward seeking professional help: stages and strategies.

flecting the nature of the phases and the participants' responses to this change.

Forgetfulness

Participants described how they realized over time that they were experiencing many episodes of forgetfulness. Although they were not able to pinpoint the exact time or the beginning of forgetfulness, retrospectively they were able to describe an increasing awareness and discomfort about forgetting appointments, and difficulty in remembering names, phone numbers, and faces. Others described how the "right word" eluded them, how figures frustrated them, and how they approached counting with trepidation. One patient described how he had difficulties in finding words to express himself and how he felt his verbal ability was diminished: "I have previously been very verbal, and now it does not work very well...you have to concentrate really hard when you are to speak with people...trying to figure out how to express yourself."

They often felt that they could not concentrate on tasks at home, and they were aware and distressed about their occasional inability to remain focused and concentrated. One participant described it this way: "I have problems concentrating...as I am doing something and all of a sudden I find myself doing something else."

Strategy for Normalizing

Early on during this stage, there was a tendency to discount and normalize what was happening to them. They described how they discounted their forgetfulness by laughing at themselves or by finding more flexible explanations for their experiences. They explained to themselves that their difficulties were caused by stress, age, or fatigue. One man thought of his problems as "a temporary blackout," so there was no good reason to start worrying or to become overly concerned.

Memory notes were frequently used by all participants, writing down appointments in calendars and keeping notebooks in strategic places around their house or at work. However, although these strategies worked for a period of time, their effectiveness slowly began to decrease. They wrote memory notes but then began to forget what they had written down, as well as where they had placed their memory notes. One woman tells of her experience:

"I keep notes of everything, but the worst thing is that when I have written it up, then I don't know where I wrote it and where I put the note. I might remember I wrote it down, but I don't know where, so there is just a big chaos anyway."

Moving from this stage into the next begins when their efforts to keep themselves functioning as normally as possible are no longer sufficient to prevent them from normalizing what is happening to them.

Something Is Wrong

Being unable to continue to normalize what is happening to them leaves the participants with a feeling that something is wrong. It is during this stage that their awareness that there is something wrong becomes more dominant in their lives. Sometimes they mentioned specific incidents at work or at home that made them realize and acknowledge the extent of their problems. One woman describes such an incident:

"I had been shopping and forgot my groceries in the store, and I didn't realize that, I didn't even realize as I came home or when I got to the car, and then I actually started wondering about myself."

Everyday surroundings may no longer be familiar to them. Some participants told of their difficulties in finding their way in well-known surroundings. One woman described how she could not find her way to the laundry room in her house. She said, "I didn't know what door led to the laundry room." One man told of how he had difficulties in finding his way to old customers whom he usually visits on his job.

Other problems were manifested in difficulties in concentrating and organizing their work, a resistance to starting new projects, and not being able to solve problems and deal with complex situations as they previously used to be able to do. They had difficulties in adapting to new routines and taking an active part in discussions.

Their experiences are no longer random or isolated incidents in their lives, which serve to raise feelings of fear and frustration. They describe the continuity, the progress, the intensity, and the pervasiveness of their suffering. One participant described how she felt about herself during this stage:

"I think it is getting worse and worse, for every day at work, like when I forget different things…it's so despairing because all of a sudden as I am working in the reception, they hand me the money and their card and I don't know what to do with it, it just disappears and it feels so embarrassing to me…so now I'm scared to death every day when I go to work…and I start crying. I am someone who usually never cries, so there is something that is not right."

During this stage, participants had an incipient sense of losing control over their own lives. They experience frustration, as they no longer feel that they are able to influence what is happening to them. They feel embarrassed when they are with other people; sometimes, they panic or are blocked when confronting situations in which they feel unsafe and unsure of themselves. One man told of how he became blocked when he confronted situations in which he had to deal with figures: "I get blocked almost immediately; there is some feeling of panicking." Another participant described her feelings as she began realizing that something was wrong:

"I have difficulties talking to other people. I am scared when I meet my neighbors. I say, 'Hello,' and walk away, as I think, 'My goodness, are they going to talk to me?' Because all of a sudden, as we stand there talking, I have lost what we are talking about and it feels so damn hard."

As their forgetfulness increases and as previously used strategies are no longer sufficient, they begin to watch out for other signs in their lives, behaviors, and environments, searching for other signs of deterioration and of reactions to such deterioration.

Strategy of Watching and Analyzing

They now start to pay more careful attention to their daily lives. In order to better understand the nature of their experiences, they begin to gather more information and data on how they are functioning. This means that they are becoming more sensitive and reflective about their own actions and abilities. Learning more about the consequences of their problems, their experiences now begin to take shape and form. One man noticed how this has made him perceive how there has been a change in him, saying that:

"There is this difference, though, of how I used to function and how I am functioning today. Before, I used to think that I just had some sort of temporary blackouts, but now I know that this is how it really is."

One participant describes how her own observations made her more aware of her increasing difficulties; she says that:

"Now there is a chaos in more areas than just one, I cannot put myself together and come up with decisions of what to do, what to do with things. I don't know what to do."

A large part of the information they gather comes from their work settings, where they feel that they can no longer meet their own and others' expectations. One man describes how he experiences a change and how this change is being confirmed by other people's reactions; he says that:

"I have always been the one who was full of ideas. It might be an overstatement to say that nothing works but...when I have an idea I decide that I will get started working with it on Monday and even though I don't get started, I still believe that I will...it is just the same thing when we are having meetings where we sit down and discuss how to plan for this week or month, and I grab those things that I think might be perfect for me. But as the meeting is over and I go into my room to start out, one feels that, damn, I can't do this either...and I can note this when assignments are being passed right over me, where there would have been no question whether they would have been mine before."

Now that their problems begin to take more shape and form, this serves to bring with it a deep concern for their future and their ability to manage their work if their problems become more severe. Thinking about his working situation, one man tells of how he feels; he says that "It can't be that you are part of a working team without things functioning. This could only last for a while when they still hope that one is able to come back to something workable," and one woman says that "I just can't keep up work if my problem continues. There is no question about that." As participants are becoming more reflective about their experiences, this stage is understood to bring with it feelings of constant worry and pervasive uncertainty, which serves to initiate the next stage, with a need to ascribe some meaning to their experiences.

Search for Meaning

As their faith in how well they have been able to normalize and hide their problems begins to waver, they begin to search for different explanations and meanings for their problems. Participants described how the well-formulated framework for understanding and managing forgetfulness begins to unravel, leaving them with an absence of meaning. One participant describes his feelings: "I don't know where this comes from. Maybe it is something hereditary, or something mixed."

They go through different processes, searching for an explanation. Some of them compare themselves with a parent who became demented, noticing some similarities. One participant tells of his way of reasoning: "Well, that's true, even if I don't walk around thinking about it, it is hard for me not to think about how my mother had almost exactly the same onset." Another woman describes her feelings, saying that, "There are days when you see those things more and more often, and it makes you so scared. Then I wonder if I will become the same" (as her mother who had dementia). Some compared their responses frequently with how they had responded to situations previously. They search for comparisons in the hope of finding no differences. One participant described how he searched for differences: "There is a difference, though, from how one was before and how one is today and the only one I can compare with is myself. I can never compare with any other person, how they used to function."

As their own efforts to find an explanation no longer provide them with a way to normalize their forgetfulness, and as new events and actions continue to confirm for them that something is wrong, they begin to see the need for help from others to provide an explanation for their situation. Before deciding to seek help, they struggle with feelings of fear and hopefulness about what may be the result of their search for an explanation. Whereas they first experience a sense of relief at having an opportunity to disclose what they are experiencing after suffering in silence and struggling on their own for a long period of time, they also approach this help opportunity with fear and trepidation about the results.

Participants also described how this milestone of seeking professional help made them pay more careful attention to their daily lives, and how they more consistently began to avoid situations in which they felt vulnerable and exposed to others.

Strategy of Avoiding and Vigilance

From paying more attention to their situation, watching, and analyzing, they now tend to be more vigilant in observing themselves and their environment, while they are constantly struggling to keep the situation under control. They constantly appraise situations, trying to decide whether to avoid them or to design a new way to deal with them. They describe how they feel off balance, as situations have dimensions that appear new to them, and they perceive that they no longer have the self-assurance to meet these situations. They then begin to search for new strategies, mainly to prevent others from discovering the change in them. They deliberately avoid situations and hide from other people because they feel unsure and vulnerable. This results in feelings that they are becoming more and more isolated, and that their world is becoming smaller as a result of their efforts to keep their problems from being recognized by other people. This statement describes one woman's experience:

> Somehow I feel how my world is shrinking...it feels distressing having too many contacts. I don't know whether I have introduced myself or not, what I said and did not say, you see...I don't know what I'm saying.

Other examples are given of how they have problems in finding words to express themselves; many of them who used to be verbal now dread situations in which they have to depend on their memories and their verbal abilities. One man talks about how he previously enjoyed making speeches to hundreds of people: "The more they asked, the more warmed up I got. This is not how it is today; today you rather want there not to be a lecture at all."

Participants described how their confidence in their own abilities was disappearing over time. More and more, even pleasurable situations were being avoided, as they felt that they had continuously to work on developing new patterns of responses, using more time and energy to cope with the new demands. More time was spent on completing activities or tasks to meet their and others' goals. This meant that they needed their weekends and their free time to supplement their working hours. Using time off to complete work that they used to complete during regular working hours was also a strategy to keep others from discovering their difficulties or problems. Participants checked and rechecked their tasks and their work for accuracy and completion, and seldom trusted themselves even after checking. Extra hours were added to their daily activities, just to maintain their ability to complete tasks.

Discussion and Reflections

The results of this study provide a first step toward understanding the early experience of memory loss from the perspective of the person so afflicted, and what it is that drives these persons toward seeking professional help. In recognizing the participants' situation as a transition with different processes and different strategies for managing memory loss, a more complete picture emerges of the source of their suffering. This knowledge does not only offer a framework for identifying the needs of younger persons suffering from memory loss, but it is also likely to contribute to a better understanding of the preclinical years that precede a dementia diagnosis.

The suffering that the participants endured was understood as an incipient sense of losing control, accompanied by a fear of continuous deterioration with no end in sight. They are frightened by these experiences, worried about what they mean, and endure them mostly alone.

To maintain a sense of competence and control in their daily lives, they develop and use different strategies that work only temporarily. They deliberately avoid situations in which they feel unsafe and vulnerable, withdrawing from social interactions by their fears of being discovered by others. A threat of social "loss of face" and humiliation increases their silence and isolation, which serves further to contribute to their suffering. The distress from a feared loss of integrity becomes the crux of their suffering.

Any threat that is directed toward personal integrity, whether painful or not, can invoke suffering (Kahn & Steeves, 1986), especially when there is an absence of meaning and when the future is unknown (Flaming, 1995). Unlike pain, suffering is not a phenomenon that can be reduced beyond the whole person, but remains a lived experience that is inseparable from a configuration of context, experience, event, and meaning (Kahn & Steeves, 1986).

In learning about the nature of the participants' suffering, this study recognizes the need for a more comprehensive approach when assessing persons with early memory loss. This is an approach that not only takes into account pathophysiological changes, as a result of which the body becomes the object of enquiry, but also includes a recognition of the meaning those experiences have for the person afflicted.

Arguing the need for a better understanding of the meaning that an illness experience has for a person, in-depth phenomenological studies have been suggested to be an important complement to traditional approaches in dementia research, because they offer a way of uncovering phenomena of lived experiences, and thereby assist health care professionals in "entering the life-world" of those persons (Kretlow, 1989; Bahro et al., 1995; Nygård, 1996).

Taking into account that the nature of an unfolding dementia disease is likely to vary over time and, thereby, also the personal meaning of those experiences, several authors have suggested the use of a more longitudinal approach in dementia research, which aims specifically at capturing the process of change over time (Conrad, 1990; Cotrell & Schulz, 1993; Keady & Nolan, 1994). From recognizing both the longitudinal and temporal characteristics of participants' experiences, we would also like to propose the use of a transitional framework, because it provides a means for capturing the process as a whole, and also offers a tool for uncovering those needs that are phase-specific by identifying vulnerable and critical points during the transitional experience (Schumacher & Meleis, 1994). By identifying different indicators of processes that are linked to health, it becomes possible to gain an insight into how the transition is proceeding, and thereby plan continuously for interventions that will assist the client during the process of change (K. L. Schumacher et al., unpublished observations).

In relating the concept of transition to the notion that early symptoms of dementia are more likely to affect persons who are still in an active part of life, and that the needs of younger sufferers will differ from those in older age groups (that is also supported by the results of this study), special care has to be directed toward uncovering the specific needs that belong to this particular group at different phases during the transitional experience.

Because there is an absence of research that is concerned with the situation of early dementia sufferers beyond traditional biomedical approaches, those needs to a large extent still remain uncovered, and are seldom responded to in clinical practice (Keady & Nolan, 1994). As a result of this limited approach, it cannot be neglected that this lack of understanding may lead to a marginalization of younger onset dementia sufferers and persons with early memory loss in terms of clinical and community care, where there otherwise might have been potential benefits from early interventions.

Finally, some methodological issues of this study need to be addressed. Because of the problem of distinguishing between normal and pathological ageing early in the disease process, there may be a chance that some of the participants in this study will not show further progress over time and can, therefore, not be considered to fulfill the criteria for a dementia disease. Because the primary concern of this study was to understand early experiences of memory loss from a sufferer's perspective, the accounts of participants' experiences are here considered to correspond with the aim of the study, and thereby, to contribute to our understanding of how early memory loss is perceived by the person so afflicted. If the primary focus of this study had been to learn from persons who already held a dementia diagnosis, it might not have been possible to capture those very early experiences of memory loss retrospectively, considering the time span that ranges from the very early manifestations of the disease and the establishment of the diagnosis, meaning that symptoms of memory loss might have been present for many years before being diagnosed and before interviews could take place.

Assuming that early symptoms of memory loss are likely to progress into a dementia disease, it becomes important to explore the impact of a continual transition in which no definitive new stability can be reached successfully. We then need to ask, what will be the result of a suffering that is not relieved, when the threat is ongoing and long-lasting, and when suffering continues together with no resolution?

Acknowledgments

The authors are grateful to all the participants in this study for their willingness to share their personal experiences. We also wish to thank the Swedish Municipal Pension Institute, Stiftelsen för Gamla Tjänarinnor, and the Einar Belven Foundation for financial support, and Neil Tomkinson for revising the text.

REFERENCES

American Psychiatric Association. (1987.) *Diagnostic and statistical manual of mental disorders* (3rd ed., rev.). Washington, DC: APA.

Bahro, M., Silber, E., & Sunderland, T. (1995.) How do patients with Alzheimer's disease cope with their illness? A clinical experience report. *Journal of the American Geriatrics Society, 43*, 41–46.

Bridges, W. (1980.) *Transitions*. Reading, MA: Addison-Wesley.

Bridges, W. (1991.) *Managing transitions: Making the most of change*. Reading, MA: Addison-Wesley.

Chick, N., & Meleis, A. I. (1986.) Transitions: A nursing concern. In P. L. Chinn (Ed.), *Nursing research methodology: Issues and implementation* (pp. 237–257). Rockville, MD: Aspen.

Conrad, P. (1990.) Qualitative research on chronic illness: A commentary on method and conceptual development. *Social Science and Medicine, 30*, 1257–1263.

Cotrell, V., & Lein, L. (1993.) Awareness and denial in the Alzheimer's disease victim. *Journal of Gerontological Social Work, 19*, 115–133.

Cotrell, V., & Schulz, R. (1993.) The perspective of the patient in Alzheimer's disease: A neglected dimension of dementia research. *The Gerontologist, 33*, 205–211.

Ekman, S. L., Robins Wahlin, T. B., Norberg, A., & Winblad, B. (1993.) Relationship between bilingual demented immigrants and bilingual/monolingual caregivers. *International Journal of Aging and Human Development, 37*, 37–54.

Flaming, D. (1995.) Patient suffering: A taxonomy from the nurse's perspective. *Journal of Advanced Nursing, 22*, 1120–1127.

Folstein, M. F., Folstein, S. E., & McHugh, P. R. (1975.) "Mini-mental state." A practical method for grading the cognitive state of patients for the clinician. *Journal of Psychiatric Research, 12*, 189–198.

Golan, N. (1981.) *Passing through transitions*. New York: Free Press.

Jansson, L., Norberg, A., Sandman, P., Athlin, E., & Asplund, K. (1993.) Interpreting facial expressions in patients in the terminal stage of Alzheimer disease. *Omega, 26*, 319–334.

Jonker, G., Launder, L. J., Hooijer, C., & Linde-boom, J. (1996.) Memory complaints and memory impairment in older individuals. *Journal of the American Geriatrics Society, 44*, 44–49.

Kahn, D. L., & Steeves, R. H. (1986.) The experience of suffering: Conceptual clarification and theoretical definition. *Journal of Advanced Nursing, 11*, 623–631.

Keady, J., & Nolan, M. (1994.) Younger onset dementia: Developing a longitudinal model as a basis for a research agenda and as a guide to interventions with sufferers and carers. *Journal of Advanced Nursing, 19*, 659–669.

Kretlow, F. (1989.) A phenomenological view of illness. *Australian Journal of Advanced Nursing, 7*(2), 8–10.

Kurz, A., Romero, B., & Lauter, H. (1990.) The onset of Alzheimer's disease. A longitudinal case study and a trial of new diagnostic criteria. *Psychiatry, 53*(2), 53–60.

Linn, R. T., Wolf, P. A., Bachman, D. L., Knoefel, J. E., Cobb, J. L., Belanger, A. J., et al. (1995.) The preclinical phase of probable Alzheimer's disease. *Archives of Neurology, 52*, 485–490.

McCormick, W. C., Kukull, W. A., van Belle, G., Bowen, J. D., Ten, L., & Larson, E. B. (1994.) Symptom patterns and comorbidity in the early stages of Alzheimer's disease. *Journal of the American Geriatrics Society, 42*, 517–521.

McKhann, G., Drachman, D., Folstein, M., Katzman, R., Price, D., & Stadlan, E. (1984.) Clinical diagnosis of Alzheimer's disease: Report of the NINCDS-ADRDA Work Group under the auspices of the Department of Health and Human Services Task Force on Alzheimer's disease. *Neurology, 34*, 939–944.

Meleis, A. I. (1991.) *Theoretical nursing: Development and progress* (2nd ed.). Philadelphia: Lippincott.

Meleis, A. I., & Tangenstein, P. A. (1994.) Facilitating transitions: Redefinition of the nursing mission. *Nursing Outlook, 42*, 255–259.

Morris, J. C., & Fulling, K. (1988.) Early Alzheimer's disease: Diagnostic considerations. *Archives of Neurology, 45*, 345–349.

Nygård, L. (1996.) Everyday life with dementia. Unpublished master's thesis, Karolinska Institute, Stockholm.

Ricoeur, P. (1971.) The model of the text: Meaningful action considered as a text. *Social Research, 38*, 529–562.

———(1976.) *Interpretation theory: Discourse and the surplus of meaning*. Fort Worth, TX: Christian University Press.

Schumacher, K. L., & Meleis, A. I. (1994.) Transitions: A central concept in nursing. *Image: Journal of Nursing Scholarship, 26*, 119–127.

Williams, O., Keady, J., & Nolan, M. (1995.) Younger-onset Alzheimer's disease: Learning from the experience of one spouse carer. *Journal of Clinical Nursing, 4*, 31–36.

Reprinted with permission from: Robinson, P., Ekman, S. L., Meleis, A. I., Winblad, B., & Wahlund, L. O. (1997). Suffering in silence: The experience of early memory loss. *Health Care in Later Life, 2*(2), 107–120.

7.8 TRANSITION TOWARDS END OF LIFE IN PALLIATIVE CARE: AN EXPLORATION OF ITS MEANING FOR ADVANCED CANCER PATIENTS IN EUROPE

PHILIP J. LARKIN
BERNADETTE DIERCKX DE CASTERLÉ
PAUL SCHOTSMANS

Abstract

Transition as a concept in health care has been explored, but there is limited empirical work that considers transition in the context of palliative care, specifically from the patient perspective. This chapter reports findings from a qualitative study designed to explore transition experiences of 100 advanced cancer patients in six European countries. Data were analyzed using the ATLAS.ti program. Findings suggest that transition is a confusing time of mixed messages, poor communication, and uncertainty, but the physical environment of the hospice offers a place of ontological security from which to address this. Transition concepts fail to capture the palliative care experience fully. Transience, as an alternative concept, is reported, although further research is needed to explore this. In clinical practice, the value given to hospice by patients suggests that clinicians must carefully balance the benefit of mainstream integration with sensitive assimilation of hospice philosophy.

Background

Transition as a concept relevant to health care is well explored in the literature. Anthropological theories describe transition as change in status for the individual, often around key life events such as birth, marriage, or death.[1–4] In health care, it has been explored in relation to a variety of therapeutic, environmental, and psychosocial topics, including the patient/client perspective on transition between health and illness.[5–8] Key to understanding the anthropological perspective has been the idea of the "limina"—a space of separation where the person undergoes a transition followed by reintegration into society.[9, 10] Hospice as a liminal space has also been explored.[11] Transition, as illustrated in the palliative care literature, relates to personal meaning in life, life/role changes, perception of end of treatment, and likelihood of death, discussed largely from the professional caregiver perspective.[12-20] However, data on the patient perspective are limited.[14, 21-30] The outcome of transition is often described in terms of an individual's resilience, reconstruction, and transformation,[31-36] although it is not clearly demonstrated how these equate to palliative care.

The close integration of palliative care with mainstream health care, earlier clinical intervention across a broad disease spectrum, and the increasing use of technology in medical palliative care practice have been criticized for obscuring the roots of modern palliative care in the British hospice movement, attributed to Cicely Saunders.[37-44] Although the British model is widely considered a foundation across Europe, many countries now favor a dynamic rehabilitative and integrated approach to palliative care in keeping with treatment, which may begin as early as disease onset.[45] When palliative care practitioners do not hold a consensus on the definition of what they purport to offer, transitions are likely to cause problems. Current interpretation of the term *palliative* is problematic, because it blurs the critical transition points that patients may experience.[43, 44] Interpreting the meaning of transition may depend on patients' understanding of shifts in clinical emphasis, and it is not clear how current transition experiences are understood by them. Given that cancer remains the predominant clinical condition in palliative care despite a shift in the international definition,[46] this study sought to address the research question, "How is the transition experience toward end of life described by European advanced cancer patients?" To answer this, three objectives were proposed: to document palliative care patients' experience at the palliative/terminal interface, to identify perceived supportive and inhibitory factors, and to analyze those common experiences in the context of current palliative care development in European terms as a means to inform practice.

Method

A phenomenological approach was used to interpret and understand contextual patterns of meanings, values, and relations that reflect the immediacy and direct nature of living.[47-53] To capture lived experiences, the method and data analysis was framed by Van Manen's[49] concept of four "life-world existentials": Lived Body, Lived Space, Lived Time, and Lived Other. These phenomenological constructs are judged to transcend individual social, cultural, or historical situations[49], and were seen to address personal experience of the transition phenomenon embedded in culture and language. Ethical approval for this study was granted by a research ethics committee (REC) in each country. Obtaining multicenter ethical approval across European countries is a complex issue[54], compounded in this study by the need to ensure that the qualitative paradigm was clearly understood by RECs more familiar with experimental designs.[55, 56]

Sample

A purposive sample[57-60] of 120 participants (20 per country) was sought from palliative care centers in six European countries: the United Kingdom (U.K.), Republic of Ireland (IRL), Italy (IT), Spain (SP), The Netherlands (NL), and Switzerland (CH). Each was recognized as a center of palliative care expertise by the national palliative care association of that country. Variation in service development across Europe (Table 7.8.1) meant that a variety of settings were used, primarily purpose-built hospices or hospital-based palliative care units (termed "palliative care centers"). Units were directly funded by statutory health services or charitable institutes, often a mix of both, dictating a variety of differing care settings. Cancer patients were the most likely recipients of care. Each country experienced specific challenges in service provision, largely related to their stage of national development.

TABLE 7.8.1 Comparison of European Union Palliative Care Services

Country	Total adult palliative care services (n)	Total inpatient palliative care units/ hospice beds (n)	Palliative care patient population with advanced cancer (estimated %)	Predominant funding source (public/ charitable)	Key challenge for the future
United Kingdom (UK)	881	2,515	95%	Both	Augment a diminishing workforce
Ireland (IRL)	49	147	95%	Both	Address structural deficiencies
Spain (SP)	287	883	95%	Public	Seek political commitment
Netherlands (NL)	128	346	80%	Public	Ensure quality of new services
Italy (I)	258	1,095	60%	Public	Seek academic recognition
Switzerland (CH)	37	NK	NK	Both	Raise awareness

Reprinted with the kind permission of Prof. Carlos Centeno and the European Association for Palliative Care Taskforce on the Development of Palliative Care in Europe. NK: not known

The suitability of research participants to participate was agreed on in consultation with the clinical director and palliative care team, based on patient awareness of cancer diagnosis and prognosis, and health status at the time of interview. Given the complexity in defining prognosis for a palliative care population,[61] the team was asked to consider patients most likely to progress to terminal care within 6 to 12 months. Patients with serious cognitive impairment that inhibited their ability to converse in their native language, and to give both written and verbal informed consent, were excluded. A senior palliative care nurse introduced the study, obtained verbal consent to participate, contacted the researcher, and arranged an interview. Written consent was obtained and reaffirmed with the patient throughout the interview.[62]

Sixteen patients were withdrawn from the study, either due to fatigue (n = 6) or judged by both interviewer and clinical team to have deteriorated significantly by the time of interview (n = 10). A further four interviews could not be completed due to treatment or communication difficulties.

Table 7.8.2 shows a relatively even distribution of the final sample (n = 100) by age and gender, with the exception of Spain, where only one female respondent was identified—an inherent weakness in the purposive sampling method.[63] For each interview group, the median length of life expectancy postinterview was calculated. Of the total sample of patients interviewed, 26.5% were still alive at the end of the study. Despite some incomplete data from Switzerland and Italy, the relatively short life expectancy overall (39.88 days) would indicate that respondents were appropriately in receipt of end-of-life management at the time of interview. In Table 7.8.3, the prevalence of breast cancer in the sample is attributed to the Italian palliative care center offering a national treatment program for the care of advanced breast disease.

> **Box 1**
>
> - Can you describe in your own words what it meant for you when you were transferred to this palliative care center?
> - Can you tell me whether there is anyone or anything that made it easier for you when you were transferred to this palliative care center?
> - Can you tell me whether there is anyone or anything that made it difficult for you when you were transferred to this palliative care center?
> - Now, has anything changed for you at all since being transferred to this palliative care center?

TABLE 7.8.2 Sample Distribution

Country	Final sample	Male patients	Female patients	Mean age (range)	Life expectancy postinterview (days)	Research centers
UK	20	8	12	72.9 (55–92 years)	41.8	2 hospices
IRL	20	10	10	72.8 49–87 years)	37.6	1 hospice
NL	15	5	10	75.8 (50–91 years)	40.5	1 hospice
I	18	5	13	59.6 (45–81 years)	48.4	1 hospital palliative care center
SP	10	9	1	64.1 (45–84 years)	32.5	1 hospital palliative care center
CH	17	8	9	79.8 (55–92 years)	38.5	1 hospice, 1 palliative care center
Total	100	45	55	70.83 years	39.88 days	8 centers

TABLE 7.8.3 Distribution of Cancer Diagnosis Across Sample

	Breast	Lung	Prostate	GIT	GU	Ovary	Brain	Other	Sample total
UK	4	4	3	5	1	1	1	1	20
IRL	3	3	3	6	3	0	1	1	20
CH	4	3	3	4	0	1	1	1	17
SP	0	4	3	0	2	1	0	0	10
I	11	2	2	0	2	0	0	1	18
NL	3	2	1	5	0	1	0	3	15
Total	25	18	15	20	8	4	3	7	100

GIT: gastrointestinal tract—colon, rectum, esophagus; GU: genitourinary—renal, bladder; Other: acute myelogenous leukemia, mesothelioma.

For this same reason, the demographic profile of the Italian sample was predominantly female and comparably younger (59.65 years) than the overall mean age range of 70.8 years (Table 7.8.2).

Data Collection

A semistructured interview[64, 65] based around four questions (Box 1) was designed to address the multilingual nature of the study, as well as the potential burden to participants. Questions were designed to be succinct, clear, and culturally appropriate. The translation process used is reported elsewhere.[66] The four questions were developed using probes to enable a description of the phenomenon and an exploration of its meaning to emerge.[67] Again, given patient frailty, interviews were conducted at one moment in time during their end-of-life management, either by the principal researcher (PJL), in English, French, and Italian, or by a palliative care nurse (Dutch and Spanish) given additional training in interviewing. Questions explored experience, associated factors, and current reflections on their transition process at this point in time. The mean length of interview was 22.05 minutes (range: 10–55 minutes). Data collection took place between April 2003 and March 2005, determined by recruitment and travel.

Psychological support was offered postinterview by qualified personnel (e.g., social worker), although no specific request was made either during or subsequent to the study.

Data Analysis

All interviews were taped using a minidisk recorder[68] and were transcribed verbatim in their country of origin. An English translation of the original script was made. The ATLAS.tihermeneutic program collated the interviews, grouped according to language, and coded to preserve anonymity.

The process of analysis is described in four stages. The first three, labeled substantive, evocative, and evaluative, are depicted in Figure 7.8.1; the fourth, termed expositional, is presented in Figure 7.8.2.

At the substantive stage, initial analysis was undertaken on the English language interviews only (U.K. and Ireland). Each interview was read and a reflection written using the respondent's own words to encapsulate their understanding of the transition experience, noting, for example, tonality, expression, and the use of silence.[67, 69] This created a series of 108 codes that provided a description of the factors that helped or hindered transition. The process was then repeated for each of the translated interviews, read alongside the original language text. A further six codes of specific relevance to the non-English-speaking countries were identified. Field notes were reviewed to add context, and a personal journal (one per country) was kept by the researcher as a supplementary resource to further inform the analysis.[70] Using the Atlas.ti program, clusters were formed for the 114 codes, which were then collapsed into 11 descriptive themes.

A collective descriptive statement of each patient group was then written, one per country. At the evocative level, these descriptive statements were analyzed in relation to Van Manen's "lifeworld existentials"[49] and compared and contrasted, resulting in four descriptions of the impact of transition—instability, impermanence, oscillation, and shift—and four patient responses—seeking stability, challenging impermanence, negotiating time, and shifting bonds.

In the affirmative stage, these results were tested for rigor in interpretation and meaning. The short life expectancy postinterview (Table 7.8.2) meant that returning data to respondents for confirmation and accuracy was not possible. Reflecting the vital role of translators and interpreters in the analysis and interpretation of qualitative data[66, 71], dialogue with translators/interviewers explored themes, language, and concepts to identify a culturally embedded representation of the respondent's story. A "critical referent" group[69] was convened, comprising experts in research methodology and clinical palliative care practice, who reviewed data analysis. They assessed the emergent findings at each stage in relation to their relevance and meaning for the clinical field, and critically considered the insights offered by the translators' and interpreters' review.

In the final expositional stage (Figure 7.8.2), through a cyclical process of reading and rereading text, theme, and descriptions, a pathway of analysis was constructed leading to an overall outcome designed to express the phenomenon as a whole. This was then again reviewed by the referent group and translators to seek congruence, and was found to be a meaningful description of shared experience across all centers. Finally, a universal draft was written to encapsulate a phenomenon described as living transiently in the shadow of death.

Results

Lived Body

Findings described a phenomenon, "seeking stability through safety and security," exemplified as: (a) the shifting complexity of their disease, (b) the emotional response to the act of transition, and (c)

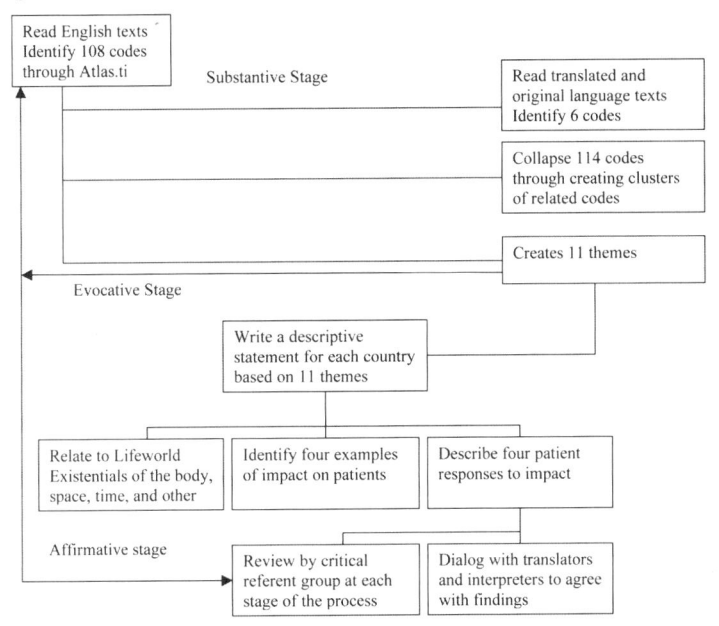

Figure 7.8.1: Substantive, evocative, and affirmative states of analysis

FIGURE 7.8.1 Substantive, evocative, and affirmative states of analysis.

the role of the hospice or palliative care center as a beacon for supportive care.

Respondents gave detailed accounts of disease progression from initial diagnosis to current prognosis, citing the limitations imposed by their advanced disease and its possible meaning:

> I don't think I'll ever be able to go home. I can't put any weight on this foot at the moment. Personally, I don't know if I'll ever be able to walk on it. I don't know.(U.K. 16)

Rapid deterioration resulting in loss of independence was a primary reason for transition to the hospice/palliative care center:

> Well, this all has happened in a very short time. Little time ago you were up; you walked a little; you even went out to the balcony with them a few months ago; and now that is impossible.(SP 3)

A variety of emotional responses to transition were described, reflecting fears and losses:

> Well, I was a bit worried about the one-way ticket system here…you come in alive and you go…as pieces of wood…I was reassured that does not happen….(U.K. 18)

> I was very emotional because I had never thought that [name of hospital] would give up on me…that I was going to die very soon and that I had to go into palliative care, and [pause] what hurt me the

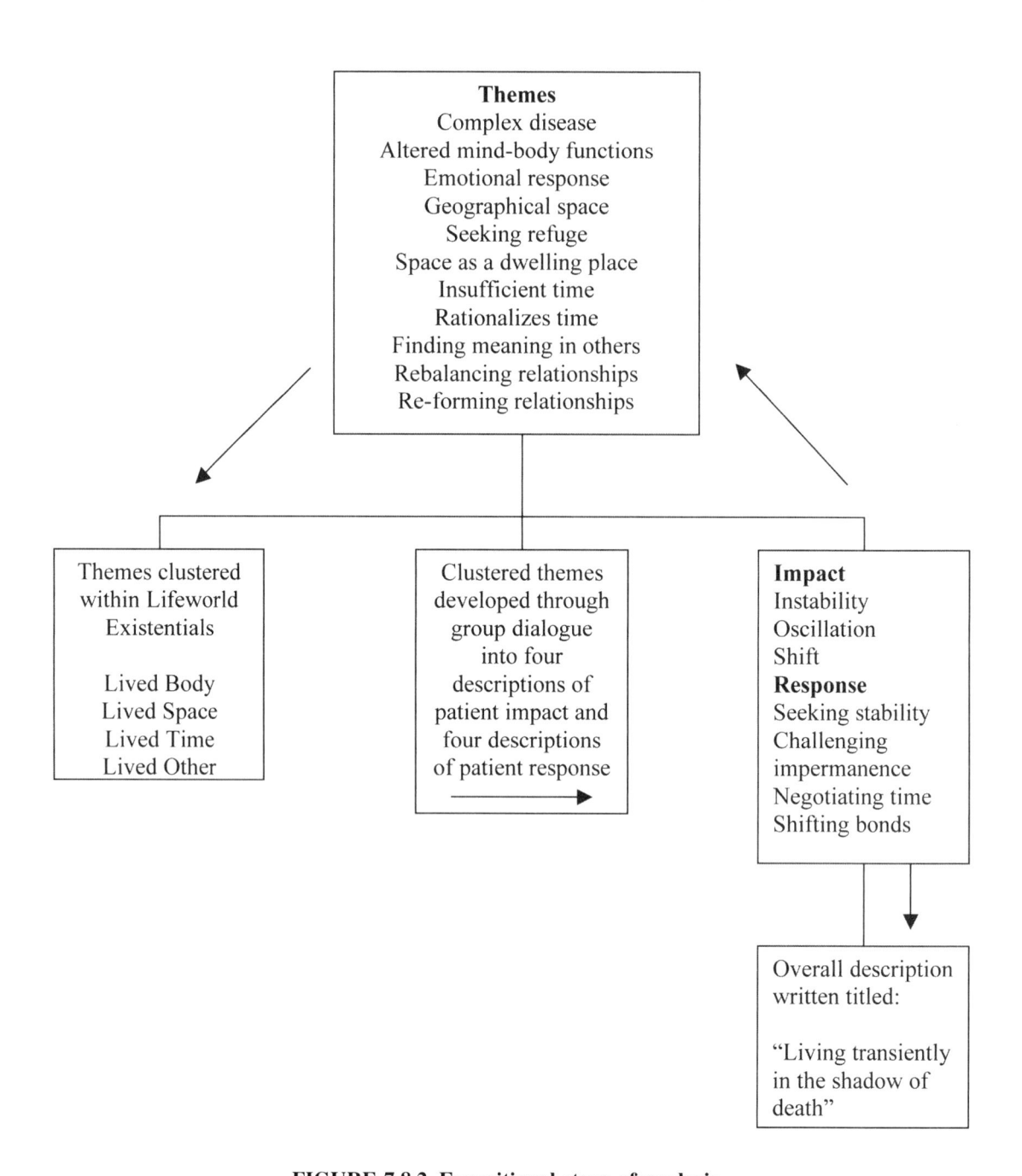

Themes
Complex disease
Altered mind-body functions
Emotional response
Geographical space
Seeking refuge
Space as a dwelling place
Insufficient time
Rationalizes time
Finding meaning in others
Rebalancing relationships
Re-forming relationships

Themes clustered within Lifeworld Existentials

Lived Body
Lived Space
Lived Time
Lived Other

Clustered themes developed through group dialogue into four descriptions of patient impact and four descriptions of patient response

Impact
Instability
Oscillation
Shift
Response
Seeking stability
Challenging impermanence
Negotiating time
Shifting bonds

Overall description written titled:

"Living transiently in the shadow of death"

FIGURE 7.8.2 Expositional stage of analysis.

most [pause] was that I found myself in a meeting with eight doctors, and what shocked me the most was that they said to me, 'To us you are merely, you are merely a scientific experiment'...I am not lying when I tell you that, [silence] their social contact is zero.[CH 8]

I didn't know what it was [palliative care]...no one told me anything...it's very, very difficult; you can't imagine what it's like...Because when I arrived here I was...[silence] How can I...lost? I felt really lost.[CH 3]

Where respondents experienced distress, the palliative care center offered the hope of safety and security at a time of emotional fragility:

Well, probably at the time I was feeling worn out. I was lying in that bed really, really like a broken person and was thinking that [transfer to a hospice] actually sounds too good to be true.[NL2]

I can assure you that I feel I am taken care of. I feel they are keeping an eye on me.[IT 15]

It would appear that, for these patients, admission to the hospice/palliative care center came at a time when the impact of multiple changes to their health status meant that they could no longer guarantee equilibrium between their life and their illness. Hence, withdrawal to the security of a hospice/palliative care center gave an opportunity to regain balance and address this instability.

Lived Space

Respondents identified three themes in relation to space as a "challenge to impermanence" through: (a) experiencing geographical space, (b) seeking a secure space as refuge, and (c) creating a dwelling space.

Geographical Space

Most, but not all, centers offered single rooms. In terms of adjustment, being able to balance privacy with proximity to staff for assistance at any time was seen as a positive factor for respondents:

...lovely in'it...smashing room...I mean...you wouldn't get better than Buckingham Palace...you wouldn't...everybody's here...you could call anybody...you know...I got a button...you gotta press that red button....[UK. 6]

Peaceful surroundings were contrasted against the limitations of multiple occupancy:

In other places, at least where I've been, it is more impersonal, like they almost cannot take care of you, there are more people in the room, more uproar, you don't have this peace, this peace, this familiarity that emerges between the center and the patient.[SP3]

Space also contributed significantly to the initial transition from one center to another:

A lovely quiet beautiful room...left alone with it to acclimatize. I found that very important because you are pushed from one environment into the other and transported in the ambulance backwards, upside down more or less, and you don't feel very well.[NL9]

Secure Space

The hospice/palliative care center was also seen as a refuge, a place of shelter and protection. One respondent had moved to live with her married daughter, and the loss of her home and new living arrangements prompted the transition to hospice:

I just got paranoid in thinking, I've outstayed my welcome because she'd got a family, she'd got three kids, a husband who works hard and I just felt it wasn't right, I should not have been there, if I'd stayed at the bungalow I would have tried harder, anyway just one thing led to another. So there was sort of arguments and upsets, so I came in here.[U.K. 10]

The room also had significance as a place to die, something only offered when close to death, an indicator of final transition. Further, respondents argued that being in the presence of others who were dying could have a positive impact on their psychological adjustment:

When I saw the room, it seemed like it was the last straw...that it was going to be the last straw because such luxury cannot be given to everyone, to any patient, this is special, I was special.[SP 8]

From the minute he came in he was bad, I knew he was...But it's something to see a man die, you know. I saw him dying slowly and I didn't see the finish because they took him out [to a single room]. I'd like to have seen it, to see what exactly happens, but he was gone.[IRL11]

Dwelling Space

Some centers invited patients to create a personal dwelling space by bringing items from home. Meaningful surroundings for the patient created a bridge between the transition from home to institutional care.

I'd rather be home, of course, but they brought things from home and when I wake up, nice, cosy, then you don't have that longing.[NL 11]

The compact space led to decisions and judgments about the significance of possessions at this time.

I have my radio here, a picture of my father and mother, a picture of my wife, I have a piece of my own home brought here. The rest I give away, they are no good to me anymore.[NL15]

Respondents who made a definitive move to the hospice/palliative care center for the remainder of their life described severance, both physically and emotionally, from the family home:

I am at home here...Even when I went out to celebrate my birthday, when I was a stone's throw from the house, we went past it. I didn't even stop. What for? To go up the stairs with great difficulty and then come down again a quarter of an hour later?...I didn't need to...I didn't go and see it because...What would I have done?...Checked for dust?[CH13]

Given the sense of instability described, it was not unexpected that the hospice/palliative care center should offer the security they sought through refuge and shelter. The space of the hospice/palliative care center offered a structure within which the shifting boundaries of home could be recreated and, in so doing, gave a sense of permanence at a time of rapid change.

Lived Time

Temporal issues emerged metaphorically as "the bomb's ticking" or, "extinguished a little more day by day." These were formulated as "negotiating time," reflecting insufficient time and rationalizing time in proximity to death.

The length of time between referral and transfer was insufficient for respondents to address its impact. They reported the urgency of agreeing to take a bed in the hospice/palliative care center, even if they were not themselves practically and emotionally ready to do so.

Monday, the GP came and said, 'Listen, they have room for you.' And they would be on the doorstep on Tuesday morning at 9 or 10 a.m. But you have to take care of things. You can't just leave like that, you have bills, you have this, you have that...[NL 6]

It was also difficult to renegotiate an admission for fear of being seen as difficult:

And then I agreed Friday with [GP]. She said, 'I have been able to agree on Thursday.' So I said OK. They were afraid that I refused. But that was not true. It just caught me by surprise. You are on a waiting list, so you don't think it will happen soon. Then you can arrange all kind of things. But the GP thought that I was refusing.[NL 2]

Respondents said their final decision to move was often based on an evaluation of their potential burden to others rather than personal choice about the perceived benefits of palliative care.

I've been a widower for 20 years. What I didn't want was to bother my family, do you understand? When I was in the other hospital, my sister-in-law was back and forth, back and forth, and the boy had to come every day.[NL15]

Respondents also described transition as temporal fatalism, the unchanging reality of death:

You're born and you die...in between, you do the best you can...and that's all there is to it...I am afraid that's the way I look at it. I've enjoyed my life...it's been wonderful. I'd like a lot more...but there you go...can't win 'em all[U.K 2]

I don't have many requests. My time has come. To lament now I am going? No, as far as that is concerned, I have had my time.[NL6]

Unsurprisingly, time was a critical descriptor of patient experience: time to undertake life tasks balanced against time left to complete them. The importance of negotiation appeared to wane over time as inevitable deterioration refocused patients toward life reflection—a shift from challenging time to rationalizing time.

Lived Other

Of all the themes identified, the shifting dynamics of relationship had the most profound effect on the respondents' ability successfully to negotiate their transition toward end of life. The degree of success appeared dependent on the balance achieved between closure of episodes of one's life and ensuring that someone could bear witness to that life, someone who was her/himself in the process of transition.

Defined as "shifting bonds," this phenomenon described: (a) finding meaningful people involved in the transition process, (b) rebalancing relationships at the end of life, and (c) relationships formed with other patients in the hospice/palliative care center. Successful transition was due to a number of relational factors, including the intervention of a thoughtful health care professional, a family friend, or relative. Yet, respondents were unable to determine how the referral process took place, nor name any key players in that process. Neither could they identify whether the key player was a palliative care professional. Variance in this respect reflected the place of palliative care services within national health systems. The more developed the palliative care system, the greater likelihood of multiple professionals being involved in planning, which led to confusion for the patient.

Transition highlighted the strengths and weaknesses of personal relationships. Family and life role were important in end-of-life adjustments:

I see them all around me: my daughter, my son, my grandson, my wife. All of them are so consistent toward me, kind, supportive, great love, because we…it's 50 years now that we have been married, this month, therefore,…I live also for these things.[IT 15]

Clinical staff held a special value for respondents as a conduit for addressing emotional isolation from family.

…this [hospice] has helped more than my whole family. I've felt free to talk about things and say—that they may not even understand. They don't understand the disease, they don't understand me, they don't understand anything [crying].[SP 5]

Equally, respondents developed strong bonds with each other, exhibited as camaraderie among patients and profound sadness at their death:

I had somebody share my room, she was a lovely lady. I noticed all the care until she passed on and I thought, well, that's very, very comforting because any time in our lives it can happen to us. I missed her. I only knew her for a few days but I felt very close to her, and I'm so pleased that she was so welcomed and so looked after by the nursing staff.[U.K 14]

It was a privilege for me to have [name] next door. She was a wonderful person. We made a joke of everything…and when she went I thought…I know it's horrible…but I wish she could stay.[U.K. 20]

The lived other experience emerged as an essence of relationship between people in enclosure—the space of the hospice/palliative care center. This relationship embodied both camaraderie and empathy for another, framed by their difference as a community apart from the world. In effect, as patients moved toward the end of their lives, there was a shift in their lifeworld as the enclosed life within the hospice/palliative care center took precedence.

Seeking the Essential Phenomenon

Phenomenological enquiry does not seek to provide empirical evidence, but rather accounts for the diversity of human experience. In order to encapsulate the commonality of that experience, given the cultural and linguistic challenges of this multicenter study, some degree of reduction is warranted. Reduction enables clarity of the phenomenon beyond obscure theoretical abstraction.[49] In this study, respondents' lifeworld descriptions incorporated a confusing time of mixed messages, poor communication, and uncertainty, reflecting an instability and impermanence that patients attempt to address through their actions and reactions. The experience was less a linear progression and more a cyclical phenomenon, a transient period of hurried admission, having to make final judgments and weigh decisions based on self-perception, complex clinical advice, and family wishes. Death was a present, but not consuming, presence in people's lives, and goals for the future were sought, albeit within the confines of failing health, as they evaluated their past and adjusted to a state of moving toward the end of their life. These descriptions were encapsulated in an essential phenomenon described as, "living transiently within the shadow of death."

> This last relapse has been a big one, but I always knew that each one was going to be worse than the one before. I've lost a lot—mobility, home, relationship. I look back and see, if somebody's not letting you die, they're also not letting you live…and I do want to live. I want to live and enjoy until the last minute, you know.[U.K. 18]

Discussion

This study did not set out to offer a comparative experience of palliative care transition between countries, but rather to determine what, if anything, was common to that experience for patients receiving a specific approach to care which is ostensibly derived from one set of founding principles[38]. The diversity of palliative care practice across Europe means that the research sites selected offered a rich and deep purposive sample, not necessarily representative of the full range of services and, therefore, of patient experiences in each country. Although rigorous efforts were made to limit the risks of potential loss of meaning with multilingual data, we acknowledge that the nature of a single interview and the presentation of those findings in English by a native English speaker have methodological limitations. However, the findings do cause us to question our current understanding of the significance of hospice/palliative care for patients at the palliative-terminal interface.

Patients appear to oscillate between their present life situation and the reality of their future. For some patients, care for the other appeared to take precedence over care for the self. Negotiation seems key to the management of transition. However, negotiation based on fear of being a burden to others puts into question assumptions that personal autonomy and choice were paramount in their decision making.

The experiences described hold some definition within transition literature, including identity shift, redefinition of self, and changing roles.[72–74] The anthropological concept of limina, as discussed earlier,[2, 10] would also seem to have relevance for the experiences described here. Time spent in the liminal space alters the quality of the social relationships of those within that space, adopting a "generic human bond"—an essential sharing between the group because they are all "wholly in becoming."[75,76] Such was evident in the findings here, particularly in relation to Lived Other descriptions of camaraderie between patients. For some, the hospice/palliative care center signified a place of ontological security.[77–82] This space offered preparation and protection: time and energy devoted to the closing of life commitments, reflection on life relationships, and ensuring the safety of family in practical and emotional terms. The recreation of home through ontological security would signify that structure and permanence held some importance in the lives of the respondents, and that a transition process could be negotiated, once boundaries were established.

That said, the findings do put into question how closely some transition outcomes described in the literature, such as reconstruction, transformation, and transcendence, fit within a palliative context.[5, 12–19, 33–36, 83] We concluded that the word, "transience," as "the action or fact of passing away," may offer a clearer description of the transition experience in this study, reflecting something of limited durability and impermanence.[84] A conceptual analysis of transience in relation to palliative care, arising from the findings of this study, is reported elsewhere.[85] Transience in this study may be attributed, in part, to a message that a hospice/palliative care center no longer equates with end-of-life care alone, but rather with a range of services aimed at improving life quality, symptom management, and discharge home. However, more data is needed to better understand the concept of transience and how this phenomenon may be reflected in the transition experiences of other patient groups.

Given the shift toward palliative units integrated within acute hospitals,[86] it remains incumbent on palliative care professionals to ensure their visibility is maintained. Where the influence of one system is evident over the other, it may threaten the values and expectations that make palliative care inherently different from their other health care experiences. The inability to recognize palliative care personnel is an example of gaps identified in this study that need to be addressed by service providers to ensure that the benefits of the acute/palliative interface are maximized.

Service planning in palliative care is clearly enhanced by incorporating the patient viewpoint into research studies that aim to improve quality of services.[87] Given that recent data suggest reluctance to include palliative care patients in research may be erroneously based on a paternalistic view of the hazards of research at the end of life,[88] further research in this field should take account of the patient and carer perspectives in the evaluation of palliative care service delivery.

Conclusions

In this chapter, we explore the experiences and meaning of transition for a distinct group of palliative care patients, and suggest that transition, as currently described in the literature, warrants further development to be clearly understood within this patient population. The successful merging of the curative-palliative interface is clearly beneficial to patients, but there is a risk that we may have unwittingly obscured the importance they place on the hospice/palliative care center as a space where they align themselves toward the inevitability of death in a safe and secure environment. Clinicians need to balance mainstream integration with sensitive assimilation of the hospice model to ensure that seamless transition proposed as a key construct in palliative care remains paramount. Further research into the professional and family perspectives on this topic would complement this patient perspective and contribute to our understanding of palliative care service delivery.

Acknowledgments

Philip Larkin is holder of the 2003 Health Research Board Fellowship In Palliative Care. This study is jointly funded by The Health Research Board of Ireland and The Irish Hospice Foundation, Dublin, Ireland.

REFERENCES

1. Van Gennep A. Rites of Passage. Chicago, University of Chicago Press, 1960.
2. Turner VW, Bruner EM, eds. The Anthropology of Experience. Urbana, Illinois: University of Illinois Press, 1986.
3. Geertz C. The Interpretation of Cultures. New York: Basic Books, 1973.
4. Draper J. Men's passage to fatherhood: An analysis of the contemporary relevance of transition theory. Nurs Inq 2003; 10: 66–78.
5. O'Connor M. Transitions in status from wellness to illness, illness to wellness. In: Payne S., Seymour J., Ingleton C. (eds). Palliative Care Nursing: Principles and evidence for practice. Buckingham: Open University Press, 2001; pp. 126–143.
6. Meleis AI, Rogers S. Women in transition: Being vs. becoming or being and becoming. Healthc Women Int 1987; 8: 199–217.
7. Schumacher KL, Meleis AI. Transitions: A central concept in nursing. Image J Nurs Sch 1994; 26: 119–127.

8. Meleis AI, Sawyer LM, Im EO, Hilfinger Messias KD, Schumacher K. Experiencing transitions: An emerging middle-range theory. Adv Nurs Sci 2000; 23: 12–28.
9. Turner VW. Dramas, fields and metaphors: Symbolic action in human society. London: Ithaca, 1967.
10. Turner V. The ritual process: Structure and antistructure. Chicago: Aldine Press, 1969.
11. Froggatt K. Rites of passage and the hospice culture. Mortality 1997; 2: 123–136.
12. Thompson GN, McClement SE, Daenick PJ. "Changing lanes": Facilitating the transition from curative to palliative care. J Palliat Care 2006; 22: 91–98.
13. Schulman-Green D, McCorkle R, Curry L, Cherlin E, Johnson-Hurzeler R, Bradley E. At the crossroads: Making the transition to hospice. Palliat Support Care 2004; 2: 351–360.
14. Friedrichsen MJ, Strang PM, Carlsson ME. Breaking bad news in the transition from curative to palliative cancer care: Patients' views of the doctor giving the information. Support Care Cancer 2000; 8: 437–438.
15. Scialla S, Cole R, Scialla T, Bednarz L, Scheerer J. Rehabilitation for elderly patients with cancer asthenia: Making a transition to palliative care. Palliat Med 2000; 14: 121–127.
16. Block SD. Perspectives of care at the close of life. Psychological considerations, growth, and transcendence at the end of life: Art of the possible. JAMA 2001; 285: 2898–2905.
17. Mak MHJ. Awareness of dying: An experience of Chinese patients with terminal cancer. Omega 2001; 4: 259–279.
18. Gordon GH. Care not cure: Dialogues at the transition. Patient Educ Couns 2003; 50: 95–98.
19. Burge FI, Lawson B, Critchley P, Maxwell D. Transitions in care during the end of life: Changes experienced following enrollment in a comprehensive palliative care program. BMC Palliat Care 2005; 4: 1–7.
20. Payne S, Sheldon F, Jarrett N, Large S, Smith P, Davis CL. Differences in understanding of specialist palliative care amongst service providers and commissioners in South London. Palliat Med 2002; 16: 395–402.
21. Schofield P, Carey M, Love A, Nehill C, Wein S. "Would you like to talk about your future treatment options?" Discussing the transition from curative cancer treatment to palliative care. Palliat Med 2006; 20: 397–406
22. Lawson B, Burge FI, Critchley P, McIntyre P. Factors associated with multiple transitions in care during the end of life following enrollment in a comprehensive palliative care program. BMC Palliat Care 2006; 5: 1–10.
23. Kristjanson L, Hanson F, Balneaves I. Research in palliative care populations: Ethical issues. J Palliat Care 1994; 10: 10–15.
24. Small N, Rhodes P. Too ill to talk? User involvement in palliative care. London: Routledge, 2000.
25. Seymour J, Ingleton C, Payne S, Beddow V. Specialist palliative care patients' experiences. J Adv Nurs 2003; 44: 24–33.
26. Kirk P, Kirk I, Kristjanson LJ. What do patients receiving palliative care for cancer and their families want to be told? A Canadian and Australian qualitative study. 2004 [cited 2006 June 20]. Available from BMJ: DOI:10.1136/bmj.38103.423576.55
27. McKinlay E. Within the circle of care: Patient experiences of receiving palliative care. J Palliat Care 2001; 17: 22–29.
28. Raynes NV, Leach J, Rawlings B, Bryson RJ. Palliative care services: Views of terminally ill patients. Palliat Med 2000;14: 169–160.
29. Yedidia MJ, MacGregor B. Confronting the prospect of dying: Reports of terminally ill patients. J Pain Symptom Manage 2001; 22: 807–819.
30. Hutchinson TA. Transitions in the lives of patients with end stage renal disease: A cause of suffering and an opportunity for healing. Palliat Med 2005; 19: 270–277.
31. Young B, Dixon-Woods M, Findlay M, Heney D. Parenting in a crisis: Conceptualizing mothers of children with cancer. Soc Sci Med 2002; 55: 1835–1847.
32. Kralik D. The quest for ordinariness: Transition experienced by midlife women living with chronic illness. J Adv Nurs 2002; 39: 146–154.
33. Kralik D, Visentin K, van Loon A. Transition: A literature review. J Adv Nurs 2006; 55: 320–329.
34. Smith JA. Reconstructing selves: An analysis of discrepancies between women's contemporaneous and respective accounts of the transition to motherhood. Br J Psych 1994; 85: 371–392.
35. Holland Wade G. A concept analysis of personal transformation. J Adv Nurs 1998; 28: 713–719.
36. Neill J. Transcendence and transformation in the life patterns of women living with rheumatoid arthritis. Adv Nurs Sci 2002; 24: 27–47.
37. Egan KA, Labyak MJ. Hospice care: A model for quality end-of-life care. In: Ferrell BT, Coyle N (eds). Textbook of Palliative Nursing. Oxford: Oxford University Press, 2001; pp. 7–26.
38. Saunders CM, Clark D. Cicely Saunders, founder of the hospice movement: Selected letters 1959–

1999. Buckingham: Open University Press, 2002.
39. Seymour JE. Using technology to help obtain the goals of palliative care. Int J Palliat Nurs 2005; 11: 240–241.
40. Skilbeck JK, Payne S. End-of-life care: A discourse analysis of specialist palliative care nursing. J Adv Nurs 2005; 51: 325–334.
41. McNamara B. Fragile lives: Death denying and care. Buckingham: Open University Press, 2001.
42. Praill D. Who are we here for? [editorial] Palliat Med 2000; 14: 91–92.
43. American Society of Clinical Oncology. Cancer care during the last phase of life. J Clin Oncol 1998; 16: 1986–1996.
44. Van Kleffens T, Van Baarsen B, Hoekman K, Van Leeuwen E. Clarifying the term "palliative" in clinical oncology. Eur J Cancer Care 2004; 13: 263–271.
45. Ventafridda V. Ten years on in EJPC. Eur J Palliat Care 1998; 5: 140.
46. World Health Organization 2002. [cited 2005, Oct 25]. Available from http://www.who.int/cancer/palliative/definition/en/print.html
47. Gadamer HG. Philosophical hermeneutics. Linghe D. (transl. & ed.). Berkeley: University of California Press, 1976.
48. Van Manen M. Practicing phenomenological writing. Phenomen Pedagogy 1984; 2: 36–69.
49. Van Manen M. Researching lived experience: Human science for an action sensitive pedagogy. London, Canada: Althouse Press, 1990.
50. Caelli K. The changing face of phenomenological research: Traditional and American phenomenology in nursing. Qual Health Res 2000; 10: 366–377.
51. Fleming V, Gaidys U, Robb Y. Hermeneutic research in nursing: Developing a Gadamerian-based research method. Nurs Inq 2003; 10: 113–120.
52. Laverty SM. Hermeneutic phenomenology and phenomenology: A comparison of historical and methodological considerations. Int J Qual Methods 2003 [cited 2005 Oct 18]. Available from: http://www.ualberta.ca/~iiqm/backissues/2_3final/pdf/laverty.pdf
53. Svenaeus F. Hermeneutics of medicine in the wake of Gadamer: The issue of phronesis. Theor Med 2003; 24: 407–431.
54. Hearnshaw H. Comparison of requirements of research ethics committees in 11 European countries for a noninvasive interventional study. BMJ 2004; 328: 140–141.
55. Carverhill PA. Qualitative research in thanatology. Death Stud 2002; 26: 195–207.
56. Clark D. What is qualitative research and what can it contribute to palliative care? Palliat Med 1997; 112: 159–166.
57. Patton MQ. Two decades of developments in qualitative inquiry: A personal experiential perspective. Qualitative Social Work 2002; 1(3): 261–284.
58. Bloor, M. Bishop Berkeley and the adeno-tonsillectomy enigma: An exploration of variation in the social construction of medical disposals. Sociology 1976; 6(10): 43–61.
59. Barbour RS. The role of qualitative research in broadening the "evidence base" for clinical practice. J Eval Clin Pract 2000; 6(2): 155–163.
60. Barbour RS. Using focus groups in general practice research. Fam Pract 1995b; 12: 328–334.
61. Maltoni M, Caraceni A, Brunelli C, Broeckaert B, Christakis N, Eychmuller S, et al. Prognostic factors in advanced cancer patients: Evidence-based clinical recommendations. A study by the Steering Committee of the European Association for Palliative Care. J Clin Oncol 2005; 23(25): 6240–6248.
62. Cutcliffe JR, Ramcharan P. Judging the ethics of qualitative research: Considering the "ethic as process" model. Health Soc Care Community 2001; 9: 358–366.
63. Robson C. Real world research. London: Blackwell, 2002.
64. Nunkoosing K. The problems with interviews. Pearls, pith, and provocation. Qual Health Res 2005; 15(5): 698–706.
65. Corbin J, Morse JM. The unstructured interactive interview: Issues of reciprocity and risks when dealing with sensitive topics. Qual Inq 2003; 9(3): 335–354.
66. Larkin PJ, Dierckx de Casterlé B, Schotsmans P. Multilingual translation issues in qualitative research: Reflections on a metaphorical process. Qual Health Res 2007; 17(4): 468–476.
67. Clare Taylor M. Interviewing. In: Holloway I (ed.). Qualitative research in health care. Buckingham: Open University Press, 2005; pp. 39–55.
68. Given LM. Mini-disc recorders: A new approach for qualitative interviewing. Int J Qual Meth 2004 [cited 2005 Oct 16]. Available from: http://www.ualberta.ca/~iiqm/backissues/3_2pdf/given.pdf
69. Pyett PM. Validation of qualitative research in the "real world". Qual Health Res 2003; 13: 1170–1179.
70. Kvale S. The social construct of validity. Qual Inq 1995; 1: 19–40.
71. Temple B, Young A. Qualitative research and translation dilemmas. Qual Res 2004; 4: 161–178.

72. Boeijea H, Duijnsteeb M, Grypdonck M, Pool A. Encountering the downward phase: Biographical work in people with multiple sclerosis living at home. Soc Sci Med 2002; 55: 881–893.
73. Young B, Dixon-Woods M, Findlay M, Heney D. Parenting in a crisis: Conceptualizing mothers of children with cancer. Soc Sci Med 2002; 55: 1835–1847.
74. Kralik D. The quest for ordinariness: Transition experienced by midlife women living with chronic illness. J Adv Nurs 2002; 39: 146–154.
75. Hockey J. The importance of being intuitive: Arnold Van Gennep's *The Rites of Passage*. Mortality 2002; 7(2): 210–217.
76. Turner V, Turner E (eds.). Blazing the trail. Way marks in the exploration of symbols. Tucson, AZ: The University of Arizona Press, 1992.
77. Bollnow OF. Lived space. Philosophy Today 1961; 5: 31–39.
78. Heidegger M. Building dwelling thinking. In: DF Krell (ed.). Martin Heidegger basic writings. San Francisco: Harper, 1992; pp. 347–363.
79. Milligan C. Location or dis-location? Toward a conceptualization of people and place in the caregiving experience. Social and Cultural Geography 2003; 4(4): 455–470.
80. Macgregor Wise J. Home: Territory and identity. Cult Stud 2000; 14: 295–310.
81. Williams A. Changing geographies of care: Employing the concept of therapeutic landscape as a framework in examining home space. Soc Sci Med 2002; 55: 141–154.
82. Gilmour JA. Hybrid space: Constituting the hospital as a home space for patients. Nurs Inq 2006; 13: 16–22.
83. Nygren B, Aléx L, Jonsén E, Gustafson Y, Norberg A, Lundman B. Resilience, sense of coherence, purpose in life and self-transcendence in relation to perceived physical and mental health among the oldest old. Aging Mental Health 2005; 9: 354–362.
84. Oxford English Dictionary 1989 [cited 2006 July 16]. Available from: http://dictionary.oed.com/cgi/entry/00181778.html 16th July 2006
85. Larkin P, Direckx de Casterlé B, Schotsmans P. Towards a conceptual analysis of transience in relation to palliative care. J Adv Nurs 2007 [in press]
86. International Expert Advisory Group Report on Palliative Care (Marymount Hospice and The Atlantic Philanthropies). Cork, Ireland, 2006.
87. Small N, Rhodes P. Too ill to talk? User involvement in palliative care. London: Routledge, 2000.
88. Terry W, Olson LG, Ravencroft P, Wilss L, Boulton-Lewis G. Hospice patients' views on research in palliative care. Intern Med J 2006; 36: 406–413.

Reprinted with permission from: Larkin, P. J., Dierckx de Casterlé, B., & Schotsmans, P. (2007). Transition towards end of life in palliative care: An exploration of its meaning for advanced cancer patients in Europe. *Journal of Palliative Care, 23*(2), 69–79.

7.9 TOWARD A CONCEPTUAL EVALUATION OF TRANSIENCE IN RELATION TO PALLIATIVE CARE

PHILIP J. LARKIN
BERNADETTE DIERCKX DE CASTERLÉ
PAUL SCHOTSMANS

Abstract

Background: *A qualitative study into palliative care patients' experiences of transition revealed a gap between current definitions of transition and their expression of the palliative care experience. Transience appears to offer a better definition, but remains conceptually weak, with limited definition in a health care context.* ***Methods:*** *A qualitative conceptual evaluation of transience was undertaken using two case examples, interview data and the literature. Multiple sources were used to identify the literature (1966–2006), including a search on Cumulative Index to Nursing and Allied Health Literature Medline, and Ovid and Arts and Humanities Index using the keywords, "transience" and "palliative care." Thirty-one papers related to transience were retrieved. Analysis and synthesis formulated a theoretical definition of transience relative to palliative care.* ***Findings:*** *Transience is a nascent concept. Preconditions and outcomes of transience appear contextually dependent, which may inhibit its conceptual development. Transience depicts a fragile emotional state related to sudden change and uncertainty at end of life, exhibited as a feeling of stasis. Defining attributes would seem to include fragility, suddenness, powerlessness, impermanence, time, space, uncertainty, separation, and homelessness.* ***Conclusions:*** *Transience is poten-*

tially more meaningful for palliative care in understanding the impact of end-of-life experiences for patients than current conceptualizations of transition as a process toward resolution. As a nascent concept, it remains strongly encapsulated within a framework of transition, and further conceptual development is needed to enhance its maturity and refinement.

Introduction

There is increasing interest in the application of qualitative approaches to concept analysis, arising largely from the critique of the positivist methods advocated by, for example, Walker and Avant (2005). It is cogently argued that reductionist stepwise approaches to concept analysis often limit the possibility of theory construction (Morse, 1995). There is a call for nursing science to move toward a more iterative and integrative approach of concept development (Morse, 1995; Morse et al., 1996b; Morse et al., 2002; Morse 2004).

Background

Conceptual Development

Conceptual development is most beneficial for extant concepts that require refinement in a specific discipline or context. Hupcey et al. (2001) advanced the concept of trust in this way. Fasnacht (2003) used similar methods to refine the concept of creativity. Both drew on a relatively strong body of literature to explore the depth and maturity of their respective concepts in relation to nursing. Finfgeld-Connett (2006) confirmed that something relatively concrete needs to exist before such an approach can be applied: "Qualitative concept development is particularly apt when constructs are *relatively* [my emphasis] immature and conceptual boundaries are difficult to identify" (p. 104).

Conceptual maturity requires critical judgment regarding the degree to which the concept can be clearly defined, adapted to different research settings, and has robust parameters or boundaries (Hupcey et al., 2001; Finfgeld-Connett, 2006). Moreover, maturity should determine the method for developing the concept (Morse et al. 1996a). Immature or nascent concepts, for example, may benefit from the use of qualitative fieldwork data to support or refute their standing. Conceptual evaluation is beneficial for such concepts, and offers criteria to undertake this procedure (Morse et al., 1996b).

The Empirical Study

In this chapter, we report a conceptual evaluation of transience applied to the discipline of palliative care (Morse et al., 1996a; Penrod, 2001). In keeping with the constructivist approach, we present data from a qualitative study into palliative care patients' experiences of transition. We addressed the research question, "How is the transition experience toward end of life described by European advanced cancer patients?" through semistructured interviews conducted with 100 palliative care patients across six European countries: United Kingdom, Ireland, Italy, Spain, Switzerland, and The Netherlands. Data were collected at one point in time from a purposeful selection of advanced cancer patients admitted to a hospice/palliative care unit (PCU) for end-of-life care. Although this was a relatively large sample in qualitative terms, we maintain that this breadth of data demonstrates particular attention to context and culture, which may not be addressed through more positivist methods of conceptual analysis (Morse, 1995; McKenna, 1997). Further, the evidence for transience in the literature enables some level of contemporaneous judgment to be made regarding its preconditions, attributes, and outcomes relative to palliative care. We use two case studies to support, define, and consolidate the emerging concept. Finally, we critically appraise how far qualitative approaches fit the examination of transience as a nascent concept, and its potential importance to palliative care.

Transience as a Concept Emerging From the Data

Concepts that arise from within practice hold greater credibility and relevance and lead eventually to stronger theory development (McKenna, 1997, p. 58). The term "transience" arose from our study exploring the different, yet not unrelated, concept, transition. Transition literature often describes overtly positive outcomes such as resilience, reconstruction, coherence, life purpose, sense of self, transcendence, and transformation (Smith, 1994; Holland Wade, 1998; Paterson et al., 1999; Block, 2001; Neill, 2002; Kralik et al., 2003; Nygren et al., 2005). Interview data did not always fit with these descriptions. Patients described having limited knowledge about the purpose and timing of transfer to the hospice/PCU, uncertainty about who instigated the transfer, limited involvement in decision making often due to rapidly increasing symptom burden and, once transferred, a sense of waiting for something to happen. We, therefore, sought other explanations to capture their experience. Concepts related to process may incur additional difficulties, termed *fuzzy boundaries*–an unclear beginning or end or variations at specific times (Kim, 1983). Given the strength of findings that suggested that transition did not clarify patients' experience satisfactorily, critical evaluation of any alternative description was warranted. In particular, we needed to test whether transience was sufficiently robust to be considered a concept per se, and what level of concept could be attributed to it (Morse, 2004). Here, we cite two cases where the richness and complexity of the transience experience is present. Names have been changed to preserve patient confidentiality. Informed consent was obtained from all patients in this study, following ethical approval procedures in each country. Data were analyzed using the ATLAS.TI program.

Selection of an exemplar is paradoxical in that, working inductively, the researcher does not yet know what the attributes of the concept are, and yet selects examples that try to demonstrate it (Morse, 1995). Clearly, the example should be explicit enough to illustrate all the possible attributes to support the case. The cases describe two respondents from different countries, in receipt of palliative care and living at the palliative care–terminal care interface of their lives. We acknowledge that the cases shown are specifically selected to demonstrate the concept in absolute terms, and that the strength of the concept in the unique and individual experiences of 100 people across a number of countries is variable. However, we identified a set of attributes from both cases and reflections on the interview data in general (Morse, 1995). These attributes were: fragility, suddenness, powerlessness, impermanence, time, space, uncertainty, separation, and homelessness. We consider these attributes to be embedded within these cases although evident in a cross-section of interviews.

In the cases presented, the impact of patients' experience describes a period of irrevocable change and an unknown future, contrasting the empowerment construct that appears to be a precondition for negotiating transitional change (Bridges, 2001). In effect, the reality of their situation was not so much in process (as would be expected from transition), but more a sense of stasis, as they rationalized past experiences with their present situation. This questioned the validity of transition as a descriptor of the totality of their experience (Table 7.9.1).

The attributes identified were then reformulated into a meaningful structure for exploration, referred to as rules of relation (Morse & Doberneck, 1995). These tentatively frame the concept, offering some preconditions and outcomes, as follows:

- A sudden and unexpected change in life circumstance
- Inability to prevent that change
- A personal shift in both time and space
- The realization of a fragile and impermanent existence
- A sense of stasis.

Search Methods

Concept Evaluation

Criteria for conceptual evaluation ascribed to Morse et al. (1996b) were then applied (Table 7.9.2). All authors agree that a review of relevant literature should be undertaken, although its focus may vary (Robinson & McKenna, 1998; Hutchfield, 1999; Morse, 2004). In all cases, the review

CHAPTER 7   HEALTH AND ILLNESS TRANSITIONS   413

TABLE 7.9.1   The Attributes of Transience Derived From Patient Interviews

Attribute	Exemplar
Powerlessness	"There was no relationship and he constantly contradicted himself, in the end you don't know what to think. When you have no experience in these matters, and you don't know anyone with this illness, you are totally lost." (Jeanne, 43, Ca Lung, Switzerland)
Fragility	"…and no-one couldn't come near me. If a doctor came near the bed, I'd say, 'Please, please, doctor, don't touch that leg, you can do anything you like with me but please don't touch that leg', and here he'd be…'I'm not going to touch you at all, I wouldn't harm you', and I'd go, 'Please don't touch the clothes,' and I was just lying in the bed and couldn't let anybody near me." (Annie, 74, Ca Breast, Ireland)
Impermanence	"I have here my radio, a picture of my father and mother, a picture of my wife, I have a piece of my own home taken here. Yes, yes, things from your own home? The rest I give away, they are no good to me anymore." (Andre, 60, Leukemia, Netherlands)
Uncertainty	"The worst thing that happened to me was the day I came for my check up and I was told the next day I was to be hospitalized…when they told me, 'Tomorrow you come in,' I asked if there was anything wrong. All I got for an answer was, 'You just come in.' The doctor didn't explain anything." (Claudio, 64, Ca Prostate, Italy)
Time	"As time goes by, the evolution of the disease progresses more, I mean I notice it much more from one day to the next. It is not like some time ago that a day or two or one week went by, and it seemed that everything was the same. And now, no. From day to day, it can be noticed, it is very different, except for certain days that are better." (Juan, 72, Ca Colon, Spain)
Space	"I'd rather be home, of course, but they brought things from home and when I wake up, nice, cosy, then you don't have that longing." (Herbert, 81, Ca Pancreas, The Netherlands)
Suddenness	"I think the thing that I noticed more than anything was the sudden transition from being at home and doing all the things that one does at home and out and about, and then coming in here and suddenly being very, very restricted." (Peter, 70, Ca Lung, U.K.)
Separation	"I am sorry I am not going to see my grandchildren grow up, obviously. You know, you promised to take care of them and bring them out and treat them, but I can't do that, because I won't be here to do that." (Claire, 68, Ca Colon, U.K.)
Homelessness	"So coming here, I don't regret it…no, because this is my home now…I haven't got nowhere else to go." (Lily, 77, Multiple Myeloma, U.K.)

should be rigorous and identify a breadth of resources to explore the concept. Multiple sources were used, including the bibliographic databases Cumulative Index to Nursing and Allied Health Literature (CINAHL) Medline and Ovid and Arts and Humanities Index. One hundred and ten papers were identified that included transience as a keyword. Of these, 79 were rejected as having limited reference to the research topic under investigation, because they described transience in the context of pure sciences only. Thirty-one papers were then retrieved, including those that offered a conceptual definition of transience, or alluded to transience as an example of other health-related phenomena.

TABLE 7.9.2 Criteria for Concept Evaluation

Is the concept well-defined?

Are the characteristics/attributes identified?

Are the preconditions and outcomes of the concept described and demonstrated?

Are the conceptual boundaries delineated?

Morse, J. M., Mitcham, C., Hupcey, J. E., & Cerdas Tasón, M. (1996). Criteria for concept evaluation. *Journal of Advanced Nursing, 24*, 385–390. Reproduced with permission.

Nineteen articles with particular relevance to our research study were selected, including philosophy (7), psychology (5), health or social science context (4), and thanatology (3). The search was then broadened to include transience in relation to the attributes identified from the case studies, using word combinations such as transience AND homelessness. A further three papers were identified. Books, texts, dictionaries, and landmark works that demonstrated the existence of the concept over time were also explored (McKenna, 1997). The body of literature identified comprised mainly clinical discussion papers, with relatively few empirically based studies. No data specifically related to palliative care were found.

Findings

Is the Concept Well-Defined?

The maturity of a concept appears proportional to the strength and reliability of its definition (Morse et al., 1996a, 1996b; McKenna, 1997; Hupcey et al., 2001; Penrod, 2001; Penrod & Hupcey, 2005a, 2005b). Although qualitative conceptual theorists consider dictionary definitions too sparse in terms of nuance, we reviewed the *Oxford English Dictionary* (1989) to ascertain properties differing from other competing concepts, such as transition. Transience was defined as, "the action or fact of passing away," reflecting a lack of permanence, something of limited durability (*Oxford English Dictionary*, 1989). Transience was evidenced in the arts, sciences, and humanities, and derived from the same etymological root as transition—transpire—to go or cross over. Transition was largely defined in terms of passage, movement, and change from one state or place to another.

Empirical literature that addresses transience in a health context is relatively sparse. Transience would appear as an attribute or consequence of larger, more mature concepts as found in psychology, medicine (including medical geography), philosophy, and social science. For example, Schacter et al. (2003) discussed transience under an investigation of the concept of self and memory. Shaw (2005) described transience as a key descriptor of the concept of spirituality. Westermeyer (1982) related transience to persistence in the experience of depression, emphasizing both cyclical and temporal characteristics to the disease. Reed et al. (1998) focused on the experiences of older people moving into care homes, and described dependency and adjustment under a heading of transience. However, transience is often used without any clear definition or expansion of its meaning or application in context, suggesting a deeper exploration of transience is timely.

Themes in the Literature and Interview Data

Themes arising from both literature and interview data were reconfigured under four specific headings: transience as an ephemeral state of being, transience as an expression of time, transience as a spatial phenomenon, and transience as a construct of home. In presenting this conceptual evaluation, we use excerpts from the case studies to ground the emerging concept within the study proper.

Transience as an Ephemeral State

Two psychoanalytical articles offered a concrete description of transience: one historical and the other contemporary. Freud's (1916/2006) seminal treatise, "On Transience," described it as an ephemeral state of existence where things once considered permanent, change. Kitayama (1998) delineated between transition and transience. He described transition as a "phenomenological description of movement," whereas transience referred to an emotional state often associated with sadness and painful feelings (p. 937). The aesthetic of transience reflects something of passing beauty, which is both joyful (as it is currently beautiful) and sad (because it is a transient experience that will pass). Important to these descriptions is a dual sense of impermanence and irreversibility associated with the transient state, a sense of wanting to hold on to something when it is not possible to do so. Barbara (case study 1) reflected on her fragility since the recent death of her husband, Martin, stating:

> I don't know what to call it but if I was to overcome…that…but I just can't see it happening because of Martin [pauses, smiles]. He was my life, soul-mate, everything, and I just can't get over him and I never will.

Case 1: Barbara. Barbara was a 49-year-old woman with colon cancer and widespread gastrointestinal metastases. She lived in a rural community with her husband until his death from prostate cancer. She cared for him at home, supported by the palliative home care team. During this time, her own diagnosis was confirmed. Barbara had one daughter who lived in a major city about 200 miles away from her. Her daughter persuaded Barbara that she should move to live with her. Barbara reluctantly agreed. Once settled with her daughter, Barbara's own home was sold at her daughter's instruction. Although she had her own room in her daughter's house, the space did not allow Barbara to bring furniture or most of her personal possessions, which were also sold. Relationships grew strained in the house, and Barbara sought admission to hospice as respite from the situation. Barbara deeply regretted the sale of her own home, and felt she was simply waiting to join her husband.

Elizabeth (case study 2), in response to a question about being in a hospice, remarked:

> "Being here [the hospice]…has made me generally a lot calmer. It gives you strength and I'm at a kind of, underpinned by it…and I said to them [her parents], 'You do realize this is where I'm going to stay to die,' and I said, 'It's important because I know I'll be looked after and I know you'll be looked after as well.' And that is important because they will be."

Case 2: Elizabeth. Elizabeth was a 58-year-old woman with a primary brain tumor. She had lived with her partner and his children in his home for a number of years. As her disease progressed, her need for assistance with personal care increased, and she required the use of a wheelchair at all times. Eventually and unexpectedly for Elizabeth, her partner told her that he was no longer prepared to care for both her and the children, and that she would have to leave the family home. Elizabeth left the home within a few days and moved in with her adult daughter from a previous relationship. The daughter was also unable to provide the necessary support needed for Elizabeth, and she was transferred to the hospice. Elizabeth never saw her partner or his children once she left the family home and, although she kept in close contact with her daughter, remained in the hospice until her death.

In these descriptions, transience would appear to reflect an emotional state where the quality of the present moment may be all the more meaningful because of its fragility and impermanence. As Freud (1916/2006) concludes:

> The beauty of the human form and face vanish for ever in the course of our own lives, but their evanescence only lends them a fresh charm. (p. 1)

Transience as an Expression of Time

Time, particularly in relation to death, is core to the expression of transience (Wilder, 1965; Wolf, 1983; Lachmann, 1985; Feifel, 1990; Johnson, 2003; Adam, 2006). Human society attempts to use time to stabilize and fix something that is essentially intangible in order to, "overcome the threat of non-existence, finitude and transience" (Adam, 2006, p. 121). Elizabeth commented:

> I do want to live. I want to live and enjoy until the last minute, you know. My daughter said we needed things to look forward to, so I had a big birthday party and it was wonderful fun.

Conversely, Barbara spent her time traveling to avoid facing difficult family situations:

> The problems were going on, I kept going away, went to Spain, I went to Canada, I went to, anywhere I could go I went, just to get out of the way, get out of their way and for me, as well.

Johnson (2003) criticized poststructuralist assumptions that all life is essentially transient, arguing that Western culture has used this assumption as a way to demean the vitality of living. He argued that, where transience has been used to define life as shaped by the imminence of death, it neglects the fact that:

> Life proceeds at its own pace, and therefore, does not slip toward death in a transient manner. (p. 210)

Both cases demonstrate positive and negative aspects of transience as time; Elizabeth describing time spent living until she dies, and Barbara describing time spent creating distance from family and her own feelings.

Transience as Spatial Phenomenon

> I think it's territorial really, dying. As my friend said, this is your manor isn't it...back to the East End...because this is where it all is. (Elizabeth)

Transience has a strong relation to social and philosophical constructs of space and home. Augé, for example, defined transience in terms of the anonymity of "non-lieu" or "non-place." (Augé, 1995, p. 104) Hospitals, and more recently hospices, fit this description by virtue of patients passing through (Reed-Danahay, 2001; Foggo, 2006).

Milligan (2003) explored the idea of home as a space of ontological security. Space as dwelling has resonance for conceptualizing transience as something fluid and intangible, which differs from space as territory, bounded and closed (Williams, 1951; MacGregor Wise, 2000; Young et al., 2002; Gilmour, 2006). The achievement of ontological security in hospice would seem to be a positive outcome for people experiencing transience in their lives:

Interviewer: "If I asked you what [name of hospice] can give you at this moment in time, what would you say?"

Elizabeth: "Safety. A feeling that I can die and it's OK. Safe to die and all the people will look after me and it's not an embarrassing thing. I don't have to apologize. I don't have to pretend."

However, dying may also be associated with "feelings of rootlessness and having to face the 'unknown' with minimal mastery" (Feifel, 1990, p. 539). In Barbara's case, her inability to accept the new space in her daughter's home left her with regret and turmoil:

> I regret selling up and moving because maybe if I'd have stuck it, well, I don't know...if I could have lived on my own or–but I wasn't given the chance. (Barbara)

Transience as a Construct of Home

Most empirical studies on transience are evidenced in the concept of homelessness (Rowe & Wolch, 1990; Pollio, 1997; Kang et al., 2000; Anderson, 2001; Lee et al., 2003; Anderson & Rayens, 2004). Homelessness is particularly associated with mental ill-health (Geissler et al., 1995; Anderson & Rayens, 2004; Muir-Chochrane et al., 2006). Pollio (1997) identified four dimensions to the concept of transience in relation to homelessness: migration, duration, intention, and involvement. Migration refers to an individual's movement from their community of origin. Duration and intention reflect the length of time spent in the new community and the reason for the initial migration. Involvement warrants considerable investment in the new community in order to create stronger community support. These descriptions, particularly shared community, may reflect the transience experience of palliative care patients coming into hospice as they seek to stabilize their emotional turbulence:

> You get that sort of rapport with people, whereas, because they understand, they do understand…we've got the same wavelength, sort of thing. (Barbara)

Radley et al. (2006), in a small ethnographic study of homeless women in London, identified that the reason for homelessness was often traumatic life events, combined with vulnerability and poverty. Family bereavement, relationship breakdown, and loss of housing contribute to the context of homelessness. Elizabeth's story is a good example of someone who became transient following the loss of her home, a decision that left her vulnerable and angry:

> When you get a death sentence, you don't get a little book of notes…to tell you how to deal with it. And he didn't want me at home…and he certainly didn't want me dying in front of his children. I didn't know where to go…and within not long I was out of the house as well…I lost my home and my relationship. I was air-brushed out of their lives. (Elizabeth)

Barbara's reaction to her loss of home was resignation and withdrawal:

> She [daughter] sees me sitting on a bed and wasting my life away. Well, as far as I'm concerned, it's what I want to do. If I could do it, I would…I would get up and go out every day and buy something and go shopping. But I've got nothing, I've got no home, that's gone from me, so there's no point. (Barbara)

It is evident that there may be specific differences between transience and being transient, which are neither discrete nor tangible. Transience has some definitional and descriptive properties, but further delineation of its characteristics and attributes is warranted.

Are the Characteristics/Attributes Identified?

Given the etymological links between transience and transition, it was important to be able to identify what differed and what, if anything, made transience unique. The main attributes emerging were fragility (of the situation and its impact on the person), impermanence (for example, the transient state of being homeless), and stasis (limitation in ability to move beyond a given situation). The overt emphasis on transition as a positive process of growth and renewal (Bridges, 2001) implies an ability to address problems of the past and move on. The inability to do so is seen as potentially harmful to well-being. Contemporary models of grief and loss refute the passage ideal in favor of a life biography-incorporation model, bringing past experiences and present situation together to create a cohesive pattern (Walters, 1996). Transience would seem to be a response by the patient to incorporate the life biography within the present. Bachelard (1955), in "The Poetics of Space," argued that:

> All the spaces of our past moments of solitude, the spaces in which we have suffered from solitude, enjoyed, desired, and compromised solitude, remain indelible within us and precisely because the human being wants them to remain so. (p. 10)

Feelings of transience and uncertainty about the future enable us to embrace the past, leading to a more authentic humanity (Wilder, 1965). Authenticity does not assume transience to be a wholly negative phenomenon, but rather real-life experience that may affect a range of responses, as demonstrated by Elizabeth and Barbara.

Are the Preconditions and Outcomes of the Concept Described and Demonstrated?

Preconditions and outcomes link concept and context, central to the qualitative approach (Morse et al., 1996a). In support of Kitayama's reflection on transience (1998), the preconditions and outcomes identified seem to arise from an emotional response to a specific set of life circumstances. However, we noted an overlying emphasis in the conceptual analysis literature on behavioral concepts (Morse, 1995; Morse et al., 1996a; Morse, 2004), and transience as a behavioral concept remains unclear. There is a need to qualify preconditions and outcomes for transience, and this gap hinders the evaluation of this concept. For example, universal characteristics and attributes should be apparent in all contexts where transience exists (Morse, 2004). This did not appear to be the case. Homeless women's experiences of transience were often precipitated by abuse or deprivation (Radley et al., 2006). This differed from the case of an older person's relocation to residential care (Reed et al., 1998). Both hold agreed properties of transience, but with mutually exclusive characteristics. Morse (2004) advises caution in developing a single concept with many similar meanings. Further exploration of the distinction between behavioral and emotional components of transience may benefit conceptual clarity.

Are the Conceptual Boundaries Delineated?

Given the description of transience as an ephemeral state of being, it is difficult to conceive of boundaries and structure in its description. Time and space, which contribute to our understanding of transience, are clearly infinitesimal. Distinction between the characteristics of transience and transition would constitute a boundary, albeit an ambiguous one. However, transience shows characteristics of uniqueness, which may separate it from other concepts. Transience clearly differs from current descriptions of transition as reconstruction and mastery (Schumacher & Meleis, 1994; Holland Wade, 1998; Bridges, 2001; Gwilliam & Bailey, 2001; Boeijea et al., 2002; Young et al., 2002; Vaartio & Kiviniemi, 2003; White, 2003; Kralik et al., 2006). Neither Barbara's nor Elizabeth's experiences suggest that it was possible to reconstruct their lives

at this point in time. This differentiation remains relatively abstract, and does not in itself offer categorical evidence for transience as a concept. Further comparative work is necessary to confirm these relationships.

Discussion

This conceptual evaluation derived from the need to explain transition experiences that current conceptual descriptions failed to capture. In choosing transience as a possible descriptor, the lack of evidence looking at transience in a palliative care context is a distinct limitation. Transience, when used to consolidate other concepts, indicates that it is an immature and underdeveloped "low-level" concept in its own right (Morse, 2004). It would be important to delineate the state of transience from the process of transition and, more specifically, to question why we seek transition as a positive outcome. Transition theory indicates potential for transformative experiences to arise out of a transition process, including the acute care–palliative care interface (Meleis & Rogers, 1987; Schumacher & Meleis, 1994; Paterson et al., 1999; Meleis et al., 2000; Kralik, 2002; Johnston, 2004; O'Connor, 2004; Schulman-Green et al., 2004; Kralik et al., 2006; Thompson et al., 2006). Transformative experience would require a, "restructuring of the illness and self in order to regain some degree of control" (Paterson et al.,1999, p. 787). It may be that we seek for transition to be transformative because the hope of a positive outcome is easier to deal with than the fragility and impermanence that transience offers. The task of understanding such relationships should form the basis of further work, particularly focusing on the transience–transition interface in relation to transience as a state of being and transition as a process of becoming (Mueller, 1943; Wilcock, 1999).

The multidisciplinary nature of palliative care means that transience can be experienced and examined by practitioners simultaneously, and yet, differently. A social worker may be more interested in transience as a consequence of homelessness. A psychologist may emphasize its impact on the self.

Thus, in the context of palliative care, transience should be seen as a multifaceted concept reflecting the complex nature of human experience. Evident from the two cases discussed here is the particular status of hospice as a place that promotes healing and maintains well-being (Williams, 1951; Gilmour, 2006). Lawton's (2000) seminal work on the experience of dying in a hospice concurs with descriptions of place based on connection, memory, and identity. In her research, connectedness to the place and community of hospice was important. This revealed itself in the experiences of Barbara and Elizabeth. Yet, the influence of biomedicine in palliative care, and the perceived use of hospice as a transient place where complex symptoms may be treated and patients then discharged, is of increasing concern (Praill, 2000; McNamara, 2001; Payne et al., 2002; Skilbeck & Payne, 2005; Foggo, 2006). This may undermine the safety and security of hospice in relation to transience for patients. Elizabeth's comments about hospice as a place where she felt safe to die is one example. Arguably, the reality of hospice as a place where people face the fragility and impermanence of life suggests that transience is an integral part of the hospice experience. The shift in clinical emphasis in hospice and PCUs risks Augé's (1995) description of transience as, "non-place," where people simply pass through.

Although a qualitative approach to evaluation has proved valuable, it is not without its problems. Qualitative conceptual development requires prior evidence of the concept and a body of literature against which that concept may be judged. There is an inherent complexity in the language and structure used. For example, the differences between defining a concept through evaluation (Morse et al., 1996b) and using higher order "principal determinants" of epistemology, pragmatism, linguistics, and logic (Penrod, 2001) seem to address the same issues and lead to similar conclusions. The difference appears based on the relative maturity of the concept under investigation, and it is difficult to judge this without firm evidence, either from the literature or the field. There are excellent examples of the different categories and uses of conceptual development methods (Finfgeld-Connett, 2006). Attempting to understand the types of approach and their various nuances can be taxing. Having rejected the stepwise approach, Morse herself has described her development of concepts using qualitative inquiry as a series of steps, albeit that the experienced analyst may be able to address those steps simultaneously (McKenna, 1997; Morse, 2004). In a state of perplexity, it may be all too easy to seek the safety of the more structured stepwise and reductionist approaches of which Morse and others are critical. Given these caveats, a qualitative approach still proves useful in determining the scope and possibilities for conceptual investigation of nascent concepts, and may be of particular interest in palliative care where tenuous and complex phenomena, like transience, exist.

Implications for Nursing

Palliative care nursing places care and comfort at the core of its practice. Palliative nursing expertise is grounded in current international definitions of palliative care and, as such, contributes to the current debate on whether palliative care should be a speciality or a generic approach to end-of-life care (World Health Organization, 2002; Skilbeck & Payne, 2005). Transience in the context of palliative care relates to understanding "social death" (Mulkay, 1993; Johnston, 2004) beyond biological or clinical definitions. Social death has been described as "the cessation of the individual person as an active agent in others' lives" (Mulkay, 1993, pp. 33–34). This description echoes the transience experience discussed in this chapter. Palliative care nurses are best placed to reorient the multidisciplinary team toward the impact of social death by virtue of their proximity to the patient and shared appreciation of the wholeness of the human being—physical, social, and spiritual—as the basis from which palliative nursing practice is derived.

Conclusions

Although the benefits of palliative care are increasingly recognized, we still need to understand more fully how it is experienced by patients. This conceptual evaluation adds to this need, offering insight into the complexity of experience faced by patients at the end of life. It challenges practitioners to reconsider the impact of living with the inevitability of death for their patients, and the importance of being able to respond to each individual and unique experience both as a nurse clinician and fellow human being.

More evidence is needed before transience can be described as a well-defined and robust concept for palliative care. Neither the literature nor the data presented can offer sufficient material on which to make a conclusive judgment. We, therefore, consider transience to be a nascent concept in need of further work to establish its credibility. Transience has some capability to describe certain experiences for palliative care patients, and it would be important to test these in other clinical areas as part of the development process. What can be concluded in the context of this study is that:

- Transience is a fragile emotional state associated with sadness or painful feelings.
- Transience can lead to the sudden realization that nothing is truly permanent.
- As such, transience has particular resonance for palliative care.

Acknowledgments

Philip Larkin is holder of the 2003 Health Research Board Fellowship in Palliative Care, and this study is jointly funded by The Health Research Board of Ireland and The Irish Hospice Foundation, Dublin, Ireland. Particular thanks are due to Dr. Jane Sixsmith for her assistance in the preparation of this chapter.

REFERENCES

Adam, B. (2006). Time. *Theory, Culture and Society, 23*, 119–138.

Anderson, D. G. (2001). Families of origin of homeless and never-homeless women. *Western Journal of Nursing Research, 23*, 394–413.

Anderson, D. G., & Rayens, M. K. (2004). Factors influencing homelessness in women. *Public Health Nursing 21*, 2–23.

Augé, M. (1995). *Non-places: An introduction to an anthropology of supermodernity* (J. Howe, Trans.). London: Verso.

Bachelard, G. (1955). *The Poetics of Space.* New York: Orion Press.

Block, S.D. (2001). Perspectives of care at the close of life. Psychological considerations, growth, and transcendence at the end of life: Art of the possible. *Journal of the American Medical Association, 285*, 2898–2905.

Boeijea, H., Duijnsteeb, M., Grypdonck, M., & Pool, A. (2002) Encountering the downward phase: Biographical work in people with multiple sclerosis living at home. *Social Science and Medicine, 55*, 881–893.

Bridges, W. (2001). *The way of transition: Embracing life's difficult moments.* Cambridge, MA: Perseus.

Fasnacht, P. H. (2003). Creativity: A refinement of the concept for nursing practice. *Journal of Advanced Nursing, 34*, 195–202.

Feifel, H. (1990). Psychology and death: Meaningful rediscovery. *American Psychologist, 45*, 537–543.

Finfgeld-Connett, D. (2006). Qualitative concept development: Implications for nursing research and knowledge. *Nursing Forum, 41*, 103–112.

Foggo, B. A. (2006). Hospice: A place to die or just passing on? *Progress in Palliative Care, 14*, 109–111.

Freud, S. (1916/2006). *On Transience* (J. Strachey, Trans.). Retrieved July 20, 2006, from http://www.freuds-requiem.com/transience.html

Geissler, L., Bormann, C. A., Kwiatkowski, C. F., Braucht, G. N., & Reichardt, C. S. (1995). Women, homelessness and substance abuse moving beyond the stereotypes. *Psychology of Women Quarterly, 19*, 65–83.

Gilmour, J. A. (2006). Hybrid space: Constituting the hospital as a home space for patients. *Nursing Inquiry, 13*, 16–22.

Gwilliam, B., & Bailey, C. (2001). The nature of terminal malignant bowel obstruction and its impact on patients with advanced cancer. *International Journal of Palliative Nursing, 7*, 474–476.

Holland Wade, G. (1998). A concept analysis of personal transformation. *Journal of Advanced Nursing, 28*, 713–719.

Hupcey, J., Penrod, J., Morse, J. M., & Mitcham, C. (2001). An exploration and advancement of the concept of trust. *Journal of Advanced Nursing, 36*, 282–293.

Hutchfield, K. (1999). Family-centred care: A concept analysis. *Journal of Advanced Nursing, 29*, 1178–1187.

Johnson, D. (2003). Why view all time from the perspective of time's end? A Bergsonian attack on Bataillean transience. *Time and Society, 12,* 209–224.

Johnston, G. (2004). Social death. The impact of protracted dying. In S. Payne, J. Seymour, & C. Ingleton, eds.), *Palliative care nursing: Principles and evidence for practice* (pp. 351–363). Maidenhead, U.K.: Open University Press.

Kang, M., Alperstein, G., Dow, A., Van Beek, I., Martin, C., & Bennett, D. (2000). Prevalence of tuberculosis infection among homeless young people in central and eastern Sydney. *Journal of Paediatrics and Child Health, 36,* 382–384.

Kim, H. S. (1983). *The nature of theoretical thinking in nursing.* Norwalk, CT: Appleton-Century-Crofts.

Kitayama, O. (1998). Transience: Its beauty and danger. *International Journal of Psychoanalysis, 79,* 937–953.

Kralik, D. (2002). The quest for ordinariness: Transition experienced by midlife women living with chronic illness. *Journal of Advanced Nursing, 39,* 146–154.

Kralik, D., Koch, T., & Eastwood, S. (2003). The salience of body: Transition in sexual identity for women living with multiple sclerosis. *Journal of Advanced Nursing, 42,* 11–20.

Kralik, D., Visentin, K., & van Loon, A. (2006). Transition: A literature review. *Journal of Advanced Nursing, 55,* 320–329.

Lachmann, F. (1985). On transience and the sense of temporal continuity. *Contemporary Psychoanalysis, 21,* 193–200.

Lawton, J. (2000). *The dying process. Patients' experience of palliative care.* London: Routledge.

Lee, B. A., Spratlen-Price, T., & Kanan, J. W. (2003). Determinants of homelessness in metropolitan areas. *Journal of Urban Affairs, 25,* 335–356.

MacGregor Wise, J. (2000). Home: Territory and identity. *Cultural Studies, 14,* 295–310.

McKenna, H. (Ed.) (1997). Building theory through concept analysis. *Nursing Theories and Models* (pp. 55–84). London: Routledge.

McNamara, B. (2001). *Fragile lives: Death denying and care.* Buckingham, U.K.: Open University Press.

Meleis, A. I., & Rogers, S. (1987). Women in transition: Being vs. becoming or being and becoming. *Health Care for Women International, 8,* 199–217.

Meleis, A. I., Sawyer, L. M., Im, E. O., Hilfinger Messias, K. D., & Schumacher, K. (2000). Experiencing transitions: An emerging middle-range theory. *Advances in Nursing Science, 23,* 12–28.

Milligan, C. (2003). Location or dis-location? Toward a conceptualization of people and place in the caregiving experience. *Social and Cultural Geography, 4,* 455–470.

Morse, J. M. (1995). Exploring the theoretical basis of nursing using advanced techniques of concept analysis. *Advances in Nursing Science, 17,* 31–46.

Morse, J. M. (2004). Constructing qualitatively derived theory: Concept construction and concept typologies. *Qualitative Health Research, 14,* 1387–1395.

Morse, J. M., & Doberneck, B. (1995). Delineating the concept of hope. *Journal of Nursing Scholarship, 27,* 277–285.

Morse, J. M., Hupcey, J. E., Mitcham, C., & Lenz, E. (1996a). Concept analysis in nursing research: A critical appraisal. *Scholarly Inquiry for Nursing Practice, 10,* 253–277.

Morse, J. M., Mitcham, C., Hupcey, J., & Tasón, M. C. (1996b). Criteria for concept evaluation. *Journal of Advanced Nursing, 24,* 385–390.

Morse, J. M., Hupcey, J. E., Penrod, J., & Mitcham, C. (2002). Integrating concepts for the development of qualitatively-derived theory. *Research and Theory for Nursing Practice, 16,* 5–18.

Mueller, G. E. (1943). On being and becoming. *Philosophy of Science, 10,* 149–162.

Muir-Chochrane, E., Fereday, J., Junedini, J., Drummond, A., & Darbyshire, P. (2006). Self-management of medication for mental health problems by homeless young people. *International Journal of Mental Health Nursing, 15,* 163–170.

Mulkay, M. (1993). Social death in Britain. In D. Clark (Ed.), *The sociology of death* (pp. 33–34). Oxford, U.K.: Blackwell.

Neill, J. (2002). Transcendence and transformation in the life patterns of women living with rheumatoid arthritis. *Advances in Nursing Science, 24,* 27–47.

Nygren, B., Aléx, L., Jonsén, E., Gustafson, Y., Norberg, A., & Lundman, B. (2005). Resilience, sense of coherence, purpose in life and self-transcendence in relation to perceived physical and mental health among the oldest old. *Ageing and Mental Health, 9,* 354–362.

O'Connor, M. (2004). Transitions in status from wellness to illness, illness to wellness. In S. Payne, J. Seymour, & C. Ingleton (Eds.), *Palliative care nursing: Principles and evidence for practice* (pp. 126–143). Maidenhead, U.K.: Open University Press.

Oxford English Dictionary. (1989). Retrieved July 10, 2006, from http://dictionary.oed.com/cgi/entry/50256265.html

Paterson, B., Thorne, S., Crawford, J., & Tarko, M. (1999). Living with diabetes as a transformational experience. *Qualitative Health Research, 9,* 786–802.

Payne, S., Sheldon, F., Jarrett, N., Large, S., Smith, P., & Davis, C. L. (2002). Differences in understanding of specialist palliative care amongst service provid-

ers and commissioners in South London. *Palliative Medicine, 16,* 395–402.
Penrod, J. (2001). Refinement of the concept of uncertainty. *Journal of Advanced Nursing, 34,* 238–245.
Penrod, J., & Hupcey, J. E. (2005a). Concept advancement: Extending science through concept-driven research. *Research and Theory for Nursing Practice: An International Journal, 19,* 231–241.
Penrod, J., & Hupcey, J. E. (2005b). Enhancing methodological clarity: Principle-based concept analysis. *Journal of Advanced Nursing, 50,* 403–409.
Pollio, D. E. (1997). The relationship between transience and current life situation in the homeless services-using population. *Social Work, 42,* 41–551.
Praill, D. (2000). Editorial: Who are we here for? *Palliative Medicine, 14,* 91–92.
Radley, A., Hodgetts, D., & Cullen, A. (2006). Fear, romance and transience in the lives of homeless women. *Social and Cultural Geography, 7,* 437–461.
Reed, J., Roskell Peyton, V., & Bond, S. (1998). Settling in and moving on: Transience and older people in care homes. *Social Policy & Administration, 32,* 151–165.
Reed-Danahay, D. (2001). This is your home now!: Conceptualizing location and dislocation in a dementia unit. *Qualitative Research, 1,* 47–63.
Robinson, D. S., & McKenna. H. P. (1998). Loss: An analysis of a concept of particular interest to nursing. *Journal of Advanced Nursing, 27,* 779–784.
Rowe, S., & Wolch, J. (1990). Social networks in time and space: Homeless women in skid row, Los Angeles. *Annals of the Association of American Geographers, 80,* 184–204.
Schacter, D. L., Chiao, J. Y., & Mitchell, J. P. (2003). The seven sins of memory implications for self. *Annals of the New York Academy of Science, 1001,* 226–239.
Schulman-Green, D., McCorkle, R., Curry, L., Cherlin, E., Johnson-Hurzeler, R., & Bradley, E. (2004). At the crossroads: Making the transition to hospice. *Palliative and Supportive Care, 2,* 351–360.
Schumacher, K. L., & Meleis, A. I. (1994). Transitions: A central concept in nursing. *Image: Journal of Nursing Scholarship, 26,* 119–127.
Shaw, J. A. (2005). A pathway to spirituality. *Psychiatry, 68,* 350–362.

Skilbeck, J. K., & Payne, S. (2005). End of life care: A discourse analysis of specialist palliative care nursing. *Journal of Advanced Nursing, 51,* 325–334.
Smith, J. A. (1994). Reconstructing selves: An analysis of discrepancies between women's contemporaneous and respective accounts of the transition to motherhood. *British Journal of Psychology, 85,* 371–392.
Thompson, G. N., McClement, S. E., & Daenick, P. J. (2006). "Changing lanes": Facilitating the transition from curative to palliative care. *Journal of Palliative Care, 22,* 91–98.
Vaartio, H., & Kiviniemi, K. (2003). Men's experiences and their resources from cancer diagnosis to recovery. *European Journal of Oncology Nursing, 7,* 182–190.
Walker, L. O., & Avant, K. C. (2005). *Strategies for theory construction in nursing.* Newbury Park, CA: Sage.
Walters, T. (1996). A new model of grief: Bereavement and biography. *Mortality, 1,* 7–25.
Westermeyer, J. (1982). Understanding the transience or persistence of depression. *American Journal of Public Health, 72,* 982–983.
White, A. (2003). Interactions between nurses and men admitted with chest pain. *European Journal of Cardiovascular Nursing, 2,* 47–55.
Wilcock, A. A. (1999). Reflections on doing, being and becoming. *Australian Occupational Therapy Journal, 46,* 1–11.
Wilder, A. N. (1965). Mortality and contemporary literature. *Harvard Theological Review, 58,* 1–20.
Williams, D. C. (1951). The myth of passage. *Journal of Philosophy, 48,* 457–472.
Wolf, E. S. (1983). Discussion: Transience or nothingness. *Psychoanalytic Inquiry, 3,* 529–542.
World Health Organization. (2002). *WHO definition of palliative care.* Retrieved February 2, 2007, from http://www.who.int/cancer/palliative/definition/en/
Young, B., Dixon-Woods, M., Findlay, M., & Heney, D. (2002). Parenting in a crisis: Conceptualizing mothers of children with cancer. *Social Science and Medicine, 55,* 1835–1847.

Reprinted with permission from: Larkin, P. J., Dierckx de Casterlé, B., & Schotsmans, P. (2007). Towards a conceptual evaluation of transience in relation to palliative care. *Journal of Advanced Nursing, 59*(1), 86–96.

Chapter 8   Organizational Transitions

8.1   ON BECOMING A FLEXIBLE POOL NURSE: EXPANSION OF THE MELEIS TRANSITION FRAMEWORK

VICTORIA L. RICH

Adequate nurse-to-patient ratios in acute-care settings have been shown to be a key factor in improving the quality of patient outcomes (Needleman, Buerhaus, Mattke, Stewart, & Zelevinsky, 2002). However, variable census and increasing fluctuations in patient acuity, coupled with the nurse shortage have made adherence to staffing ratios increasingly more difficult, and have demanded considerable efforts by nurse administrators to devise flexible and creative staffing approaches. Common solutions to address staffing issues include the use of per diem agency nurses, 13-week contract nurses, overtime compensation and incentives, and internal, flexible pool nurses. These strategies have allowed mechanisms by which nurse leaders can assure safe staffing levels and respond to fluctuating patient census and acuity, and changes in the nursing workforce.

The importance of safe nursing staffing captured national attention in 2004 with the issuing of a hallmark report by the Institute of Medicine entitled "Keeping Patients Safe: Transforming the Work." This seminal publication based on the work of Aiken, Clarke, Cheung, Sloane, and Silber (2003) and other influential leaders in health care suggested that registered nurses employed and internal to the organization provide safer care and better continuity for patients than nurses from external agencies who work sporadically in hospital settings. Additionally, current research has also demonstrated that improved patient outcomes and decreased mortality are related to lower nurse-to-patient ratios, higher educational preparation of the nurse, and years of experience (Aiken et al., 2003).

Based on compelling research and consensus regarding safe nursing staffing, an internal, flexible pool of nurses entitled "Staffing for All Seasons" (SFAS) was created at the Hospital of the University of Pennsylvania in 2004. The SFAS program's guiding principles address: (a) *recruitment strategies,* by offering flexibility in scheduling for nurses needing alterations in life–work balance at different times in their career life span; (b) *retention strategies,* by offering experienced nurses who desire different growth experiences in their professional careers without leaving the institution; and (c) *patient safety and outcome strategies,* by employing nurses with unit-specific competencies and flexible staffing practices to assure adequate nurse-to-patient ratios.

Five years after the implementation of this program, SFAS has over 80 registered nurses who practice in specific areas of the hospital in need of supplemental staffing and who deliver expert nursing care. Clinical specialty teams for SFAS nurses have been developed to recruit nurses interested in and committed to care of diverse patient populations. Examples of these teams include (a) medical-surgical, (b) critical care, (c) maternal/child, (d) emergency department, (e) ambulatory and office-based practice, (f) perioperative, (g) home care, and (h) private duty. A differential pay scale has been implemented that is graded and leveled based on factors such as vacancy rates, required staffing expertise, and coverage for weekends, off-shifts and unplanned call-outs.

Page (2008) has suggested in a chapter written for "Patient Safety and Quality: An Evidence-Based Handbook for Nurses" that more research is needed surrounding flexible staffing models, such as the types of nurses that practice in this model, the impact on patient outcomes, and the effect on nurse recruitment and retention. Considering these complex, multifactoral issues, the Chief Nurse Executive at the Hospital of the University of Pennsylvania, a 730-bed academic medical center, designed a survey methodology to explore the personal and professional characteristics of the organization's internal, flexible pool nurses, SFAS, to measure the developmental transitions that occur as the nurse evolves from having a defined unit identity and specialty practice to a flexible nursing practice and a redefined identity.

The emerging middle-range theory of transitions by Meleis and colleagues was used as a framework for conducting a pilot evaluation and guiding the construction of research instruments to capture nurses' perceptions and work fulfillment (Meleis, Sawyer, Im, Messias, & Schumacher, 2000). This framework is graphically depicted in Figure 8.1.1. Three broad dimensions are components of the model: nature of transitions, transition conditions, and patterns of response. The *nature of transitions* refers to the type and patterns of the transitions, as well as the properties of the transition process. Because they are complex and multidimensional, essential properties involve awareness of the transition, engagement in the transition process, identifying change and differences between the old and new states, a time span, and critical points and events that mark the transition process.

Transition conditions refer to the personal and social context in which the transition occurs, with emphasis on factors that may facilitate and/or inhibit the transition process. Personal background meanings, attitudes, and beliefs attached to the transition process are examples of this domain. Social conditions refer to social factors in both the local and broader social environments that facilitate or inhibit the change process.

Patterns of response refer to the process and to the outcome indicators that the transition has occurred. The transition is complete when the person demonstrates mastery of new skills and behaviors applicable to the new situation and demonstrates the integration and reformulation of a new identity (Meleis et al., 2000). Various process indicators along the way such as successful coping, the gaining of confidence, identification with the new role, and feeling part of a new community of shared experiences serve as process indicators that the transition is on course.

The intent of this pilot study was to expand the transitions framework's applicability to the population of registered nurses employed in acute-care hospitals and to validate the utility of survey questions to assess the transitional process.

Methods

A qualitative methodology with semi-structured items and an open-ended format was used to investigate how SFAS registered nurses arrived at decisions to join an internal, flexible pool and how they viewed their practice, influence on patient care, peer relationships and collegiality, and loyalty to the organization. Survey questions were developed to reflect the fundamental principles of transition processes, and to capture the essence of an identity with an internal, flexible nurse's team. Content validity for each survey question was established by an independent PhD psychologist rater, who evaluated the relevance of the questions to the domains of transitions.

A sample ($N = 82$) of SFAS registered nurses were invited to participate by e-mail from the CNE and were asked to respond to an opinion survey about the SFAS program (Table 8.1.1). The nurse leader of the SFAS Internal Flexible Team also encouraged the nurses to complete the survey. The survey form was then distributed to willing participants by e-mail, and was made available in paper form in the central SFAS central office. No further contact was made with the respondents. Anonymity was assured and participants were not required to identify themselves on the survey form. After the participants had completed the anonymous survey, all forms were returned to the investigator for analysis.

All responses to the survey form were transcribed, collated, and reviewed by the investigator and the PhD psychologist, who served as an independent content validity expert. Data clusters for similar responses were compiled, and emerging

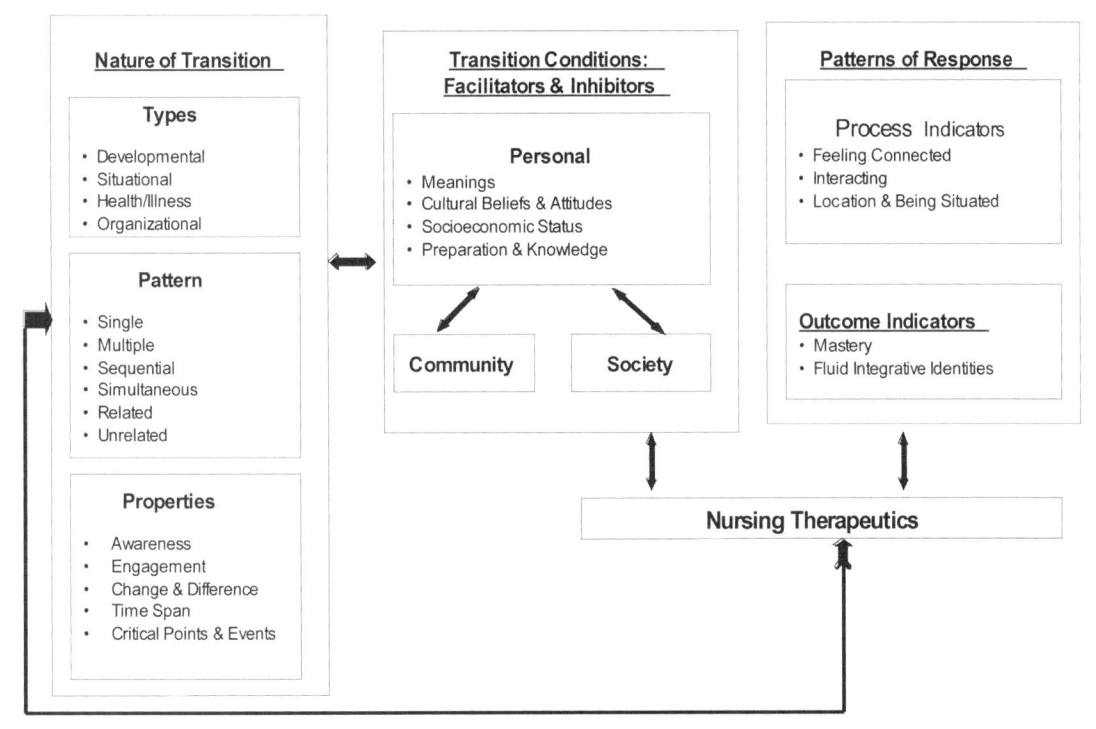

FIGURE 8.1.1 Transitions: A middle-range theory.
Reprinted from *Advances in Nursing Science* with permission of Lippincott, Williams and Wilkins
(Meleis, Sawyer, Im, Messias, & Schumacher, 2001).

themes were identified and categorized. Because the survey questions were designed to elicit personal descriptions of the transitional process, the investigator and content expert independently evaluated the data themes and confirmed the relevance of responses to the data themes. Patterns for the responses were then validated by the content expert to assure that the clusters of responses and emerging themes were aligned with the contextual underpinnings of Meleis and colleagues' (2000) framework.

Table 8.1.2 displays the demographic characteristics of the respondents; 72% of the SFAS nurses completed the survey.

Findings

Nature of the Transitions

As Meleis and colleagues (2000) suggest, transitions do not occur in isolation, but in the context of other transitions. Becoming an SFAS nurse involved not only a personal and professional developmental transition, but also transitional changes in life situations such as work schedule, family interactions and dynamics, and social network changes. Additionally, the SFAS program involved a transition in the way the organization staffed units and the consistency of the environment in which the nurses worked. For our purposes, however, this investigation focuses on the developmental transition of the SFAS nurse.

The data suggest that the SFAS transition involved multiple patterns. Answers to open-ended questions related to the process of being an SFAS nurse were categorized into three domains: easy or seamless, difficult, or mixed. Nurses with prior experience as a "traveler" or "float" nurse found the transition process to be seamless, and the experience was exactly what they had expected. For them, adapting to each unit's policies and procedures was the most difficult task. But others found the transi-

TABLE 8.1.1   Transitions Survey Questions

- Describe the process of your transition or adjustment to SFAS.
- What did you feel that you lost by becoming an SFAS nurse?
- What did you feel you gained by becoming an SFAS nurse?
- Which factors, people, events, or situations were supportive of this decision?
- Which factors, people, events, or situations were not supportive of this decision?
- How would you describe your ability to provide professional nursing care, both before and after the transition to SFAS? If possible, give an example.
- Describe your greatest strengths and weaknesses as an SFAS nurse.
- How have your specific competencies and experiences in nursing practice assisted you and/or the patients on a particular unit or specialty area?
- In your opinion, how has SFAS affected patient care in the areas you practice?
- What have you learned about yourself?
- What have you learned about nursing practice and/or the profession?
- What have you learned about patient-care outcomes?
- Has MAGNET status influenced your role and/or identity as an SFAS nurse?
- Do you believe the SFAS program has improved or diminished the efficacy and importance of quality patient care and outcomes?

TABLE 8.1.2   Demographic Characteristics of Respondents ($n = 59$)

Age
Average: 35.45 years
Range: 25–55 years
Median: 35 years

Gender
Male: 6   10%
Female: 53 90%

Tenure for SFAS
Average: 2.96 years
Range: 3 months–5 years
Median: 3 years

RN Years of Experience
Average: 11.2 years
Range: 3 years–28 years
Median: 9 years

---

tion difficult. While mentioning that learning each unit's policies and procedures was a challenge, adjusting each unit's "culture" and "climate" was also challenging. Some perceived the unit nurses as welcoming and supportive, while others perceived that they were isolated and resented. Some mentioned difficulty in establishing trust with fellow nurses that they did not know well, and in adjusting to the expectations of different nurse managers. These nurses were acutely aware of their limitations in servicing some units in the beginning of the transition.

In addition, a third pattern emerged that suggested that the transition was either easy or difficult depending on the situation or unit. Previous nursing experience made assignments to congruent units less taxing than working in units for which their previous experience provided little background.

Almost all SFAS nurses described the engagement in the transition process as a methodical, thorough, on-the-job training experience of learning to diagnose their strengths and weaknesses relative to the area in which they were working, of developing new skills, of adjusting to the different climates/cultures and the procedures of each unit, and then becoming comfortable in their new role. The role required them to be "more attentive and careful" in their nursing practice, to be in a "constant state of learning," to be "constantly researching" different patient illnesses, complications, potential drug interactions, and in general to "work harder" than the unit nurses. Adapting to a "change is constant" working environment was described as ongoing, and becoming comfortable with that realization was challenging at first.

Transition Conditions: Facilitators and Inhibitors

Factors that facilitated or inhibited the transition were easily classified into three domains: personal, social, and material. Nurses described factors such as "increased control" over self and the various domains of their life, the excitement of encountering new challenges and change each day, and the need to be constantly learning and growing as prime supporters of the transition to an SFAS nurse. Personal growth in terms of broader experience and knowledge base, confidence related to improved problem solving and nursing skills, the ability to function autonomously, and becoming more open and flexible was mentioned almost uniformly as factors that changed their perception of themselves personally and as a practicing nurse. Personal fulfillment related to their mastery of their new role was self-validating.

Most SFAS nurses described the love and social support of family and friends as being invaluable through the transition. Also mentioned by most participants was the support of supervisors and fellow nurses. The SFAS nurse manager, in particular, was mentioned specifically as being extremely important during the process.

Past nursing experiences (preparation and knowledge) with different units, areas of expertise, and specialty skills were reported to be easily transferable to the new role. Pride in educating unit nurses about specific conditions and procedures derived from their previous nursing experiences reinforced these attitudes.

A number of nurses also viewed the increased pay and flexible schedules as incentives for becoming an SFAS nurse.

Inhibitors of the transition process revolved around loss, self-doubt, and social rejection. Nurses reported grieving over the loss of "a home base" and "close relationships." Now, there is no one to remember and celebrate your birthday or other events; there is no home base to go to when you are feeling alienated. Also, perceptions of eroding specialty skills were expressed by some as resulting from working in a variety of units.

When first encountering units in which they had little or no previous nursing background, some nurses worried about their ability to function effectively. This self-doubt served to undermine their self-confidence early in the process.

The majority of nurses perceived unit nurses as welcoming and accepting of them and their role, while others perceived the opposite and therefore perceived themselves to be "an outsider," "resented," "not part of the team," and "picked on" by being given the most difficult and unpleasant nursing tasks. Nurses that reported social rejection were more likely to perceive the transition as difficult.

Patterns of Response

As mentioned previously, most nurses reported a slow process in becoming an SFAS nurse: Adapting to the new role, becoming aware of strengths and weaknesses regarding each assignment, developing new problem-solving and nursing skills, and experience in expanded areas of nursing. Uniformly, the nurses reported becoming more confident in themselves and nursing practice. Their knowledge base was broadened, they believed themselves to be able to treat a wider variety of patients, and they, themselves, had become more "well-rounded" and "holistic." Words such as "adaptable," "flexible," "less judgmental," "more patient," "more independent," and "autonomous" were used to describe the changes that had taken place during the transition. Nurses reported changes in attitude such as "being more goal-oriented," "more attentive and careful," and "more patient-centered," as a result of the SFAS experience. Because each day and each unit is different, an increased ability to focus on the patients and their needs was reported as being necessary.

Although some of the nurses reported that they had always given excellent nursing care, and now still do, most believed that, as a result of the SFAS experience, they now provide better and more efficient care. All reported high nursing satisfaction and generally being very happy with their choice.

One nurse wrote, "happy nurses = positive outcomes" to express her opinion that the SFAS nurses are helping to achieve better patient outcomes. Much of this improvement they attribute to the better nurse-to-patient ratios that their presence on the unit creates. But many also appear to believe that they are held to a higher standard than the regular nurses, and that this drives better patient care, as does their broader knowledge, self-confidence, and attitude. Clearly, all the SFAS nurses surveyed believe that they have mastered their new role and have solidified the personal changes into a new identity at both the personal and professional level.

Discussion

The purpose of the present pilot study was to identify and describe the transitional process that occurs when nurses change roles and practices in the hospital setting, more specifically, the transition from being a unit-based specialty nurse to that of an internal, flexible pool nurse. Using Meleis and colleagues' (2000) Theory of Transitions as a framework, this pilot study used a survey format to survey 59 nurses from the SFAS program.

The findings suggest that although the patterns of the transition may have differed, similar properties of the transition emerged. Aware of being new to the units and outsiders, the SFAS nurses described a process of engaging in various personal adaptations to learn the climate and the culture of the different units. A process of on-the-job training occurred in which they had to become more careful and attentive in their nursing practice. The new role required them to quickly diagnose their strengths and weaknesses relative to the unit of the day, to be in a constant state of learning and researching, and generally to work harder than the regular unit nurses. This process was quicker for those that had previous experience as a pool nurse. Likewise, previous experience and background made the adaptation to experience-congruent units easier than experience-incongruent units. One respondent said it this way:

> I now provide better care than I did before. I am more diligent when it comes to understanding the disease process and clinical picture. As a staff nurse I saw the same patients and knew them fairly well. It was therefore easy to understand their surgery and disease. As a SFAS nurse I may not know about a certain surgery or disease process. This lack of knowledge forces me to do greater research and ask more questions of my colleagues.

Various personal and social factors were identified that either facilitated or inhibited the change process. The transition was facilitated by beliefs in increased personal control, the excitement of encountering new challenges every day, the self-validation of mastering new skills and problems, and perceived positive changes in personality such as feeling more independent, competent, and more open and flexible. Being able to provide expertise and education in areas of previous special skill was also validating. While it may have taken some time, most SFAS nurses now feel respected by their unit colleagues. The positive social support from family, friends, colleagues, and supervisors was reported to be invaluable.

But the transition was not always smooth. Some nurses reported grieving the loss of a home unit with the close relationships and social support system that it entails. Additionally, not all nurses felt accepted by the unit nurses and instead reported feeling like an outsider and being given the most unpleasant nursing tasks.

> I have found that there are bad apples no matter where you go. With recent awareness of the budget, I have found that resource nurses have been replacing overtime on almost every floor. This has left a sour taste in most people's mouths. I can sense this. Some floors have certain nurses who already had a problem with SFAS. I am not sure if it is our higher salary, schedule flexibility, or what. They appear to try to give us the "bad" or "heavy" assignments. I just smile and accept the assignment knowing I will leave at the end of my shift satisfied with my work and knowing that my patients didn't know anything was wrong.

Indications that the transition from unit-based nurse to internal, flexible pool nurse was complete were the expressions of positive nurse satisfaction, pride, confidence, and other positive personal changes reported by almost all of the SFAS nurses. They all felt more competent, knowledgeable, holistic, confident, and possessed pride in their identity as an SFAS nurse. Although there is no independent verification, most SFAS nurses believe that they now provide better care having gone through this transitional process and because of the experiences that they had and continue to have. Of note, only a few of the SFAS nurses viewed external recognition from professional organizations and U.S. regulatory bodies as important in transition to their new role and identity.

Limitations

Even though the survey was anonymous, respondents were aware that the study was conducted by the CNE. This may have resulted in bias towards more favorable responses or limited the ability of respondents to feel comfortable expressing their perceptions and opinions honestly. These factors may have, to some degree, affected the results and may pose a threat to the internal and external validity of the findings. Additionally, not all of the survey questions provided useful information, and there were still some elements of the transitional process that were not explored to the fullest extent. Refinement of the survey is needed for future studies.

Implications

As a pilot study with an in-house sample, these findings obviously need to be replicated and cross-validated with independent samples. Reports of high satisfaction and positive outcomes may be questioned because of the nature of the study. However, descriptions of the process and the facilitating and inhibiting conditions are less so because of a clear lack of right or wrong answers. Hence, this study may provide valuable insights for nurse administrators on the types of issues and adoptive mechanisms internal, flexible pool nurses address and manage on a shift to shift basis. Their candid insights provide opportunities for nurse leaders to maximize internal, flexible pool nurses to not only provide professional bedside care, but to function in roles such as mentor, educator, patient safety officer, and evidence-based leader.

The findings also infer the importance of onboarding strategies for newly hired internal, flexible pool nurses based on the Meleis *Transitional Framework* (Meleis et al., 2000). Suggestions include explaining the stages of transition that the nurse can expect and timely intervention sessions with mentors and peers to discuss feelings, concerns, opportunities, and solutions to the various stages. The acceptance and awareness that becoming an internal, flexible pool nurse is a transitional process with available supportive interventions occurring within a shared process should be viewed as a key factor for the success of the practicing nurse, the internal pool program, and patient care.

Overall, the SFAS nurses in the study reinvented their self-perception by assimilating this alteration in their professional view of nursing practice and the nursing profession. Such a transition can be summarized as "an inner reorientation and self-redefinition" (Bridges, 2004).

Hence, the research implications of "becoming a flexible pool nurse" are rich in unanswered questions and questions not yet discovered. Queries to be considered include:

- How does internal, flexible pool nursing affect patient care?
- Is there a selection profile for a nurse who can adapt best to a flexible staffing model?
- Are internal, flexible pools cost-effective?
- Do internal, flexible-pool programs influence vacancy and turnover rates?
- Does the patient's family have a right to know a nurse is a flexible pool nurse?

Acknowledgments

The author thanks Alexander Rich, PhD, Professor Emeritus, Indiana University of Pennsylvania, for his independent content validation of common themes and concepts that were derived from the survey, and also thanks Rosemary Polomano, PhD, RN, FAAN, Associate Professor of Nursing, University of Pennsylvania, for her expertise and thoughtful comments and additions to this chapter.

REFERENCES

Aiken, L. H., Clarke, S. P., Cheung, R. B., Sloane, D. M., & Silber, J. H. (2003). Educational levels of hospital nurses and surgical patient mortality. *Journal of the American Medical Association, 290*(12), 1617–1623.

Bridges, W. (2004). *Transitions: Making sense of life's changes.* Cambridge, MA: Da Capo Press.

Meleis, A. I., Sawyer, L. M., Im, E., Messias, D. K., & Schumacher, K. (2000). Experiencing transitions: An emerging middle range theory. *Advances in Nursing Science, 23*(1), 12–28.

Needleman, J., Buerhaus, P., Mattke, S., Stewart, M., & Zelevinsky, K. (2002). Nurse-staffing levels and the quality of care in hospitals. *New England Journal of Medicine, 346*(22), 1715–1722.

Page, A. E. K. (2008). Temporary agency and other contingent workers. In R. G. Hughes (Ed.), *Patient safety and quality: An evidence-based handbook for nurses.* (Prepared with support from the Robert Wood Johnson Foundation.) (AHRQ Publication No. 08-0043.) Rockville, MD: Agency for Healthcare Research and Quality.

8.2 THE EXPERIENCE OF ROLE TRANSITION IN ACUTE CARE NURSE PRACTITIONERS IN TAIWAN UNDER THE COLLABORATIVE PRACTICE MODEL

WEI-CHIN CHANG
PEI-FAN MU
SHIOW-LUAN TSAY

Abstract

The role of the acute-care nurse practitioner in Taiwan has changed significantly since the 1990s due, in significant part, to a shortage of interns and resident physicians in acute-care settings. The first year of professional practice represents an important transitional year during which new professionals develop their competence to provide high-quality care to hospitalized patients. Because the actual experience of individuals undergoing this transitional process into their new role has yet to be fully explored, this research studied and categorized the experiences of acute-care nurse practitioners during their first year of role transition under the collaborative model of practice. We used a qualitative inquiry method with in-depth interviews to investigate the relevant experiences of 10 acute-care nurse practitioners working at a medical center in Taiwan. Results show that the experience of expert nurses in their transition to acute-care nurse practitioners passed through three phases during the first year under the collaborative practice model. These phases include role ambiguity, role acquisition, and role implementation. Each phase contains a set of subthemes that describe the multiple dimensions of this experience. This chapter highlights the experiences, stresses, and accomplishments of acute-care nurse practitioners during their initial year of advanced practice.

Introduction

Rises in the cost of health care, consumer demands for accountability, a shortage of new medical residents resulting from a shift away from tertiary care in favor of primary care, and increases in the number of medically vulnerable patient admissions requiring complex and comprehensive care have all greatly changed the landscape of health care in Taiwan (Tsai et al., 2003). Concurrent with this change has been pressure to decrease the amount of time that patients receive acute care in order to reduce fiscal pressures on Taiwan's universal National Health Insurance program. Acute-care nurse practitioners (ACNPs) were first introduced into hospital settings around the year 2000 to serve as advanced-practice nurses capable of efficiently and effectively meeting new hospital demands (Tsai et al., 2003). ACNPs have an expanded scope of practice that incorporates medical and advanced nursing functions and responsibilities, and provides care in collaboration with other healthcare professionals (Tsai et al., 2003). In other words, ACNPs have extended their role into medical practice to provide direct, comprehensive care that often includes documenting patient histories, conducting physical examinations, performing medical diagnoses, identifying and initiating diagnostic tests and procedures, and performing specialty-specific procedures (Klein, 2004). This expanded scope of practice is considered beneficial to patients in acute-care institutions (Green & Davis, 2005; Hoffman, Tasota, Zullo, Scharfenberg, & Donahoe, 2005).

The nurse practitioner (NP) is a new position classification in Taiwan, and many hospitals still use terms such as Clinical Nurse Specialist or Senior Nurse in lieu of the ACNP title. Because the government does not yet issue NP licenses, many trained nurses are working as nurse practitioners. Most NPs work in acute-care settings. As the number of acute-care nurse practitioners (ACNPs) entering the work force increases, it is crucial to understand and facilitate the role transition that takes place as nurses move into their new position as ACNPs. The first year of professional practice is an important transitional time during which new professionals develop competence in providing high-quality health care to hospitalized patients (Brown & Olshansky, 1997, 1998; Talarczyk & Milbrandt, 1988). Challenges faced during the initial year of practice for primary care nurse practitioners were explored by Brown and Olshansky (1998). However, little is known about the experience in the role transition of acute-care nurse practitioners under the collaborative practice model in acutecare institutions. Therefore, we designed this study to explore the role transition of novice ACNPs during their first year of acute-care practice.

Even an experienced nursing expert may perform as a novice when entering a new working environment or position. This seeming decline in competence by nurses in new positions sometimes results in a loss of confidence in knowledge and a high level of anxiety (Benner, 2001). An individual must adapt to new ways of thinking, absorb new knowledge, and change personal behavior and orientation within the social structure during role transition (Meleis, 1975). If a nurse shows incompatibility in personal values, self-concept, and expected role behavior, or her capability cannot match the responsibility she should assume, it will likely result in role strain and a failure to perform to potential. It could further result in role conflict with other members of the professional team due to differences in role expectations, thus leading to opposition or discrimination, disruption of the working atmosphere and organizational efficiency, and, as a result, decreases in health-care quality (Benner, 2001).

Role theory helps to explain both how an individual plays a specific role and, under a particular set of circumstances, what kind of behavior model might be expected (Conway, 1978). The two principal role theories related to the health-care profession include the structural-functionalist paradigm and the symbolic-interactionist model. The structural-functionalist paradigm emphasizes the link between an individual and the social system, with each behavior model differing based on the position a particular nurse holds in the societal structure. Therefore, social structure is considered an important factor molding and determining an individual's behavior. As a social structure changes over time, the value and norm of the position held adjusts accordingly. The symbolic-interactionist model focuses on the interaction between people in a societal system, meaning that the action and symbol represented are based on behaviors selected and the roles constructed by individuals (Burr, Leigh, Day, & Constantine, 1979). Under conditions of effective communication, symbols hold the same meaning to both interacting sides. Both recognize the shared meaning of symbols in order to perform associated role behavior (Hardy, 1978). Both perspectives are applicable to the nursing profession because the organizational structure possesses high functionality. The structural function viewpoint is very helpful to the research of formalized nursing roles, while the symbolic interaction point of view is common in literature investigating the essence of interdependence in nursing roles or defining some specific nursing role behavior (Creasia & Parker, 1991).

Collaborative practice is the method that physicians and nurses use to work together to share and solve patient problems and initiate decision-making responsibilities to care for patients (Baggs & Schmitt, 1998; Cummings, Fraser, & Tarlier, 2003). Fagin (1992) pointed out that the collaborative model for patient care is almost unavoidable due to the complexity of patient healthcare needs. This kind of collaboration also provides physicians a chance to understand the roles and viewpoints of advanced-practice nurses (Marfell, 2002). In order to achieve an effective collaborative practice, in addition to strengthening education, training, active participation, and learning (Whitehead, 2001), nurses need to trust and respect each other in their profession; then, the care of patients can be more efficient and qualitative (Kleinpell et al., 2002).

According to Schumacher and Meleis (1994), the role transition of an NP is influenced by factors and levels of motivation in an ever-changing process. These factors include: transition to personal meaning; level of prior preparation; medical environment supportiveness; personal knowledge and skills; and personal and organizational expectations regarding the new role. Hamric and Taylor (1989) used a questionnaire to inquire about 100 primary care NPs with various numbers of years of work experience. They found that nurses with fewer than three years of work experience generally experienced an orientation phase, a frustration phase, and an implementation phase. Characteristic behavior during the orientation phase included enthusiasm, optimism, and a focus on mastering necessary clinical skills. In the frustration phase, nurses had feelings of conflict, maladaptation, frustration, and anxiety. In the implementation phase, nurses responded through role modification after interaction with other people. Moreover, Brown and Olshansky (1998) applied grounded theory to study the first-year role transition experience of 35 new primary care NPs and constructed a theoretical model to represent the transition to a primary care nurse practitioner role. This model consists of a process dubbed "from limbo to legitimacy" and encompasses four major categories: laying the foundation, launching, meeting the challenge, and broadening the perspective.

In summary, current literature focuses on the role transition undergone by primary care nurse practitioners and lacks adequate studies on the experiences of new acute-care nurse practitioners as they make the transition to their new roles under the collaborative practice model in acute-care settings. Therefore, this study attempts to describe the experiences of novice acute-care nurse practitioners during their initial year of practice.

Methods

Research Design

The aim of the study was to explore the role transition experiences of ACNPs in the first-year trainee collaborative practice model. This study used a qualitative inquiry method with in-depth interviews to collect data. Content analysis was then used to analyze collected data to profile the experiences of ACNPs during their first year of role transition under the physician and nursing collaborative model. Qualitative research is a systematic and subjective research method used to describe experience and convey its meaning (Burns & Grove, 1999). The purpose is to understand the psychological process in a subjective world (Lee et al., 1996). Furthermore, content analysis uses an objective, systematic, and qualitative research technique to describe and display the contents of communications (Berelson, 1954). The qualitative research technique is also a method that objectively analyzes key topic data.

The Sample

The selection criteria for nurse practitioners in this study included: completion in Taiwan of a standardized ACNP education and training program; current service in his/her first year as an ACNP; current practice under a collaborative model; and a job description mainly focused on direct patient care, patient consultation, or education.

Ethical Considerations

Prior to the formal study, approvals were received from the university and the hospital Human Subjects Committee. Potential participants were informed of the content and scope of the study and asked to sign a consent form to confirm their willingness to participate. In addition, potential participants were informed that they could decide at any point in time to discontinue the study with no adverse consequences.

Data Collection

The first author served as data collector. After consent by study participants, interviews were conducted and tape-recorded based upon an open-ended question format, such as "Describe your experience making the transition to nurse practitioner." Interviews were discontinued when data reached a saturation point. Each interview was transcribed verbatim for data analysis.

Data Analysis

Qualitative data analyses followed Burnard's (1991) content analysis procedures. Researchers carefully read and reread written transcripts to single out significant elements. Several themes, identified while comparing transcript results, were categorized (Miles & Huberman, 1984). Further data were collected to verify or modify the initial data analysis. The significant themes identified were verified by two qualitative researchers. Data was considered "saturated" when no new data could be identified and themes were coherent.

The rigorousness of data collection was addressed according to the four-criteria assessment proposed by Lincoln and Guba (1985), which addressed credibility, fittingness, auditability, and confirmability. In terms of "credibility," the first author, a trained acute-care nurse practitioner, was involved in the creation of NP positions at the hospital targeted by this research. Researchers also had profound personal experience and an understanding of role development and job descriptions. In terms of "fittingness," all the data collected from the interviews were faithfully transcribed and similar themes were categorized to allow readers afterward to grasp the real situation at that time and understand the nature of the data. In terms of "auditability," a tape recorder was used during research to insure the data analysis procedure was properly preserved and recorded in detail, as well as to provide the opportunity for independent review of the accuracy of the research process. Finally, in terms of "confirmability," complete records and related material were retained for future examination, including tapes, original transcripts, observation records, an interview diary, and analyzed records.

Results

Ten acute-care nurse practitioners, all women ranging in age from 33 to 44 (mean 36.7) years, comprised the sample population of this study. The sample included new ACNPs from five different acute-care specialties: general surgery, neurologic surgery, plastic surgery, genitourinary surgery, and obstetrics-gynecology. The majority had practiced as registered nurses for at least 13 years before beginning their advanced-practice role.

Through descriptions provided by study participants on their role transition experience, the following three transition phases were identified: role ambiguity; role acquisition; and role implementation.

The Role Ambiguity Phase

Participants, uncertain regarding the expectations of their new ACNPs role prior to beginning work, found their new position to be totally different from their previous nursing positions. Four subthemes were apparent in this phase:

Expectations and Fighting Alone for the New Role. Participants felt their personal competence was recognized by their having passed the selection criteria and were full of expectation and confidence regarding their new roles. One participant expected to perform differently in her new position based on her significant clinical experience in the past. Nevertheless, when another NP began work in her clinical practice, she felt under great pressure to relearn and adapt to a totally different work environment. In addition, as a senior nurse, no one would think of giving guidance, so she felt entirely on her own in adapting to and succeeding in an unfamiliar working environment. Nurse I said,

> Apart from not needing to give injections, I always feel that being an ACNP would not be too different from being a nurse. although, I will still do those things when necessary. When transiting to the new position, I felt I had a lot of experience. I was competent and the ACNP position would not be too difficult for me. But I now know that I was too confident in myself…We all thought we were selected by the test as the most suitable candidates; at least, I thought this way myself, so at the beginning I was full of confidence.

The Change of Professional Practice and Its Unclear Duty Boundaries. After beginning their ACNP role within a physician and nursing collaborative model, nurse practitioners found their knowledge and skills insufficient to work closely with physicians. In the beginning, no one knew how to separate ACNP and physician responsibilities. In the process of clarifying responsibilities, conflicts erupted between ACNPs and physicians. Nurse E said,

> I found that not only do I have to know my nursing theories, but also the physician's knowledge and skills. Therefore, I have to review anatomy and I have to refresh my knowledge about all aspects of diagnosis and treatment. I feel that I have to know all of them because sometimes doctors will tell me they want to discuss issues or hand over work to me.

Self-Directed Learning. When in a new position, the ACNP will begin working with a primary doctor immediately. In addition to handling her own significant workload, the ACNP is responsible for facing emergent problems and issues proactively. Nurse B said,

> I bring patient name lists home and review each case for their health history, current condition, and treatment. In other words, the main purpose is to gradually accumulate information and put everything in order for the case and review it repeatedly. There are some more regular norms and clinical diseases that I have to familiarize myself with as well…otherwise, I will face too many things, giving me even more stress on top of the stress of my new working environment.

Lack of Nursing Staff Recognition of the New Role and Status of ACNPs. The nursing staff was not familiar with the job descriptions of the nurse practitioners when the latter began practicing in the ward. Some nurses were of the opinion that nurse practitioners were exceeding their authority by taking on physicians' duties. Nurse practitioners also lacked good communication with their supervisors. Both supervisors and nursing staff questioned whether nurse practitioners could issue medical orders or whether they were involved in ancillary medical behaviors only. Again this reflected the opinion that ACNPs were infringing on physicians' authorities, and even acting like doctors. Nurse A said,

> Primarily…everyone thinks that you should do these things, but you do not. Finally, when you issue a medical order for others to carry out, like a doctor, they think you are snobbish like a doctor.

The Role-Acquisition Phase

Role acquisition began when an individual started to realize the extent of the categories, content, and characteristics of her new position, and gradually understood and grasped the direction she should strive for to achieve position objectives. The experiences related to this phase are summed up in the following five subthemes:

Gradually Emerging Work Patterns. New ACNPs began to appreciate that, although their duties to take care of patients directly had diminished, work responsibilities had expanded and had become more complex, and one was required to develop autonomy in practice. Acute-care nurse practitioners must represent the doctor to resolve hospitalized patients' problems and must gradually develop autonomous coping methods that include being able to evaluate the level of immediacy of individual problems, limitations in implementing their role and authority, and identifying and securing resources necessary to ensure their responsibilities can be fully carried out. Nurse C said,

> As an acute care nurse practitioner, in the beginning I found the nature of our work to be totally different from that of clinical nurse. I was responsible for handling all the check-ups and examinations, as well as other tasks when a patient was hospitalized.

Emphasizing Personal Competency in Decision Making. As an ACNP, participants found that they were no longer able to simply find a doctor to solve problems they encountered. Acute-care nurse practitioners need to judge and evaluate patient problems independently, and then provide active and integrated care. They have to think independently and not just follow doctors' orders. Nurse D said,

> I can no longer be like a nurse and, when things happen, just call the doctor for a solution. You have to think first and then find the resources necessary to solve the problems. I feel resources are very important. When something happens to a patient, but the resident doctor is in surgery, you cannot be like a nurse anymore and call the doctor and ask what to do. You have to find resources on your own and solve the problem.

Understanding the Professional Growth Direction. Owing to changes in the work model, acute-care nurse practitioners feel they have assumed much heavier responsibilities and are perceived as being required to possess relatively more advanced and specialized professional knowledge, as well as the capability to communicate and coordinate. They can then properly handle patients' problems and earn the respect of others. Nurse E said,

> What is different from the past is that you contact more people, so the ability to communicate and coordinate is more important than before when you were a nurse. We just stayed at the same unit before.

> If you were a leader, you would do your best to lead your co-workers and, if you were a team member, you just took good care of your patients ... Now we contact patients from different departments and colleagues from different wards...

The New Role Gradually Identified by Patients. Because acute-care nurse practitioners always accompany the primary doctor to check on patients, they are familiar with patient status and treatment regimens. Patients think that acute-care nurse practitioners are more authoritative than nurses, so quite often they are mistaken as doctors. Nurse C said,

> They think that you may be the doctor's assistant. You know many things. They may not show additional respect in the way they treat you, but they understand your role. I personally feel that patients' families have different feelings with you and they think of you as doctors, as members of the medical care team, which has some distinction with nurses.

Setting Up a New Work Support System. Acute-care nurse practitioners felt that they received support from the head nurse, because the head nurse typically helps to coordinate when ACNPs encounter problems. In addition, talking to peers about their complaints, comforting each other, consulting, and giving guidance on clinical problems all provided significant spiritual/moral support. Nurse E said,

> When you did not do things well, the primary doctor would think that both of us didn't coordinate the shift transition well. At that time, I thought it was my entire fault and I was so sorry and I would talk to my peers.

The Role-Implementation Phase

Role implementation indicates a gradual familiarization with the practice model and a growing concern regarding the orientation and implementation of job descriptions. This phase can be summed up in terms of the following three themes:

New Nurse–Physician Relationships in the Changed Work Model. The primary doctor is responsible for medical decision-making. An acute care nurse practitioner can participate in a discussion, but generally follows the physician's opinions. Work prioritization also follows the primary physician's recommendations. The new work model increases the interactions between, and closeness of, acute-care nurse practitioners and physicians and develops mutual trust among team members. Nurse G said,

> At the beginning it is much simpler, but then finally, no matter what, the primary doctor or resident doctor will rely on the acute-care nurse practitioners very much and they will assign and share a lot of their work to you because they think you are trustworthy. This is what I think.

A Nursing Role Deeply Relied Upon by the Other Nurses. As the acute-care nurse practitioner's practice model and responsibilities became generally understood, interactions with other nurses improved. In addition, the acute-care nurse practitioner knows where the physicians are and can always get in touch with them, which regularly helps resolve patient problems. In the event of an emergency, the acute-care nurse practitioner is equipped to handle it immediately. They also have a role to play in providing clinical guidance to new nurses. Because of their efficiency and competence, acute-care nurse practitioners are gradually relied upon by the other nurses. Nurse C said,

> Some colleagues in the ward sometimes also have situations that they cannot handle by themselves and they cannot find the doctor. The first thing they think is to find us. I feel that if they are willing to seek you out to solve their problems, this indicates they think you are pretty competent. I think if I am capable of managing it, I will help as much as I can.

Demonstrating the Importance of the Acute-Care Nurse Practitioner to Patients and Their Families. Because the ACNP fully understands the patient's therapy regimen and can provide effective methods and in-depth explanations to handle problems faced by the patients and their families, the acute-care nurse practitioner fulfills a role as communicator and coordinator among patients, doctors, and nurses. Nurse D said,

> The patient felt the care here was very good. Everything was clearly explained regarding the disease and the kinds of things and examinations that would be done during hospitalization. Sometimes patients will also ask what kind of problems they have and which doctor or which department to see.

Discussion

Study data supports the role theory and Benner's (2001) view as a framework for the experience of entering a new practice situation in the collaborative practice model as an acute-care nurse practitioner. Study results indicate that, in the early stage of professional development, the novice acute-care nurse practitioner lacks the experience necessary to feel competent and confident. These findings highlight the process of ACNPs' challenges and accomplishments during their first year in their new position.

This study indicated that acute-care nurse practitioners in the physician and nursing collaborative model underwent three phases during their first year of duty. The first phase, defined by role ambiguity, challenges the new ACNP to face the gap between their idealized role and the reality of their new position. Although most ACNPs are senior nurses with significant experience and confidence in their previous roles, they must relearn and readjust to people and duties in their new acute-care nurse practitioner role. In addition, ACNPs must partially assume the work of resident doctors, forcing them to face their lack of knowledge and skills on specific medical issues. All these challenges combine to frustrate the new ACNP in her initial ability to work and perform. Meanwhile, the boundaries separating the ACNP's work from that of the resident physician and other nurses are ill-defined, and frequently cause friction and conflict. All these further heighten the new ACNP's feelings of anxiety. A similar result was indicated by Benner's research (2001, p. 21), which found that even persons with expert skills exhibited lower competence levels when facing the unfamiliar demands and expectations of a new work environment or position. Hamric and Taylor (1989) also identified that nurses underwent orientation and frustration phases when changing professional positions.

During the second phase identified in this research, the role acquisition phase, the acute-care nurse practitioner gradually clarifies the new position's requirements, understands what needs to be done to strengthen knowledge and skills, establishes a work support system, recognizes that in the new role one must develop autonomy and make critical decisions rather than awaiting a doctor's advice during emergencies. In short, responsibility grows with autonomy, reflecting the need for a much stronger foundation for knowledge and skills development and clinical decision making. Because Hamric and Taylor's (1989) study and Brown and Olshansky's (1998) findings do not indicate the presence of a role acquisition phase, this appears to be a unique experience in Taiwan, perhaps due to the unique role development experience faced by acute-care nurse practitioners in Taiwanese hospitals.

In the third phase, the role implementation phase, the role of acute-care nurse practitioners has gradually emerged following the development of the physician and nursing collaborative practice model. Inter-relationships between medical team members exhibit greater positive adjustment because of the involvement of the acute-care nurse practitioners. Once the nursing staff realizes and accepts the responsibilities of the acute-care nurse practitioner, their interaction with the ACNP is greatly improved. Because of her outstanding work performance, the acute-care nurse practitioner not only becomes a working partner upon which doctors and the nursing staff rely, she also provides comprehensive services to patients and increases patient satisfaction with the medical care received. This achievement indicates a solid step forward in the realization of a physician and nursing collaborative model. The essence of the implementation phase has also been found in the studies of both Hamric and Taylor (1989) and Brown and Olshansky (1998).

Our data supports the successful transition of expert nurses to acute-care nurse practitioners during the first year under the collaborative practice model. Role transition occurs in three phases, namely the role ambiguity, role acquisition, and role implementation phases. Although we defined three phases, our findings agree with Brown and Olshansky (1997), who identified four phases of role development during the first year of primary-care ACNP practice. The role ambiguity phase in our findings is analogous to Brown and Olshansky's foundation laying phase, while our role acquisition phase is analogous to their launching phase, and our role implementation phase covers both their meeting the challenge and broadening the perspective phases. Both studies represent comparable progressions through a series of common experiences for the family nurse practitioner or acute-care nurse practitioner.

There are some primary differences between this study and the relevant literature. Most research participants could not clearly describe their own job descriptions during the first year of practice. Questions regarding the NP role increased conflict within the medical team and demonstrated that, before transferring to the new role, participants lacked a clear recognition and understanding of the scope and responsibilities of the new NP position. In addition, study participants often indicated that they lacked guidance in their work and that it was necessary to learn many things on their own. Workshops or in-services designed according to ACNP needs during the transition may assist their adaptation to their new role. Study participants felt deeply the importance of problem solving and having the capacity to make correct decisions. These are actually the critical elements that are required of a nurse practitioner (Davies & Hughes, 1995).

The role transition of an ACNP under a collaborative model has been explored only rarely in the literature. This study investigated role transition under this model in an acute-care setting where subjects believe in their ability to function largely independently as an NP, albeit in consultation with a physician, if needed. Study results highlight key issues involved in NP role transitions and provide data critical to further developing regulations related to educational requirements and practices in Taiwan.

Conclusion

We found that experienced nurses transitioning into new roles as acute-care nurse practitioners undergo three phases during their first year under the collaborative practice model. These phases include role ambiguity, role acquisition, and role implementation. ACNPs in our study progressed through each role transition phase at her own pace. Each phase incorporates a set of subthemes that describe the multiple dimensions of the experience. This chapter highlights both the distresses felt and the accomplishments achieved during the initial year of advanced practice, as well as the nature of ACNP role transition in Taiwan.

A constantly changing health-care climate, challenges to the legitimacy of the newly created acute-care nurse practitioner practice from the established hierarchy, and working conditions that are particularly stressful during the initial year of practice for ACNPs all have a devastating effect on the development of competence and confidence among new ACNPs. Therefore, it is crucial to identify factors that enhance the initial role transition in order that appropriate interventions can be designed to support new ACNPs.

A limitation of this study is the involvement of only a small number of acute-care nurse practitioners who were all purposely sampled from one medical center. As a result, research results may not reflect conditions generally experienced at other institutions. Multi-angled investigations will help achieve an overall understanding of the ACNP experience in role transition.

In summary, this study makes three contributions. First, it develops a descriptive profile of the role transition of the acute care nurse practitioner during the first year of practice, providing anticipatory guidance for prospective ACNPs. Secondly, the study identifies barriers to the effective development of the ACNP practice, providing data essential to developing effective strategies to facilitate the roles of new ACNPs, ACNP preceptors, and administrators. Third, this study delivers a clear message to government officials and professional organizations regarding the need to establish standards and regulations related to the ACNP practice.

Acknowledgments

The authors would like to thank the acute-care nurse practitioners who participated in this study.

REFERENCES

Baggs, J. G., & Schmitt, M. H. (1998). Collaboration between nurses and physicians. *IMAGE: The Journal of Nursing Scholarship, 20,* 145–149.

Benner, P. (2001). *From novice to expert: Excellence and power in clinical nursing practice.* Menlo Park, CA: Addison-Wesley.

Berelson, B. (1954). Content analysis. In G. Lindzey (Ed.), *Handbook for social psychology: Theory and method.* Reading, MA: Addison-Wesley.

Brown, M. A., & Olshansky, E. F. (1997). From limbo to legitimacy: A theoretical model of the transition to the primary care nurse practitioner role. *Journal of Advanced Nursing, 46*(1), 46–51.

Brown, M. A., & Olshansky, E. F. (1998). Becoming a primary care nurse practitioner: Challenges of the initial year of practice. *Nurse Practitioner, 23*(7), 46, 52–58, 61–66.

Burns, N., & Grove, S. K. (1999). *Understanding nursing research* (2nd ed.). Philadelphia: W. B. Saunders.

Burnard, P. (1991). A method of analyzing interview transcripts in qualitative research. *Nurse Education Today, 11,* 461–466.

Burr, W. R., Leigh, G. K., Day, R. D., & Constantine, J. (1979). Symbolic interaction and the family. In W. R. Burr, R. Hill, F. I. Nye, & I. L. Reiss (Eds.), *Contemporary theories about the family,* Vol. II. New York: The Free Press.

Conway, M. E. (1978). Theoretical approaches to the study of roles. In M. E. Hardy & M. E. Conway (Eds.), *Role theory: Perspectives for professionals* (pp. 17–27). Norwalk, CT: Appleton-Century-Crofts.

Creasia, J. L., & Parker, B. (1991). *Conceptual foundations of professional nursing practice.* St. Louis, MO: Mosby.

Cummings, G. G. M., Fraser, K., & Tarlier, D. S. (2003). Implementing advanced nurse practitioner roles in acute care: An evaluation of organizational change. *Journal of Nursing Administration, 33*(3), 139–345.

Davies, B., & Hughes, A. M. (1995). Clarification of advanced nursing practice: Characteristics and competencies. *Clinical Nurse Specialist, 9*(3), 156–160.

Fagin, C. M. (1992). Collaboration between nurses and physicians: No longer a choice. *Academic Medicine, 67*(5), 295–303.

Green, A., & Davis, S. (2005). Toward a predictive model of patient satisfaction with nurse practitioner care. *Journal of the American Academy of Nurse Practitioners, 17*(4), 139–148.

Hamric, A. B., & Taylor, J. W. (1989). Role development of the CNS. In A. B. Hamric & J. A. Spross (Eds.), *The clinical nurse specialist in theory and practice* (2nd ed., pp. 41–82). Philadelphia: W. B. Saunders.

Hardy, M. E. (1978). Role stress and role strain. In M. E. Hardy & M. E. Conway (Eds.), *Role theory: Perspectives for professionals* (pp. 73–109). Norwalk, CT: Appleton-Century-Crofts.

Hoffman, L. A., Tasota, F. J., Zullo, T. G., Scharfenberg, C., & Donahoe, M. P. (2005). Outcome of care managed by an acute-care nurse practitioner/attending physician team in a subacute medical intensive care unit. *American Journal of Critical Care, 14*(2), 121–129.

Klein, T. A. (2004). Scope of practice and the nurse practitioner: Regulation, competency, expansion, evolution. *Topics in Advanced Practice Nursing, 4*(4), 6–12.

Kleinpell, R. M., Faut-Callahan, M., Lauer, K., Kremer, M. J., Murphy, M., & Sperhac, A. (2002). A collaboration practice in advanced practice nursing in acute care. *Critical Care Nursing Clinics of North America, 14*(3), 307–313.

Lee, S., Shu, L. W., Lee, J. T., Chiou, E. W., Lee, T. F., Rae, Z. L., et al. (1996). *Nursing research: Principles and practice.* Taipei, Taiwan: Far-Seeing.

Lincoln, Y. S., & Guba, E. G. (1985). *Naturalistic inquiry.* Newbury Park, CA: Sage.

Marfell, J. A. (2002). Clinical practice opportunities for advanced practice nurses. *Critical Care Nursing Clinics of North America, 14,* 223–229.

Meleis, A. I. (1975). Role insufficiency and role supplementation: A conceptual framework. *Nursing Research, 24*(4), 264–272.

Miles, M. B., & Huberman, A. M. (1984). *Qualitative data analysis: A sourcebook of new methods.* Beverly Hills, CA: Sage.

Schumacher, K. L., & Meleis, A. I. (1994). Transitions: A central concept in nursing. *IMAGE: The Journal of Nursing Scholarship, 26*(2), 119–127.

Talarczyk, G., & Milbrandt, D. (1988). A collaborative effort to facilitate role transition from student to registered nurse practitioner. *Nursing Management, 19*(2), 30–32.

Tsai, J. S., Yu, Y. M., Hung, J. S., Cheng, Y. C, Yu, L. H., Tsay, S. L., et al. (2003). *Nurse practitioner: A proposal for education and practice regulations.* Taipei, Taiwan: National Health Research Institute.

Whitehead, D. (2001). Applying collaborative practice to health promotion. *Nursing Standard, 15*(20), 33–37.

Reprinted with permission from: Chang, W. C., Mu, P. F., & Tsay, S. L. (2006). The experience of role transition in acute care nurse practitioners in Taiwan under the collaborative practice model. *Journal of Nursing Research, 14*(2), 83–91.

8.3 GUIDING THE TRANSITION OF NURSING PRACTISE FROM AN INPATIENT TO A COMMUNITY-CARE SETTING: A SAUDI ARABIAN EXPERIENCE

ELAINE SIMPSON
MOLLIE BUTLER
SHAYDA AL-SOMALI
MARY COURTNEY

Abstract

The purpose of this chapter is to provide an overview of the Transitional Practise Model, which was used as the educational learning program to guide the transition of two Saudi nurses from an acute inpatient environment into a community setting. This model is informed by Benner's "novice to expert" concept and is grounded in experiential learning and critical thinking. The aim was to enhance knowledge and skills by providing opportunities for learning in order to make an effective transition from an acute inpatient environment to community nursing. The model was effective in guiding and bridging the gap for nurses to undertake a transition from a hospital inpatient environment to a community setting. The use of preceptors was invaluable in providing an understanding of the nature of professional practise through learning opportunities, mentoring, and support.

Introduction

Hospital patient care in Saudi Arabia is influenced by the services of the Joint Commission on Accreditation of Healthcare Organizations (JCAHO, 1993) in the United States for the purposes of accreditation and is provided by skilled professionals from more than 30 nations. Although the majority of patients and their families speak Arabic, most professionals communicate in English and many do not speak Arabic. More frequently than not, care is navigated using interpreters who act as intermediaries between patients, families, and providers. Saudi nurses have an edge over their foreign counterparts because they understand the culture and social norms and can communicate in Arabic.

In July 2001, a Home Health Care (HHC) program in a 550-bed Saudi Arabian tertiary hospital employed two Saudi nurses with Bachelor of Science degrees in nursing, who had practised in inpatient hospital settings for 4 years: 2 years in medical–surgical units, and 6 months each in orthopedics, pediatrics, gynecology, and oncology wards. They were keen to expand their clinical practise to include community nursing. Initially, HHC collaborated with the Nursing Education Center at the hospital to discuss an educational learning program in order to upgrade the nurses' knowledge, skills, and attitudes in this field of care. Given that the majority of patients in the HHC program comprised patients from the medical-surgical, oncology, gynecologic (inpatient), wound, and diabetic clinics (outpatients), HHC also collaborated with head nurses in these clinical areas to elicit their support.

The objectives were to: (i) provide clinical placements for these nurses in the aforementioned clinical units; (ii) formulate learning objectives for each clinical placement; (iii) complete clinical competencies in each area prior to moving onto the next clinical placement; and (iv) "buddy" with preceptors in all the selected clinical areas, including HHC.

The purpose of this chapter is to provide an overview of the Transitional Practise Model, which was used as the educational learning program to guide the transition of two Saudi nurses from an acute inpatient environment to a community setting. This model was informed by Benner's (1984) "novice to expert" concept. The aim was to enhance nursing practise by providing opportunities for learning in order to make an effective transition to community nursing. The Transitional Practise Model and process are explained below.

Transitional Practise Model and Process

This model is grounded in experiential learning and critical thinking, and is diagrammatically presented in Figure 8.3.1. The model is divided into three components: dimensions, domains of practise, and evaluation. The term "dimensions" relates to the stages of development on a continuum from novice to expert (Benner, 1984), which was used to guide the Saudi nurses' professional development. The "domains of practise" relate to growth and development as the practitioners move through stages 1–5 of the model. "Evaluation" consists of interviews, reflective documentation, the development and presentation of case studies, completion of all clinical competencies in each selected clinical area, and initiating research.

The educational learning program commenced with an orientation period of 2 weeks in HHC and the community at large. The inpatient practicum period followed, and comprised: (i) 7 weeks in a medical–surgical unit; (ii) 2 weeks in the wound clinic; (iii) 3 weeks in the diabetic clinic; (iv) 4 weeks in a gynecology unit; and (v) 10 weeks in oncology/palliative care because a large number of patients in the HHC population typically received oncology/palliative care. The Saudi nurses "buddied" with their respective preceptors in stages 1, 2, and 3 of the conceptual model.

Materials and Methods

Stages of the Transitional Practise Model

Stage 1. Novice: Familiarizing Oneself With the Community. The Saudi nurses held a Bachelor of Science degree in nursing, with at least 3 years post-registration experience in areas such as medical-surgical, pediatrics, orthopedics, and gynecology. Additionally, they brought with them a sound

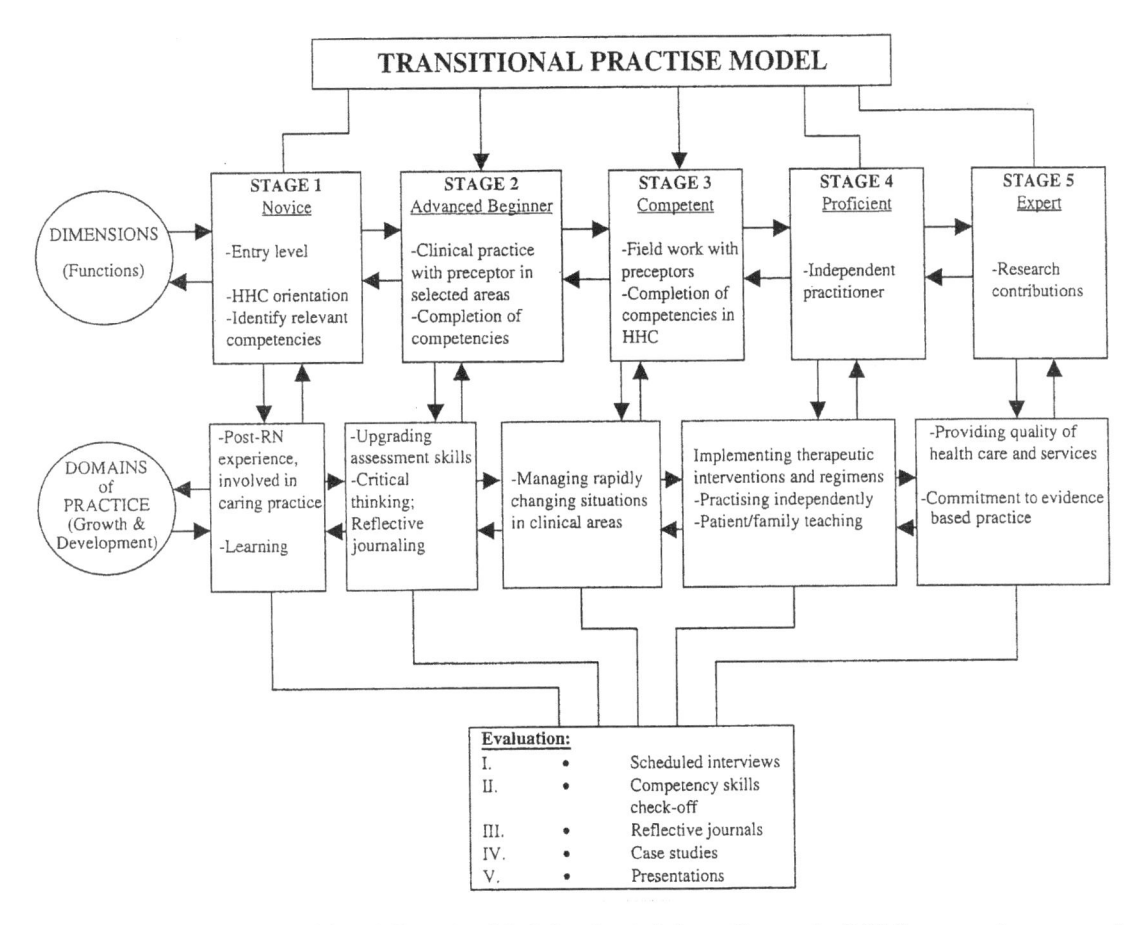

```
                        TRANSITIONAL PRACTISE MODEL

    ┌──────────┐   STAGE 1         STAGE 2            STAGE 3           STAGE 4          STAGE 5
    │DIMENSIONS│   Novice          Advanced Beginner  Competent         Proficient       Expert
    │(Functions)│
    └──────────┘   -Entry level    -Clinical practice -Field work with  -Independent     -Research
                                    with preceptor in  preceptors        practitioner     contributions
                   -HHC orientation selected areas    -Completion of
                   -Identify relevant -Completion of   competencies in
                   competencies    competencies       HHC

    ┌──────────┐   -Post-RN        -Upgrading         -Managing rapidly Implementing     -Providing quality of
    │ DOMAINS  │    experience,     assessment skills  changing situations therapeutic     health care and services
    │    of    │    involved in    -Critical           in clinical areas interventions and
    │ PRACTICE │    caring practice thinking;                            regimens         -Commitment to evidence
    │ (Growth &│                    Reflective                           -Practising       based practice
    │Development)│  -Learning       journaling                           independently
    └──────────┘                                                         -Patient/family
                                                                         teaching

                                   Evaluation:
                                   I.    • Scheduled interviews
                                   II.   • Competency skills
                                           check-off
                                   III.  • Reflective journals
                                   IV.   • Case studies
                                   V.    • Presentations
```

FIGURE 8.3.1 The Transitional Practise Model, adapted from Benner's (1984) research, was used to guide the nurse's professional development from novice to expert.
HHC = home health care.

knowledge of disease processes, which they could apply to their community practise.

At the outset an in-depth orientation to the HHC was provided, during which time visits to a range of patients in the community were undertaken. The Saudi nurses buddied with a community nurse for 2 days at a time, giving them an overall exposure to about 100 patients in five areas, located within a 50-km radius serviced by the HHC program. The Saudi nurses completed competency assessments in areas such as fire and safety protocols, lifting and handling, medication administration, and patient assessment. The Saudi nurses observed how the preceptors cared for the patients and how they engaged in teaching patients and their families via interpreters. They also noted the difficulties encountered by the expatriate nurses in trying to communicate with limited Arabic language and using interpreters. They also were taught how to acquire equipment and resources (e.g., beds, oxygen concentrators) relevant to the patients' needs. After gaining an insight into the community environment and typical patient population, the Saudi nurses commenced their clinical practise in the in/outpatient units.

Preceptors played a vital role in the development of these Saudi nurses. Therefore, it was important to select preceptors who had the ability to:

1. Communicate and demonstrate knowledge and skills clearly to the learner while remaining open and respectful.
2. Motivate the learner by emphasizing a problem-solving approach.
3. Connect information to broader concepts in order for the learner to apply the information to other clinical situations.
4. Foster a pleasant and stimulating learning environment using humor and enthusiasm (Tumulty, 1993; Whitman, 1996).

These characteristics were discussed with the head nurses in the medical-surgical, wound, diabetic, gynecology, oncology/palliative, and community units. They utilized these guidelines to select the appropriate preceptors.

Stage 2. Advanced Beginner: Inpatient Field. As the Saudi nurses moved through the selected in/outpatient units with their preceptors, the nurses were encouraged to:

1. Engage in case studies and to give presentations of their experiences.
2. Be involved in reflective practise through journal documentation.
3. Utilize critical-type thinking/questioning to stimulate their thinking processes in order to make clinical judgments, based on factual information, and to obtain better patient outcomes.

The preceptors provided guidance in helping the nurses to assess patients skillfully and to link the assessment to their case-study projects. The preceptors arranged weekly and/or biweekly case-study presentations, in which nurses in other units were invited to interact and participate. The HHC head nurse and education coordinator attended several meetings conducted with the HHC head nurse, education coordinator, preceptors, and head nurses of the respective clinical areas. As the nurses completed their clinical competencies, they moved on to the next identified clinical placement. Head nurses within each unit reminded the nurses that they could extend their practicum if they had more learning needs to fulfill. On completion of their clinical practise in all the selected in/outpatient units, they moved into the community.

Stage 3. Competent: In the Community. Two senior HHC nurses were selected as preceptors for the Saudi nurses. For the first 2 weeks, the Saudi nurses observed their preceptors, who pressed them with questions. They were encouraged to document their experiences in their journals. Each day on return to the HHC center, the Saudi nurses and their preceptors sat together to discuss their patients with the physicians (a physician consulted with HHC nurses on a daily basis about the patients' health status and concerns). This interaction gave the nurses the opportunity to ask questions about their observations and to be involved in designing new interventions. At the end of each week, the HHC head nurse, preceptors, and preceptees met to discuss their progress. Timely and constructive feedback was provided about their progress and they were encouraged to interact without feeling threatened.

In the third week of their community experience, the preceptors encouraged the Saudi nurses to take an active role in terms of communicating with the patients and/or their families, perform physical assessments, make clinical judgments, and report their findings. The Saudi nurses also were encouraged to telephone the physician(s) as required. When the preceptors were confident that their preceptees were safe and competent, the preceptors took a step back and observed as the Saudi nurses took on their roles as independent practitioners.

Stage 4. Proficient. Within 7 months, the Saudi nurses became independent practitioners, interacting with patients and their families and providing the much-needed patient teaching that the expatriate nurses struggled to accomplish because of the need to use interpreters. The Saudi nurses also were effectively networking with allied health professionals, physicians, and their peers to ensure the patients' holistic needs were provided.

Throughout the stages of learning, the head nurse in HHC and the education coordinator followed up with the preceptors in order to monitor the Saudi nurses' progress and provided a non-threatening environment in which the nurses could discuss or clarify any issues/problems.

Stage 5. Expert. The Saudi nurses had grown and developed in their knowledge, skills, and attitudes since completing this educational learning program. They demonstrated a keen interest toward research in that they volunteered to participate as subjects of this chapter and in compiling articles for the hospital's monthly nursing magazine. Furthermore, they regularly utilized the internet to obtain best-practise information, which was not a typical practise before they embarked on this educational learning program.

Results and Discussion

Evaluation

Besides the weekly interviews/meetings, the two Saudi nurses were keen to express and share their learning experience, and a focus group interview was conducted with the Saudi nurses, the HHC head nurse, and the education coordinator. It is reported as follows:

Interviewer: How do you feel about working in the community following the clinical practise experience that was provided for you?

Saudi nurses: We realized that we needed to upgrade our knowledge, skills, and attitudes, and we are more competent, having learned from the preceptors, who were very knowledgeable and skilled practitioners. The encouragement from our preceptors to present our case studies was helpful as we were nervous at first. By the time we did a few, we became confident and felt competent. Journal documentation helped us to reflect on our practise. All of this made learning and completing competencies more meaningful.

Interviewer: Tell us about the environment in the community as distinct from the inpatient field.

Saudi nurses: In the inpatient units, there is always someone, for example, colleagues, the head nurse, and so forth, that you can turn to. In the community, you are basically practising independently and have to think on your feet —use all the facts and findings to make purposeful clinical judgments in order to implement effective interventions and provide quality care. Primarily, you have to think critically and ask questions, such as what, when, why, how, what if (prediction). This was the big challenge.

Interviewer: How did you feel about that?

Saudi nurses: We developed our critical thinking skills very rapidly—it was a steep learning curve. Besides, we have to deal directly with the family and communicate effectively and diplomatically so that they understand our purpose and their responsibilities. We also have to ensure that one member of the family takes responsibility and is capable to care for the patient in the absence of the HHC nurse, which is pivotal to the ongoing well-being of the patient. Then, we had to assess for resources—a lot of things to do. Time management and organizational skills was also something that we learned to do very quickly and become good at it. This was another challenge.

Interviewer: What is the best thing about working as a community nurse?

Saudi nurses: The 10 weeks that we spent in the oncology and palliative care unit was invaluable as it prepared us to deal with issues such as death and dying and grieving. When we know that the patient is close to death, we

	stay with the patient in order to be a support for the family and take over so that the burden on the family is lessened. We always call the next day and follow up 3 days later and then a week later, or sometimes earlier, depending on the family situation, to see if they need further assistance or a visit. This provides closure to our work. The other aspect was journal documentation. It was always helpful to refer to our journals and reflect on our practise. It is a useful document.
Interviewer:	Is there anything else you would like to comment on or share about your recent learning and experiences?
Saudi nurses:	Yes, using the model gave us direction as to where, how, and what our experiences were going to be. The model was flexible because it gave us the opportunity to move back and forth within the stages if we needed to do more learning. This is a good aspect of the model, as there was no pressure or stress on us. The use of preceptors, clinical competencies, clinical assessments, journaling, case studies, and presentations was effective for our learning needs. The preceptors were role models and always gave us constructive feedback, which boosted our self-esteem.
Interviewer:	What changes would you like to make within the model that was used to guide your transition, or any other aspects that would assist nurses wishing to make this same transition?
Saudi nurses:	Basically, keep up with frequent meetings to discuss progress and/or concerns and receive feedback . . . we have no changes to make.
Interviewer:	What advice would you like to give other Saudi nurses?
Saudi nurses:	Make sure they have a strong medical-surgical background. We spent 2 years in these units after we graduated, which gave us a sound understanding of the disease processes and much-needed practical experience, which made it easier to transfer theory into practise

The model, which consisted of three major components, namely, dimensions, domains of practise, and evaluation, was effective in guiding Saudi nurses and bridging the gap for them to undertake a transition from an inpatient environment to a community setting. These nurses expressed their feelings of confidence, especially with the use of preceptors, and stated that the varied experiences in the clinical areas prepared them to understand and deal more competently with the typical disease processes. The model also provided flexibility, whereby the nurses could move from one unit to the next when they were confident and when their respective preceptors felt that they were competent.

Summary

The commitment provided by in/outpatient and HHC preceptors helped the nurses broaden their understanding of patients' disease manifestations, especially regarding issues relating to death and dying. Timely, constructive feedback given by the preceptors and frequent meetings enabled these nurses to identify practise gaps and apply new knowledge, skills, values, and attitudes competently. The preceptors also encouraged reflective thinking, critical thinking, and learning as a means to reinforce practical knowledge and skills.

The team effort afforded by health professionals, such as preceptors, head nurses, nurse educators, doctors, and others, provided guidance, support, ongoing learning opportunities, as well as collegial support, for the Saudi nurses.

Recommendations

1. The importance of having substantial medical and surgical clinical practise (2 years) provides the grounding to understand the different disease processes.

2. The use of preceptors is invaluable in that a preceptor, as an experienced nurse, can provide an understanding of the nature of professional practise through learning opportunities, mentoring, and support (International Council of Nurses, 2003).
3. The use of a model to provide structure and guidance is indispensable.

REFERENCES

Benner P. *From Novice to Expert: Excellence and Power in Clinical Nursing Practice.* Menlo Park, CA: Addison-Wesley, 1984.

International Council of Nurses. *An Implementation Model for the ICN Framework of Competencies for the Generally Nurse.* Geneva: International Council of Nurses, 2003.

Joint Commission of Accreditation of Healthcare Organizations. *Accreditation Manual for Hospitals.* Oakbrook, IL: Joint Commission of Accreditation for Health Care Organizations, 1993.

Tumulty P. *Effective Clinician.* Philadelphia: W. B. Saunders, 1993.

Whitman N. *Creative Medical Teaching.* Salt Lake City, UT: University of Utah School of Medicine, 1996.

Reprinted with permission from: Simpson, E., Butler, M., Al-Somali, S., & Courtney, M. (2006). Guiding the transition of nursing practice from an impatient to a community-care setting: A Saudi Arabian experience. *Nursing and Health Sciences,* 8(2), 120–124.

8.4 IMPLEMENTING AN INTERDISCIPLINARY GOVERNANCE MODEL IN A COMPREHENSIVE CANCER CENTER

PATRICIA REID PONTE
ANNE H. GROSS
ERIC WINER
MARY J. CONNAUGHTON
JAMES HASSINGER

Interdisciplinary collaboration, in which decision making and accountability are shared by members of different disciplines, is a central feature of oncology clinical practice, but it rarely is built into the governance and management structures that oversee oncology clinics. In many ambulatory settings, decisions affecting clinic operations are made centrally by those removed from day-to-day activity. Front-line nurses, physicians, and other staff who are most familiar with patient care and operational issues have less input.

In the late 1990s, ambulatory oncology services at the Dana-Farber Cancer Institute (DFCI), a comprehensive cancer center affiliated with Harvard Medical School, began to experience extraordinary growth in patient volume. Like other cancer care providers, DFCI witnessed steady growth as a result of the aging of the general population and improvements in cancer diagnosis. A joint venture with nearby Brigham and Women's Hospital intensified the growth. As patient volume and acuity surged, the ambulatory practices at DFCI were increasingly challenged to keep up with demand and were pressured by patients and referring providers to ensure timely access to appointments.

As the practices struggled to accommodate the needs of patients and referring physicians, the chief executive officer (CEO) and DFCF's other senior leaders considered the Institute's clinical infrastructure and determined that its operational systems and governing structure needed to be evaluated. They realized that, over time, the organization's culture and management style had become more controlled and less inclusive; they believed that a more responsive governance and management model—one that placed decision making and responsibility for change in the hands of those most familiar with day-to-day operations—would benefit the Institute, its staff, and the patients it served.

In December 2001, the CEO, the senior vice president for patient care services, and the chief nurse appointed a multidisciplinary task force to design a new governance and management structure for ambulatory operations. The goal of the task force was to achieve effective, locally based decision making in each of the Institute's 12 disease centers. As part of their deliberations, the task force considered what needed to be in place to achieve that goal and identified two essential criteria: the knowledge and perspectives of the different disciplines involved in care operations must be represented in the decision-making process, and members of each discipline must feel responsible for the implementation and outcomes of decisions that are made.

Such interdisciplinary collaboration was familiar to the task force, given that it is integral to the Institute's care-delivery model and its quality-improvement and patient-safety programs. Collaboration also is a key characteristic of the leadership structure for inpatient oncology care as evidenced by the registered nurse (RN)/medical doctor (MD) leadership teams that have overseen the inpatient units since 1994. Although interdisciplinary collaboration was valued by the ambulatory nurse managers, structures to promote its practice were not built into the ambulatory services governance model then in place. The task force agreed that in designing a new governance model, interdisciplinary collaboration would be a cornerstone that informed not just the new model's structure but also the processes used to make decisions and manage operations on a daily basis.

In this chapter, the interdisciplinary governance model developed by the task force will be described, the process used to design and implement the model will be reviewed, and how the model ensures accountability, communication, and collaboration among disciplines and how it has helped DFCI achieve substantial improvements in clinic operations will be discussed.

Collaboration and Teamwork in Health Care

The value of interdisciplinary collaboration in health care has been examined by many health-care researchers and practitioners. A number of investigators have assessed its effect on patient care and the education of health-care practitioners, and have demonstrated benefits for a range of patient and student populations (see Table 8.4.1). The importance of interdisciplinary collaboration to quality improvement has been underscored by two landmark reports from the Institute of Medicine (IOM). The first, *To Err Is Human: Building a Safer Health System* (IOM, 2000), cites the essential role that interdisciplinary teams play in efforts to improve patient safety. A follow-up report, *Crossing the Quality Chasm: A New Health System for the 21st Century* (IOM, 2001), cites the teams' fundamental importance to all improvement efforts.

The management literature also describes the importance of interdisciplinary collaboration by discussing how teamwork favorably affects organizational performance (Kouzes & Posner, 1995) and by highlighting the success of corporations that embrace the principles of self-managing work teams (Katzenback & Smith, 1993). Today's health-care organizations, which contend with numerous and complex external factors and rely on the knowledge of a broad range of constituencies, providers, and professions, arguably need to develop governance models that engage all key stakeholders and apply the principles of partnership, equity, and accountability (Porter-O'Grady, Hawkins, & Parker, 1997). Despite the recommendations, interdisciplinary collaboration rarely is a feature of the leadership and governance models employed by ambulatory oncology practices, not because those who oversee such settings do not value collaboration, but because a structure to facilitate collaboration and ensure its practice are not built into the governance model's design.

Former Management Structure

The task force charged with designing a new governance model for ambulatory services at DFCI consisted of representatives from a broad range of departments and disciplines, including managers and staff from nursing, social work, pharmacy, clinical laboratories, radiology, finance, quality improvement, and clinical operations, as well as physician representatives from medical, surgical, radiation, and psychosocial oncology. A patient from DFCI's Patient and Family Advisory Council (Ponte et al., 2003) was also a member of the group. The chief nurse and two physicians, one from medical oncol-

```
                    ┌─────────────────────┐         ┌──────────────────────┐
                    │  Medical Oncology   │         │ Nursing and Patient  │
                    └──────────┬──────────┘         │   Care Services      │
                               │                    └──────────┬───────────┘
                    ┌──────────┴──────────┐                    │
                    │  Disease centers    │                    │
                    │      (N=12)         │         ┌──────────┴───────────┐
                    └──┬────────┬─────────┘         │  Nurse managers      │
        ┌──────────┐   │        │                   │  Social workers      │
        │          │   │        │                   │  Pharmacists         │
   ┌────┴─────┐ ┌──┴───┴──┐ ┌───┴──────────┐        │  Respiratory         │
   │ Teaching │ │Research │ │ Clinical Care├────────┤  therapists          │
   └──────────┘ └─────────┘ └───┬──────────┘        │  Clinic facilitators │
                               │                    │  Clinic assistants   │
                    ┌──────────┴──────────┐         └──────────────────────┘
                    │  Physicians         │
                    │  Clinical and research nurses │
                    │  New patient coordinators     │
                    └───────────────────────────────┘
```

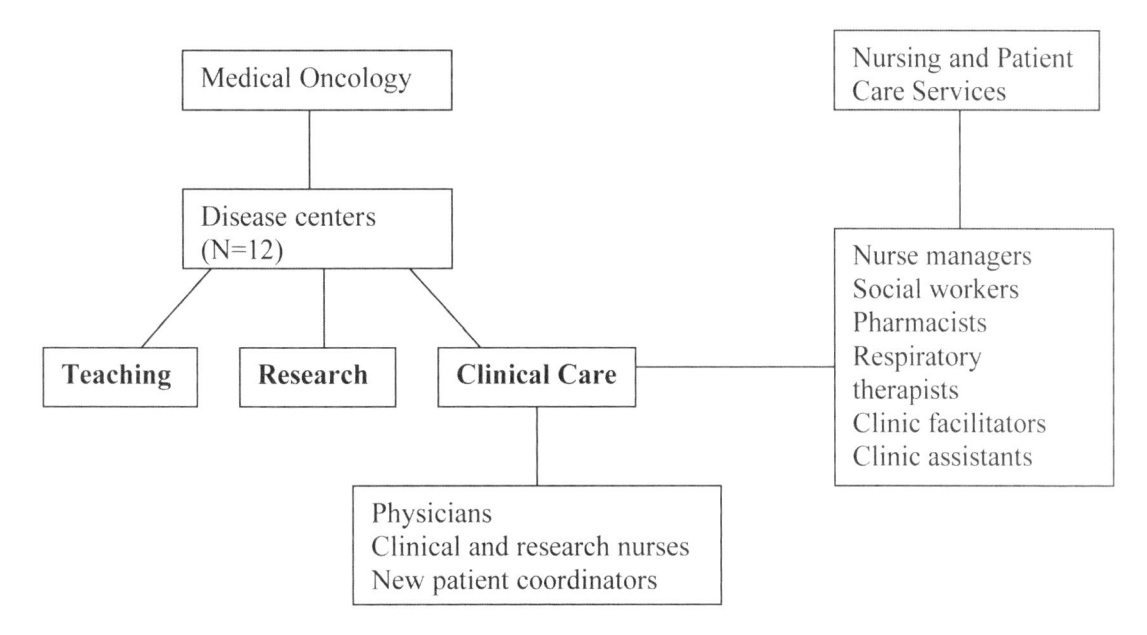

FIGURE 8.4.1 Ambulatory governance: Old model.

ogy and the other from surgical oncology, led the group. The task-force leaders realized that they were embarking on a major management change that would require a significant time commitment. Given the situation, they opted to engage the support of two management consultants who were familiar with DFCI and had expertise in leadership, management structures, and organizational change.

The task force began by reviewing the strengths and weaknesses of the ambulatory governance model in place at the time (see Figure 8.4.1). Under the model, clinical services were administered through 12 disease centers, each dedicated to a specific area of oncology (e.g., gynecologic cancers, neuro-oncology, breast cancer). A physician leader was responsible for each center's research, teaching, and clinical care activities. The physician leader also supervised some of the staff providing care in the disease center, including the physicians, nurse practitioners (NPs), program nurses (staff nurses who work with MDs and NPs to coordinate patient care), and new patient coordinators. The remainder of the staff, including the nurse manager, social workers, pharmacists, respiratory therapists, clinic facilitators, and clinic assis-

tants, reported to the Nursing and Patient Care Services (NPCS) department.

The parallel reporting structure created a number of problems. For example, the disease centers' physician leaders believed that they had little control over or accountability for many administrative functions that affected clinic operations, such as budget monitoring, patient scheduling, and management of front-line support staff, whereas the nurse managers had difficulty overseeing some of the nursing staff, such as NPs and research nurses, who had a stronger alliance with the physician leaders. In addition, effective "bridging" structures were lacking, making collaboration among the disease centers difficult, and complicating efforts by the NPCS department to introduce changes affecting clinic operations.

Because of the problems with the management model, decisions regarding ambulatory operations often were triaged to the chief nurse, chief operating officer (COO), or chief medical officer (CMO), who were responsible for all patient care provided by the Institute, including the care provided through the inpatient service, pediatric oncology, and 12 disease centers. Over time, the centralized and often

TABLE 8.4.1 Interdisciplinary Collaboration in Patient Care and Academia

Investigators	Area of Focus	Findings
Patient Care		
Abrahm et al., 1996	Impact of multidisciplinary hospice consultation team on the care of veterans with advanced cancer	The team identified a large number of new medical/nursing and psychosocial/spiritual problems and was able to resolve many of the problems it identified.
August et al., 1995	Satisfaction among patients treated at a comprehensive breast center	Overall, satisfaction was high and was influenced by staff concern for patients, opportunity for "one-stop shopping," and medical thoroughness.
Baggs et al., 2004	A review of research on the role of interdisciplinary teams in the care of the dying patient in the intensive care unit (ICU)	Researchers demonstrated improvements in ICU care stemming from collaboration, but concluded that additional studies involving more than one unit, unit comparisons, and randomized trials are needed.
Chang et al., 2001	Recommendations for patients with breast cancer	A case review by a multidisciplinary team resulted in treatment recommendations that differed from those of outside physicians for 43% of women studied.
Preparation of health care professionals		
Blazer et al., 2005	Genetic cancer-risk counseling	A program of intensive training in genetic cancer risk counseling designed to simultaneously train clinicians from different disciplines (e.g., genetic counselors, oncology nurses, physicians) led to an increase in cancer genetics knowledge, increased professional self-efficacy, and changes in practice.
Chang et al., 2005	Cancer Prevention Fellowship Program	The fellowship program draws on multiple disciplines to prepare students for interdisciplinary research.
Siegrist, 2004	Public health nursing experiences in baccalaureate nursing education	A partnership model involving a public health department, academic nursing program, and community agencies increased student skills related to interdisciplinary team work, program development, and cultural competency.

"siloed" decision-making process hampered the flexibility and responsiveness of individual disease centers, contributing to senior leadership's determination that a significant change in the ambulatory governance and management structure was needed.

As the task force considered the structure of ambulatory operations, the members recognized its strengths and weaknesses. On the positive side, the disease center structure allowed clinicians with expertise in particular areas of cancer care to work closely with one another, benefiting research and care delivery. The problems lay with the structure that was used to govern and manage operations within and among disease centers. That structure, the task force determined, was ineffective and required a redesign.

A New Governance Model for Clinic Operations

Before defining a new governance model, task force members identified the following principles to guide its design:

- Representatives from nursing, medicine, and administration—the groups most integrally involved in day-to-day clinical operations—must play a role in guiding decisions and be held accountable for their outcomes.
- Leadership roles, including individual and shared accountabilities, must be defined clearly.
- The model must promote care that is efficient, safe, and patient- and family-centered by fostering timely and effective communication among caregivers and the coordination of care among programs, departments, and practice settings.
- The model's effectiveness would be assessed by metrics evaluating patient and staff satisfaction, operational efficiency and productivity, and clinical quality and safety.

Over a nine-month period, the task force outlined a new governance model to meet the criteria. During that time, they met frequently with a larger, multidisciplinary advisory group to obtain input on the evolving model and held multiple open forums for all clinical staff in which they presented the new model's proposed design and sought input on its structure. They also kept the Institute's executive team informed of their progress through regular reports. At the end of the nine months, the executive team approved the proposed governance model and sanctioned its implementation. The new model (see Figure 8.4.2) focuses on redefining the governance and management of clinical services for the 12 disease centers. By design, the model does not affect the research and teaching arms of the disease centers.

Under the new model, each disease center is overseen by an interdisciplinary team composed of a clinical physician director and a nurse program leader, both supported by a program administrator. (When the new model was introduced, the nurse manager title was changed to nurse program leader to make it commensurate with the physician leader's title.) The physician and nurse leaders share responsibility for all aspects of operational decision making and are accountable for managing and improving systems, managing the budget associated with capital and clinic operations, and meeting clinical, operational, and financial targets. They also collaborate on managing the disease center's personnel budget, even though certain employee groups are located in other cost centers (e.g., patient care assistants and nurse managers are located in the NPCS cost center; NPs and physicians are located in the cost center for the medical oncology, surgical oncology, and radiation oncology departments).

The physician and nurse leaders are responsible for guiding the performance of staff and addressing personnel and performance issues. Working together, they provide input into physician evaluations conducted by the chair of medical oncology and into the evaluations of nurses and NPs that now are conducted by the nurse program leader. (Although NP positions still are located in the department of medical oncology's cost center, performance is evaluated by the nurse program leader rather than the physician clinical director. That change has been viewed as logical by the NPs, and they have readily accepted it.) The nurse and

```
┌─────────────────────┐                              ┌─────────────────────┐
│ Medical oncology    │                              │ Nursing and Patient │
│ Surgical oncology   │                              │ Care Services       │
│ Radiation oncology  │                              │                     │
└─────────────────────┘                              └─────────────────────┘
           \                                                    /
            \              ┌───────────────────┐               /
             \             │ Multidisciplinary │              /
              \            │ Clinical Services │             /
               \           │ Committee         │            /           ┌──────────────────────┐
                \          └───────────────────┘                        │ Social Work          │
┌─────────────────────┐                                                 │ Care coordination or │
│ **Disease Centers** │                                                 │ case management      │
│ **(n = 12)**        │                                                 │ Pharmacy             │
│ Research program    │                                                 │ Respiratory therapy  │
│ Teaching Program    │                                                 └──────────────────────┘
│ Clinical care program│
└─────────────────────┘
                         ┌──────────────────────────────┐
                         │ **Disease center clinical**  │
                         │ **practice operations (N=12)**│
                         │ Clinical physician director  │
                         │ Nurse program leader         │
                         │ Program administrator        │
                         │ Interdisciplinary care team  │
                         └──────────────────────────────┘
```

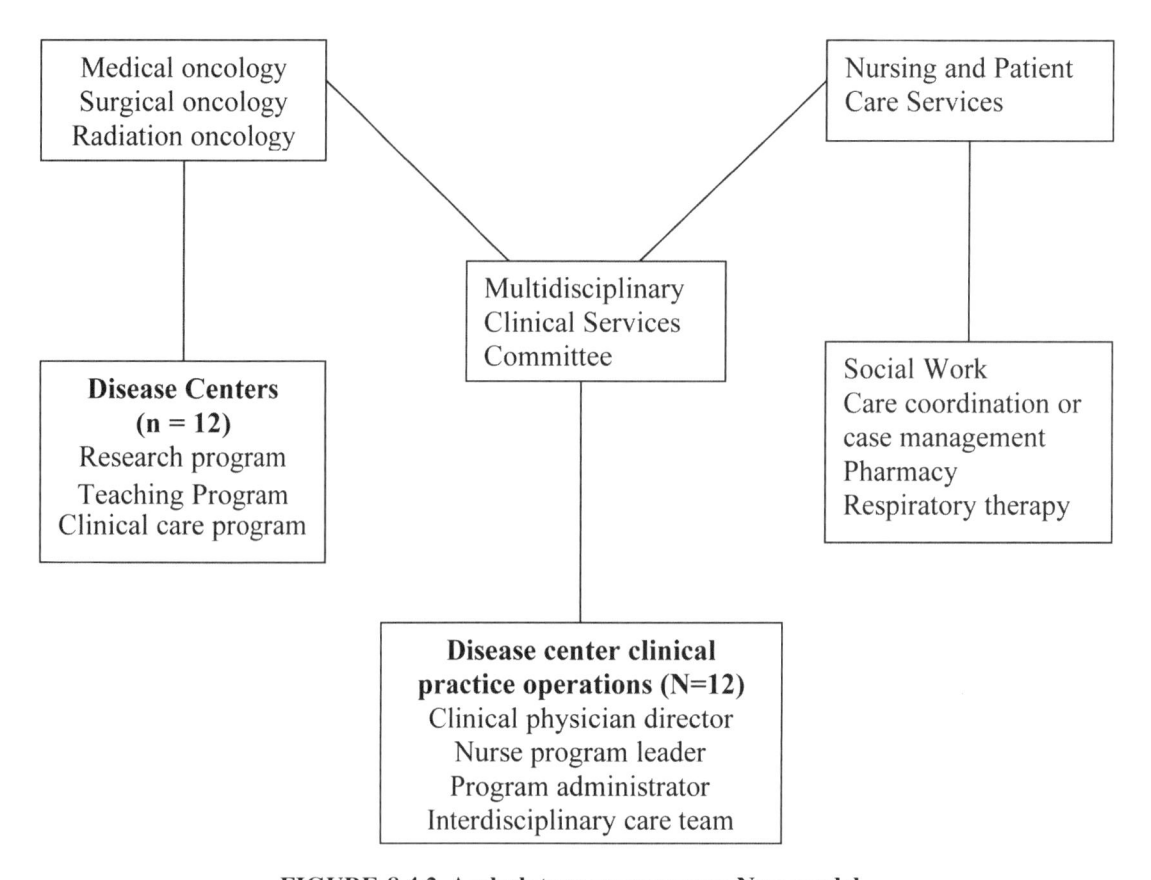

FIGURE 8.4.2 Ambulatory governance: New model.

physician leaders also provide input into the evaluations of many clinicians outside the disease centers, including clinicians in surgical oncology, radiation oncology, social work, pharmacy, and other disciplines that provide care among the disease centers and report to the chiefs of their respective disciplines. The chiefs look to the disease centers' physician and nurse leaders for input on whether the clinicians work as members of the team and adhere to practice standards.

Overall, accountability for care that is delivered in a disease center is shared by members of the center's care team. Although each clinician is accountable on an individual level for the care delivered, the care team, along with the disease center's clinical physician director and nurse program leader, is accountable for the outcomes of care delivery in that center and for the quality of the systems that affect and support care.

The clinical physician director and nurse program leader meet regularly with the disease center's staff, a multidisciplinary group that includes nurses, physicians, new patient coordinators, practice coordinators, and clinic assistants. During the meetings, the leadership team obtains input on improvement priorities and initiatives and reviews evaluation metrics. The meetings ensure that the clinicians and support staff in a disease center have input into clinical operations, and that the disease center reaps the benefit of the perspective, knowledge, and skills brought by different disciplines.

Promoting Collaboration Among Disease Centers

Several structures ensure collaboration among disease centers. Collaboration among disease centers that share the same floor (and, in some instances, the same clinic space) is ensured through a floor-level leadership structure. All of the disease centers on a floor have the same nurse program leader, who works closely with a designated clinical physician director to coordinate floor-level operations and address shared systems issues.

Collaboration and coordination among all 12 disease centers are promoted through the Multidisciplinary Clinical Services Committee (MCSC). The committee reports to the Institute's primary clinical departments (i.e., NPCS and medical, surgical, and radiation oncology) and is co-chaired by a senior nursing leader (the vice president of adult ambulatory services and director of adult ambulatory nursing) and a senior physician leader (the vice chair of medical oncology and director of the Breast Oncology Center), who have incorporated the committee and its work into their leadership roles. The committee's membership includes the physician clinical directors, nurse program leaders, and operations managers of each disease center, who work to establish operational priorities for ambulatory services as a whole, discuss and evaluate policies, share information and best practices, and engage in joint problem solving.

The MCSC also serves as a way for centralized departments, such as social work and pharmacy, to provide input into disease center operations. The directors of those departments attend committee meetings and work through the group to introduce changes that affect multiple disease centers. Patient and family input is ensured through the participation of a member of the Institute's Patient and Family Advisory Council, who attends all committee meetings.

Implementation of the New Governance Model

As part of its work to define a new governance model, the design task force considered behaviors and attributes that RN and MD leaders and staff would need to demonstrate for interdisciplinary collaboration to occur and for the new model to be successful. Among those deemed especially important were respect for other disciplines, a willingness to share information and listen to others' opinions, and a tolerance for disagreement. As part of its effort to promote respect among disciplines, DFCI was engaged in a patient safety initiative focused on adopting principles of a fair and just culture and a blame-free systems approach to error investigation and risk management. The initiative complemented the task force's efforts to introduce the new governance model and helped underscore the importance of key behaviors. Although most of the clinicians and staff at the Institute valued the needed attributes, the task force knew that helping leaders and staff members put them into action would be a primary challenge of the model's implementation. That challenge was highlighted by concerns such as those expressed by patient care assistants and others that, too often, decisions in the disease centers were made unilaterally and that staff affected by the decisions were left out of the decision-making process.

The physician and nurse leaders of each disease center were appointed soon after the new interdisciplinary governance model was approved. Although they had a comprehensive job description and had been informed of their new responsibilities, many leaders were uncertain where to begin. The MCSC, which began meeting monthly in September 2002, played a significant role in helping them get started.

During the committee's first meetings, the committee co-chairs guided the disease center leaders through a series of discussions that resulted in the identification of operational priorities and goals for the next fiscal year and changes that had to be implemented to achieve them. The goals targeted specific and persistent problems with clinic operations and aimed to:

- Reduce the amount of time patients wait on the days of their appointments
- Improve patient and family satisfaction with waiting time
- Improve billing efficiency by reducing the incidence of missing charge data.

The MCSC also identified outcome metrics that would be monitored to track the disease centers' progress toward meeting each goal. For example, a data-collection system was established to monitor the amount of time that patients wait in each disease center. Patient satisfaction with waiting time was tracked using the patient satisfaction survey that was already in place, and billing efficiency was assessed by counting the number of appointments that did not have a charge linked to them 15 days after service was rendered.

Perhaps the most important goal identified by the MCSC was establishing a collaborative way of working, one that involved members of each discipline in effecting change and improving clinic operations. Toward that end, the MCSC co-chairs met regularly with each disease center's leadership team to help them form strategies to implement changes and address other issues in their clinical areas. The disease center leaders, in turn, met with their staff members and clinicians to discuss what the goals meant for them, to seek their suggestions for changes, and to assign tasks and responsibilities for next steps. By working with each disease center's leadership team to establish shared goals and design initiatives to improve operations, the MCSC co-chairs helped instill a sense of empowerment and accountability in the disease center leaders. More important, they served as role models for the collaborative, interdisciplinary leadership style that was now an expectation.

Results

During the first year, progress toward forming strong interdisciplinary leadership dyads and meeting the goals established by the MCSC varied among programs and floors. To some extent, this reflected variations in the leadership skills of each dyad. Those who quickly grasped the scope of their roles and who were more skilled in working collaboratively with co-leaders and staff accomplished more than those who were reluctant to assume responsibility or who were unaccustomed to working as members of a team. In addition, several of the leadership teams experienced turnover once individuals began to understand their roles and determined that the changes did not match their interests or skills.

In time, the leadership teams became comfortable with their new roles and began to make noteworthy progress toward achieving many of the operational goals. For example, the percentage of appointments with missing charge data dropped substantially, from 8.59% in 2002 to 2.15% by mid-2005. Since 2005, improvements in that area have been sustained but with a slight drop-off in performance caused, in part, by increased clinic activity. Implementation of an electronic charge system now is under way. Waiting time also was reduced in two of the larger disease centers and one infusion unit. In addition, the entire ambulatory service collaborated to implement an online medical record, improve the reporting of laboratory results, and improve patient access on holidays, weekends, and evenings. All of the improvements were accomplished even though the clinic and infusion volume continued to increase at a rate of approximately 5% per year.

Today, 4 years after the new leadership structure was introduced, interdisciplinary governance, which had long been accepted by the Institute's CEO, COO, CMO, chief nurse, and other senior executives, is firmly in place at the disease center and floor levels. As a result, the process used to make decisions, define priorities, and plan and implement improvements has changed dramatically. Before the new model was implemented, efforts to change clinic processes and systems often were met with resistance by clinicians and staff in the disease centers. Under the new governance model, in which the RN and MD leaders are accountable for making operational decisions and achieving agreed-upon goals, change is accomplished more readily.

A qualitative evaluation of the model's impact that captured the perspectives of many of the Institute's leaders and staff highlights how the model has affected the work environment. Among the evaluation's findings was the observation that many staff believed that a culture shift occurred after the model's introduction and that a more effective work environment—one that promotes accountability, communication, respect, and collaboration—has been established.

Lessons Learned

Leaders at DFCI learned many lessons while developing and implementing the new governance model. Lessons that might be most helpful to those interested in changing governance structures at their institutions follow.

Lesson 1. Go Slow to Go Fast

Taking time at the beginning of the change process—to articulate guiding principles, specify priorities for design and implementation, and obtain input from the Institute's faculty and staff—facilitated more rapid implementation of the new model and increased the likelihood of its acceptance by clinicians and other staff. People are more apt to support what they help create, which underpins not only the model but also the processes used to design and implement it. Although using a top-down change process may have been faster in the short run, it would have run counter to the institution's philosophy and could have created resistance that would have derailed the change effort or made it more drawn out.

Lesson 2. Align Group Purpose, Accountability, and Membership

The design and implementation phases of a change process often require the involvement of two very different kinds of groups. Too often, a change effort fails because its purpose is not perceived to be compelling by those who will be affected or implementation is left to a group without the proper authority and accountability to shepherd it through.

To develop the new governance model, a diverse group representing a wide range of disciplines and roles was convened. Group members were asked to shape the model's design based on their firsthand knowledge of the organization and broad experience with clinical work. Involving such a group in the design phase was essential because it ensured that the rationale for change was compelling and that the model designed by the group would lend itself to successful implementation. In contrast, accountability for implementation was given to the leaders of the disease centers and the MCSC. Those individuals had the authority to effect the necessary changes and the ability to influence senior executives to provide the resources and support that were required.

Lesson 3. The Importance of Executive Leadership

The executive team is responsible for creating a climate that inspires possibilities and fosters productive exchange. At DFCI, overall accountability for clinical operations and decisions related to strategic priorities reside with the chief nurse, CEO, COO, and CMO—a model that is particularly effective for a complex academic medical environment. The involvement of each member of the executive triad was essential to the successful implementation of the new governance model.

During the early stages of implementation, the executive team relied on the disease center leaders to encourage dialogue and keep staff informed about the progress of implementation. Over time, they realized that their expectation was unrealistic because the disease center leaders were just beginning to understand the implications of the new model and had difficulty representing the progress of implementation. As the executive team became involved more actively, they began to appreciate the important role they played in responding to the fear and resistance that inevitably occurs when a new management structure is introduced.

Wise leaders always manage expectations. During the implementation of the new governance model at DFCI, leaders quickly learned that if the implementation of some aspect of the model was to be delayed, they had to thoroughly communicate the information and reasons behind it to avoid disappointment and, possibly, cynicism by those eager to see change. By maintaining an ongoing dialogue with those who have a vested interest in preserving the status quo and engaging them in the change process, executive leaders can help staff appreciate how involving others benefits clinical operations, patient safety, patient and employee satisfaction, and the organization as a whole.

Lesson 4. Use Data to Drive Decisions

Using data to drive decisions can help to defuse much of the emotion that may be attached to decision making and allows the use of benchmarks to gauge progress. The MCSC co-chairs realized substantial benefits from using a data-driven approach. By using data about operational processes and outcomes to formulate goals and evaluate the effects of various initiatives, the co-chairs kept the RN and MD leaders and staff focused on improving performance and gave each disease center the ability to assess the effectiveness of their improvement efforts.

Lesson 5. Be Patient

Organizational change of the magnitude described herein takes time. Companies that have introduced self-directed work teams have found that teams often need several years to function independently; most health-care organizations will find that they are no different. Only with time can leaders in a new governance structure begin to appreciate the responsibilities associated with their roles and develop and refine the required skills. Over time, small successes build on one another and become the most effective argument for the model's continuation. The model has been accepted when staff at all levels view it simply as the right way to do business and the way in which patient- and family-centered care will be ensured.

REFERENCES

Abrahm, J.L., Callahan, J., Rossetti, K., & Pierre, L. (1996). The impact of a hospice consultation team on the care of veterans with advanced cancer. *Journal of Pain and Symptom Management, 12*(1), 23–31.

August, D.A., Ehrlich, D., & Carpenter, L.C. (1995). Patient evaluation of care within a multidisciplinary breast care center. *Quality Management in Health Care, 3*(3), 1–15.

Baggs, J.G., Norton, S.A., Schmitt, M.H., & Sellers, C.R. (2004). The dying patient in the ICU: Role of the interdisciplinary team. *Critical Care Clinics, 20,* 525–540.

Blazer, K.R., MacDonald, D.J., Ricker, C., Sand, S., Uman, G.C., & Weitzel, J.N. (2005). Outcomes from intensive training in genetic cancer risk counseling for clinicians. *Genetics in Medicine, 7*(1), 40–47.

Chang, J.H., Vines, E., Bertsch, H., Fraker, D.L., Czerniecki, B.J., Rosato, E.F., et al. (2001). The impact of a multidisciplinary breast cancer center on recommendations for patient management: The University of Pennsylvania experience. *Cancer, 91,* 1231–1237.

Chang, S., Hursting, S.D., Perkins, S.N., Dores, G.M., & Weed, D.L. (2005). Adapting postdoctoral training to interdisciplinary science in the 21st century: The Cancer Prevention Fellowship Program at the National Cancer Institute. *Academic Medicine, 80,* 261–265.

Institute of Medicine. (2000). *To err is human: Building a safer health system.* Washington, DC: National Academies Press.

Institute of Medicine. (2001). *Crossing the quality chasm: A new health system for the 21st century.* Washington, DC: National Academies Press.

Katzenback, J.R., & Smith, D.K. (1993). *The wisdom of teams.* Boston: Harvard Business School Press.

Kouzes, J.M., & Posner, B.Z. (1995). Foster collaboration: Promoting cooperative goals and mutual trust. In *The leadership challenge* (pp. 151–179). San Francisco: Jossey-Bass.

Ponte, P.R., Conlin, G., Conway, J., Grant, S., Medeiros, C., Nies, J., et al. (2003). Making patient-centered care come alive: Achieving full integration of the patient's perspective. *Journal of Nursing Administration, 33*(2), 82–90.

Porter-O'Grady, T., Hawkins, M.A., & Parker, M.L. (1997). Whole-systems shared governance: A model for integrated health care systems. In T. Porter-O'Grady, M.A. Hawkins, & M.L. Parker (Eds.), *Whole-systems shared governance: Architecture for integration* (pp. 35–68). Gaithersburg, MD: Aspen.

Siegrist, B.C. (2004). Partnering with public health: A model for baccalaureate nursing education. *Family and Community Health, 27,* 316–325.

Reprinted with permission from: Ponte, P., Gross, A. H., Winer, E., Connaughton, M. J., & Hassinger, J. (2007). Implementing an interdisciplinary governance model in a comprehensive cancer center. *Oncology Nursing Forum, 34*(3), 611–616.

IV
Nursing Therapeutics

Nurses have helped clients, families, and communities to cope with transitions by anticipating responses, providing anticipatory guidance, ameliorating symptoms, enhancing health and well-being, and supporting the development of self-care actions. We have selected three types of nursing therapeutics that nurses use in their practice for individuals, patients, and families experiencing transitions. These three types of therapeutics have conceptual bases, established longevity, and have been reviewed and evaluated extensively in the literature. Each nursing therapeutic is supported by research evidence,

I recommend that the reader consider each nursing intervention with healthy skepticism for its conceptual bases and the research evidence provided, because it is through such skepticism that we can continue to advance our knowledge. Therefore, it is imperative that you, the reader, may want to amass other writings about each nursing intervention, propose studies to test other hypothesis related to each intervention modality, and perhaps even indentify transitions and milestones in the transition trajectory to evaluate the effectiveness and the efficacy of each intervention.

In addition, it is imperative that these interventions be viewed as examples of nursing therapeutics used during transitions and not as totally exhaustive of all possible interventions for transitional experiences and responses. The three interventions selected for highlighting in this book are the transitional care, role supplementation, and debriefing, which are explored in chapters 9, 10, and 11, respectively.

The transitional care model is well described in an introductory chapter that was written especially for this book by Dr. Mary Naylor and Janet Van Cleave. This nursing therapeutic was developed to test intervention care at the time of predischarge and continues with the daily availability of nurses in person or by phone for vigilant assessment and monitoring inside and outside the hospital walls (Brooten et al.,, 1988). This intervention was used for patients ranging from newborns to elderly. More recently, members of The New Courtland Center for Transitions and Health at the University of Pennsylvania, specifically Dr. Naylor, the Director of the Center, and her colleagues who began focusing on older adults as well as the older adults with heart failure. Dr. Barbara Riegel, a member of this Center, outlines how she connects her focus on older adults with heart failure with the development of self-care practices to support patients in complex transitions. I have put Dr. Riegel's contribution in chapter 7 as it also reflects the health-and-illness transition. The articles by Drs. Dorothy Brooten, Mary Naylor (Brooten & Naylor, 1999; Naylor et al., 2004), and Drs. Kathy McCauley and M. Brian Bixby (McCauley, & Bixby, 2006) provide comprehensive descriptions and evidence on how to develop transitional environments and how advanced nursing practice can enhance outcomes and reduce health care costs. This nursing therapeutic has amassed research that provides evidence of the positive outcomes that result from using this nursing intervention.

Role supplementation as a nursing therapeutic has been used to enhance a healthy transition, and is one of many nursing strategies considered in clinical care. It is another model used as a nursing therapeutic for transitions that I developed in the late 1960s. When recovery is viewed to include role transition, a program is designed to cope with the transitional roles to achieve healthy outcomes.

This program included opportunities provided by nurses to clarify the different roles expected during and after recovery with opportunities for the rehearsal of the new and the old roles, an invitation for others to model new roles, and to develop supportive relations for healthy roles during recovery processes and to achieve healthy roles as outcomes. This brings me full circle from where I started this journey as I attempted to highlight the centrality of transitions in using knowledge and for nursing actions. Facilitating transitions by employing a role supplementation program has been used for new mothers, for patients and spouses rehabilitating from myocardial infarctions, for the elderly who are in transition to institutional care, and for battering parents during their recovery transition.

Role supplementation was defined as any deliberate process whereby role insufficiency or potential role insufficiency is identified by the role incumbent and significant others. It includes the components of role clarification and role taking. It is both preventative and therapeutic. To be able to help people and their significant others understand the new roles and the new identities that they need to develop, nurses may provide role clarification and facilitate their abilities to empathetically assume each others' roles.

The strategies needed to create these complementary healthy and dynamic roles and identities were defined as role modeling and role rehearsal. These were based on my clinical observations of the health-oriented groups created by nurses and by individuals who were part of the self-help movement. Members were provided with opportunities to watch and speak with others who had successfully gone through an illness or developmental transition. New mothers and fathers were bought into groups of people anticipating being new mothers and fathers. A patient who had successfully undergone mastectomy surgery was invited to dialogue with newly diagnosed groups of women with breast cancer who were anticipating mastectomies. A group of colostomy patients discussed and practiced colostomy management and shared different coping strategies.

Hence after much conceptual thinking, and with reliance on a framework inspired by Ralph Turner's work on roles (Turner, 1962), I labeled the strategies used in these groups as role taking, role modeling, and role rehearsal. All of these processes that I observed were only possible within the context of dialogues among groups of supporting individuals who were undergoing similar illness conditions. Therefore I identified and defined the main process that makes all of these strategies possible to be the central process of communication.

Subsequently, role supplementation as a nursing therapeutic has been used in a number of research projects. The major questions in each research project sought to further define the components, the processes, and the strategies related to role supplementation and to answer the question of whether it made a difference or not in helping patients complete a healthy transition. At that time I defined health as mastery, and in different research projects mastery was tested through such proxy variables as fewer symptoms, perceived well-being, and/or ability to assume new roles. Examples of the research projects based on role supplementation are provided.

Role Supplementation was used to help couples assume the new role of parenting (Meleis & Swendsen, 1978) and to help past myocardial infarction patients develop an at-risk identity that led to compliance with a rehabilitation regimen (Dracup, Meleis, Baker, & Edlefsen, 1984). It was also used to describe how the elderly maintained their sexuality (Kass & Rousseau, 1983) and in acquiring parental caregiving roles effectively (Brackley, 1992). Similarly it was used to ease the caregivers' roles for Alzheimer's patients (Kelly & Lakin, 1988). The framework was also used to better describe women who were not successful in becoming mothers and who manifested role insufficiency (Gaffney, 1992).

One of the well-researched interventions used at times of transitions is "debriefing." In some ways nurses used this caring intervention even before it was named as a concept, defined, operationalized, and subjected to many tests. Nurses "chatted," dialogued, and asked questions of patients after birthing, trauma events, disasters, surgical procedures, new admissions, or at discharge. They engaged in dialogues about each of these events, asked questions, provided patients and families with the opportunity to process the events and the aftermath of them. By not naming these pointed dialogues as debriefing the impetus for testing its effect on patients and families was not provided. Nurses and patients considered these dialogues as conversations between friends and acquaintances rather than as between a professional and a client. Once these conversations were named "debriefing," they were conceptually described, operationalized, and tested.

Debriefing is defined as a process of communicating to others the experiences that a person or group has encountered around a critical event. The narrator may relive the story emotionally, relate to it cognitively, describe it, interpret meanings, reflect on its effect on him/herself or others, and/or share feelings. The story usually includes the context and the before, during, and after responses related to the experience.

REFERENCES

Brackley, M. H. (1992). A role supplementation group pilot study: A nursing therapy for potential parental care givers, *Clinical Nurses Specialist, 6*(1), 14–19.

Brooten, D., Brown, L. P., Munoro, B. H., York, R., Cohen, S. M., Roncoli, M., et al. (1988). Early discharge and specialist transitional care. *Image: Journal of Nursing Scholarship, 20*, 64–68.

Brooten, D., & Naylor, M. D. (1999). Transitional environments. In A. S. Hinshaw, S. L. Feetham, & J. L. F. Shaver (Eds.), *Handbook of clinical nursing research* (pp. 641–653). Thousand Oaks, CA: Sage.

Dracup, K., Meleis, A. I., Baker, K., & Edlefsen, P. (1984). Family-focused cardiac rehabilitation: A role supplementation program for cardiac patients and spouses. *Nursing Clinics of North American, 19*(1), 113–124.

Gaffney, K. F. (1992). Nursing practice model for maternal role sufficiency. *Advances in Nursing Science, 15*(2), 76–84.

Kass, M. J., & Rousseau, G. K. (1983). Geriatric sexual conformity: Assessment and Intervention. *Clinical Gerontologist, 2*(1), 31–44.

Kelly, L. S., & Lakin, J. A. (1988). Role supplementation as a nursing intervention for Alzheimer's disease: A case study. *Public Health Nursing, 5*(3), 146–152.

McCauley, K., & Bixby, M. B. (2006). Advanced practice nurse strategies to improve outcomes and reduce cost in elders with heart failure. *Disease Management, 9*(5), 302–310.

Meleis, A. I., & Swendsen, P. A. (1978). Role supplementation: An empirical test of a nursing intervention. *Nursing Research, 27*, 11–18.

Naylor, M., Brooten D. A., Campbell R. L., Maislin G., McCauley K. M., & Schwartz, J. S. (2004). Transitional care of older adults hospitalized with heart failure: A randomized, controlled trial. *Journal of the American Geriatrics Society, 52*(5), 675–684.

Turner, R. (1962). Role taking: Process vs. conformity. In A. Rose (Ed.), *Human behavior and social processes*. Boston: Houghton-Mifflin.

Chapter 9 Transitional Care Model

9.1 THE TRANSITIONAL CARE MODEL FOR OLDER ADULTS

MARY D. NAYLOR
JANET VAN CLEAVE

TL, a 78-year-old African American man, was admitted to the hospital for the third time in 6 months for an acute episode of heart failure. TL also is coping with six other chronic conditions, including hypertension, diabetes, and coronary artery disease.

Current Care: By day 3 of his hospitalization, TL is medically stable. He is discharged to his home with a plan of care that does not reflect his goals, needs, literacy level, or learning style. His wife, and primary caregiver, was not involved in developing this plan or in the teaching about new medications and dietary modifications provided to her husband the morning of his discharge. The clinicians involved in his hospital care carefully managed his acute medical event but did not address the "root cause" of his multiple, recent hospitalizations. TL was rehospitalized for severe chest pain within 2 months after his discharge. These experiences reinforced his growing distrust of the health care system.

Although this scenario repeats itself regularly in communities across the United States, an alternative, evidence-based approach is available. Tested and refined over 20 years by a multidisciplinary team at the University of Pennsylvania, the Transitional Care Model (TCM) targets the growing population of chronically ill older adults at high risk for poor and costly outcomes. This chapter provides an overview of the Transitional Care Model, a description of its effect on quality of patient care and health care costs, and a summary of ongoing efforts to promote widespread use of this evidence-based approach to care.

Background

Transitional care is a term that encompasses a broad range of time-limited services, and environments designed to ensure health care continuity and avoid preventable poor outcomes among at-risk populations as they move from one level of care to another, among multiple providers, and/or across settings (American Geriatrics Society, 2003). In 1981, a multidisciplinary model of transitional care delivered by advanced practice nurses (APNs) was developed at the University of Pennsylvania, School of Nursing, Philadelphia. Initially, this health care innovation was designed to enable earlier hospital discharge of vulnerable low-birth-weight infants by substituting a portion of hospital care with home care, followed up by APNs (Brooten et al., 1986). The quality cost model of APN transitional care (hereafter referred to as the Transitional Care Model) was subsequently tested with several vulnerable groups, including women who underwent unplanned cesarean births and pregnant women with diabetes and hypertension. In response to national trends for earlier hospital discharge, the TCM focuses on improving the care and outcomes of high-risk, high-cost, and high-volume patient groups. Chronically ill older adults represent one such group.

Significance of TCM for Older Adults

High-quality transitional care is especially important for vulnerable groups of older adults coping with multiple, complex chronic conditions because these patients typically are cared for by multiple providers and move frequently among health care settings. Poorly executed transitions are common among these patients because of incomplete communication between providers and across settings, inadequate patient and caregiver education and involvement in decision making, limited continuity of care, and decreased access to essential services. Language barriers, literary issues, and cultural differences further exacerbate the problem (Naylor, 2006). Ineffective transitions have been linked to adverse events, serious unmet needs, and poor satisfaction with care (Naylor, 2006).

Rehospitalization rates among recently hospitalized older adults are very high; one quarter to one third are considered preventable (Naylor, 2006). In 2007, the Medicare Payment Advisory Commission (MedPAC) estimated that nearly 18% of Medicare beneficiaries admitted to a hospital are readmitted within 30 days of discharge. The rate is higher among beneficiaries with multiple chronic conditions. MedPAC calculated that this "churning" of patients accounts for an estimated $15 billion in spending (MedPac, 2007). The cycle of repeated, avoidable hospital readmissions has tremendous human as well as economic consequences (Naylor, 2006).

Application of TCM for Older Adults

The TCM provides comprehensive discharge planning and home follow-up care for chronically ill high-risk older adults admitted to the hospital for common medical conditions and surgical procedures. Central to this model is the relationship established among patients, family caregivers, and the transitional care nurse (TCN). In testing the model, the TCN has been a masters-prepared APN with advanced knowledge and skills in the care of chronically ill elders. The TCN follows patients from the hospital into their homes, providing evidence-based services designed to meet the patient and family caregiver goals, improve health outcomes and quality of life, and interrupt patterns of frequent use of acute care. Although the TCM is nurse led, this care model engages all members of the patient health care team in the implementation of proven protocols, with a unique focus on increasing patient and caregiver ability to manage the frequent transitions in health that characterize chronic illness trajectory.

For the millions of Americans who suffer multiple chronic conditions and complex therapeutic regimens, the TCM emphasizes coordination and continuity of care, prevention and avoidance of complications, and close clinical treatment and management—all accomplished with the active engagement of patients and their family caregivers and in collaboration with the patient's physicians and other health care team members. The TCM targets older adults with two or more risk factors, including history of recent hospitalizations, multiple chronic conditions or medications, and poor self-health ratings. See Exhibit 9.1.1 for the 10 essential elements of the model.

Effect on Quality, Cost, and Value

The research team of the University of Pennsylvania has attempted to address gaps in knowledge regarding the unique challenges of acutely ill older adults and their caregivers and to create effective strategies to address their needs systematically. Focus groups and pilot studies have preceded every large scale, randomized clinical trial (RCT). Across three National Institute of Nursing Research (NINR)–funded RCTs completed to date (Naylor et al., 1994, 1999, 2004). When compared with standard care, the TCM has demonstrated improved quality and cost outcomes for high-risk, cognitively intact older adults:

- **Reductions in preventable hospital readmissions for primary and coexisting conditions.** Additionally, among those patients who require rehospitalization, the time between their index hospital discharge and readmission was increased and the number of inpatient days was decreased (Figure 9.1.1).
- **Improvements in health outcomes after discharge.** In the most recently reported RCT

EXHIBIT 9.1.1. Ten Essential Elements of the Transitional Care Model

1. TCN as the primary coordinator of care to assure continuity throughout acute episodes of care;
2. In-hospital assessment, collaboration with team members to reduce adverse events and prevent functional decline, and preparation and development of an evidenced-based plan of care;
3. Regular home visits by the TCN, with available ongoing telephone support (7 days per week) through an average of 2 months postdischarge;
4. Continuity of medical care between hospital and primary care providers facilitated by the TCN accompanying patients to first follow-up visits;
5. Comprehensive, holistic focus on each patient's goals and needs, including the reason for the primary hospitalization, as well as other complicating or coexisting health problems and risks;
6. Active engagement of patients and caregivers, with focus on meeting their goals;
7. Emphasis on early identification and response to health care risks and symptoms to achieve longer term positive outcomes and avoid adverse and untoward events that lead to readmissions;
8. Multidisciplinary approach that includes the patient, family caregivers, and health care providers as members of a team;
9. Physician–nurse collaboration across episodes of acute care; and
10. Communication with, between, and among the patient, family caregivers, and health care providers.

Note. TCN = transitional care nurse.

(Naylor et al., 2004), short-term improvements in physical health, functional status, and quality of life were reported by patients who received care using the TCM.
- **Enhancement in patient satisfaction.** Overall, patient satisfaction increased among patients who received care using the TCM.
- **Reductions in total health care costs.** Total and average reimbursements per patient have been reduced in TCM-focused RCTs (Figure 9.1.2).

Continuing to Advance the Science

The University of Pennsylvania team is testing the effects of use of the TCM among hospitalized, cognitively impaired older adults (National Institute on Aging, R01-AG023116; Marian S. Ware Alzheimer's Program, 2005-2010). For this patient group, the impact of serious gaps in care across acute episodes of illness can be devastating. High rates of medical errors and avoidable hospital readmissions are common (Naylor et al., 2007). Medicare costs for cognitively impaired patients are three times higher than that for other older adults (Bynum et al., 2004). The primary goal of this project is to assess the clinical and economic outcomes achieved by nurse-led interventions of varying intensities, each designed to improve transitions in care for these patients and their caregivers. Findings from this study will contribute to our understanding of the unique needs of cognitively impaired elders and their caregivers across an episode of acute illness, offer evidence-based solutions to enhance their care and outcomes, and position the University of Pennsylvania team to make the case for improving the standards of care for these vulnerable groups.

Another ongoing study, Health Related Quality of Life (HRQoL): Elders in Long-Term Care, is helping to make the case to expand the application of the TCM among elders receiving long-term care (National Institute on Aging and the National Institute of Nursing Research, R01-AG025524, Marian S. Ware Alzheimer's Program, 2006-2011). Frail older adults receiving long-term care services are arguably the most vulnerable of patient groups. Currently, these older adults experience frequent, often avoidable transitions between the acute and long-term-care (LTC) sectors of the health care system, which have vastly different goals and few bridges to connect them. Consequently, their transitions are characterized by serious breakdowns in care, with human and economic tolls that are not fully appreciated. The HRQoL study is the first attempt to document the experiences of frail elders, including those with cognitive impairment, as they navigate these very challenging care transitions. This longitudinal study is assessing changes in health and quality of life over time among approximately 500 English- and Spanish-speaking elders newly transitioned to long-term care; comparing changes in these domains among elders who chose

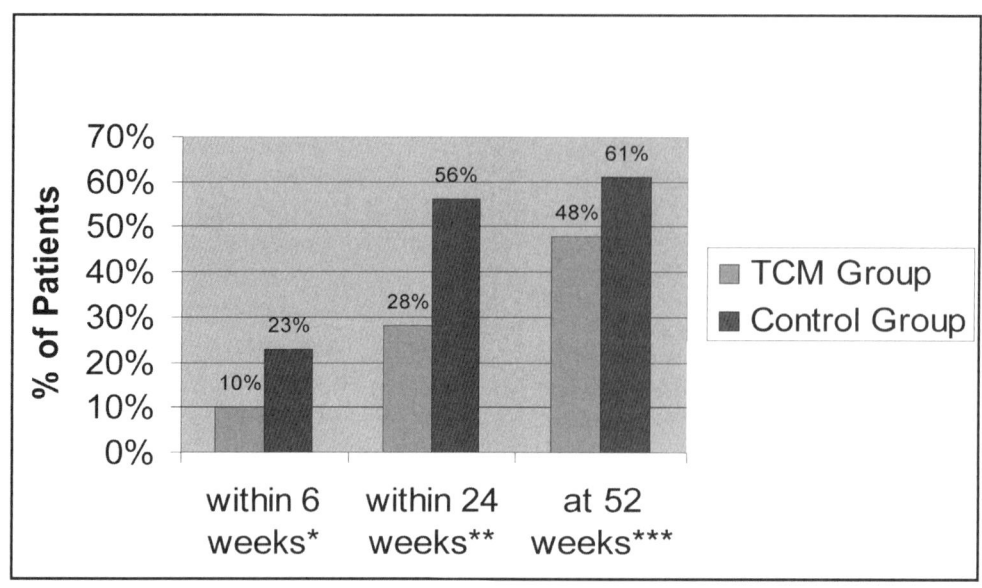

[Bar chart showing TCM's impact on readmission rates: within 6 weeks — TCM Group 10%, Control Group 23%; within 24 weeks — TCM Group 28%, Control Group 56%; at 52 weeks — TCM Group 48%, Control Group 61%.]

*Naylor et al., 1994; **Naylor et al., 1999; ***Naylor et al., 2004*

FIGURE 9.1.1 TCM's impact on readmission rates after index hospitalization.

to receive long-term care at home, in assisted-living facilities, or in nursing homes; and assessing the impact of transitions between long-term care and hospitals for this group. Frail elders in this study will be followed until their deaths.

Translating Research Into Practice

Despite the rich base of evidence establishing the link between the TCM and enhanced value, a number of organizational, regulatory, financial, and cultural barriers have prevented the adoption of the model. In response to these challenges and with the support of The Commonwealth Fund and the Jacob and Valeria Langeloth Foundation, the research team of the University of Pennsylvania formed a partnership with leaders of the Aetna Corporation (Aetna) to translate and integrate the TCM for use in everyday practice and promote widespread adoption of the model by demonstrating its effectiveness with a high-risk Medicare managed-care population in the mid-Atlantic region. As a result of the findings of this translational research effort, Aetna leaders have identified the TCM as a high-value proposition, and, as a result, spread of this model to Aetna markets with high Medicare penetration is planned for 2009. Additionally, based on the improvements in health outcomes, member and physician satisfaction and the reduction in the number of hospital readmissions and in total health care costs observed in this project, the University of Pennsylvania Health System (UPHS) has adopted the TCM as a service, and, early in 2009, local insurers are expected to reimburse UPHS for delivery of the TCM to their members.

A potential barrier to widespread adoption of this care model, raised by members of a National Advisory Committee (NAC) overseeing the translational efforts of the University of Pennsylvania team, is the availability of qualified APNs. NAC members also have questioned whether the use of APNs is the most efficient method to achieve the goals of this evidence-based approach to care. To address these important questions and concerns, and with the support of the John A. Hartford Foundation, Jacob and Valeria Langeloth Foundation,

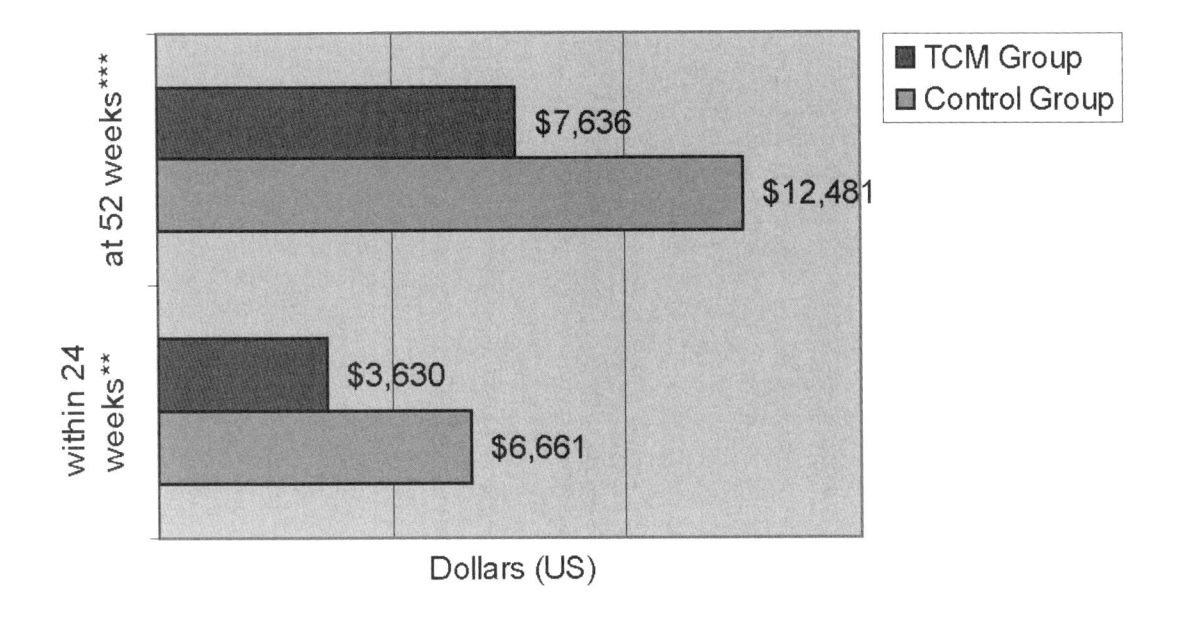

[Bar chart showing TCM's impact on total health care costs:
- At 52 weeks***: TCM Group $7,636; Control Group $12,481
- Within 24 weeks**: TCM Group $3,630; Control Group $6,661]

FIGURE 9.1.2 TCM's impact on total health care costs.

Note. Total costs were calculated using average Medicare reimbursements for hospital readmissions, ED visits, unscheduled acute care physician visits, and care provided by visiting nurses and other health care personnel. Costs for APN care were added to intervention group total. **Naylor et al., 1999; ***Naylor et al., 2004.

the Gordon and Betty Moore Foundation and the California Health Care Foundation, the University of Pennsylvania team formed a partnership with leaders of Kaiser Permanente. In addition to providing an entirely different organizational context to evaluate the translation and diffusion use of the TCM, the partnership with Kaiser Permanente offered the unique opportunity to determine whether the goals of this model could be achieved using nurses with varying educational backgrounds and skill sets, among elders hospitalized at Kaiser Permanente–owned and contract sites. Analyses of findings from this effort are ongoing. Kaiser Permanente leaders have agreed to consider adoption of TCM based on evaluation of the findings.

Conclusion

Given the expected increase in the number of older adults coping with complex chronic conditions, rapidly rising health care costs, and a projected shortfall in the Medicare Trust Fund, there is an urgent need to promote older adults' access to high-quality, cost-effective, and efficient services such as those provided via TCM. In addition to continued efforts to advance the science related to transitional care and promote rapid translation and dissemination of the TCM, the University of Pennsylvania team and others are promoting policy changes needed to accelerate access to evidence-based transitional care models. Prominent among these are policies that (a) emphasize geriatrics, transitional and palliative care, interdisciplinary care, and engagement of family caregivers in the educational preparation of the existing and future health care workforce, (b) promote performance monitoring and reporting systems that measure effective transitional care, (c) align financial incentives to stimulate effective and efficient transitional care, and (d) reform eligibility rules, quality monitoring systems, criteria for reimbursement, and funding streams within and among public and private health insurance benefits.

The recent recommendations of MedPAC encouraging public reporting of hospital readmission rates, payment reform to financially encourage lower readmission rates, and adoption by hospitals of readmission-reducing strategies have resulted in a swift cascade of policy reforms (MedPAC, 2007). The Centers for Medicare and Medicaid Services (CMS) recently emphasized reducing readmission rates through its Quality Improvement Organization (QIO) Program, transparency initiatives (e.g., public reporting of 30-day risk standardized readmission rates for heart failure), and value-based purchasing activities (e.g., proposed incentives to hospitals and home health providers to reduce avoidable readmissions). The TCM is a validated approach to reducing high hospital readmission rates and, therefore, an effective response to these policy reforms.

Ultimately, however, the best measure of the value of the TCM is its impact on each patient served by this model. A case in point is TL's experience when he was enrolled in the TCM during his fourth hospitalization in the fall of 2007.

Care of TL under the TCM. *The TCN learns that TL does not take any of his 14 prescribed medications because the drugs are "too costly" and "only make me feel worse." In addition, he refuses to complete follow-up physician visits because "no one is interested in listening to my problems." The TCN collaborates with the attending cardiologist to develop a simplified discharge plan. At discharge, the patient is prescribed only three medications for heart failure and agrees to adhere to the protocol for 1 month. The TCN helps the patient enroll in a Veteran's Affairs (VA) Clinic, where he receives his medications with minimal out-of-pocket costs, TL's medication costs are reduced. TL complies with a follow-up physician visit accompanied by the TCN within 1 week of hospital discharge.*

Before this year, TL was very active maintaining a large community garden. TL's major goal was to return to this satisfying work. His TCN requested a physical therapy evaluation during hospitalization and then worked with TL to implement the plan of care, gradually adding more activity to his routine while closely monitoring his response. TL is gardening daily for short periods by the time the TCM intervention is complete.

TL's wife reported serving a "near-perfect diet" despite ample evidence of high-sodium foods in the kitchen. Because TL's wife did all cooking and grocery shopping, the TCN directs her teaching toward reading labels and dietary principles. Using teach-back, TL's wife is able to demonstrate her understanding of basic concepts such as avoiding adding salt at the table, avoiding high-sodium foods when selecting menu items from a favorite restaurant, and limiting fluid intake.

TL received 10 home visits and two physician office visits with his TCN and eight telephone calls during the course of his 2-month involvement with the TCM. At 12 months postenrollment, he remains adherent to his treatment plan and is in close follow-up with the cardiologist. He has had no subsequent rehospitalizations. TL and his wife both express a high level of satisfaction with their health care.

REFERENCES

American Geriatrics Society Health Care Systems Committee, Coleman, E. A., & Boult, C. (2003). Improving the quality of transitional care for persons with complex needs. Position statement of The American Geriatrics Society Health Care Systems Committee. *Journal of the American Geriatrics Society, 51,* 556–557.

Brooten, D., Kumar, S., Brown, L. P., Butts, P., Finkler, S. A., Bakewell-Sachs, S., et al. (1986). A randomized clinical trial of early discharge and home follow-up of very low birthweight infants. *New England Journal of Medicine, 315,* 934–939.

Bynum, J. P., Rabins, P. V., Weller, W., Niefeld, M., Anderson, G. F., & Wu, A. W. (2004). The relationship between a dementia diagnosis, chronic illness, medicare expenditures, and hospital use. *Journal of the American Geriatrics Society, 52*(2), 187–194.

MedPAC. (2007, June). *Promoting greater efficiency in Medicare.* Washington, DC: Author.

Naylor, M. D. (2006). Transitional care: A critical dimension of the home healthcare quality agenda. *Journal for Healthcare Quality, 28,* 48–54.

Naylor, M. D., Brooten, D., Jones, R., Lavizzo-Mourey, R., Mezey, M., & Pauley, M. (1994). Comprehensive discharge planning for the hospitalized elderly. *Annals of Internal Medicine, 120,* 999–1006.

Naylor, M. D., Brooten, D., Campbell, R., Jacobsen, B. S., Mezey, M.D., Pauley, M.V., et al. (1999). Comprehensive discharge planning and home follow-up of hospitalized elders: A randomized clinical trial. *Journal of the American Medical Association, 281,* 613–620.

Naylor, M. D., Brooten, D. A., Campell, R. L., Maislin, G., McCauley, K. M., & Schwartz, J. S. (2004). Transitional care of older adults hospitalized with heart failure: A randomized, controlled trial. *Journal of the American Geriatrics Society, 52,* 675–684.

Naylor, M. D., Hirschman, K. B., Bowles, K. H., Bixby, M. B., Konick-McMahan, J., & Stephens, C. (2007). Care coordination for cognitively impaired older adults and their caregivers. *Home Health Care Services Quarterly, 26*(4), 57–78.

9.2 TRANSITIONAL ENVIRONMENTS

Dorothy Brooten
Mary Duffin Naylor

Abstract

The science supporting environments that provide transitional care and that optimize out-comes is sparse and relatively recent. Although some empirical data are available, much of the reported literature is anecdotal, descriptive, and lacks reported outcomes. This chapter (a) defines transitional environments and the research issues that have arisen in the literature on transitional care, (b) describes the major current and emerging models of transitional care reported in the literature, and (c) summarizes gaps in the current science in this area and offers recommendations for future research.

Definitions and Issues

Transitional environments are those environments in which a transitional care service is provided. These services, however, are defined and implemented differently. Transition implies an in-between period. Therefore, the nature of transitional services is that they are not long-term services but temporary short-term services, which are different from long-term home care. Most commonly, transitional care refers to care and services required in the safe and timely transfer of patients from one level of care to another (e.g., acute to subacute) or from one type of health care setting to another (e.g., hospital to home) (Brooten, 1993). Therefore, transitional care environments may include the hospital, home, nursing home, rehabilitation center, home care agency, and hospice. Some authors differentiate subacute care from transitional care (Micheletti & Shlala, 1995; Robinson, Mead, & Boswell, 1995; Stahl, 1994); others use the terms interchangeably (Ellis & Mendlen, 1995; Heller & Walton, 1995; Hyatt, 1995). Those who do differentiate view subacute care as a unit or component of inpatient care in an acute care hospital, skilled nursing facility, or freestanding medical or rehabilitation center. Transitional services ideally end with normal functioning and recovery, functional independence, or stabilization of the patient's condition (Brooten, 1993).

The number of transitional care services has increased exponentially during the past 15 years in response to changes in the delivery of health care services—mainly the shortening of hospital duration of stay and the increase in acuity levels of patients cared for at sites other than hospitals. One indicator of the growth of transitional care services is the increase in the number of home care agencies from approximately 1,100 in 1963 to 17,561 in 1995 (National Association for Home Care [NAHC], 1995). In evaluating transitional care services that optimize patient outcomes, issues affecting research include determination of the nature and necessary duration of the service, the profile of patients who require the service, the type and level of providers needed, and the costs for the services.

Determining the Nature and Necessary Duration of Services

Features of transitional care include discharge planning from one site of care to another, coordination of postdischarge services at the new site of care, provision of short-term in-home services, and continued health care follow-up. The most important features of transitional care services are continuity of care across sites, communication of the plan of care among the providers, and matching patient needs and the knowledge and skills of the care providers (Brooten, 1993).

Transitional care services most often begin with discharge planning from an acute care setting. Discharge planning should begin on the day of patient admission. This is essential in this time of very short hospital stays and increased patient acuity, for only then can services be projected and referrals made (Morrow-Howell & Proctor, 1994; Naylor, 1993; Prescott, Soeken, & Griggs, 1995). However, this is an ideal. Currently, discharge planning is fragmented (Haddock, 1991; Prescott et al., 1995; Roe-Prior, Watts, & Burke, 1994). Often, discharge planning is conducted using protocols developed for use across all patient groups, with little or no modification to meet the needs of specific patient groups (Naylor, 1993). In addition, there is institutional variability in the criteria used to determine which patients receive more than cursory discharge planning and follow-up services (Prescott et al., 1995; Winograd, 1990). There is also institutional variability in the preparation and expertise of the persons conducting the discharge planning (Anderson & Helms, 1993; Findeis, 1994; Naylor, 1990; Prescott et al., 1995; Roe-Prior et al., 1994; Winograd, 1990). One panel of experts in the care of elderly individuals rated the quality of current planning for care after discharge as very poor. A study of more than 900 Medicare-certified hospitals revealed that only 9% of elderly patients were discharged with plans for further care, and, of that 9%, only half actually received the care (U.S. General Accounting Office [GAO], 1987).

The duration of transitional care services should vary with the specific needs of the patient or group of patients. However, data indicating the most effective and cost-efficient end point for receipt of these services for specific patient groups or subgroups are not available. In today's era of health care cost containment, transitional care services end with as much home care or service as is reimbursable.

Determining Which Patients Require Transitional Care Services

There is general agreement (nonempirically based) that vulnerable groups, such as elderly individuals, technologically dependent individuals, disabled persons, and some high-risk infants and children, should receive transitional care services (Berk & Berstein, 1985). Yet, as many researchers have noted, not everyone within these groups may require the full complement of services or services over the same duration or with the same level and type of provider (Brooten, 1993; Patterson, Leonard, & Titus, 1992).

Research in providing early hospital discharge and advanced practice nurse (APN) transitional care services to women with unplanned cesarean births showed that women who experienced infections required an average of 40 more minutes during home visits and 20 more minutes during hospital admission than women without infections. However, many women without infections also consumed much APN time during home visits and during telephone follow-up. This time was used to teach infant care and parenting and to making referrals to community resources (Brooten, Knapp, et al., 1996).

Data suggest that not all elders admitted to the hospital are at risk for poor postdischarge outcomes. Many elders and their families who receive effective preparation while in the hospital do well after discharge and do not require transitional care services. Naylor (1990) and Neidlinger, Scroggins, and Kennedy (1987) have shown this. Research findings have helped to identify those patients who will require transitional care services. The group includes elders with major mental and functional deficits, those without family or friends able or willing to help them, and those with complex medical problems (Naylor, 1993).

Decisions regarding which patients should receive transitional services are based on patient functional ability, presence of available caretakers at home, ethnicity, geography, age, sociodemographics, history of hospital admissions, and dependence on technology (Bakewell-Sachs & Porth, 1995; Corrigan & Martin, 1992; Gilmartin, 1994; Helberg, 1994; Prescott et al., 1995). The decision that a patient requires discharge planning and follow-up services is often based on patient ability to perform activities of daily living (Branch et al., 1988; Cox et al., 1990; Helberg, 1994; Kemper, 1992). However, no uniform method exists to evaluate patient functional ability during hospital admission.

Reed, Pearlman, and Buchner (1991) reported that the only two measures of functional ability consistently recorded on the medical record were ability to ambulate and orientation. In a study of 737 elderly patients discharged from 15 Illinois hospitals, Jones, Densen, and Brown (1989) found that 63% of elders with an identified deficit in one or more activities of daily living at the time of hospital discharge did not receive a referral for home services, and, of these patients, 60% reported that no one at the hospital asked them how they would be able to manage after discharge. Prescott et al. (1995) reported that hospital personnel were fairly adept at identifying the most impaired patients in need of postdischarge services. However, clinicians failed to identify a subgroup of patients in need of transitional care services who had less severe functional impairment but a greater number of diagnoses. Clearly, functional ability, though predictive of a patient's need for transitional care services, should not be the only criterion used to make that determination.

Presence or absence of a family member, assumed to provide caretaking, also is often used to determine who receives follow-up transitional care services. Living with someone frequently excludes the patient from receiving essential services after hospital discharge. The study by Furstenberg and Mezey (1987) reported that 94% of patients who lived alone were visited by a discharge planner; however, only 40% of those who lived with someone else received a similar visit. One of the patients not visited was an 89-year-old woman who accurately reported that she lived with someone—her 91- and 93-year-old sisters, who were not capable of providing postdischarge care.

Duration of acute care stay may also determine who receives transitional care services. Shorter durations of acute care stays may result in the staff's having insufficient time to identify patients who would benefit from transitional care services (Magilvy & Lakomy, 1991). Shorter duration acute care stays may also prevent staff from adequately preparing the patient and the family for postdischarge treatment. Several investigators have suggested links between readmissions to acute care hospitals with lack of adherence to therapeutic regimens because of inadequate patient education before discharge (Ghali, Kadakia, Cooper, & Ferlinz, 1988; Vinson, Rich, Sperry, Shah, & McNamara, 1990). Even when discharge teaching has been provided, patients may be too anxious to absorb the information or the quantity of information is too overwhelming to be absorbed at one time (O'Brien & McCluskey-Fawcett, 1993). Ethnicity also was a factor in who received which type of transitional services. Falcone, Bolda, and Leak (1991) reported that elderly Black patients were more likely to face a delay in hospital-to-nursing home placement than White patients, even after controlling for the complexity of care necessary and the type of insurance coverage. The researchers suggest that the delay may be attributable to nursing home policies of "race matching" elders in semiprivate rooms, which is in violation of antidiscrimination laws. Mui and Burnette (1994) reported that there were ethnic differences related to the use of in-home, community-based, and nursing home services. They found that White elders were more likely than Blacks or Hispanics to use in-home and nursing home services. In contrast, Black and Hispanic individuals were more likely to rely on informal support networks and community-based services. Kemper (1992) found race to be the only important sociodemographic factor to have a large effect on the amount or type of home care used. Blacks and Hispanics were more likely than White patients to depend on informal care, both resident and visiting, to meet home care needs. These ethnic differences in the use of transitional care services may reflect variations in acceptability of the services, awareness of availability of the services, and differences in accessibility because of economic or geographic reasons.

As with other health care services, communication among providers of the service is an important factor in who receives adequate transitional care services. A study that evaluated the adequacy of communication between a hospital's discharge planners and home health agencies found that patient records contained only slightly more than half the information necessary to ensure continuity of patient care (Anderson & Helms, 1993). Significantly more patient data were communicated to the receiving agency when patient information was collected by a liaison nurse employed by the home care agency. The results of the study indicate that, even when discharge planning occurs, essential information may not be relayed to the providers of the next level of service and this may have a negative effect on patient outcomes. Similar findings were reported by others (Harrington, Lynch, & Newcomer, 1993; Hazlett, 1989; Meara, Wood, Wilson, & Hart, 1992; Patterson et al., 1992; Williams, Greenwell, & Groom, 1992).

The type of health institution, insurer, and the patient's distance from care sites also influence which patients receive transitional care. In a national study designed to document the types and quantity of transitional care provided by psychiatric hospitals, Dorwart and Hoover (1994) reported that the provision of transitional care was inadequate and uneven. Urban psychiatric hospitals with residency programs were more likely than general hospitals to provide aftercare services and to use case management to ensure continuity of care. Others reported that, even when a service was available locally, insurers might dictate that care be received at a distant site and restrict access to certain providers and services (Fox, Wicks, & Newacheck, 1993; Harrington et al., 1993).

Determining Type and Level of Providers of Transitional Care

The providers of transitional care are as varied as the programs and services (Brooten, 1993; Schwartz, Blumenfield, & Perlman Simon, 1990), and there is disagreement about who should provide the care (Kornowski, 1995; Rich, 1995; Roselle & D'Amico, 1990). The work of Brooten (Brooten et al., 1994; Brooten et al., 1986; Brooten et al., 1995), Naylor (1994), and others (Thurber & DiGiamarino, 1992; York et al., 1997) using APNs to provide transitional care for high-risk groups has consistently shown improved patient outcomes, with reduced health care costs for the patient groups followed up. Nurses specialize at the masters level; therefore, use of a masters-prepared nurse specialist assumes that the nurse has advanced knowledge and skill in the care of the specific patient groups followed up, an assumption that cannot be made of a nurse generalist. Using a masters-prepared nurse also avoids the great variability in preparation (diploma, associate degree [AD], bachelor of science in nursing [BSN]) of the nurse generalist. Masters-prepared nurse specialists with advanced knowledge and skills can function under general protocols, with less-detailed instructions for procedures and protocols and direct supervision than do personnel with less educational preparation. Finally, the average annual national salaries of masters-prepared nurses in nonadministrative roles is only approximately $5,500 higher than that of a registered nurse (American Nurses Association, 1994). When this cost is divided among the number of patients followed up, the added cost is negligible. Whether masters-prepared nurse specialists are necessary for all patient populations has yet to be evaluated (Brooten et al., 1995).

Patterson et al. (1992) reported that home care provided by professional nurses decreased the negative psychosocial effect on parents caring for medically fragile children at home, especially as the number of nursing hours increased. In this study, care by a home health aide was associated with a greater negative psychosocial affect on the family. Improved patient outcomes from home care provided by RNs have also been reported by Hazlett (1989) with ventilator-dependent children, by McCorkle et al. (1994) with oncology patients, and by Bull (1994) with elders.

Many authors (Katz, 1993; Landefeld, Palmer, Kresevic, Fortinsky, & Kowal, 1995; Rich, 1995; Sivak, Cordasco, & Gipson, 1983; Wong, 1991) have advocated a multidisciplinary model to implement discharge planning and ensure the successful transition of patients from one level of care to another. However, this model is not routinely used in most institutions because of cost. The diversity of individuals providing transitional care ranges from individuals with little health care training to masters-prepared nurses and includes a variety of providers who offer specialized services, such as respiratory therapy, physical therapy, occupational therapy, and social work services. Transitional care is most successful using a multidisciplinary approach from the hospital to the many community agencies and resources needed by the patient and family. However, a member of the multidisciplinary team must coordinate the care.

Determining Costs for Transitional Care Services

Managed care and capitated reimbursement have changed the system of delivery of care, the focus of care, and the window of opportunity for evaluating patient outcomes and costs. Evaluating cost and outcome in one setting (e.g., hospital or home) provides one snapshot but does not capture outcome and cost over a period of transitional care or over a period of insured care. In addition, cost and outcome data that are focused on one site of care do not capture cumulative effects of system changes, such as those resulting from shortened hospital stay; on cost and outcomes in other sites of care; or on the family unit. The issues in collecting valid and meaningful data on cost across sites of care include which costs can be collected, whether the costs can be collected across all sites of care, and who is responsible for absorbing these costs.

Which Costs Can Be Collected

Estimation of true costs of health care resources consumed in transitional care is problematic. In some studies, charges are used as reasonably good proxies for resource costs. However, the health care market shows severe distortions, such that, charges for services often have little relationship to resource costs. Various mechanisms have been used in studies to improve the validity of estimates of health care resource costs, including: cost–to–charge ratios (subject to accounting artifacts and problems of aggregation); time and motion studies (limited by high cost of collecting information, sampling error, and generalizability of results); and cost estimates derived from managed care payments, which often consider only payer costs.

A major issue in attempting to cost out transitional care is what should be included in calculating the cost and whether the investigators were able to cost out all the factors that should be included. Items commonly included in calculating costs include personnel time (salary and benefits), administrative costs, supplies, and indirect costs (space, heat, electricity). Costs for personnel time are often measured based on actual or average salary and fringe benefits for the personnel plus time involved for the task. This approach may work well when a single person can be identified with tasks or similar types and levels of patient need. However, when a number of types and levels of staff are involved (such as in transitional care), cost allocation and association with specific outcomes becomes more difficult.

Charge data have been commonly used in studies as a proxy for the costs of hospital and physician care (Carey, 1996). Charges for hospital stay and physician services are obtained from patient bills, acquired either through the hospital or agency or from patients themselves. In today's cost-cutting environment, many hospitals and agencies have become very resistant to providing patient bills, making the cost estimates for comparing types of transitional services difficult. Although charges are not the same as costs, they can serve as a reasonable proxy. Use of charge information is adequate to uncover *relative* changes in cost-in studies. Given the use of sensitivity analysis, this approach can provide adequate information to generate useful comparisons of study results.

The limitations of using charges as a proxy for costs should be acknowledged in studies on transitional care that use this method. Charges include fixed and variable costs. Fixed costs may not decrease as output is reduced. Furthermore, methods of cost allocation may not accurately assign costs to the patients who consumed specific resources.

"Microcosting," a method considered superior to the use of charge information, has been used in a few studies that compared transitional services. In this approach, specific data collection is undertaken for every element of resource consumed. Microcosting has been successfully used in clinical situations that are very narrow and limited in scope (such as the study of the administration of one particular drug); however, it is less feasible for studies that include the costs of an entire hospital stay. The many aspects of cost that should be evaluated make such studies prohibitive, given most hospital cost-accounting systems and the resources required.

Resource units, or health service resource use, is another approach to measure costs in studies of transitional care services. Here, all major health care resources consumed are collected and the various resource units are converted to estimates of costs (Horn et al., 1996). Resources consumed include the number of hospital admissions (duration of stay and unit within the hospital), physician services, nursing services, allied professional services, ancillary services, postdischarge nursing services, and vendor services. Costs are then summarized overall and by type of service and component. This approach allows evaluation of the effect of an intervention—for example, on total costs—and provides insight into how and where cost savings may be achieved.

Allowable insurer costs (the allowable cost on which payments by insurer and patient are calculated) are often used as proxies for costs to convert resource use to estimates of costs. Allowable costs based on national providers (e.g., Medicare) provide an enhanced level of generalizability for comparing study results. In today's era of health care cost containment, comparisons of the most efficient and cost-effective transitional care services are especially difficult given the differences in cost-accounting methods in documenting health care costs across sites of care.

Finally, any evaluation of cost for transitional care must include evaluation of the shift in cost burden from hospitals and insurers to patients and families. As duration of hospital stay has decreased, costs for care normally incurred by hospitals have shifted to the family unit. Nonreimbursable costs for supplies and caregiver time and loss of employment and leisure time are costs that should be documented and compared. Documented costs of home care include an increase in the charges on utility bills in homes with ventilator-dependent children, insufficient funds for home care services, loss of employment, and an increased occurrence of physical illnesses in family caretakers (Hazlett, 1989; Sevick et al. 1992).

Although the costs for transitional services are calculated in some studies, indirect costs, such as prevention of hospital readmission, acute care visits, decreased employment, and burden on family caregivers, are less well documented. These data are important in evaluating the overall cost benefit or cost-effectiveness of transitional care services.

Models of Transitional Care

Home Health Care

The fastest growing site of transitional care services is home health care. Several types of agencies provide home services: public agencies (operated by the state or local government); private not-for-profit agencies (freestanding and privately operated); proprietary agencies (freestanding and operated for profit); hospital-based agencies; and dedicated units or departments operated by a hospital. In the past, public health agencies were the major providers of home care. Since the revision of the Medicare home payment law in 1987, hospital-based and proprietary agencies have supplanted public health agencies (NAHC, 1995) as the largest providers of this service.

Expansion in home care is also a result of cost-containment efforts to substitute home health care for acute care stays. With fewer acute care beds occupied, hospitals have entered the home care field to provide a safety net for their patients and as another source of revenue (Keenan & Fanale, 1989; Stahl, 1995b). Some authors note differences in the patient population and the services provided based on the type of home care agency. Public agencies are more likely to serve Medicare patients or the indigent. Proprietary agencies are more likely to serve the relatively well-insured. Hospital-based agencies substitute home care for inpatient days (Williams, 1991).

Home Health Care From Community Nursing Services

Community or public health nurses have historically provided home follow-up care to high-risk patients with complex health needs. Their services are well known and accepted by the general public and health care providers. Nurses working within the community are also familiar with community resources, health care needs, and the values and culture of the community residents. Unfortunately, over the past 10 to 15 years, budget reductions of community nursing services have virtually eliminated home follow-up services to many patient groups. Programs focused on prevention and well-child care, for example, were curtailed to provide services to more acutely ill patients, mainly elders, now discharged to home earlier and still recovering (Bull, 1994; NAHC, 1995). More recently, services for less stable, more acutely ill newborns and pregnant and women newly delivered of a newborn have been added (NAHC, 1995).

The challenges for community nursing services include updating the specialty knowledge and skills of agency nurses with a generalist preparation, maintaining continuity of patient care from the hospital to the home, and providing sufficient services to maintain good patient outcomes while insurers are reimbursing for fewer services (Brooten, 1995). To provide service to a more high-risk group of patients, agencies have been providing continuing education for their nurses, using masters-prepared clinical nurse specialists and nurse practitioners with advanced practice skills as consultants (Zelle, 1995) or, in agencies with sufficient caseloads, hiring APNs to provide direct care in the home. Attempts to improve continuity of care to high-risk groups have included predischarge hospital visits to patients by a community nurse and having a community liaison nurse on site in the hospital (Dawson, 1994). Some agencies now provide 7-days-a-week 24-hour-a-day nurse coverage and expanded use of ancillary personnel, including homemaker–home health aides.

Hospital Home Care Services and HMO Follow-Up Services

As reimbursed length of stay for even high-risk patients decreases, hospitals' need for improved discharge planning and postdischarge home care services for these groups increases. Documented discharge planning is mandatory for hospitals, and many have hired discharge planners to facilitate earlier discharge. Some hospitals contract with community nursing services or independent home care agencies to provide home care services for high-risk patients. An increasing number of hospitals are establishing home care services. In some instances, this home care is provided by hospital nursing staff from units on which bed occupancy has decreased, thus reducing the number of nursing staff needed on the units. As Dahlberg and Koloroutis (1994) note, one of the greatest advantages of a hospital-based program is the internal availability of knowledgeable and skilled nursing staff. Physicians are more likely to refer patients to a program that is staffed with nurses they know and trust from the hospital setting (Dahlberg & Koloroutis, 1994). In other hospitals, home care services are provided by a nursing staff hired and managed by the hospital home care department (Brooten, 1995).

HMOs have a clear financial incentive for discharging patients early and for preventing costly rehospitalizations. Case managers and nurses with specialty knowledge and skills are used to review patient discharge and home care needs. Because realizing a profit is essential to HMOs, the HMO approach has been one of minimal hospital duration of stay and postdischarge services. The number of visits provided, the type of nurse provider (nurse generalist or specialist), and length of follow-up vary for home follow-up services. More than the routine allowable number of home visits may be reimbursable for a patient; however, this must be negotiated between provider and insurer.

Entrepreneurial Services

Over the past decade, many entrepreneurial groups have established services to provide home care to patients (Eaton, 1994). Usually these groups are not involved in discharge planning but do provide home care services on a fee-for-service or contractual basis. The services provided may be determined by the company medical advisory board or by the contracting agency and reviewed and approved by the company medical advisory board. Nurses providing services may be full-time employees or temporary nursing staff who may or may not have specialty preparation and skills in caring for the patient groups they are following up.

Research Models of Transitional Services

Quality Cost Model of Advanced Practice Nurse Transitional Care

Responding to national trends in earlier hospital discharge of vulnerable patient groups, an interdisciplinary model of transitional care (comprehensive discharge planning and home follow-up) delivered by APN specialists was developed by Brooten et al. in 1981 (Brooten et al., 1988; Brooten et al., 1986) and has undergone further evaluation and refinement over the past 16 years (Brooten et al., 1994; Hollingsworth, Cohen, Finkler, Rubin, & Morgan, in review; Naylor et al., 1994; Thurber & DiGiamarino, 1992; York et al., 1997). The model uses masters-prepared APNs (clinical nurse specialists and nurse practitioners) for reasons of quality and cost.

The model was originally designed for early discharge of patients from the hospital by replacing a portion of hospital care with a comprehensive program of transitional care delivered by APN specialists whose specialty preparation matched the patient groups they followed up. *Transitional care* was defined as comprehensive discharge planning developed for each specific patient group plus home follow-up care through the period of normally expected recovery or stabilization (Brooten et al., 1988).

Using the model, patients are discharged early, provided they meet a standard set of discharge criteria agreed on by the physician and nurse specialist. Criteria include physical, emotional, and informational patient readiness for discharge and an environment supportive of convalescence at home. The APN prepares the patient for discharge and coordinates discharge planning with the patient, physician, hospital nursing staff, and, where appropriate, social service staff, community resource groups, and equipment vendors. The APN also coordinates or provides patient teaching, helps establish a timeframe for the day of discharge, coordinates plans for medical follow-up, and makes referrals to community agencies as needed.

After discharge, the APN specialist conducts a series of home visits and is frequently in touch with patients and their families by telephone. The number and timing of home visits varies with the patient group being followed up. APNs were available to patients and families by telephone from 8 a.m. to 10 p.m. Monday through Friday and from 8 a.m. to noon Saturday and Sunday. After 10 p.m. on weekdays and during the afternoon on weekends, patients were asked to call their private physician or hospital emergency room should immediate care be needed (Brooten et al., 1988).

The APNs assess and monitor the physical, emotional, and functional status of the patient, provide direct care as needed, assist in obtaining services or other resources available in the community, and provide group-specific and individual teaching, counseling, and support during the period of convalescence. If complications arise, the nurse specialist consults with the backup physician for a plan of immediate and most effective treatment.

The model was designed to provide data on the quality of care as reflected in patient outcomes, cost of care, and thorough documentation of nursing functions. It was developed for use with any patient population, from frail infants to frail elders. It was designed to provide data on physical and psychosocial patient outcomes, including mortality, morbidity (e.g., hospital readmissions, emergency room visits, incidence of infection), return of patients to normal activities, patient satisfaction with care, and outcomes important to specific patient groups.

The model was also constructed to provide data reagarding the cost of transitional follow-up care by APN specialists, compared with routine care and discharge. Cost data include charges for initial hospital stay, hospital readmissions, and physician services, and, in an early discharge group, it includes the cost of the services of the APN specialist, as well as time lost from employment by family members who assume care of the patient during the period of early discharge (Brooten et al., 1988).

Using a randomized clinical trial, the model was originally tested with very-low-birth-weight (VLBW) (< 1500 g) infants (Brooten et al., 1986). One group was discharged earlier from the hospital and received the APN intervention; a second group received usual care and was discharged after the standard time. Both groups were followed up for 18 months postdischarge. Study results demonstrated no significant differences in infant outcomes (rehospitalizations, number of acute care visits, infant growth and development) between the groups; however, cost savings were significant in the early-discharge group (more than $18,000 per infant).

The model was next tested with three high-volume, high-risk, or high-cost groups of women. In a randomized clinical trial, women who underwent unplanned cesarean deliveries were enrolled after the birth and followed up for 8 weeks. Study results showed that women who received the APN intervention were discharged a mean of 30.3 hours earlier than usual ($p < .001$), were significantly more satisfied with their care. There was also a significantly greater number of infants immunized, a 29% reduction in health care costs, and no maternal hospital readmissions (vs. three in the control group). No significant differences were found between the groups in regard to maternal affect, self-esteem, and overall functional status (Brooten et al., 1994).

In a randomized clinical trial with pregnant women with diabetes (gestational and pregestational) during pregnancy, women were followed up from diagnosis to 8 weeks postpartum. In the APN intervention group, there were significantly fewer rehospitalizations ($p < .05$), fewer LBW infants (8.3% vs. 29%), and 38% lower total hospital charges than in the control group. No significant differences were found between groups in regard to outcomes of affect, self-esteem, return to function, satisfaction with care, and infant immunization (York et al., 1997).

In the randomized trial of women who underwent abdominal hysterectomy, women were followed up from surgery to 8 weeks after discharge. In the APN intervention group, women were discharged a mean of 12 hours earlier, were significantly more satisfied with their care, and had a savings in health care costs of 6%. The number of acute care visits and rehospitalizations was similar for both groups, but the mean rehospitalizations charges for the control group were $2,153, compared with $609 for the APN-followed group (Hollingsworth et al., in review).

In a randomized clinical trial of elders with cardiac medical and surgical diagnosis-related groups (DRGs), Naylor et al. (1994) evaluated the comprehensive discharge planning portion of the model without the home visit component. The intervention consisted of comprehensive discharge planning conducted by the APNs, APN hospital visits, and 2-week APN telephone follow-up. Study results showed that, in the APN intervention group, the number of readmissions was significantly reduced for subjects in medical DRGs in the first 6 weeks, and postdischarge hospital readmission charges were reduced 20.5%, compared with the control group during this same period. There were no statistically significant differences in other patient and family outcomes.

Ongoing work by Naylor et al. is testing the full model, incorporating the home visit component with elders with common medical and surgical DRGs who are at high risk for poor outcomes. Ongoing work by Brooten et al. focuses on women with medically and socioeconomically high-risk pregnancies. This effort substitutes half of prenatal care normally delivered in the clinic or physician office with prenatal care delivered in the woman's home by APNs. Pilot work by Medoff-Cooper is evaluating the model with earlier discharge of smaller, more vulnerable infants than those involved in the original work.

Subacute Care Units

Another rapidly growing transitional care setting is the subacute care unit (Stahl, 1994, 1995a). These units are designed to meet the needs of medically stable patients who no longer require acute care services but whose needs for licensed skilled nursing care exceed the abilities of skilled nursing facilities or nursing homes (Micheletti & Shlala, 1995; Stahl, 1994; Walsh, 1995). Patients referred to subacute care units include those who are technology dependent, those who require frequent respiratory or physical therapy, and those with complex nursing needs.

To serve these patients, hospital beds are being converted to subacute beds, free-standing subacute care hospitals are being established, and skilled nursing facilities are adding subacute care units (Ellis & Mendlen, 1995; Micheletti & Shlala, 1995). The incentive for the establishment of these units is economic. Care is provided in a less expensive setting, hospital beds are freed for severely ill patients, and unoccupied hospital beds are converted into a revenue source (Ellis & Mendlen, 1995; Stahl, 1994).

In-hospital subacute care units have been reported to improve patient outcomes for selected patient populations, including the elderly (Brymer et al., 1995; Landefield et al., 1995), ill infants and children (Goldson: 1981; Grebin & Kaplan, 1995), and ventilator-dependent individuals (Gilmartin, 1994; Gracey, et al., 1995; Make, 1986). The success of the units has been partially attributed to a multidisciplinary approach. Not all of these reports are research based.

The concept for subacute care units builds on the experience of transitional or step-down units, which have existed in many institutions for years. Transitional units have long been established for acutely ill newborns, cardiac patients, and so on, patients who now need less acute hospital care (Goldson, 1981; Whitby, 1983a, 1983b). Many of these transitional care units have also served as sites where family members are taught postdischarge care of patients and as a point of postdischarge contact for patients and family members with questions and concerns. These services can facilitate home management of patients rather than transfer to other institutional facilities (MacLeod & Head, 1994).

Integrated Health Care Systems

Managed care has fueled the formation of integrated health care delivery systems that provide all levels of service delivery, from acute care to home care, skilled nursing facilities, nursing homes, outpatient clinics, durable medical suppliers, and subacute care units (Heller & Walton, 1995; Stahl, 1995b). These systems provide "one-stop shopping" for managed care organizations. Theoretically, integrated systems provide continuity of care for patients by having them remain within the same health care delivery system (Frasca, 1986; Stahl, 1995b). Such systems also have the potential for coordination of health services and good communication between care providers in the various settings. Despite the use of case management and other coordination mechanisms, much fragmentation of care across systems remains (Fox, 1993; Harrington et al., 1993).

Robinson et al. (1995) discussed the efforts of one center to provide continuity of care in a vertically integrated system that included an acute care hospital, a subacute ward, a nursing home unit, domiciliary care, ambulatory care, and extended care programs, including adult day health care. The hospital hired hospital-based APNs to coordinate and plan care between and among the various care settings. The APNs were also responsible for collaborating with community-based home care agencies and nursing homes to which the patients were transferred. Provider communication and consultation reportedly improved, resulting in less duplication of services by providers from different disciplines. Hospital admissions and lengths of stay also decreased.

Nurse Case Management

Case management by nurses to coordinate the delivery of care to patients across settings may be an effective method of reducing fragmentation and improving patient and cost of care outcomes. One model of nurse case management was developed at Carondelet St. Mary's Hospital and Health Center, Tucson, Arizona, to assist high-risk elderly patients in managing their health care and accessing needed services in a timely and effective manner (Lamb, 1992). The professional nurse case manager (PNCM) is at the hub of the nursing network, the integrated system of nursing care at Carondelet St. Mary's (Ethridge & Lamb, 1989). Network components include acute care inpatient services, extended care or long-term care services, home care services, hospice, and ambulatory care services. The PNCMs work with clients across acute and long-term care settings and in the home (Lamb, 1992) and are responsible for facilitating patient movement through the components of the nursing network (Etheridge & Lamb, 1989).

Research conducted with Carondelet St. Mary's clients revealed that elders who worked with a PNCM had greater confidence in self-care, experienced improved symptom management, and used hospital and emergency room services less frequently (Lamb, 1992). Analysis of cost data revealed that nurse case management also resulted in decreased length of stay (Etheridge & Lamb, 1989).

Gaps and Recommendations

As noted previously, transitional environments are a relatively new dimension in the continuum of health care services. Consequently, the gaps in science to support this increasingly important component of care are considerable, and many have been identified throughout this chapter. Additional research is necessary to determine the nature, intensity, and length of transitional care services needed to optimize patient and family outcomes; the profile of patients who would benefit most from these services; and the type and level of providers needed to deliver these services and the costs of the services. Continued study of models of transitional care is also necessary to determine which of these models achieves the highest quality, most cost-effective outcomes.

Research findings suggest that the core components of transitional care for patients discharged from the hospital to home are comprehensive discharge planning and home follow-up. Furthermore, study findings suggest that, for selected patient groups (or subgroups), discharge planning and home care protocols designed to meet their unique needs are more effective than the general protocols designed for all patients that are used by many hospitals and home care agencies. Targeted protocols should be derived from empirical data regarding the unique needs of specific patient groups and their caregivers after hospital discharge. Transitional care protocols should be based on an empirical understanding of the nature of the patients' and caregivers' needs (e.g., lack of knowledge, complexity of therapeutic regimen); the strengths (e.g., supportive family) or barriers (e.g., language) to meeting needs; the timing of needs (e.g., 24 hours after discharge); the most cost-effective strategy to meet needs (e.g., telephone contact vs. home visit); and the length of follow-up needed. Unfortunately, for many patient groups, this research base is limited. For these patient groups, research efforts should be focused first on identifying patient and caregiver needs and subsequently on the design and testing of interventions to meet these unique needs.

Rigorous testing of transitional care protocols is necessary not only to determine the efficacy of the protocols, but also to determine which patient groups (or subgroups) will benefit the most from these services. As noted previously, evidence suggests that not all patient groups (or subgroups) require transitional care services to achieve stabilization or functional recovery. An important scientific gap is the profile of patients who are at high risk for poor outcomes and for whom transitional care is essential. What is the constellation of sociodemographic, clinical, and health care system factors that contribute to these poor outcomes? Equally important is the need to identify patients who are at low risk for poor outcomes and who do not require transitional care services. Researchers have only begun to address these knowledge gaps. The design and testing of profiling techniques to assess the relative risk of patients for positive and negative outcomes after a major change in health status (e.g., pregnancy or an episode of illness) is essential to advance the knowledge base related to transitional care.

Transitional care services have only recently been incorporated into the health care system; therefore, it is not surprising that little research has been conducted on the issue of access to these services. As noted previously, some evidence suggests that level of awareness about services, race, culture, ethnicity, economics, and geography may influence use of such services. Research is necessary to identify factors that promote access and serve as barriers to transitional care. The relatively rich information base about factors influencing access to primary care services should be used to advance this important component of the transitional care research agenda.

A number of approaches have emerged to guide the delivery of transitional care services. However, only a few are research models of transitional care. There is a need for additional evaluation of models of transitional care, with particular attention to their effectiveness in responding to continued pressures within the health care system to further decrease lengths of stay and prevent the use of more costly health services, such as hospitals. Furthermore, studies are necessary that compare models of transitional care, focusing on differences in processes and outcomes of care. Knowledge generated from studies of these models would contribute to the ongoing discussion and debate about which providers are most effective and efficient in coordinating transitional care services and providing continuity of care for patients and their caregivers. Study findings would also advance understanding about effective ways to engage a multidisciplinary team of providers in transitional care services. Finally, the knowledge generated from this research would help improve the processes of care that data suggest are important to positive patient outcomes: assessing, communicating, clinical decision making, teaching, collaborating, referring, monitoring, and evaluating.

A number of methodological issues must be considered as part of the recommended research agenda for transitional care services. For example, which outcomes are important to evaluate in measuring the effectiveness of transitional services? When and for how long should they be measured? The methodological issues related to the measurement of costs were explored previously in this chapter. Because of the nature and durations of the service, transitional care provides a unique opportunity to evaluate the contributions of different providers (i.e., processes of care) to patient and family outcomes. Brooten et al. are taking advantage of this opportunity by evaluating the relationship between APN functions and patient outcomes in the delivery of transitional care services to five different patient groups.

Transitional care is emerging as a critical component of the U. S. health care system. At this stage in its evolution, opportunities abound for significant research contributions spearheaded by nurse scholars in advancing the knowledge base related to the needs of patients and caregivers during this phase of care and in the design and evaluation of clinical interventions and models of care to optimize outcomes while decreasing costs of care.

REFERENCES

American Nurses Association. (1994). *Today's registered nurse: Numbers and demographics.* Washington, DC: Author.

Anderson, M. A., & Helms, L. (1993). An assessment of discharge planning models: Communication in referrals for home care. *Orthopedic Nursing, 12*(4), 41–49.

Bakewell-Sachs, S., & Porth, S. (1995). Discharge planning and home care of the technology-dependent infant. *Journal of Obstetric, Gynecologic and Neonatal Nursing, 24*(1), 77–83.

Berk, M., & Bernstein, A. (1985). Home health services: Some findings from the national medical care expenditure survey. *Home Health Care Services Quarterly, 6,* 13–23.

Branch, L. G., Wetle, T. T., Scherr, P. A., Cook, N. R., Evans, D. A., Hebert, L. E., et al. (1988). A prospective study of incident comprehensive medical home care use among the elderly. *American Journal of Public Health, 78*(3), 255–259.

Brooten, D. (1993). Assisting with transitions from hospital to home. In S. Funk, E. Tornquist, M. Champagne, & R. Wiese (Eds.), *Key aspects of caring for the chronically ill: Hospital and home.* New York: Springer.

Brooten, D. (1995). Perinatal care across the continuum: Early discharge and nursing home follow-up. *Journal of Perinatal and Neonatal Nursing, 9*(1), 38–44.

Brooten, D., Brown, L., Munro, B., York, R., Cohen, S., Roncoli, M, et al. (1988). Early discharge and specialist transitional care. *Image: The Journal of Nursing Scholarship, 20*(2), 64–68.

Brooten, D., Knapp, H., Borucki, L., Jacobsen, B., Finkler, S., Arnold, L., et al. (1996). Early discharge and home care after unplanned cesarean birth: Nursing care time. *Journal of Obstetric, Gynecologic and Neonatal Nursing, 25*(1), 595–600.

Brooten, D., Kumar, S., Brown, L., Butts, P., Finkler, S., Bakewell-Sachs, S., et al. (1986). A randomized clinical trial of early discharge and home follow-up of very low birth weight infants. *New England Journal of Medicine, 315,* 934–939.

Brooten, D., Naylor, M., York, R., Brown, L., Roncoli, M., Hollingsworth, A., et al. (1995). Effects of nurse specialist transitional care on patient outcomes and cost: Results of five randomized trials. *American Journal of Managed Care, 1*(1), 35–41.

Brooten, D., Roncoli, M, Finkler, S., Arnold, L., Cohen, A., & Mennuti, M. (1994). A randomized clinical trial of early hospital discharge and home follow-up of women having cesarean birth. *Obstetrics and Gynecology, 84,* 832–838.

Brymer, C. D., Kohm, C. A., Naglie, G., Shekter-Wolfson, L., Zorzitto, M. L., O'Rourke, K., et al. (1995). Do geriatric programs decrease long-term use of acute care beds? *Journal of the American Geriatrics Society, 43,* 885–889.

Bull, M. J. (1994). Use of formal community services by elders and their family care givers 2 weeks following hospital discharge. *Journal of Advanced Nursing, 19,* 503–508.

Carey, T. (1996). Outcomes and costs of care for acute low back pain among specialties: Implications for managed care. *American Journal of Managed Care, 11*(4), 409–413.

Corrigan, J. M., & Martin, J. B. (1992). Identification of factors associated with hospital readmission and development of a predictive model. *Health Services Research, 27*(1), 81–101.

Cox, C. L., Wood, J. E., Montgomery, A. C., & Smith, P. C. (1990). Patient classification in home health care: Are we ready? *Public Health Nursing, 7*(3), 130–137.

Dahlberg, N. L. F., & Koloroutis, M. (1994). Hospital-based perinatal home-care program. *Journal of Obstetric, Gynecologic and Neonatal Nursing, 23*(8), 682–686.

Dawson, B. (1994). "Special care" in the community: Role of the community neonatal liaison sister. *Professional Nurse, 10*(2), 78–80.

Dorwart, R. A., & Hoover, C. W. (1994). A national study of transitional hospital services in mental health. *American Journal of Public Health, 84*(8), 1229–1234.

Eaton, D. G. (1994). Perinatal home care: One entrepreneur's experience. *Journal of Obstetric, Gynecologic and Neonatal Nursing, 23*(8), 726–730.

Ellis, S., & Mendlen, J. (1995). Teaming up with hospitals. *Provider, 21*(3), 35–36.

Etheridge, P., & Lamb, G. S. (1989). Professional nursing case management improves quality, access and cost. *Nursing Management, 20*(3), 30–35.

Falcone, D., Bolda, E., & Leak, S. C. (1991). Waiting for placement: An exploratory analysis of determinants of delayed discharges of elderly hospital patients. *Health Services Research, 26*(3), 339–374.

Findeis, A., Larson, J. L., Gallo, A., & Shekleton, M. (1994). Caring for individuals using home ventilators: An appraisal by family care givers. *Rehabilitation Nursing, 19*(1), 6–11.

Fox, H. B., Wicks, L. B., & Newacheck, P. W. (1993). Health maintenance organizations and children with special needs. A suitable match? *American Journal of the Disabled Child, 147*(5), 546–552.

Frasca, C., & Christy, M. W. (1986). Assuring continuity of care through a hospital-based home health agency. *Quality Review Bulletin, 12*(5), 167–171.

Furstenberg, A., & Mezey, M. (1987). Mental impairment of elderly hospitalized hip fracture patients. *Comprehensive Gerontology, 1,* 80–86.

Ghali, J. K., Kadakia, S., Cooper, R., & Ferlinz, J. (1988). Precipitating factors leading to decompensation of heart failure: Traits among urban Blacks. *Archives of Internal Medicine, 148,* 2013–2016.

Gilmartin, M. (1994). Transition from the intensive care unit to home: Patient selection and discharge planning. *Respiratory Care, 10*(4), 456–480.

Goldson, E. (1981). The family care center: Transitional care for the sick infant and his family. *Children Today, 10*(4), 15–20.

Gracey, D. R., Naessens, J. M., Viggiano, R. W., Koenig, G. E., Silverstein, M. D., & Hubmayr, R. D. (1995). Outcome of patients cared for in a ventilator-dependent unit in a general hospital. *Chest: The Cardiopulmonary Journal, 107*(2), 494–499.

Grebin, B., & Kaplan, S. (1995). Toward a pediatric subacute care model: Clinical and administrative features. *Archives of Physical Medicine and Rehabilitation, 76*(Suppl. 12), SC16–SC20.

Haddock, K. S. (1991). Characteristics of effective discharge planning programs for the frail elderly. *Journal of Gerontological Nursing, 17*(7), 10–14.

Haffey, W. J., & Welsh, J. H. (1995). Subacute care: Evolution in search of value. *Archives of Physical Medicine and Rehabilitation, 76*(12 Suppl.), SC2–SC4.

Harrington, C., Lynch, M., & Newcomer, R. J. (1993). Medical services in social health maintenance organizations. *Gerontologist, 33*(6), 790–800.

Hazlett, D. E. (1989). A study of pediatric home ventilator management: Medical, psychosocial, and financial aspects. *Journal of Pediatric Nursing, 4*(4), 284–294.

Helberg, J. L. (1994). Use of home care nursing resources by the elderly. *Public Health Nursing, 11*(2), 104–112.

Heller, J. F., & Walton, J. R. (1995). The postacute link. *RT: The Journal for Respiratory Care Practitioners, 8*(1), 153–155.

Hollingsworth, A., Cohen, S., Finkler, S., Rubin, M., & Morgan, M. (in review). A randomized trial of early hospital discharge and home follow-up discharge and home follow-up of women having hysterectomy.

Hyatt, L. (1995). The Feds focus on subacute. *Nursing Homes, 44*(1), 11.

Jones, E. W., Densen, P. M., & Brown, S. D. (1989). Posthospital needs of elderly people at home: Findings from an eight-month follow-up study. *Health Services Research, 24*(5), 643–664.

Katz, K. S. (1993). Project Headed Home: Intervention in the pediatric intensive care unit for infants and their families. *Infants and Young Children, 5*(3), 67–75.

Keenan, J. M., & Fanale, J. E. (1989). Home care: Past and present, problems and potential. *Journal of the American Geriatrics Society, 37,* 1076–1083.

Kemper, P. (1992). The use of formal and informal home care by the disabled elderly. *Health Services Research, 27*(4), 421–451.

Kornowski, R., Zeeli, D., Averbuch, M., Finkelstein, A., Schwartz, D., Moshkovitz, M., Weinreb, B., Hershkovitz, R., Eyal, D., Miller, M., Levo, Y., & Pines, A. (1995). Intensive home-care surveillance prevents hospitalization and improves morbidity rates among elderly patients with severe congestive heart failure. *American Heart Journal, 129*(4), 762–766.

Lamb, G. S. (1992). Conceptual and methodological issues in nurse case management research. *Advances in Nursing Science, 15*(2), 16–24.

Landefeld, C. S., Palmer, R. M., Kresevic, D. M., Fortinsky, R. H., & Kowal, J. (1995). A randomized trial of care in a hospital medical unit especially designed to improve the functional outcomes of acutely ill older patients. *New England Journal of Medicine, 332*(20), 1338–1344.

MacLeod, F., & Head, D. (1994). Transitional care: Filling the gap for older patients. *Leadership in Health Services, 3*(6), 28–32.

Magilvy, J. K., & Lakomy, J. M. (1991). Transitions of older adults to home care. *Home Health Care Services Quarterly, 12*(4), 59–70.

Make, B. J. (1986). Long-term management of ventilator-assisted individuals: The Boston University experience. *Respiratory Care, 31*(4), 303–310.

McCorkle, R., Jepson, C., Malone, D., Lusk, E., Braitman, L., Buhler-Wilkerson, K., & Daly, J. (1994). The impact of posthospital home care on patients with cancer. *Research in Nursing and Health, 17,* 243–251.

Meara, J. R, Wood, J. L., Wilson, M. A., & Hart, M. C. (1992). Home from hospital: A survey of hospital discharge arrangements in Northamptonshire. *Journal of Public Health Medicine, 14*(2), 145–150.

Micheletti, J. A., & Shlala, T. J. (1995). Understanding and operationalizing subacute services. *Nursing Management, 26*(6), 49, 51-52, 54–56.

Morrow-Howell, N., & Proctor, E. (1994). Discharge destinations of Medicare patients receiving discharge planning: Who goes where? *Medical Care, 32*(5), 486–497.

Mui, A. C., & Burnette, D. (1994). Long-term care service use by frail elders: Is ethnicity a factor? *The Gerontologist, 34*(2), 190–198.

National Association for Home Care. (1995). *Basic statistics about home care 1995.* Washington, DC: Author.

Naylor, M. (1990). Comprehensive discharge planning for hospitalized elderly: A pilot study. *Nursing Research, 39*(3), 156–160.

Naylor, M., & Brooten, D. (1993). The roles and functions of clinical nurse specialists: State of the science. *Image: The Journal of Nursing Scholarship, 25*(2), 99–104.

Naylor, M., Brooten, D., Jones, R., Lavizzo-Mourey, R., Mezey, M., & Pauly, M. (1994). Comprehensive discharge planning for hospitalized elderly: A randomized clinical trial. *Annals of Internal Medicine, 120*(12), 999–1006.

Neidlinger, S. H., Scroggins, K., & Kennedy, L. M. (1987). Cost-evaluation of discharge planning for hospitalized elderly: The efficacy of a clinical nurse specialist. *Nursing Economics, 5*(5), 225–230.

Patterson, J. M., Leonard, B. J., & Titus, J. C. (1992). Home care for medically fragile children: Impact on family health and well-being. *Developmental and Behavioral Pediatrics, 13*(4), 248–255.

Prescott, P. A., Soeken, K. L., & Griggs, M. (1995). Identification and referral of hospitalized patients in need of home care. *Research in Nursing and Health, 18,* 85–95.

Reed, R. L., Pearlman, R. A., & Buchner, D. M. (1991). Risk factors for early unplanned hospital readmission in the elderly. *Journal of General Internal Medicine, 6,* 223–228.

Rich, M. W., Beckham, V., Wittenberg, C., Leven, C. L., Freedland, K. E., et al. (1995). A multidisciplinary intervention to prevent the readmission of elderly patients with congestive heart failure. *New England Journal of Medicine, 333*(18), 1190–1195.

Robinson, D. K., Mead, M. J., & Boswell, C. R. (1995). Inside looking out: Innovations in community health nursing. *Clinical Nurse Specialist, 9*(4), 227–229, 235.

Roe-Prior, P., Watts, R. J., & Burke, K. (1994). Critical care clinical specialist in home health care: Survey results. *Clinical Nurse Specialist, 8*(1), 35–40.

Roselle, S., & D'Amico, F. J. (1990). The effect of home respiratory therapy on hospital readmission rates of patients with chronic obstructive pulmonary disease. *Respiratory Care, 35*(12), 1208–1213.

Schwartz, P., Blumenfield, S., & Perlman Simon, E. (1990). The interim home care program: An innovative discharge planning alternative. *Health and Social Work, 15,* 152–160.

Sevick, M. A., Zucconi, S., Sereika, S., Puczynski, S., Drury, R., Marra, R., Mattes, P., & Taylor, J. (1992). Characteristics and health service utilization patterns of ventilator-dependent patients cared for within a vertically integrated health system. *American Journal of Critical Care, 1*(3), 45–51.

Sheikh, L., O'Brien, M., & McCluskey-Fawcett (1993). Parent preparation for the NICU to home transition: Staff and parent perceptions. *Children's Health Care, 22*(3), 227–239.

Sivak, E. D., Cordasco, E. M., & Gipson, W. T. (1983). Pulmonary mechanical ventilation at home: A reasonable and less expensive alternative. *Respiratory Care, 28*(1), 42–49.

Stahl, D. A. (1994). Subacute care: The future of health care. *Nursing Management, 25*(10), 34, 36, 38–40.

Stahl, D. A. (1995a). Maximizing reimbursement for subacute care. *Nursing Management, 26*(4), 16–19.

Stahl, D. A. (1995b). Integrated delivery system: An opportunity or a dilemma. *Nursing Management, 26*(7), 20, 22–23.

Thurber, F., & DiGiamarino, L. (1992). Development of a model of transitional care for the HIV positive child and family. *Clinical Nurse Specialist, 6*(3), 142–146.

U. S. General Accounting Office. (1987). *Post-hospital care: Discharge planners report increasing difficulty in planning for medicare patients* (GAO/PMED 87-5BR). Washington, DC: Author.

Vinson, J. M., Rich, M. W., Sperry, J. C., Shah, A. S., & McNamara, T. (1990). Early readmission of elderly patients with congestive heart failure. *Journal of the American Geriatrics Society, 38,* 1290–1295.

Walsh, M. B., & Wilhere, S.P.G. (1988). The future of teaching nursing homes. *Geriatric Nursing, 9*(6), 354–356.

Whitby, C. A. (1983a). Moving forward in neonatal care–transitional care. *Midwives Chronicle, 96*(Suppl. 1149), 17–18.

Whitby, C. A. (1983b). Transitional care of low birth weight infants. *Journal of Nurse-Midwifery, 28*(5), 25–26.

Williams, B. C., MacKay, S. A., & Torner, J. C. (1991). Home health care: Comparison of patients and services among three types of agencies. *Medical Care, 29*(6), 583–587.

Williams, E. I., Greenwell, J., & Groom, L. M. (1992). The care of people over 75 years old after discharge from hospital: An evaluation of timetabled visiting by health visitor assistants. *Journal of Public Health Medicine, 14*(2), 138–144.

Winograd, C. H. (1991). Targeting strategies: An overview of criteria and outcomes. *Journal of the American Geriatrics Society, 39*(Suppl.), 25S–35S.

Wong, D. L. (1991). Transition from hospital to home for children with complex medical care. *Journal of Pediatric Oncology Nursing, 8*(1), 3–9.

York, R., Brown, L. P., Samuels, P., Finkler, S., Jacobsen, B., Armstrong, C., Swank, A., & Robbins, D. (1997). A randomized clinical trial of early discharge and nurse specialist transitional follow-up care of high-risk childbearing women. *Nursing Research, 46*(5), 254–261.

Zelle, R. S. (1995). Follow-up of at-risk infants in the home setting: Consultation model. *Journal of Obstetric, Gynecologic and Neonatal Nursing, 24*(1), 51–55.

Reprinted with permission from: Brooten, D., & Naylor, M. D. (1999). Transitional environments. In A. S. Hinshaw, S. L.

Feetham, & J. L. F. Shaver (Eds.), *Handbook of clinical nursing research* (pp. 641–653). Thousand Oaks, CA: Sage Publications, Inc.

9.3 TRANSITIONAL CARE OF OLDER ADULTS HOSPITALIZED WITH HEART FAILURE: A RANDOMIZED, CONTROLLED TRIAL

Mary D. Naylor
Dorothy A. Brooten
Roberta L. Campbell
Greg Maislin
Kathleen M. McCauley
J. Sanford Schwartz

Abstract

Objectives: *To examine the effectiveness of a transitional care intervention delivered by advanced practice nurses (APNs) to elders hospitalized with heart failure.* ***Design:*** *Randomized, controlled trial with follow-up through 52 weeks postindex hospital discharge.* ***Setting:*** *Six Philadelphia academic and community hospitals.* ***Participants:*** *Two hundred thirty-nine eligible patients were aged 65 and older and hospitalized with heart failure.* ***Intervention:*** *A 3-month APN-directed discharge planning and home follow-up protocol.* ***Measurements:*** *Time to first rehospitalization or death, number of rehospitalizations, quality of life, functional status, costs, and satisfaction with care.* ***Results:*** *Mean age of patients (control n = 121; intervention n = 118) enrolled was 76; 43% were male, and 36% were African American. Time to first readmission or death was longer in intervention patients (log rank 2 = 5.0, p = .026; Cox regression incidence density ratio = 1.65, 95% confidence interval = 1.13–2.40). At 52 weeks, intervention group patients had fewer readmissions (104 vs. 162, p = .047) and lower mean total costs ($7,636 vs. $12,481, p = .002). For intervention patients, only short-term improvements were demonstrated in overall quality of life (12 weeks, p < .05), physical dimension of quality of life (2 weeks, p < .01; 12 weeks, p < .05) and patient satisfaction (assessed at 2 and 6 weeks, p < .001).* ***Conclusion:*** *A comprehensive transitional care intervention for elders hospitalized with heart failure increased the length of time between hospital discharge and readmission or death, reduced total number of rehospitalizations, and decreased health care costs, thus demonstrating great promise for improving clinical and economic outcomes.*

A growing body of science suggests that older adults coping with multiple comorbid conditions and complex therapeutic regimens are particularly vulnerable during the transition from hospital to home. A review of 94 studies reported between 1985 and 2001 revealed that the transition of older adults from hospital to home is associated with high rates of preventable poor postdischarge outcomes.[1] Individual factors contributing to negative outcomes include multiple comorbid conditions, functional deficits, cognitive impairment, emotional problems, and poor general health behaviors. System factors associated with poor outcomes include breakdown in communication between providers and across health care agencies, inadequate patient and caregiver education, poor continuity of care, and limited access to services. As a result, at least one third of all patients and caregivers report substantial unmet needs and high levels of dissatisfaction. Rehospitalization rates for these patients are high, with one quarter to one third of hospital readmissions considered preventable.[2,3]

Elders with heart failure have the highest rehospitalization rate of all adult patient groups, with estimated annual total direct health care expenditures exceeding $24.3 billion.[4] This patient group is representative of the growing segment of the U. S. population living longer with chronic health problems and experiencing breakdowns in care during multiple transitions from hospital to home that negatively affect quality of life and consume substantial health care resources. Similar to most chronically ill elders, these patients typically have multiple comorbid medical conditions, numerous disabling symptoms, complex medication regimens, and limited self-management skills.[5] Comorbidity contributes substantially to increased rehospitalization rates and health care costs for elders with heart failure.[6-8] Therefore, attention to the comprehensive care management needs of this patient group has the potential to reduce total health care costs.

Although reports of randomized, controlled trials (RCTs) have yielded important information regarding the management of adults hospitalized for heart failure,[9-12] little is known about the effectiveness of care management strategies for elders experiencing an acute episode of heart failure complicated by multiple other chronic health conditions. Only two single-site RCTs have tested multidisciplinary, nurse-directed, home-based interventions specifically targeting hospitalized older adults (aged 65 years) and including patients with diastolic failure (approximately 50% of elders) and coexisting chronic conditions (which account for approximately 40% of rehospitalizations of older patients).[13,14] Both studies showed only short-term reductions in rehospitalizations resulting from heart failure and no effect on readmissions owing to comorbid conditions. Evidence suggests that a multidimensional, individualized approach that targets patients and their caregivers and emphasizes the needs associated with acute heart failure and coexisting conditions is the most clinically relevant and potentially effective intervention. Given the established association between breakdown in care during the transition from hospital to home and poor postdischarge outcomes, such an intervention must continue through the postdischarge period to ensure longer term improvements in patient and caregiver outcomes.

The objective of this RCT was to evaluate the sustained effect of a 3-month comprehensive transitional care intervention (discharge planning and home follow-up) directed by advanced practice nurses (APNs) for elders hospitalized with heart failure on time to first readmission or death, total rehospitalizations, readmissions owing to heart failure and comorbid conditions, quality of life, functional status, patient satisfaction, and medical costs. This study presents, on a spectrum of clinical and economic outcomes, the first multisite assessment of a transitional care intervention targeting the comprehensive set of serious health problems and risk factors common in elders throughout an acute episode of heart failure.

Methods

Study Sample

The study was conducted at six Philadelphia academic and community hospitals. All patients 65 years of age and older admitted to study hospitals from their homes between February 1997 and January 2001 with a diagnosis of heart failure (diagnosis-related group 127 validated at discharge) were screened for participation. Eligible patients had to speak English, be alert and oriented, be reachable by telephone after discharge, and reside within a 60-mile radius of the admitting hospital. Elders with end-stage renal disease were excluded because of their access to unique Medicare services. Of 641 patients screened, 37.3% were enrolled, a percentage comparing favorably with RCTs involving a similar population.[14,15] Enrollees ($n = 239$) and nonenrollees ($n = 402$) were similar in regard to mean age (76 vs. 77 years, $p = .089$), race (64% vs. 69% White, $p = .20$) and gender (57% vs. 59% female, $p = .804$). The primary reasons for nonenrollment were residency outside the defined service area radius; patient discharge before consent could be obtained; and patient or family member refusal, most often because of an established relationship with a home health agency.

Study Design

The University of Pennsylvania institutional review board approved the study protocol. After screening patients within 24 hours of hospital admission for eligibility and obtaining informed consent, research assistants (RAs) blind to study aims and groups obtained baseline sociodemographic and health status data and notified the project manager, who assigned patients to study groups using a computer-generated, institution-specific block 1 to 1 randomization algorithm.

Control Group

Control group patients received care routine for the admitting hospital, including site-specific heart failure patient management and discharge planning critical paths and, if referred, standard home agency care consisting of comprehensive skilled home health services 7 days a week. Standards of care for all study hospitals include institutional policies to guide, document, and evaluate discharge planning. The discharge planning process across hospital sites was similar. The attending physician was responsible for determining the discharge date, and the primary nurse, discharge planner, and physician collaborated in the design and implementation of the discharge plan. Standards and processes of care for the primary home care sites were also similar. These included use of liaison nurses to facilitate referrals to home care; availability of comprehensive, intermittent skilled home care services in patient residences 7 days per week; and on-call registered nurse availability 24 hours per day. Fifty-eight percent (71/121) of the control group received referrals for skilled nursing or physical therapy after the index hospital discharge.

Intervention Group

In collaboration with patient physicians, three APNs implemented an intervention extending from index hospital admission through 3 months after the index hospital discharge. The intervention included all of the following components:

1. A standardized orientation and training program guided by a multidisciplinary team of heart failure experts (composed of a geropsychiatric clinical nurse specialist, a pharmacist, a nutritionist, a social worker, a physical therapist, and a board-certified cardiologist specializing in the treatment of heart failure) to prepare APNs to address the unique needs of older adults and their caregivers throughout an acute episode of heart failure
2. Use of care management strategies foundational to the quality–cost model of APN transitional care,[16,17] including identification of patient and caregiver goals, individualized plans of care developed and implemented by APNs in collaboration with patient physicians, educational and behavioral strategies to address patient and caregiver learning needs, and continuity of care and care coordination across settings and the use of expert nurses to deliver and manage clinical services to high-risk patient groups
3. APN implementation of an evidence-based protocol, guided by national heart failure guidelines[18,19] and designed specifically for this patient group and their caregivers with a unique focus on comprehensive management of needs and therapies associated with an acute episode of heart failure complicated by multiple comorbid conditions.

The protocol consisted of an initial APN visit within 24 hours of index hospital admission, APN visits at least daily during the index hospitalization, at least eight APN home visits (one within 24 hours of discharge), weekly visits during the first month (with one of these visits coinciding with the initial follow-up visit to the patient physician), bimonthly visits during the second and third months, additional APN visits based on patient need, and APN telephone availability 7 days per week (8 a.m. to 8 p.m., weekdays; 8 a.m. to noon, weekends). If a patient was rehospitalized for any reason during the intervention period, the APN resumed daily hospital visits to facilitate the transition from hospital to home, but the length of time devoted to the intervention for such patients did not extend beyond 3 months postdischarge from index hospital. Although the study protocol guided patient management and specified a minimum number of APN hospital and home visits, it allowed the APN considerable flexibility to individualize care.

Masters-prepared nurses with general expertise in the management of conditions common in older adults were recruited. Their knowledge and skills in the management of elders with heart failure were assessed. The APNs participated in a 2-month orientation and training program focused on developing their competencies related to early recognition and treatment of acute episodes of heart failure in elders, with particular attention to how it complicates and is complicated by common comorbid conditions, such as diabetes mellitus or depression. Content and clinical experiences included review of relevant evidence-based guidelines, case study discussions led by multidisciplinary team members, and participation in clinical rounds. Particular attention was paid to educating APNs regarding optimal therapeutic management (e.g., medications, exercise). The training program emphasized application of educational and behavioral strategies in the home to address patient and caregiver unique learning needs. Finally, APNs were prepared to implement the study protocol using the constellation of care management strategies identified previously herein. After patient enrollment began, APNs had access to multidisciplinary team members via e-mail or phone for consultation on the most challenging cases.

After completion of the training program, APNs assumed responsibility for discharge planning while the patient was hospitalized and substituted for any visiting nurse services that might have been ordered at discharge during the 3 months after hospital discharge. During patient hospitalization, a comprehensive patient assessment, using valid and reliable instruments, was conducted and addressed the following: patient and caregiver goals; nature, duration, and severity of heart failure and comorbid conditions; physical, cognitive, and emotional health status; general health behaviors and skills; and availability and adequacy of social support.

A major focus of APN intervention during hospitalization was collaboration with physicians and other providers to optimize patient health status at discharge, design the discharge plan, and arrange for necessary home care services. Special emphasis was placed on preventing functional decline and streamlining medication regimens. APNs were able to provide input to the nursing staff regarding the discharge needs of patients and caregivers, thus maximizing the time staff nurses devoted to these areas. APNs worked with discharge planners to prevent duplication of postdischarge services and coordinate the ordering of essential medical supplies.

After patients were discharged to home, APNs conducted targeted assessments to identify changes in patient health status. APN involvement throughout the transition from hospital to home provided a safety net designed to prevent medication and other medical errors and ensure accurate transfer of information. As a result of advanced physical assessment skills, including expertise in evaluating responses to therapy, APNs were able to identify early signs of problems, such as impending volume overload, and, in collaboration with patient physicians, implement strategies to prevent the onset of symptoms or to minimize their effects. Unless working under specific guidelines unique to a treating physician, APNs collaborated with each patient's physician regarding adjustments in medications and other therapies.

Face-to-face interactions with the patient's physician during hospitalization and the initial follow-up visit (aimed at promoting continuity of care) helped to foster collaborative relationships. APN expertise in management of heart failure and common comorbid conditions, coupled with the APN ability to coordinate care, nurtured these relationships and provided patients with increased access to symptom management tools. For example, in collaboration with physicians, APNs were able not only to teach patients and caregivers about early symptom recognition, but also to coach them regarding effective treatment, such as the use of as-needed diuretics. Positioning patients and caregivers to manage their symptoms was a goal for all intervention group patients.

Patient goals were the primary sources of motivation to promote adherence to therapies and behavioral change. Although approaches to achieve these goals were based on patient and caregiver identification of strategies that worked best for them, all patient teaching was audiotaped, with tapes and recorders left for patients and caregivers to review throughout the intervention period. If applicable, videocassette recorder tapes featuring management of common comorbid conditions (e.g., diabetes mellitus) were also left with patients and caregivers to review. At the conclusion of the intervention, APNs provided patients, caregivers, physicians, and other providers with summaries of goal progression, unresolved issues, and recommendations.

Outcome Measures

Research assistants, blind to study aims and groups, conducted standardized patient telephone interviews at 2, 6, 12, 26, and 52 weeks after index hospital discharge to obtain information about rehospitalizations and unscheduled acute care visits to physicians, clinics, and emergency departments; quality of life (assessed using the Minnesota Living With Heart Failure questionnaire[20]); and functional status (measured using the Enforced Social Dependency scale[21]). Patient satisfaction was assessed (using an investigator-developed instrument) at 2 and 6 weeks postindex hospitalization. Prior testing of this instrument revealed that, for control patients who did not receive home follow-up, the hospital experience was too far removed for accurate recall and the generation of reliable data.

Data on number of, timing of, and reasons for hospital readmissions, unscheduled acute care visits, and care provided by visiting nurses or APNs and other health care personnel were abstracted from patient records and bills were requested by the project manager via telephone calls and letters to physicians, hospitals, and home care agencies. All records from physician offices and records from remote hospitals and home care agencies were copied and mailed or sent by facsimile to the research offices at the University of Pennsylvania. RAs traveled to local hospitals and home care agencies and copied records on site. Two cardiologists specializing in the treatment of heart failure (blind to study group) validated reasons for rehospitalizations and categorized them as *index related, comorbid* (diagnoses abstracted from medical records during index hospitalization), or *new health problem*. Resource costs were estimated using standardized Medicare reimbursement for services used.[22] The cost of the intervention, including time devoted by APNs to the preparation of patient education materials, was calculated by assessing the intervention-related effort of APNs and multidisciplinary team experts (from detailed logs) and applying representative annual salaries for APNs and individual team members plus benefits. Cost of pharmaceuticals, over-the-counter drugs, other supplies, and indirect costs were not collected.

Statistical Analysis

The primary end point was time to first rehospitalization or death.[10,11,13] Patients alive and not hospitalized were censored at study completion (190/239 [79.5%]). Patients not completing follow-up (49/239 [20.5%]) were censored at withdrawal. Based on previous results,[14] it was estimated that 102 patients per group were necessary to achieve 80% or greater power to detect a control to intervention group hazard ratio of 1.61.[23] Enrollment ended with 118 intervention group and 121 control group participants, allowing for loss to follow-up, statistical adjustment for institution, and other a priori risk factors. Secondary analyses defined death as a censoring event (24/239 [10%]).

Group-specific Kaplan-Meier survival curves[24] were constructed. Intervention effectiveness was assessed using proportional hazards regression,[25] adjusting for institution and a priori baseline prognostic factors, including self-rated health, number of hospitalizations during previous 6 months, and living arrangement.[14] Confounding factors that changed the risk ratio by more than 15%[26] and prognostic factors with $p < .05$ were added to the a priori model. The proportional hazards assumption was evaluated using time-dependent covariates. Intervention and covariate effect sizes were expressed using incidence density ratios (IDRs) with 95% confidence intervals (CIs).[25]

Secondary end points included time to first rehospitalization, cumulative days of rehospitalization, mean readmission length of stay, number of unscheduled acute care visits after discharge, other measures of health care use, cost of postindex hospitalization medical services, quality of life, functional status, and patient satisfaction. All analyses were performed using the intention-to-treat principle.[27]

Resource utilization comparisons (including acute care visits, home visits, and hospital readmissions) were evaluated overall and by resource category over four periods (0–12, 0–3, 3–6, and 6–12 months). Descriptive statistical comparisons were performed using Wilcoxon rank sum tests, dividing by follow-up days to adjust for unequal observation periods. Standardized unit costs were assigned to each service and aggregated across services within patients and groups. Group-specific average total intervention costs were adjusted for incomplete follow-up using the method of Lin et al.[28] This method involved incorporating the Kaplan-Meier survival estimates of the conditional survival probabilities into the computation of average cost per patient. Ninety-five percent nonparametric percentile CIs and two-sided p values of group differences were derived from a bootstrap empiric sampling distribution (1,000 iterations).[29,30] This method involved randomly selecting, with replacement from the intervention and control samples, 118 and 121 observations, respectively, reestimating the group-specific Kaplan-Meier survival curves for each bootstrap sample, recomputing the Lin et al. estimates of average treatment costs separately for each group, and then recomputing difference in mean total costs.

Tertiary analyses compared quality of life, functional status, and patient satisfaction over time using Wilcoxon rank sum tests. Quality-of-life and functional status comparisons must properly account for missing values[31] because the mechanism generating missing values is not ignorable,[32] therefore making analyses restricted to complete cases biased. To this end, measures were transformed to ordinal scales by assigning a score of 0 to patients who died (which was carried forward to subsequent time periods) and 1 to patients who were hospitalized during scheduled assessments. Nonmissing scores were grouped into quartiles, with the lowest quartile receiving a score of 2 and the top quartile receiving a score of 5. Patients with a missing value who did not die or become hospitalized but who had prior and subsequent nonmissing values were assigned the score from the prior nonmissing time. The Wilcoxon test for patient satisfaction outcome was based on raw scores and did not incorporate categories for deaths and hospitalizations.

Result

All baseline sociodemographic characteristics were similar between the intervention and control groups. With the exception of hypertension, there were no statistically significant differences, and, overall, the groups were clinically similar (Table 9.3.1). Mean age was 76 years; 43% were male, and 36% were Black. Forty-six percent of the control group experienced diastolic failure, compared with 40% of the intervention group (p = .434). The primary physician for 50% (60/121) of the control group and 43% (51/118) of the intervention group was a board-certified cardiologist; physician generalists (internal or family medicine) cared for the other 50% (61/121) of the control group and 57% (67/118) of the intervention group throughout the episode of acute heart failure. Of the 121 control-group patients, 39% (48/121) were prescribed an angiotensin-converting enzyme inhibitor, as were 37% (44/118) of intervention-group patients.

Twenty-four patients (10%) died by 52 weeks postdischarge (13 control vs. 11 intervention, p = .830). Study follow-up did not differ significantly between control and intervention groups (mean = 281 vs. 279 days; p = .871). The 31% attrition owing to death or withdrawal (37/121 control; 36/118 intervention, p = .99) was consistent with another RCT that involved a similar patient population.[14,15] Most of the attrition (32/239) occurred at the 52-week data collection point (17 intervention group; 15 control group) because patients moved and could not be located, did not answer the telephone despite multiple calls, or did not want to be bothered. There were no significant differences in

TABLE 9.3.1 Baseline Sociodemographic and Health Characteristics (N = 239)

Characteristic	Intervention (n = 118)	Control (n = 121)	p-value
Age, mean ± SD	76.4 ± 6.9	75.6 ± 6.5	.355
Gender, n (%)			
Male	47 (40)	55 (44)	
Female	71 (60)	66 (56)	.433
Race, n (%)			
Black	40 (34)	46 (38)	
White	78 (66)	75 (62)	.59
Education, n (%)			
< High school	52 (44)	54 (44)	
> High school	66 (56)	67 (55)	1.00
Retired or unemployed, n (%)	98 (82)	109 (90)	.178
Social support, n (%)			
Spouse	48 (41)	51 (42)	
Other relative or friend	27 (23)	30 (25)	
No one	43 (36)	40 (33)	.879
Income, U.S. $, n (%)			
< 10,000	34 (29)	45 (37)	
10,000–19,999	31 (26)	33 (27)	
≥ 20,000	18 (15)	20 (17)	
Missing	35 (29)	23 (19)	.792
Insurance, n (%)			
HMO	42 (36)	52 (43)	
Medicare only	13 (11)	10 (8)	
Medicare + Medicaid	9 (7)	10 (8)	
Medicare + supplemental	54 (46)	49 (41)	.636
Type of admission to hospital, n (%)			
Elective	24 (20)	19 (15)	
Emergency	92 (78)	100 (83)	
Transfer	2 (2)	2 (2)	.544
Index duration of stay, mean ± SD	5 ± 2.9	4.6 ± 2.3	.245
Patient subjective health rating,[33] n (%)			
Excellent/good	4 (3.4)	2 (1.7)	
Fair	87 (74)	92 (76)	
Poor	27 (23)	27 (22)	.877
No. physician visits (within past 6 months), mean ± SD	6.2 ± 3.6	6.6 ± 5.6	.726
No. hospital admissions (within past 6 months), mean ± SD	1.1 ± 1.6	1.1 ± 1.3	.991
No. hospital discharges (within past 30 days), mean ± SD	0.3 ± 0.6	0.2 ± 0.4	.177
Functional status,[21] mean ± SD			
Personal	17.1 ± 5.8	16.9 ± 5.8	.815
Social	8.4 ± 2.6	8.6 ± 2.6	.719
Total	25.5 ± 8	25.4 ± 7.8	.629
Quality of life,[20] mean ± SD			
Emotional	6.6 ± 7.4	6.4 ± 7.4	.823
Physical	21.7 ± 10.8	20.8 ± 9.5	.55
Total	38.0 ± 20.9	36 ± 19.5	.476
No. daily prescription medications, mean ± SD	7 ± 3.1	6.5 ± 2.7	.262

(continued)

TABLE 9.3.1 *(continued)*

Number health conditions,[a] mean ± SD	6.4 ± 2.5	6.4 ± 2	.748
Coronary artery disease, n (%)	62 (53)	54 (45)	.22
Hypertension, n (%)	54 (46)	71 (59)	.046
Atrial tachycardia, n (%)	45 (38)	39 (32)	.339
Diabetes mellitus, n (%)	44 (37)	46 (38)	.887
Pulmonary disease, n (%)	41 (35)	30 (24)	.093
Type of heart failure (as documented in the medical record), n (%)			
Systolic	70 (59)	65 (53)	
Diastolic	48 (40)	56 (46)	.434
Documented ejection fraction, n (%)	88 (72)	98 (80)	
< 20%	12 (14)	17 (17)	.755
20 to < 25%	10 (11)	9 (9)	.760
25 to < 35%	28 (32)	30 (30)	.914
35 to < 45%	26 (30)	28 (28)	.942
≥ 45%	12 (14)	14 (14)	1.00

[a] Active health problems requiring therapy as reported by patients and documented in the medical record.
Note. SD = standard deviation.

the severity of illness between control-group patients (24/121) and intervention-group patients (25/118) lost to follow-up, as assessed using baseline ejection fraction, number of hospitalizations in the 6 months before index hospitalization, number of comorbid conditions, and number of prescription medications.

Rehospitalization and Death

The number of rehospitalizations or deaths at 52 weeks were lower in the intervention group (56/118 [47.5%] vs. 74/121 [61.2%], adjusted $p = .01$). The distribution of times to first readmission or death was similarly shifted toward longer time intervals in the intervention group than in the control group (Kaplan-Meier log rank $\chi^2 = 5.0$, $p = .026$). The estimated proportions ± standard error of patients in the intervention group remaining alive and with no hospital readmission at 30, 60, 90, 180, and 365 days postdischarge were 0.869 ± 0.033, 0.750 ± 0.043, 0.071 ± 0.045, 0.600 ± 0.047, and 0.445 ± 0.050, respectively. These proportions were significantly lower in control patients: 0.737 ± 0.041, 0.621 ± 0.046, 0.558 ± 0.047, 0.444 ± 0.047, and 0.321 ± 0.046, respectively. Similarly, the estimated median event-free survival of patients in the APN intervention and control groups was 131 and 241 days, respectively. There were no statistically significant group differences (at $p < .05$) by time interactions whether time was defined as an interval variable ($p = .472$) or dichotomized at 2, 6, 12, or 26 weeks. The crude IDR from the simple Cox regression was 1.48 (95% CI = 1.05–2.09, $p = .027$). Only number of daily medications at admission had $p = .05$ when added to the a priori multivariable model ($p = .014$). The final multivariate model–adjusted IDR was 1.65 (95% CI = 1.13–2.40, $p = .001$) (Table 9.3.2). Relative efficacy did not vary by institution. When follow-up was censored at death, the unadjusted and adjusted IDRs were 1.44 (95% CI = 1.00–2.07) and 1.58 (95% CI = 1.07–2.34), respectively.

Readmissions and Hospital Days at 1 Year

Fewer intervention group patients were rehospitalized after discharge from index hospital than control group patients (44.9% vs. 55.4%, $p = .12$) (Table 9.3.3). There were 104 readmissions of intervention

TABLE 9.3.2 Time to First Rehospitalization or Death by Patient Characteristic (Multivariate Cox Proportional Hazards Model)

Variable	Incidence Density Ratio (95% CI)	p-value
Control group versus intervention group	1.65 (1.13–2.40)	.001
Fair or poor self-rating versus good or excellent self-rating	1.29 (0.83–2.00)	.263
Number of prior hospitalizations within the past 6 months	1.19 (1.06–1.35)	.005
Living with spouse versus relative or friend[a]	0.81 (0.51–1.29)	.376
Living alone versus with relative or friend[a]	0.59 (0.35–0.98)	.043
Daily medications	1.09 (1.02–1.16)	.014
Site[b]		.176

[a]Likelihood ratio test for prior living arrangements $\chi^2 = 4.262$, $df = 2$, $p = .119$.
[b]Likelihood ratio test for site differences $\chi^2 = 7.663$, $df = 5$.
Note. CI = confidence interval.

TABLE 9.3.3 Rehospitalizations and Hospital Days 1 Year After Index Hospitalization Discharge

Variable	Intervention (n = 118)	Control (n = 121)	p[a]	Relative Risk (95% CI)
Patients rehospitalized, n (%)				
> 1 time	53 (44.9)	67 (55.4)	<.121	1.24 (0.95–1.60)
> 2 times	34 (28.8)	44 (36.4)	<.218	1.20 (0.89–1.60)
Rehospitalizations, n				
Index related	40	72	<.184	
Comorbidity related	23	50	<.013	
New health problem	41	40	<.881	
Total	104	162	<.047	
Rehospitalizations per patient/year[b]	1.18	1.79	<.001	
Total hospital days, n	588	970		
Per patient, mean ± SD	5.0 ± 7.3	8.0 ± 12.3	<.071	
Per rehospitalized patient, mean ± SD	11.1 ± 7.2	14.5 ± 13.4	<.411	

[a]Wilcoxon rank sum tests used to compare the distribution of per-patient rates for number of rehospitalizations and hospital days; χ^2 analysis for proportion of patients rehospitalized.
[b]Rehospitalization rate per patient per year: total rehospitalizations/total nonhospital days times 365.
Note. CI = confidence interval; SD = standard deviation.

group patients versus 162 control group patients ($p = .047$) (readmission rate per nonhospitalized year 1.18 vs. 1.79; IDR = 0.66; $p < .001$). Of rehospitalizations, 23 of 104 (22%) in the intervention group versus 50 of 162 (31%) in the control group were related to comorbidity ($p = .013$), 40 (38%) versus 72 (44%) for heart failure ($p = .184$) and 41 (39%) versus 40 (24%) for new health problems ($P = .881$). Hospital days were fewer in the intervention group (588 days vs. 970 days, $p = .071$). Forty-three intervention patients versus 40 control patients had two or fewer rehospitalizations ($p = .77$) and 11 intervention patients versus 28 control patients had three or more rehospitalizations ($p < .001$).

Effect Persistence

Although results were similar regardless of time interval evaluated, the intervention effect decreased as the time after intervention increased. Relative differences between groups in index-related (11 vs. 35) and comorbidity-related (12 vs. 28) rehospitalizations were greatest during the 3 months postdischarge active-intervention period. Additional APN group reductions were observed for index- (11 vs. 22) and comorbidity-related (4 vs. 13) rehospitalizations in Months 3 through 6, although the incremental benefit of the intervention group was less than in Months 0 through 3. Although preexisting study group differences were sustained, there were no additional decreases between groups in rates of rehospitalization 6 to 12 months post-index hospitalization discharge (index-related, 18 vs. 15; comorbidity-related, 7 vs. 9).

Cost Analyses

Total and mean costs (reimbursements) per patient were lower in the intervention group than in the control group (Table 9.3.4). Mean 52-week total costs adjusted for unequal follow-up were $7,636 for the intervention group and $12,481 for the control group, yielding an estimated mean cost savings of $4,845 per patient (nonparametric bootstrap 95% CI of true difference in mean total costs $8,975.84–$1,301.02; $p = .002$). Although adjusted mean number of and estimated costs for home visits for the 52 weeks after index hospitalization discharge were higher for the intervention group, these increased costs were offset by reductions in heart failure- and comorbidity-related rehospitalizations within the first 6 months after discharge from the index hospital.

Quality of Life, Functional Status, and Patient Satisfaction

The intervention group reported greater overall quality of life at 12 weeks ($p < .05$) and in the physical dimension at 2 weeks ($p < .01$) and 12 weeks ($p < .05$) (Table 9.3.5). Satisfaction with care was greater in patients in the intervention group at 2 and 6 weeks after discharge ($p < .001$) (Table 9.3.6). Statistically significant group differences in functional status did not emerge; however, less dependency was, on average, observed (Table 9.3.7).

Discussion

In this multisite RCT, a comprehensive intervention directed by APNs experienced in the care of older adults and management of heart failure and working in close collaboration with patient physicians increased time to first readmission or death through 1 year after index hospital discharge, reduced the total number of rehospitalizations, and decreased medical costs of elders hospitalized with systolic and diastolic heart failure. Overall quality of life and the physical dimension of quality of life were improved at only one (12 weeks) and two (2 and 12 weeks) of the five follow-up points, respectively. Patient satisfaction, assessed only through 6 weeks, was also enhanced.

The study confirms previous results about the short-term effectiveness of such interventions in improving heart failure-related outcomes in older adults.[9–14] Additionally, this study is the first to show reductions in the number of rehospitalizations caused by comorbid conditions and reductions in overall number of hospitalizations and costs for elderly patients hospitalized with systolic and diastolic heart failure.

Unlike many disease-management interventions, a flexible protocol guided APNs, enabling them to individualize the schedule and content of patient care to manage heart failure, comorbid conditions, and other health and social problems that contribute to poor outcomes. This approach is especially important because exacerbation of coexisting conditions cause 40% of rehospitalizations of elders with heart failure.[6–8] In this study, patients had a mean of six active, comorbid problems. Absolute reductions in the number of rehospitalizations owing to heart failure ($n = 32$) and comorbid conditions

TABLE 9.3.4 Costs (Reimbursements) for Rehospitalizations, Acute Care Visits, and Home Visits for 52 Weeks After Index Hospitalization Discharge

Parameter	Control (n = 121) Mean No. Visits ± SD	Cost, $	Intervention (n = 118) Mean No. Visits ± SD	Cost, $	p No. Visits	Cost
Rehospitalizations						
Index related		314,955		175,960		.152
Comorbidity related		498,110		175,840		.015
New health problem		246,134		235,453		.997
Total hospitalizations		1,065,927		587,253		.088
Rehospitalizations						
0–3 months		489,420		236,144		.010
0–6 months		841,164		381,725		.030
6–12 months		218,035		205,528		.235
Acute care visits						
Physician's office	0.8 ± 1.6	5,169	0.8 ± 1.5	4,549	.609	.636
Emergency room	0.3 ± 1.2	5,650	0.1 ± 0.4	1,780	.116	.105
Home visits						
Visiting nurse	6.3 ± 13.2	64,531	1.1 ± 4.9	11,837	<.001	<.001
Advance practice nurse	0	0	12.1 ± 6.7	104,019*	—	—
Physical therapists	1.0 ± 4.4	10,918	0.7 ± 3.0	7,120	.703	.708
Social workers	0.0 ± 0.4	534	0.0 ± 0.1	178	.678	.678
Home health aides	1.1 ± 5.1	11,081	0.9 ± 5.5	9,167	.286	.286
Total home visits	9.5 ± 19.0	97,883	± 12.2	138,649	<.001	<.001
Totals		1,163,810		725,903		.404
Per patient		9,618		6,152		
Lin estimate		12,481		7,636		.002

*Includes costs of multidisciplinary team member services.
Note: Visits and costs are aggregate values. Visits and costs were standardized for unequal follow-up by converting to costs per day in the study before significance testing. SD = standard deviation.

(n = 27) were similar. In contrast, previous reports of nurse-directed interventions designed specifically for older adults resulted in substantial short-term reductions in the number of readmissions owing to heart failure but in no significant difference in readmissions for other causes.[13,14]

This intervention did not simply delay hospital readmissions but avoided them, with significant reductions in total readmissions persisting through 52 weeks postindex discharge (9 months post intervention). The greatest reductions in the number of index hospital and comorbidity-related rehospitalizations were observed during the 3-month intervention (23 vs. 63). Rehospitalizations were further reduced, but at a lower rate, during the 3 months immediately after the intervention (15 vs. 35). Although previous differences in the cumulative number of rehospitalization rates were sustained beyond 3 months after intervention (study Months 6–12), the number of index hospital and comorbidity-related rehospitalizations were not further reduced (25 vs. 24).

Themes identified in case studies maintained by APNs for all intervention patients suggest that, although many patients demonstrated growth in their ability to manage their health needs, the progressive nature of heart failure and other long-term conditions, severity of resulting symptoms, and in-

TABLE 9.3.5 QOL Comparing Intervention and Control Groups

	QOL Total Score Category[a]				QOL Physical Dimension Category[b]		QOL Emotional Dimension Category[c]	
	APN		Control		APN	Control	APN	Control
	n	Mean ± SD	n	Mean ± SD	Mean ± SD			
Baseline	117	2.4 ± 0.7	118	2.3 ± 0.7	2.8 ± 0.9	2.8 ± 0.9	3.3 ± 1.3	3.3 ± 1.2
2 weeks	114	3.0 ± 1.2*	112	2.7 ± 1.2	3.5 ± 1.2**	3.0 ± 1.2	3.6 ± 1.3***	3.3 ± 1.4
6 weeks	99	3.1 ± 1.3	109	2.9 ± 1.4	3.6 ± 1.4	3.3 ± 1.5	3.5 ± 1.5	3.3 ± 1.6
12 weeks	89	3.2 ± 1.5****	100	2.7 ± 1.5	3.6 ± 1.4****	3.1 ± 1.6	3.6 ± 1.6	3.2 ± 1.7
26 weeks	86	2.9 ± 1.6	92	2.6 ± 1.5	3.3 ± 1.6	3.0 ± 1.7	3.2 ± 1.7	3.1 ± 1.8
52 weeks	75	2.8 ± 1.8	74	2.6 ± 1.7	3.1 ± 1.9	2.9 ± 1.9	3.1 ± 1.9	3.0 ± 1.9

[a] 0 = Died; 1 = hospitalized; 2 = 1st quartile score (> 35); 3 = 2nd quartile score (> 18 to = 35); 4 = 3rd quartile score (> 7 to = 18); 5 = 4th quartile score (= 7) highest QOL.
[b] 0 = Died; 1 = hospitalized; 2 = 1st quartile score (> 21); 3 = 2nd quartile score (> 12 to = 21); 4 = 3rd quartile score (> 4 to = 12); 5 = 4th quartile score (= 4).
[c] 0 = Died; 1 = hospitalized; 2 = 1st quartile score (> 6); 3 = 2nd quartile score (> 1 to = 6); 4 = 3rd quartile score (> 0 to = 1); 5 = 4th quartile score (= 0).
Difference between groups: *p = .07; **p < .01; ***p = .094; ****p < .05.
Note: The Minnesota Living with Heart Failure questionnaire has 21 items and provides a total score (range 0–105) and two subscales. Each item is self-rated on a 0- to 5-point scale. The physical and emotional subscales are subset sum scores with 8 and 5 items each, with ranges from 0 to 40 and 0 to 25, respectively. Higher scores reflect lower QOL. APN = advanced practice nurse; QOL = quality of life; SD = standard deviation.

TABLE 9.3.6 Patient Satisfaction Comparing Intervention and Control Groups

	Patient Satisfaction Score Category n (mean ± SD)	
	APN	Control
2 weeks	99 (83.0 ± 10.3*)	97 (74.6 ± 10.4)
6 weeks	92 (83.1 ± 9.6*)	91 (77.8 ± 11.2)

Note: The Patient Satisfaction score is an investigator-developed and -tested instrument with 25 items self-rated on a 0- to 4-point scale, with a range of 44 to 100. Higher scores reflect greater satisfaction. APN = advanced practice nurse; SD = standard deviation.
Difference between groups: *p < .001.

creasing frailty of elders (i.e., increased functional or cognitive deficits) may necessitate some level of ongoing APN involvement. Therefore, an extended intervention may provide additional reductions in the number of rehospitalizations over time, but the incremental benefits and cost-effectiveness of such an intervention must be rigorously evaluated.

Compared with other reported interventions for the management of heart failure,[9–12] the protocol used in this study was unique in that it was directed by APNs; substituted for traditional postdischarge skilled nursing follow-up; and focused on the complex care of older adults coping with heart failure, multiple comorbid conditions, and other risk factors. It seems that its success largely was derived from two factors: (a) the continuity of care provided by the same APN who coordinated the patient's hospital discharge plan and implemented it in the patient's home and (b) the use of highly skilled APNs who are prepared to use a holistic approach to address the complex needs of patients and their caregivers and whose skills in collaboration and coordination enable them to navigate an intricate, often disjointed care system to promote continuity of care.

Although assessment of the relative contributions of various intervention components is necessary to optimize cost-effective clinical programs, such evaluation strategies generally do not capture the synergy achieved by a multidimensional approach and do not adequately account for variation

TABLE 9.3.7 Functional Status Scores Comparing Intervention and Control Groups

	Total Dependency Category[a]				Personal Dependency Category[b]		Social Dependency Category[c]	
	APN		Control		APN	Control	APN	Control
	n	Mean ± SD	n	Mean ± SD	Mean ± SD			
Baseline	117	3.3 ± 1.1	120	3.3 ± 1.1	3.3 ± 1.1	3.4 ± 1.1	3.5 ± 1.1	3.5 ± 1.1
2 weeks	111	3.4 ± 1.2	112	3.3 ± 1.2	3.4 ± 1.2	3.3 ± 1.3	3.6 ± 1.2	3.4 ± 1.2
6 weeks	99	3.4 ± 1.3	109	3.1 ± 1.4	3.4 ± 1.3	3.1 ± 1.4	3.5 ± 1.4	3.2 ± 1.4
12 weeks	97	3.5 ± 1.3	104	3.1 ± 1.4	3.5 ± 1.4	3.2 ± 1.6	3.6 ± 1.4	3.3 ± 1.5
26 weeks	92	3.3 ± 1.3	97	3.0 ± 1.5	3.3 ± 1.6	3.0 ± 1.7	3.6 ± 1.6	3.2 ± 1.7
52 weeks	76	3.1 ± 1.5	71	2.9 ± 1.6	3.0 ± 1.7	2.9 ± 1.9	3.3 ± 1.8	3.0 ± 1.9

[a] 0 = Died; 1 = hospitalized; 2 = 1st quartile score (> 30); 3 = 2nd quartile score (> 23 to = 30); 4 = 3rd quartile score (> 17 to = 23); 5 = 4th quartile score (= 17) highest function.
[b] 0 = Died; 1 = hospitalized; 2 = 1st quartile score (> 20); 3 = 2nd quartile score (> 15 to = 20); 4 = 3rd quartile score (> 11 to = 15); 5 = 4th quartile score (= 11).
[c] 0 = Died; 1 = hospitalized; 2 = 1st quartile score (> 10); 3 = 2nd quartile score (> 8 to = 10); 4 = 3rd quartile score (> 6 to = 8); 5 = 4th quartile score (= 6).
Note: The Enforced Social Dependency scale consists of twelve 6-point scales (4 for each capacity). Total scores (range, 12–72) and subscores (range, 4–24) are computed. Higher scores reflect greater dependency. QOL and function, missing values owing to deaths, and hospitalizations were incorporated into transformed ordinal scales. Distributions were compared between groups using Wilcoxon rank sum tests. APN = advanced practice nurse; QOL = quality of life; *SD* = standard deviation.

between patients in components needed and used. Nonetheless, the absolute and incremental effect of such interventions must be assessed by type of heart failure, type of physician–nurse provider team, and case mix. Such studies will require significantly larger sample sizes.

The higher direct costs of the intervention ($115,856 vs. $64,531) resulting from the increased mean number of APN home visits relative to routine home care (13.2 vs. 6.3 visits), higher salaries commanded by APNs, and involvement of multidisciplinary heart failure experts (limited to their participation in APN training and individual consultation on less than 10% of intervention cases) were more than offset by savings from reductions in the number of other home visits ($16,465 vs. $22,533), acute care visits to physicians or the emergency department ($6,329 vs. $10,819), and hospitalizations ($587,253 vs. $1,065,927). The net result was a 37.6% reduction in total costs over the 12-month study period ($725,903 vs. $1,163,810, $p < .002$; $6,152 vs. $9,618 per person).

These study findings substantially enhance understanding of patient management strategies necessary to improve clinical outcomes for a growing population of elders living longer with multiple, debilitating conditions while reducing overall costs. The findings suggest the potential benefit of a comprehensive, multidisciplinary, individualized intervention directed by clinical nurse experts that spans the entire episode of acute illness and bridges the transition from hospital to home.

Transitional care programs such as this have typically not been adopted because of lack of Medicare reimbursement, the absence of effective marketing forces, the challenges such care present to the culture of current medical practice, which is characterized by the organization of care into distinct and separate silos (i.e., hospital and home care), and limited meaningful longitudinal integration of physician and nursing care to support patient needs throughout an acute episode of illness.

Although further research is necessary to define the relative effectiveness and cost-effectiveness of alternative intervention designs and components, to define the optimal duration and intensity of interventions, and to further evaluate the generalizability of findings across a broader spectrum of geographic and care settings, the clinical and economic effectiveness of these interventions support the value of their more widespread use.

Acknowledgment

The authors thank the APNs for their extraordinary commitment to accomplishing the goals of this study. Special recognition is given to M. Brian Bixby, MSN, CRNP, CS, Joanne Konick-McMahan, RN, MSN, CCRN, and Catherine McKenna, RN, MSN. The support provided by a group of dedicated research assistants was deeply appreciated. Finally, the authors thank Lenore Wilkas, MALS, for her assistance in the completion of this manuscript.

REFERENCES

1. Naylor MD. Transitional care of older adults. *Annu Rev Nuts Res.* 2003;20:127–147.
2. Vinson J, Rich M, Sperry J, et al. Early readmission of elderly patients with congestive heart failure. *J Am Geriarr Soc.* 1990;38:1290–1295.
3. Oddone EZ, Weinberger M, Horner M, et al. Classifying general medical readmissions: Are they preventable? *J Gen Intern Med.* 1996;11:597–607.
4. American Heart Association. *Heart Disease and Stroke Statistics—2003 Update.* Dallas: Author. 2003.
5. Happ MB, Naylor MD, Roe-Prior P. Factors contributing to rehospitalization of elderly patients with heart failure. *J Cardiovasc Nurs.* 1997;11:75–84.
6. Krumholz HM, Wang Y, Parent EM, et al. Quality of care for elderly patients hospitalized with heart failure. *Arch Intern Med.* 1997;157:2242–2247.
7. Stevenson WG, Stevenson LW, Middlekauff HR, et al. Improving survival for patients with advanced heart failure: A study of 737 consecutive patients. *J Am Coll Cardiol.* 1995;26:1417–1423.
8. Digitalis Investigation Group. The effect of digoxin on mortality and morbidity in patients with heart failure. *N Engl J Med.* 1997;336:525–533.
9. Stewart S, Pearson S, Horowitz JD. Effects of a home-based intervention among patients with congestive heart failure discharged from acute hospital care. *Arch Intern Med.* 1998;158:1067–1071.
10. Stewart S, Vandenbroek AJ, Pearson S, et al. Effects of a multidisciplinary, home based intervention on unplanned readmissions and survival among patients with chronic congestive heart failure: A randomized controlled study. *Lancet.* 1999;354:1077–1083.
11. Krumholz HM, Amatruda J, Smith GL, et al. Randomized trial of an education and support intervention to prevent readmission of patients with heart failure. *J Am Coll Cardiol.* 2002;39:83–89.
12. Blue L, Lang E, McMurray JJV, et al. Randomized controlled trial of specialist nurse intervention in heart failure. *BMJ.* 2001;323:715–718.
13. Rich MW, Beckham V, Wittenberg C, et al. A multidisciplinary intervention to prevent the readmission of elderly patients with congestive heart failure. *N Engl J Med.* 1995;333:1190–1195.
14. Naylor MD, Brooten D, Campbell R, et al. Comprehensive discharge planning and home follow-up of hospitalized elders: A randomized clinical trial. *JAMA.* 1999;281:613–620.
15. Naylor M, Brooten D, Jones R, et al. Comprehensive discharge planning for the hospitalized elderly: A randomized clinical trial. *Ann Intern Med.* 1994;120:999–1006.
16. Brooten D, Brown L, Munro B, et al. Early discharge and specialist transitional care. *Image J Nutr Sch.* 1986;20:64–68.
17. Brooten D, Naylor MD, York R, et al. Lessons learned from testing the quality cost model of advanced practice nursing (APN) transitional care. *J Nutr Scholarsh.* 2003;34:369–375.

18. ACC/AHA Task Force on Practice Guidelines. Committee on Evaluation and Management of Heart Failure. Guidelines for the evaluation and management of heart failure. *J Am Coll Cardiol.* 1995;26:1376–1398.
19. Konstam MA, Dracup K, Baker DW, et al. *Heart Failure: Evaluation and Care of Patients With Left Ventricular Systolic Dysfunction* (Clinical Practice Guideline, no. 11, Publication no. 94–0612). Rockville, MD: Agency for Health Care Policy and Research. 1994.
20. Rector TS, Kubo SH, Cohn JN. Patients self-assessment of their congestive heart failure. Part 2: Content, reliability and validity of a new measure, the Minnesota Living with Heart Failure Questionnaire. *Heart Fail.* 1987;3:198–215.
21. Moinpour C, McCorkle R, Saunders J. Measuring functional status. In: Frank Stromberg M, ed. *Instruments for Clinical Nursing Research.* Boston: Jones and Bartlett, 1992:385–401.
22. Health Care Financing Administration. Bureau of Data Management and Statistics. From the 100% MEDPAR Inpatient Hospital Fiscal Year, 1998.
23. Elashoff JD. Query Advisor, Version 4.0. User's Guide. Los Angeles: Dixon Associates, 2000.
24. Kaplan EL, Meier P. Nonparametric estimation from incomplete observations. *J Am Star Assoc.* 1958;53:457–481.
25. Cox DR. Regression models with life-tables. *J R Star Soc.* 1972;66:188–190.
26. Mickey RM, Greenland S. The impact of confounder selection criteria on effect estimation. [erratum in *Am J Epidemiol.* 1989;130:1066]. *Am J Epidemiol.* 1989;129:125–137.
27. Knickerbocker RK. Intent to treat analyses. In: Chow S-C, ed. *Encyclopedia of Biopharmaceutical Statistics.* New York: Marcel Dekker. 2000: 271–275.
28. Lin DY, Feuer EJ, Etzioni R, et al. Estimating medical costs from incomplete follow-up data. *Biometrics.* 1997;53:419–434.
29. Efron B, Tibshirani RJ. *An Introduction to the Bootstrap.* New York: Chapman & Hall. 1993.
30. Mooney CZ, Duval RD. Bootstrapping: *A Nonparametric Approach to Statistical Inference.* Newbury Park, CA: Sage. 1993.
31. Diehr P, Patrick D, Hendrick S, et al. Including death when measuring health status over time. *Med Care.* 1995;33:164–172.
32. Rubin DB. Inference and missing data. *Biometrika.* 1976;63:581–592.
33. Maddox GL. Self-assessment of health status: A longitudinal study of selected elderly subjects. *J Chronic Dis.* 1964;17:449–460.

Reprinted with permission from: Naylor, M., Brooten, D. A., Campbell, R. L., Maislin, G., McCauley, K. M., & Schwartz, J. S. (2004). Transitional care of older adults hospitalized with heart failure: A randomized, controlled trial. *Journal of the American Geriatrics Society, 52*(5), 675–684.

9.4 ADOLESCENTS WITH TYPE 1 DIABETES: TRANSITION BETWEEN DIABETES SERVICES

KATE VISENTIN
TINA KOCH
DEBBIE KRALIK

Abstract

Aim: The research aimed to develop a sustainable and coordinated approach to facilitating the transition between diabetes services for adolescents. The objectives were to: (a) involve key diabetes health delivery stakeholders in expressing their concerns and issues about current service delivery and ways to improve same, and (b) reveal from the perspective of the adolescents living with type 1 diabetes their experiences surrounding the process of transition. **Background:** This chapter presents research that sought to identify the major concerns and issues that stakeholders had about transition and to reveal the experience of transition for the adolescent with type 1 diabetes. Key representatives from seven public diabetes services in Adelaide, South Australia, worked collaboratively to answer the objectives of this inquiry. *Approach:* Interview data were generated and analysed using a response focus framework provided by fourth generation evaluation research. In this study, the focus was on common concerns, claims, and issues raised by health care professionals (n = 21) and adolescents (n = 10) aged between 15 and 18 years about transferring from child to adult diabetes services. **Findings:** Data revealed education and dietetic advice was reactive rather than proactive and that the paediatric *model of care is philosophically and practically different to the adult model of diabetes care. Three phases of transition were identified: preparation, formal transition, and evaluation. Our findings indicated that these stages of transition were not being fully implemented in health units.* **Conclusion:** *The project findings have set the scene to establish a multidisciplinary working party to work collaboratively across agencies to develop effective transition pathways.* **Relevance to Clinical Practice:** *The role of diabetes nurse educators and dietitians in South Australia is underused throughout the transition process. Diabetes nurse educators are in an ideal position to prepare, coordinate, and evaluate transitional processes.*

Introduction

It has been previously reported that adolescents who live with type 1 diabetes may experience the transition from the child to the adult health service as an additional burden over and above the everyday challenges of becoming a young adult (Frank, 1992; Blum, 1994; Fleming et al., 2002; McGill, 2002). Clinicians working in child and adult services raised concerns that young people transferring from child services were falling through service gaps. It was thought that many were not receiving adequate follow-up until a crisis forced them back into the system. These concerns were also reflected in the literature around the topic of transition from child to adult services (Viner, 1999; Fleming et al., 2002; Kipps et al., 2002). In response to these concerns, key representatives from seven public diabetes services in South Australia were involved in the study, which sought to identify the major concerns and issues that stakeholders hadabout transition and to reveal the experience of transition for the adolescent with type 1 diabetes.

Background

Type 1 diabetes is the most common metabolic disease in children (Christian et al., 1999) and occurs when the pancreas is unable to produce insulin. Treatment consists of at least twice-daily insulin injections to prevent serious short- and long-term complications. In addition, children and their families must ensure that an appropriate diet is followed and blood glucose levels are closely monitored (Christian et al., 1999).

Adolescents with diabetes and living in South Australia either make the transition from a major children's hospital to an adult health service or they move from a children's department to the adult department within the one institution. Transition in this context was defined by Blum et al. (1993, p. 570) as "the purposeful, planned movement of adolescents and young adults with chronic physical and medical conditions from child-centred to adult-orientated health care systems." It was recognized by diabetes nurse educators that each diabetes service had different processes to facilitate this transition. Although there was collaboration between the two major health services, other services had limited communication.

District nurse consultants (diabetes) were previously funded for a pilot study that explored the experiences of transition with four young adults with type 1 diabetes. The pilot study raised questions about service delivery in South Australia because it was evident a lack of uniformity existed across service providers. The study reported in this chapter enabled the research team to further explore service delivery issues by interviewing key diabetes health professionals and adolescents who had not yet made the transition to adult services.

A systematic review by Fleming et al. (2002) highlighted the need for collaboration between child and adult services particularly in the light of the well-documented differences between adult and child services (Schidlow & Fiel, 1990; Eiser et al., 1992; Frank, 1992; Sawyer et al., 1997). Although it is necessary for the child and adult services to have different foci, collaboration is necessary to bridge the gap so that transition is smoother (Frank, 1992; Fleming et al., 2002). South Australia has a population of approximately 1 million people; therefore, the health services are ideally situated to work collaboratively toward a coordinated approach to transition.

Literature

Transition to adult services has been the subject of much discussion for not only adolescents with diabetes, but also for other long-term conditions such as cystic fibrosis. Although the conditions may be different, the literature suggests that the issues are similar. A search of the literature identified articles from Australia, the United Kingdom, and United States of America, which all called for national policies for transition (Blum, 1994; Sawyer et al., 1997; Viner, 1999; Fleming et al., 2002; Rosen et al., 2003). Authors recommended that transition should be planned and coordinated (Blum, 1994; Sawyer et al., 1997; Fleming et al., 2002; Rosen et al., 2003).

Transition to adult services is difficult for myriad reasons. The most reported concern is the notable differences in the approach to care between child and adult diabetes services. Child services focus on the whole family, whereas the adult sectors take a more individual approach (Eiser et al., 1992; Sawyer et al., 1997). In addition, adult services expect a much greater degree of independence from young people and encourage communication without parents being present. It may be difficult for adolescents to adapt to this type of relationship, particularly when they have had a long-standing relationship with their paediatrician (Frank, 1992).

Adult service staff may make the assumption that the adolescent has the necessary skills and maturity to plan his or her future and has the insight to understand the consequences if he or she chooses not to undertake diabetes self-care (Frank, 1992; Fleming et al., 2002). Viner (1999) argued that adolescents are not served well by either model of diabetes care because the children's clinic may not acknowledge the adolescent's growing independence, whereas the adult clinic may not acknowledge the adolescent's growth, development and family concerns. It has been recommended that transition be "a family affair" (Schidlow & Fiel, 1990) and it has been suggested that transition in health care is only one aspect of a broader life transition that adolescents move through (Viner, 1999).

If the transition process is not meeting the needs of adolescents then they might choose to "drop out of the system." A general practitioner may be accessed to prescribe insulin. However, a multidisciplinary approach to diabetes care provides optimal management (Strategic Plan for Diabetes in South Australia, 1999; Parsons et al., 2000). If diabetes is poorly managed, young adults are at an increased risk of micro- and macrovascular complications and life-threatening severe complications, such as diabetic ketoacidosis (DCCTRG, 1993).

The demands of diabetes may be difficult during the adolescent years; it has been documented that glycaemic control deteriorates (Frank, 1992; Bryden et al., 2001; Fleming et al., 2002; Silink et al., 2003–2004). The deterioration in gylcaemic control is thought to be related to an increase in insulin resistance that relates to physiologic changes in puberty coupled with the psychosocial pressures associated with this period of life (Bryden et al., 2001; Silink et al., 2003–2004). Observations by clinicians were supported in the literature by results of studies that showed higher rates of nonattendance at clinic appointments after transition from child to adult services (Frank, 1992; Blum et al., 1993; Fleming et al., 2002). Of further concern, glycaemic control in young people in the 16- to 25-year age group was poorer than at other times during the life span (Wills et al., 2003).

Although the literature outlined principles for successful transition and made suggestions for develop of a model, research that provided outcome data to support one model over another was limited (Viner, 1999; Kipps et al., 2002; Rosen et al., 2003). A study undertaken in the United Kingdom compared different modes of transfer within one region using data generated through interviews and retrospective case note review (Kipps et al., 2002). Findings suggested that transfer to a young adult clinic was preferable to direct transfer to an adult-only clinic. Another U. K. study (Eiser et al., 1992) surveyed adolescents who were attending the clinic for persons under 25 years of age. Interestingly, a high number of adolescents did not report difficulties with transition; however, they did feel it would have been helpful to have visited the clinic before transfer.

A study undertaken in Australia (Court, 1993) surveyed adolescents 15 to 18 years of age. The author concluded that a specific transition clinic can provide an important link and that transition must be a gradual process. Schidlow and Fiel (1990) discussed a transition clinic established in the United States, where the paediatrician and adult physician conducted joint clinics in paediatrics as a stepping stone to the adult clinic. Unfortunately, there was no reported evaluation of this service.

Scant qualitative research has explored how adolescents experience transition. One recent Australian study researched the experiences of six young adults with cystic fibrosis using in-depth interviews (Brumfield & Lansbury, 2004). The aim was to reveal the factors that contributed to the experience of transition and potential outcomes. A number of strategies were outlined that might improve the transition process with this client group. These included seeing a familiar face at adult clinics, conducting orientation tours, and providing written and verbal information as part of the transition program.

The Study

Aims

The aim was to develop a sustainable and coordinated approach to facilitating the transition between diabetes services for adolescents. The objectives were to (a) involve key diabetes health delivery stakeholders in expressing their concerns and issues about current service delivery and ways to improve same and (b) reveal from the perspective of adolescents living with type 1 diabetes their experiences in the process of transition.

Method

Using principles from fourth-generation research (Guba & Lincoln, 1989; Koch, 1993; Lewis et al., 1997; Mitchell & Koch, 1997), we collaborated with key diabetes health professionals and adolescents. Fourth-generation research aims to include all stakeholders in the evaluation process by enabling them to present their concerns, claims, and issues (Koch, 1994). For this research, the stakeholders referred to diabetes health professionals and to adolescents.

Participation and collaboration are central to fourth-generation research because it is based in the constructivist paradigm (Koch, 1994). A claim is any assertion that a stakeholder introduces that is favourable. A concern is any assertion that a stakeholder introduces that is unfavourable about a local situation, that is, within their own health service. An issue is any assertion that a stakeholder introduces that refers to a situation wider than the local service and, therefore, requires multiple partners or organizations to address the problems identified.

Ethical Issues

Ethics approval was obtained from seven South Australian Health services before data generation. Informed consent was obtained from health professionals and adolescents before interviewing.

Recruitment

Recruitment for this group of young people proved difficult. The initial aim was for recruitment to occur via snowballing through diabetes educators. Flyers were developed and a personalized recruitment process was undertaken in which individuals were invited to participate. Adolescents who had not made the transition to adult services did not perceive that there was an issue because they had not experienced the transition. During the project, it was realized that it may have been useful to also interview parents because they often held concerns about transition; however, because of funding constraints, the interviewing of parents was not within the scope of this project.

Permission was obtained for the researcher to be present in the children's clinics and to approach parents and adolescents to participate in the interview during clinic time. This was the main method of recruitment for this project (n = 8). Two interviews were undertaken in participant homes (n = 2), at their request.

Participants

Interviews were performed with 21 diabetes health professionals (n = 21) and 10 adolescents (n = 10) between 15 and 18 years of age and who had been diagnosed with type 1 diabetes a minimum of 12 months previously. Eleven (n = 11) health professionals were also part of the project management team and met monthly to discuss and direct the project. This allowed participation and collaboration, which are essential to fourth-generation research methods. Adolescents were recruited from two major child services located in metropolitan Adelaide. Of the health professionals, seven were medical consultants: endocrinologists, paediatricians, paediatric endocrinologists and physicians (n = 7), 10 were diabetes nurse educators (n = 10), three were dietitians (n = 3), and one was a psychologist (n = 1). All interviews with health professionals were conducted at the health service site at which they worked. Eight interviews with adolescents were conducted at the diabetes clinic and two were undertaken in their own home. The time taken for all interviews ranged from 15 minutes to 1 hour, with the average being half an hour. Interviews were audiotaped and transcribed verbatim and analysed by the first and second authors.

Data Generation

The project manager conducted the interviews between February 2004 and June 2004. The interviews with health professionals used questions framed as concerns, claims, and issues. Refer to Table 9.4.1 for a list of the questions asked.

Data Analysis

Following established protocols (Koch, 1993; Lewis et al., 1997; Mitchell & Koch, 1997), data from the interviews with health professionals were categorized under concerns, claims, and issues. Data were analysed concurrently by the project manager and the research director, who provided oversight of the process. Agreement on common claims, issues, and concerns was reached by the research team. Data from both sources were merged to give shape to this chapter.

Findings

The data showed that health professionals were concerned about young people becoming "lost" in the health care system. A link was made between being lost in the system and having an increased risk for long- and short-term complications. These concerns were based on anecdotal observations because there was no tracking system or reporting mechanism in place after transfer from child to adult diabetes services. Table 9.4.2 summarizes the main claims concerns and issues raised by health professionals.

A minority of the 10 adolescent participants were concerned about the transition to adult diabetes services: most stated that it was a process that must occur. Although the adolescents were not particularly concerned about the transition process, very few understood the differences between the two services.

For the purpose of this chapter, we chose one concern and two issues to discuss in depth because these areas had the most relevance for an international audience. The other concerns, claims, and issues are local to South Australian diabetes health services. The findings reported herein include merged data from health professional and adolescent groups.

Education and Dietetic Advice Was Reactive Not Proactive

Many health professionals believed educational services were working in a reactive rather than a proactive and preventative model of care. The routine assessment of an adolescent was undertaken by the paediatrician at 3 monthly intervals and often excluded other health care professionals until a crisis occurred. This "band aiding" approach to service provision and involvement of other members of the

TABLE 9.4.1 List of Interview Questions

Health Professionals	Adolescents
What is working well?	What health services are you receiving now? How do you find these services? Is there a special person that you identify with?
Do you have any concerns about the structures and processes related to transition within your health unit?	Is it important to meet the staff from the new service to transition?
Are there any issues when working with other health units when adolescents are making the transition?	Would you prefer clinics set up for young adults only?
What do you think the main problems are for adolescents making a transition?	Are you interested in receiving a booklet about transition?
Can you think of any ways in which current services for transition could be improved?	Which educational activities have you accessed or would like to access in the future?
	Would you be interested in a support group? How are you feeling about the transfer to adult services and the increased level of responsibility expected?
	What, in your opinion, is the best age for transferring from children to adult services?

TABLE 9.4.2 Main Claims, Concerns and Issues

Claims	Concerns (Local Health Service Level)	Issues (Wider Health System)
The major paediatric and adult service has set up a formalized transition process.	Education and dietetic advice is often reactive not proactive.	Some clients get lost in the system and, consequently, are at an increased risk for complications.
Highly specialized and quality services are provided to this client group.	There is a lack of communication and collaboration between some services.	The paediatric model is different from the adult model of care.
There is collaboration and communication between services and health professionals.	Current systems are underresourced.	Not all phases of the transition process are being adequately addressed (preparation, formal transition, and evaluation).
Clients are prepared for transition by the paediatrician/endocrinologist.		There are access and equity issues around service provision for consumers from rural and metropolitan areas both.
Continuity and consistency are maintained in services for which paediatric and adult diabetes clinics are colocated.		

diabetes health service team was reported to occur because of multiple factors. Reasons given were inadequate staffing, inadequate recall systems, and medical paediatric clinics being run off site. Of the four adolescents who were about to transition to adult services, only one underwent a dietitian review during the past 5 years. Two stated that they had not received a formal education review since diagnosis, and the other two said that they had some contact with the diabetes nurse educator. A number of health professionals provided examples of young people who did not have the skills for adequate self-management, as highlighted by a diabetes nurse educator:

> . . . young adults who are in their early 20s and they hadn't actually been retaught anything about their diabetes so they had no idea what sick days were or what to do. They didn't know much about ketoacidosis and had . . . dated ideas, around food and exercise and that sort of thing. . . . Lots of issues around obviously that they just haven't been reeducated. They've just run off the information that their parents had given them and that seemed very "hit and miss." That seemed to be only if they had problems; that wasn't very proactive. So, the endocrinologist would refer only if they were a problem.

Highlighted by this quote are the possible consequences if adolescents only have access to education if diabetes instability is evident or if a crisis occurs. Creating a problem focus for adolescents rather than a preventive model of care may inhibit the promotion of self-care. Of the four child services, only one had a recall system established to offer adolescents regular education updates at designated intervals. Similarly, only one of the adult services had an established pathway to ensure that all adolescents were offered dietitian and diabetes nurse educator appointments at the time of transition. Furthermore, health professionals reported poor uptake of these appointments.

Adolescents focused on the medical transfer of care during transition. The focus on medical care may be because many adolescents did not regularly see any other health professional. When asked by the researcher, adolescents stated that they were interested in being introduced to the diabetes nurse educator and dietitian at the adult services.

The Child Model Is Different From the Adult Model

Health professionals perceived differences between the child and adult model of care: the environment, the role of parents, levels of expected responsibility and support, and medical approach to diabetes management. The data were incongruent between the concerns of adolescents and health professionals.

One of the differences assumed by health professionals was that adolescents feel uncomfortable waiting in adult diabetes clinics. Many health professionals expressed concern about exposing adolescents to older clients with type 2 diabetes, particularly if those older clients experienced obvious complications of diabetes, such as amputation. Interestingly, adolescents claimed that such exposure was not really an issue, and comments such as "everybody deserves the same respect as everybody else" were made. However, it was agreed that the environment in an adult service was less friendly and more formal.

A major difference between child and adult services was the role of parents. Part of the preparation for transition is to encourage adolescents to attend appointments solo. Contrary to this, nearly all of the adolescents interviewed continued to attend paediatrician appointments accompanied by a parent. This was the case even for those adolescents who were planning to transition within the next 3 to 12 months. An assumption exists that independence will be promoted parents no longer accompany the adolescents to appointments.

Responsibility referred to the day-to-day requirements of diabetes self-care, which included managing appointments. Health professionals revealed that adult service clients were less likely to be "chased" if they did not attend appointments. Health professionals reported that the adult service does not automatically rebook client appointments for those who do not attend. The onus in the adult system is on the individual to telephone the clinic and make another appointment. However, adolescents were perceived by health professionals to be "babied" in the child service. The aim of the adult model is one "where adolescents are encouraged to take more control." A paediatrician said:

> The paediatric model is quite different from the adult model of care in that if they don't come to clinic...we chase them, whereas in the adult field...it is up to them to do the chasing...the adult model is...here is the information, do with it what you will. In the paediatric scene...we don't...give up on them...they're babied, you know.

Adult services do not provide standard appointment rebookings should a young adult not attend, and this difference in approach was seen by some health professionals as problematic. A diabetes nurse educator said, "I can see that being a problem for the person themselves because they become quite frustrated and upset with the service and feel that nobody's caring here as such."

Although adolescents may not take on the responsibility of making appointments at the diabetes clinic, adolescents revealed that they strongly believed they were responsible for their day-to-day diabetes management:

> Over the past few years, I can control my insulin. So if I must take more or less or things like that, I've learnt to do that by myself. This is a good way of being independent.

One other difference was that adult endocrinologists claimed that they had a larger "complication" focus in their diabetes care:

> . . . We are much more geared towards complications screening than the [child service] have had to be...because they're much too early. Whereas by the time they get to us, we're really looking towards complications screening, blood pressure monitoring, lipids monitoring, and starting them on a whole range of other medications.

Endocrinologists claimed that they attempted to make the transition less confrontational by establishing a rapport with the young adult before making changes to medical treatment.

Not All Phases of the Transition Process Are Adequately Addressed

The Australian Clinical Practice Guidelines: Type 1 diabetes in Children and Adolescents (2003) described three phases of transition: preparation, formal transition, and evaluation. Our findings indicated that these stages of transition were not fully implemented in health units. Health professionals agreed that young people must be better prepared for the transition to adult services. The guidelines recommend that the preparation phase commence at 12 years of age. Although adolescents were prepared early for the physical aspects of the transfer, the preparation for increased responsibility was lacking. One major limitations of the current system was that preparation for transition seemed to be carried out entirely by the paediatrician or paediatric endocrinologist, with little input from the diabetes nurse educator or the dietitian.

Health professionals made references to the promotion of self-care by using terms such as "they're a partner" and "they're in the driving seat," but the ways in which adolescents were prepared for independent self-care were unclear. Health professionals agreed that adolescents could receive further self-care preparation in a wide range of areas, such as nutrition, insulin adjustment, sick-day management, and life skills associated with moving through adolescence into adulthood.

Discussion around adolescents making life transition, or learning to be an adult, was taking place alongside independence in diabetes self-care. Health professionals raised the idea of preparation for transition to an adult diabetes service occurring side by side with the young person's life transition. Preparation must be more inclusive of issues relevant to adolescents and must sett the scene for independence and transfer to the adult setting. The aim would be to "create a person that is ... confident enough when they actually go to an adult clinic, to demand or to request ... to know exactly what is needed for them to maintain a degree of well-being."

Three adolescents talked with their paediatrician about transition to adult services and reported that they felt supported because they were able to remain in the child service until they had finished their secondary schooling and until their diabetes was stable. One participant described the contents of a letter she received that stated that it was nearing time for transfer. This letter was sent to those between 17 and 18 years of age, encouraging them to speak with their paediatrician about transition and make an appointment with the diabetes nurse educator. In the past, information nights and activity days have been held, with a focus on transition. These were reported by a parent as helpful, especially when it came to preparing her daughter for decision making. Adolescents thought that written information describing the process and options for transition was something they would use; however, none of those interviewed received written information about transition.

There was debate about the most suitable age for transfer to the adult service. The Australian Clinical Practice Guidelines: Type 1 Diabetes in Children and Adolescents (2003) recommended that the transition phase occur between the ages of 16 and 18 years. Most health professionals agreed that adolescents should be transferred near the age of 18. Four adolescents preferred the transfer age be 18 years, giving completion of schooling as the reason. One adolescent said, "as soon as possible—so you can get used to it quicker and its not all coming on to you while you're half way through study or anything like that." Another adolescent was aware that the time for transition was near but, "I want to stay here but I don't because there's all the little kids and I'm too old."

Although a formal transition process consisting of a medical-to-medical referral occurs between some services, it could be further enhanced. One option to smooth the transition process would be to provide opportunities for adolescents to meet the adult service providers before transfer. This was suggested by health professionals, and adolescents embraced this initiative.

The evaluation phase posttransition is important (Silink et al., 2003–2004). Follow-up and confirmation of the effectiveness of the transition process should be part of that evaluation. One health professional said, "at the moment, there's no follow-up of whether the transition has worked smoothly or not." Health professionals identified that this lack of a systematic client tracking system and ability to evaluate is a problem across all services.

Discussion

The notion that transition is more than a physical transfer to adult services and, as such, must be well planned and coordinated has been widely acknowledged in the literature (Blum, 1994; Sawyer et al., 1997; Rosen et al., 2003). Transition is about a passage of change (Kralik, 2002). Meleis and Trangenstein (1994) proposed that a central focus of nursing is the facilitation of clients, families, and communities through transition. They write that nursing "is concerned with the process and the experiences of human beings undergoing transitions where health and perceived well-being is the outcome" (Meleis & Trangenstein, 1994, p. 257). Adolescents in transition from child to adult diabetes services are involved in a period of critical, but forced, change. We acknowledge that there are variations in the way adolescents engage or fail to engage in transitional processes. Adaptation to change involves a process of trial and error (Kralik, 2002).

Dalton and Gottlieb (2003) explored the concept of readiness to embrace change, which they argued was often linked with a person's compliance to a medical regimen. However, previous research revealed that living with long-term illness seems to be about incorporating the consequences of illness into everyday life (Kralik, 2002; Kralik et al., 2004). Dalton and Gottlieb (2003) provided an alternative view that conceptualized readiness as a process of *becoming* ready over time. Readiness to change was embedded within a process of learning. Baker and Stern (1993) described a process of readiness that involved making the illness a part of life and coming to terms with self-care teaching and having a sense of control. Relationship-building between health professionals and adolescents, as a means of mapping individual context and identifying shifting values over time and dealing with difference and miscommunication, is maybe the first step toward facilitating this transition.

A number of studies found that adolescents were keen to receive written and verbal information about transition and that they wanted to be provided opportunities to meet the new team before transition (Eiser et al., 1992; Court, 1993; Kipps et al., 2002; Brumfield & Lansbury, 2004). A transition model is necessary that takes into account the stakeholders (professionals, parents, and clients) views. Transition literature from the diabetes and cystic fibrosis fields agrees that there is a lack of outcome data that can clearly support one model over another (Viner, 1999; Fleming et al., 2002; Rosen et al., 2003). Suggestions such as young adult clinics, stepped transition, joint clinics with paediatricians, and adult clinic physicians and transition nurses have all been described in the literature.

Health professionals and adolescents in this study highlighted that transition is frequently focused on the medical transfer of care, with the allied health teams playing a minor role. The ramifications are that adolescents are not receiving holistic preparation for transition in terms of developing the self-management skills necessary for adaptation to an adult health setting. Similarly, adolescents were keen to be given opportunities to meet staff before and receive written information. We would argue that, if adolescents were informed about what to expect from the adult service and how it may differ from their current service, transition might be easier.

Limitations of the research included the omission of the parental voice, the small number of adolescent participants, and lack of opportunity for one-off interviews. Parents often play a pivotal support role for children and adolescents living with diabetes, and their experiences and perception of the period of transition may have enhanced effects. One-off interviews with adolescents may have precluded thoughtful responses. Follow-up interviews may have yielded greater insight into the experience of transition. A recommendation for future research is to follow adolescents through the transition process. Parents must be included in such a study.

Implications for Nursing

Data from health professional and adolescents indicate that transition to adult services is based on the medical model. Transition must be viewed holistically instead of focusing solely on the referral from one medical doctor to another. A problem-focused or reactive approach to diabetes care effectively relinquishes the potential for independence and control for the adolescent. If nurses and dietitians are only involved during periods of diabetes instability, adolescents may not be provided the opportunity to learn self-care skills. Type 1 diabetes is often a family issue, with reliance on parents for information and advice. It is important that diabetes nurses and dietitians become involved in working with adolescents toward self-care because many were diagnosed as children and may never have received first-hand information about diabetes. In the current study context, resources limited the involvement of diabetes nurse educators and dietitians in the preparation and care of adolescents in transition.

The role of diabetes nurse educators in preparation and facilitation of the transition process and follow-up has not been fully realized. Preparation must be expanded so that there is a larger focus on developing self-care skills. This would assist individuals in taking on the extra responsibilities expected by adult services. Frank (1992) stated that a gradual preparation of youth and parents is an important principle for transition. Blum et al. (1993) argued that the notion of transition should be discussed as early as diagnosis. One of the transition principles advocated by Rosen et al. (2003) is to have a designated health professional coordinate the transition process between child and adult diabetes services. Diabetes nurse educators are in an excellent position to undertake this role.

Conclusion

The concerns, claims, and issues that have been raised by health professionals can provide a basis for services to address the needs of those adolescents who are making the transition to adult services. The project findings set the scene to establish a multidisciplinary working party to work collaboratively across services. The aim will be to implement a transition program that works across multiple sites, ensuring uniformity of approach to service and the ability for diabetes nurse educators and dietitians to review children and adolescents at milestone ages. Heads of departments are in the process of negotiating further funding for the ongoing implementation of the proposed transition program.

REFERENCES

Baker, C., & Stern, P. (1993). Finding meaning in chronic illness and the key to self care. *Canadian Journal of Nursing Research, 25*, 23–36.

Blum, R. (1994). Transition to adult health care: Setting the stage. *Journal of Adolescent Health. 17*, 3–5.

Blum, R., Garell, D., Hodgman, C., Jorissen, T., Okinow, N., Orr, D., et al. (1993). Transition from child-centred to adult health-care systems for adolescents with chronic conditions. *Journal of Adolescent Health, 14*, 570–576.

Brumfield, K., & Lansbury, G. (2004). Experiences of adolescents with cystic fibrosis during their transition from paediatric to adult health acre: a qualitative study of young Australian adults. *Disability and Rehabilitation, 26*, 223–234.

Bryden, K., Peveler, R., Stein, A., Neil, A., Mayou, R., & Dunger, D. (2001). Clinical and psychological course of diabetes from adolescence to young adulthood: A longitudinal cohort study. *Diabetes Care, 24*, 1536–1540.

Christian, B., D'Auria, J., & Fox, L. (1999). Gaining freedom: Self-responsibility in adolescents with diabetes. *Pediatric Nursing, 25*, 255–266.

Court, J. (1993). Issues of transition to adult care. *Journal Paediatric Child Health, 29*, S53–S55.

Dalton, C., & Gottlieb, L. (2003). The concept of readiness to change. *Journal of Advanced Nursing, 42*, 108–117.

DCCTRG (1993). The effect of intensive treatment of diabetes on the development and progression of long-term complications in insulin-dependent diabetes mellitus. *New England Journal of Medicine, 329*, 977–986.

Eiser, C., Flynn, M., Green, E., Havermans, T., Kirby, R., Sandeman, D., et al. (1992). Coming of age with diabetes: Patients' views of a clinic for under-25 year olds. *Diabetic Medicine, 10*, 185–289.

Fleming, E., Carter, B., & Gillibrand, W. (2002). The transition of adolescents with diabetes from the child health care service into the adult health care service: A review of the literature. *Journal of Clinical Nursing, 11*, 560–567.

Frank, M. (1992). Rights to passage: Transition from paediatric to adult diabetes care. *Beta Release, 16*, 85–89.

Guba, E., & Lincoln, Y. (1989). *Fourth generation evaluation.* Thousand Oaks, CA: Sage Publications.

Kipps, S., Bahu, T., Ong, K., Ackland, F., Brown, R., Foxt, C., et al. (2002). Current methods of transfer of young people with type 1 diabetes to adult services. *Diabetic Medicine, 19*, 649–654.

Koch, T. (1993). *Towards fourth generation evaluation: listening to the voices of older patients. A hermeneutic inquiry.* Manchester, UK: University of Manchester.

Koch, T. (1994). Beyond measurement: Fourth-generation evaluation in nursing. *Journal of Advanced Nursing, 20*, 1148–1155.

Kralik, D. (2002). The quest for ordinariness: Transition experienced by midlife women living with chronic illness. *Journal of Advanced Nursing, 39*, 146–154.

Kralik, D., Koch, T., Price, K., & Howard, N. (2004). Chronic illness self-management: Taking action to create order. *Journal of Clinical Nursing, 13*, 259–267.

Lewis, C., Bridge, K., Koch, T., & Zadoroznyj, M. (1997). *A new negotiated career structure for level 3 nurses: RDNS pilot project study.* Glenside, South Australia: Royal District Nursing Service Research Unit, RDNS Foundation.

McGill, M. (2002). How do we organize smooth, effective transfer from paediatric to adult diabetes care? *Hormone Research, 57*, 66–68.

Meleis, A., & Trangenstein, P. (1994). Facilitating transitions: Redefinition of the nursing mission. *Nursing Outlook, 42*, 255–259.

Mitchell, P., & Koch, T. (1997). An attempt to give nursing home residents a voice in the quality improvement process: The challenge of frailty. *Journal of Clinical Nursing, 6*, 453–461.

Parsons, J., Wilson, D., & Scardigno, A. (2000). *The impact of diabetes in South Australia. The evidence.* On behalf of the South Australian Diabetes Health Priority Area Advisory Group. Adelaide, Australia: South Australian Department of Human Services.

Rosen, D., Blum, R., Britto, M., Sawyer, S., & Siegel, D. (2003). Transition to adult health care for adolescents and young adults with chronic illness. *Journal of Adolescent Health, 33*, 309–311.

Sawyer, S., Blair, S., & Bowes, G. (1997). Chronic illness in adolescents: Transfer or transition to adult services. *Journal Paediatric Child Health, 33*, 88–90.

Schidlow, D,. & Fiel, S. (1990). Transition of chronically ill adolescents from pediatric to adult health care systems. *Medical Clinics of North America, 74*, 1113–1120.

Silink, M., Clarke, C., Couper, J., Craig, M., Crock, P., Davies, R., et al. (2003–2004) Adolescent health. In *Clinical practice guidelines: Type 1 diabetes in children and adolescents* (p. 176). Australia: Department of Health and Ageing, Australian Government.

Strategic Plan for Diabetes in South Australia. (1999). Department of Human Services. Australia.

Viner, R. (1999). Transition from paediatric to adult care. Bridging the gaps or passing the buck? *Archives of disease in childhood, 81*, 271–275.

Wills, C., Scott, A., Swift, P., Davies, M., Mackie, A., & Mansell, P. (2003). Retrospective review of care and outcomes in young adults with type 1 diabetes. *British Medical Journal, 327*, 260–261.

Reprinted with permission from: Visentin, K., Koch, T., & Kralik, D. (2006). Adolescents with type 1 diabetes: Transition between diabetes services. *Journal of Clinical Nursing, 15*(6), 761–769.

9.5 ADVANCED PRACTICE NURSE STRATEGIES TO IMPROVE OUTCOMES AND REDUCE COST IN ELDERS WITH HEART FAILURE

KATHLEEN M. MCCAULEY
M. BRIAN BIXBY
MARY D. NAYLOR

Abstract

The aim of this study was to investigate whether, in a randomized controlled trial (RCT) of vulnerable elders with heart failure (HF), advanced practice nurses (APNs) who were coordinating care in the transition from hospital to home could improve outcomes, prevent rehospitalizations, and reduce costs, when compared with usual care. The APN strategies focused on improving patient and family or caregiver effectiveness in managing their illnesses, strengthening the patient–provider relationship, and managing comorbid conditions while improving overall health. The results were positive. By capitalizing on the patient's desire to achieve their identified goals, APNs successfully educated patients about the meaning of their symptoms and appropriate self-management strategies; improved patient–provider communication patterns; and marshaled caregiver and community resources to maximize patient adherence to the treatment plan and overall quality of life. While HF was the primary reason for enrollment in the study, optimal health outcomes demanded a strong focus on integrating management of comorbid conditions and other long-standing health problems. Specific strategies used by the APN to achieve these positive outcomes are addressed in this report. These strategies are compared with nursing interventions used in other RCTs of HF home management. Directions for future research are explored (Disease Management, 2006).

Introduction

Research evaluating the problems elders face during transition from hospital to home has shown that elders are at increased risk for poor outcomes (including preventable rehospitalizations) because of ineffective self-management and poor interprovider and provider–patient communication.[1] Elders at highest risk for postdischarge problems include those with multiple chronic and comorbid conditions, disabling symptoms, highly complicated management protocols, and inadequate self-management skills.[2] A growing body of research has provided clear evidence that an advanced practice nurse (APN), who coordinates care collaboratively with the patient's healthcare team while the patient is hospitalized and during the immediate period postdischarge to home, will prevent complications and errors and improve outcomes while reducing the cost of care.[3–6]

A recently completed randomized controlled trial (RCT) from our team's program of transitional care research[6] showed that, for elders with heart failure (HF), the APN intervention was effective in increasing the length of time between hospital discharge and readmission or death, in reducing the number of readmissions, and in decreasing overall healthcare costs. Intervention patients also experienced some improvement in quality of life, physical function, and patient satisfaction. Similar reductions in rehospitalization rates were seen in our team's previous studies of patients with various medical conditions and patients who underwent surgical procedures, with shorter intervention times.[3,4] The most recent RCT was conducted because, for elders with HF, the positive effects of delayed or prevented rehospitalizations were not sustained beyond the 1-month intervention period.[4] By extending the length of time of the home care intervention to 3 months and recruiting APNs with significant HF expertise, we showed that this comprehensive, nurse-directed, collaborative, home-based management program improved outcomes for up to 52 weeks follow-up after an acute episode of HF.[6]

The original analysis of this research did not include detailed identification of the strategies that the APNs used with the 118 intervention patients to achieve these outcomes. The purpose of this chapter is to evaluate interventions used by APNs to improve patient or caregiver self-management skills, provider understanding of patient needs, and overall management of HF and comorbid conditions.

Methods

During the RCT, APNs followed a protocol that directed them to visit the hospitalized patient daily, collaborate with the patient's healthcare team and family to ensure optimum discharge planning, and visit the patient in the home within 24 hours of discharge, at least weekly for the first month and at least bimonthly for the next 2 months.[6] Patients and caregivers had telephone access to APNs between visits. APNs had complete flexibility to visit or phone the patient as often as needed to achieve care goals. Guided by national evidence-based practice guidelines available at the time, such as the 1994 heart failure guideline from the Agency for Health Care Policy and Researchs,[7] APNs focused on identifying and managing patients' unique needs related to HF and comorbid conditions. They wrote detailed progress notes describing patient assessment findings, problems and needs, provider interactions, and APN interventions. Summary case studies also were completed. APNs had access to experts in HF, pharmacology, and nutrition. They discussed challenging cases in bimonthly conferences attended by the domain expert of the issue to be discussed. Therefore, subject case summaries, notes from case conferences, APN summaries of major issues, and APN interviews comprised the data sources for this report. The authors were actively engaged in all aspects of this project, serving as the study principal investigator (M.D.N.); intervention APN (M.B.B.); and coinvestigator in charge of clinical protocol development and APN training and the case conference leader (K.M.M.).

Statistical Analysis

In the original RCT group, specific Kaplan-Meier survival curves and proportional hazards regression were used to assess group differences in rehospitalization rates and factors such as comorbid conditions that affected the number of rehospitalizations.[6]

Results

The analysis revealed that APN interventions focused on three domains: patient and family or caregiver effectiveness; the patient–provider relationship; and management of comorbid conditions and improving overall health. Although the primary focus of the study was management of HF, the majority of patients had multiple, active, comorbid conditions that complicated the HF and put them at risk for poor outcomes. APNs were particularly effective in reducing the number of rehospitalizations related to these comorbid conditions ($p < .013$).[6]

Patient and Family/Caregiver Advanced Practice Nurse Interventions

APN activities focused predominantly on individualized patient assessment, enhanced patient–provider communication, targeted interventions to improve self-management, and improved access to resources. Comprehensive assessment included identification of the patient's specific constellation of HF signs and symptoms and the contribution of any comorbid conditions to the patient's symptom profile. Sources and strength of social support were assessed, including the patients' caregiver networks, access to and use of services available for elders in the community, and access to transportation, supermarkets, pharmacies, and other services. The environmental safety assessment included risk for falls and neighborhood safety.

Patient education began with an assessment of knowledge base, learning capabilities, and learning styles. With up to 3 months to influence learning and behaviors, the APN was able to plan knowledge and skill development over time. APNs had the option of audiotaping patient education sessions and leaving the tape with the patient for later review. If patients did not have access to a tape recorder, one was provided, as was a digital scale to support monitoring of daily weight. Videotapes and pamphlets from recognized sources, such as the American Heart Association, were given to patients. The focus of education was on learning comprehension and behavioral change. To this end, all patients participated in the development of two management plans: their overall plan for managing their HF and comorbid conditions, and a "911 plan," which covered actions that should be taken if symptoms were to worsen. The goal was to educate patients in detecting subtle worsening of their specific symptoms and in intervening before emergency care were needed. Patients were taught how to access their physician, which physician to contact for which symptoms, and when and how to move quickly to receive emergency care.

Significant barriers to adherence and behavioral change were encountered. Although overt cognitive impairment made a patient ineligible for the study, more subtle cognitive changes interfered with some patients' learning. Other barriers included inadequate reading skills, poor visual acuity, lack of ability or interest in cooking with consequent eating at a restaurant or poor nutrition, and lack of access to medication. Nonadherence to medication regimens was related to the cost of medication, patient inability to leave home to go to a pharmacy, lack of pharmacy delivery systems, and lack of a system to organize medications with reminders to take them. An overarching barrier that affected self-management was some patients' lack of acceptance that they had chronic conditions. After patients felt better it was common for them to stop adhering to their management plan. APNs were instrumental in helping patients see connections between behavior and symptoms, such as taking diuretic medications as prescribed and improved exercise tolerance or increased sodium intake and worsening ankle edema.

Therefore, APNs used multiple strategies to improve patient self-management, including education about the chronic nature of the patient's illnesses; practical solutions, such as pill organizers and patient-specific prompts to remember to take them; and detailed nutrition counseling sessions with the patient or whoever does the cooking. The APNs took patients to grocery stores to teach them to read food labels and make healthier choices within their budget constraints, collected menus from local restaurants to teach patients to choose foods more wisely, and focused on helping patients see the relationship between worsening HF symptoms and recent food choices or nonadherence to medication regimens. Community resources such as Meals on Wheels and medication financing systems were used. Pharmacies that delivered were identified, and a relationship between the patient and a particular pharmacist was established. Patients were taught to identify signs and symptoms of improvement versus worsening HF and other illnesses. Based on the patient's specific situation, his or her management plan included a list of symptoms that could be managed with behavioral change, such as further salt and water restriction, and those that necessitated physician notification or even emergency care.

Because APNs worked out of home care agencies affiliated with the RCT, they had access to social workers, physical therapists, and psychiatric clinical nurse specialists for consultation about planning patient care and for patient referral, as needed.

Patient Goals as Key Motivator

The connection between symptoms and recent patient behaviors were made whenever possible, with the goal of enabling patients to gain control over their illness. This desire for control was strengthened by identification of the patient's goals. These goals became the primary motivator for behavioral change. The APNs determined from the patients what the patients wanted, what would bring them happiness, and used these goals to improve patient self-management. For example, one patient with HF, diabetes, and sleep apnea had not been off the second floor of her home in months; yet, she had a strong desire to go to church. The APN used this goal to enhance patient participation in diet management, medication adherence, and a gradual increase in walking endurance. Other patients wanted to avoid nursing home placement and become more functional within their own homes. Taking the focus from the APN and physician goals for the patient and helping the patient to see the connection between behavioral change and achieving his or her own goals proved to be the most powerful strategy used by the APNs.

Family and Community Resources

Subjects in this study came from poor inner city communities, wealthier suburbs, and isolated rural areas. Family and caregiver support ranged from highly involved, and sometimes overprotective, relatives to weak family support but a few caring neighbors. One patient required a weekly injection; however, nearby family members refused to learn how to administer the injection. The patient's insurance company denied coverage for home care nurses because the patient was not homebound and could theoretically travel to her physician's office for the injection. This plan, however, necessitated that the patient take two buses and proved exhausting. The APN was able to identify a neighbor who was willing to learn to administer the injection and the problem was resolved. Another patient whose wife had dementia had difficulty focusing on learning to manage his own problems because he was overwhelmed with his wife's care. The APN arranged for the wife to attend a community agency that provides day care for elders with dementia for several hours per week, which provided the patient with a needed respite. The APN timed his visits to coincide with times when the patient was relieved of caregiver responsibilities.

Strategies to Strengthen the Patient–Provider Relationship

For the RCT described herein, patients were recruited from six hospital sites and five home care agencies. Therefore, APNs needed to establish relationships with multiple physicians, most of whom had little experience with this particular APN role. Physician consultants were identified in each hospital and used to learn about the physician structures in place, for advice on establishing relationships with physicians, and to communicate the overall goals of the study. However, the APNs were responsible for educating individual physicians about the goals and benefits of the study and for establishing the relationships necessary to enhance patient care. This was most effectively accomplished by accompanying patients to their first postdischarge physician office visit. During this visit, the APNs learned about the physician's plan for the patient, demonstrated their ability to influence the patient in participating more effectively as a partner in management, and coached the patient to communicate more effectively with the physician. APN communication during this visit was effective in establishing the partnership between the patient, the physician, and the APN.

Several challenges emerged. APNs worked with patients who made conscious decisions not to take medications as prescribed (e.g., reducing diuretic doses or skipping doses on days when an activity was planned) and who refused to share this information with the physician. APNs guided patients in understanding how they would benefit from a management plan based on best practice and open communication that considered their individual needs. They coached patients to communicate their needs and actions to the physician and they worked with physicians to develop greater insight into the broader needs of patients and become more flexible and creative in management strategies. Sometimes the treatment regimen caused worsening of symptoms (e.g., initiation of carvedilol) and increased risk for rehospitalization. APNs and physicians collaborated by increasing the frequency of APN home visits to monitor and support patients and by identifying a plan for managing worsening symptoms. The authors of this chapter discussed these challenges during case conferences and sought the opinion of relevant experts. Ultimately, the authors found that this experienced group of APNs possessed the knowledge and skill to work effectively and enhance patient and provider communication. With rare exceptions, APNs found physicians to be superb partners in care. The physicians quickly realized that with APN support difficult patient management problems had potential for resolution.

Management of Comorbid Conditions and Improving Overall Health

The challenges presented by the patients' comorbid conditions and the need to improve overall health outcomes emerged as the third domain of this analysis because, although the study was begun to improve outcomes in HF, it was quickly learned that elders must manage HF within the context of other illnesses and health problems. Many patients with HF also had diabetes, chronic lung disease, atrial fibrillation, or arthritis. APNs worked closely with patients and their caregivers to identify the meaning of symptoms, and they became close partners with physicians in identifying optimum treatment strategies. For example, APNs helped patients who had HF and chronic lung disease become more adherent in their use of prescribed inhalers and used physical assessment skills to sort out the contribution of HF versus lung disease in interpreting worsening shortness of breath. Diabetes patients faced enormous challenges in managing the complexities of a diet that addressed both health problems. APNs helped patients use diet diaries to track food intake, taught them to make better choices within their food preferences, and enabled them to see the connections between what they ate and drank and their symptoms and blood glucose levels. By accompanying the patient to select physician office visits, they coached the patient in communicating progress, needs, and preferences and partnered with the physician in enabling the treatment plan to become part of the patient's lifestyle.

Problems with substance abuse emerged as a significant health concern. Excessive alcohol intake, continued smoking, and long-standing use of prescribed antianxiety and narcotic pain agents contributed to patient symptoms and interfered with achieving optimal function. Many times, neither the patient nor the physician understood why the patient was taking antianxiety or narcotic agents. Evaluating the cause and influence of symptoms of depression was complicated by use of these agents. APNs were effective at working with physicians and patients to reduce dosages gradually or to discontinue the drug and initiate the use of antidepressant agents, if necessary.

The study showed that many patients' functional status was hampered by long-standing effects of deconditioning owing to poor exercise habits that now were exacerbated by HF symptoms and the effects of aging. Improving functional status and exercise performance became a goal for most patients. APNs were able to help patients see that enhanced function was related to achieving many of their goals. In collaboration with the patients' physicians, the study authors were able to refer some patients to outpatient cardiac rehabilitation programs; however, for most patients, gradually increasing walking and other muscle strengthening exercises in the home became the primary focus.

Discussion

This analysis revealed that APN effectiveness may be related to their knowing their patients as individuals, developing an understanding of how patient goals will motivate them to learn to care for themselves more effectively and to persist in effective self-management over time, and improving patient–provider communication. It became clear that the strength of the intervention lay in the APN's attention to all the physical, psychosocial, and financial problems these frail patients face. Their holistic approach considered the interconnectedness of problems and the need for a collaborative, individualized management approach that capitalized on and strengthened patient capabilities and support systems. Research has increasingly shown the positive effect of nursing interventions on patient outcome and resource use during the transition from hospital to home. The outcomes and nursing interventions of several of these RCTs in HF are described in Table 9.5.1. Common themes include a strong focus on patient education, symptom identification, and promotion of adherence to the treatment plan.

In previous publications this research team described APN interventions using content analysis of APN documentation of subjects with a wide range of medical and surgical conditions,[8] an overview of medical and nursing care of patients with HF,[9] case study reports of patients with HF,[10] and an overview of the transitional care model as applied across the entire author program of research.[11] Davidson and colleagues recently published a narrative analysis of clinical notes of nurses caring for patients with HF in the home.[12] They identified seven strategies, including symptom monitoring, enhancing patient self-management, collaborating with health professionals to manage clinical deterioration, helping patients avoid institutionalization, dealing with psychologic problems, and helping patients and families cope with dying. The interventions described in these reports and the interventions noted in the RCTs described in Table 9.5.1 are congruent.

In the analysis described herein, the study authors identified other strategies that might account for the successful outcomes and warrant evaluation in future research. First, identification of the patients' unique goals and connecting achievement of these goals to health-related behaviors proved to be a powerful force in gaining patient and caregiver partnership in sustained behavioral change. Second, the APNs worked actively to gain the support of the patient physicians as partners in designing the optimum treatment plan and as partners with patients in sustained behavioral change. Research that shows effective strategies in establishing ongoing physician–patient partnerships is necessary. Some of the educational strategies used (e.g., supermarket visits to teach label reading and healthy food choices, giving patients audiotapes of the teaching session) warrant further investigation and may influence future educational programs. The three domains of APN influence described herein (i.e.. patient and family or caregiver effectiveness; the patient–provider relationship; management of comorbid conditions and improving overall health) may provide a useful framework for future research designed to improve patient outcomes and identify the specific nursing interventions responsible for those outcomes.

This author team is extending this research in two important directions. They have been funded by the National Institute of Aging and the Ware Family Foundation to test the transitional care model among elders with cognitive impairment. This funding builds on previous funding from the Alzheimer's Association that enabled these authors to design and pilot test a cognitive impairment management protocol. Secondly, the authors of this study are collaborating with several national insurance companies to translate this model into the real world of managed health care. The combined effect of these efforts will be to test strategies for effective, collaborative management of the most vulnerable elders in a real-world practice setting.

This chapter summarizes the interventions of APNs in optimizing health outcomes of high-risk elders in a cost-effective manner. The problems these patients face test the creativity and knowledge base of highly experienced APNs. It remains to be shown whether appropriately prepared nurses without graduate nursing education could achieve similar outcomes. The authors' current program of research promises to provide insight into this question.

TABLE 9.5.1 Randomized Clinical Trials Testing Nursing Interventions in Heart Failure (HF) Patients' Transition From Hospital to Home

Reference/Design/ Participants	Intervention	Outcome	Specific Nurse Interventions
Rich et al., 1995[13] RCT testing a nurse-directed multidisciplinary intervention for high-risk elders (= 70 years) hospitalized with HF. Intervention group $n = 142$, control group $n = 140$. Control patients received all standard care and services ordered by their physicians. Patients were followed up for 90 days after discharge. Quality of life was assessed at baseline and 3 months in 126 patients.	Experienced cardiovascular research nurse implemented program of intensive HF education, use of a teaching booklet, patient consultation with dietician and social worker, medication analysis by gerontology cardiologist to eliminate unnecessary medications/simplify regimen, routine home care plus visits by study specialists.	For subjects who survived initial hospitalization, improved survival rates were seen in the intervention group (66.9% vs. 54.3%, $p = .04$), fewer single ($p = .03$) and multiple ($p = .01$) readmissions, total readmissions ($p = .02$) and readmissions for HF ($p = .04$) were seen. Quality of life improved for both groups but significantly more for the intervention group ($p = .001$). Rate of readmission was significantly higher in the control group ($p = .03$).	Focus of intervention: • Reinforce patient education, ensure compliance with medications and diet • Identify recurrent symptoms that should be treated during outpatient care • Simplifying regimen and ensuring compliance
Stewart et al., 1998[14] RCT testing the effect of an HBI on readmission and death rates in high-risk HF patients discharged after HF admission. Intervention $n = 49$, usual care $n = 48$. Subjects were followed up for outcome measures for 6 months.	Inpatient visit by study nurse for education about treatment regimen, importance of compliance, and reporting symptoms. One-week after discharge, visit by study nurse and pharmacist for knowledge and compliance assessment and targeted education. Communication with patient primary physician regarding patient progress, needs, and ongoing plan.	HBI group: fewer unplanned readmissions ($\geq .03$), fewer total days of hospitalization ($p = .05$), fewer multiple (= 3) readmissions ($p = .02$), fewer emergency department visits ($p = .05$). Cost of hospital care was lower in HBI group but not statistically significant.	Educational focus: • Remedial counseling • Reminder systems to ensure medication compliance • Use of weekly medication dosage systems • Improved caregiver monitoring • Medication information and reminder cards • Referral to community pharmacist for ongoing education/support • Referral to physician if clinical deterioration
Jaarsma et al., 1999[15] RCT testing of educational program for elders with HF during hospital stay and at home 1-week after discharge on self-care behaviors and resource use. Intervention $n = 84$, control $n = 95$. Subjects were followed up for 9 months for outcome measurements.	Inpatient visit by study nurse for education about consequences of HF in daily life. Standard nursing care plan used. One-week after discharge, visit by study nurse for ongoing education. Intervention duration: hospital admission to 10 days after discharge	Both groups' self-care behaviors improved at 1 month over baseline ($p < .001$) but greater improvement seen in intervention ($p = .001$). Both groups decreased self-care behaviors over time but greater compliance at 3 months ($p = .005$) and between baseline and 9 months ($p < .001$) in intervention.	Educational topics: • Warning symptoms of worsening HF, sodium restriction, fluid balance, compliance. • Patient's individualized problems addressed. • Family/caregiver included. • Nurse available by telephone between hospital discharge and home visit; patient advised to call physician after that.

TABLE 9.5.1 *(continued)*

Reference/Design/Participants	Intervention	Outcome	Specific nurse interventions
Harrison et al., 2002[16] RCT testing a 12-week nurse-led intervention using a structured protocol compared with usual home care. Intervention n = 92, usual care n = 100. Outcomes measured at baseline, 2, 6, and 12 weeks.	The same hospital and home care nurses delivered care to both groups. Intervention patients received care via structured protocol emphasizing transitional care and self-management. Usual care patients received assessment, monitoring, health teaching, and direct care from home care nurses.	Improved MLHFQ total scores for transitional care intervention group at 6 weeks (p = .002) and 12 weeks (p < .001) Improved physical dimension at 6 weeks (p = .001) and 12 weeks (p < 0.001) Improved emotional dimension at 6 weeks (p = .006). Intervention patients had fewer emergency department visits (p = .003).	In addition to usual discharge planning and care, intervention patients received an evidence-based, structured protocol that guided supportive care, education for self management, linkages between hospital, home care nurses, patients, families, and providers. Also provided a patient workbook, an educational workbook, an educational map/plan and a patient documentation tool
Riegel et al., 2002[17] RCT testing the effect of a 6-month telephonic case management intervention about hospital readmissions and cost. Intervention n = 130, usual care n = 228. Outcomes measured at 3 and 6 months.	Registered nurse telephonic case management using a decision support software program (Pfizer, Inc.) that emphasized management of factors predicting rehospitalization and guided education, data collection, and documentation; organized clinical information and included evidence-based guidelines. Mean number of phone calls = 17.	HF hospitalization rates were 45.7% lower in intervention group at 3 months (p = .03) and 47.8% at 6 months (p = .01). All-cause hospitalization rates were 25.6% lower at 3 months and 28.2% lower at 6 months (p = .03). Improved patient satisfaction at 6 months (p = .01).	Intervention patients contacted by phone within 5 days of discharge. Software program directed future calls based on patient symptoms, needs and knowledge. Nurses spoke with family members, physicians, and other professionals; sent updated reports and treatment guidelines to physicians; mailed patients educational materials.
Stewart and Horowitz, 2002[18] RCT of multidisciplinary HBI. Intervention n = 149, usual care n = 148, followed up for median of 4.2 years.	After an admission for acute HF, individuals in HBI group received structured home visit by pharmacist or nurse within 7–14 days after discharge. Some patients received repeated home visits and some patients received additional education about their condition.	Intervention subjects: • 30% reduction in readmission or death (p < .01) • Increased probability of remaining event free (p < .05). Greatest effect on preventing readmission occurred in first 6 months (p < .001), no difference in 6–24 months but significant (p < .05) effects thereafter. Reduced cost of readmissions (p < .01), compared with usual care.	Structured home visit to optimize management of illnesses and to facilitate rapid recognition and treatment of health problems Physical examination Assessment of patient adherence to treatment plan Adequacy of social support Identification of factors likely to produce readmission or death Report with recommendations to patient's physician Nurse coordination of management

Note: HBI = Home-based intervention; HF = heart failure; MLHFQ = Minnesota Living with Heart Failure questionnaire; RCT = randomized controlled trial.

Acknowledgments

This work was supported by the National Institute of Nursing Research, Department of Health and Human Services, Public Health Service (research grant 5-R01-NR-04315 to M. D. N.). This work was presented in abstract form at the 58th Annual Scientific Meeting of the Gerontological Society of America, November 21, 2005, Orlando, Florida.

REFERENCES

1. Naylor MD. Transitional care of older adults. Annu Rev Nurs Res 2003;20:127–147.
2. Happ MB, Naylor MD, Roe-Prior P. Factors contributing to rehospitalization of elderly patients with heart failure. J Cardiovasc Nurs 1997;11:75–84.
3. Naylor M, Brooten D, Jones R, Lavizzo-Mourey R, Mezey M, Pauly M. Comprehensive discharge planning for the hospitalized elderly. A randomized clinical trial. Ann Intern Med 1994;120:999–1006.
4. Naylor MD, Brooten D, Campbell R, et al. Comprehensive discharge planning and home follow up of hospitalized elderly: a randomized clinical trial. JAMA 1999;281:613–620.
5. Naylor MD, McCauley KM. The effects of a discharge planning and home follow-up intervention on elders hospitalized with common medical and surgical cardiac conditions. J Cardiovasc Nurs 1999;14:44–54.
6. Naylor MD, Brooten DA, Campbell RL, Maislin G, McCauley KM, Schwartz JS. Transitional care of older adults hospitalized with heart failure: a randomized, controlled trial. J Am Geriatr Soc 2004;52:675–684. [Erratum in J Am Geriatr Soc 2004;52:1228.]
7. Konstarn MA, Dracup K, Baker DW, et al. Heart failure: evaluation and care of patients with left-ventricular systolic dysfunction. Clinical practice guideline, no. 11. (AHCPR publication no. 94–0612). Rockville, MD: U.S. Department of Health and Human Services, Agency for Health Care Policy and Research, Public Health Service.
8. Naylor MD, Bowles KH, Brooten D. Patient problems and advanced practice nurse interventions during transitional care. Public Health Nurs 2000;12:94–102.
9. Campbell RL, Banner R, Konick-McMahon J, Naylor MD. Discharge planning and home follow-up of the elderly patient with heart failure. Nurs Clin North Am 1998;33:497–513.
10. Bixby MB, Konick-McMahon J, McKenna CG. Applying the transitional care model to elderly patients with heart failure. J Cardiovasc Nurs 2000;14:53–63.
11. Naylor MD. A decade of transitional care research with vulnerable elders. J Cardiovasc Nurs 2000;14:1–14.
12. Davidson P, Paull G, Rees D, Daly J, Cockburn J. Activities of home-based heart failure nurse specialists: a modified narrative analysis. Am J Crit Care 2005;14: 426–433.
13. Rich MW, Beckham V, Wittenberg C, Leven CL, Freedland KE, Carney RM. A multidisciplinary intervention to prevent the readmission of elderly patients with congestive heart failure. N Engl J Med 1995;333:1190–1195.
14. Stewart S, Pearson S, Horowitz JD. Effects of a home-based intervention among patients with congestive heart failure discharged from acute hospital care. Arch Intern Med 1998;158: 1067–1072.
15. Jaarsma T, Halfens R, Huijer Abu-Saad H, et al. Effects of education and support on self-care and resource utilization in patients with heart failure. Eur Heart J 1999;20:673–682.
16. Harrison MB, Browne GB, Roberts J, Tugwell P, Gafni A, Graham ID. Quality of life of individuals with heart failure: a randomized trial of the effectiveness of two models of hospital-to-home transition. Med Care 2002;40:271–282.
17. Riegel B, Carlson B, Kopp Z, LePetri B, Glaser D, Unger A. Effect of a standardized nurse case-management telephone intervention on resource use in patients with chronic heart failure. Arch Intern Med 2002;162:705–712.
18. Stewart S, Horowitz JD. Home-based intervention in congestive heart failure: long-term implications on readmission and survival. Circulation 2002;105:2861–2866.

Reprinted with permission from: McCauley, K., Bixby, M. B., & Naylor, M. D. (2006). Advanced practice nurse strategies to improve outcomes and reduce cost in elders with heart failure. *Disease Management*, 9(5), 302–310.

Chapter 10 Role Supplementation Models

10.1 PREVENTIVE ROLE SUPPLEMENTATION: A GROUNDED CONCEPTUAL FRAMEWORK

AFAF I. MELEIS
LESLEE SWENDSEN
DELORAS JONES

Abstract

One of the major issues confronting nursing today is whether nursing will survive the many turmoils with which it is beset. Questions raised around the profession of nursing continue. What are the goals of nursing? Does nursing possess a body of knowledge? How different is that body of knowledge from that of other health professions? Is what nursing offers unique? Although we will not and could not possibly answer these questions in this chapter, we will demonstrate an aspect of a systematic body of knowledge in nursing. A conceptual framework with potential for focused research in nursing has been operationalized and implemented in a clinical situation. The conceptual framework was reported theoretically (Meleis, 1975) and empirically (Meleis & Swendsen, 1978; Swendsen, Meleis, & Jones, 1978). This chapter presents all parts of the framework clinically. Other clinical situations could use the framework.

The major assumption here is that conceptual frameworks offer structure for nursing knowledge. Without such frameworks, knowledge of various phenomena cannot be interrelated and fractions of knowledge may be isolated and, most likely, lost. Thus, an integrative framework is essential to the development of a body of knowledge encompassing theory, practice, and research.

Chin (1962) views models as an orientation to practice, to be used for diagnosis and treatment (or assessment and interventions). Even though many practitioners question the utility of a model for practice, Chin maintains that no one can observe without a preconceived notion of the elements to be observed and how those elements can be interpreted. Such preconceived notions, when systematized, are referred to as *conceptual models*. Inkles (1964) maintains that a scientist needs a mental image of how a realm is "put together and how it works." Without such preconceived images, a scientist could not raise appropriate questions.

Models are essential for practitioners in diagnosing and treating (assessment and intervention), for teachers in classifying phenomena, and finally, for researchers in asking and interpreting questions and establishing a "foundation for continuing development of relevant research and significant utilizations of investigatory findings" (Rogers, 1970). We will show how a conceptual framework can suggest and help structure a particular nursing intervention. Although many practicing nurses shrug away the notion of using nursing models, the mere fact that they observe, assess, intervene, and ask questions evidences the fact that they are guided by "a mental image." Public health nurses and maternal-child health nurses, for example, are often involved in preventive role supplementation, although their work may not have been conceptually organized to provide a framework for nursing intervention and research. This presentation is rooted in the conviction that nursing practice must flow from theory and substantive knowledge.

In the course of a lifetime, an individual undergoes many transitions that entail extensive mobilization of personal resources to cope with resulting stresses. Therefore, the loss of some roles and the acquisition of new ones are of particular significance to nurses. The developmental stages of a life cycle, along with health and illness, are the occasions for a number of important role changes. To demonstrate preventive role supplementation (Meleis, 1975), a number of couples expecting their first child were chosen. As will become apparent, many other types of clients, such as chronically ill patients, parents of a handicapped child, mastectomy patients, and others could also benefit from role supplementation.

LeMasters (1969), in his study of middle-class couples, confirmed that the birth of a first child constitutes a crisis event, and that most couples find the transition to parenthood difficult. This finding was confirmed by Dyer (1969), who said a majority of the couples he studied experienced extensive or severe crisis. The conflict aspects of adaptation to early parenthood and the association with severe stress have been described by many (James & Benedick, 1970; Sheresfsky & Yarrow, 1974).

During crisis, the normal coping mechanisms of individuals are inadequate. In this study, the nurse clinicians used preventive role supplementation to augment the expectant parents' adaptive capacity during the transitional crisis. Whether transitions are viewed as mere developmental stages or as crisis periods would not affect the proposed framework. It is assumed that the situation of the unit of study (be it a family or group) will determine whether a crisis model or a transition model is more suitable. Because preventive role supplementation is an interactional conceptual framework, the perspective of the clients will help determine the most appropriate content included.

The conceptual basis of nursing intervention discussed in this chapter is that of preventive role supplementation as proposed by Meleis (1975). It is defined as "the information or experience necessary to bring the role incumbent and significant others to full awareness of the anticipated behavior patterns, units, sentiments, sensations, and goals involved in each role and its complement" (Meleis, 1975). Preventive role supplementation may be a means to achieve role mastery for the novice who is to acquire and master the appropriate behaviors and sentiments by learning: (a) the behaviors that are expected, (a) the sentiments and goals appropriate to the role, and (c) the costs and rewards to be anticipated, including whether or not significant others provide negative or positive reinforcement. Preventive role supplementation can be a way in which significant others clarify roles for persons *anticipating* transition, and through which the individual can master the anticipated transition by means of role rehearsal and role modeling.

The goal of the preventive role supplementation program (ROSP) (ROSP is the acronym used to refer to the preventive role supplementation program as outlined by Meleis [1975]) is to prevent the development of *role insufficiency*. Role insufficiency is defined by Meleis (1975, p. 266) as behavior that indicates "...any felt disparity in fulfilling role obligations or expectations of significant others' roles in a health-illness situation. It denotes the incongruency of the self-concept and the role anticipations of others." Further, role insufficiency characterizes an ego confronted with expectations that it cannot articulate.

Concept of Role

A *role* is a set of behaviors or expected behaviors, as well as a sentiment or goal that provides unity to a set of potential actions (Turner, 1962). More recently, Turner (1967) has suggested:

> In any interactive situation, behavior, sentiments, and motives tend to be differentiated into units, which can be called roles; once roles are differentiated, elements of behavior, sentiments, and motives which appear in the same situation tend to be assigned to the existing roles.

Thus, role, as used in the development and conceptualization of role supplementation, will be based on the symbolic interactionist use of the concept (Morris, 1934). Role in this sense is conceptualized as a way of coping with an imputed other role (Cottrell, 1942; Turner, 1967).

Components of ROSP

In this section, each component of ROSP, as outlined by Meleis (1975), is presented as a concept, followed by a discussion of an implementation program with expectant parents and examples drawn from actual experience with the program. It must be emphasized that a "viable role supplementation program should capitalize on the importance of a significant other and/or others in reinforcing new roles and counter roles" (Meleis, 1975).

The program was developed within the, "context of an appropriately designated reference group involving the self and appropriate significant others" (Meleis, 1975). On this basis, 12 couples expecting their first child were invited to participate in ROSP. Their ages ranged from 19 to 32 years. Their ethnic backgrounds included White, Black, Oriental, and Spanish American. Their education ranged from high school to postgraduate. They included blue-collar workers and professionals, working and nonworking mothers, and those who planned their pregnancies, as well as those who did not. The members held varied opinions and interest in natural childbirth. They were divided into two groups. Starting around the beginning of the third trimester, each group attended 2-hour group meetings each week for 8 weeks.

Because roles develop in pairs to complement each other, it was essential to include both wives and husbands in the group meetings and in the individual family sessions with the nurse clinician. Therefore, only couples in which both husbands and wives could attend most of the sessions were invited to take part.

The content and the process of ROSP were derived directly from the conceptual framework mentioned previously. The components are discussed next.

Communication and interaction are central concepts in the symbolic interactionist school, and are "...important components of role supplementation, because it is through open and clear communication of symbols that roles evolve" (Meleis, 1975).

Interaction was emphasized as the means whereby feelings were explored, uncertainties were discussed, information was gathered, and expectations about the parental role were aired. The interaction occurred among and between all the couples, between the couples and the nurse clinicians, and between the individual husbands and wives. Open communication was encouraged as the basis for incorporating the various components of role supplementation in the program as it functioned.

Planning and Implementing of Role Supplementation

Reference Groups

The *reference group* is a group whose viewpoint is used as a frame of reference. Reference groups are essential in providing the means by which a person's identity is formed. In such groups, alternative ways of coping with life changes and divergent viewpoints are explored, discussed, and, through a reflective process, adopted or discarded. In this environment, positive and negative reinforcements are provided for an individual's values and beliefs. Through reference groups, an individual can identify the range of normal behavior in a certain role and ascertain his or her position on the continuum.

Each preventive role supplementation reference group should be organized with individuals of similar developmental stages, even though these same individuals may exhibit a wide range of perspectives. Reference groups in cultures are formed informally, but because of the many social variables in this society (numerous subcultures, lateral and vertical mobility, residential mobilities, and alienation and apathy), there is a need to consciously and formally organize appropriate reference groups.

Aside from the many sociological and educational advantages of reference groups cited in the literature, a reference group has the advantage of providing a social function for its incumbents. It also is easier to change behaviors in a group setting than in an individual setting. Group members can reinforce, clarify, and support one another during the transition process.

The reference groups are a major component of ROSP. In this program, reference groups serve as forums for obtaining knowledge and exploring alternatives so that clients will have a basis for formulating their own decisions. Several couples said they joined the program to find out whether their own values, attitudes, and feelings were similar or dissimilar to those of other couples in the same situation. Many felt the need to verify the normalcy of their experience. Several prospective fathers suggested the establishment of a father's reference group to focus on paternal feelings and concerns. Most couples wished to continue to meet after delivery.

The weekly meeting provided opportunities to talk and work out feelings and plans about pregnancy, labor, delivery, and parenting. Members discussed their feelings about the pregnancy, their physical complaints, emotional changes, fears for the baby and themselves, and resulting changes in lifestyle. The women were relieved to find that other mothers had the same complaints. After they learned to understand the physiological basis for many of their problems, they shared suggestions for relieving discomforts. They were reassured that their mood changes were normal when they heard of similar experiences from other members of the group and expressed relief to find that others had the same concerns. They shared ideas about reasons for fears and coping mechanisms. Many expressed apprehension about labor and delivery and the anticipated pain.

Another major area of concern and topic of discussion was the father's presence during labor and delivery. Alternative father roles were presented by both the group leaders and the parents. Much of the discussion centered on this controversial area and formed the basis for what evolved as *this* group's standard of behavior and expectations about the father's role during labor and delivery. His presence was expected, although he might or might not be responsible for pain control through coaching. Feelings about the father's role in labor coaching varied among the couples. A feeling of helplessness was expressed in the beginning, but after discussion, most expectant fathers clarified the roles with which they were most comfortable. Some even said they had already discussed with other expectant fathers their notions of what to expect and what their role toward their wives could be. Many said their coworkers expressed astonishment and even some ridicule that they chose to be with their wives in labor and delivery. These men were relieved to find support in the reference group. One father did not perceive his role to be with his wife during labor and delivery, but he hesitated to express this in the group meetings. He preferred to share and discuss his concerns with the nurse clinician, whom he saw as a significant other. The reference group helped this father to become aware of some of his concerns and of his need to clarify them with the help of a significant other. He did not feel pressure to conform to the standard of the reference group; he was already an accepted group member.

The reference groups provided a forum for sharing concerns about parenthood and an opportunity to explore alternative parenting styles. One of the most important functions of the reference group was to help new parents develop ongoing cooperative relationships for future reference. After the weekly classes had ended and each couple had delivered, many called each other to report the birth and to exchange information and ask questions. Mothers who delivered earliest gave anticipatory guidance to those whose babies came later. Soon they called each other to confer about questions that arose. Many said they received support from other couples in making decisions about infant care.

Significant Others

Roles are formed and imputed through a process of definition and redefinition in interaction with significant others. The responses of significant others are important to the self-concept and for the support an individual needs. The support of significant others is highly important in judging and reducing the anxiety of an incumbent. Some significant others may already be intimately related to the role incumbent, whereas others may become influential in the course of role assumption, such as nurses, teachers, priests, and social workers.

ROSP was designed to allow each client family an opportunity to confer with an expert clinician who could become a significant other and provide support during the role-transition process.

The nurse clinician helped the families explore many viewpoints, alternatives, and possible consequences of decisions they had to make, but ultimately left the responsibility for the final decision to the family. The nurse clinician's role was not only to offer alternatives, but also to help each family feel more confident of its ability to make decisions and to orient it to the health care system. One couple said they had decided to take their 7-day-old baby shopping. The mother said they were confident in making the decision based on the knowledge she had gained learning the problem-solving approach. She said, "I didn't feel I had to read a book or that I had to call anyone to ask if it was all right to take my baby out. I felt we could decide that for ourselves and that felt good." They had received reinforcement of their ability to solve problems systematically from significant others. This confidence helped them approach other significant decisions. In discussing the shopping incident with the nurse clinician (her significant other), this mother was seeking reassurance about her problem-solving and parenting abilities.

The nurse clinician also served as a source of technical assistance. Many of the expectant mothers "did not want to bother a physician with their questions or concerns," and were more comfortable discussing their concerns with the nurse clinicians. These transactions often took place during the group meetings, although such discussions also occurred during prenatal home visits and in the course of client-initiated telephone calls to the nurse clinicians.

The first postpartum visit, scheduled within 24 hours after delivery, offered the couples an opportunity to discuss in detail their recent labor and delivery experience with the nurse clinician. Sharing a birth experience with a significant person seems to be a most important step. It was observed that all couples must describe the birth experience before they can focus on the next developmental stage of parenthood, such as infant care, plans for hospital discharge, and so forth.

At each subsequent postpartum visit, the parents sought reassurance about their infant care techniques by asking questions or by describing what they had done.

Role Taking

Role taking is a key concept in the symbolic interactionist theory of George Herbert Mead (Morris, 1934). The individual plans and enacts his or her role by vicariously assuming the role of another. As Turner (1970) indicates, individuals learn roles in pairs and not in isolation.

Role taking is defined as "imaginatively assuming the position or point of view of another person" (Lindesmith & Strauss, 1956). Thus, in order to develop any form of cooperative activity, each individual must have the ability to take on the role of another. The incorporation of a role-taking component in the ROSP is based on the assumption that (Meleis, 1975):

> Effective role transition is theoretically less difficult for persons who have learned to enact a role and counter role imaginatively and if the other understands the salient components of the transitions as they involve each of them.

Couples were introduced to the different behaviors and feelings of the roles and the counter roles they would encounter during the transitional period. Even though roles might (and most probably would) be modified in the course of actual interaction, the salient features of roles unique to each couple could be anticipated, constructed, and communicated before the actual transition was to occur.

Successful transition to the parental role depends on sensitivity and awareness of the feelings and behavior of each spouse. The importance of open communication between the two was emphasized as essential to the role-taking process, and the significance of role-taking ability was explored.

The group members explored potential changes in the mother's mood as a result of physiological changes associated with pregnancy, and of emotional responses to her anticipated role changes. The father was encouraged to acknowledge and understand these changes so that he might become more sensitive to her needs.

Similar changes were anticipated in the behavior of prospective fathers with stresses unique to fatherhood. At first, some fathers were reluctant to share such feelings in the group setting; however, they did so before the series of group meetings was over.

Various incidents that might be stressful to the new parents were explored. Alternative approaches to coping and their effect on interactions in the family were discussed and explored. Several other anticipated situations were discussed in the reference group, including postpartum depression. The couples were encouraged to attempt to role take the feelings of the spouse, especially when they observed behaviors indicating stress in the other, and to be supportive in an attempt to alleviate the stress. As a result of the emphasis on role taking, many fathers took on tasks they had not done before, such as grocery shopping, cooking, dishwashing, and house cleaning. Husbands took turns getting up with the baby during the night. One husband offered his wife frequent back rubs—something he had not done previous to the delivery. Some wives noticed signs of stress in their husbands and discussed with them their feelings and concerns about having to work as well as adapting to the new baby. Some husbands offered to care for the baby occasionally during the first three weeks after delivery so that their wives could leave the house to visit friends or go shopping. Couples' frequent use of role taking to empathize with and assist the spouse was one of the most rewarding aspects of the program for the participants.

Both parents were encouraged to "role try out" the experience of the newborn baby to anticipate some of his needs. They were helped to become aware of the baby's intrauterine life, security, feeding, environment, position, and experience through labor and delivery. Using this as a guide, they could anticipate and plan for the baby's needs, their own counter needs, and probable coping mechanisms.

Role Clarification

Role clarification is the identification of role-linked behaviors, sentiments, and goals associated with a role vis-à-vis significant others in the context of particular situations. As was indicated earlier, in the course of a lifetime a person must discard old roles, assume new ones, and modify existing roles or simultaneously manage several roles involving incompatible demands. Furthermore, "One develops competency in a role as one acquires the knowledge and resources to carry out that role" (Shaw, 1974).

The nurse helped the parents during pregnancy to understand better their roles as expectant parents by helping them identify and become aware of their feelings and thoughts and the significance of these feelings and thoughts in shaping behavior. During group sessions, the nurses and couples discussed their experiences during pregnancy and how these were similar to or different from the way they expected pregnancy to be. The role of both the husband and wife in labor and delivery were explored. The nurses guided the couples through the process, encouraging them to think about what would be happening to the wife, then how her husband, as her significant other, might best support and assist her. The explorations and sharing included his role behaviors (such as giving her a back rub or wiping her face with a wet washcloth) and their meaning to his wife. The husbands were especially encouraged to experience their wives' roles in an attempt to heighten their awareness of what the wives were to experience and how the fathers might complement this experience.

Besides discussing feelings and expectations, role clarification was enhanced when the group leaders shared knowledge about physiological changes in the mother and fetus during pregnancy, thereby providing a rationale and prognosis for the discomforts the mothers were having. Further clarification of present and anticipated role behavior called for information on the processes of labor and delivery. Further, along with prenatal experiences and breathing techniques for labor and delivery, analgesia and anesthesia were explained. A film showing a couple's labor and delivery, a tour of the hospital, and slides showing characteristics of the newborn helped provide information for role clarification. Although such information has always been part of prenatal classes, the reason for including it in this program was derived from the framework under discussion. The information and exploration of role expectations and feelings gave each couple an opportunity to anticipate more appropriately the transition to a parental role.

Couples were most concerned about infant care behaviors. Most had never held a baby, and their anxiety was evident in their repeated questions about how to pick up a baby, feed him, bathe him, and change his diaper. The nurses demonstrated these actions during the group sessions, and explained that all couples would have rooming-in in the hospital so that the father and mother could learn these activities with their own infant under the direction of the nursing staff. After the rooming-in experience and the postpartum home visit by the nurse, all couples said that they felt confident. Nevertheless, their initial hesitancy, before rooming-in, about whether they would be able to care adequately for the infant led us to believe that some role rehearsal with a doll helped relieve some anxiety.

In addition to infant care, the group members discussed the changes a baby might bring about in their lives. Each mother and father attempted to identify changes that they expected in lifestyle and to discuss how they would adapt to these changes. Most couples talked about their social activities outside of the home; they discussed how they would have to plan to take the baby with them or find a baby sitter. Finding a baby sitter would require more planning ahead than many were used to. Group members also discussed anticipated changes in sleeping patterns with night feedings and crying periods. The discussions centered on feelings they might anticipate as parents of a newborn. They discussed anger, resentment of the infant, guilt, joy, and happiness. This was an attempt to clarify the range of emotions new parents have and to demonstrate that these were considered to be "normal."

Postpartum depression, its manifestations, some possible causes, the length of time, and prognosis were identified. After one such discussion, a husband asked whether or not a similar depression might be encountered by prospective fathers. A discussion was then aimed at clarifying behaviors, sentiments, and potential role changes of new fathers.

A major portion of the program dealt with expectations one has of self as a parent. Members of the group identified their own notions of good and bad parenting and behaviors and feelings associated with each. They then compared their expectations of themselves with identified criteria. Thus, in addition to role identification, couples also identified counter-role expectations. The discussion centered on the idea that each expected his or her spouse to be what he or she considered to be a good parent. The prospective parents were especially concerned about the way their spouses might discipline a child. One mother said she was concerned that her expectations of her husband were unrealistic when she saw him discipline his niece during a recent visit. She felt he might be a stricter disciplinarian than she had expected or believed necessary. She said that they needed to discuss their views, and this discussion led later to clarification with each other.

One mother phoned four days after hospital discharge to ask that the nurse help her husband cope with his feelings after he had become angry with the baby for crying incessantly the night before. He felt extremely guilty about his anger. When the nurse arrived, he said, "I now realize that I was angry at myself for my inability to comfort him in his distress. The guilt was so heavy I didn't realize that I could become so angry at my helpless little son whom I love so much." The discussion went on from there and enabled the father to see his feelings of guilt in proper perspective as a part of the range of feelings parents experience.

The example just discussed demonstrates the need for follow-up home care on an individual basis to fully implement ROSP, especially when the follow up is designed to alleviate a crisis. The example also illustrates the importance of such intervention in enabling the individual to resume an adult role with minimal disruption after a crisis. Unless the client is able to work through feelings in relation to the role, he or she will be unable to resume other more familiar roles adequately.

Role Modeling

Role clarification and role taking may be accomplished through role modeling and role rehearsal. Both techniques facilitate the process of communication. In order to practice role modeling and role rehearsal with relative ease, it is essential that the actor be able to identify appropriate significant others and reference groups, as ROSP is intended and designed to do.

Sometimes the reference group as a whole served as a role model, as each member discussed ideas and thoughts on a particular topic. The role model might be the nurse who demonstrated a procedure such as diapering, feeding, or holding a baby. The nurse also acted as a role model while leading the discussion on role expectations and demonstrating how the father and mother could facilitate communication between themselves. Members of the group served as role models for each other. Members also discussed the experiences of friends and relatives, who thus served indirectly as role models.

Significant role models in the ROSP program were a couple who had recently had a baby. They were invited to the group to discuss their labor and delivery experience, as well as their experiences as new parents. They shared their feelings of ineptness, awkwardness, helplessness, and, finally, competence. Group members raised such questions as, "What changes has the baby made in your lives?" and, "How do you feel about those changes?" These two new parents enabled the prospective role incumbents to anticipate some of the experiences and to understand how others might cope with certain situations. This served to broaden the alternatives available to potential role incumbents.

Role models are essential to the process of role transition. A few of the couples mentioned that they did not know anyone who had a baby. One couple said that they had two friends who had recently had babies, who were well prepared for childbirth, and who believed they had had a wonderful experience during labor and delivery, but "it had been a horror ever since, with a dependent creature who interrupted their lives in many ways." The couple thus questioned the wisdom of their decision to conceive and expressed the need to explore these feelings with those who could be their role models. It became apparent to the members of the group that each had formulated ideas about their own experience based on input they had received from others who were significant in their lives.

There are many advantages in using both the nurse and the new parents as role models. The couples in the group provided an opportunity to identify and share their experiences with each other. The couples generally provided some, but not all, alternatives for a situation, whereas the nurse could provide many more based on professional knowledge. Members of the group explained what the experience was like for them; the nurse helped interpret the situational meaning and the implications and raised questions about feelings, behavioral effects on partners, and parameters of the range of experiences in any given situation. Many couples had no other role models aside from the reference group and the nurse.

Role Rehearsal

Role rehearsal as a concept refers to internal activity preceding overt interaction, in which the individual fantasizes, imagines, and mentally enacts how an encounter might take place and how a role might evolve. In other words, the individual mentally acts out the role, anticipating in imagination the responses of significant others.

Role rehearsal thus serves a crucial function in anticipating and planning the course of future actions, and is an important prelude to role taking. Role rehearsal does not proceed on the assumption that roles will be rigidly structured. The roles that will finally evolve in actual enactment may be quite different from those rehearsed in fantasy. However, rehearsal enables the individual and others to anticipate behavior and sentiments associated with the roles rehearsed.

Various aspects of the transition to parenthood were explored through role rehearsal. These included labor and delivery, hospitalization, the temporary assumption of a "sick" role, and early parenting.

The first night home with a new baby was taken as an example of role rehearsal for early parenting. A situation such as the following was described to the families, who were then asked to imagine how they would feel about it and to respond to it: "It's the first day home with the baby, who is three days old. He or she slept a great deal of the time in the hospital, and the baby's few needs were easily satisfied by feeding and changing diapers. Actually, the mother seldom even needed to ask the nurse for help. Now home, the baby suddenly begins to cry unceasingly, rejects the mother's breast, and will not nurse."

Another role rehearsal dealt with a family situation when the baby was a few weeks old and focused not only on the specific situation, but also on the changing relationship between the husband and wife. "The father has had a rather frustrating day at work. He has been trying to concentrate on his work again after being preoccupied with the birth of his baby. It has been a long, tedious day, and he is looking forward to a relaxing, quiet dinner at home with his wife. When he arrives, the baby is crying and will not take a feeding; the mother is irritable; dinner is not ready; everything he says to her receives a sharp, curt, cutting remark from her." The parents were asked how they would respond and what feelings they could anticipate having toward each other. Various realistic coping strategies were presented and explored.

Implications for Nursing

Nurses have always been involved in group teaching and in anticipatory guidance, principally aimed at providing knowledge and information to health care recipients. Parts of ROSP have been offered in fragments. A holistic program deduced from a conceptual framework has not been reported in the literature. A review of nursing literature points out the richness of work on conceptualizing nursing care and the paucity of adequate operational schema.

The insecurity inherent in the professional status of nursing could be ameliorated when clients of nursing care are able to articulate nursing interventions. This, in turn, could be promoted when nurses provide interventions that are systematically organized and empirically tested. The potential for a systematic testing increases when nurses use conceptual frameworks to guide the nursing process. This chapter presents an implementation of a conceptual framework into nursing practice. The same preventive framework could be used for episodic care.

The framework provides a direction for patient care and, hence, provides a way to organize knowledge for teaching and curriculum implementation, and for the systematic inquiry desperately needed for research in nursing. Each component of ROSP might lend itself to several testable hypotheses. ROSP, as a whole, also involves a number of testable hypotheses. Accumulated knowledge and data related to each research problem area could provide a scientific basis for nursing care.

REFERENCES

1. Chin, R.: The utility of system models and developmental models for practitioners. In Bennis, W. G., Benne, K. D., & Chin, R., editors: The planning of change, New York, 1962, Holt, Rinehart and Winston, Inc., pp. 200–215.
2. Cottrell, L. S.: The adjustment of the individual to his age and sex roles. Am. Sociol. Rev. 7(5):617–620, 1942.
3. Dyer, E.: Parenthood as crisis. In Parad, H. J., editor: Crisis intervention: Selected readings. New York, 1969, Family Services Association of America.
4. Inkles, A.: What is sociology? Englewood Cliffs, N.J., 1964, Prentice-Hall, Inc., pp. 28–61.
5. James, A. E., & Benedick, T.: Parenthood, its psychology and psychopathology. Boston, 1970, Little, Brown & Co.

6. LeMasters, G. G.: Parenthood as crisis. In Parad, H. J., editor: Crisis intervention: selected readings. New York, 1969, Family Services Association of America.
7. Lindesmith, A. R., & Strauss, A.: Social psychology. New York, 1956, Holt, Rinehart & Winston, Inc.
8. Meleis, A. I.: Role insufficiency and role supplementation: A conceptual framework. Nurs. Res. 24(4): 264–271, 1975.
9. Meleis, A. I., & Swendsen, L.: Does nursing intervention make a difference? A test of the ROSP. Communicating Nurs. Res. 81:208–324, 1977.
10. Meleis, A. I., & Swendson, L.: Role supplementation–An empirical test of a nursing intervention. Nurs. Res. 27(1):11–18, 1978.
11. Morris, Charles W., editor: George Herbert Mead, Mind, self and society: From the standpoint of a social behaviorist. Chicago, 1934, University of Chicago Press.
12. Rogers, M.: An introduction to the theoretical basis of nursing. Philadelphia, 1970, F. A. Davis Co.
13. Shaw, N. R.: Teaching young mothers their role, Nurs. Outlook 22:695–698, 1974.
14. Sheresfsky, P. M., & Yarrow, L. J.: Psychological aspects of a first pregnancy and early postnatal adaptation. New York, 1974, Raven Press.
15. Swendsen, L., Meleis, A. I., & Jones, D.: Role supplementation: A means of role mastery. Am. J. Maternal Child Nurs. 3(2):85–91, 1978.
16. Turner, R.: Role taking: Process vs. conformity. In Rose, Arnold M., editor: Human behavior and social processes. Boston, 1962, Houghton Mifflin Co., pp. 10–40.
17. Turner, R.: The self-conception in social interaction. In Gordon, Chad, & Gergen, Kenneth J., editors: The self in social interaction. New York, 1967, John Wiley & Sons, Inc.
18. Turner, R.: Family interaction. New York, 1970, John Wiley & Sons, Inc.

Reprinted with permission from: Meleis, A. I., Swendsen, L., & Jones, D. (1980). Preventive role supplementation: A grounded conceptual framework. In M. H. Miller & B. Flynn (Eds.), *Current perspectives in nursing: Social issues and trends* (Vol. 2, pp. 3–14). St. Louis, MO: C.V. Mosby.

10.2 ROLE SUPPLEMENTATION FOR NEW PARENTS—A ROLE MASTERY PLAN

LESLEE A. SWENDSEN
AFAF I. MELEIS
DELORAS JONES

Nurses have traditionally considered teaching patients about health care an important part of their responsibility. In maternal child health, nurses have conducted prenatal infant care and prepared childbirth classes, to enable both mothers and fathers to become more confident and competent as parents. However, expectant parents need more than knowledge to make the transition to parenthood successfully. They need an opportunity to express their concerns and feelings, and to explore ways of maximizing their new role.

A role is a set of actual or expected behaviors and feelings or goals demonstrating unity in action. Roles develop as a result of a relationship with another individual. To be a parent, for example, one must have a child; to be a wife, one must have a husband.

This means that every individual role has a corresponding complementary role.

The crisis associated with assuming the role of parent is well documented in the literature.[1-6] In interacting with patients through the nursing process, the nurse provides care and support to expectant parents facing this crisis. One integrative conceptual framework for supporting and caring for couples in parental role transition is role supplementation. This concept in nursing intervention was proposed by Afaf Meleis. She defined it as:

> The information or experience necessary to bring the role incumbent and significant others to full awareness of the anticipated behavior patterns, units, sentiments, sensations, and goals involved in each role and its complement. In short, such an approach assists parents-to-be in moving toward role mastery.[7]

A program for first-time parents demonstrating role supplementation as a conceptual framework was conducted at Kaiser Permanente Medical Center in San Francisco. Two nurses conducted the program, which is called preventive role supplementation (ROSP). Eight weekly two-hour group meetings are held in the third trimester of pregnancy under the program. Each meeting is in the evening, so both fathers and mothers can attend. The first 90 minutes consist of didactic presentation and discussion; the last half hour is devoted to teaching exercises for labor and delivery.

Group Activities and Purposes

The meetings provide a *reference group*, a group whose standpoint is used as a frame of reference for participants. Providing such a group through which members can form their own identities is an overall strategy of the program. In the group, viewpoints are explored, discussed, and adopted or discarded. Comments and views of the group members and leaders act as either positive or negative reinforcement of each individual's values and beliefs. The discussion also identifies a normal range of behavior in certain situations or roles.

Three basic principles are established with the group at the very beginning:

- There are no right or wrong ideas or feelings. Each person has the right to express himself and others can agree or disagree. Each thought is valued as important to the person expressing it.
- The group is meant to explore ways of problem solving and decision making. There are many alternatives involved in making decisions, and thoughtful pursuit of the consequences of each alternative assists a person to make his own decision. A main function of the program is to enable each couple to make their own decisions and to feel confident about their ability to do so.
- The group, rather than the leaders, is to set its own objectives for the sessions. If disagreement arises over the discussion topics, each idea is pursued in whatever order the group establishes. The leaders merely make suggestions as needed.

The reference group, then, provides an opportunity for interchange and exploration of various alternatives among group members. Factual knowledge about pregnancy, labor and delivery, and child care are also given during the sessions. This allows participants to anticipate the experiences they will be encountering, and thus, to determine and clarify their roles. The birth films, visual aids, and hospital tour are a part of this aspect of the sessions.

Role clarification, the identification of the knowledge and behaviors associated with a role, is a major strategy of the program and guides the educational process. How the physiological changes involved in childbearing, the mechanisms of labor and delivery, and infant care-taking activities, for example, will influence one's feelings in these situations and how one might respond are, therefore, also covered.

Expectations of oneself and of one's spouse during the process of becoming a parent and later as a parent are discussed. Parents-to-be are encouraged to think of how their spouses might be feeling and how they could best support the other.

Couples are very concerned about infant care activities, such as bathing and diapering. We found that reassuring the couples that they would have rooming-in after delivery, with experienced maternity nurses to demonstrate these activities, was not helpful to the couples before the birth. They needed demonstrations in the classes and did not seem ready to go on to other topics until that need was met. Another important focus in the group discussions is the change a new infant brings to the individual lives of a couple, the feelings of each spouse, and alternatives for handling the anticipated changes.

Individual Family Visits

In conjunction with the discussions during the weekly sessions, individual home visits help the nurse group leaders in assessing the needs of each couple. The nurses continually revise their nursing plans to meet these needs as they emerge. Before delivery, at least two home visits are made, and one hospital visit and at least two home visits—the first between 24 and 48 hours after discharge from the hospital, the other 5 to 6 days later—are made after delivery. Additional visits are scheduled if the couple or the nurse feels they would be beneficial.

The nurse group leaders are also on call 24 hours a day both before and after delivery, should the couples have questions or concerns between visits or classes. Surprisingly, very few calls are actually made; most families indicate that just knowing they can call is reassuring. Calls that are made concern immediate matters, and parents indicate that the quick feedback reduces their anxiety greatly.

The purpose of the hospital visit, made within 24 hours after delivery, is to give the couple an opportunity to discuss their labor and delivery experiences, which seems to be a vital psychological and developmental need. We have found that until mothers can describe these experiences in detail, they are unable to focus on restoring themselves and accepting and caring for the infant outside of the womb. The hospital visit also provides continuity of care, since a consistent nurse is involved during the prenatal, childbirth, and postnatal experiences. As such, the visit is a crucial part of the overall ROSP program.

Through rooming-in, which this particular hospital provides for all mothers, parents receive further help in mastering their roles. Both father and mother may care for their infant, while hospital staff provides infant care classes and individual teaching, and is constantly available to give assistance or to answer questions.

Modeling and Rehearsal

Throughout all aspects of the ROSP program—group meetings, home visits, and the hospital experience—two other strategies besides providing a reference group and role clarification are used. One of these strategies is *role modeling*. A role model is an individual who knows and uses the behaviors, knowledge, and values expected in a specific role. The ROSP nurses themselves serve as very significant role models, in that they actively discuss problems and explore alternatives. The expectant parents are learning from this example or model (see Figure 10.2.1).

At the same time, however, each family has its own internal role models—parents, relatives, friends, professionals. Most couples come to the program with ambiguous feelings and expectations about parenthood, since they have received several different messages about its problems and joys. It is, therefore, very important for the nurses in the program to assess each couple's various role models, including other group members, and their significance.

Especially influential on parents-to-be is the example of people who are currently in the parenting role. We, therefore, try to arrange a visit to the group by a couple who recently have had their first child to relate their experiences and discuss their ideas about handling the minor crises that occurred along the way. All program participants valued this visit highly.

"If that couple could enjoy being new parents, so could I," one parent said. "The way they seemed to think everything through and come to their own conclusions was impressive. I was afraid I'd have to be calling someone every five minutes to ask them how to do something," another parent confided.

Still another very effective strategy of the program is *role rehearsal*. Role rehearsal is a practice in which an individual fantasizes, imagines, or enacts an experience that may take place in a role. He literally acts out his role mentally and/or physically and anticipates the responses of significant others. In our program, short case studies or situations are presented to the group, and the couples discuss how they each might respond and react in the situation. The two situations that evoke the most discussion are labor and delivery and the first night home from the hospital with a baby who cries incessantly.

Role rehearsal does not imply that roles are rigidly structured. Rather, preliminary enactment gives the individual some feel for working through the role and identifying different ways of dealing with specific situations before they occur. This serves a crucial function in planning the course of future actions and is an important prelude to role taking.

Communication—not only between nurses and parents and among couples, but between husband and wife—is the underlying thread of the ROSP program. Communication and interaction are "important components of role supplementation, because it is through open and clear communication of symbols that roles evolve."[7] Couples are especially encouraged throughout the program to talk freely with spouses, because such interchange is essential to role adaptation. The nurses discuss ex-

Figure 10.2.1: Components and Process of Preventive Role Supplementation Program (ROSP)

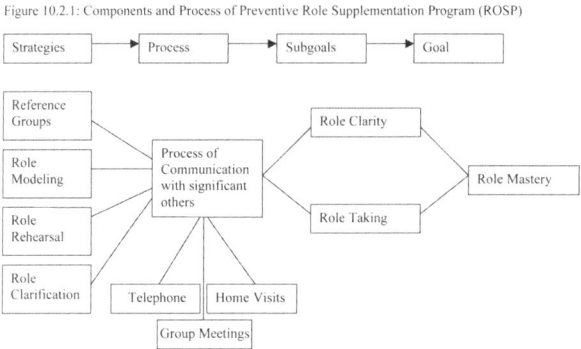

See also "Role Supplementation: An Empirical Test of a Nursing Intervention in January/February 1976, Nursing Research, p. 14

FIGURE 10.2.1 Components and process of preventive Role Supplementation Program (ROSP).

pressing concerns and feelings, including anger and anxiety, as a part of open communication.

Support from highly valued persons during the stress of role transition can serve to increase confidence in the new role and reduce anxiety, thus influencing self-concept in the new role. The nurses conducting the ROSP program become significant others for the participants and offer support in addition to that of spouse, family, friends, and physician.

Achieving Role Mastery

Actual integration or internalization of the parenting role must take place within each individual, and the process will vary according to the individual's own experiences, feelings, and needs. After one attains a clear picture of a role, role taking is another important aspect of integrating that role. Role taking is imaginatively assuming the position or point of view of another. In order to develop any form of cooperative activity, each individual must have the ability to take on the other's role.

Couples are prepared for this final step in mastering their roles as parents through all the strategies of ROSP. (See Components and Process of the ROSP program for illustration of the entire program.) They discuss their own perspective of the current and anticipated events; then they are asked to think of how the spouse might be feeling and describe how they could best assist and support the other as well as meet their own needs. They are also asked to take the role of the infant, a newborn coming from a warm, secure womb into a foreign, cold world where the experiences of hunger and pain are all too real. The couples then discuss how they might assist their infant in meeting his needs.

One couple's ability to role take is demonstrated by the following incident. Related by a mother in our program, it occurred three weeks postpartum.

> "The day was awful. I felt so confined and restricted and I began to wonder what I had gotten myself into. The baby seemed to cry nonstop all day and I was feeling blue and tied down. Finally, in desperation, I called Robert at the office, and he arranged to come home early.
>
> When he arrived, he put his arms around me and said, 'Honey, you need to go out, you've been here for three weeks. I'll stay with the baby and you go out. Do whatever you would like. In case you want to go shopping, here is some money.'
>
> I went shopping and relaxed. It felt so good to feel 'free' again. I guess I spent about three hours doing what I wanted. When I returned, I felt wonderful

and the baby was asleep. Robert hugged me and told me I was a good mother. We shared our feelings about the baby and what he has been to our lives. It was a good happy evening.

The father later revealed he was responding to ideas about role taking that he had gotten in the reference group. He admitted he had never been very empathetic before, and that he might have even responded in disgust to his wife's behavior had it not been for the program. The above example also demonstrates how couples can learn to make decisions and problem solve effectively through the ROSP program.

Two Couples' Experiences

We do not attempt to differentiate among cultural, socioeconomic, or religious backgrounds when we establish a ROSP reference group. Each couple seems to take from the program what they need or want to adapt to their new role. We have had couples from 19 to 32 years of age, professionals and laborers (all were employed), and several ethnic groups—Spanish American, Asian, Black, and white—in the group. This fostered a richness of life experiences and interchange, giving all a variety of alternatives for dealing with various situations.

Program Assumptions and Premises

1. Clients can participate in making decisions about their own health care. This participation can help them gain confidence in their ability to cope with a new role. Such participation depends on:

   - An orientation to the formal and informal structure of the health care system through which they are to work;
   - Knowledge of when and how to use each component of the system;
   - Knowledge of alternatives available to them;
   - Recognition of their rights as health care consumers;
   - Awareness of resources available to them.
2. Changes on the health–illness continuum will influence the individual's response to health–illness and will be reflected in his interaction with others.
3. Clients should be aware of the contingencies of role transition in order to achieve mastery of their roles. Awareness can be enhanced by knowing:

   - The specifics of role changes;
   - The stresses and ecstasies involved in role transition;
   - Expectations of oneself in relation to others and vice versa.
4. Interaction will facilitate role transition. Adequate and open interaction will enhance sensitivity and awareness of a client's own role and others' complementary roles.
5. Clients can, with appropriate support and assistance, resume adult functioning with minimal disruption after transition to a new role.

To illustrate how different couples responded to the program, we will present two case studies. Nancy and Joe were both 19 years old, and had been high school sweethearts. He was an automobile mechanic and she was a clerk for a large business firm. They had married because of the pregnancy, which was unplanned. Hilary and John were 29 and 30 years of age, respectively, and had been married for five years. He operated heavy equipment; she was a secretary. During their years together, they had traveled, purchased a home, and done most of the things they had wanted to do before having a family. They both enjoyed classical music and art, which they pursued as a joint hobby. The pregnancy was definitely planned.

In the Reference Group

During group meetings, the four individuals seemed responsive and interested. All were friendly and verbalized questions and responses, but none monopolized the discussion. Each couple attended regularly; each mother came to the group alone on one occasion because her husband was unable to attend.

Joe and Nancy asked "how to" questions—how to bathe a baby, how to make a formula, how to get one's figure back in shape after delivery. They did not otherwise share feelings or express concerns. Nancy often talked about a friend who had just had a baby. She remarked on several occasions "my girl friend says…." They never expressed their feelings about the reference group or what the ROSP program meant to them.

John and Hilary, on the other hand, asked very few "how to" questions. Their interest seemed to lie with changes the infant would bring to their lives, and how they would respond and deal with the more general aspects of parenthood. They readily expressed their concerns, and asked others in the group if they had similar feelings.

For example, Hilary said that she was working and was afraid that she would become bored and depressed staying home after the baby was born. She and John had decided that she would stay home with the baby for the first year; then she would go back to work if she felt the need. She expressed her conflict about wanting to be with the baby and also to continue enjoying the stimulation of work. She asked the other mothers if they had similar thoughts and how they either planned to adapt to being at home or why they had decided to return to work.

John stated emphatically on the first night the reference group met that he did not want to go into the delivery room with his wife. In elaborating, he said the men with whom he worked (strong role models) thought childbirth was a matter for the woman and her doctor alone. He then asked the other fathers, who were expressing a desire to go into the delivery room, why they wanted to be there.

Joe and Nancy seemed to be searching for some authority to tell them the "right way," while Hilary and John used the reference group to explore their own ideas and concerns. All four, however, learned from the group and found strong role models in it.

Individual Role Modeling

Nancy's friend who had recently had a baby was her strongest role model. Unfortunately, the nurse did not recognize this fact until after delivery, although Nancy referred to her friend often in the reference group. Nancy's expectations of her own birth process were exactly what her friend had experienced—a short, easy labor and delivery. Nancy's was long and difficult.

Afterward, she confided that she had not been prepared for the terrible pain, the length of time, and the "horrible" experience. It was apparent she had not internalized the many aspects of labor and delivery, including pain control, which had emerged during the program. The nurses could have been more helpful had they discussed with Nancy her self-expectations and helped her to understand more realistically the range of possibilities.

After delivery, Nancy asked one of the nurses to visit her at home to give a bath demonstration. This seemed important to her, and afterward, she revealed for the first time some of her lack of confidence in herself as a mother. These feelings were discussed at length during the visit, and she expressed relief and increased confidence at the end of the discussion and during the next week.

Unlike Nancy, neither Hilary nor John had close friends or family with infants. They stated several times that they knew of no one outside the ROSP program who could help them learn to care for their baby. Accordingly, their most significant role models were the nurses and other parents in the group.

After John made his initial announcement that he would not go into the delivery room, he listened attentively as other fathers explained their reasons for wanting to be there. One father told the group that all aspects of his baby's development were important to him and he felt it was important to be a part of the delivery. He also commented that he did not know what labor and delivery would be like, and that he was in the program to learn what was going to take place and how he could help his wife (role clarification).

No one tried to talk John into being present at delivery, but as the sessions progressed and he learned the father's role, he gave thoughtful consideration to the prospect. Finally, after the scheduled visit to the group by a couple who had just recently had an infant, he announced he was ready to go into the delivery room with Hilary and that he looked forward to the experience. "I feel competent now to handle the whole trip," he commented.

Unfortunately, Hilary had a cesarean section after several hours of labor, so John was unable to attend the delivery. He expressed his disappointment at the turn of events, but he had been prepared for possible complications, too, so they had a most pleasant and satisfying labor experience just the same. At home again, the couple explained how they were caring for the baby and mother, and sought only validation and support from the nurses rather than demonstrations or lessons. They seemed relaxed and confident.

Role Rehearsal Activity

Nancy and Joe indulged in role rehearsal only when it was initiated by someone else in the reference group or by the nurse during a home visit, not when they were alone together. They liked the rehearsal sessions and were attentive to others when they were rehearsing a specific situation, but they themselves responded only when others directly asked their opinion about what to do. When they did respond, however, they did so eagerly. The response was usually "I don't know for sure, but I think I might...." Role rehearsal was a new experience for them.

Nancy and Joe never practiced their exercises for labor and delivery at home, either. During the home visit prior to delivery, however, they asked the nurse to go through the exercises with them to be sure "we are doing them right." They also wanted to review the hospital admission procedure and how to tell when it was time to go to the hospital.

Hilary and John actively participated in all role rehearsal sessions, offering their opinions, expressing their concerns, and listening attentively to what others were saying. During the home visit prior to delivery, they rehearsed the labor experience to the point of physically acting it out with the nurse as onlooker. Hilary went through all the exercises, discussing when in labor they were used. John described and demonstrated how he could support and coach his wife, what comfort measures he would use, when he would call the nurse, etc.

Hilary had compiled the labor and delivery handouts from the ROSP program into a booklet to take with them to the hospital. Throughout the book she had written love notes to John such as "I love you" "Hang in there. I need you," and "You're doing great!"

Achieving Role Clarification

Both couples were eager to learn about the processes of pregnancy, labor and delivery, and infant care. Hilary asked many questions about why physiological changes were occurring, why labor was painful, and so forth. The others accepted the information presented, showing very little desire to know why.

Nancy and Joe did not seek to gain an understanding about the role of the parent. Whatever the nurse said their role was, they seemed to accept and willing to comply. Obviously this had been their life experience; they had identified and related to new roles by whatever the significant other or role model said it should be. It seemed foreign to them to think through the alternatives and arrive at an answer for themselves, but they began to master this ability as the program progressed.

Hilary and John seemed from the beginning to explore their new role with others, to seek alternatives and validation for their feelings and behaviors. John grew to want to attend delivery when he understood what his role in the process would be. He received role clarification from the other fathers-to-be who modeled that there is a place for the father in the delivery room.

Role Mastery: Arriving There

The goal of the ROSP program is role mastery. To achieve that goal, one must first attain role clarity (an understanding of one's role) and the ability to role take (empathize with significant others in their roles). Nancy and Joe did not feel they achieved role mastery in labor and delivery. The experience was very different from what they had expected. He did not feel he was able to assist her, and she did not feel his attempts were helpful. They had not internalized the information activities from the ROSP program for this aspect of the experience; Joe did not realize or understand either role taking or role clarity.

The couple did, however, demonstrate role mastery in the first month of parenting. Both father and mother felt they enjoyed the baby; both fed her because she was bottle-fed. They fed her on demand and felt they knew when to feed and how much. When she cried, they could cope and knew how to comfort her. They seemed able to problem solve and make decisions regarding her care without asking the nurse how they should do it.

In short, they felt competent in meeting her needs and very pleased with themselves over it. They also felt able to cope with other aspects of their lives, and that they had resources to go to when the nurse would eventually terminate the relationship with them four to six weeks after the baby's birth.

Hilary and John showed evidence of role mastery throughout the entire experience, regardless of the fact that they had expressed high anxiety and a feeling of incompetence in adequately caring for a child. After they started the ROSP program, many physical complaints that Hilary had suffered disappeared. She slept better, ate better, and stated she felt better. She said that after attending the reference group discussions, she felt much more in control, and her confidence to deal with each stage was enhanced. Both Hilary and John felt that ROSP was a "lifesaver," because neither had been prepared either to care for a child or to cope with the changes in their life until they were able to explore them with others.

The labor experience was a successful and valuable one for both, and afterward they shared in the care of the child. They felt very positive toward the baby, and very little anxiety about their ability to care for her. They mentioned they felt comforted by the fact they could call the nurse at any time to ask questions or to receive assistance, but Hilary called only once, expressing some concern about the baby's stools.

An instance showing both role clarity and role taking on the couple's part was when John returned from work one day two weeks after delivery to find Hilary tired. He suggested that she lie down while he fixed dinner. They ate and he washed the dishes. Then he suggested she take a warm bath and climb into bed, after which he gave her a long, relaxing back rub.

She later commented, "I was so touched by his concern and care for me. He had never spent so much time and energy trying to make me comfortable. It made me feel so good that he and I and our baby were a family." He commented, "I never realized how good it could make me feel to be in tune to Hilary's feelings and needs. I felt I was a real husband and father."

ROSP as Seen by the Families

As different as the two families are, their evaluations of the program were similar. Basically, both couples' perception of the program was:

- It helped them in becoming more aware of the changes in the life of a couple with the birth of a child, and provided them with alternative ways to cope with these changes;
- The group approach and freedom in discussion helped them realize that they were not alone in some of their concerns;
- Although the group experience was great and rewarding, they definitely enjoyed the individual attention from the nurses through phone calls and visits;
- The program helped in changing views of husband (father) toward his responsibilities;
- It helped them understand each other's feelings and needs and those of the baby and how to cope with them;
- Role playing and role modeling brought them close to the reality of the situation, and they cited these strategies with enthusiasm.

Evaluating the Program

Research conducted to evaluate the effects of the ROSP program is reported elsewhere. The responses by the two couples discussed here, however, do indicate the program's effect in these individual cases. The ROSP program is best described as an attempt to help families actualize their own needs at their own pace, by providing the means by which those goals are articulated and the media through which they can be achieved. Role mastery and integration are not an end point, but a continuum. Families with different capabilities and different research profiles achieve different levels of role mastery and integration, as did Nancy and Joe and Hilary and John.

Role supplementation may be used with any client undergoing role change, not just with expectant parents. Among other clients who may benefit from such a program are those who are in transition from illness, especially psychiatric disorders, to wellness; wellness to chronic illness; active work to retirement; childhood to adolescence; adolescence to adulthood; and single to married life.

Nursing is in dire need of systematic, theoretical frameworks upon which to base sound nursing practice. Role supplementation offers a framework for nursing assessment and intervention in one very crucial and commonly occurring area of need, making the transition from one role to another. We believe offering help to clients based on this framework can lead to their mastering of their new roles. When new parents are concerned, this can make the difference between a happy, well-adjusted family and a discontented, maladjusted one.

REFERENCES

1. Benedick, T. Parenthood during the lifecycle. In *Parenthood: Its psychology and psychopathology*, ed. by A. E. James & T. Benedick. Boston: Little, Brown and Company, 1970.
2. Colman, A. D., & Colman, L. L. *Pregnancy: The psychological experience*. New York: Seabury Press, 1972.
3. LeMasters, E. E. Parenthood as crisis. In *Crisis intervention: Selected readings*, ed. by H. J. Parad. New York: Family Service Association of America, 1965, pp. 111–117.
4. Dyer, E. D. Parenthood as crisis: A re-study. In *Crisis intervention: Selected readings*, ed. by H. J. Parad. New York: Family Service Association of America, 1965, pp. 312–323.
5. Rossi, A. S. Transition to parenthood. *J. Marriage Fam.* 30:26–39, Feb. 1968.
6. Shereshefsky, P. M., & Yarrow, L. J. *Psychological aspects of a first pregnancy and early postnatal adaptation.* New York: Raven Press, 1974.
7. Meleis, A. I. Role insufficiency and role supplementation: A conceptual framework. *Nurs. Res.* 24:2, 1975.

Reprinted with permission from: Swendsen, L., Meleis, A. I., & Jones, D. (1978). Role supplementation for new parents: A role mastery plan. *American Journal of Maternal Child Nursing,* 3(2), 84–91.

10.3 A ROLE SUPPLEMENTATION GROUP PILOT STUDY: A NURSING THERAPY FOR POTENTIAL PARENTAL CAREGIVERS

MARGARET H. BRACKLEY

Abstract

This pilot study addressed the question: Will transition support for midlife women during role transition into the caregiver or care manager role for their parents lead to role adaptation? A systematic sample of 30 women between the ages of 30 and 60 was drawn from a pool of employees of a large health science center in the Southwest; their mothers were also asked to volunteer as research subjects. A before–after group with random assignment design was used to determine the effects of a CNS-led support group on role adaptation of midlife women during role transition. Role adaptation was measured by correlating the scores of mother and daughter pairs on the Brackley Concerns of Aging Scale. The level of depression as an indicator of role insufficiency was determined by score on Zung's Self-Rating Depression Scale. The independent variables were social support and the CNS-led group. A two-way analysis of covariance was calculated to test each hypothesis. Hypothesis 1, which predicted a decrease in role insufficiency following transitional nursing support, was rejected. Support was found for Hypothesis 2, which specified an increase in role adaptation following transitional nursing support. Alpha was set at p = 0.05.

Providing nursing support to family caregivers is an urgent need because of increases in the aging population. Demographic data illustrate this increase: some 11% of the U.S. population is 65 years of age or older. The group of elders 85 years and older (2.8 million in 1986) is growing the fastest.

Despite the myth of abandonment, the family has traditionally provided for the care and support of its members, including care of the elderly. Some 95% of the elderly live in the community, whereas only 5% are institutionalized at any one time (Butler & Lewis, 1982). Although the elderly consume 29% of the nation's health dollar, 85% of elderly people prefer to have home care by family members (Pegels, 1981). The health care system has failed to respond to this desire, as evidenced by designating only 1% of health care costs for home health care (Archbold, 1982). Although families deliver 80% of all home health care (USDHHS, 1987), they receive no aid in their role as caregivers.

The traditional role of caregiver in modern society, whether for children, the sick, or the elderly (Brody, 1981; Hooyman, 1990; USDHHS, 1987), is assumed primarily by women. Today, women provide care for more dependents at either end of the age continuum (Brody, Johnson, Fulcomer, & Lang, 1983), primarily because of recent population trends. Archbold (1982) has identified two distinct caregiving roles: direct caregiver and care manager.

The direct caregiver is usually an older female with numerous health problems and limited financial resources. The caregiver experiences symptoms directly related to caregiving activities, such as back strain, sleep disruption, social isolation, and depression. Even while sleeping, the caregiver must often remain guarded in case her "patient" wanders or cries out for help in the night (Archbold, 1982).

In contrast, the role of care manager (i.e., one who controls the caring situation from a distance) results in role conflict, guilt, disruption of lifestyle, and depression (Archbold, 1982). Often the care manager, a daughter living across town or in another state, manages the care of her elderly parents via telephone calls (Archbold, 1982). Care management usually occurs as an addition to job and household responsibilities. The care manager often finds herself feeling guilty for not doing enough; to borrow Friedan's phrase (1981), the care manger tries to be a "super woman."

In response to the increased elder care responsibilities of families, nurses are being called upon to offer supportive care. Group methods have been particularly popular, although little scientific evidence supports the effectiveness of this methodology (see Clark & Rakowski, 1983, for a review of such groups). The National Support Center for Families of the Aging (1984) identified 60 ongoing support groups for caregivers of the elderly, yet only one of these groups was involved in evaluation research.

Steuer (1984) posited that although some empirical evidence exists on the benefits of educational and support groups for caregivers, no data are available on possible harmful effects. Steuer hypothesized that increased awareness about the caregiving situation that results from participation in such groups can lead to potentially harmful effects of increased depression, anxiety, and feelings of hopelessness and anger. Because denial has been identified as the defense mechanism most used by caregivers in an attempt to adapt to their situations (Steuer, 1984), awareness of the reality of caregiving could lead to increased levels of depression and feelings of hopelessness.

Research on what constitutes effective nursing support for these caregiving families remains minimal. Consequently, studies need to be undertaken to evaluate nursing interventions for family caregivers. A pilot study was conducted to address the following research question: Will support for women during transition into the caregiver or care manager role for their parents lead to role adaptation?

Review of the Literature

Although the strain of caregiving has been studied for the past two decades, successful caregiving has yet to be described except in terms of avoiding institutionalization of the elderly person or continuing the caregiving relationship. Surveys and clinical work indicate that most adult children are willing to assume the caregiver role; this is the first step toward role adaptation (Shanas, 1979; Sussman, 1965; USDHHS, 1987). Role adaptation involves role taking, similar to empathy and role making, which means creating a personal definition of the role (Albert, 1990; Hardy & Conway, 1978). Successful adaptation to the caregiver role would probably entail a tolerable level of stress for the caregiver and an increased ability to cope with problems as they arise (Johnson & Catalano, 1983). Although adaptation to the caregiving role is desirable, no socialization process exists to assist elderly parents and their adult children in adapting to new roles in later life (Brody, 1985; Johnson & Bursk, 1977).

Zarit, Reever, and Bach-Peterson (1980) found no difference in perceived, "burden of caregiving" when they compared spouse and daughter caregivers. Furthermore, feelings of burden were not associated with the number of behavior problems exhibited by care recipients with dementia; however, feelings of burden correlated with the social supports available to the household.

Feelings of guilt and depression are common emotions associated with caring for parents (Drummond, 1984; Poulshock & Deimling, 1984; Silverstone & Hyman, 1982). Although these feelings are commonplace, no studies address why they prevail. Likewise, nursing therapies for these responses have not been addressed in any depth in nursing literature, and supportive nursing actions for families assuming caregiving roles have not been identified. Meleis (1975) suggests using role supplementation as an intervention for preventing and treating role insufficiency, i.e., the, "perception of role performance as inadequate" (p. 266). Meleis defined role supplementation as a deliberate process of conveying information or experience in an effort to increase the awareness of anticipated behavior patterns, sentiments, sensations, and goals involved in each role. Although group methods have been used extensively to deliver role supplementation to potential parental caregivers, this practice is not based on empirical evidence of its effectiveness (Clark & Rakowski, 1983).

Theoretical Perspective

The theoretical perspective for studying support for family caregivers was derived from symbolic interactionism. From this perspective, all behavior has meaning, and human beings act in relation to each other. Fawcett (1984) outlined the characteristics of an interaction model for nursing as including social acts and relationships, perception, communication, role, and self-concept. From this perspective, actual or potential problems of interpersonal relationships are foci of nursing interest.

For this pilot study, the author used the method of concept synthesis as described by Walker and Avant (1987) to develop a concept of transition support. *Webster's Third International Dictionary* defines transition as "passage from one state, condition or place to another." Thus transition support refers to that support available to the person during developmental, situational, and health–illness passages that require an alteration in the definition of self. Support is those aspects of the internal and/or external environment of the individual that provide the strength necessary to meet the tasks at hand. Support may come from within the person (as in self-support and/or self-care capabilities), from the person's external environment (as in social support), or from professional sources (as in nursing support).

Theoretically, if a person faced with transition to caregiver has enough support from various sources to meet the demands for redefinition of self and life roles, then the transition process will be smooth and without harmful side effects of role insufficiency, such as depression, anxiety, and feelings of inadequacy (Meleis, 1975). The professional nurse can use the concept of transition support to guide practice with caregiving families as the nurse assists them with functional role adaptations.

Several assumptions are specific to this study regarding the effects of transition support as a guide for nursing practice with caregiving families. First, the literature supports the assumption that the role of direct caregiver or care manager contains inherent stress and strain. Second, role insufficiency will occur during role transition if role adaptation fails to occur. Third, depression is an empirical referent of role insufficiency in the caregiver. Fourth, role taking (empathy) is assumed to be the first step in role adaptation (Hardy & Conway, 1978).

Statement of the Problem

The following hypotheses were tested in the study:

1. The adult child who reports high levels of social support and who receives nursing support in the form of a role supplementation group (RSG) will demonstrate less depression.
2. The adult child who reports high levels of social support and who receives nursing support in the form of an RSG will demonstrate higher levels of role adaptation, as measured by the Concerns of Aging Scale (CAS).

Methodology

This study compared two groups of potential caregivers before and after an intervention to test transition support as a preventive measure. Subjects were randomly assigned to groups. The study focused on women and their responses to transition support before assuming the caregiver role. This particular group of women was studied so that any harmful effects of the nursing therapy could be identified before using transition support with women already caught up in the complexities of caring for elderly parents.

Experimental Treatment

Transition support was provided through an RSG, which met for 4 weeks and consisted of four $1^{1}/_{2}$-hour group sessions for caregivers led by two nurses with Master's degrees, a geriatric clinical nurse specialist, and a psychiatric/mental health (PMH) clinical nurse specialist. Each group session consisted of 30 minutes of didactic content (Table 10.3.1), followed by 1 hour of group process. Essential content was identified through a literature search. The sessions focused on group members acquiring active listening and communication skills in order to negotiate the caregiver role with the elderly parent. Topics addressed the multiplicity of roles for midlife women; aging, death, and dying; and assertiveness with health care professionals, as well as with aging parents. Subjects were encouraged to talk to their mothers about the content of group sessions in order to develop empathy through communication, and to assess how well the didactic content in the sessions applied to individual mothers.

Sample

The sample of 30 women resulted from randomly picking a name from among the 7800 employees listed in the directory of a large Southwestern academic health science center. Every 77th name was selected after that to ensure at least 100 names. We knew that at least 50% of the names could be male and not all subjects would meet the following criteria:

1. The adult child and elderly parent lived in separate housing.
2. The adult child was a female over the age of 30 years.
3. Both members of the dyad understood and spoke English.
4. The elder parent was female.
5. The daughter agreed to attend four group sessions.
6. The subject's mother agreed to participate in the study by completing a questionnaire she re-

TABLE 10.3.1   Content of RSG

Week 1	Women in the middle
	  A. Population trends
	  B. Myth of the empty nest
	  C. Shrinking of contemporary families
	  D. Multiplicity of midlife woman's roles/responsibilities

Week 2	Normal adult development
	  A. Film: "Everyone Rides the Carousel, Part III" (Pyramid Films), an animated representation of Erikson's stages of adult development
	  B. Death and dying
	  C. Stages of grief
	  D. Impact of multiple loss
	  E. Physical symptoms of unresolved grief
	  F. Awareness of parental aging as reminder of personal aging

Week 3	Communication as basis of role negotiation
	  A. Basic skills of active listening
	  B. Role play mother–daughter communication

Week 4	Listening with elderly parents
	  A. Build on active listening tried during week
	  B. Simulated communication exercises centered on role negotiation

ceived via the postal service. By volunteering for a research project on aging mother/adult daughter relationships, the subject pairs presumably felt a need to explore this aspect of daily life.

The first subject was randomly assigned to a group by the toss of a coin; the other subjects were assigned by alternating between experimental and control groups. After all 30 subjects had been assigned, subjects were mailed consent forms to sign and a packet of scales to complete. The daughter-subjects were asked to complete the CAS, the Social Support Questionnaire (SSQ), and the Self-Rating Depression Scale (SDS), and the mother-subjects were asked to complete the CAS. The experimental subjects attended the treatment group, and the control subjects received no intervention. At the end of four weeks, control and experimental daughter-subjects were again asked to complete the CAS and the SDS. Experimental subjects who missed one group session were sent audiotape and written materials for the didactic portion of the group. If two sessions were missed, the subject was dropped from the study.

Instruments

The CAS involves ranking a deck of cards, with each card containing one of the top 20 common concerns about growing old. The scale was examined for content validity by 10 elderly people and 2 geriatric nurse experts. Both mothers and daughters were asked to rank cards, with the daughter responding from what she thought would be her mother's perspective (Brackley, 1986). Responses were correlated using a Spearman Rank correlation for each mother–daughter pair. Test–retest reliability was $r = 0.80$ when pretested with eight mother-daughter pairs, whereas internal consistency for the same group varied from $r = 0.75$–0.85.

The SSQ measured social support for daughter-subjects. Social support includes interpersonal transactions exhibiting one or more of the following: expression of positive affect of one person toward another, affirmation or endorsement of another's behavior, giving of symbolic or material aid (Kahn, 1979). The instrument is a Likert-type scale and was developed for use by nurses during clinical assessment. Norbeck, Lindsey, and Carrieri (1981) found test–retest reliability to be $r = 0.85$–0.92, whereas internal consistency varied between $r = 0.89$–0.98. Normative testing indicates 281 is a likely score, with a range of 48–567 possible findings.

The SDS was developed by Zung (1974) for use in measurement of depression. It consists of 20 common symptoms of depression with four categories that, when checked, identify the frequency with which a symptom is experienced. Test–retest reliability was reported as $r = 0.85$–0.92, and internal consistency was $r = 0.89$–0.98. A score of 50–59 indicates mild to moderate depression.

TABLE 10.3.2 Spearman Rank Order Correlation Coefficients for CAS

	Median	Range
Pre/post daughter scores		
All SS	0.637	0.94–0.161
Exper.	0.530	0.94–0.161
Control	0.676	0.83–0.295
Pre daughter score with mother's ranks		
All SS	0.551	0.825–0.075
Exper.	0.218	0.614–0.075
Control	0.599	0.825–0.124
Post daughter ranks with mother's ranked concerns		
All SS	0.417	0.730–0.022
Exper.	0.415	0.641–0.040
Control	0.519	0.730–0.022

TABLE 10.3.3 Mean, Low, and High Scores for the SSQ

Subjects	SSQ
Total sample	
M	284
Low	78
High	485
Experimental	
M	195
Low	78
High	450
Control	
M	−300
Low	162
High	485

CAS

For each mother–daughter pair, three correlation coefficients were calculated. A Spearman $\rho\tilde{n}$ for each daughter before and after treatment was calculated, as were coefficients for pretreatment daughter score with mother's score and the posttreatment daughter score with the mother's score. Spearman correlation coefficients are displayed in Table 10.3.2.

SSQ

The subjects in this study had a mean score of 284 with scores varying from a low of 78 to a high of 485. Table 10.3.3 shows mean, low, and high scores on the SSQ.

SDS

At the beginning of the study, the scores on the SDS for the total sample varied from 38 to 54, with a median score of 45 and a mode of 50. The experimental group varied from 38 to 53, with a median of 45 and was bimodal at 42 and 45. The control scores ranged from 41 to 54, with a median of 48 and mode of 50. At the beginning of the study, seven subjects (five in the control group and two in the experimental) scored as mildly depressed. After treatment, five remained mildly depressed. Three control subjects improved their scores to within normal range. Table 10.3.4 displays SDS scores.

Results

Of the original 30 mother–daughter pairs, 10 in the experimental group and 12 in the control group completed the pilot study. Subjects who dropped out cited work demands as their reason for not completing the study.

Daughters ranged in age from 30–60 years, with a mean age of 40.18 years (and a standard deviation of 8.43 years). Ten (45%) of the subjects fell within the 30–35 age bracket, whereas five (23%) were in the 46–50 age bracket. Thirteen (59%) of the women were married, whereas nine (41%) were single, never married, divorced, or widowed.

Daughters' education level ranged from 12–21 years, with a mean of 15.72 years. Twenty-four subjects were Caucasian, with the rest being African American (1), Hispanic (2), and Native American (3).

TABLE 10.3.4 Median, Mode, and Range for SDS

	Median	Mode	Range
Total Sample	45	50	38–54
Experimental	45	42–45	38–53
Control	48	50	41–54

TABLE 10.3.5 Two-Way Analysis of Variance for Depression by Group and Level of Social Support

Source of Variance	Sum of Squares	df	Mean Square	F	Probability
Social Support	8.296	1	8.296	1.90	0.3556
Group	8.296	1	8.296	1.90	0.3556
Interaction	1.024	1	1.024	0.11	1.7429
Error	166.133	18	9.229		

Significant $F = 4.41$, $p = 0.05$.

No change in scores on the depression scale as an indicator of role insufficiency was found in subjects who received the RSG and who reported high levels of social support (see Table 10.3.5), thus Hypothesis 1 was rejected. This finding was not totally unexpected. Steuer (1984) has warned of the potential negative effects of raising awareness of the caregiver's plight through educational and support groups. Denial may be one of the primary defense mechanisms caregivers use to continue to meet uncomfortable role demands; when they develop insight into their present situation, depression can occur. The current study has no direct data with which to support or reject Steuer's concern. Due to the small sample size, absence of changes in depression should be viewed with caution.

The level of role adaptation increased in subjects in the RSG when social support was held as a covariant (see Table 10.3.6), and Hypothesis 2 was accepted. When the effects of social support were removed from the dependent variable role adaptation, the subjects in the RSG had higher levels of role adaptation than those subjects who did not attend the treatment group. Support for Hypothesis 2 was an expected finding both from a theoretical perspective (Meleis, 1975) and from a review of published literature (Biegel & Blum, 1990). Meleis (1975) wrote that role supplementation during periods of role transition was one form of support nurses could give clients to help them adapt to their new role. Support for this strategy was found in this pilot study and warrants additional testing in future studies.

Discussion

When Lazarus, Stafford, Cooper, Cohler, and Dysken (1981) conducted group sessions with relatives of elderly Alzheimer's patients, they identified three goals the families hoped to achieve. These goals were to find help, to find new ways of relating to their loved ones, and to find new ways of coping with problems. The approach used in the RSG in the present study focused on communication and problem solving. An RSG that addressed the goals listed above was found to be an effective means of increasing the daughter's adaptation to the caregiver role.

Van Servellen (1984) identified supportive and change agent functions as roles nurse group

TABLE 10.3.6   Two-Way Analysis of Covariance[a] for Role Adaptation[b] by Group

Source of Variance	Sum of Squares	df	Mean Square	f	Probability
Group	0.23073	1	0.23073	4.58[c]	0.049
1st Cover	0.24421	1	0.24421	4.85[c]	0.044
Error	0.75599	15	0.05040		
R	0.00085	1	0.00085	0.05	0.825
RG	0.00852	1	0.00852	0.50	0.488

[a] Measured by the CAS.
[b] Social support as covariant.
[c] Significant $F = 4.41$.

leaders used most often. The RSG employed these functions in an attempt to meet the stated goals discussed by Lazarus et al. (1981). The RSG provided help for potential caregivers through emotional support and creating an environment that encourages change. Change in how the caregiver relates to the care recipient was explored through active listening exercises and content on aging concerns. New ways of coping were suggested through group process.

Increased congruence between mother's CAS and daughter's CAS reflects an increase in understanding between the concerns of aging by the mother and the daughter's perception of these concerns. Thus, this pilot lends support to the idea that an RSG can effectively increase dyadic understanding.

The collaboration between the geriatric and PMH CNSs in the RSG added extra dimensions to this nursing therapy. The geriatric CNS added a depth and breadth of knowledge about aging and concerns of the mother, whereas the PMH CNS focused on the daughter's concerns in role adaptation. Thus, both parties in the caregiving dyad were given voice.

Family caregivers must be considered in any discussions of health care for the elderly (Hooyman, 1990). This person provides a vital service to a health care industry that would certainly collapse under the weight of caring for all elderly persons currently receiving care at home. The caregiver sacrifices time, money, competing demands, and often health as the care recipient requires more and more care.

CNSs in their roles of expert clinician, consultant, educator, administrator, and researcher are in key positions to aid the caregiver. This study has described one therapy that CNSs can use in their quest for quality care for elders and their families.

As the population of persons over age 75 increases, the need for nursing support of family caregivers will also continue to increase. This pilot study has provided tentative support for the idea of using group process to promote role adaptation during role transition to caregiver. The CNS role has traditionally encompassed both client teaching and group process. Thus, role supplementation for family caregivers using this methodology clearly falls within the purview of advanced nursing practice.

REFERENCES

Albert, S. M. (1990). The dependent elderly, home health care, and strategies of household adaptation. In J. F. Gubrium, & A. Sankar (Eds.), *The home care experience: Ethnography and policy.* Newbury Park, CA: Sage Publications.

Archbold, P. G. (1982). All-consuming activity: The family as caregiver. *Generations*, Winter, 12–14.

Biegel, D. E., & Blum, A. (1990). *Aging and caregiving: Theory, research and policy.* Newbury Park, CA: Sage Publications.

Brackley, M. H. (1986). Role adaptation in the employed adult female caregiver following transitional nursing support. (Doctoral dissertation, Texas Woman's University, 1986). *Dissertation Abstracts International, 47*, 3292-B.

Brody, E. M. (1981). Women in the middle and family help to older people. *The Gerontologist, 21*, 471–480.

Brody, E. M. (1985). Parent care as a normative family stress. *The Gerontologist, 25*(1), 19–29.

Brody, E. M., Johnson, P. T., Fulcomer, M. C., & Lang, A. M. (1983). Women's changing roles and help to elderly patients: Attitudes of three generations of women. *Journal of Gerontology, 38*(5), 597–607.

Buckwalter, K. (1990). *Alzheimer's and caretakers*. Paper presented at State of the Art and Science of Psychiatric Nursing Conference, National Institute of Mental Health, Bethesda, MD.

Butler, R. N., & Lewis, M. I. (1982). *Aging & mental health: Positive psychosocial and biomedical approaches*. St. Louis, MO: Mosby.

Clark, N. M., & Rakowski, W. (1983). Family caregivers of older adults: Improving helping skills. *The Gerontologist, 23*(6), 637–642.

Drummond, G. (1984). A support group for caring relatives. *Health Visitor, 57*, 201–202.

Fawcett, J. (1984). *Analysis and evaluation of conceptual models of nursing*. Philadelphia: F. A. Davis.

Friedan, B. (1981). *The second stage*. New York: Summit.

Hardy, M. E., & Conway, M. E. (1978). *Role theory: Perspectives for health professionals*. New York: Appleton-Century-Crofts.

Hooyman, N. Z. (1990). Women as caregivers of the elderly: Implications for social welfare policy and practice. In D. E. Biegel & A. Blum (Eds.), *Aging and caregiving: Theory, research, and policy*. Newbury Park, CA: Sage Publications.

Johnson, E. S., & Bursk, B. J. (1977). Relationships between the elderly and their adult children. *The Gerontologist, 17*(1), 90–95.

Johnson, E. S., & Catalano, D. J. (1983). A longitudinal study of family supports to impaired elderly. *The Gerontologist, 23*(6), 612–618.

Kahn, R. L. (1979). Aging and social support. In W. M. Wiley (Ed.), *Aging from birth to death: Interdisciplinary perspectives*. Boulder, CO: Westview Press.

Lazarus, L. W., Stafford, B., Cooper, K., Cohler, B., & Dysken, M. (1981). A pilot study of Alzheimer patients' relatives discussion group. *The Gerontologist, 21*(4), 264–271.

Meleis, A. I. (1975). Role insufficiency and role supplementation: A conceptual framework. *Nursing Research, 24*(4), 264–271.

National Support Center for the Families of the Aging. (1984). *Help for families of the aging: Survey of support services*. Swarthmore, PA: National Support Center for Families of the Aging.

Norbeck, J. S., Lindsey, P. A., & Carrieri, V. L. (1981). The development of an instrument to measure social support. *Nursing Research, 30*(5), 264–269.

Pegels, C. C. (1981). *Health care and the elderly*. Rockville, MD: Aspen.

Poulshock, W. S., & Deimling, G. T. (1984). Families caring for elders in the residence: Issues in the measurement of burden. *Journal of Gerontology, 39*(2), 230–239.

Shanas, E. (1979). The family as a social support system in old age. *Gerontology, 19*(2), 169–175.

Silverstone, B., & Hyman, H. K. (1982). *You and your aging parent*. New York: Pantheon Books.

Steuer, J. (1984). Caring for the caregiver. *Generations*, Winter, 56–58.

Sussman, M. B. (1965). Relationships of adult children with their parents in the United States. In E. Shanas & G. Streib (Eds.), *Social structure and the family: Generational relations*. Englewood Cliffs, NJ: Prentice Hall.

U.S. Department of Health and Human Services (1987). *Caregivers of the frail elderly: A national profile*. U.S. Government Printing Office, 181–345:60026.

Van Servellen, G. M. (1984). *Group and family therapy: A model for psychotherapeutic nursing practice*. St. Louis, MO: Mosby.

Walker, L., & Avant, K. (1987). *Strategies for theory construction in nursing*. Norwalk, CT: Appleton-Century-Crofts.

Zarit, S. H., Reever, K. E., & Bach-Peterson, K. (1980). Relatives of the impaired elderly: Correlates of feelings of burden. *The Gerontologist, 20*(6), 649–655.

Zung, W. K. (1974). The measurements of affects: Depression and anxiety. In P. Pinchot (Ed.), *Psychological measurements in psychopharmacology* (Modern Problems in Pharmacopsychiatry Series 7). Paris: Karger.

Reprinted with permission from: Brackley, M. H. (1992). A role supplementation group pilot study: A nursing therapy for potential parental caregivers. *Clinical Nurse Specialist, 6*(1), 14–19.

10.4 ROLE SUPPLEMENTATION: AN EMPIRICAL TEST OF A NURSING INTERVENTION

AFAF IBRAHIM MELEIS

LESLEE A. SWENDSEN

Abstract

This study tested the effect of role supplementation, as a preventive nursing intervention, on families who were experiencing a transition from a dyadic to a triadic relationship through the birth of a first child. Three groups—experimental (N = 12), control (N = 36), and FamCap (N = 10)—participated. Participation in the role supplementation program did not sharpen communication skills, increase skill in role taking, or increase the congruency in role perceptions. The intervention did help experimental group wives to have lower anxiety scores postdelivery than other wives in the study, although anxiety increased in all subjects. Through role supplementation intervention, experimental wives showed significant differences in their perceptions and attitudes toward ignoring the infant, protectiveness of the infant, and responsiveness to infant's needs.

Life change has the potential of producing stress, which, in turn, may give rise to consequences such as anxiety, depression, inability to cope, or psychiatric problems. To experience a number of stressful experiences without knowledge of, or preparation in, social skills needed to cope with new roles and new responsibilities may lead to physical or mental illness. This study explored effects of a preventive nursing intervention on families who were anticipating changes in their life styles, that is, were experiencing a transition from a dyadic to a triadic relationship through the anticipated birth of their first child.

The research project stemmed from the belief that systematic accumulation of nursing knowledge takes place only if conceptualizations precede empirical testing of resulting propositions. It was based on the assumptions that conceptual framework offers structure for nursing knowledge and that, without such framework, knowledge of various phenomena cannot be interrelated. Findings related to various phenomena may become fragmented and lost, unless bound together with an integrative framework. Findings that are interrelated provide a sense of history and a potential for the future, through further exploration of related phenomena or replication of already-explored phenomena. Thus, an integrative framework is essential to the development of a body of knowledge that encompasses theory, practice, and research.

This investigation explored whether role supplementation, as a nursing intervention, affected criterion variables that are considered important in the practice of nursing.

Conceptual Framework

The conceptual framework in this study was that of role theory and the work of symbolic interactionists such as Herbert Blumer (1969), Charles Horton Cooley (1922), John Dewey (1922), George Herbert Mead (1934), and Ralph Turner (1962).

Specifically, the study tested propositions that evolved from using role supplementation in a transitional situation as a conceptual framework for nursing practice. Role supplementation was defined as any deliberative process whereby role insufficiency of potential role insufficiency is identified by the role incumbent and significant others, and the conditions and strategies of role clarification and role taking are used to develop a preventive or therapeutic intervention to decrease, ameliorate, or prevent role insufficiency. Role supplementation is further defined as the conveying of information or experience necessary to bring the role incumbent and significant others to full awareness of the anticipated behavior patterns, units, sentiments, sensations, and goals involved in each role and its complement (Meleis, 1975, p. 267).

Role supplementation was operationalized into process, components, and strategies. Process was identified as that of communication, the components were role clarification and role taking, and the strategies were reference groups, role rehearsal, and role modeling. The main goal of the role supplementation program was that of role mastery, through development of congruency between perceived roles by role incumbent and imputed roles by significant others. The conceptual assumption underlying the use of role supplementation in this research was that, if conditions and processes surrounding role transitions were well defined and well rehearsed, and if resources to facilitate the transition were identified, role transition might be accomplished more smoothly and with as little psychosocial discomfort as possible.

To test the effect of role supplementation on clients who were undergoing transitions, situational transition was chosen as a determining condition for the selection of the sample. Situational transitions, "involve the addition or the subtraction of persons in a preexisting constellation of roles and complements" (Meleis, 1975 p. 265). The addition of a new member to a family constellation represents only one example of situational transition.

Rationale for Using the Condition of Situational Transition

"The commitment to parenthood, more than the nuptial vows, implies a decision for lifetime" (Jessner et al., 1970, pp. 211–212). Both pregnancy and infant care bring about changes in the lives of couples that can produce intense stress, anxieties, and conflicts, and call for emotional adjustment to adapt to the situational transition. Fantasies and old conflicts may surface in couples as they move through the process of pregnancy and early parenthood. The degree to which they can adapt and adjust to the parental transition depends on their previous life experiences and subsequent emotional intactness (Benedick, 1970; Caplan, 1961; Colman & Colman, 1971; Grimm, 1967; Jessner et al., 1970; Rossi, 1968).

LeMasters (1965), in his study of middle-class couples, noted that most couples found the transition to parenthood difficult and that the birth of a first child constituted a crisis event. Caplan (1961) found pregnancy and the development of the mother–child relationship stressful. Dyer (1965) indicated that the majority of the couples in her sample experienced a severe crisis. Shereshefsky and Yarrow (1973), in studying the psychological aspects of the first pregnancy and postnatal adaptation, observed that members of their study population needed psychological support during this period.

Nurses have been leaders in assisting couples with crises of pregnancy, childbirth, and infant care, individually and in groups. More recently, nurses have recognized the importance of the individual concerns and feelings of patients. Nurses' responsibilities now extend not only to patient education, but also to assessment of psychosocial needs and implementation of interventions according to the needs (Acton, 1973; Banasiak & Corcoran, 1973; Chinn, 1974; Feldman, 1974; Fitzpatrick et al., 1971; Littlefield, 1973). As Acton pointed out, "The nurse acts as the patient advocate, teacher and counselor concerned with the total experience of childbearing and childrearing" (p. 294).

Anxiety

Gould and Kalb (1974, p. 30) defined anxiety as a reaction of apprehension from uneasiness to complete panic, preceded by a real symbolic condition of threat that the subject perceives diffusely. Transitions in lifestyles increase the potential for perceived anxiety as a reaction to emotionally charged symbols. Anxiety has the potential of a detrimental effect on ability to cope with new situations or on learning (Lucas, 1952). Harry Stack Sullivan (1953) indicated that anxiety in mothers and fathers "induces anxiety" in infants (p. 41).

Prenatal and Postpartum Reactions

Prenatal responses to pregnancy can predetermine parents' postnatal response and responses of the infant. The works of Schaefer (1959) and Schaefer and Manheimer (1960) were used in this study. Pre- and postnatal reactions were conceptualized in terms of attitudinal and psychosomatic reactions to both pregnancy and the delivery of the baby.

Role Perceptions

Numerous variables affect changes in role definitions in families, yet such definitions are always based on reinforcements by significant others and reference groups. Because roles, in the conceptual framework guiding the study, are defined vis-à-vis significant others, role definitions should be considered through perception of both ego and his significant other. The more congruent the role definition between ego and his significant other, and the more congruent the definition of a relationship by partners, the less interference there is with effective family interactions and the lower the potential for stressful transitions.

Expectant parents who participated in role supplementation were assisted in focusing on their interaction patterns with each other, as well as with others. In doing so, expectant parents were able to clarify roles and, consequently, either positively or negatively reinforce each role. The program strove to increase the congruency in role perceptions of participants by having as a more practical goal the maintenance of role perceptions at the same level that existed prior to the change to a triadic relationship.

Problems of the Study

The research specifically asked:

1. Does participation in role supplementation, as a nursing intervention, result in lower anxiety postdelivery for both husbands and wives?
2. Does participation in role supplementation, as a nursing intervention, increase the congruency between husbands' and wives' role perceptions of their dyadic relationship?
3. Is there a relationship between the use of role supplementation as a nursing intervention, and postpartum reactions to pregnancy and delivery as perceived by wives?

Hypotheses

Four major hypotheses were postulated:

1. There will be no significant differences between experimental and control groups (both husbands and wives) in initial measurements of religion, education, occupation, length of marriage, or results of the Pregnancy Research Inventory.
2. There will be no significant differences in role perception scores of husbands or of wives in experimental, FamCap, and control groups pre-experimental program and predelivery, but there will be significant differences in role perception scores of husbands and wives among the three groups postexperimental program and postdelivery.
3. There will be no significant differences in the anxiety scores of wives and of husbands in experimental, FamCap, and control groups, pre-program and predelivery, but there will be significant differences in the anxiety scores of wives and of husbands among the three research groups, postprogram and postdelivery; There will be significant differences among experimental, control, and FamCap groups in the attitudes toward self and infant, as manifested in scores of the Postnatal Research Inventory.

Methodology

Setting

The study took place at the Kaiser-Permanente Hospital, San Francisco, California.

Sample

Subjects in this study were normal couples experiencing a first pregnancy, who were accepted for obstetric care in the hospital. Criteria were:

Mother was a low-risk primigravida.
Residence was in Marin or San Francisco Counties, California.
The couples were English-speaking.
Mother and father lived together at the inception of the study.
There was not a wide gap in cultural backgrounds of husband and wife (any racial or cultural background was accepted).
Neither husband nor wife suffered from physical handicap or deformity.

Age of the mother was between 18 and 34 years; Mothers were in the fourth gestational month when accepted to the study.

All prenatal records at the hospital were screened, and all clients who met the criteria were invited to participate in the study. They were admitted to the sample at the beginning of the fifth month of pregnancy.

Three groups were included: experimental (role supplementation), control, and a third group, isolated from the control group because of their involvement in FamCap, a special program of individualized care and early hospital discharge offered by clinical nursing specialists.

The experimental program included subjects who consented to participate in the study and who, after research visit 1, consented to role supplementation.

FamCap, one of the options of prenatal preparation programs available at Kaiser-Permanente Hospital, is a program that allows mother and child to be discharged from the hospital as early as 12 hours after delivery. Parents who choose FamCap are visited at least once prenatally by a maternity nurse practitioner to discuss the program and the family's resources for caring for mother and infant on discharge. Parents also attend a group meeting one month prior to delivery to discuss discharge plans; they also attend the prenatal program offered by the hospital.

The control group included all subjects who did not participate in the role supplementation or FamCap programs. These subjects took part in other prenatal programs offered by Kaiser-Permanente Hospital, such as Lamaze classes.

Although the goal was to incorporate a similar number in all groups, this was not possible, because of prohibitive cost and length of time required to accommodate and complete the treatment program. The experimental group, therefore, included 12 couples; the control group, 46 couples. When 10 FamCap families were placed in a separate group, the control group was reduced to 36. Care was taken to ensure that differences among research groups did not result from preexisting differences in demographic characteristics.

Application of Underlying Concepts to Experimental Group

Role Supplementation[1]

Role supplementation involves the attempt to develop role-clarity and role-taking skills in clients, and to provide them with a framework for the continuous analysis of new experience and identification of roles and counterroles in a transition situation. The underlying process is communication. Clients exposed to this program were encouraged to practice open and honest communication, using such methods as feedback and reinforcements. The sentiment in the group was that of acceptance of all ideas, correction of false ideas, provision of alternative ways for action, reinforcement of assets, and assistance in the development of skills that are essential for the transition in roles.

Three major strategies were used to facilitate achievement of the goal of nursing action during a role transition, which is the acquisition of a sense of integration in the roles associated with the transition (role clarity) and mastery (the degree differs with different people) of sentiments and skills associated with such roles (Figure 10.4.1). Strategies were.

• The **reference group** was a group of individuals whose standpoints were used as a frame of reference. The program included formation of a group consisting of husband–wife teams who were expecting their first child. Organized and led by two nurse clinicians, members of the reference group presented their viewpoints; ideas were explored, discussed, adopted, or discarded. The group members had an opportunity to understand the normal range of feelings, fears, idiosyncracies, and experiences that were being experienced by others in similar circumstances. Group members tested ideas on and received reinforcements from each other. Leaders also were significant others who gave guidance, clarification, reinforcement, alternatives, and referrals when needed. The group met once a week.

---

[1]For more information, see Swendsen et al. (1978).

- **Role modeling** was provided by an individual or individuals who knew and used the behaviors, knowledge, and values expected in the role. The expectant parents learned from examples set by others who were or had been in the role. They also learned from professionals who knew the behaviors and expectations of the role. Each couple had its own set of role models, i.e., family, friends, physicians, and nurses. In the reference group, the couples discussed role models for parenting, ideas they had received from them, and how they intended to use those ideas in their own parenting. The role supplementation nurses served as role models because of their knowledge about the role. The nurses also brought to one of the group meetings a couple who had recently had an infant. This couple shared their experiences of pregnancy, labor and delivery, and infant care, and became strong role models for the experimental families.
- **Role rehearsal** was the mental enactment, fantasy, or image of what the role would be like. Each participant imagined himself or herself in the role, and anticipated or planned his or her responses to situations. The nurses facilitated role rehearsal by describing a case study or a situation that might occur in labor and delivery or in infant care, such as what the mother and father might be doing during labor. Couples were then asked to think about and explain how they might handle the situation. They explored alternatives as each person explained what his or her reaction and response might be.

The nurses recognized and stressed that roles and situations are not rigid, and that other circumstances or consequences may occur in the real-life situation. Therefore, the role rehearsal served to help persons learn to be cognizant of their potential responses in a variety of situations.

Two components provided the content for the program: role clarification and role taking. Role clarification is the identification of the knowledge and behaviors associated with the role. Examples of areas to help clarify roles associated with pregnancy, delivery, and child rearing were identified, using knowledge in physiology of pregnancy, labor, and delivery; knowledge of care of parents and the infant throughout the changes, growth, and development; expectations of parents of each other; normal disappointments encountered, and so on. Research findings in those and similar areas were translated into simple language and references were given where appropriate. Films and hospital tours were provided; pregnancy, labor, and postpartum exercises were practiced.

The second component was role taking. Role-taking skills help a person construct the world of significant others and act accordingly. Games to facilitate the development of such skill were provided (Figure 10.4.1).

Data Collection

Families were tested preprogram, predelivery, postprogram, and postdelivery. Research visits were made to each family, and various variables and research tools were used in each visit.

All subjects were contacted by phone and briefly told of the ongoing research project and invited to participate. Contact was made by research assistants, who did not know the treatment program or the families in the experimental group. Subjects who consented by phone to participate were recontacted by a research assistant to schedule the first visit. Research visit I was made at the beginning of the third trimester. A consent form, approved by the University of California Human Rights Committee, was presented to each subject, explaining the nature of the study, the meaning of participation in it, and the number and the length of future visits. The form also explained that couples had an option to withdraw from the study at any point. After the form was signed by both husband and wife, research visit I questionnaires were given and interviewing took place. Consent for each subsequent research visit was sought by telephone before the actual visit was made.

All participants were revisited two to four weeks predelivery. (For experimental group members, research visit II was done after the role supplementation intervention, but predelivery.) All research visits were made by research assistants who were not involved in the treatment program.

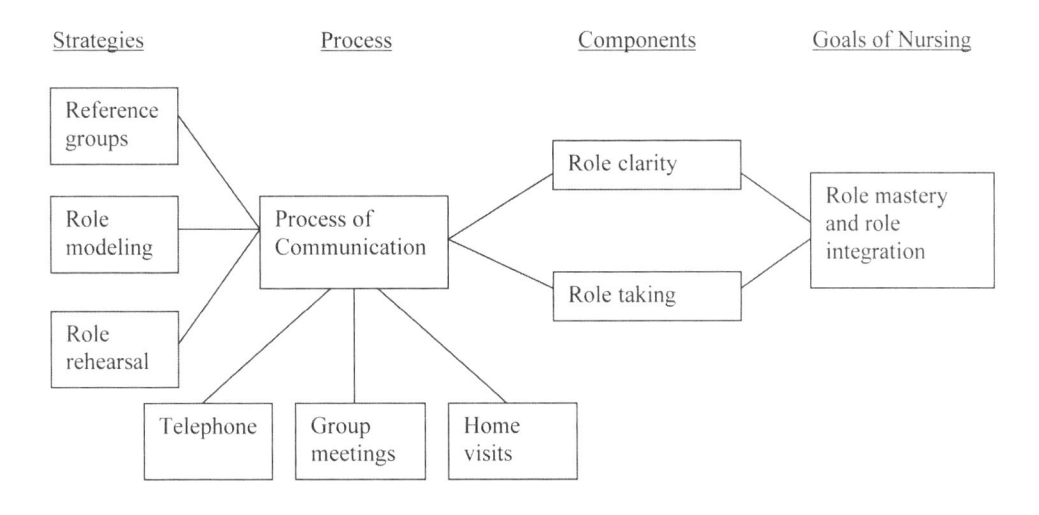

FIGURE 10.4.1 Clinical paradigm of a Preventive Role Supplementation Program.

Research visit III was made to all subjects one week postpartum. Research visit IV was made to all subjects six weeks postpartum. All subjects were mailed a research visit V protocol.

The rationale for selection of variables and research instruments for each visit was: research visit I was conducted to acquire preprogram baseline data for comparison with postprogram and postdelivery data. That the visit take place three to four months predelivery was essential so that subjects could participate and complete the role supplementation program.

Two experimental group couples failed to return the research visit V protocol, but completed all other research visits. All FamCap families completed the study. Twenty-one of the 36 control group couples completed all research visits.

Role Supplementation Visits

After research visit I, subjects were contacted by the clinical specialists, a short description of role supplementation was given, and subjects were asked whether both prospective parents were interested in participating.[2] The clinical specialist used the same procedure used by the hospital in inviting subjects to participate in hospital programs. Those who consented were entered in the experiment. This was continued until a sample of 12 couples was achieved. These subjects were then visited by the clinical specialist for orientation to role supplementation.

Two prenatal home visits were made to each couple in the experimental sample—the first to explain the program and enroll the couple; the second, after group meetings had ended but before delivery, to discuss individual questions and concerns. Eight weekly 2-hour group meetings were held during the last trimester of pregnancy. The meetings included dyadic material and discussion. The last half hour of each class was devoted to prenatal exercises and breathing techniques used in labor.

Two clinical nurse specialists conducted the classes, and one nurse made all the home visits. Couples were instructed to call one of the nurses after delivery. Wives made a hospital visit with their husbands and one of the nurses to discuss the labor and delivery experience and its meaning. Two home visits were made: one 24 to 48 hours after hospital discharge, and one 5 to 6 days later. The clinical specialists were on call 24 hours before and after delivery. Other home visits were made according to the needs and desire of the families,

---
[2]The research visits and the experimental (role supplementation) procedure were conducted by two different teams.

TABLE 10.4.1 Nurse–Family Contact for the Role Supplementation (Experimental) Group Families

Number and Topics of Classes Missed	Total Classes Attended	Telephone Calls to Patients Before Delivery	Telephone Calls to Patients After[1] Delivery	Telephone Calls to Nurse Before Delivery	Telephone Calls to Nurse After[2] Delivery	Home Visits Before[3] Delivery	Home Visits After Delivery	Hospital Visits
—	8	3	2	3	3	3	3	1
#5 Hospital tour; husband's role in labor and delivery	7	1	3	2	3	3	7	2
#1 Introduction #3 Pregnancy #4 Labor and delivery	5	0	1	0	1	2	2	1
#6 Newborn	7	0	1	0	2	2	3	1
#5 Hospital tour; husband's role in labor and delivery	7	0	1	0	2	1	2	1
#6 Newborn	7	0	3	2	3	2	3	1
#3 Pregnancy #6 Newborn	6	0	2	0	2	2	3	1
—	8	0	2	0	2	2	2	1
—	8	0	2	1	2	2	2	1
#6 Newborn	7	0	1	1	1	2	2	1
#4 Labor and delivery (Husband only attended one class because of work)	7 (wife only)	0	1	0	0	2	2	1
#2 Pregnancy #4 Labor and delivery	6	0	2	1	1	2	2	1

[1] Does not include telephone calls to arrange for home visits only.
[2] Includes call to inform nurse of the birth.
[3] Includes first visit to orient husband and wife to role supplementation program.

and termination generally took place about four weeks postpartum, after the couple had visited a pediatrician or pediatric nurse specialist. From three to ten visits were made on each subject.

Table 10.4.1 outlines nurse–family contact for the role supplementation group.

Instruments

Tools used in this study are indicated in Table 10.4.2. Demographic data, education, ethnic background, occupation, and age were obtained by questionnaire, through interviewing, and by self-report.

The Pregnancy Research Inventory (Schaefer & Manheimer, 1960) is composed of 68 statements denoting attitudes of mothers toward themselves, pregnancy, husband, and future baby. Fourteen factors were selected for this study, based on the need to establish lack of difference between experimental and control groups. The factors examined: fears for self, fears for pregnancy, dependency, fears for infant, irritability and tension, maternal feelings, depression and withdrawal, psychosomatic anxiety, sleep disturbance, nausea and vomiting, combined score of health problems during pregnancy, problems of menstruation, combined score of menstrual problems, and combined score of health and menstruation problems.

The Postnatal Research Inventory, also developed by Schaefer and Manheimer (1960), is composed of 91 statements concerning behaviors and

TABLE 10.4.2 Research Design for the Complete Role Supplementation Study[1]

Procedure	Pretest	Predelivery	Research	Visit 1	Posttests
		Predelivery		Postdelivery	
		Research Visit 2	Research Visit 3	Research Visit 4	Research Visit 5
Time	3–4 months pre-EDC	Postprogram and 2–3 weeks (pre EDC)	7–14 days Postdelivery	6–8 weeks Postdelivery	4–5 months Postdelivery
Variables	1) Interactions (H,W)[2] (Role perceptions)	1) Attitudes toward ROSP[3], FAMCAP—Prenatal program (H,W)	1) Depression (W)	1) Perception of changes (H,W)	1) Anxiety (H,W)
	2) Anxiety (H,W)	2) Perceptions of major components of program (Role clarity, reference group, etc.) (H,W)	2) Powerlessness (H,W)	2) Coping styles with changes (H,W)	2) Interactions (H,W)
	3) Powerlessness (H,W)	3) Anticipated role changes (H,W)	3) Perception of delivery experience and changes in life style (H,W)	3) Perception of baby's health (H,W)	3) Perceptions of baby's growth and development (H,W)
	4) Role identity of wife (by H,W)	4) Perception of each other's roles (H,W)	4) Congruency between anticipated and actual role changes (H,W)	4) Perception of role changes (H,W)	
	5) Number of stressful events (H,W)			5) Congruency in quantity and quality of roles (H,W)	5) Baby's health (H,W)
Research instruments	1) Interactions (Dunn, 1960, 1963) (H,W)1) Open-ended interview[4] (H,W)	1) Depression (MMPI) (W)	1) Baby's Health Inventory (Schaefer & Manheimer, 1960) (H,W)	1) Anxiety scale (Taylor, 1953) (H,W)	
	2) Anxiety scale (Taylor, 1953) (H,W)	2) Role Strain and Congruency (Hurvitz, 1960) (H,W)	2) Powerlessness (Seeman & Evans, 1962) (H,W)	2) Who Am I (Kuhn & McPartland, 1954) (W)	2) Interaction (Dunn, 1960, 1963) (H,W)
	3) Powerlessness (Seeman, 1962) (H,W)		3) Adjective mood list (H,W)	3) Perception of role adequacy[4] (H,W)3) Questionnaires[4] (H,W) a. Growth and development b. Role adequacy c. Role changes d. Change in recent events	

TABLE 10.4.2 *(continued)*[1]

Procedure	Pretest	Predelivery	Research	Visit 1	Posttests
		Predelivery		Postdelivery	
		Research Visit 2	Research Visit 3	Research Visit 4	Research Visit 5
	4) Perceptions of Roles (Meleis, 1974; Kuhn & McPartland, 1954) (H,W) 5) Schedule of recent events (Holmes & Rahe, 1967) (H,W) 6) Demographic data[4] (H,W) 7) Open-ended interview[4] (H,W) 8) Pregnancy Research Inventory (Schaefer & Manheimer, 1960) (H,W)	5) Open-ended interview[4] (H,W)	4) Baby's Health Inventory (Schaefer & Manheimer, 1960) (H,W)	4) Open-ended interview[4] (H,W) 5) Baby's Health (Schaefer & Manheimer, 1960) (H,W)	4) Who Am I (Kuhn & McPartland, 1954) (W)

[1] Not all tests shown in Table 10.4.2 pertain to the study described in this chapter. Table 10.4.2 presents the test design for the complete study.
[2] H = husband, W = wife.
[3] ROSP = role supplementation.
[4] The interview and questionnaire were developed for this study.

reactions of mothers related to the postpartum period. The inventory was subjected to factor analysis. The 26 factors used in this study were those related to the mother—depression and irritability, and those related to the relationship to the baby—ignoring, protecting, and responsiveness. They were happiness, need for assistance, irritability, positive perception of others, fear or concern for baby, negative aspects of childbearing, acceptance, intrapunitive, ignoring, need for showing experience, protectiveness, extrapermissive, responsiveness to infant's needs, convalescence, denial, need for consultation, fear for self, need for responsiveness, depression, mothering, confidence, disposition, convalescence, need for consultation, confidence.

The Taylor (1953) Manifest Anxiety Scale is a revised form of 50 true–false Minnesota Multiphasic Personality Inventory items, judged by a panel of experts as being indicative of manifest anxiety. The scale measures such anxiety feelings and symptoms as nervousness, inability to sleep or concentrate, fatigue, and loss of appetite. Test–retest reliability and validity have been established (Taylor, 1953, pp. 288–289) for the tool.

The Marriage Role Inventory (Dunn, 1960, 1963) is an exploratory pencil-and-paper test that evaluates and compares what is expected of self and of partner in seven years of marriage. Areas covered by the 71 items are authority, homemaking, care of children, personal characteristics, social participation, education, employment, and support. Re-

TABLE 10.4.3 Participation and Attrition of Study Sample

Factors	Study Groups			Total Participants
	Experimental	Control	FamCap	
Complete stillborn	0	1	0	1
Refusal to complete research	0	4	0	4[a]
Moved	0	7	0	7[b]
Failure to return research visit 5 tests	2	2	0	4
Completed visits	10	22	10	42
Total	12	36	10	58

[a] Following research visits 1 and 2.
[b] Following research visits 1 (3), 2 (1), and 4 (3).

spondents answer in terms of agreement, uncertainty, or disagreement with statements that describe marital behaviors and attitudes indicating a companionship egalitarian relationship, or a traditional patriarchal relationship to a marriage partner. The inventory was used in this study preexperiment, postexperiment, and poststudy.

Results and Discussion

Participation and attrition in the study are shown in Table 10.4.3.

Hypothesis I

There were no significant differences among experimental, control, or FamCap groups in mean age of wives, mean age of husbands, religious characteristics of husbands, educational characteristics of wives and husbands, length of marriage, or husband's occupation. All but two of the mothers who participated in the study worked, with the majority involved in sales, clerical, or craft-type jobs, as opposed to professional, labor, or service jobs.

A significant difference was found among groups regarding wives' religion ($p = .05$). On the whole, differences among the groups did not result from preexisting differences in demographic characteristics. When group differences in the means of the 14 variables in the Pregnancy Research Inventory were calculated and an F-ratio test was employed, no significant differences were found among groups. Fears for self, fears for pregnancy, fears for baby, psychosomatic problems and complaints were among the 14 variables tested.

Hypothesis II

To test this hypothesis, the Marriage Role Expectation Inventory was administered several times to husbands and wives. There were significant differences among mean scores of wives in experimental, FamCap, and control groups in interaction (role perceptions) prior to their participation in the research groups (Table 10.4.4). In other words, wives who had a more egalitarian perception of their marriage roles sought to participate in special prenatal programs, i.e., in FamCap and in the role supplementation programs. They agreed to commit themselves and their husbands to cooperation and participation through the delivery and postpartum periods.

A similar pattern was manifested by husbands. There were significant differences among inventory scores of husbands who participated in the three groups (Table 10.4.4). However, unlike the wives, the actual birth of the infant helped to improve the role perception of husbands (to more egalitarian perceptions) more than did participation in role supplementation or FamCap programs.

TABLE 10.4.4 Role Perception Inventory Mean Scores on Marriage Role Expectation Inventory for Husbands and Wives Pre- and Postdelivery for Experimental (N = 10), Control (N = 20), and FamCap (N = 10) Groups

Groups	Scores	
	Husbands[1]	Wives[2]
Predelivery		
Experimental	57	61
Control	51	50
FamCap	56	63
Postdelivery		
Experimental	61	62
Control	54	53
FamCap	62	64

[1] Predelivery: $F = 4.42$, df = 2/34, $p = .02$; postdelivery: $F = 2.31$, df = 2/34, pre–postdelivery, $F = .15$, df = 2/34.
[2] Predelivery: $F = 10.00$, df = 2/37, $p = .0003$; postdelivery: $F = 8.83$, df = 2/37, $p = .0007$; pre–postdelivery: $F = .18$, df = 2/37.

TABLE 10.4.5 Anxiety Scores for Husbands and Wives in Experimental (N = 9), FamCap (N = 10), and Control (N = 19) Groups Predelivery and Postdelivery

Groups	Scores	
	Husbands[1]	Wives[2]
Predelivery		
Experimental	15.10	14.00
FamCap	7.00	13.00
Control	10.25	14.75
Postdelivery		
Experimental	11.00	15.75
FamCap	7.75	17.10
Control	10.50	18.10

[1] Predelivery: $F = 5.05$, df = 2/36, $p = .01$; postdelivery: $F = .85$, df = 2/36; pre–postdelivery: $F = 3.85$; df = 2/36, $p = .03$
[2] Predelivery: $F = .23$, df = 2/35; postdelivery: $F = .31$, df = 2/35; pre–postdelivery: $F = .034$, df = 2/35.

Participation in the role supplementation program, it had been anticipated, would sharpen communication skills, increase skill in role taking, and increase the congruency in role perceptions. FamCap families, especially husbands, however, showed the greatest change in role perceptions.

Hypothesis III

There were no significant differences in anxiety scores among wives of the three research groups at the onset of the investigation (Table 10.4.5). Mean anxiety level of experimental group wives was considerably lower after the study than that of control or FamCap groups, though not statistically significant. Findings indicated role supplementation may have prevented increase in the level of postdelivery anxiety, so that although role supplementation did not lower wives' anxiety, it may have helped them maintain a level of anxiety.

The picture for husbands was different. Husbands who consented to participate in the role supplementation program originally manifested a significantly higher level of anxiety than the control or the FamCap groups. Following the nursing intervention, the anxiety level of experimental group husbands was significantly ($p = .01$) lower and the mean anxiety level for all groups became comparable (Table 10.4.5).

Anxiety level increased during the study in all participants, especially women, except in experimental group husbands; role supplementation succeeded in lowering the level of anxiety in husbands.

Hypothesis IV

All wives who participated in the study were given the Postpartum Research Inventory to determine whether participation in the role supplementation program resulted in differences in general feelings and attitudes toward self and infant during the postpartum period. No differences were found among groups on variables that explored attitudes toward self, such as need for consultation, confidence in self, acceptance of delivery, happiness, or feelings of irritability. When variables relating to the infant were explored, three major differences were detected. Among the three research groups there were significant differences in the wives' perceptions and attitudes toward ignoring the baby ($F = 6.3650$, $df = 2/42$, $p = .01$), protectiveness of the baby ($F = 8.4439$, $df = 2/42$, $p = .01$), and responsiveness to infants' needs ($F = 5.9835$, df $= 2/42$, $p = .01$), indicating that participation in role supplementation might have been responsible for such differences. Further exploration of the differences in the group means indicated that experimental and FamCap group mothers manifested less ignorance and more cognizance of the needs of their infants than did control group mothers. Control group mothers demonstrated more protective behavior and more nonintegrative (nonappropriate) responsiveness to the infant than the others. In other words, although the prenatal programs of role supplementation and FamCap appeared to have influenced mothers toward more positive attitudes toward their infants, they did not significantly affect attitudes of mothers toward self.

Limitations

Limitations were recognized in this study. A larger sample would have made interpretations more valid. Ideally, matched experimental and control samples would have decreased the chance that extraneous variables might have caused the statistical differences in the analysis. Expectant date of delivery presented a problem in matching samples. Before the study is replicated, the validity and reliability of a number of the tools should be ensured.

Implications

Despite limitations, research implications of a conceptual framework, its components, and the methodological definitions of its concepts were demonstrated. Results of using such a framework on changes or prevention of changes in couples who participated in the experiment were shown. In home visits, group meetings, and telephone conversations, the nurse acted as a role model, a significant other, and was accountable for her actions. She was there when needed. But more significantly, she delivered nursing care that could be articulated and tested.

REFERENCES

Acton, R. L. Initiating the nursing process. In *Maternity Nursing Today*, ed. by J. P. Clausen et al. New York: McGraw-Hill Book Co., 1973, pp. 293–320.

Banasiak, P. A., & Corcoran, M. M. Preparation for childbirth. In *Maternity Nursing Today*, ed. by J. P. Clausen et al. New York: McGraw-Hill Book Co., 1973, pp. 367–388.

Benedick, T. Parenthood during the life cycle. In *Parenthood, Its Psychology and Psychopathology*, ed. by E. J. Anthony, & T. Benedick. Boston: Little, Brown & Co., 1970, pp. 185–206.

Blumer, H. *Symbolic Interactionism: Perspective and Method*. Englewood Cliffs, NJ: Prentice-Hall, 1969.

Caplan, G. *An Approach to Community Mental Health*. New York: Grune & Stratton, 1961.

Chinn, P. L. *Child Health Maintenance*. St. Louis, MO: C. V. Mosby Co., 1974.

Colman, A. D., & Colman, L. *Pregnancy: The Psychological Experience*. New York: Seabury Press, 1971.

Cooley, C. H. *Human Nature and the Social Order*, rev. ed. New York: Charles Schribner's Sons, 1922.

Dewey, J. *Human Nature & Conduct: An Introduction to Social Psychology*. New York: Henry Holt & Co., 1922.

Dunn, M. S. Marriage role expectations of adolescents. *Marriage & Fam Liv*, 22:99–111, May 1960.

Dunn, M. S. *A Marriage Role Expectation Inventory*. New York: Family Life Publications, 1963.

Dyer, E. D. Parenthood as crisis: A re-study. In *Crisis Intervention: Selected Readings*, ed. by H. J. Parad. New York: Family Service Association of America, 1965, pp. 312–323.

Feldman, M. Cluster visits. *Am J Nurs*, 74:1485–1491, Aug. 1974.

Fitzpatrick, E. et al. *Maternity Nursing*, 12th ed. Philadelphia: J. B. Lippincott Co., 1971.

Gould, J., & Kalb, W. L. *A Dictionary of Social Sciences*. New York: Free Press of Glencoe, 1974.

Grimm, E. Psychological and social factors in pregnancy, delivery and outcome. In *Child Bearing—Its Social and Psychological Aspects*, ed. by S. A. Richardson, & A. F. Guttmacher. Baltimore: Williams & Wilkins Co., 1967, pp. 1–52.

Holmes, T. H., & Rahe, R. H. Social readjustment rating scale. *J Psychosomatic Res*, 11 (2):213–218, 1967.

Hurvitz, N. Marital roles inventory and the measurement of marital adjustment. *J Clin Psychol*, 16:377–380, 1960.

Jessner, L. et al. The development of parental attitude during pregnancy. In *Parenthood, Its Psychology and Psychopathology*, ed. by E. J. Anthony, & T. Benedick. Boston: Little, Brown & Co., 1970, pp. 209–244.

Kuhn, M. H., & McPartland, T. S. Empirical investigation of self-attitude. *Am Soc Rev*, 19:68–76, Feb. 1954.

LeMasters, G. G. Parenthood as crisis. In *Crisis Intervention: Selected Readings*, ed. by H. J. Parad. New York: Family Services Association of America, 1965, pp. 111–117.

Littlefield, V. Emotional consideration for pregnant family. In *Maternity Nursing Today*, ed. by J. P. Clausen et al. New York: McGraw-Hill Book Co., 1973, pp. 389–432.

Lucas, J. D. The interactive effects of anxiety, failure, and intraserial duplication. *Am J Psychol*, 65:59–66, Jan. 1952.

Mead, G. H. *Mind, Self and Society*. Introduction by C. W. Morris. Chicago: University of Chicago Press, 1934.

Meleis, A. I. Self-concept photograph: A research tool. *Videosociology*, 2:46–62, Dec. 1974.

———. Role insufficiency and role supplementation: A conceptual framework. *Nurs Res*, 24:264–271, July–Aug. 1975.

Rossi, A. S. Transition to parenthood. *J Marriage & Fam*, 30:26–39, Feb. 1968.

Schaefer, E. S. A circumplex model for maternal behavior. *J Abnorm Soc Psychol*, 59:226–235, Sept. 1959.

Schaefer, E. S., & Manheimer, H. *Dimensions of Prenatal Adjustments*. Paper presented at the Eastern Psychological Association, New York, NY, Apr. 6, 1960. (Unpublished)

Seeman, M., & Evans, J. W. Alienation and learning in a hospital setting. *Am Soc Rev*, 27:772–782, Dec. 1962.

Shereshefsky, P. M., & Yarrow, L. J. *Psychological Aspects of a First Pregnancy and Early Postnatal Adaptation*. New York: Raven Press, 1973.

Sullivan, H. S. *The Interpersonal Theory of Psychiatry*, ed. by H. S. Perry, & M. L. Gawel. New York: W. W. Norton & Co., 1953.

Swendsen, L., Meleis & Jones. Role supplementation for new parents: A means to role mastery. *MCN Am J Matern Child Nursing*, 3(2):84-91, Mar-Apr 1978.

Taylor, J. A. A personality scale of manifest anxiety. *J Abnorm Soc Psychol*, 48:285–290, Apr. 1953.

Turner, R. Role taking: Process vs. Conformity. In *Human Behavior and Social Processes*, ed. by A. M. Rose. Boston: Houghton Mifflin Co., 1962, pp. 20–40.

Reprinted with permission from: Meleis, A. I., & Swendsen, L. (1978). Role supplementation: An empirical test of a nursing intervention. *Nursing Research, 27,* 11–18.

10.5 GROUP COUNSELING IN CARDIAC REHABILITATION: EFFECT ON PATIENT COMPLIANCE

KATHLEEN DRACUP
AFAF IBRAHIM MELEIS
SUZANNE CLARK
ARLINE CLYBURN
LINDA SHIELDS
MARILYN STALEY

Abstract

A multicenter clinical trial was conducted to evaluate the effects on compliance of a group counseling program for cardiac patients and spouses. The sample comprised 58 couples, in which one of the partners had documented atherosclerotic heart disease and was enrolled in an outpatient cardiac rehabilitation program. The experimental intervention involved a 10-week series of group sessions based on symbolic interactionist role theory. The research used a quasi-experimental, three-group, time-series design: Experimental group 1 consisted of 17 patients and their spouses who participated in group counseling; experimental group 2 consisted of 22 patients and their spouses, but only the patients participated in the group series; the control group consisted of 19 patients and their spouses who did not participate in the experimental program. Data were collected at baseline, 10 weeks, and 6 months on 4 cardiac risk factors: weight loss, blood pressure, exercise, and smoking. Repeated measures analysis of variance showed a significant difference (p < 0.01) in mean body fat among treatment groups, with experimental group 2 having the greatest decrease over time. Patients in both experimental groups demonstrated lowered blood pressure, with a significant decrease (p < 0.05) in systolic blood pressure. Again, the largest decrease was in experimental group 2. Changes in weekly exercise level were not significantly *different among groups, although the highest compliance was reported by experimental group 1 patients. Results support the efficacy of group counseling based on an interactionist role theory framework to increase compliance. The anticipated effect of spouse participation was not confirmed.*

Introduction

The extent to which an individual's behavior coincides with a prescribed medical regimen is surprisingly low. Investigators have consistently documented that compliance with therapeutic medication regimens averages 50%, and falls dramatically with the passage of time; compliance with short-term preventive regimens (e.g., immunizations) is 75% and falls to 50% with long-term regimens (e.g., rheumatic fever prophylaxis); and patients keep 45% of appointments made for them by nurses and physicians.[1,2] The lowest compliance rates are recorded for lifestyle regimen, (e.g., weight control, exercise programs, and smoking cessation). At 6 months, compliance rates fall to approximately 20%.[2-4]

During the past 15 years, a number of investigators have conducted randomized clinical trials to test the effects of various strategies on patient compliance. Contrary to expectations, many of these strategies have proved ineffective. For example, teaching patients about their illness or their prescribed medications makes them more knowledgeable, but does not necessarily increase their adherence to prescribed regimens[5-7]; neither does making health care more accessible by bringing it to the work setting improve adherence.[7,8]

In contrast, three strategies have yielded positive results in experimental trials. These are: (a) behavioral contracting aimed at cuing and reinforcement of compliant behavior;[9-11] (b) simplification of medical regimens with respect to complexity, duration, and cost;[5,12] and (c) enlistment of family members to support prescribed regimens.[13-15]

Two problems have hampered efforts in both the descriptive and experimental phases of compliance research. The first of these is methodological. The methods employed to measure adherence have been admittedly inadequate. As noted by Gordis,[16] this deficiency is particularly true for medication compliance. Pill counts and even serum and urine tests are not necessarily valid indicators. Moreover, patients and health professionals are subject to conscious (and unconscious) pressures to report more adherence to a regimen than actually exists.[17,18] Thus, self or physician reports may provide an overestimation of compliance rates.

The second area of concern is conceptual. In general, research efforts have been atheoretical, either examining patient characteristics to predict compliance/noncompliance or testing clinical strategies recommended in the anecdotal literature. Neither of these types of research has been based on appropriate explanatory (structural) and predictive conceptual models.

As noted by Stone,[19] the few theories that have been developed and tested have failed to take into account the myriad of variables known to affect compliance. For example, the quality of interaction between patient and health care professional and the relationship of the patient with significant others (potential supporters of the medical regimen) are two variables noted previously as important in the development of compliance behavior. Yet neither is included in the best-known compliance models/theories, namely, the medical model, the health belief model, or control theory.

Theoretical Model

Interactionist role theory was proposed by Dracup and Meleis[20] as a potential framework for defining the phenomenon of compliance, delineating the antecedents of compliant behavior, and determining effective interventions. It has the advantage of including all the agents involved in a compliance interaction—patient, health professional, significant other(s)—as well as the individual variables related to each actor and to the medical regimen.

Briefly stated, symbolic interactionism holds that roles are constantly being formulated and redefined on the basis of interactions with others. These others enact complementary or reciprocal roles (e.g., husband/wife, patient/nurse, employer/employee) and provide cues regarding the appropriateness of behaviors for a given role.[21-23] Roles, then, are not based on positions with attendant rights and duties, but are fluid in nature. They evolve and are personalized through interactions with significant others.

The two roles pertinent to a discussion of compliance are the sick role and the at-risk role. The former is well described by Parsons.[24] The latter provides a new dimension to our understanding of compliance behavior. This role assumes that the patient or client is no longer acutely ill but, by virtue of chronic illness or identifiable risk factors, is at high risk for a catastrophic illness.[25] For example, the patient who has suffered a myocardial infarction is at greater risk for a second myocardial infarction or a sudden-death event than the rest of the population.

Both the sick role and the at-risk role demand complementary roles. For instance, cardiac patients need to modify what they eat, how much they exercise, what medications they do or do not take, and what degree of stress they allow in their lives. Spouses, in turn, are asked to support these lifestyle changes and are encouraged to make similar changes.

Using symbolic interactionist theory, four components can be delineated for an analysis of compliance behavior: (a) the individual's self-concept, (b) the behaviors that are demanded in a prescribed regimen (and are appropriate for the sick role or at-risk role), (c) the counterroles played by significant others, and (d) the periodic evaluations of roles enacted both by the individual and by those in reciprocal roles.[26] Dracup and Meleis[20] suggested seven propositions based on these four components. Two of the propositions were: (a) compliance is enhanced if the sick or at-risk role is reinforced by significant others and other reference groups; (b) compliance is enhanced when relevant other roles are congruent or complementary, or both, with client roles. These two propositions were tested in the present study as hypotheses. The purpose of our study was twofold:

1. To evaluate the effect of a group counseling intervention based on the above four components on the compliance of cardiac patients.
2. To evaluate the effect of increased involvement of spouses within the context of a group counseling intervention on the compliance of cardiac patients.

Hypotheses

1. Patients who participate in a group counseling program will have greater compliance than will patients who do not participate.
2. Patients whose spouses also participate in a group counseling program will have greater compliance than will patients who participate without spouses.

Methods

Sample

All patients attending four outpatient cardiac rehabilitation centers during the period of data collection were asked to participate in the study. Patient eligibility criteria for inclusion in the study were enrollment in an outpatient cardiac rehabilitation program, documented coronary heart disease, married or currently living in the same household with a partner, and consent of the private physician. Of 63 couples originally enrolled, 4 dropped out within the first week after completing baseline testing, and another couple separated and were lost to follow-up after completing the role supplementation program but before the 6-month testing. The study sample thus comprised 116 subjects (58 patients and their spouses), with approximately equal representation from each center. The four centers are located in a large Western metropolitan city and are similar in philosophy, admission criteria, and treatment protocols. Patients in all four centers attended the cardiac rehabilitation program three times weekly for one hour of exercise training. They also received information on various topics related to coronary heart disease. Prior to participation in this study, none of the centers had included spouses in the rehabilitation program beyond an initial interview.

The subjects ranged in age from 33 to 73 years (mean 57 years). All but one of the couples were married, with the mean duration of marriage being 28 years. Couples in the sample scored in the upper three levels of socio-economic class on the Hollingshead Four Factor Index of Social Status.[27] Eleven subjects were Asian; the remainder were Caucasian. Fifty-two (90%) of the patients were male.

Although all patients had documented atherosclerotic heart disease, their medical histories differed. Clinical status was assessed in terms of: (a) number of documented myocardial infarctions, (b) number of coronary revascularization operations, (c) number of surgical grafts required during last coronary revascularization, (d) highest metabolic equivalent (MET) achieved on most recent treadmill test, and (e) functional class. The last variable was based on the New York Heart Association's categories:

Functional class I: Ordinary activity does not cause symptoms;
Functional class II: Patients experience slight limitation of physical activity. Ordinary physical activity causes fatigue, dyspnea, palpitation, or angina pectoris;
Functional class III: Patients have marked limitation of activity and experience symptoms with less than ordinary activity. They do not have symptoms at rest;
Functional class IV: Patients cannot engage in any physical activity without symptoms and have symptoms at rest.

Twenty-eight patients were referred to cardiac rehabilitation because of a recent myocardial infarction, whereas the remaining 30 had recent coronary revascularization surgery. Two patients experienced both a heart attack and surgery within the preceding three months. The majority of patients achieved exercise levels higher than six METs on their most recent exercise stress test. All but 4 of the 58 patients were classified in functional classes I or II.

Procedures

Patients and their spouses signed a consent form prior to participation and were assigned to one of three groups according to a time series design:

1. Experimental group 1 comprised 17 cardiac patients and their spouses who participated in a group counseling program (the experimental treatment).
2. Experimental group 2 comprised 22 cardiac patients and their spouses, but only the patients participated in a group counseling program (the modified experimental treatment).
3. The control group comprised 19 cardiac patients and their spouses, none of whom attended the role supplementation program.

Each of the study centers offered the two experimental interventions and the control condition in a consecutive series, with the sequence of the experimental groups determined by coin toss. This design reduced the potential for contamination of subjects during exercise periods.

The experimental intervention consisted of a 10-week series of group discussions, each lasting 90 minutes. The initial session was designed to acquaint the participants with the concepts of role transition and the at-risk role. Patients (and spouses in experimental group 1) introduced themselves by reviewing their coronary events and the ways in which their lives and relationships had changed because of their illness. Sessions 2 and 3 focused on the anxiety experienced in a role transition period, and the group leaders presented a systematic approach to problem solving aimed at clarifying alternatives and decreasing anxiety. In the fourth session, a couple who had already completed the cardiac rehabilitation program were invited to discuss their experiences. They served as role models for the group in their ability to master the at-risk role (and its complement) and to make adjustments in their other roles. The fifth and sixth sessions focused on stress reduction as a specific component required of the at-risk role. The participants were taught a relaxation technique and were given appropriate homework assignments to practice. They also were encouraged to role-play stressful situations in the group. Sessions 7 through 10 were devoted to discussing general areas of stress: social, sexual, physical, or those related to conforming to the at-risk role by reducing cardiac risk factors. The final session also included a summary and general critique of the group.

The groups met at the cardiac treatment center one evening a week. Two nurses, one the coordinator of the cardiac rehabilitation program at each center, and the second a nurse with a master's degree in nursing and special expertise in group dynamics, served as group facilitators. The experimental protocol was based on the assumption that both patients and spouses experience a period of role transition upon entry into a cardiac rehabilitation program. It was hypothesized that patient compliance would increase as patients incorporated the at-risk role in their self-concept and as this new role was supported by those in reciprocal roles. The group facilitators used the techniques and processes of role supplementation, including role modeling, role rehearsal, role clarification, and the use of reference groups.[28,29] The same protocol was followed in both experimental groups.

Compliance Measures

Four dependent variables were identified as measures of compliance to a cardiac risk-factor regimen: smoking, blood pressure, body weight, and weekly exercise. Data about smoking and weekly exercise (defined as the amount of time spent exercising at a prescribed target heart rate) were obtained by means of two interview questions. These were asked in the presence of spouses in an attempt to increase the truthfulness of the self-report.

Systolic and diastolic blood pressures were obtained using the standard auscultatory methods defined by the American Heart Association.[30] The same sphygmomanometer was used throughout the duration of the study and was calibrated weekly. To circumvent the minor fluctuations that occur from arm to arm, each subject's measurements were made in the same arm.

A decrease in fatfold measurements was considered an indirect measure of weight loss. The procedure consists of measuring a double layer of skin and subcutaneous fat at a specific body site with skinfold calipers.[31] The most common sites used are subscapular and the triceps, the latter having the advantage of being more accessible. In this study, triceps skinfold measurements were obtained by use of a Harpenden skinfold calipers. Three readings were taken, and the average was used as a final value. The site of measurement was the left triceps, halfway down the arm between the tip of the acromion and the top of the radius. The skinfold was picked up in a line passing directly up the arm from the tip of the olecranon process. A measuring tape was used to establish the midpoint for measurement. All measurements were taken with the subject's arm hanging relaxed at his/her side. Reported accuracy of this measurement is ± 5% with repeated measures.[32]

These same four compliance outcomes were measured for spouses in all three treatment groups to determine whether (and to what extent) spousal support for cardiac risk factor modification extended to actual changes in the spouses' cardiac risk factors, as well. Spouse data were not related to hypothesis testing, but were collected to gain insight into the dynamics of the role-taking process.

Data were collected at baseline, at 10 weeks, and at 6 months. One researcher collected all data to eliminate interobserver variation of blood pressure and skinfold measurements. All testing took an average of 40 minutes.

Results

Preliminary Data Analyses

Preliminary analyses were conducted to test the comparability of the three research groups and the four centers on nine demographic variables. A two-way ANOVA using group and center as factors established no significant differences ($p > 0.05$) for patients or spouses for age, years married, number of children, number of children in residence, or

TABLE 10.5.1 Medical Status of Patient Sample by Treatment Group

Characteristic	Experimental group 1: patients and spouses (n = 17) No.	%	Experimental group 2: patients only (n = 22) No.	%	Control group (n = 19) No.	%
Myocardial infarction*						
0	11	64.7	11	50.0	8	42.1
1	5	29.4	10	45.5	8	42.1
1	1	5.9	1	4.5	3	15.8
CABG†						
0	5	29.4	11	50.0	6	31.6
1	12	70.6	10	45.4	12	63.2
1	0	0	1	4.5	1	5.2
	Mean	Range	Mean	Range	Mean	Range
Grafts‡	3.0	1–5	2.8	1–5	2.0	1–5
MET level§	7.6	4–14	8.5	3–12	9.1	4–14
Functional class	2.1¶	1–3	1.7	1–3	1.4	1–3

*Number of documented myocardial infarctions.
†CABG = number of coronary artery bypass graft procedures performed.
‡Number of surgical grafts required during last coronary revascularization.
§Highest MET achieved on most recent treadmill test.
¶Significantly greater than in the other two groups ($p < 0.05$).

income. Patients in experimental group 2 had a mean of two more years education than the other two groups ($F = 5.04$, $df = 2$, $p < 0.05$). Chi-square analyses revealed no differences for occupation, religion, or sex among research groups.

With the exception of MET, the medical characteristics of patients were analyzed using chi-square (Table 10.5.1). MET levels were compared among groups using a one-way ANOVA. There were no significant differences among study groups on any of the clinical variables with the exception of functional class. More experimental group 1 patients were in functional class III than were those in the other two treatment groups (chi-square = 9.427, $df = 4$, $p < 0.05$). Although the difference was not significant, the patients in this group also achieved lower treadmill MET levels than did patients in the other two groups.

Hypothesis Testing

The three groups in each center were analyzed on the basis of their differences over time by means of a repeated measures analysis of variance. To reduce the chance of a type 1 error occurring from multiple testing, the Greenhouse-Geisser[33] method for determining probability values was used, with significance set at $p < 0.05$. The two factors used in the analysis were group and center. There were no center interactions, attesting to the homogeneity of the sample across the four research settings.

Smoking behavior was not significantly different over time among groups for either patients or spouses. In the patient sample, only 2 of the 58 subjects smoked upon entry into the study, 1 in the control group and 1 in the experimental group 2, although 36 subjects had a recent (less than 1 year) smoking history. Both continued to smoke at 6-month follow-up. The remaining 56 patients had maximum compliance on this variable.

The number of hours per week that the patient and spouse exercised over the study period are presented in Table 10.5.2. Although the changes are consistent with the study hypotheses, i.e., patients and spouses who participated in a group counseling program showed the greatest compliance at six-

TABLE 10.5.2 Hours Exercised per Week by Treatment Group Over Time

Time	Experimental group 1 Mean	SD	Percent change*	Experimental group 2 Mean	SD	Percent change*	Control group Mean	SD	Percent change*
Patients									
Baseline	3.45	1.00	—	3.64	0.58	—	3.09	0.94	—
10 weeks	3.50	0.86	+1.45	3.82	0.50	+4.95	3.05	1.35	−1.29
6 months	3.53	1.18	+2.32	3.50	0.74	−3.85	2.68	1.29	−13.27
Spouses									
Baseline	1.95	1.91	—	1.68	1.70	—	1.81	1.81	—
10 weeks	2.17	1.72	+11.28	1.81	1.60	+7.73	1.26	1.59	−30.39
6 months	1.94	1.78	−0.51	1.57	1.66	−6.55	0.95	1.43	−47.51

*Calculated from baseline.

month follow-up; whereas patients who participated without spousal involvement showed greater compliance than did patients in the control group, the differences among the three groups were not statistically significant (patients: $F_{4,92} = 0.08$, $p < 0.05$; spouses $F_{4,86} = 0.48$, $p < 0.05$).

As noted in Table 10.5.3, there was a significant difference among groups regarding changes in body fat, as indicated in lower triceps skinfold measurements over the six months ($F_{4,92} = 3.39$, $p < 0.01$). Patients who met with their spouses had a mean decrease at 6 months of 12.57%, and patients who met without spouses had a mean decrease of 17.37%. These positive compliance outcomes were in marked contrast to the control group. Initially, control patients had a similar decrease, but these changes were not maintained at six months. In fact, the control group had a 1.79% mean increase in skinfold measurements from baseline to 6 months. Thus, the experimental intervention seemed to be effective in achieving long-term weight loss (hypothesis 1).

The data, however, do not support hypothesis 2. Despite the fact that spouses in experimental group 1 were the only spouses to have a decrease in their skinfold measurements ($F_{4,86} = 2.37$, $p = 0.06$) from baseline to 6 months (indicating the efficacy of their participation in the group sessions), these effects were not reflected in the patient data.

The largest decrease for patients was seen in the patient-only group, in which spouses had a consistent increase in triceps skinfold measurement over the six months.

Changes in patients' systolic and diastolic blood pressure measurements over the six-month period are summarized in Table 10.5.4. A significant difference among groups occurred in systolic pressure ($F_{4,92} = 2.61$, $p < 0.05$). In reviewing the data, it is clear that the most significant decrease again occurred for patients who met without their spouses. Patients whose spouses participated also showed a decrease, but it was less marked. Patients in the control group had a marked increase. Similar patterns emerge for diastolic blood pressure measurements, although the differences among groups were not statistically significant ($F_{4,92} = 1.42$, $p < 0.05$).

The changes in spouses' blood pressure measurements mirrored those of the patient sample (Table 10.5.5). The largest decreases were seen in spouses whose mates had attended the group series, with similar but less dramatic decreases in spouses who had participated in the experimental program with their mates. Control-group spouses had relatively little change. The differences among groups were not statistically significant.

In reviewing the blood pressure data, it can be seen that the patients who experienced the most

TABLE 10.5.3   Triceps Skinfold Measurements (mm) by Treatment Group Over Time

Time	Experimental group 1 Mean	SD	Percent change[*]	Experimental group 2 Mean	SD	Percent change[*]	Control group Mean	SD	Percent change[*]
Patients									
Baseline	15.75	6.27	—	13.59	3.36	—	15.05	7.39	—
10 weeks	14.56	5.95	−7.56	11.55	3.10	−15.01	12.74	4.05	−15.35
6 months	13.77	6.00	−12.57	11.23	3.21	−17.37	15.32	6.80	+1.79
Spouses									
Baseline	22.00	7.00	—	18.64	6.98	—	20.10	6.77	—
10 weeks	20.56	6.58	−6.55	19.20	4.74	+3.00	19.53	6.65	−2.84
6 months	20.94	7.15	−4.82	20.33	6.26	+9.07	20.84	6.86	+3.68

[*]Calculated from baseline.

TABLE 10.5.4   Blood Pressure Measurements (mmHg) by Treatment Group Over Time

Time	Experimental group 1 Mean	SD	Percent change[*]	Experimental group 2 Mean	SD	Percent change[*]	Control group Mean	SD	Percent change[*]
Systolic									
Baseline	125.85	17.89	—	128.73	16.37	—	125.52	20.81	—
10 weeks	123.89	18.79	−1.56	120.32	11.59	−6.53	132.42	28.90	+5.50
6 months	124.71	14.12	−0.91	119.18	22.07	−7.42	129.63	24.32	+3.27
Diastolic									
Baseline	76.65	12.97	—	77.27	8.76	—	74.52	11.88	—
10 weeks	73.22	9.61	−4.47	73.73	6.85	−4.58	74.11	9.46	−0.55
6 months	71.00	8.13	−7.37	71.86	9.21	−7.00	75.68	11.29	+1.56

[*]Calculated from baseline.

significant decreases in blood pressure were those who participated in the formal reference group provided by the group series (hypothesis 1). Hypothesis 2 was not supported, in that patients in both experimental interventions experienced significant decreases. Spouse participation did not yield a particular advantage. However, it should be noted that patients' and spouses' mean blood pressure changes were similar across groups. This finding does support the interactive nature of compliance behaviors.

Although this study documents the beneficial effects of a group-counseling intervention based on role theory, it does not indicate whether such a program affects ultimate morbidity and mortality. If the true incidence of 1-year mortality for post-myocardial infarction patients is 5%,[34] it would take a sample of 16,000 patients to have a power of 0.80 in detecting such differences at a 0.05 level of significance (one-sided). Within the sample of 58 patients, 3 were rehospitalized. One patient suffered a second myocardial infarction; a second patient was hospitalized for chest pain, but a myocardial infarction was ruled out. A third patient was hospitalized for complications related to his previous

TABLE 10.5.5 Spouses' Blood Pressure Measurements (mmHg) by Treatment Group Over Time

	Experimental group 1			Experimental group 2			Control group		
Time	Mean	SD	Percent change*	Mean	SD	Percent change*	Mean	SD	Percent change*
Systolic									
Baseline	129.50	21.55	—	136.82	22.50	—	133.20	27.02	—
10 weeks	129.11	19.41	−0.30	128.00	14.88	−6.45	132.21	23.99	−0.74
6 months	121.06	18.15	−6.52	123.76	20.20	−9.55	133.47	25.61	+0.20
Diastolic									
Baseline	75.80	13.78	—	78.64	11.64	—	75.10	12.97	—
10 weeks	74.67	9.23	−1.49	77.65	12.11	−1.26	73.90	9.51	−1.60
6 months	70.35	10.37	−7.19	72.81	12.83	−7.41	73.21	11.63	−2.52

*Calculated from baseline.

coronary artery bypass graft surgery. Interestingly, all three patients were in the control group. None of the patients who participated in the experimental groups were hospitalized before the six-month follow-up. None of the subjects had died at 6-month follow-up.

In summary, the group-counseling series did appear to have a positive effect on the course of the patients' disease. This conclusion must be viewed with caution, however, given the small sample size and the relatively short period of follow-up

Discussion

The study findings support the positive effects of a role-oriented, group-counseling intervention on cardiac risk-factor compliance. Both experimental groups had significantly lower blood pressures and decreased triceps skinfold measurements at six-month follow-up. This finding is in contrast to the data of Adsett and Bruhn[35] and Ibrahim and associates.[36] Neither found positive compliance changes (decreased blood pressure or weight loss) in postmyocardial infarction patients who attended a series of open-ended group-therapy sessions.

These current findings support the view of compliance as being dependent on interactional processes. The at-risk role, like all roles, is created, defined, stabilized, and modified as an outgrowth of interactions with one or more relevant others.

The experimental protocol provided a framework for interactions that enhanced the assumption of the at-risk role. Turner[23] has suggested that a person's tendency to merge a new role with the self increases as the individual invests more time and effort in learning to play a role. The data from this study suggest that the experimental treatment, which emphasized cardiac risk-factor reduction and acknowledged the difficulties inherent in altering behaviors, provided a critical ingredient not present in previously tested open-ended discussion groups for cardiac patients. Comparison of experimental and control data also indicates that participation in a cardiac rehabilitation program is, of itself, not enough to affect long-term compliance. The control data are similar to the large body of compliance research that has documented high dropout and recidivism rates for lifestyle regimens.

An unexpected finding in this investigation was that smoking was not a useful outcome variable. Among those patients who had smoked before entering the rehabilitation program, none had resumed at 6-month follow-up. This result is in marked contrast to previous studies involving noncardiac subjects. In their evaluation of a variety of antismoking programs, Hunt and Bespalec[37] found a six-month recidivism of 80%. Perhaps cardiac patients experience effective pressure from families and friends to quit permanently, because smoking is probably the most visible of the risk factors that such patients are asked to control. It is also true that data on smoking were obtained by self-report. Reliability could have been enhanced considerably by the use of serum thiocyanate and expired air carbon monoxide samples.[38]

A number of studies have documented the importance of spousal support as a predictor of patient compliance.[13,39,40] Based on these findings and the dynamics predicted by symbolic interactionist role theory, we hypothesized that patients who met in groups with their spouses would manifest the greatest compliance. No such advantage was noted except in the area of exercise, and these differences were not statistically significant. In terms of blood pressure and body fat reduction, patients who met alone had equivalent or superior compliance when compared with patients who met with their spouses. Several explanations for these unexpected findings can be posed.

The first explanation is that the theory suggested by symbolic interactionists is incorrect. Roles do not require a complementary role; they do not develop in pairs. Yet the patterns in this data set are quite clear. With few exceptions, patient and spouse compliance behaviors changed in the same direction, thus indicating a reciprocity in the development of the at-risk role. The findings of this study support the view that family members can have an enabling or inhibitive effect on patient compliance. They may apply pressure to conform (or not to conform) to a specific regimen. They may communicate their support and thereby enhance the importance of compliance, or they may themselves serve as role models for health-promoting lifestyles.

A second explanation lies in the differences between the two groups. Although both experimental groups at each center had the same group leaders and functioned under an identical protocol, a review of written process recordings from the sessions indicates that the two groups developed characteristics quite distinct from each other. The patient-spouse groups focused on emotion-laden topics, for example, fear of death and disability, resentment toward family, and alterations in sexuality. Many of these topics were initiated by wives. In contrast, the patient-only groups were information-oriented. Members posed numerous questions about diet, activity, medications, and the value of risk-factor modification. In their written evaluations, participants in the patient-spouse groups most frequently listed "universality of feeling" as the most valuable characteristic of the group series, whereas participants in the patient-only groups cited "information received."

Given previously cited data on the relationship of knowledge and compliance, it does not seem plausible that the information received by patients was the critical factor. We propose that it was the dynamic within the reference group. The patient-only groups were competitive in nature, with individual patients competing against each other for higher exercise levels, decreased weight, etc. For example, one patient, an engineer, came to each meeting with a histogram of his weekly weight loss. This dynamic was also described by Adsett and Bruhn[35] and by Ibrahim and colleagues[36] in their groups of male cardiac patients. Thus, expectations for compliance existed within the patient-only groups, and these apparently served as a stronger force for compliance than did spouse support.

In summary, one of the primary goals of cardiac rehabilitation is to provide support to patients and their family members in a manner that fosters successful cardiac risk-factor reduction. Understanding the role transitions that occur within the context of a cardiac rehabilitation program is a complex task that needs more systematic study. The protocol we used needs to be replicated in future studies using a wider range of compliance variables (e.g., diet, serum cholesterol, and medication) for evaluation. The results of this study can, however, serve as an impetus for future research on the development of the at-risk role as it affects patient compliance.

Acknowledgments

This research was supported by grants from the graduate division of the University of California, San Francisco, and from the academic senate, University of California at Los Angeles. We thank Dr. Jan Tillisch for consultation about the measurement of cardiac clinical status.

REFERENCES

1. Lauck BW, Bigelow DA. Why patients follow through on referrals from the emergency room and why they don't. *Nurs Res* 1983; 32:186–187.
2. Sackett DL. Is there a patient compliance problem? If so, what do we do about it? In: Lasagna L, ed. *Controversies in therapeutics.* Philadelphia: W.B. Saunders, 1980:552–558.
3. Dunbar J. Adhering to medical advice: A review. *Int J Ment Health* 1981; 9:70–87.
4. Oldridge NB. Compliance and exercise in primary and secondary prevention of coronary heart disease: A review. *Prev Med* 1982; 11:56–70.
5. Clinite J, Kabat H. Improving patient compliance. *J Am Pharmacol Assoc* 1976; 16(18):74–76.
6. Hecht AB. Improving medication compliance by teaching outpatients. *Nurs Forum* 1974; 13:112–129.
7. Sackett DL, Haynes RB, Gibson ES, et al. Randomized clinical trial of strategies for improving medication compliance in primary hypertension. *Lancet* 1975; 1:1205–1207.
8. Alderman MA, Miller KF. Blood pressure control: The effect of facilitated access to treatment. *Clin Sci Mol Med* 1978; 55:349–351.
9. Aragona J, Cassady J, Drabman RS. Treating overweight children through parental training and contingency contracting. *J Appl Behav Anal* 1975; 8:269–278.
10. Levy RL, Yamashita D, Pow G. The relationship of an overt commitment to the frequency and speed of compliance with symptom reporting. *Med Care* 1979; 17:281–284.
11. Steckel SB, Swain MA. Contracting with patients to improve compliance. *J Am Hosp Assoc* 1977; 51:81–84.
12. Brand F, Smith R, Brand P. Effect of economic barriers to medical-care on patients' noncompliance. *Public Health Rep* 1977; 92:72–78.
13. Brownell KD, Heckerman CL, Westlake RJ, et al. The effect of couples training and partner cooperativeness in the behavioral treatment of obesity. *Behav Res Ther* 1978; 16:323–333.
14. Green LW, Levine DM, Wolle J, Deeds S. Department of randomized patient education experiments with urban poor hypertensives. *Patient Couns Health Educ* 1979; 1:106–111.
15. Zitter RE, Fremouw WJ. Individual versus partner consequation for weight loss. *Behav Ther* 1978; 9:808–813.
16. Gordis L. Conceptual and methodological problems in measuring patient compliance. In: Haynes RB, Taylor DW, Sackett DL, eds. *Compliance in health care.* Baltimore: Johns Hopkins University Press, 1979:23–45.
17. Roth HP, Caron HS. Accuracy of doctors' estimates and patients' statements on adherence to a drug regimen. *Clin Pharmacol Ther* 1978; 23:361–370.
18. Sheiner L, Rosenberg B, Marathe V, Peck C. Differences in serum digoxin concentrations between outpatients and inpatients: An effect of compliance? *Clin Pharmacol Ther* 1974; 15:239–246.
19. Stone G. Patient compliance and the role of the expert. *J Soc Issues* 1979; 35:34–59.
20. Dracup KA, Meleis AI. Compliance: An interactionist approach. *Nurs Res* 1982; 31:31–36.
21. Mead GH. *Mind, self, and society.* Chicago: University of Chicago Press, 1934.
22. Turner RH. *Family interaction.* New York: John Wiley & Sons, 1970.
23. Turner RH. The role and the person. *Am J Sociol* 1978; 84:1–23.
24. Parsons T. Illness and the role of the physician: A sociological perspective. *Am J Orthopsychiatry* 1951; 21:452–460.
25. Baric L. Recognition of the "at risk" role: A means to influence health behavior. *Int J Health Educ* 1969; 12:24–34.
26. Lindesmith AR, Strauss AL. *Social psychology.* 3rd ed. New York: Holt, Rinehart & Winston, 1968:276–298.
27. Hollingshead AB. Four factor index of social status. (Monograph.) New Haven: Department of Sociology, Yale University, 1975.
28. Meleis AI. Role insufficiency and role supplementation: A conceptual framework. *Nurs Res* 1978; 27:11–18.
29. Dracup KA, Meleis AI, Baker K, Edlefsen P. Family-focused cardiac rehabilitation: A role supplementation program for cardiac patients and spouses. *Nurs Clin North Am* 1984; 19(1):113–114.
30. Kirkendall WM, Feinleib M, Freis ED, Mark AL. Recommendations for human blood pressure determination by sphygmomanometers. *Circulation* 1980; 62:1146A–1155A.
31. Frisancho AR. Triceps skinfold and upper arm muscle size norms for assessment of nutritional status. *Am J Clin Nutr* 1974; 27:1052–1058.
32. Tanner JM. The measurement of body fat in man. *J Br Nutr Soc* 1959; 18:148.
33. Greenhouse SW, Geisser S. Methods in the analysis of profile data. *Psychometrika* 1954; 24:95–112.
34. Theroux P, Watters DD, Halphon C, et al. Prognostic value of exercise testing soon after M.I. *N Engl J Med* 1979; 301:341–345.

35. Adsett C, Bruhn J. Short-term group psychotherapy for post-myocardial infarction patients with their wives. *Can Med Assoc J* 1968; 99:577–584.
36. Ibrahim M, Feldman JG, Sultz HA, et al. Management after myocardial infarction: A controlled trial of the effects of group psychotherapy. *Int J Psychiatr Med* 1974; 5:253–268.
37. Hunt WA, Bespalec DA. An evaluation of current methods of modifying smoking behavior. *J Clin Psychol* 1974; 30:431–438.
38. Hymowitz N. Behavioral approaches to preventing heart disease: Risk factor modification. *Int J Ment Health* 1980; 9:27–69.
39. Mann GV, Garrett HL, Farhi A, et al. Exercise to prevent coronary heart disease. An experimental study of the effects of training on risk factors for coronary heart disease in men. *Am J Med* 1969; 46:12–27.
40. Saccone AJ, Israel AC. Effect of experimenter versus significant other controlled reinforcement and choice of target behavior on weight loss. *Behav Ther* 1978; 9:27.

Reprinted with permission from: Dracup, K., Meleis, A. I., Clark, S., Clyburn, A., Shields, L., & Staley, M. (1985). Group counseling in cardiac rehabilitation: Effect on patient compliance. *Patient Education and Counseling, 6*(4), 169–177.

10.6 FAMILY-FOCUSED CARDIAC REHABILITATION: A ROLE SUPPLEMENTATION PROGRAM FOR CARDIAC PATIENTS AND SPOUSES

KATHLEEN DRACUP
AFAF IBRAHIM MELEIS
KATHERINE BAKER
PATRICIA EDLEFSEN

Abstract

A nursing intervention based on interactionist role theory is currently being used in cardiac rehabilitation centers to meet the special needs of coronary patients and their spouses. The intervention consists of 10 weekly, 90-minute group sessions for married couples, one of whom has had recent acute coronary event; that is, either a myocardial infarction or coronary artery bypass graft surgery. The protocol was developed and initially tested at four cardiac rehabilitation centers in the Southern California area. A total of 62 couples participated. The data from this study, which are reported elsewhere,[9, 10] support the view that role supplementation is an important adjunct to the physical conditioning provided in outpatient cardiac rehabilitation programs. The purpose of this chapter is fourfold: (a) to identify the need for this type of nursing intervention in a cardiac rehabilitation setting, (b) to describe briefly the theory on which it is based, (c) to outline the protocol used in the group sessions, and (d) to summarize its therapeutic benefits.

Identifying the Need

The hospital course of the patient who experiences an acute coronary event is characterized by severe emotional distress. The patient's self-image changes from feeling whole to feeling damaged, from feeling competent and self-sufficient to feeling incompetent and dependent on others. In the intensive care unit, these changes are manifested by feelings of anxiety, depression, and fear of death in approximately 80% of patients.[3, 7, 13, 15]

Such patients use a variety of coping mechanisms to decrease the attendant emotional pain, for example, intellectualization, repression, denial, and projection.[13, 27] Indeed, excessive denial, sexually aggressive behavior, and hostile-dependent conflicts with staff have been documented in approximately 20% of coronary care unit patients.[6, 14] All such behaviors can be viewed as attempts on the part of the patient to regain control over his or her life and deal with the awesome anxiety experienced in this unfamiliar environment. These attempts not withstanding, the majority of patients are preoccupied with the limitations imposed by their cardiac illness and experience fears of death, pain, dysrhythmias, and future heart attacks.

Besides its effect on a patient, an acute coronary event presents a massive disruption in the psychodynamic balance of the family, as well. Anxiety, depression, sleep and appetite disturbances, and psychosomatic symptoms have been documented in interviews with spouses of coronary patients during the time of acute hospitalization.[2, 16, 23, 24] Spouses share their husbands' or wives' fear of death and disability, but often have fewer resources to assist them. They are also faced with the added burden of maintaining their families, for example, arranging for child care during visits to the hospital, paying bills, and performing essential household chores.

Nursing has attempted to meet the special needs of these family members in a variety of ways: by providing specialized "spouse care plans" in the intensive care unit,[11] by holding educational classes once the patient is out of the intensive care unit,[22] and by having informal support groups in waiting-room areas.[17, 18] These nursing interventions, however, are only a first step, because the emotional distress experienced by both patient and family continues, and in some cases intensifies, upon discharge to home. Dramatic role changes occur. Patients are temporarily at home all day and are faced with the problems of domestic routines. They deal with oversolicitous, anxious spouses, often while coping with the noise and conflicts of their children. In view of these domestic problems, which are usually combined with a multitude of lifestyle changes related to coronary-risk-factor modification, it is not surprising that emotional problems continue to be experienced by both the cardiac patient and the spouse.

A number of investigators have documented that emotional problems do exist up to two years following a coronary event. Specifically, 88% of patients have described themselves as anxious and depressed at 3 months following discharge,[27] 50% at 6 months,[17] and 20% at 6 to 12 months.[25] In a study reported by Wishnie and colleagues,[27] all 18 of the postmyocardial infarction patients interviewed with their family members reported moderate-to-severe family disturbances secondary to emotional disequilibrium and role changes. In later studies, wives of postmyocardial infarction patients have described feeling severe emotional distress at 1-year follow-up, and 20% reported a deterioration in their marriages.[8, 16, 24]

If nurses are to be effective in helping patients and their families achieve the goals of rehabilitation, they must take into account the nature and severity of the problems experienced by cardiac families, and provide an appropriate nursing intervention beyond the intensive care setting. A review of the pertinent literature suggests that a major source of psychosocial discomfort experienced by both patients and spouses during hospitalization and convalescence is a result of role changes and alterations in self-concept. Therefore, role theory was used as the theoretic basis for the patient-spouse groups described here.

Role Transition and Cardiac Rehabilitation

The term "role transition" refers to the process of moving in and out of roles in a social system.[5] Meleis suggests three categories of role transitions:

1. Developmental transitions, which occur in the normal course of growth and development;
2. situational transitions, which involve the addition or subtraction of persons in a preexisting constellation of roles and complements; and
3. health-illness transitions, which occur when an individual moves from a well state to an acute or chronic illness state, or from an illness state to a well state.[19]

Entry into a cardiac rehabilitation program demands a period of role transition for both the patient and his or her family that falls into the third category. The patient must relinquish the sick role and resume many of his previous roles, roles that demand a high degree of independence and autonomy.

A rehabilitation program also requires the acquisition of a new role for the patient. It is not a "sick role," and yet it is not really a "well role," because coronary artery disease is a chronic condition. Baric has called this role the "at risk" role.[1] The patient is identified as being at high risk for experiencing a future myocardial infarction, and as such, he or she is exhorted to modify all coronary risk factors. Such modification presents a number of lifestyle changes for both patients and spouses. Patients have to modify what they eat, how much they exercise, what medication they do or do not take, and what stressors they allow in their lives. Spouses, in turn, are asked to support their mates in these lifestyle changes and are strongly encouraged to make similar changes in their own risk factors. (In the groups, in fact, spouses complained frequently about the fact that they were under great pressure to modify their own lifestyle when they did not have the illness.)

The "at risk" role is an extremely difficult one for cardiac patients to acquire and for spouses to support appropriately by complementary roles, because the role demands changes in almost every aspect of one's life. Moreover, the patient and spouse know that these changes must be permanent.[12]

The unique needs of patients and spouses during this period of role transition are only partially met in a traditional cardiac rehabilitation program. Spouses rarely come to the center and are left to grapple with altered life goals and expectations by themselves. A nursing intervention of role supplementation can assist couples to develop role clarification and role rehearsal skills, and to sharpen their styles of coping.[20, 21] It provides them with a framework for the continuous analysis of new experiences and encourages them to communicate their concerns and fears to each other.

The processes and components of a role supplementation program are based on interactionist role theory. According to this theory, every role is created, defined, stabilized, and altered based on interactions with others in complementary roles (for example, husband–wife, teacher–student, nurse–patient).[4, 26] The theory suggests a variety of strategies that can be used to assist couples to assimilate and integrate new roles, for example, role modeling, role clarification, reference groups, and role rehearsal. The theoretic basis for these strategies has been described previously by Meleis.[19] Their use in this particular program is exemplified in the protocol for the group sessions.

Protocol for Group Sessions

The content of the 10 group sessions is described in Table 10.6.1. The majority of the sessions are structured to provide approximately 30 minutes of didactic presentation by the group leaders (or, in Session 4, by the guest couple invited to speak to the group) and 60 minutes of discussion. In three of the sessions, audiovisual aids are used as part of the didactic material.

In each setting, two group leaders are responsible for facilitating the group process. The first leader is the cardiovascular nurse coordinator of the rehabilitation program, and the second is a nurse consultant who holds a master's degree in psychiatric nursing. The nurse coordinator sees the patient and his or her spouse for an extensive assessment interview at the initiation of the cardiac rehabilitation program. The nurse also sees the patient three times a week in exercise sessions, and therefore, has a significant amount of data on which to base his or her interventions within the role supplementation program. Given the limited duration of the couples' program (10 weeks), it was hypothesized that the nurse coordinator's relationships with patients might prove an asset in decreasing the amount of time required for trust building in the group sessions and, ultimately, might increase the effectiveness of the experimental intervention.

The second group leader brings knowledge and skills in the areas of group dynamics and crisis theory. Thus, both nurses serve critical but complementary functions because of their knowledge of clinical cardiology and psychologic issues. They are able to answer questions about diet, medications, effects of exercise, and pathophysiology, as well as to identify and explore the sources of anxiety expressed by patients and spouses.

The inclusion of spouses in group sessions is critical for several reasons.

1. Such inclusion provides a reference group for spouses, as well as opportunities for role modeling and role rehearsal for the reciprocal roles required of them. The reference group is an important source of support for spouses, most of whom are

TABLE 10.6.1 Protocol of the Role Supplementation Program

Session 1: Clarifying Roles
Content:

Introduction of group facilitators and participants

Discussion of program purpose and "ground rules" (e.g., confidentiality, attendance)

Review of 10-session content

Review of coronary risk factors

Identification of changes in roles and relationships by participants since coronary event

Identification of commonalities and differences in problems resulting from coronary event

Audiovisual:

Written schedule of 10 sessions

Discussion questions:

What changes have occurred with the assumption of the "at risk" role?

How have these changes affected your feelings about yourself?

How do your partners feel about these changes?

What do you see as your major problems at this point?

How do you view the group helping with these?

Session 2: Overcoming Fear

Discussion of common emotional response to coronary heart disease (i.e., anxiety, depression, anger)

Identification of major sources of anxiety for both patient and spouse

Discussion regarding gaining control over one's life

Identification of ways to set new goals

Audiovisual:

16 mm film, "Pack Your Own Chute" (Ramie Productions)

Discussion questions:

What don't you like about having coronary heart disease?

How have you felt since discharge from the hospital?

What do you do when you start to feel anxious?

What changes would you like to make in your lives?

Session 3: Problem-Solving I
Content:

Review of the five-step problem-solving process

Identification of the importance of taking time to gather data, generate alternative solutions, and examine different points of view before making decisions

Application of process to example situations (role rehearsal)

TABLE 10.6.1 (continued)

Homework assignment: couple to apply problem-solving process to a mutual problem experienced during the week

Audiovisual:

Written summary of problem-solving process

Discussion questions:

What problems have arisen since your coronary event?

How can we use this process to solve one of them?

When do you feel most frustrated? Can you identify a problem in these situations?

What problems can you anticipate because of the new "at risk" role?

Do we always need to be perfect?

What problems arise from this need?

Session 4: Problem Solving II
Content:

Introduction of couple who has successfully completed cardiac rehabilitation program

Discussion of ways in which this couple dealt with role transition

Discussion of strategies to increase communication within family

Audiovisual:

None

Discussion questions:

What kinds of problems described by the couple are similar to those of the group?

What strategies seemed to work for them?

What problems do husbands and wives of cardiac patients face that the patient doesn't share?

What problems do patients have that the spouse doesn't share?

Session 5: Stress Management I
Content:

Review of physiologic changes during stress

Presentation of Benson's relaxation response

Homework assignment: couple to practice relaxation response twice daily during week

Audiovisual:

Film-audiocassette "Stress and the Relaxation Response" (Trainex Corporation)

Stress dots (Communications Unit)

Written summary of relaxation response

TABLE 10.6.1 *(continued)*

Discussion questions:

How can you know when you feel stressed?

What is the difference between distress and eustress?

What is the physiologic response to stress?

How do you feel after the relaxation response exercise?

How can you incorporate this exercise into your day, e.g., times, place, etc.?

Session 6: Stress Management II

Content:

Review of participants' experience with relaxation response

Identification of sources of stress for each couple

Review of other alternatives to stress management: (a) exercise; (b) transcendental meditation; (c) yoga; (d) effective communication; (e) assertive techniques

Audiovisual:

None

Discussion questions:

What were your experiences with the relaxation response during the week?

What stressors did you identify during the past week?

What other strategies have you used to decrease stress?

Do you feel stressed when you want to say no to a request?

What strategies can you use in this situation?

Session 7: Relationships With Family

Content:

Identification of role changes in family relationships since cardiac event

Identification of problems in maintaining "at risk" role

Facilitation of communication between spouses

Audiovisual:

None

Discussion questions:

What has been the family's reaction to the patient's illness?

How has it affected their lives?

Do you (patient) expect anything different from your family because of your cardiac status?

TABLE 10.6.1 *(continued)*

Do you (spouse) expect anything different from your husband/wife because of his/her cardiac status?

How have your roles changed within the family?

Do you (spouse) feel responsible for your partner?

Do you ever feel resentment about the changes in the family since the cardiac event?

Where do you both get your support?

Session 8: Communication Through Sex

Content:

Review of information about resuming sexual activity following a cardiac event

Identification of common postcoronary sexual problems

Identification of common fears and misconceptions

Audiovisual:

16 mm. movie "Sex and the Heart Patient" (Synthesis Communication, for Burroughs Wellcome Co.)

Discussion questions:

What fears have you had about resuming sexual activity?

Did you receive any information to help you?

What questions or concerns do you have now?

Session 9: Dealing With the "At Risk" Role

Content:

Review of behavior changes on part of patient and spouse related to the "at risk" role

Identification of changes in attitudes and relationships related to role transitions

Open agenda to allow participants to discuss issues and feelings related to role transition

Audiovisual:

None

Discussion questions:

What changes have occurred in your relationship since you began the cardiac rehabilitation program?

What risk factors are most difficult to alter?

Do you have any concerns or fears related to your coronary heart disease?

Session 10: What Now?

Content:

Review of material presented in group sessions

Identification of participants' feelings and perceptions about group process

TABLE 10.6.1 *(continued)*

Open agenda to deal with termination issues

Audiovisual:

None

Discussion questions:

Have the groups been helpful? How?

What changes have occurred within your family since you began the group sessions?

What are your plans for the future?

---

relatively isolated in their anxiety and fear, and feel uniquely incompetent to deal with the changes required of them.

2. Patients in cardiac rehabilitation programs are asked to make many lifestyle changes that profoundly affect their daily lives. Enlisting the support of spouses provides the day-to-day positive reinforcement required if such changes are to occur and be maintained.

3. A common dynamic frequently seen in cardiology is the assignment of the spouse to a "watchdog" role. He or she is covertly asked to make certain that the patient complies with all aspects of the "at risk" role. The spouse then becomes accountable for the patient and any transgressions that may occur from the prescribed medical regimen. This dynamic increases stress and needs to be discussed in a group setting, in which both patient and spouse can clarify their responsibilities and roles.

The couples are recruited by signs posted in the rehabilitation center announcing the purpose, content, and starting date of the sessions. The nurse coordinator also describes the program to each couple during their initial interview upon entry into the rehabilitation program. If couples express concern that the sessions might be "psychotherapy," the nurse coordinators emphasize that the groups are supportive and educational in nature. The minimal and maximal sizes of the groups are set at four and six couples, respectively, to facilitate the group process.

Themes and Therapeutic Benefits

The couples' groups have been conducted at the participating rehabilitation center for 3 years. In reviewing our experience with these series of groups, we have identified recurring themes that have served as therapeutic benefits for the couples. These themes provide at least a partial answer to the question, "How does a role supplementation program help?" Although stylistic clarity demands that they be discussed singly, the discriminations are, in actuality, quite arbitrary, and many occur and function in an interdependent fashion.

Imparting of Information

This category, "imparting of information," encompasses the didactic instruction about coronary atherosclerotic disease and cardiac-risk-factor management given by the group leaders, as well as the advice, suggestions, or direct guidance about life problems offered either by the leaders or other paticipants. As in other types of groups (for example, group psychotherapy), information transfer often functions as the initial binding force in the groups until other therapeutic benefits become operative.[28] In part, however, explanation and role clarification are effective in their own right. As participants clarify misconceptions and identify the behaviors appropriate to the "at risk" role (and its complementary role), anxiety decreases.

The need to dispel uncertainty with factual information has been exemplified in each group by the recurring theme of diet. Although this topic is not covered in any of the didactic material presented by the group leaders, questions about the importance of maintaining a low-sodium, low-cholesterol diet constantly are raised. This repetition undoubtedly reflects the lack of clarity on dietary restrictions provided in the media and by physicians, and the participants frequently seek clarification from the nurse leaders.

Direct advice from the group members also occurs in every group. Patients and/or spouses present difficulties related to their role transitions, for example, how to tell a son or daughter with young children that a two-week visit would be too stressful, given the recent coronary event. Responses from the group members are often in an advice-giving mode, being preceded by such phrases as, "Why don't you...," or "What worked for us was...." The specific suggestion may or may not be helpful, but they are interpreted as mutual caring and interest and contribute to group cohesiveness.

Instillation of Hope

The role-modeling component of the experimental intervention provides the participants with a feeling of hopefulness that, in itself, is therapeutically effective. The groups invariably contain individuals who are at different points in their mastery of new roles. Participants have an opportunity to hear about problems very similar to their own and about how other patients/spouses have successfully coped with them. In the fourth meeting, a guest couple discusses their "passage" through the cardiac rehabilitation program and provides something of a testimonial to the positive outcomes they experienced. The effects of such role-modeling processes are evidenced in new attitudes of hopefulness and conviction on the part of the participants.

Redefinition of Wellness

As the groups progress through the 10 sessions, the patients begin to redefine what it means to be healthy. Prior to their coronary events, wellness meant the absence of disease. As they discuss their changing lifestyles, necessitated by the diagnosis of coronary atherosclerosis, they frequently talk about changing their values to incorporate the health-seeking behaviors promoted by the cardiac rehabilitation program personnel. The majority had smoked, worked long hours under stress, and led sedentary lifestyles. Many are overweight. They encourage and support each others' changes in modifying these risk factors. Wellness is now measured by weight loss, the ability to reduce stress, and new prescriptions for exercise at higher target heart rates. For example, one subject (an engineer) brought a histogram to a last group session that showed his weekly weight loss. Wellness is redefined by the majority of patients as an absence of coronary risk factors and the ability to do regular aerobic exercise without cardiac symptoms.

In a very early discussion of role change, Burr described role transition as a process of disintegration of the old self and a redefinition and reconstruction of a new self.[5] In the couples' groups, each patient seeks cues from significant others as to the kinds of changes to make in his or her attitudes and behaviors to achieve health. By integrating and stabilizing the new behaviors related to risk-factor modification, the patients receive cues from both the health professionals involved in their care and from their family members that they are achieving a "well state." Thus the goals, values, and behaviors of the "at risk" role are integrated into the patients' perceptions of themselves as healthy.

Reference Group

"Reference group" refers to a group of people with whom an individual can identify and from whom he or she can derive values and emotional support.

In a final written evaluation of the program, many subjects have expressed the most important benefit of the groups as being the recognition that their feelings and concerns are shared by others. The confirmation by members of a reference group that their feelings are not unique is a powerful source of relief. Despite the complexity of problems each couple faces in adjusting to a chronic illness, certain common denominators are evident. Patients resent being stereotyped a "cardiac" by family, friends, and employers. Couples openly discuss fears of sudden death, which in our experience are more common for spouses than patients. Although these two themes appear paradoxic, they reflect one reality. The cardiac patient appears no different externally and often feels physically well, despite the occurrence of a cardiac event. He or she resents being relegated to invalid status by others, because it is a reminder of the heart damage suffered but now not felt. Despite the frequent lack of symptomatology, cardiac patients (and their spouses) are also acutely aware of their increased risk for sudden death. The first premonition of one's mortality is a painful experience, and the concern of significant others often serves as a poignant reminder for the cardiac patient.

Confusion about changes in roles within the family system are also discussed, and solutions are offered by other members of the group. For example, one patient described his mixed feelings when his wife came to the coronary care unit and told him that his 12-year-old son had put his wedding ring on the first night of the hospitalization and assured her that now he would take care of her. The group focused on the patient's loss of self-esteem with these shifts in roles and supported the patient's need to reassert his paternal role during this transitional period.

Humor is often used by the groups to defuse feelings of anguish and uncertainty. For example, one patient, who was an author by profession, admitted to the group that he had not been able to use the word "deadline" since his myocardial infarction. As patients and spouses perceive their similarity to others in the group, they benefit from the humor expressed by others and the accompanying catharsis. The ultimate acceptance by other members of the reference group, then, is a major force in the patients' ability to redefine wellness in an appropriate and meaningful manner.

Altruism

Altruistic acts often set healing forces in motion within a group setting. Throughout the course of the program, subjects offer support, suggestions, reassurance, and insights to other group members. The self-absorption that has characterized much of the couples' interactions since the coronary event is slowly replaced by concern for others in the group. As the subjects begin to experience their contributions to the group as worthwhile, self-esteem increases.

Summary

A review of the literature yields general agreement among investigators regarding the responses of both patients and spouses to a cardiac event. Anxiety, depression, low self-esteem, marital and sexual dysfunction, and psychosomatic symptoms have been consistently documented up to 1 year following a myocardial infarction or cardiac surgery. Although the patient's physiologic status sets limits on the potential level of recovery, psychosocial variables are now recognized as playing a critical role in the rehabilitation process for both patients and their families.

Our 3-year experience with patient-spouse groups supports the view that spouses must be involved throughout the rehabilitative process, and that effective participation is provided within the context of a role supplementation program. Such a program facilitates direct and consistent communication, as well as flexibility within and between roles. Both end points are critical to the re-establishment of family equilibrium and the ultimate recovery of the cardiac patient.

Acknowledgment

The authors would like to acknowledge the following individuals who served as group leaders in the experimental study: Suzanne Clark, RN, MS; Arline Clyburn, RN, MN; Mary Kattus, RN, M.; Pam Rosenberg, RN, MN; Linda Shields, RN, BS; Marilyn Staley, RN; and Mary Wilson, RN, MN.

REFERENCES

1. Baric, L.: Recognition of the 'at risk' role: A means to influence health behavior. Int. J. Health Educ., *12*:24–34, 1969.
2. Bedsworth, J. A., & Melon, M. T.: Psychological stress in spouses of patients with myocardial infarction. Heart Lung, *11*:450–456, 1982.
3. Bigos, K. M.: Behavioral adaptation during the acute phase of a myocardial infarction. West. J. Nurs. Res., *3*:150–171, 1981.
4. Blumer, H.: Symbolic interactionism: Perspective and method. Englewood Cliffs, N.J.: Prentice-Hall, 1969.
5. Burr, R.: Role transitions: A reformulation of theory. J. Marriage Fam., *34*:407–416, 1972.

6. Cassem, N. H., & Hackett, T. P.: Psychiatric consultation in a coronary care unit. Ann. Intern. Med., 75:9–14, 1971.
7. Cassem, N. H., & Hackett, T. P.: Psychological rehabilitation of myocardial infarction patients in the acute phase. Heart Lung, 2:382–388, 1973.
8. Croog, S. H., & Fitzgerald, E. F.: Subjective stress and serious illness of a spouse: Wives of heart patients. J. Health Soc. Behav., 19:166–178, 1978.
9. Dracup, K.: The effect of a role supplementation program for cardiac patients and spouses on mastery of the at-risk role. Unpublished doctoral dissertation. University of California, San Francisco, 1982.
10. Dracup, K.: Influence of a role supplementation program on the psychosocial adaptation of cardiac patients and spouses. Circulation, Suppl. 2, 66:280, 1982.
11. Dracup, K., & Breu, C. S.: Using nursing findings to meet the needs of grieving spouses. Nurs. Res., 27:212–216, 1978.
12. Dracup, K., & Meleis, A. I.: Compliance: An interactionist approach. Nurs. Res., 31:31–36, 1982.
13. Froese, A., Hackett, T. P., Cassem, N. H., et al.: Trajectories of anxiety and depression in denying and nondenying acute myocardial infarction patients during hospitalization. J. Psychosom. Res., 18:413–420, 1974.
14. Gentry, W. D., Foster, S., & Haney, T.: Denial as a determinant of anxiety and perceived health status in the coronary care unit. Psychosom. Med., 34:39–43, 1972.
15. Gundle, M. J., Reeves, B. R., Tate, S., et al.: Psychological outcome after coronary artery surgery. Am. J. Psychiatry, 137:1591–1594, 1980.
16. Mayou, R., Foster, A., & Williamson, B.: The psychological and social effects of myocardial infarction on wives. Br. Med. J., 1:699–701, 1978.
17. McGrath, F., & Robinson, J.: The medical social worker in the coronary care unit. Med. J. Aust., 2:1113–1116, 1973.
18. McLane, M., Krop, H., & Mehta, J.: Psychosexual adjustment and counseling after myocardial infarction. Ann. Intern. Med., 92:514–519, 1980.
19. Meleis, A. I.: Role insufficiency and role supplementation: A conceptual framework. Nurs. Res., 24:264–271, 1975.
20. Meleis, A. I., & Swendsen, L. A.: Role supplementation: An empirical test of a nursing intervention. Nurs. Res., 27:11–18, 1978.
21. Meleis, A. I., Swendsen, L. A., & Jones, D.: Preventive role supplementation. In Flynn, B. C., & Miller, M. H. (eds): Current perspectives in nursing: Social issues and trends. St. Louis, MO: C. V. Mosby 1980.
22. Scalzi, C. C., Burke, L. E., & Greenland, S.: Evaluation of an inpatient educational program for coronary patients and families. Heart Lung, 9:84–853, 1980.
23. Skelton, M., & Dominian, J.: Psychological stress in wives of patients with myocardial infarction. Br. Med. J., 14:101–103, 1973.
24. Stern, M. J., & Pascale, L.: Psychosocial adaptation postmyocardial infarction: The spouse's dilemma. J. Psychosom. Res., 23:83–87, 1979.
25. Stern, M. J., Pascale, L., & McLoone, J.: Psychosocial adaptation following an acute myocardial infarction. J. Chronic Dis., 29:513–526, 1976.
26. Turner, R. H.: The role and the person. Am. J. Sociol., 84:1–23, 1978.
27. Wishnie, H. A., Hackett, T. P., & Cassem, N. H.: Psychological hazards of convalescence following myocardial infarction. J.A.M.A., 215:1292–1296, 1971.
28. Yalom, I. D.: The theory and practice of group psychotherapy. New York: Basic Books, 1970.

Reprinted with permission from: Dracup, K., Meleis, A. I., Baker, K., & Edlefsen, P. (1985). Family-focused cardiac rehabilitation: A role supplementation program for cardiac patients and spouses. *Nursing Clinics of North America, 19*(1), 113–124.

10.7 ROLE SUPPLEMENTATION AS A NURSING INTERVENTION FOR ALZHEIMER'S DISEASE: A CASE STUDY

LISA SKEMP KELLEY
JEAN A. LAKIN

Abstract

With a long-term chronic illness, family structure and functioning often become impaired. Family members require assistance in understanding the nature and progression of the illness, and in assuming new roles to preserve the stability of the family unit. This case study describes how a community health nurse used role supplementation to assist one family effectively to cope with the changes associated with Alzheimer's disease.

When individuals and families experience changes due to chronic illness, the functioning of the family system may be upset. Roles are often altered and redefined because chronically ill persons can no longer participate in the manner once expected of them. The community health nurse can play a significant role in helping families adjust to these changes. This chapter describes the use of role supplementation as a nursing intervention to promote effective adaptation, functioning, and growth in one family in which a member had Alzheimer's disease. Role theory was used to assess family structure and functioning, and to implement care strategies.

Conceptual Framework

Roles and Role Transition

Roles are the expected attitudes, values, skills, and knowledge associated with various positions (Biddle & Thomas, 1966). They are largely derived from the expectations of others, although individuals may choose to accept, reject, or transform their meaning according to personal interpretation of events (Mead, 1972). Throughout the life span, individuals may change or modify their roles with different events such as marriage, divorce, childbearing, employment, and chronic/debilitating illness. To perform new roles, the individual must experience role transition.

Role transition is the process of learning behaviors necessary to carry out a new role effectively. The ease of this process is affected by the congruity between past and future roles (Louis, 1980; Minkler & Biller, 1979) and the anticipation of the role change. Anticipation of the change is further influenced by the individual's degree of choice in taking on the new role, previous experience in anticipating similar change, and degree of readiness for the new role (Allen & van de Vliert, 1984).

During transition, role stress and strain may become apparent (Doehrman, 1984), although it is possible that few adverse effects may occur (Glaser & Strauss, 1971), based on individual's perception of the change as positive or negative. If the individual chooses a new role and has an opportunity to prepare for it, there is less strain (Minkler & Biller, 1979). In addition, the ease of transition is facilitated by appropriate anticipation of the new expectations (Mederer, 1984; Minkler & Biller, 1979).

Role Insufficiency

Role insufficiency occurs when an individual has unclear expectations of the knowledge, attitudes, values, and skills essential to performing a new role. With this state, stress may occur and manifest itself in physical and/or psychologic strain such as grief, mourning, powerlessness, depression, anxiety, withdrawal, apathy, frustration, unhappiness, aggression to self or others, or symptoms of physiologic stress response (Allen & van de Vliert, 1984; Meleis, 1975). Role supplementation is an intervention that can be used to reduce role stress and decrease, ameliorate, or prevent role insufficiency.

Role Supplementation

Role supplementation was defined by Meleis (1975) as "the conveying of information or experience necessary to bring the role incumbent and significant others to full awareness of the anticipated behavior patterns, units, sentiments, sensations, and goals involved in each role and its complement. It includes necessary knowledge and experience that emphasizes heightened awareness of one's own roles and other's roles and the dynamics of the interrelationships" (p. 267) It is made operational through several strategies, including role modeling (demonstrating behaviors associated with particular roles), role rehearsal (mental enactment, fantasy, or image of what the role would be like), role play (practicing appropriate behaviors for simulated real-life situations), and reference group interactions (interactions with others who are experiencing similar role transitions, such as support groups) to facilitate role clarification (appropriate identification of new role behaviors) and role taking (effective demonstration of appropriate role behaviors) (Meleis & Swendsen, 1978; van Ments, 1983). The goal of supplementation is to achieve role mastery. Mastery becomes apparent when the individual and others involved achieve mutual expectations and behaviors.

Role supplementation was originally studied as a nursing intervention for role insufficiency in families undergoing transition due to childbirth, and was found to facilitate an increased understanding of life changes, an awareness of new responsibilities, and the sharing of anxieties between husband and wife (Meleis & Swendsen, 1975; Swendsen, Meleis, & Jones, 1978). Although it has not been reported elsewhere in the nursing literature, it appears to be applicable to families who are experiencing role changes, such as occur when a member has Alzheimer's disease.

Alzheimer's Disease

The steady deterioration of mental functioning associated with Alzheimer's disease can be demonstrated through three behavioral phrases that occur over a number of years: forgetfulness, confusion, and dementia (Gwyther & Matteson, 1983; Hayter, 1974; Pinel, 1975). Forgetfulness is characterized by progressive memory loss, especially for recent events (e.g., loss of commonly used articles); changes in personality; withdrawal from social contact; lack of spontaneity; difficulty with previously known/simple tasks; impaired reading, writing, and language; loss of motor coordination and disequilibrium; and neglect of personal appearance.

Confusion may be manifested by loss of knowledge for current and recent events; inability to handle finances; overreactions to known inabilities (e.g., depression and/or verbal/physical abuse); emotional lability; dysarthria; difficulty choosing proper clothing; wandering, restlessness; repetitious behavior; constant or agitated pacing; slow, shuffling, wide-based gait; agnosia (inability to recall commonly used objects); and incapacity to remember addresses, or names and relationships of family members.

Dementia is characterized by paraphasia (use of words in wrong and senseless combinations), irritability, loss of ability to speak, seizures or tremors, inability to recognize and interpret complex sensory stimuli, incontinence, prosopagnosia (inability to recognize significant others or self), and hallucinations. Ultimately, the individual becomes completely incapacitated and bedridden.

This loss of normal functioning is emotionally trying to family members. It necessitates continual adaptation to preserve effective family operation and concomitant coping with the progressive cognitive, emotional, and behavioral deterioration of their loved one.

Family Assessment

Seventeen visits were made to the family over an 11-month period. Initially, they were made every week. The early visits provided the time to understand the family's needs, help them meet imminent physical and safety needs, and develop a therapeutic and trusting relationship with the wife and husband. As role transition proceeded and other problems were resolved, visits were gradually decreased to every other week, and eventually, every third week. This pattern of visitation allowed the wife time to "try on" her new and expanded role as spouse caregiver, develop alternative support systems, and increase control of the situation although knowing that assistance was available at any time between visits.

The following assessment data were obtained during the initial visits. The husband, Joseph, an 83-year-old, retired professional man, was previously very active with community service, many hobbies, and traveling. He had noninsulin-dependent diabetes mellitus that was controlled by Glucotrol. He was diagnosed with Alzheimer's disease (confusional phase) after an extensive medical work-up for the symptoms of agitation, extreme forgetfulness, and mild ataxia. Other than these two conditions, he had no other major physical health problems.

On questioning, Joseph said he had no problems with memory and had not had an evaluation for forgetfulness. When his wife, Ruth, remarked that he had had a work-up for forgetfulness, Joseph retorted that she was crazy and imagining things, and that there was nothing wrong with him. Other behaviors that Joseph demonstrated included pacing and intermittent repetitious questioning. Whereas he was detached from the objective and specific aspects, he was very sensitive to the emotional atmosphere. For example, he did not understand how to carry out everyday tasks such as making out the budget, but would become very agitated if Ruth showed any frustration while she did it.

Ruth, 75 years of age, had worked as a secretary before marrying Joseph 55 years previously. Since then, her primary roles consisted of home manager, wife, and mother to their only child, Tom. Ruth's medical diagnoses included ataxia due to a brain stem stroke five years earlier, and labile hypertension. In the last year, she had also begun to experience severe esophageal burning approximately three to five times per day, which was relieved by medication. When questioned, Ruth stated that she felt fine, and the esophageal burning was something the doctor said she had to live with. Loss of appetite, dizziness, and headaches had also become more frequent since her husband's diagnosis of Alzheimer's disease.

Significant findings on physical assessment included blood pressure 172/86, pulse 80, height 5 feet 2 inches, and weight 103 pounds, which was 15 pounds less than the previous year. On visual inspection, Ruth demonstrated tension and guardedness by her clenched hands, tense facial muscles, and intermittent tapping movements of her left leg.

Ruth expressed little awareness of the progression of Alzheimer's disease. Her sister had cared for her husband until he died of some type of dementia. Ruth stated that she was not aware of how bad things had become until her sister had a nervous breakdown, and she did not want that to happen to her.

Ruth explained that her relationship with Joseph had altered drastically during the past year. Problems within their interaction were clearly evident during early home visits. For example, when she expressed concerns, such as Joseph not driving the car because of his forgetfulness, he reacted with agitation and verbal aggressiveness toward her. In response, she initially tried to convince Joseph that he sometimes forgot where he was going and got lost. He announced that she was crazy and told her to be quiet. In turn, Ruth became quiet and teary-eyed, and demonstrated more muscle tension. Joseph often began pacing the floor, repeatedly stating she was crazy, and eventually would leave the room for a short period of time.

Ruth's receptivity to available support systems was limited. Their son lived approximately one hour away, and visited or called occasionally. He did not wish to become involved in his father's care because of his own family and professional responsibilities. Ruth whispered to the nurse at one of the early visits that they did not talk about Joseph's disease or want other people to witness his condition because it was "uncomfortable for our friends." Consequently, the couple had become quite isolated from friends and past associates.

Ruth and Joseph had not anticipated any long-term or debilitating illness during their retirement years. There was a great deal of discontinuity between her prior roles and her new role of caregiver. Previously, she found meaning in the discussions she had with her husband and from his support of her. Now discussions between them were very stressful. With Joseph's progressive forgetfulness, Ruth attempted to manage the budget, housework, yard work, and family care with little emotional or physical support from him or others. She did not know how to anticipate the changes that might occur in Joseph or how to cope with them. She had no prior experience in caring for a family member with Alzheimer's disease; however, she believed it was her responsibility to care for Joseph as long as possible.

Nursing Diagnosis

These assessment data indicate that the family's role expectations were changing. In the past, Joseph managed the house and yard, was the sole breadwinner, and was a supportive and nurturing husband. Their past communication pattern was one of discussing problems until mutual decisions were reached. Now Joseph was unable to carry out these roles and became angry if Ruth attempted to discuss anything with him. Consequently, their communication was severely curtailed, and Ruth no longer perceived Joseph as supportive and nurturing.

The primary nursing diagnosis for the family was alterations in coping (family and individual) related to role insufficiency, secondary to Joseph's progressive irreversible dementia (Alzheimer's type), evidenced by increased forgetfulness, pacing, repeated questioning, denial of problem, and occasional panic look (Joseph); and physical and psychologic manifestations of strain (Ruth). Other diagnoses were as follows:

1. Potential for physical injury related to cognitive deficits associated with progressive dementia, manifested in wandering, ataxia, forgetfulness, and refusal to stop driving the car despite repeated incidences of becoming lost (Joseph).
2. Potential for physical injury related to physiologic stress response, manifested in increased blood pressure, dizziness, headaches, muscle tension, decreased appetite, and epigastric distress (Ruth).
3. Sleep pattern disturbance related to nocturnal wandering, evidenced by sleep pattern reversal (Joseph); interrupted sleep (Ruth); dark circles under eyes, frequent yawning, expressionless face (Ruth and Joseph).
4. Moderate anxiety related to change in family functioning secondary to Alzheimer's disease as manifested by expressed feelings of unfocused apprehension (Ruth); restlessness, tremors, increased muscle tension, narrow focus of attention, and sleeping and eating disturbances (Joseph and Ruth).

Plan

Sensitivity to client readiness is a key element in planning the specific interventions for role supplementation. For example, Ruth initially was receptive to reading about other people's experiences with caring for family members with Alzheimer's disease. After about 2 months she expressed interest in reading the book, *The 36-Hour Day* (Mace & Rabins, 1981), and stated later that it was very helpful, although she could not have read it earlier. It was approximately 4 months before she was ready to read informational brochures from the Alzheimer's Disease and Related Disorders Association.

Joseph was in the confusional phase of the Alzheimer's process, which was confounded with denial and anger. Because of his fear, anger, and progressive memory loss, it was unrealistic to work directly with him or expect that he could voluntarily change his behavior. Therefore, to promote effective family functioning, it was essential to modify his environment. The primary aspect of his surroundings on which this plan was based focused on Ruth's attitudes and behaviors toward him. It seemed feasible to assist her in assessing Joseph's needs as well as her own, and help her identify ways to meet those needs in a healthy manner.

The primary treatment goal, identified in collaboration with Ruth, was to develop effective coping strategies during role transition from spouse to spouse caregiver. Ruth stated the goal as "I want to know how to handle this so we can live our last years together in happiness."

The plan included continually identifying and clarifying current family roles, needs, and problems; developing knowledge of the Alzheimer's disease process; reclarifying individual and family goals; delineating behaviors that facilitated family functioning, and that were congruous with Ruth's value system and abilities; identifying the methods by which Ruth could best learn and find meaning within the evolving role of spouse caregiver; and facilitating her ability to make continuing decisions regarding alternative choices in dealing with this life change. By conveying the information and experiences essential to the caregiver role and its complement, Ruth's personal power would be strengthened as she continued assuming the role.

The home visits were designed so that the first portion was used to assess each client's health status and discuss nonthreatening concerns with them together. A short exercise period was then held for

Ruth and Joseph, consisting of a short walk outside or use of a stationary indoor bicycle. After this Joseph was usually ready to lie down and rest, and the remaining time was spent with Ruth discussing ways to implement her caregiver role. The intervention of role supplementation was used to promote her clarity on and taking of the role.

Intervention: Role Supplementation

The strategies of role clarification, role modeling, role rehearsal, and reference group interactions were used to implement role supplementation and facilitate role taking.

Role Clarification

To clarify her role, past and present family roles were discussed, and knowledge of the process and problems associated with Alzheimer's disease were provided at Ruth's readiness. Previous roles in the family were discussed, and behaviors associated with them were delineated. The roles were then evaluated as to their effectiveness, so that they could be redefined as needed to meet individual and family needs. To facilitate her understanding of viable options, information on available resources was provided and discussed. Throughout this process, it was continually emphasized that Ruth had choices in the roles she accepted.

Between visits Ruth kept a diary, making entries in it as she felt necessary. She described difficult episodes, such as specific behaviors displayed by Joseph and herself, their reactions to each other, and how she felt. The journal was an excellent method of promoting recall, not only of behavioral patterns, but also the attitude and value conflicts that she had for each event. During home visits, entries from the journal were reviewed, areas of uncertainty clarified, and alternatives for managing them discussed and practiced through several strategies.

Role Modeling

Role modeling was provided by the first author during interactions with Joseph and Ruth. For example, when Joseph would become upset, the author would demonstrate alternative ways to manage him, such as acknowledging his concerns and feelings, and gently shifting his focus of attention to a nonthreatening topic or activity. Ruth observed this and was able to see behaviors that more effectively managed her husband's fear and agitation.

Role Rehearsal

Role rehearsal was implemented by using mental imagery and role play, so that Ruth could experiment with new behaviors during simulations of previous experiences. Specific behaviors were established for her to use if difficulties arose between visits. After she learned this strategy, she was able to use it independently to prepare for new events.

Reference Group Interactions

Ruth initially declined the use of reference group interactions, such as an Alzheimer's disease support group, stating that she never was a group person and just did not like them. After about eight months, however, she began to establish a modified reference group by sharing concerns with a neighbor whose husband also had had an irreversible dementia and recently died.

Role Taking

Some of the specific roles that Ruth was eventually able to change included improving her interactions with Joseph, managing yard maintenance (by hiring a volunteer from a local aging agency), and accepting budgetary assistance from her son and emotional support from friends.

The following chronology illustrates Ruth's readiness to participate in role-supplementation strategies. Initially, she was receptive to role modeling. She felt comfortable observing the first author demonstrate effective interactive behaviors with Joseph. After about two months, she expressed readiness to participate in role-rehearsal strategies. It was approximately eight months before she was ready to participate in a modified reference group interaction.

Evaluation

Ruth's mastery of the spouse caregiver role was evaluated by assessing her physiologic stress response and obtaining feedback from her on family functioning and how she and Joseph were coping.

Ruth's physiologic status was altered over the course of the home visits, although none of her medications had changed. She became more physically active due to regular (three to five times/week) exercise periods, no longer had problems falling asleep at night, and was more relaxed during the day. Her blood pressure ranged between 132/64 and 138/68, which was lower than readings during the first months of nursing care. She had no further weight loss, her appetite was good, and she denied any headaches for over two months. The epigastric burns had decreased to 1 every 7 to 10 days, and usually occurred when she ate something that she knew would disagree with her.

Ruth and Joseph's interactive pattern was no longer as conflict-ridden, and they had not argued for a long time. Ruth did not confront or disagree with Joseph. By acknowledging his feelings and refocusing his attention, confrontation, anger, and frustration were minimized. She expressed that, although she was not laughing at Joseph, sometimes his behaviors and her reactions to them made her giggle. She reestablished some of her close friendships and realized that the disease did not have to be kept, "hidden in a closet." She was engaged in daily activities to promote her own health and prevent current and future loneliness and isolation.

Following are some events that were identified as problematic, how they were managed, and Ruth's statements of the effectiveness of the role change.

The Worn-Out Pajamas

Joseph routinely took a morning shower, and Ruth hung his pajamas in the closet for him to wear the next night. At times, however, he refused to wear these pajamas, wanted clean ones, became angry, and refused to get ready for bed. Ruth tried to convince him that he had only worn the pajamas a few times, but he ignored her or became more angry. Then she became upset and yelled at him or cried. Ruth identified that this became a major problem for them because of the cost of new pajamas and the frustration it caused both of them.

Ruth modified her behavior by not arguing. Instead, she waited until Joseph had his shower and then took his pajamas, refolded them, and placed them in the dresser drawer. She told herself that he could not be reasoned with and this was the best way to handle the problem.

At first she felt that she was not being honest with Joseph, but she came to realize that, through the strategy of role supplementation and daily experiences, this type of interaction prevented fear, frustration, and anxiety for Joseph, and consequently, for herself. Ruth stated, "Joseph even put his hand on my shoulder, in a caring way, the other night. He hasn't done that for years. Our relationship is more important than my not telling him about the pajamas. To be honest, the other day as I was putting them in the drawer I even got the giggles…the giggles are much nicer than yelling or being frustrated."

Repeated Behaviors and Questioning

Joseph frequently became anxious and exhibited repeat behaviors or asked numerous repetitious questions; for example, when strangers stopped by the house, when he received telephone calls requesting donations, or when Ruth was upset. The principal way this was managed was to help Ruth recognize that repetition was a way that Joseph handled his anxiety. She learned to accept his repeated behaviors and did not try to convince him to feel differently. Instead, she attempted to change his activity either by joking with him, or encouraging him to go for a walk with her, wash the windows, or ride the exercise bike.

Ruth's evaluation of how she managed this problem can be seen in this example. One evening, Joseph put on his coat, went to the garage to check that the garbage was out, came back into the house, and took off his jacket. He repeated this routine five times. Ruth said that she sat in a chair with her book so that she could keep an eye on him. Each time when he came back in the house, she asked him whether he would like to watch television. He ignored her the first four times, but when he came in the last time he seemed to be getting tired, so she asked him to rub her neck and started joking with him. He rubbed her neck and then went to bed. Ruth stated, "Didn't that work out well? I'm really proud of myself. In the past I would have gotten so upset, yelled at him, and been so frustrated."

Driving the Car

When they were ready to go somewhere Joseph expected to drive. Ruth was very nervous about this because he got lost and did not pay attention to the traffic. If Ruth told him he could not drive or that she would, he became angry and refused to let her drive.

Ruth managed this by never disagreeing with Joseph or asking him about driving. Instead, she agreed with what he wanted, but as they went to the car she got into the driver's seat and drove. He did not question this.

Summary

This case study was not designed as a research study to test the effectiveness of role supplementation as an intervention. However, the response to this conceptual approach demonstrated individual and family coping, and effective role transition. Ruth expressed that she was much happier because she understood how to live with Joseph. She now saw that there were day-to-day events to cope with, and that the time might come when she would have to make some major decisions about his care. These statements suggest that the Alzheimer's disease no longer controlled the family, and that Ruth had acquired personal power in her perception of their life together, and how to make the everyday changes and those the future might demand. She had reached her goal of caring for Joseph at home and living her life to the fullest, as evidenced by the following comment made on one of the last home visits:

> I can't believe how well things are going. I know the changes I've made are right. We are both so much calmer, I can see it in his eyes that he feels safer. We both sleep so much better...he doesn't pace nearly as much or yell at me.
>
> I've changed how I feel about talking with my friends. I used to think I should keep it quiet and no one should know. Since I know you won't be coming to see me much longer, I'm talking with a friend whose husband died of Alzheimer's, she is very helpful to me now. It's so nice to have someone to talk with so I can manage Joseph better. I talk more with Tom. I think he's not so frightened about all of this either.
>
> We can't do anything that takes concentration, but we can be together without all the frustration. I used to think Alzheimer's was hopeless—it still is, he may some day have to go to a nursing home, but I have so much hope because we can be together now and have some happy times.

REFERENCES

Allen, V. L., & van de Vliert, E. (1984). *Role transitions: Explorations and explanations*. New York: Plenum Press.

Biddle, B. J., & Thomas, E. J. (1966). *Role theory: Concepts and research*. New York: John Wiley & Sons.

Doehrman, S. R. (1984). Stress, strain, and social support during a role transition. In V. L. Allen & E. van de Vliert (Eds.), *Role transitions: Explorations and explanations* (pp. 253–262). New York: Plenum Press.

Glaser, B. G., & Strauss, A. L. (1971). *Status passages*. Chicago: Aldine.

Gwyther, L. P., & Matteson, M. A. (1983). Care for the caregivers. *Journal of Gerontological Nursing*, 9(2), 92–110.

Hayter, J. (1974, February). Patients who have Alzheimer's disease. *American Journal of Nursing*, 74, 1460–1563.

Louis, M. R. (1980). Surprise and sense making: What newcomers experience in entering unfamiliar organizational settings. *Administrative Science Quarterly*, 25, 226–251.

Mace, N. L., & Rabins, P. V. (1981). *The 36-hour day*. Baltimore: Johns Hopkins Press.

Mead, G. (1972). *Mind, self, and society* (18th ed.). Belmont, CA: Wadsworth.

Mederer, H. (1984). The transition to a parent-caring role by adult children. In V. L. Allen & E. van de Vliert (Eds.), *Role transitions: Explorations and explanations* (pp. 301–314). New York: Plenum Press.

Meleis, A. I. (1975, July–August). Role insufficiency and role supplementation: A conceptual framework. *Nursing Research, 24*(4), 265–271.

Meleis, A. I., & Swendsen, L. A., (1978, January–February). Role supplementation: An empirical test of a nursing intervention. *Nursing Research, 27*(1), 11–18.

Minkler, M., & Biller, R. P. (1979). Role shock: A tool for conceptualizing stresses accompanying disruptive role transitions. *Human Relations, 32*, 125–140.

Pinel, C. (1975). Alzheimer's disease. *Nursing Times, 71*(3), 105–106.

Swendsen, L. A., Meleis, A. I., & Jones, E. (1978). Role supplementation for new parents—A role mastery plan. *American Journal of Maternal Child Nursing, 3*(2), 84–91.

van Ments, M. (1983). *The effective use of role-play: A handbook for teachers and trainers.* London: Kogan Page.

Reprinted with permission from: Kelley, L. S., & Lakin, J. A. (1988). Role supplementation as a nursing intervention for Alzheimer's disease: A case study. *Public Health Nursing, 5*(3), 146–152.

10.8 TRANSITION ENTRY GROUPS: EASING NEW PATIENTS' ADJUSTMENT TO PSYCHIATRIC HOSPITALIZATION

KAREN AROIAN
MARITA PRATER

Newly hospitalized psychiatric patients experience two kinds of crises: the personal crisis that brought them into the hospital and the generic crisis of being hospitalized. This generic crisis involves facing what it means to be a psychiatric patient, confined in a novel and confusing environment and confronted by staff expectations that patients will adapt quickly to their new environment.

Patients commonly respond to psychiatric hospitalization by feeling removed from normal routines and abandoned by family and friends. They also experience failure and guilt over not being able to function outside of the hospital, and anticipate being socially stigmatized for having been treated in a psychiatric hospital. Patients must cope with their subordinate status and sense of powerlessness, and they may feel vulnerable and dependent on a structure and staff that are unfamiliar to them.

Patients may also perceive treatment as pressure to relinquish defenses and as a threat to self-control. Consequently, they may distrust staff and display anger toward them, manifest ambivalence about the need to be hospitalized, and question if and how the hospital can help them. These reactions may be more severe in involuntary patients who continue to deny or minimize their psychiatric difficulties.

Transition Entry Group Goals and Organization

Transition entry groups were developed at Charles River Hospital, a private 58-bed facility in Wellesley, Massachusetts, to address problems commonly experienced by new patients during their adjustment to psychiatric hospitalization. The groups' goals are to help reduce the anxiety newly admitted patients experience during the initial transition period of psychiatric hospitalization, to provide information about hospital rules and procedures, and to establish the expectation of individual responsibility for the course of treatment. The groups also provide an opportunity for staff to evaluate patients' patterns of interaction and motivations for treatment.

Transition entry groups are led by master's-level psychiatric nurses, and meet for 50 minutes each day Thursday through Sunday. The group is open, and new members join at each session. Patients who have been admitted one hour to one day before any session in the four-day sequence are eligible to attend that session, and to continue in the group through the last session on Sunday. This scheduling provides patients with specialized interventions soon after admission. Each week's group thus includes patients admitted to the hospital during the period from Wednesday through Sunday.

This design specifically accommodates patients admitted late in the week or during weekends. During the first few days of their hospital stay, these patients have fewer opportunities to attend psychotherapy sessions, and fewer staff available to respond to their difficulties in adjustment, than do patients admitted on Mondays and Tuesdays.

The groups include adults and adolescents with a wide range of diagnoses and disturbed behavior. The size of the group varies from 2 to 10 patients. The sessions are held in a hospital conference room, outside the hospital's units. Patients are excluded from the group only if they are so seriously disturbed that they would endanger themselves or others if they left the unit.

Prescreening is based on the admission evaluation, and on the judgment of the milieu staff and the group leader about the patient's safety off the unit. If the patient had been admitted to the hospital on Wednesday or Thursday, additional information may be available from the primary therapist. More often, however, the groups are initiated before a primary therapist has been assigned to the patient.

Therapeutic Techniques

Transition entry groups can help diminish the anxiety associated with psychiatric hospitalization, and help establish the expectation of individual responsibility for the course of treatment. However, in meeting these goals, each group is challenged by several factors, including the fluctuation in its membership, the disparity in patients' ages, diagnoses, and precipitants of illness, and the variation in the severity of patients' pathology and in the intensity of their anxiety.

Several techniques are used by the therapist to assist the group in overcoming these obstacles. The group leader begins the session by encouraging patients to focus on why they have been hospitalized, and by asking patients to share their reasons for and reactions to hospitalization. The leader then calls attention to any common themes that emerge from the patients' responses. This technique increases the patients' sense of commonality and decreases their shame.

The leader provides accurate information about hospital regulations and patients' rights and explains the rationale for the restrictiveness of hospital rules. The leader also encourages group members who have previously been hospitalized, or who have attended earlier group sessions, to assume responsibility for imparting information. This technique promotes group participation and decreases patients' sense of helplessness.

Patients' feelings of loss of control are usually expressed in the groups through rebellion, struggles for dominance, and hostility toward the group leader, the hospital, and other group members. The leader encourages patients to express such conflicts, points out that they are normal reactions to hospitalization, and reinterprets them as signs that patients are attempting to resume control over their lives.

Patients may react to the varying ages and diagnoses of the group members with feelings of vulnerability or lack of control. The group leader addresses these reactions by describing the range of symptoms that patients may express and the variety of developmental tasks facing them. The leader also listens for and presents the common themes among the seemingly different problems and concerns of the group members. In addition, the group leader helps decrease the anxiety associated with the differences within the group by role modeling empathic and effective ways for group members to interact with and support their fellow patients. Group members are also encouraged to confront each other about appropriate ways of interacting. These techniques help increase the patients' interpersonal skills, enhance their feeling of control, and improve their sense of altruism. They also help establish the expectation that individual patients have the ultimate responsibility for their own treatment and recovery.

When patients begin to feel more comfortable in the group, they reveal their hopes and fears about the course of their problems and the outcome of their hospitalization. Patients who have been hospitalized previously are encouraged to discuss the outcome of earlier hospitalizations as a means of generating hope or providing advice. These discussions also serve to foster altruism and help restore patients' morale.

The final task for the group leader is helping the group to terminate effectively by acknowledging, during the end of the third meeting, that the next session will be the last. At the last session, the leader encourages patients to express sadness and loss, and facilitates the review of group process by asking members to recall their thoughts and feelings at the start of the group, and to identify the ways they have changed since joining the group. This technique summarizes and terminates the group's experience.

Reprinted with permission from: Aroian, K., & Prater, M. (1988). Transitions entry groups: Easing new patients' adjustment to psychiatric hospitalization. *Hospital and Community Psychiatry, 39,* 312–313.

Chapter 11   Debriefing Models

11.1   A SURVEY OF POSTNATAL DEBRIEFING

ANNE-MARIE STEELE
MARY BEADLE

Abstract

Background: *The evidence for postnatal debriefing generally lacks clarification of what postnatal debriefing constitutes. This is true of the recommendation in the United Kingdom for midwives to undertake, "active postnatal debriefing" (Department of Health, 1999).* **Aim:** *The study aimed to explore current practice and describe the provision of postnatal debriefing in two health regions of England.* **Methods:** *A descriptive survey using cohort sampling was undertaken using a self-report questionnaire that was sent to each maternity unit in the two regions (n = 46). A response rate of 93% (n = 43) was obtained. The questionnaire collected information about the maternity units and their provision of postnatal debriefing. A list of debriefing descriptors formed the basis of the questionnaire, and comprised activities that various authors had included in their definitions of debriefing.* **Results:** *Responses indicated that 38 (88%) maternity units offered women an opportunity to debrief by discussing their experiences of maternity care. The provision of this service fell into three distinct subgroups: first, those who provided a service that is in keeping with debriefing, however, not all the maternity units actually called their service debriefing; second, those who provided a service that is fundamental postnatal care, usually called routine postnatal care; third, those who provided a service that was inconsistent and neither debriefing nor postnatal care. This inconsistency was also reflected in the names chosen for the service.* **Conclusions:** *The findings of this study support previous claims that confusion about postnatal debriefing continues. Recommendations for practice are made with the intention of promoting a consistent approach; this would also enable further research and evaluation to be conducted.*

Introduction

The concept of debriefing has attracted international interest, with papers originating from Norway (Dyregrov, 1989), the United Kingdom (U.K.) (Smith & Mitchell, 1996; Alexander, 1998), the United States (U.S.) (Affonso, 1977; Stolte, 1986), and Australia (Small et al., 2000). In order to explore the concept of debriefing, a literature review was undertaken using a number of electronic databases: EBSCO Academic Search Elite, CINAHL, BIOMED, MIDIRS, Medline, and Cochrane. The following key words were used: debriefing, postnatal debriefing, postnatal, nondirective counseling, posttraumatic stress disorder, and postnatal depression. References from the papers and texts then provided further direction for obtaining additional literature that might add to the evidence. The literature search was not limited by exclusion criteria such as dates, and not confined to postnatal debriefing or maternity care settings. The total number of papers/chapters reviewed was 79.

When reviewing the literature it appears that the evidence for postnatal debriefing is, at best, inconclusive, and at worst, demonstrates potentially negative effects both for service users and providers (Kenardy et al., 1996; Alexander, 1998; Benbow,

2000; Small et al., 2000). Some of the ambiguity appears to arise from the adaptation of psychological debriefing for survivors or those bereaved following critical incidents, accidents, or disasters. The appropriateness of comparing and associating childbirth with an abnormal event is questionable. Similarly, the application of psychological debriefing to maternity services requires scrutiny of the relevance and underpinning evidence. Such scrutiny of the application and implementation of debriefing in the childbirth setting prompted the study reported in this chapter.

There appears to be growing recognition that childbirth can be associated with short- and long-term psychological morbidity, including posttraumatic stress and depression. Strategies to prevent or reduce psychological morbidity range from unstructured discussion (Abbott et al., 1997) to structured psychological interventions (Hagan et al., 1999). Although significant variation exists in the strategies adopted, the name given is often the same, postnatal debriefing. Different authors have identified different approaches to debriefing. The literature offers some evidence and guidance (Wessely, 1998) about what debriefing might or should entail. However, this is often limited by the lack of clarity (Alexander, 1998).

Very few randomized controlled trials of debriefing following childbirth have been undertaken. These include those by Small et al. (2000) and Hagan et al. (1999), and both of these reported no beneficial effect of postnatal debriefing on postnatal depression or well-being. Furthermore, it was not possible to rule out the possibility that debriefing contributed to poorer emotional health (Small et al., 2000). However, both studies lack clarity in what the debriefing intervention involved. For example, in the brief description offered by Small et al. (2000), the debriefing intervention provided women with an opportunity to discuss their labor, birth, and postdelivery events and experiences. Stallard (2000) questions whether this intervention is actually debriefing, and cautions against using the term inappropriately.

The majority of postnatal debriefing definitions are quite simple, usually comprising an unstructured process, such as the woman describing her experiences and feelings and receiving information. Broader definitions tend to originate from outside childbirth. These generally comprise a structured process starting with describing experiences and feelings, then moving on to other activities, such as confirming normality and exploring sensory perceptions. The range of descriptions of postnatal debriefing found in the literature is shown in Table 11.1.1.

Given the continued debate about the evidence underpinning debriefing, communication, and postnatal care (Benbow, 2000; Singh, 2000), it was surprising that recommendations were made by the U.K. Department of Health (DOH) for midwives to undertake "active postnatal debriefing" (DOH, 1999). The recommendations included little detail about what active postnatal debriefing constitutes. The implementation of postnatal debriefing, therefore, remains open to wide interpretation. The purpose of this study was to find whether the maternity units provided a debriefing service and what this actually entailed.

The Study

Aims

The study was conducted between June 2000 and December 2001 following the DOH recommendations (DOH, 1999), and aimed to explore current practices and describe the provision of postnatal debriefing within two health regions. The study objectives were to:

- describe the provision of postnatal debriefing in two Health Authority regions in England;
- clarify the meaning of the term postnatal debriefing;
- make recommendations on the provision of postnatal debriefing.

Method

The method used was a descriptive survey of the maternity units in two regions of England ($n = 46$).

TABLE 11.1.1 Potential Postnatal Debriefing Descriptors

Descriptor	Source
1. Woman describes the details of her experience	Dyregrov (1989); Charles & Curtis (1994); Abbott et al. (1997); Lavender & Walkinshaw (1998); Hagan et al. (1999); Small et al. (2000)
2. Woman discusses feelings around the experience	Dyregrov (1989); Charles & Curtis (1994); Abbott et al. (1997); Lavender & Walkinshaw (1998); Hagan et al. (1999); Small et al. (2000)
3. Information is given to the woman	Dyregrov (1989); Abbott et al. (1997); Hagan et al. (1999)
4. Rationale for management/care is given	Abbott et al. (1997)
5. Identification and referral to supporting agencies	Dyregrov (1989)
6. Discussion around how the woman may feel in the future	Dyregrov (1989)
7. Confirmation of normality of the woman's experience	Dyregrov (1989); Hagan et al. (1999)
8. Focus around sensory perceptions, smells, visions, noises, etc.	Dyregrov (1989)
9. Identification of the worst thing about what happened	Dyregrov (1989)

Based on the literature, we designed a self-report questionnaire to collect information about all the maternity units and their provision of postnatal debriefing.

From the debriefing definitions in the literature, the activities and/or events that commonly take place during debriefing were amalgamated into a list of potential postnatal debriefing descriptors (see Table 11.1.1). The descriptors ranged from activities associated with informal or unstructured debriefing to those associated with structured psychological debriefing. For example, descriptors 1–4 included the woman describing her experiences, discussing her feelings, receiving information, and being provided with some rationale for the care she received. This definition of postnatal debriefing is offered by Abbott et al. (1997). However, Alexander (1998) disagrees, and claims that debriefing operates at a different level.

Dyregrov (1989) provides a more encompassing definition of debriefing that expands on descriptors 1–3 and includes descriptors 5–9; identification and referral to supporting agencies, discussion about how the woman might feel in the future, confirming normality, focus on sensory perception, and identification of the worst thing that happened. It is suggested by Dyregrov (1989) that debriefing is a structured psychological intervention that should be facilitated by an appropriately trained person. Descriptor 4, the rationale for management/care given, does not feature in Dyregrov's work. This work is a reflection of debriefing being used for survivors of accidents and disasters, rather than in health care or maternity settings.

According to the United Kingdom Central Council for Nursing, Midwifery and Health Visiting (UKCC), the fifth descriptor, identification and referral to supporting agencies, is an essential aspect of midwifery practice. This is a recognized role and responsibility of the midwife (UKCC, 1998) and an identified midwifery competency in the U.K. (UKCC, 2000). We suggest that descriptors 1–5 constitute nothing more than the fundamental aspects of postnatal care.

The list of descriptors formed the basis of the questionnaire, and was included in one of the initial questions seeking to define the service each maternity unit provided. The remainder of the questionnaire focused on the practicalities of providing a debriefing service. One open-ended question was included to identify the purpose of the debriefing service. The questionnaire ended by inviting any additional comments the participants wished to make on postnatal debriefing.

The questionnaire, consisting of 17 multiple-choice questions, was pilot-tested with several midwives who were not involved in the study itself, and minor amendments were made to the wording of questions to improve clarification. The choice of responses provided for each question were taken from the findings of the literature review. Each question also had an "other" option to allow for any responses that had not been anticipated.

Sample

The final version of the questionnaire was then mailed to all the maternity units ($n = 46$) in two randomly selected English health regions. The questionnaire was sent to every Head of Midwifery in the two regions, and an accompanying letter requested that it be completed for each maternity unit by the most appropriate member staff. One reminder was sent out after 8 weeks, following which only three units did not complete the questionnaire. The final response rate was 93% ($n = 43$).

Ethical Considerations

Approval to undertake the study was obtained from the Director of Nursing for each maternity unit and a Multicenter Research Ethics Committee (MREC). Participants were assured that all details from the questionnaire would remain anonymous and confidential. Names and contact numbers were requested, but only for verification purposes and access should a follow-up qualitative study be undertaken. Most participants volunteered this information, and explicitly requested feedback on the findings of the study.

Data Analysis

Responses to the multiple-choice questions were entered into a database and analyzed using the Statistical Package for the Social Sciences, version 10. Descriptive analyses including frequencies and cross tabulations were carried out.

Results

Participants were asked, "Does the maternity unit offer an opportunity for women to discuss their experiences of maternity care?" Responses indicated that 38 (88%) maternity units offered women this opportunity.

The next question asked, "Which elements of care best describes the service available to women in the maternity unit?" The multiple-choice options provided to answer this were the nine postnatal debriefing descriptors in listed in Table 11.1.1. None of the participants identified activities or care outside these descriptors, and responses fell into three distinct subgroups, which are described in the following.

Group A

In this group, all participants (14%, $n = 6$) selected all nine descriptor statements; the service provided by the maternity units in this subgroup can be identified as debriefing. The names given to the service offered by this group were debriefing: 4 (10%), birth reflections: 1 (2%), and birth afterthoughts: 1 (2%). The majority of participants (12%, $n = 5$) identified that the service was evaluated separately from other maternity services, using a number of evaluation tools. Only one maternity unit in this group (2%) did not evaluate their service.

Group B

In this group, all participants (28%, $n = 12$) selected only descriptor statements between 1 and 5 from

Table 11.1.1. We suggest that the service provided by this group simply constitutes postnatal care. Indeed, the name used by many of the participants (16%, n = 7) was routine postnatal care. The remaining participants (12%, n = 5) gave a combination of names, but all included routine postnatal care as part of their combination. Eight (19%) participants reported that the service was not evaluated separately.

Group C

In this group, all participants (58%, n = 25) selected combinations of descriptor statements from Table 11.1.1. Because of the number of variations in the responses of this group, it is not possible to identify any consistency in what the service entailed. However, analysis revealed that, unlike Group A, they did not offer a full debriefing service, but included descriptors that extended beyond postnatal care (descriptors 1–5; Table 11.1.1), for example, a focus on sensory perceptions.

The service was inconsistent, and this was reflected in the names chosen for the service: birth afterthoughts (5%, n = 2); debriefing (14%, n = 6); routine postnatal care (19%, n = 8); and postevent support (2%, n = 1). The remainder of this group (16%, n = 7) gave more than one name for their services, all of which included in their combination, "routine postnatal care." The service was not evaluated separately by 10 (23%) of this group. Those who evaluated the service did so using a range of tools, but most frequently, a client satisfaction survey (19%, n = 8).

Barriers to Providing the Service

The most frequently encountered barriers to providing the service were finance, staffing levels, and training of staff. Given the current debate about the shortage of health care professionals and funding of the National Health Service (NHS) in the U.K., it is not surprising that staffing was identified as a barrier by 30 (70%) and finance by 14 (33%) of the sample.

Purpose of Debriefing

Participants were given the opportunity to identify the purpose of their service. From the narrative data collected, it was possible to identify the following themes:

- to answer questions
- to aid understanding
- provide explanations and rationale for care
- to provide information
- to listen to the women
- to help the women to come to terms with the experience.

Discussion

Limitations

The sample studied is limited in terms of how representative it might be of other geographical areas, but the high response rate (93%) indicates that the findings are highly representative of the two health regions involved.

In order to reduce the possible limitations imposed by multiple-choice questions, each question had an "other" option allowing participants to include answers outside the provided options. This option was used in response to many of the questions, and participants offered further details, for example, names of the service. This option was particularly important in the question designed to describe what type of "debriefing" service the maternity unit offered. Participants were invited to provide any other descriptors of their service, and so identify any deficiencies in the potential postnatal debriefing list (Table 11.1.1). No further descriptors were added by any of the participants.

Debriefing: Group A

Group A provided a service that included all nine postnatal debriefing descriptors (Table 11.1.1). This structured psychological intervention could be accurately defined as debriefing (Dyregrov, 1989);

however, not all the maternity units called their service debriefing.

The results of this survey support the earlier work of Hammett (1997), which identified staffing as an area of concern. The health care professionals providing the debriefing service were mainly midwives, obstetricians, and psychologists. Hammett (1997) claims that midwives already possess the skills relevant to labor debriefing, but may wish to enhance or develop them further. However, Dyregrov (1989) suggested that professionals such as psychologists, psychiatrists, and psychiatric nurses would require specific debriefing training. Authors such as Benbow (2000) and Parkinson (1993) support this assertion, arguing that this structured psychological intervention is outside the skill and expertise of most midwives. The need for very specifically trained personnel is, therefore, advocated (Parkinson, 1993; Benbow, 2000). The training of health care professionals for this work would be a useful area to explore in more depth in a future study.

Group A did not place any restrictions on when the service could be accessed before or after birth. Parkinson (1993), Hobbs et al. (1996), and Wilson et al. (2000) all recommend that debriefing is undertaken within 48 hours of the event/incident, whereas Dyregrov (1989) cautions against debriefing on the same day, giving time first for physical recovery. This subgroup also did not restrict the time available for each debriefing session, or the number of occasions a woman might attend debriefing. The evidence is inconclusive about attendance for postnatal debriefing. Authors such as Lavender and Walkinshaw (1998), Wilson et al. (2000), and Charles and Curtis (1994) advocate that restrictions should be placed on the number of occasions and the length of each session. However, Rose et al. (1999) and Wessely et al. (2000) question the usefulness of brief, single sessions in preventing posttrauma symptoms. Providing a service without any restrictions has workload and cost implications, and ultimately may be unrealistic. It also raises questions about whether those who feel a need to attend for prolonged periods require additional psychological support and referral.

The debriefing service was provided by face-to-face and telephone contact with professionals. During data analysis, consideration was given to whether telephone contact might be the initial self-referral by the woman, after which a face-to-face meeting could be arranged, as recommended by Charles and Curtis (1994). Further analyses of the data found that not all the maternity units offering a telephone service indicated that women could self-refer. This suggests that some units actually provided a telephone debriefing service; there does not appear to be any evidence to support or refute the use of such a telephone service. Advertisement in the press was identified as one way to notify women of the service, regardless of when they delivered.

The maternity units providing a debriefing service did not always evaluate their service, either separately or as part of other quality assurance systems, and this is a matter of concern. The units that did evaluate the debriefing service used client satisfaction survey, risk management tools, audit, or a combination of these. It is recommended that all care be evaluated. Given the concerns raised by Kenardy et al. (1996), Benbow (2000), and Alexander (1998) about the possible harmful effects of debriefing for both users and providers, evaluation by all those involved is essential. Furthermore, because debriefing involves emotional and psychological well-being, the tool used should be selected accordingly. The use of audit and risk management tools could, therefore, be questioned.

Postnatal Care: Group B

Group B did not provide a debriefing service like that of Group A; instead, their service was more limited and was essentially postnatal care. Inappropriate use of other terms, such as defusing and debriefing, should be avoided (Stallard, 2000). Effective postnatal care must include psychological care of women and their families (Benbow, 2000). We suggest that attempts to meet such needs should include the provision of care that is in keeping with descriptors 1–5 (Table 11.1.1). Group B placed restrictions on when women could access the service, which was available up to 28 days after delivery. This is in keeping with the postnatal period and the time in which women routinely receive postnatal care in the U.K.

There is a focus in the literature on postnatal debriefing to address incidents arising during labour and delivery (Axe, 2000; Niven & Murphy-Black, 2000). However, incidents causing anxiety or stress can arise at any point during maternity care, for example, undergoing antenatal screening. If professionals provide maternity care focusing on psychological well-being at every contact, women would have the opportunity to fill in the missing pieces in their experiences that they either cannot recall or understand (Affonso, 1977). This may also screen and possibly identify women who require more structured psychological care and allow for appropriate referral.

The importance of access to mental health professionals with specialist knowledge and skills is emphasized in the most recent confidential enquiry into maternal deaths in the U.K. It also revealed that psychiatric disorders caused or contributed to 12% of maternal deaths (DOH, 2001). If women are screened and referred appropriately, then there is the potential to reduce the numbers who develop more serious mental health problems. However, this could also lead to an increase in the reported numbers requiring additional support from health/social services and family. The availability of such support needs to be considered. In the long term, there is also the potential to reduce the need identified by Friend (1996) for women to access a debriefing service many years after delivery.

It was interesting to find that some maternity units in Group B that had identified themselves as providing routine postnatal care identified staff training to be a barrier. One might question why the professionals, namely the midwife, health visitor, and GP, would require such training, because they are part of the primary care team and, therefore, are routinely involved in providing postnatal care.

Evidence of Confusion: Group C

Group C, the largest subgroup, provided a varied and inconsistent service that was not debriefing, but extended beyond the fundamental aspects of postnatal care. The evidence available does not appear to support the effectiveness or safety of this kind of service. The study highlights the need to recognize the difference between:

- **postnatal care,** which was described by Group B, and constitutes descriptors 1–5 (Table 11.1.1). This should be available to all women, and definitely should not be called postnatal debriefing
- **postnatal debriefing,** which was described by Group A, and constitutes descriptors 1–9. This may be helpful for specific women whose psychological needs have not been met by postnatal care. It is recommended that specific training be undertaken by health care professionals to undertake this psychological intervention.

Conclusions

This study supports the existing evidence that identifies that confusion surrounding postnatal debriefing continues. In the two health regions of England, three variations in the provision of postnatal debriefing were identified. The largest subgroup was inconsistent in their approach and the name used for the service. There is no evidence to support that this service constitutes postnatal debriefing. Furthermore, the effects for both service users and providers are unknown.

The second largest group had a consistent approach, but we consider that this service is simply effective postnatal care, which:

- recognizes the importance of the psychological well-being of women and their families
- should be available to all women throughout their contact with the maternity services
- includes the referral of women who require debriefing or other psychological interventions
- does not require a separate name
- is not an extension of the midwife's role.

Effective postnatal care should recognize the importance of psychological well-being of women. This involves opportunities throughout the period of contact for the woman to describe her experiences, discuss her feelings, and receive information and a rationale for the care she receives. Such care may help to identify those who require referral to professionals with specialist mental health knowledge. These are fundamental aspects of postnatal care, and recognized responsibilities of the midwife. It might be more appropriate, for most of the women and families, for midwives to focus on providing effective maternity care, rather than expanding the midwife's role into psychological interventions such as postnatal debriefing.

The final group offered a true debriefing service, as described in Table 11.1.1. Our findings indicate that this list of postnatal debriefing descriptors provides an acceptable and accurate description of postnatal debriefing, although further research into its effectiveness and evaluation is required. This structured approach may be suitable for women whose emotional and psychological needs have not been met. Consideration must be given to which professionals should provide postnatal debriefing and the training necessary. Debriefing is a structured psychological intervention, for which a clear and consistent framework or model should used. This would help to reduce the number of maternity units providing an inconsistent approach. It would also enhance the rigor of future research into the safety and effectiveness of postnatal debriefing.

Acknowledgments

We were grateful to receive funding to cover stationery from three companies: Proctor & Gamble, Daniels Healthcare Ltd., and Rehabilicare (U.K.) Ltd. We would like to thank all the participants, as well as Annie Macleod and Professor Roger Watson, for their advice, support, and encouragement during this study.

REFERENCES

Abbott H., Bick D., & McArthur C. (1997). Health after birth. In *Essential midwifery* (Henderson C., & Jones K., eds), Mosby, London, pp. 285–318.

Affonso D. (1977). Missing pieces a study of postpartum feelings. *Birth and The Family Journal* 4, 159–164.

Alexander J. (1998). Confusing debriefing and defusing postnatally: The need for clarity of terms, purpose and value. *Midwifery* 14, 122–124.

Axe S. (2000). Labour debriefing is crucial for good psychological care. *British Journal of Midwifery* 8, 626–631.

Benbow P. (2000). Listening to women following birth. In *Midwifery practice in the postnatal period* (Royal College of Midwives, ed.), Royal College of Midwives, London, pp. 39–40.

Charles J., & Curtis L. (1994). Birth afterthoughts: A listening and information service. *British Journal of Midwifery* 2, 331–334.

Department of Health. (1999). *Making a difference*. Department of Health, London.

Department of Health. (2001). *Why mothers die 1997–1999: The confidential enquiries into maternal deaths in the United Kingdom*. RCOG, London.

Dyregrov A. (1989). Caring for helpers in disaster situations: Psychological debriefing. *Disaster Management* 2, 25–34.

Friend B. (1996). Thoughts after birth. *Nursing Times* 92, 24–25.

Hagan R., Priest S., Evans S., et al. (1999). Stress debriefing after childbirth: Maternal outcomes [abstract A 84]. Third Annual Congress of the Perinatal Society of Australia and New Zealand. http://128.250.188.72/psanz/Melbourne/Tuesday.htm

Hammett P. (1997). Midwives and debriefing. In *Reflections on midwifery* (Kirkham M., & Perkins E., eds.). Bailliere Tindall, London, pp. 135–159.

Hobbs M., Mayou R., Harrison B., & Worlock P. (1996). A randomised controlled trial of psychological debriefing for victims of road traffic accidents. *British Medical Journal* 31, 1438–1439.

Kenardy J., Webster R., Lewin T., Carr V., Hazell P., & Carter G. (1996). Stress debriefing and patterns of recovery following a natural disaster. *Journal of Trauma Stress* 1, 37–49.

Lavender T., & Walkinshaw S. (1998). Can midwives reduce postpartum psychological morbidity? A randomised trial. *Birth* 25, 215–219.

Niven C.A., & Murphy-Black T. (2000). Memory for labour pain: A review of the literature. *Birth* 27, 244–253.

Parkinson F. (1993). *Post trauma stress*. Sheldon Press, London.

Rose S., Brewing C., Andrews B., & Kirk M. (1999). A randomised controlled trial of individual psychological debriefing for victims of violent crime. *Psychological Medicine* 29, 793–799.

Singh D. (2000). Postnatal care needs are not being met. *British Journal of Midwifery* 8, 472–474.

Small R., Lumley J., Donohue L., Potter A., & Waldenstrom U. (2000). Randomised controlled trial of midwife led debriefing to reduce maternal depression after operative childbirth. *British Medical Journal* 321, 1043–1047.

Smith J.A., & Mitchell S. (1996). Debriefing after childbirth: A tool for effective risk management. *British Journal of Midwifery* 4, 581–586.

Stallard P. (2000). The effectiveness of psychological debriefing: A more sophisticated approach is required. *British Medical Journal Electronic Response.* http://www.bmj.com/cgi/eletters/321/7268/1043

Stolte K. (1986). Postpartum 'missing pieces': Sequela of a passing obstetrical era? *Birth* 13, 100–103.

UKCC. (1998). *Midwives' rules and code of practice.* UKCC, London.

UKCC. (2000). *Requirements for pre registration midwifery registration programmes.* UKCC, London.

Wessely S. (1998). Commentary: Reducing distress after normal childbirth. *Birth* 25, 220–221.

Wessely S., Rose S., & Bisson J. (2000). Brief psychological interventions (debriefing) for trauma related symptoms and the prevention of post traumatic stress disorder (Cochrane Review). In *The Cochrane Library*, Issue 3, Oxford: Update Software Ltd.

Wilson J., Raphael B., Meldrum L., Bedosky C., & Sigman M. (2000). Preventing PTSD in trauma survivors. *Bulletin of the Menninger Clinic* 64, 181–196.

Reprinted with permission from: Steele, A. M., & Beadle, M. (2003). A survey of postnatal debriefing. *Journal of Advanced Nursing, 43*(2), 130–136.

11.2 THE LONGITUDINAL EFFECTS OF MIDWIFE-LED POSTNATAL DEBRIEFING ON THE PSYCHOLOGICAL HEALTH OF MOTHERS

ROSEMARY SELKIRK
SUZANNE MCLAREN
ALISON OLLERENSHAW
ANGUS J. MCLACHLAN
JULIE MOTEN

Abstract

To assess the effect of midwife-led postpartum debriefing on psychological variables, 149 women were recruited in the third trimester of their pregnancy and were randomly assigned to treatment and control conditions. Women in the treatment group received midwife-led postpartum debriefing within three days postpartum, whereas women in the control group did not receive formalized debriefing. Background information and psychological variables were assessed prepartum, and birthing information was gathered two days postpartum. The psychological variables, plus a measure of birth trauma, were re-assessed at one month, and again, together with a measure of parenting stress, at three months postpartum. Although the majority of women reported positively on their debriefing experience, statistical analyses indicated that only on the measure of dyadic satisfaction was there some suggestion that debriefing was effective. There were no significant differences between the treatment and control groups on measures of personal information, depression, anxiety, trauma, perception of the birth, or parenting stress at any assessment points postpartum. On the other hand, the effect of medical intervention on women's perceptions of their birthing was evident, with women who experienced more medical intervention reporting more negative perceptions of their birthing than women who had experienced less medical intervention. Surprisingly, this difference was more marked among the women who had been debriefed than among the control group. Generally, the results did not support midwife-led debriefing as an effective intervention postpartum.

Significant life events and experiences that are generally regarded positively may also be a potential source of psychological stress and distress through the life span (Raphael & Prague, 1996). In particular, there appears to be a potential risk of psychological damage for women following childbirth (Raphael-Leff, 1991; Simkin, 1991), despite childbirth being generally perceived as a major and positive life event (Boyce & Condon, 2000). Empirical evidence indicates that some women's memories and perceptions of childbirth have been associated with significant adverse psychological effects, including lack of birth satisfaction (Green, 1993), negative birth perceptions (Cranley et al., 1983), and deterioration in mood and self-esteem (Fisher et al., 1997). There is also evidence that assisted delivery (Astbury et al., 1994) and difficult childbirth (Bergant et al., 1999) are associated with postnatal depressive symptoms.

Postnatal depression (PND) refers to a range of depressive symptoms of varying severity and prolongation that may be experienced by the mother up to two months after childbirth, and persist for a year or longer (Albright, 1993). Women suffering from PND have been found to experience elevated levels of anxiety (Green, 1998), reduced levels of satisfaction with partner, and lack of enjoyment and positive attitude towards the infant (Webster et al., 1994). Current indicators suggest the incidence of PND ranges between 3% and 27% (Milgrom & McCloud, 1996), depending upon the measures employed to study the population characteristics. Various factors associated with childbirth have been linked with the development of PND. Biological (Harris, 1994), medical/obstetric (Burger et al., 1993), and psychiatric and psychological (McMahon et al., 2001) factors have been implicated in the condition, as well as specific aspects of personal history (sexual abuse; Rhodes & Hutchinson, 1994) and psychosocial characteristics (dyadic satisfaction; Webster et al., 1994).

Post traumatic stress disorder (PTSD) is another psychological disorder that may occur after childbirth. PTSD may have a smaller incidence rate, but can be as disruptive as PND. Two British studies suggest that between 5 and 10% of women may experience a high level of distress one month after delivery, with a similar percentage experiencing a medium level of PTSD-type distress at this time (Allen, 1999; Lyons, 1998).

The evolution of midwife-led postnatal debriefing, as a tool for assisting women after childbirth, has grown from its uncritical acceptance as a useful psychological technique to its considered use as one possible adjunct during postnatal care. Originally developed as a group process for emergency personnel after exposure to a critical incident or disaster, psychological debriefing has been transferred to the individual context. The main aim of psychological debriefing is to prevent the development of permanent emotional injury, by enabling normalizing cognitive appraisal and emotional processing of the traumatic experience (Kaplan et al., 2001). Debriefing provides the opportunity to acknowledge grief, vent emotion, and construct a coherent whole of the experiences. The process appears to be beneficial in increasing morale and self-esteem (Rose, 1997).

Postnatal debriefing has been defined in different ways. Authors such as Ball (1988), for example, suggested that providing women with the opportunity to integrate their birth experience through education about that experience might be beneficial in strengthening psychological processes. Raphael-Leff (1991) proposed that re-examining the birth would help women evaluate and integrate this extraordinary event into their particular everyday life experience. For the purposes of this study, postnatal debriefing refers to a midwife-led, semistructured interview with the mother around three days postpartum.

Anecdotal evidence abounds that postnatal debriefing is valued by those who choose it (Charles & Curtis, 1994; Smith & Mitchell, 1996; Westley, 1997). Early evidence suggested it may be a valid method of reducing psychological morbidity (Snaith & Zigmond, 1994), however, the current empirical evidence relating to the efficacy of debriefing is conflicting. A study by Lavinder and Walkinshaw (1998) provides support for the proposal that postnatal debriefing is associated with positive psychological outcomes. In this study, debriefing comprised a 30–120-minute interactive, midwife-led interview whereby women spent as much time as needed discussing their labor, asking questions, and exploring their feelings. They found that women who received debriefing were less likely to have elevated anxiety and depression three weeks postnatally than those mothers who did not receive debriefing.

These findings contrast with the research of Henderson et al. (1998), who found no significant differences in levels of depression at 2, 6, and 12 months postpartum between those women who received midwife-led debriefing and those who did not. In this study, debriefing consisted of a single structured stress debriefing conducted by a trained midwife. Similarly, a study by Small et al. (2000) found no differences in depression following midwife-led debriefing for women who experienced operative childbirth. In this study, the debriefing intervention, which lasted up to 1 hour in duration, provided women with an opportunity to discuss their birthing with a midwife who was experienced in talking with women about their birth, was an emphatic listener, and was knowledgeable about the common concerns and issues of women who had experienced operative deliveries. The content of the debriefing session was determined by the woman's own experiences and concerns (Small et al., 2000). More recently, Priest et al. (2003) found no significant differences on posttraumatic stress and depression between those women who received debriefing and those who did not, when they were assessed at 2, 6, and 12 months postpartum. This study was also unable to detect any major differences in the proportion of women who were diagnosed with stress disorder or with major or minor depressions at 1-year postpartum. The debriefing intervention comprised a single, standard debriefing session led by trained midwives, and based upon a seven-stage critical incident stress debriefing model which had been adapted for use in postpartum debriefing sessions. Each debriefing session lasted between 15 minutes and 1 hour in duration.

Several reasons exist for the apparent inconsistencies in the findings: failure to control for variability in prepartum conditions, variability in the birth and postpartum experience, and employment of differing postpartum measures. The present study controls for variables that have been identified in previous research as confounding variables, including antenatal psychological health, levels of depression and anxiety, and dyadic adjustment. To our knowledge, this is the first study of its kind to investigate trauma, anxiety, and depression simultaneously; to add measures of dyadic adjustment and parenting stress; and to control for a wider range of psychological variables, both pre- and postpartum.

Method

Participants

Participants were recruited to the study from a large regional hospital in Victoria, Australia, over a 3-month period between January and April 2001. Ethics approval was granted from the hospital and tertiary institution from which the study was being conducted. Initially, 180 women were approached to participate in the study. In total, 149 women (83%) agreed to participate and were recruited to the study in the third trimester (= 28 weeks) of their pregnancy. At this time, participants were randomly allocated to treatment and control groups, in order of the receipt of their completed informed consent forms. Each participant's completed consent form was numbered as it arrived. Those participants with an odd number were allocated to the treatment group, and those participants with an even number were allocated to the control group. A sticker was placed on the medical file of each participant, alerting midwifery staff of mothers who were to be debriefed before discharge from the hospital.

Measures

Background Information Questionnaire. A 27-item questionnaire was designed by the researchers to gain information about the birth and parenting expectations, previous psychological history (depression and anxiety), and demographic details.

Symptom Checklist 90-R (SCL 90-R). Designed by Derogatis (1994), the SCL-90-R is a measure of psychological symptomology. The 90-item self-report inventory is rated on a five-point scale of distress (0 = "not at all"; 4 = "extremely"). The SCL-90-R yields nine primary symptom dimensions: (a) somatization, (b) obsessive-compulsion, (c) interpersonal sensitivity, (d) depression, (e) anxiety, (f) hostility, (g) phobic anxiety, (h) paranoid ideation, and (i) psychoticism. In addition, a single summary score, the Global Severity Index, indicates the current level or depth of disorder.

Internal reliability coefficients range from $\alpha = 0.77$ to $\alpha = 0.90$ for the 9 primary symptoms, and test–retest reliability at 10 weeks for these symptoms range from $\alpha = 0.68$ to $\alpha = 0.83$. The SCL-90-R has been used as a measurement of change in clinical cohorts, and as outcome measures of psychotherapeutic, psychopharmacology, and other treatment research (Derogatis, 1994). In this study, the Cronbach α coefficient ranged from $\alpha = 0.73$ to $\alpha = 0.87$ for the nine primary symptoms.

Dyadic Adjustment Scale (DAS). The DAS is a 32-item self report questionnaire developed by Spanier (1989) to measure dyadic relationship or adult partnership quality. Items are rated on a six-point scale (0 = "always disagree"; 5 = "always agree"), with higher scores indicating a better relationship.

Strong internal reliability has been reported, with the total score for dyadic adjustment being $\alpha = 0.96$, and the subscales ranging from $\alpha = 0.73$ to $\alpha = 0.94$ (Spanier, 1989). The scale has been shown to have good criterion-related validity when comparing divorced and married groups of people (Spanier, 1989). In the present study, the Cronbach α coefficient for dyadic adjustment was also strong, $\alpha = 0.93$, with the subscales ranging from $\alpha = 0.66$ to $\alpha = 0.91$, and a median of $\alpha = 0.81$.

State-Trait Anxiety Inventory (STAI). Spielberger (1983) designed the STAI as a two-dimensional measure of trait and state anxiety. The STAI comprises 40 items, with the first 20 items measuring state anxiety, and items 21–40 measuring trait anxiety. Items are rated on a four-point scale (1 = "not at all"; 4 = "very much so"), with higher scores indicating higher levels of anxiety.

Vines and Williams-Burgess (1994) reported strong internal reliability ($\alpha = 0.88$) in a study of mothers at high or low risk for child abuse using the STAI. Mercer and Ferketich (1990) reported strong internal reliability coefficients, ranging from $\alpha = 0.92$ to $\alpha = 0.95$ for state anxiety, and from $\alpha = 0.90$ to $\alpha = 0.93$ for trait anxiety, when using the STAI as part of a battery of tests seeking predictors of parental attachment. In the current study, the Cronbach α coefficient was also strong, $\alpha = 0.93$ for state anxiety and $\alpha = 0.94$ for trait anxiety.

Edinburgh Postnatal Depression Scale (EPDS). Developed by Cox et al. (1997), the EPDS is a 10-item self-report measure of postnatal depressive symptoms, scored on a four-point rating scale (0 = "as much as I ever did"; 3 = "not at all"). Higher scores on the EPDS represent greater levels of depression.

The validity of the EPDS is generally reported in terms of sensitivity (the percentage of true depressed cases identified), specificity (the percentage of true nondepressed cases identified), and positive predictive value (the percentage of all cases positively identified as depressed correctly identified as such). Cox et al. (1987) reported EPDS sensitivity of 86%, specificity of 78%, and positive predictive value of 73%.

Strong validity for the scale has been reported worldwide, with sensitivity and specificity rates ranging from 67.7% (Murray & Carothers, 1990) to 100% (Boyce et al., 1993). The scale has also been validated for use with nonpostnatal women, yielding satisfactory sensitivity (79%) and specificity (85%) (Cox et al., 1996). Boyce et al. (1993) validated the EPDS for an Australian sample of 103 postpartum women, using the Diagnostic Interview Schedule. They reported EPDS sensitivity of 100%, specificity of 95.7%, and positive predictive value of 69.2% for this sample. In this study, the Cronbach α coefficient was $\alpha = 0.87$.

Perception of Birth Scale (POBS). Marut and Mercer (1979) designed this 29-item questionnaire to measure maternal perceptions of the labor and delivery experience. The women used a five-point rating scale (1 = "not at all"; 5 = "extremely") with higher scores indicative of fewer problems and a more positive perception of the birth experience.

Internal reliability coefficients of the instrument have been reported at α = 0.83 for 50 cases (Marut & Mercer, 1979), and α = 0.86 for 360 cases (Fawcett et al., 1992). Fawcett and Knauth (1996) conducted an exploratory factor analysis of the scale that demonstrated strong reliability of α = 0.85 for a 25-item version of the questionnaire with 320 women. In this study, the Cronbach α coefficient was also strong at α = 0.86.

Intrapartum Intervention Scale (IIS). The IIS was developed by Clement et al. (1999) and consists of 20 items (yes/no responses) relating to medical procedures associated with the labor and delivery. IIS scores were only collected at Assessment Point 2 (2 days postpartum). Two levels of this scale were used in the analysis, low and high levels of intervention, based on a median split of the sample. Participants scoring 28 or less were defined as having less medical intervention (low intervention), and those scoring more than 29 were defined as having more medical intervention (high intervention).

Impact of Events Scale (IES). Designed by Horowitz et al. (1979), the IES comprises 15 items requiring participants to respond to statements about stressful life events using a rating scale ranging from 0 to 5 (0 = "not at all"; 5 = "often"). High scores on this measure signified that the event, in this case the birth, had a significant effect on the mother.

Lee et al. (1996) found mean scores on the Intrusion and Avoidance subscales of women following miscarriage to be similar to those reported by Horowitz et al. (1979) for a sample of people suffering with stress response syndromes. Horowitz et al. (1979) reported split-half reliability for the total score as $r = 0.86$. Internal consistency of the subscales was high for Intrusion (α = 0.78) and Avoidance (α = 0.82). Test–retest reliability at 1 week was satisfactory for Intrusion ($r = 0.89$), Avoidance ($r = 0.79$), and for the total score ($r = 0.87$). Other research has confirmed the test's reliability (e.g., Turner & Lee, 1998). In this study, the Cronbach α coefficient was high for the subscales Intrusion (α = 0.80) and Avoidance (α = 0.82), and for the total IES score (α = 0.88).

Parenting Stress Index Short Form (PSI). The PSI is a 36-item questionnaire designed by Abidin (1995) to measure participants' responses to parenting by circling one of five response categories, ranging from "strongly agree" to "strongly disagree." Again, a high score on this index was associated with higher levels of stress.

Abidin (1995) reports strong test–retest reliability at the 6-month interval and internal reliability coefficients for the PSI, with α = 0.84 (test–retest) and α = 0.91 (internal reliability) obtained for the Total Stress score. Test–retest reliability for the three subscales ranges from α = 0.68 (parent–child dysfunctional interaction) to α = 0.85 (parental distress). Similarly, strong internal reliability has also been demonstrated for the three subscales, ranging from α = 0.80 (parent–child dysfunctional interaction) to α = 0.87 (parental distress). Internal reliability was strong in this study, with the Cronbach α coefficient for the PSI being α = 0.94 for the total score, and α = 0.90 for each of the three subscales.

Feedback after Debriefing Questionnaire (FAD). The 20-item FAD was designed by the researchers to gain information about the women's perceptions of, feelings about, reactions to, and satisfaction with, their postnatal debriefing. Using a five-point scale (0 = "not at all"; 4 = "extremely"), participants were asked to respond to items such as how important it was for women to have debriefing, how useful they found debriefing, and how intrusive they thought it was.

Procedure

The procedure for the study involved the collection of self-report questionnaires at four assessment points. The sequence effect of questionnaire presentation was controled by using a Latin square design. At the first assessment point, all participants completed the Background Information Questionnaire, SCL 90-R, the DAS, the STAI, and the EPDS, between the 28th week of gestation and their delivery. At the second assessment point, a day or two after giving birth, all participants completed the POBS and the IIS. At the third assessment point, one month after giving birth, all participants completed the EPDS, STAI, POBS, and the IES, and at the fourth and final assessment point, three months postpartum, all participants completed the EPDS, DAS, STAI, POBS, IES, and the PSI. Participants in the treatment group, who had been debriefed in hospital, also received a FAD questionnaire.

On the second or third day after delivery, around the second assessment point, women in the treatment group received midwife-led postnatal debriefing of between 30 and 60 minutes duration. The hospital midwife specifically employed for debriefing and parenting craft conducted the debriefings in a separate, private room. The debriefing session was consistent with the participating hospital's protocols and followed the guidelines outlined in the hospital's debriefing workshop manual. Each debriefing session consisted of 8 distinct phases, summarized as follows: Phase 1, "Introduction": The mother is told that debriefing is confidential, nonjudgmental, and allows her access to her labor and delivery information. Phase 2, "Fact Phase": The mother is invited to summarize her birth experience. Phase 3, "Thoughts Phase": The mother is asked to describe her thoughts about her birthing. Phase 4, "Feelings Phase": The midwife enquires after the mother's feelings during labor, delivery, and now, including reactions to physical sensations and unexpected occurrences. Phase 5, "Symptoms Phase": The midwife asks the mother to describe her current experience. Phase 6, "Education Phase": The midwife explains to the mother that it is normal and natural to experience a variety of signs, symptoms, and emotional reactions to the birth experience. The midwife clarifies events and myths surrounding the birth, and shares information from the partagraph and delivery notes. Phase 7, "Re-entry Phase": The midwife summarises the mother's overall emotional reactions and response to her birthing expectations. The mother is given the opportunity to convey comments to management regarding the service provided during her birth. Phase 8, "Final Phase": Closure and information. Any further questions the mother has are answered, and information is provided on support services available (if necessary).

Results

Preliminary Group Comparisons: Prepartum and Postdelivery Measures

A series of chi-square analyses of demographic variables comparing the treatment and control groups at the commencement of the study confirmed that the randomization process had been successful. The two groups were similar in regards to marital status ($\chi^2 = 1.27, p > 0.05$), educational level ($\chi^2 = 2.34, p > 0.05$), employment status ($\chi^2 = 0.88, p > 0.05$), expectations of returning to work ($\chi^2 = 0.50, p > 0.05$), and financial security ($\chi^2 = 0.57, p > 0.05$). The groups also did not differ with respect to previous pregnancy and obstetric factors [first pregnancy ($\chi^2 = 0.08, p > 0.05$), first birth ($\chi^2 = 0.21, p > 0.05$), normal pregnancy ($\chi^2 = 0.46, p > 0.05$), delivery type ($\chi^2 = 0.11, p > 0.05$), birth plan ($\chi^2 = 1.50, p > 0.05$)] perceived support factors [family ($\chi^2 = 0.01, p > 0.05$), and friends ($\chi^2 = 1.80, p > 0.05$)], and history of psychiatric illness [depression ($\chi^2 = 2.78, p > 0.05$), anxiety ($\chi^2 = 0.46, p > 0.05$)]. Two *t*-tests also revealed that both groups were of similar age (treatment group, $M = 28.43, SD = 4.70$; control group, $M = 28.85, SD = 4.65, t(147) = 0.54, p > 0.05$) and had similar psychological symptomatology as measured by the Global Severity Index subscale of the SCL-90R (treatment group: $M = 0.57, SD = 0.50$; control group: $M = 0.51, SD = 0.39, t(147) = 0.81, p > .05$).

Efficacy of Treatment

Means and standard deviations for the treatment and control groups for each dependent variable can be seen in Table 11.2.1.

A series of split plot analyses of variance (SPANOVA) were conducted to test for the efficacy of the treatment. All analyses involved the two between subject variables, Condition (treatment/

TABLE 11.2.1 Descriptive Statistics for the Dependent Variables Over Time

	Treatment group				Control group			
	Low[a]		High[b]		Low[a]		High[b]	
Time[c]	M	(SD)	M	(SD)	M	(SD)	M	(SD)
EPDS								
1	7.48	(5.78)	7.35	(4.38)	7.41	(5.49)	6.33	(4.24)
3	6.41	(6.10)	6.45	(4.41)	6.50	(5.32)	6.97	(4.51)
4	6.69	(5.27)	6.13	(5.67)	5.25	(4.98)	5.57	(4.51)
STAI								
1	71.00	(25.23)	68.64	(18.36)	66.13	(22.09)	61.97	(15.56)
3	67.59	(24.10)	65.77	(18.29)	65.44	(21.91)	65.00	(15.34)
4	66.55	(24.60)	63.21	(20.12)	59.50	(18.63)	60.10	(16.71)
POBS								
2	106.00	(13.69)	92.97	(15.18)	100.25	(16.06)	97.03	(17.07)
3	111.31	(15.54)	93.03	(19.45)	99.72	(18.30)	98.60	(18.85)
4	109.86	(17.03)	89.92	(22.70)	96.19	(17.66)	92.83	(23.13)
DAS								
1	114.28	(18.00)	119.81	(14.80)	113.74	(15.64)	121.14	(13.69)
4	113.06	(19.81)	118.59	(14.92)	111.71	(16.15)	112.86	(20.26)
IES								
3	8.76	(10.67)	11.90	(11.76)	6.25	(7.87)	9.80	(8.60)
4	6.72	(8.55)	9.20	(10.10)	5.47	(8.58)	6.53	(7.31)
PSI								
4	62.36	(19.36)	64.02	(17.35)	61.00	(16.75)	67.50	(19.54)

[a]Low level of medical intervention.
[b]High level of medical intervention.
[c]Time Period: 1 = prepartum; 2 = 1/2 days postpartum; 3 = 1 month postpartum; 4 = 3 months postpartum.

control) and Medical Intervention (high/low), and most incorporated within the subject variable of Time. The levels of the last variable differed across analyses, depending on the occasions at which the dependent variables were administered (prepartum, 1/2 days, 1 month, and 3 months postpartum). In the case of parental stress, Time was not included in the analysis, as this was measured only once at 3 months postpartum. Results can be seen in Table 11.2.2.

As is evident from Table 11.2.2, results generally failed to show a main effect for Condition (postnatal debriefing), nor was it involved in any interaction except with Medical Intervention, in the case of POBS (perceived problems with birth), and to a limited extent with Time, in the case of DAS (dyadic satisfaction).

The interaction ($p = 0.06$) between Condition and Time in the measure of Dyadic Satisfaction emerged as debriefed mothers showed a small and insignificant loss of satisfaction with their partners from prepartum ($M = 117.25$) to 3 months postpartum ($M = 116.02$), whereas mothers who were not debriefed showed a significant loss of satisfaction over the same period (prepartum: $M = 117.49$; 3 months postpartum: $M = 112.29$).

The interaction between Condition and Medical Intervention for the POBS can be seen in Figure 11.2.1. A Tukey HSD post hoc analysis showed that women who had high levels of medical intervention and were debriefed ($M = 91.90$) had more negative perceptions of the birth, compared with women who had low levels of intervention and were debriefed ($M = 109.10$). There was no difference be-

TABLE 11.2.2 Split Plot ANOVA Analyses of the Effects of Condition, Medical Intervention, and Time on EPDS, STAI, DAS, and IES

Measure	df	F	Partial η^2	p
EPDS				
Between-subjects effects				
Condition (Treatment/Control)	1, 127	0.29	0.00	0.59
Medical Intervention	1, 127	0.04	0.00	0.84
Condition x Medical Intervention	1, 127	0.01	0.00	0.94
Within-subjects effects				
Time[a]	1.85, 234.47	5.24	0.04	0.01
Condition x Time[a]	1.85, 234.47	1.49	0.01	0.23
Medical Intervention x Time[a]	1.85, 234.47	0.63	0.01	0.52
Condition x Med Int x Time[a]	1.85, 234.47	0.77	0.01	0.46
STAI				
Between-subjects effects				
Condition (Treatment/Control)	1, 126	1.73	0.01	0.19
Medical Intervention	1, 126	0.38	0.00	0.54
Condition x Medical Intervention	1, 126	0.04	0.00	0.85
Within-subjects effects				
Time[a]	1.89, 238.10	5.13	0.04	0.01
Condition x Time[a]	1.89, 238.10	1.18	0.01	0.31
Medical Intervention x Time[a]	1.89, 238.10	0.30	0.00	0.73
Condition x Med Int x Time[a]	1.89, 238.10	0.45	0.00	0.62
POBS				
Between-subjects effects				
Condition (Treatment/Control)	1, 126	1.07	0.01	0.30
Medical Intervention	1, 126	10.92	0.08	0.00
Condition x Medical Intervention	1, 126	5.96	0.05	0.02
Within-subjects effects				
Time[b]	1.67, 210.52	5.40	0.04	0.01
Condition x Time[b]	1.67, 210.52	2.31	0.02	0.11
Medical Intervention x Time[b]	1.67, 210.52	1.40	0.01	0.25
Condition x Med Int x Time[b]	1.67, 210.52	1.88	0.02	0.16
DAS				
Between-subjects effects				
Condition (Treatment/Control)	1, 134	0.35	0.00	0.55
Medical Intervention	1, 134	3.42	0.03	0.07
Condition x Medical Intervention	1, 134	0.06	0.00	0.81
Within-subjects effects				
Time[c]	1, 134	9.18	0.06	0.00
Condition x Time[c]	1, 134	3.51	0.03	0.06
Medical Intervention x Time[c]	1, 134	2.21	0.02	0.14
Condition x Med Int x Time[c]	1, 134	2.21	0.02	0.14

TABLE 11.2.2 *(continued)*

Measure	df	F	Partial η²	p
IES				
Between-subjects effects				
Condition (Treatment/Control)	1, 127	2.25	0.02	0.14
Medical Intervention	1, 127	3.24	0.03	0.07
Condition x Medical Intervention	1, 127	0.03	0.00	0.86
Within-subjects effects				
Time^d	1, 127	6.62	0.05	0.01
Condition x Time^d	1, 127	0.04	0.00	0.84
Medical Intervention x Time^d	1, 127	0.85	0.01	0.36
Condition x Med Int x Time^d	1, 127	0.28	0.00	0.60
PS1				
Between-subjects effects				
Condition (Treatment/Control)	1, 141	0.12	0.00	0.73
Medical Intervention	1, 141	1.80	0.01	0.18
Condition x Medical Intervention	1, 141	0.63	0.00	0.43

Note: The Greenhouse–Geisser adjustment correction was used for tests of within-subjects effects.
Time^a = Scores collected at three assessment points (prepartum, and 1 and 3 months postpartum).
Time^b = Scores collected at three assessment points (1/2 days, and 1 and 3 months postpartum).
Time^c = Scores collected at two assessment points (prepartum and 3 months postpartum).
Time^d = Scores collected at two assessment points (1 and 3 months postpartum).

tween high ($M = 96.20$) and low ($M = 98.7$) intervention groups when no debriefing occurred.

There was a significant main effect of Medical Intervention for the POBS, and a strong suggestion of the effect for DAS and IES. Women who experienced more medical intervention during the birth of their child reported less positive perceptions of the birth, less satisfaction with their partners, and greater stress.

A statistical main effect of Time was evident on the EPDS, STAI, POBS, and IES, as indicated in Table 11.2.2. All participants reported significantly fewer symptoms of depression and less anxiety, over time, from prepartum to one month postpartum and to three months postpartum. Participants also showed declining levels of stress from one to three months postpartum. Perceptions of the birth were not quite as consistent, being more positive at one month postpartum compared with two days postpartum, but were less positive at three months compared with one month postpartum.

Women's Feedback Following Debriefing

FAD scores for both treatment and control groups at assessment point 4 (3 months postpartum, $n = 111$), were not significantly different, indicating that all participants rated their postnatal debriefing in a similar fashion, whether it took place 2 days or 3 months after delivery ($t(109) = 1.07, p = 0.29$). Over 90% of all participants rated their debriefing positively, and indicated that debriefing was not threatening (97.5%) or intrusive (91.5%), and that it was very (21.0%) or extremely (73.1%) important for all women to have the chance to be debriefed. Almost all women (95.7%) indicated that they had received information that was moderately to extremely useful, and over 80% of women felt willing to talk about their birthing, and were comfortable talking with the midwife.

Discussion

The results of this study found women who were debriefed were no less likely to develop symptoms of PND (using the EPDS) than women who did not receive debriefing. This finding confirms the results of previous Australian studies (Henderson et al., 1998; Priest et al., 2003; Small et al., 2000), which used the same measure. The tendency for debriefed women to report more depression than nondebriefed women, noted by Small et al. (2000), was not evident in the current sample. EPDS scores decreased steadily over time for all participants.

PND is an individual response, with multiple possible contributing factors from biological (Harris, 1994), psychological (McMahon et al., 2001), and psychosocial characteristics (Webster et al., 1994), according to the biopsychosocial model. The role of postnatal debriefing in the prevention of PND is to minimize the effect of exacerbating factors, relevant to the birth experience, which may influence the development of depressive symptoms. However, other contributing factors still exist within the context of the woman's life, and a woman may be at risk of PND due to a variety of factors unrelated to the birth experience, which postnatal debriefing does not and cannot address. Boyce and Condon (2001), in their criticism of the Small et al. (2000) study, in fact question whether a single session of debriefing could have an impact on PND, when other psychosocial variables contribute perhaps more significantly to its onset. It is to be noted, however, that this study measured EPDS responses at one and three months postpartum, whereas the two previous studies measured EPDS responses at six months. PND may develop up to six months postpartum, so the current study does not allow for women who may have developed PND between three and six months postpartum.

No differences were evident between women in the control and treatment groups on levels of anxiety, as the state anxiety level of all participants decreased over time regardless of treatment condition. Given that Green (1998) has shown that state STAI scores correlate strongly with EPDS scores at both prepartum and postpartum, and that there were no significant differences on PND, this result is consistent with previous findings.

Interestingly, there were some differences between women in the treatment and control groups on their levels of dyadic satisfaction (as measured by the DAS) over time. Although debriefed mothers showed no loss of dyadic satisfaction from pre- to postpartum, mothers in the control condition did. As dyadic satisfaction is a strong predictor of PND (Webster et al., 1994), the impact of debriefing on dyadic satisfaction but its failure to affect PND is puzzling.

A partial answer to the puzzle may be evident in the effect of debriefing on perceptions of birth. High levels of medical intervention were found, not surprisingly, to adversely affect perceptions of birth. This finding is consistent with that of Cranley et al. (1983), who found less positive perceptions of birth among women who were delivered by caesarean. However, there was an additional and unexpected finding in relation to perceptions of the birth. Results indicated that women who experienced high levels of medical intervention during the birth of their children and who were debriefed had more negative perceptions of the birth, compared with women who had low levels of medical intervention and who were debriefed. Such results raise the possibility that postnatal debriefing may be harmful for women who experience a difficult birth. This would be consistent with Small et al.'s (2000) suggestion of a negative effect of postnatal debriefing on traumatised women, though the Small et al. study focused on women with operative delivery only. Given that the present study included all births, the capacity for debriefing to actually exacerbate negative perceptions among mothers who experience high levels of intervention might account for the small and limited effect of debriefing more generally. Thus, only on the measure of dyadic satisfaction, a measure not directly concerned with the birthing experience, did debriefing show signs of arresting the decline in satisfaction with partner that typically coincides with the birth of a child.

Levels of parental stress (as measured by the PSI) did not differ at one and three months postpartum between women in the treatment and control groups. Milgrom and McCloud (1996) have shown that women with PND rate their infant, and their relationship with their infant, more negatively than controls. Debriefed women in this study did not rate their infant or their relationship with their infant differently from women in the control group.

Finally, it should be noted that all participants' level of trauma generally decreased over time, regardless of condition. This is consistent with previous writings (e.g., Stuhlmiller & Dunning, 2000; Turton et al., 2001) concerning the high spontaneous reduction in symptoms over time among trauma survivors who receive no treatment.

Despite the lack of clear statistical evidence supporting the benefits of postnatal debriefing, women who were debriefed rated the experience positively. This is consistent with previous research (Henderson et al., 1998; Small et al., 2000) and anecdotal evidence. Allen (1999), for example, in a study of 61 women, reported that a number of participants with a high score on the EPDS or the IES spoke of the benefit of talking to, or the need to talk to, others, including health professionals, about their experience. Women perceive the discussion of their birthing, and the sharing of information that takes place, to be helpful, and report positively on the experience. The majority of women on the maternity ward of the participating hospital accepted the opportunity of debriefing when it was offered. Women who have been debriefed after a previous birthing asked when their debriefing for the current birthing would take place.

In summary, this study has confirmed the results of previous studies that recognized that women appreciate the opportunity to talk and gain information about their birthing. The study has also provided support for previous research that concluded that postnatal debriefing does not significantly affect psychological variables related to depression, anxiety, or trauma symptoms following childbirth. However, it has provided some indication that debriefing may arrest declines in dyadic satisfaction.

Several years ago, Alexander (1998) highlighted the lack of clarity of terminology with respect to postnatal debriefing, along with the lack of its systematic evaluation. It seems evident that women appreciate the opportunity to review their birth experience and clarify events with a midwife (Bondas-Salonen, 1998; Charles & Curtis, 1994; Henderson et al., 1998; Small et al., 2000). Whether this review should comprise "psychological debriefing" or some other form of self-reflection requires further examination. It may be that a birthing review, as an opportunity for women to gain information about their birthing, constitutes appropriate quality of care in its own right for those women who experience less medical intervention, regardless of measurable psychological benefits. However, for those women who experience more medical intervention, other protocols may need to be developed and implemented.

This study is limited by statistical, methodological, and extraneous or confounding variable considerations. First, statistically, the number of measures used ideally requires a larger population to sustain the number of analyses performed at the 0.05 level of significance. Second, only self-report measures were used; there was no clinical assessment of depression, anxiety, or birth trauma. However, given that the measures used (EPDS, STAI, SCL-90R, IES, and POBS) have been consistently reported in the literature as having good psychometric properties and have been widely used in previous research, combined with the broad investigative nature of the study, it was reasoned that their use was appropriate. Finally, the study may have been inadvertently affected by confounding or extraneous variables, such as different delivery staff, and factors relating to the debriefing midwife (the midwife in this study was also responsible for parenting craft in the hospital).

As Raphael and Wilson (2000) point out, the use of the term debriefing has powerful connotations that presume an activity with a formalized structure that has been derived from a militaristic model of intervention. The widespread use of the term "debriefing" to cover all potential psychological interventions in association with life experience must be a cause for concern, as is any suggestion of widespread use of this type of intervention for what is, in the majority of instances, a normal and joyful experience. The recovery from childbirth should be facilitated and not pathologized. "Normal" recovery from this experience may include the forgetting of trauma and the spontaneous remission of trauma symptoms over time, perhaps providing understanding relevant to normal recovery from other major life experiences.

Recommending debriefing for all women presupposes that childbirth is traumatic for all women, rather than potentially traumatic for some women. The term "birth review" is preferable, both semantically and practically, as it carries with it no dramatic connotation. The results of this study indicate that whereas having the opportunity to discuss their birthing experience is regarded positively by women, and that debriefing may have some limited impact on dyadic satisfaction, there is little empirical support for its routine use to reduce PND, anxiety, trauma, or parenting stress. Indeed, there is some evidence to suggest that such a procedure may be harmful for women who experience a difficult birth.

REFERENCES

Abidin, R. (1995). *Parenting stress index professional manual*. Charlottesville, VA: Psychological Assessment Resources.

Albright, A. (1993). Postpartum depression: An overview. *Journal of Counseling & Development, 71,* 316–319.

Alexander, J. (1998). Confusing debriefing and defusing postnatally: The need for clarity of terms, purpose and value. *Midwifery, 14,* 122–124.

Allen, H. (1999). "How was it for you?" Debriefing for postnatal women: Does it help? *Professional Care of Mother and Child, 9,* 77–79.

Astbury, J., Brown, S., Lumley, J., & Small, R. (1994). Birth events, birth experiences and social differences in postnatal depression. *Australian Journal of Public Health, 18,* 176–184.

Ball, J. (1988). Mothers need nurturing, too. *Nursing Times, 84,* 29–31.

Bergant, A., Heim, K., Ulmer, H., & Illmensee, K. (1999). Early postnatal depressive mood: Associations with obstetric and psychosocial factors. *Journal of Psychosomatic Research, 46,* 391–394.

Bondas-Salonen, T. (1998). New mothers experiences of post-partum care—A phenomenological follow-up study. *Journal of Clinical Nursing, 7,* 165–174.

Boyce, P., & Condon, J. (2000). Traumatic childbirth and the role of debriefing. In B. Raphael & J. P. Wilson, (Eds.), *Psychological debriefing: Theory, practice and evidence* (pp. 272–280). New York: Cambridge University Press.

Boyce, P., Stubbs, J., & Todd, A. (1993). The Edinburgh Postnatal Depression Scale: Validation for an Australian sample. *Australian and New Zealand Journal of Psychiatry, 27,* 472–476.

Burger, J., Mccue Horwitz, S., Forsyth, B., Leventhal, J. M., & Leaf, P. J. (1993). Psychological sequelae of medical complications during pregnancy. *Pediatrics, 91,* 566–571.

Charles, J., & Curtis, L. (1994). Birth afterthoughts: A listening and information service. *British Journal of Midwifery, 2,* 331–334.

Clement, S., Wilson, J., & Sikorski, J. (1999). The development of an intrapartum intervention score based on women's experiences. *Journal of Reproductive and Infant Psychology, 17,* 53–62.

Cox, J. (1986). *Postnatal depression: A guide for health professionals*. New York: Churchill Livingstone.

Cox, J., Chapman, G., Murray, D., & Jones, P. (1996). Validation of the Edinburgh Postnatal Depression Scale in non-postnatal women. *Journal of Affective Disorders, 39,* 185–189.

Cranley, M., Hedahl, K., & Pegg, S. (1983). Women's perceptions of vaginal and cesarean deliveries. *Nursing Research, 32,* 10–15.

Crompton, J. (1996). Post-traumatic stress disorder and childbirth. *British Journal of Midwifery, 4,* 290–294.

Da Costa, D., Larouche, J., Dritsa, M., & Brender, W. (2000). Psychosocial correlates of prepartum and postpartum depressed mood. *Journal of Affective Disorders, 59,* 31–40.

Derogatis, L. R. (1994). *SCL-90-R symptom checklist-90-R: Administration, scoring and procedures manual*. Minneapolis, MN: National Computer Systems.

Fawcett, J., & Knauth, D. (1996). The factor structure of the perception of birth scale. *Nursing Research, 45,* 83–86.

Fawcett, J., Pollio, N., & Tully, A. (1992). Women's perceptions of cesarean and vaginal delivery: Another look. *Research in Nursing and Health, 15,* 439–446.

Fisher, J., Astbury, J., & Smith, A. (1997). Adverse psychological impact of operative obstetric interventions: A prospective longitudinal study. *Australian and New Zealand Journal of Psychiatry, 31,* 728–738.

Gotlib, I., Whiffen, V., Wallace, P., & Mount, J. (1991). Prospective investigation of postpartum depression: Factors involved in onset and recovery. *Journal of Abnormal Psychology, 100,* 122–132.

Green, J. M. (1993). Expectations and experiences of pain in labour: Findings from a large prospective study. *Birth: Issues in Perinatal Care and Education, 20,* 65–72.

Green, J. (1998). Postnatal depression or perinatal dysphoria? Findings from a longitudinal community-based using the Edinburgh postnatal depression scale. *Journal of Reproductive and Infant Psychology, 16,* 143–155.

Harris, B. (1994). Biological and hormonal aspects of postpartum depressed mood. *British Journal of Psychiatry, 164,* 288–292.

Henderson, J., Sharp, J., Priest, S., Hagan, R., & Evans, S. (1998, March–April). *Postnatal debriefing: What do women feel about it?* Paper presented at the Perinatal Society of Australia and New Zealand Conference, Alice Springs, Australia.

Horowitz, M., Wilner, N., & Alvarez, W. (1979). Impact of event scale: A measure of subjective stress. *Psychosomatic Medicine, 41,* 209–218.

Lavender, T., & Walkinshaw, S. (1998). Can midwives reduce postpartum psychological morbidity? A randomised trial. *Birth: Issues in Perinatal Care and Education, 25,* 215–219.

Kaplan, Z., Iancu, I., & Bodner, E. (2001). A review of psychological debriefing after extreme stress. *Psychiatric Services, 52,* 824–827.

Lee, C., Slade, P., & Lygo, V. (1996). The influence of psychological debriefing on emotional adaption in women following early miscarriage: A preliminary study. *British Journal of Medical Psychology, 69,* 45–58.

Lyons, S. (1998). A prospective study of post traumatic stress symptoms 1 month following childbirth in a group of 42 first-time mothers. *Journal of Reproductive and Infant Psychology, 16,* 91–105.

Madsen, L. (1994). *Rebounding from childbirth: Toward emotional recovery.* Westport, VA: Bergin and Garvey.

Marut, J. S., & Mercer, R. T. (1979). Comparisons of primiparas' perceptions of vaginal and cesarean births. *Nursing Research, 28,* 260–266.

McMahon, C., Barnett, B., Kowalenko, N., Tennant, C., & Don, N. (2001). Postnatal depression, anxiety and unsettled infant behaviour. *Australian and New Zealand Journal of Psychiatry, 35,* 581–588.

Mercer, R. T., & Ferketich, S. L. (1990). Predictors of parental attachment during early parenthood. *Journal of Advanced Nursing, 15,* 268–280.

Milgrom, J., & McCloud, P. (1996). Parenting stress and postnatal depression. *Stress Medicine, 12,* 177–186.

Murray, L., & Carothers, A. (1990). The validation of the Edinburgh postnatal depression scale on a community sample. *British Journal of Psychiatry, 157,* 288–290.

Priest, S. R., Henderson, J., Evans, S. F., & Hagan, R. (2003). Stress debriefing after childbirth: A randomised controlled trial. *Medical Journal of Australia, 178,* 542–454.

Raphael, B., & Sprague, T. (1996). Mental health and prevention for families. *Family Matters, 44,* 26–29.

Raphael, B., & Wilson, J. P. (Eds.) (2000). *Psychological debriefing: Theory, practice and evidence.* Cambridge, U.K.: Cambridge Press.

Raphael-Leff, J. (1991). *Psychological processes of childbearing.* London: Chapman & Hall.

Rhodes, N., & Hutchinson, S. (1994). Labour experiences of childhood sexual abuse survivors. *Birth: Issues in Perinatal Care and Education, 21,* 213–220.

Rose, S. (1997). Psychological debriefing: History and methods. *Counselling, 8,* 48–51.

Simkin, P. (1991). Just another day in a woman's life? Women's long-term perceptions of their first birth experience. *Birth: Issues in Perinatal Care and Education, 18,* 203–210.

Small, R., Lumley, J., Donohue, L., Potter, A., & Waldenstrom, U. (2000). Randomised controlled trial of midwife-led debriefing to reduce maternal depression after operative childbirth. *British Medical Journal, 321,* 1043–1047.

Smith, J., & Mitchell, S. (1996). Debriefing after childbirth: A tool for effective risk management. *British Journal of Midwifery, 4,* 581–586.

Snaith, R. P., & Zigmond, A. S. (1994). *The hospital and anxiety depression scale manual.* Windsor: NFER-Nelson.

Spanier, G. (1989). *Manual for the dyadic adjustment scale.* North Tonawanda, NY: Multi-Health Systems.

Spielberger, C. D. (1983). *State-trait anxiety inventory for adults.* Redwood City, CA: Mind Garden.

Stuhlmiller, C., & Dunning, C. (2000). Concerns about debriefing: Challenging the mainstream. In B. Raphael, & J. P. Wilson (Eds.), *Psychological debriefing: Theory, practice and evidence* (pp. 305–317). New York: Cambridge University Press.

Turner, S., & Lee, D. (1998). *Measures in post traumatic stress disorder. A practitioner's guide.* Berkshire, U.K.: NFER-Nelson.

Turton, P., Hughes, P., Evans, C., & Fainman, D. (2001). Incidence, correlates and predictors of post-traumatic stress disorder in the pregnancy after childbirth. *British Journal of Psychiatry, 178*, 556–560.

Vines, S. W., & Williams-Burgess, C. (1994). Effects of a community health nursing parent-baby (ad)venture program on depression and other selected maternal-child health outcomes. *Public Health Nursing, 11*, 188–195.

Webster, M. L., Thompson, J., Mitchell, E. A., & Werry, J. S. (1994). Postnatal depression in community cohort. *Australian and New Zealand Journal of Psychiatry, 28*, 42–49.

Westley, W. (1997). "Time to talk." Listening service. *Midwives, 110*, 30–31.

Reprinted with permission from: Selkirk, R., McLaren, S., Ollerenshaw, A., McLachlan, A., & Moten, J. (2006). The longitudinal effects of midwife-led postnatal debriefing on the psychological health of mothers. *Journal of Reproductive and Infant Psychology, 24*(2), 133–147.

11.3 PERCEIVED EFFECTIVENESS OF CRITICAL INCIDENT STRESS DEBRIEFING BY AUSTRALIAN NURSES

JILLIAN O'CONNOR
SUE JEAVONS

Abstract

This chapter examines the perceived effectiveness of stress debriefing by a sample of 129 Australian hospital nurses, and the relationship of their perceptions to demographic variables, such as qualifications and work area. The survey generally showed debriefing as helpful, but lack of helpfulness was also recognized because of time taken from personal lives and adverse group processes. Factor analysis identified five scales; three helpful ("Understanding," "Sharing," and "Cohesion"), and two unhelpful ("Procedure" and "Dynamics"). Results suggested that helpfulness of debriefing was unrelated to demographic differences. Although further research is required to replicate these findings, they suggest that replacing the current ad hoc forms of debriefing available at the hospital with a standardized model would overcome shortcomings identified by respondents.

Introduction

The earliest description of critical incident stress debriefing (CISD) in nursing literature appeared in 1988, when Jimmerson described a program modeled on Mitchell's (1983) prototype. This was seen as a turning point for emergency nurses, because they could acknowledge the psychological impact of their work. According to Jimmerson (1988, p. 44A), the experience of CISD had eroded the view of the emergency nurses being "unhurtable superbeings" and "pillars of strength."

In the following decade, the value of CISD in mitigating critical incident stress (CIS) experienced by nurses was recognised by the nursing profession (Cudmore, 1998; Jefferson & Northway, 1996; Wright & Casier, 1996; Laws & Hawkins, 1995; Appleton, 1994; Martin, 1993). Martin (1993) considered that implementation of critical incident stress management (CISM) programs in hospitals provided caregivers with a way of countering the insidious, cumulative effects of emotional trauma because "medical/surgical nurses, oncology nurses, neonatal nurses—all nurses involved in traumatic events" could benefit from them. (Martin, p. 39) Following the categorization of critical incidents experienced by the nurses in her study, Appleton (1994) suggested that debriefing could be useful in assisting nurses to cope with CIS, and recommended the availability of peer support groups and counseling for all acute care agencies.

Laws and Hawkins (1995) argued that debriefing was essential, but lamented the lack of wide recognition of CIS in Australian hospitals and the sparsity of CISD facilities for nurses. Lam et al. (1999) also identified the urgent need for support services such as debriefing and counseling. Jefferson and Northway (1996) reported that CIS was real for nurses, occurred regularly in hospitals, and the time for ignoring potential short- and long-term effects of such stress for health care workers was long past. Wright and Casier (1996) proposed CISM as an effective, inexpensive, and collaborative approach to mitigating the impact of traumatic events. Similarly, Cudmore (1998) considered developing a policy/protocol for instigating debriefing following critical incidents to circumvent potentially harmful effects of cumulative stress and CIS for accident and emergency staff.

Despite adoption of CISM programs by the nursing profession throughout the 1990s, a few articles appeared in the literature reflecting doubts about the efficacy of debriefing (Macnab et al., 2000; Northcott, 1998; Hudson, 1995). Northcott (1998), citing studies critical of debriefing (Bisson, 1997; Brom et al., 1993; McFarlane, 1988), stated that the effectiveness of debriefing in reducing psychological stress and preventing posttraumatic stress disorder (PTSD) was unconfirmed, or possibly, made no difference. She recommended treating any problems that occurred with prolonged therapy, claiming, "the right culture and relationships can do much more to ensure well being after traumatic events than the reactive strategies that are so often mobilised" (p. 32). Hudson (1995) reported that admonitions that one must be debriefed or suffer a posttraumatic stress syndrome were false, because research had demonstrated that 77% of individuals who suffered acute stress disorder went into spontaneous remission. Furthermore, she suggested that debriefing could exacerbate stress. Cotterill (2000) suggests that CISM is only one option for dealing with CIS, and proposes clinical supervision as an alternative.

Of the few published studies evaluating the efficacy of debriefing, three supported the value of debriefing for hospital nurses (Burns & Harm, 1993; Mitchell, 2001; Robinson & Mitchell, 1993), one was inconclusive (Roffey-Mitchel & Jeavons, 1998). Burns and Harm (1993) found that only 32% of nurses surveyed about debriefing had ever participated in debriefing and, of those, 88% reported the process helpful in reducing stress.

Robinson and Mitchell (1993) evaluated debriefing with mainly emergency service personnel, but a small sample of welfare/hospital personnel, including 17 nurses, was included. Of the latter group, 84% found debriefing helpful, and 44% were happy with the process. Emergency personnel reported more cognitive stress, such as sleep disturbances, flashbacks, preoccupation with the incident, and fear of the future than welfare/hospital personnel who reported more emotional distress (sad, weepy, numb, feeling horrified, fearful, enraged, uneasy, and shocked). Robinson and Mitchell (1993) suggested that occupation and gender were both relevant to understanding the stress response, and further work was required to separate these variables.

This controversy about the efficacy of debriefing highlights the need for further investigation of Australian nurses' experiences. The usefulness or not of debriefing for nurses would provide valuable support for its introduction in hospitals and identify necessary modifications. The hospital in which this study was undertaken did not, at the time, have a formal debriefing program, although the staff counselor had been trained in the procedure, so may have offered it to individuals. Some staff may also have experienced debriefing at previous places of employment. The objectives of this study were to determine (a) nurses' perceptions of the effectiveness of stress debriefing, and (b) whether their perceptions of stress debriefing were associated with any of the demographic variables: gender, age, nursing qualifications, method of obtaining initial practising certificate, number of years postregistration, current area of work, and years of experience in that area.

Method

Participants

This study formed the second part of a broader study into CIS in a 750-bed metropolitan teaching and research hospital (O'Connor & Jeavons, 2002). The sample represented 59% of full-time registered nurses (RNs) from the whole study who had attended one or more debriefing sessions in the course of their work. It comprised 129 nurses (88% female)

TABLE 11.3.1 Highest Qualifications of RNs (n = 129)

Qualification	Sample numbers	Sample (%)
Hospital certificate	10	7.8
Diploma	4	3.1
Degree	38	29.4
Master's degree	5	3.9
Postgraduate certificate/diploma	55	42.6
Other qualification	17	132
Total	129	100.0

TABLE 11.3.2 Areas of Work of RNs (n = 129)

Area of Work	Sample Numbers	Sample (%)
Aged care	2	1.6
Intensive care	13	10.1
Oncology	4	3.1
Psychiatry	17	13.2
Coronary care	2	1.6
Medical	11	8.5
Spinal care	3	2.3
Pediatric	2	1.6
Emergency department	7	5.4
Neurology	5	3.9
Surgical	23	17.8
Operating theatre	9	6.9
Mixed medical/surgical	10	7.8
Other	21	16.2
Total	129	100.0

with a mean age of 32.6 years (SD = 8.5 years). The original study targeted all full-time RNs, with a response rate of 40%. This was lower than expected, possibly because it was conducted pre-Christmas and during major hospital restructuring.

Participants had practised full-time-equivalent nursing for nine years (SD = 6.4 years), and worked in their particular area for four-and-a-half years (SD = 3.6 years). Fifty-eight percent had obtained their initial practising certificate by college diploma and university degree (22% and 36%, respectively). Highest qualifications and areas of work are shown in Tables 11.3.1 and 11.3.2, respectively. Designated titles of the nurses (Table 11.3.3) show the largest category of nurses were Division 2 RNs (enrolled nurses) (35%).

Data Collection and Measures

Following ethics committee approval, data were collected using a survey questionnaire that asked for demographic and debriefing information.

Debriefing Questionnaire (DQ). This section contained 20 statements relating to helpfulness or lack of helpfulness of debriefing. It was designed by the authors, based on earlier studies by Burns and Harm (1993) and Robinson and Mitchell (1993). Reliability and validity information was not used for this type of measure, but factor analysis indicated the extent to which the items in the scale

TABLE 11.3.3 Designated Titles of RNs (n = 129)

Title	Sample number	Sample (%)
RN Division 1	8	6.2
RN Division 2 (EN)	45	34.9
RN Division 3	4	3.1
Associate Nurse Unit Manager (ANUM)	21	16.3
Nurse Unit Manager (NUM)	14	10.8
Clinical Nurse Specialist/Nurse Educator (CNS/NE)	24	18.6
Other	13	10.1
Total	129	100.0

represented consistent concepts. Debriefing was defined as a structured group meeting, emphasizing ventilation of feelings, discussion of reactions to the event, and education and information about coping strategies. The wording of some statements was altered to obtain equal positive (meaning statements that said it was helpful) and negative (statements that said it was not helpful) items in the scale. These were randomly ordered to avoid biased responding.

Respondents were asked to rate level of agreement to statements: 0, neutral; 1, strongly disagree; 2, disagree; 3, agree; 4, strongly agree. The neutral category gave respondents the option of non-commitment. Participants were asked whether debriefing should be voluntary and what other interventions they considered appropriate following a critical incident.

Analysis

Data obtained for the study were analysed using Statistical Package for Social Sciences 6.1 (SPSS). Descriptive statistics summarised the characteristics of respondents and DQ responses.

Factor analysis of the DQ was undertaken first to determine the factor structure of the scale. Principal components analysis (PCA) with oblimin rotation was performed because it was assumed that all items on the DQ would be correlated with each other, because they reflected aspects of helpfulness and lack of helpfulness of debriefing (see West 1991, p.139).

The second purpose was to reduce nurses' responses to a small number of factors, to study the relationship between their debriefing experiences and demographic variables. This was analysed using multivariate analysis (MANOVA) using the five PCA scales as dependent variables. Four potential independent (demographic) variables were reduced (qualifications, from seven to four levels; basis for obtaining initial practising certificate, from three to two categories; current area of work, from 15 to 6 areas; title, from 8 to 5 titles) to increase numbers of respondents in cells. Gender was unaltered. Correlations were then obtained between the independent variables with the averaged five scales. Finally, relationships between the effects of the demographic variables and the DQ scales were investigated in a four-way MANOVA.

Results

Results of the Descriptive Analysis

Although respondents identified the process as helpful in alleviating distress (Table 11.3.4), rea-

TABLE 11.3.4 Ranked Responses for Helpfulness of Debriefing by Respondents ($n = 129$)

Debriefing Statement	Mean Likert Scale Score
1. Being part of the group that had also experienced the incident.	3.3
2. Talking with others about the event.	3.3
3. Hearing others talk about the incident.	3.3
4. Hearing how others were handling the stress.	3.2
5. Realizing I was not alone.	3.0
6. Understanding my situation.	2.9
7. The group gained solution, support, and direction.	.5
8. It promoted departmental cohesion.	2.2
9. Understanding myself.	2.2
10. My stress levels were less intense.	2.1
11. Learning about stress from the leaders.	2.0
12. The independent forum was helpful.	1.7

Note: Although items were altered in order to obtain an equal number of positive and negative items on the DQ and to enable random ordering, items are presented in this table as statements for helpfulness of debriefing according to their item source. Rankings based on mean scores on a 5-point Likert scale in response to whether respondent considered the statement helpful: 0, neutral; 1, strongly disagree; 2, disagree; 3, agree; 4, strongly agree.

sons for lack of helpfulness were also strongly endorsed (Table 11.3.5). The items that received low mean Likert scale scores do not indicate that these factors were unhelpful (in the case of helpful items), merely that some respondents did not feel that this item had been important to them. As the neutral option was scored 0, this could reduce mean scores. Helpful themes were: communication, sharing with others who had experienced the same incident, group cohesion, and self-understanding/stress education. Lack of helpfulness related to poor timing and duration of the debriefing, discomfort with the group process, and poor leadership qualities. Most believed that attending debriefing should be voluntary, and many selected alternatives or supplements such as support group and/or stress management classes.

TABLE 11.3.5 Ranked Responses for Lack of Helpfulness of Debriefing by Respondents ($n = 129$)

Debriefing Statement	Mean Likert Scale Score
1. I resented the time the debriefing took from my personal life.	3.0
2. I was not comfortable discussing the event in a group.	2.7
3. It was too soon after the event to be helpful.	2.5
4. The leaders had no relevant experience.	2.4
5. The leader did not seek discussion from participants who would not open up.	2.3
6. It was too long after the event to be helpful.	2.3
7. It was too short to be helpful.	2.1
8. There were people present in the group with whom I was uncomfortable.	2.1

Note: Although items were altered in order to obtain an equal number of positive and negative items on the DQ and to enable random ordering, items are presented in this table as statements for lack of helpfulness of debriefing according to their item source.
Rankings based on mean scores on a 5-point Likert scale in response to whether respondent considered the statement lacked helpfulness: 0, neutral; 1, strongly disagree; 2, disagree; 3, agree; 4, strongly agree.

Results of Factor Analysis

The sample size of 129 for the 20-item DQ met the desired number of cases to variable ratio for the PCA (Tabachnick & Fidell, 1996). The correlation matrix indicated that a considerable number of correlations exceeded 0.3, and thus, the matrix was suitable for factoring. The factorability of these items was further supported because the Bartlett Test of Sphericity was significant, and the Kaiser Meyer Olin measure of sampling adequacy was greater than 0.6 (0.7).

Analysis of the DQ produced six factors with eigenvalues greater than one. However, inspection of the scree plot (Tabachnick & Fidell, 1996) indicated that a five-factor solution was most appropriate. The eigenvalues for these factors were 4.03, 2.24, 1.72, 1.34, and 1.13, and the factors accounted for 20.15%, 11.19%, 8.64%, 6.71%, and 5.65% (total 52.3%) of the total variance.

The pattern matrix is shown in Table 11.3.6. Individual factor loadings of at least 0.40 were taken as the criterion for deciding whether an item was retained in the construction of the DQ. At this magnitude, all items but one (Item 18) loaded on only one factor. Items that loaded on the first, second, and fourth factors reflected helpful aspects of debriefing. The five items that loaded on the first rotated factor denote an "Understanding" dimension. The five items that loaded on the second rotated factor suggest a "Sharing" dimension. Although the three items that have a loading on the fourth factor suggest a "Cohesion" dimension, the loading of one item ("It was not helpful because the leader did not seek discussion from participants who would not open up.") appears to indicate that respondents were responding more to the cohesion aspect of debriefing than to its helpfulness, and needs further clarification.

Only one item ("realising that I was not alone") has a dual loading on DQ factors, indicating that participants may have considered this at both a social support and cognitive level. They may have experienced debriefing as helpful because they understood that they were not alone and, concomitantly, gained an appreciation that others were similarly affected by the incident through sharing their experience of the incident.

The third and fifth factor items reflected lack of helpfulness. The three items on the third factor appear to denote unhelpful aspects of "Procedure:" timing, duration, and leadership. Items on the fifth factor appear to denote adverse aspects relating to the group "Dynamics."

To further the analysis, five scales were constructed by summing equally weighted scores of the items identified as loading significantly on respective factors. The correlations between the Understanding and Sharing factors was −0.11; Sharing and Dynamics factors, −0.22; Procedure and Dynamics factors, −0.17; and between the Cohesion and Dynamics factors, 0.25. Scales of Sharing, Procedure, and Cohesion were effectively independent,

TABLE 11.3.6 Pattern Matrix of Debriefing Questionnaire Items

Factor Loadings (Loadings Less than 0.40 Not Reported)

Item	Factor 1	Factor 2	Factor 3	Factor 4	Factor 5
20	Learning about stress from the leaders was helpful.	0.72			
17	My stress responses less intense.	0.64			
09	The group gained solution, support, and direction.	.55			
15	It was helpful in understanding myself.	0.51			
07	It was helpful in understanding my situation.	0.49			
11	Being part of a group that had also experienced the incident was helpful.		−0.78		
03	Talking with others about the incident was helpful.		−0.77		
10	Hearing others talk about the incident was helpful.		−0.63		
18	Realising that I was not alone was helpful.	0.47	−0.56		
02	Hearing how others were handling the stress was helpful.	−0.55			
12	It was too short to be helpful.			−0.78	
14	It was too long after event to be helpful.			−0.74	
05	The leaders had no relevant experience.			−0.49	
16	It was helpful because it promoted departmental cohesion.	0.76			
01	It was not helpful because the leader did not seek discussion from participants who would not open up.				0.52
13	The independent forum was helpful.				0.47
08	Not comfortable discussing event in a group.				0.74
04	There were people present in the group with whom I am uncomfortable.				0.72
06	I resented the time debriefing took from personal life.	0.57			
19	Too soon after event to be helpful.				0.45

Extraction Method: Principal Components Analysis; Rotation Method: Oblimin with Kaiser Normalisation; Rotation converged in 13 iterations.

as their intercorrelations were less than 0.1. Table 11.3.7 records scale means, standard deviations (SD) and the Cronbach alpha (α) coefficients of internal consistency for the scales.

As can be seen, the potential range for Understanding, Sharing, and Dynamics is moderate, and for the remaining scales, low. The relatively high negative skew for the Sharing scale indicates that it is more helpful than the other helpful scales. Apart from the Cohesion scale, which shows low reliability (0.40), the remaining scales show moderate reliability.

TABLE 11.3.7 Means: Standard Deviations, and Cronbach Alphas for the Five Scales Constructed From the Factor Analysis of the Debriefing Questionnaire (DQ)

Scales	Number of Items (range)	Number of Cases	Mean	SD	Cronbach α
Understanding	5 (0–16)	127	11.71	3.93	0.58
Sharing	5 (0–20)	127	16.18	2.99	0.74
Procedure	3 (0–12)	127	6.80	3.14	0.66
Cohesion	3 (0–12)	127	6.30	2.93	0.40
Dynamics	4 (0–16)	127	10.31	3.26	0.62

Finally, in order to compare the means of the DQ scale, a repeated measures ANOVA was conducted, where the dependent variables were the averaged mean scores of the items. Using Wilks' criterion, inspection of means indicated that the Sharing scale was the most significant of the five scales on the DQ [$F(4, 120) = 41.10, p < 0.000$], and was significantly greater than the other scales that did not differ significantly from each other.

Results of Multivariate Analysis

Significant findings were obtained for the DQ scales (Table 11.3.8), and confirm the factor analysis findings that the five scales of the DQ are interdependent. However, no significant relationships were found between any of the variables of age of respondents, full-time equivalent postregistration nursing practice, and years in current area.

Results of the four-way MANOVA revealed a significant multivariate main effect for only Qualifications [$F(15, 121), = 1.923, p = 0.020$]. There were no significant interaction effects. Univariate tests were conducted to identify which Qualification was specifically related to Understanding. Findings suggested that nurses with postgraduate qualifications ($n = 61$, mean $= 2.12$) and nurses with hospital certificate qualifications ($n = 10$, mean $= 3.02$) accounted for significance with that factor ($p < 0.05$). The former nurses experienced the Understanding obtained from debriefing as "moderately helpful," whereas the latter group experienced it as "considerably helpful." However, because a series of analyses were examined for statistical significance, this result needs to be treated as tentative.

No significant ($p < 0.05$) correlations were found between gender and experiences of debriefing.

Discussion

Survey respondents identified the most helpful aspects of debriefing as being part of a group who had also experienced the incident, hearing others talk about it, realising they were not alone, and hearing how others were handling their stress. Lack of helpfulness items receiving strongest endorsement were "resented the time debriefing took from their personal lives" and "felt uncomfortable discussing the event in a group." Some respondents also endorsed poor leadership issues.

Resentment about the time debriefing took from their personal lives suggested that those respondents had attended debriefings outside of work hours. This encroachment on nonwork time may also have worked against their active participation in the group and reduced the potential value of debriefing. Furthermore, defusing, a shortened form of debriefing, provided prior to staff leaving work, will often eliminate the need for a full critical incident debriefing and reduce the overuse of debriefings (Westerink, 1995). Education of all staff, especially nurse unit managers, about appropriate times to use defusing or debriefing, and goals and advantages of each, could allay resentment, especially if scheduled before staff left work.

The greatest consensus between this sample and Burns and Harm's (1993) concerned talking to others and hearing them talk about the incident and reduction of stress. However, the greatest disparity

TABLE 11.3.8 Correlations of Debriefing Scales (DQ)

Scales	Number of Respondents	Pearson Product–Moment Correlation	Probability
Sharing by Procedure	126	0.27	0.002
Sharing by Cohesion	122	0.20	0.032
Sharing by Dynamics	126	0.31	0.001
Procedure by Cohesion	125	0.31	0.000
Procedure by Dynamics	127	0.38	0.000
Cohesion by Dynamics	125	0.51	0.000

occurred for lack of helpfulness, represented by resentment of the time debriefing took from their personal life, feeling uncomfortable discussing the event in a group, and the debriefing being conducted too soon after the event. Variations in findings were probably due to different modes of scoring, differences in sampling procedures, and social context. However, when the two levels of helpfulness indicated in this study were combined, reasons for helpfulness roughly equated those of Burns and Harm (1993). In contrast, when the two levels of agreement for lack of helpfulness were combined, a large disparity was evident. For example, this sample more strongly endorsed "resenting the time debriefing took from their personal life" and "felt uncomfortable discussing the event in a group," compared with low endorsement by Burns and Harm's (1993) sample. Low endorsement concerning resentment of the time the debriefing took by the USA sample suggested that the debriefing model had been integrated into the work environment, and was an accepted procedure for postcritical incident management. Even though only 32% of Burns and Harm's (1993) sample had participated in debriefings, services available would very likely have been consistent with the CISM model based on its popularity within the nursing profession in the USA at the time. Emergency nurses were, therefore, likely to use the service during their work time. Furthermore, the lower endorsement by them of other statements regarding lack of helpfulness indicated that they received debriefing from those trained in its application, and were likely to have been acquainted with the debriefing model (CISD) for longer than Australian counterparts.

The five DQ scales offered a parsimonious explanation of the 20 statements relating to helpful and unhelpful aspects of debriefing: three related to helpfulness: Sharing, Understanding and Cohesion; two scales, Procedure and Dynamics, to lack of helpfulness. With regard to the helpful scales, the majority endorsed Sharing, which represented aspects of communication and social support, followed by Understanding. Low correlation of the Cohesion scale with the other DQ scales suggested that its items should be interpreted individually. Understanding, a cognitive process whereby participants reappraised or reframed their role in the incident as a result of information from other participants at the debriefing, was the only scale related to a demographic variable. Nurses with hospital certificates found its aspects more helpful compared with nurses with university qualifications, which suggests that the former group benefited from educational aspects offered by debriefing possibly because of lack of exposure to stress management during their training, in contrast to their university-educated colleagues.

The Sharing and Understanding scales comprised elements identified by Everly and Mitchell (1998) as essential to trauma recovery. For example, Sharing included items associated with communication and social support that reflected verbalisation and normalisation of the trauma through discussion, and appreciation that others at debriefing experienced similar reactions (Everly & Mitchell,

1998). "Understanding" items related to other essential elements for trauma recovery, mobilisation, and stress management. Mobilisation occurred when individual and group strengths were recognised and used to assist recovery.

The Cohesion scale was represented by two helpful items (promotion of departmental cohesion and independent forum), and one item reflecting lack of helpfulness (leader not seeking discussion from participants who would not open up). One explanation was that respondents focused on the cohesion aspect of the scale, and their belief that failure of the leader to encourage participants to speak up worked against cohesion. Alternatively, respondents might have experienced being in the group but not being pushed to talk as beneficial when they had the opportunity to listen and learn from the reactions of others. This would be consistent with normalization. With regard to lack of helpfulness scales, more respondents endorsed "Dynamics" rather than "Procedure." The former reflected personal discomfort, such as with discussing the event in a group; the latter, adverse aspects such as leader's lack of relevant experience. Evidently, personal factors about the process were of greater concern than aspects related to the application of debriefing. It is likely that high endorsement of statements concerning Dynamics were consistent with national characteristics. Generally, Australians are less likely to disclose personal information, particularly in a work setting, because they fear evaluation as "not coping," which could jeopardise job security. This possibly reflected lack of education and familiarity with an appropriate debriefing model.

There are some limitations to this study. These findings are specific to a relatively small sample of full-time RNs working at an Australian metropolitan hospital. The survey was conducted prior to introduction of CISD/CISM in the hospital to explore nurses' experiences and use the findings to modify the proposed program. Although this study attempted to capture the essence of debriefing according to the study on which it was based (Burns & Harm, 1993) by providing a specific definition of the process, many respondents may have applied their own interpretation to its meaning. Nonetheless, the generally positive findings regarding debriefing are promising, because they suggest that replacing the various ad hoc forms currently available with a standardised model would not only improve the quality of service at the hospital, but overcome shortcomings identified by respondents. A standardised approach would also ensure that providers would receive appropriate training and staff members, pre-incident education about CIS, and various types of intervention.

Conclusions

These findings provide an initial description of Australian nurses' perceptions of their experiences of debriefing in a hospital setting. For future research, the distinction and definition of the type of debriefing being evaluated by a study, as well as the training of the people providing it and the population to whom the process is applied, remain essential. Otherwise, the issue of what is being evaluated will remain unclear and lead to inaccurate results. These distinctions would enable researchers to discover which method of debriefing led by what type of leader is effective, and with which population. In addition, a combined quantitative/qualitative research design is recommended to assist the identification of helpful processes of debriefing.

REFERENCES

Appleton, L. 1994. What's a critical incident? *The Canadian Nurse*. September: 23–26.

Burns, C., & Harm, N. J. 1993. Emergency nurses' perceptions of critical incidents and stress debriefing. *Journal of Emergency Nursing*. October: 431–436.

Cotterill, W. S. 2000. Debriefing in the intensive care unit: A personal experience of critical incident stress. *Nursing in Critical Care*. March–April. 5:82–86.

Cudmore, J. 1998. Critical incident stress management strategies. *Emergency Nurse*. 6:22–27.

Everly, G. S., & Mitchell, J. T. 1998. A new era in crisis intervention. Key concepts in critical incident stress management. Frontieres. Hiver Printemps: 43–46.

Hudson, S. 1995. New responses to stress and trauma. *Australian Nursing Journal.* 2:13.

Jefferson, R., & Northway, T. 1996. Staff helping staff–Establishment of a critical incident stress management team in a tertiary care centre. *Canadian Association of Critical Care Nurses.* 7, Spring: 19–22.

Jimmerson, C. 1988. Critical incident stress debriefing. *Journal of Emergency Nursing.* 14:43–45A.

Lam, L. T., Ross, F. I., Cass, D. T., Quine, S., & Lazarus, R. 1999. The impact of work related trauma on the psychological health of nursing staff: A cross sectional study. *Australian Journal of Advanced Nursing.* March–May, 16(3):14–20.

Laws, T., & Hawkins, C. 1995. Critical incident stress. *Australian Nursing Journal.* February: 32–34.

Macnab, A. J., Russell, J. A., Lowe, J. P., & Gagnon, P. 1999. Critical incident stress intervention after loss of an air ambulance: Two year follow up. *Prehospital and Disaster Medicine.* 14:8–12.

Martin, K. R. 1993. Critical incidents: Pulling together to cope with the stress. *Nursing.* May: 39–41.

Mitchell, G. J. 2001. A qualitative study exploring how qualified mental health nurses deal with incidents that conflict with their accountability. *Journal of Psychiatric and Mental Health Nursing.* 8:241–248.

Mitchell, J. T. 1983. When disaster strikes: The critical incident stress debriefing process. *Journal of Emergency Medical Services.* 8(1):36–39.

Northcott, N. 1998. Don't accept the debrief. *Nursing Times.* 94(10):32.

O'Connor, J., & Jeavons, S. 2003. Nurses' perceptions of critical incidents. *Journal of Advanced Nursing.* 41:53-62.

Robinson, R. C., & Mitchell, J. T. 1993 Evaluation of psychological debriefings. *Journal of Tranmatic Stress.* 6:367–382.

Roffey-Mitchel, K., & Jeavons, S. 1998. An evaluation of debriefing for nurses in a hospital setting. *Critical Times.* 1:4–5.

Tabachnick, B. G., & Fidell, L. S. 1996. Principal components and factor analysis. In *Using multivariate analysis.* 2nd ed. New York: Harper and Row.

West, R. 1991. *Computing for psychologists.* Amsterdam: Harwood Academic Publishers.

Westerink, J. 1995. Developing critical incident stress management programs. *The Australian Counselling Psychologist.* 11:19–25.

Wright, C., & Casier, S. 1996. Critical incident stress management: Navigating through crisis in critical care. *Canadian Association of Critical Care Nurses.* 7:25–29.

Reprinted with permission from: O'Connor, J., & Jeavons, S. (2003). Perceived effectiveness of critical incident stress debriefing by Australian nurses. *Australian Journal of Advanced Nursing,* 20(4), 22–29.

11.4 CRITICAL INCIDENT STRESS DEBRIEFING: APPLICATION FOR PERIANESTHESIA NURSES

MAUREEN IACONO

The hallmark quality of perianesthesia nurses—what sets experts apart—may well be the management of emergent, unexpected incidents with numerous patients in rapid succession. We care for vulnerable patients, frequently without the benefit of patient history, a chart to review, or a knowledgeable resource for pertinent information. We move on to the next patient, the next challenge, smoothly and automatically. Our focus on real or potential problems, with assessment skills and critical care competencies, assists us to ease the transitions patients undergo while in our units. We handle stressful situations for our patients and ourselves. We are constantly challenged with critical issues, such as preempting emergencies and recognizing subtle and overt signs of patient instability. At the same time, we deal with patient flow issues such as, "turnover time" and, "unavailable postoperative beds" in critical care and clinical nursing units. We also deal with colorful personalities and interesting communication styles from professional colleagues.

The impressive expertise of perianesthesia nurses is often taken for granted by both nursing staff and medical colleagues. We expect patients under our care to do well, and we clearly expect to be able to handle any problems or crises during a routine shift. But how do we manage when things go wrong? How do we deal with staff feelings of angst and self-doubt? Perhaps we miss a significant patient problem or a nursing error occurs. A patient outcome may be worse than anticipated, or a critical incident is not handled well. A nurse may be berated and intimidated by criticism and comments made by coworkers, physicians, and other colleagues. In addition, nurses are toughest on themselves, and may have great difficulty in getting past the personal trauma, guilt, and negative self-talk that occurs.

There are clear mechanisms within our institutions to document and handle outcome variances. Continuous quality improvement tools, occurrence reports, root cause analyses, sentinel event review, and individual counseling with corrective action may be used as necessary to evaluate and process incidents occurring in our units. These are formal means of ensuring appropriate management and follow-up of significant problems or untoward outcomes.

Many critical incidents, however, do not require formal follow-through. Even if a formal mechanism is necessary, individualized support of staff is essential to promote learning, growth, and healing. Active listening to staff concerns regarding patient care, individual actions and reactions, and preferred patient outcomes is essential on an ongoing basis to show support and advocacy for nursing staff.

Nurse managers and caring perianesthesia colleagues can do more, however, than active listening. We can borrow strategies from colleagues in emergency nursing, psychosocial science, and the military to adapt the tenets of critical incident stress debriefing (CISD) for nurses in perianesthesia settings. We can encourage staff to improve skills and coping strategies in dealing with stress. We can create a support mechanism to provide "critical help" to those involved in the incident.

Posttraumatic Stress

Disasters of all types can leave hidden damage in individuals who have survived. Anxiety, fear, and distress may last for a long time after the actual disaster or incident. The effects of the trauma can also spread to family, friends, and coworkers. "Posttraumatic stress is the development of certain symptoms or reactions, following an abnormal event. The event is abnormal in that it is life threatening or extremely disturbing, and can be anything from a minor accident to a major disaster."[1] Life events, such as divorce, death of a family member or friend, and serious illness can be the cause of the stress. Certainly, riots, war, fatal accidents, and community disasters may cause this type of stress.

In perianesthesia units, posttraumatic stress might be precipitated by a crisis that was managed poorly. It might be that the early clues were missed in a patient with pulmonary embolus, sepsis, or anaphylaxis. Perhaps a medication error occurred or a written order was overlooked for a specific diagnostic test. Preoperative laboratory results may not have been related to colleagues in a timely manner, causing delays in OR start time or untoward patient outcomes. A nurse may be so involved in the care of an unstable, critical patient that time is not taken to see the whole picture, and a significant omission occurs. In the frenzy of a critical incident, harsh words and angry sentiments may be used in frustration. Physicians may be at odds regarding the management of a patient's care, with the nurse in the middle of the opposition. A patient may be transferred to a clinical unit from the postanesthesia care unit (PACU) and suffer a cardiac or respiratory arrest within hours of discharge from PACU. These incidents cause significant stress and self-doubt for PACU staff.

The stress, or critical incident, ". . . disturbs our normal life beliefs and turns our world upside down, causing confusion, disbelief, feelings of vulnerability, a loss of meaning and purpose in life, and a change in self-image or self-esteem."[1] Each nurse brings her or his character, personality, and previous experiences to bear with each encounter in the clinical arena. These factors, coupled with a critical event, will determine how the nurse reacts during the incident and afterward.

The military model of psychological debriefing is based in part on the value of group survival. Caring for individuals who are involved in military conflicts and at war, when an express need is voiced or recognized, is essential for individual soldiers and for the group. The effectiveness of debriefing depends on leadership and the management of morale. A belief in the dignity of the individual and his or her importance to the broader social group is basic. This belief can be applied in the context of the PACU. We need to recognize high levels of stress within our units, particularly after critical incidents, and structure an intervention to support staff to help modify reactions, heal, and move forward.

The military literature suggests a "PIE" method: proximity, immediacy, and expectancy.[2] Encourage discussion of the critical event close to the battlefield, in our case, the clinical unit where the stress or critical incident occurred. Treat it immediately, as close to the incident or event as possible. Establish the clear expectation that individuals and staff will recover fully after rest, reassurance, support, and activities that restore confidence. Debriefing can be spiritually purging and can help build morale. The focus can be on lessons learned and what is to be done next.

Critical Incident Stress Debriefing

CISD was articulated by Jeffrey T. Mitchell, PhD, in 1983 to help emergency service personnel who were routinely exposed to trauma in their work.[3] The goal was to reduce psychological "casualties" among emergency personnel. "Critical incident stress involves any situation faced by emergency personnel that causes them to experience unusually strong emotional reactions having the potential to interfere with their ability to function at the scene or later."[3] CISD consists of semistructured interventions designed to decrease initial distress and prevent ongoing concerns, and negative or destructive behaviors. Staff may experience emotional numbing, hostility, anger, withdrawal, or sleep problems. CISD promotes emotional processing through ventilation (verbal acknowledgement) and normalization of reactions to trauma, stress, disasters, and critical incidents. It also prepares the staff for possible future experiences. The focus is on how the individual is reacting now.[4] CISD provides peer support and encouragement, and opens communication between helpers and involved nurses. It gives legitimacy to the stress, so that the staff feels more comfortable coming forward with concern and anxiety related to the event. It can improve the culture of your unit and increase awareness of staff strength and cohesiveness.

The seven phases of CISD described in the following are based on the work of Dyregov, in 1989.[3] His work enhanced the original phases described by Mitchell to include sensory factors related to the critical incident.[3]

1. Introduction

Make it a priority to intervene to help a staff member or nurse colleague after a critical incident. Establish a safe environment for discussion and the sharing of the experience. The debriefer states the purpose of the process—to review the involved nurse(s) reactions to the incident, discuss them, and identify methods of dealing with them to prevent future problems. No information goes into personnel files; no reports are made. The leader (debriefer) who manages the session should have firm self-control, confidence, and competence. Questions that may stimulate discussion include: Why are you here? What was your role for the patient? What was your assignment? Clarify that this session is confidential and will focus on the nurses' impressions and reactions to the incident. The primary purpose of the session is to restore nurses to their routine lives and roles.

2. Expectations and Facts

Encourage discussion of exactly what happened during the critical incident. Elicit details, acts, and circumstances of the event; impressions and emotional reactions to the event should be separated and dealt with after the facts are stated. The focus of this phase is to obtain individualized, factual information. Questions might include the following: Did it happen the way you expected? Did you respond as you thought you would? Are you secure with your knowledge of ventriculostomy setup, the biphasic defibrillator, and the malignant hyperthermia cart and mixing dantrolene? If reviewing the incident of a patient's death after cardiac arrest, ask the nurse, did you know the advanced cardiac life support (ACLS) algorithm? Was there adequate intravenous access? Was the patient ventilated appropriately, and were medications given correctly? Do you understand what caused the critical incident?

3. Thoughts and Impressions

Once the facts are stated, the debriefer offers constructive support, perhaps sharing anecdotes of nurses' past experiences, personal struggles, or from the collective wisdom of other perianesthesia nurses. Questions asked might be as follows: What were you thinking as you cared for the patient? What thoughts did you have as you found the patient (in ventricular tachycardia, in respiratory arrest, with an arterial bleeder, with a flail chest, found the airway occluded, etc.)? What did you do? What did you see, hear, or touch? What did the patient's skin feel like? What was your reaction to the pulse of the unit at the time? Was your perception that there was no one to help you, that you were alone and sinking? Did you ask for help, access your resources? This phase helps the individual personalize the incident with meaningful recollection.

4. Emotional Reaction

This phase is concerned with the psychological and physical aftereffects of the incident. This phase may take the longest of all phases. The release of emotions reflects the internal conflict the nurse has been suffering. Fear of failure, self-reproach, anger, guilt, anxiety, and depression are common feelings. Helpful questions include the following: What was the worst part of the incident? How did you react to this? The nurse may say, "I can't do this job; I'm not measuring up." "That patient might have died if…" "I don't want any more craniotomy patients." This phase must be dealt with, but it must also end with compassionate leadership and encouragement.

5. Normalization

The debriefer facilitates the acceptance of emotions. Unless the shared emotional response is exaggerated, reinforce that the emotions are normal and universal. Reinforce what went well during the incident; discuss activities to restore confidence and security for the nurse. Talk about what might happen later, the next time a patient decompensates in this manner or a cardiac arrest occurs. What resources will the nurse use? Discourage detachment from coworkers and irritability; encourage esprit de corps and camaraderie. Review stress management strategies. Questions should focus on: What techniques work for you? In what ways can you communicate more effectively? What support will you seek next time?

6. Future Planning and Coping

Focus on managing symptoms of stress. The debriefer should assess the emotional reactions of the involved nurse and offer further help if required. Questions that may help include the following: What steps will you take if you feel overwhelmed like this in a future critical incident? Do you need help now to cope with any unresolved feelings? What kind of external support can you expect from your family and friends? Encourage more discussion if needed.

7. Disengagement

Seek help for the nurse if there has been no resolution. Professional counseling may be called for if there are unresolved feelings, fears, and worries. Family and health stressors may have an enormous impact on the coping skills of the individual nurse after critical incidents. Critical incident debriefing does not duplicate or replace ongoing professional counseling; its value is to alleviate symptoms created by a critical incident.

    Perianesthesia nurses take pride in astute recognition and intervention to prevent complications in their patients. Stress management and maintaining calm in the midst of chaos may be routine in our clinical setting. However, there are instances in which things just go wrong. CISD is a valuable tool that can be applied in our specialty practice. Caring for our colleagues includes shielding them from additional stress, assisting them to mobilize resources, and helping them to see the "big picture." Debriefing a critical incident will lower the tension level in your unit, help individual nurses achieve relative emotional control, and improve behavioral interactions. It will allow nurses to obtain a complete picture of what took place, put closure on it, and let it go.

(Please note: There is no intent to minimize the significance of military engagement or to imply that a community disaster can be compared with one critical incident in a PACU. Rather, with utmost respect and admiration for colleagues in the field, perianesthesia nurses can learn more adaptive behavior from mentors who have practiced CISD.)

REFERENCES

1. Parkinson, F: *Post-trauma stress: A personal guide to reduce the long-term effects and hidden emotional damage caused by violence and disaster.* Tucson, AZ: Fisher Books, 2000.
2. U.S. Army: *Soldier and family support, United States Army Medical Department Center and School correspondence subcourse.* Washington, DC: U.S. Army, 1995.
3. Rubin, J: Critical incident stress debriefing: Helping the helpers. *J Emerg Nurs* 16:255–258, 1990.
4. Foa, E: *Effective treatments for PTSD.* New York: The Guilford Press, 2000.

SUGGESTED READINGS

Antai-Otong, D: Critical incident stress debriefing: A health promotion model for workplace violence. *Perspectives in Psychiatric Care* 37:125–132, 2001.

Scott, M, & Palmer, S: *Trauma and posttraumatic stress disorder.* London: Cassell Academic, 1999.

Reprinted with permission from: Iacono, M. (2002). Critical incident stress debriefing: Application for perianesthesia nurses. *Journal of PeriAnesthesia Nursing, 17*(6), 423–426.

V
Epilogue (Frequently Asked Questions)

Epilogue

Over the years, I received many inquiries about "transitions." I have selected 13 commonly asked questions and included answers to these questions. The goal for sharing the questions and answers is to stimulate a dialogue to use as an example for generating more questions and to inspire better answers. Theories are constructed to guide research and practice, to be refuted, to be extended, and to be modified. Providing this epilogue with questions also serves to remind readers that all the writings about transitions are tentative, dynamic, and constantly changing.

The questions posed are not exhaustive and are works in progress. None of the answers is definitive. Use the questions to stimulate additional questions of your own and use the answers as a catalyst toward constructing your own answers. I want to extend my deep appreciation for those who take the time to ask questions, and for the authors of the questions I use here, sometimes almost verbatim. I have not included the authors' names for two reasons: first, to protect them and second, because I use some of the questions as prototypes and as patterns of questions.

FREQUENTLY ASKED QUESTIONS

Q1: What are the focuses of your transition model?

A1: There are two major parts to transition theory. The first is an intervention made by a nurse to facilitate transition and promote well-being and mastery of the changes that result from the transition. What this includes conceptually is providing support through significant others as well as a care team of advanced practice nurses. Through home visits and telephone conferences the care team attempts to clarify what the person in transition may be going through and will go through during the transition to recovery; the team then provides knowledge, skills, strategies, self-care, and psychosocial competencies to help the person deal with the transition experience.

The second most important part of transition theory is having an understanding of the transition experience itself, which is defined as the experience of losses and gains, changes and transformations, and a passage from one state to another. However, these experiences and responses are defined by whether the transition is the result of normal development, changes in health and illness, acute or chronic diagnoses, going in or out of hospitals, divorce, or organizational changes. The experience is also mediated by whether the person is going through single or multiple transitions, the meaning of the transition to the person undergoing it, and what else is occurring in the life of the person. There are so many conditions that act to exacerbate or ameliorate responses to these personal, immediate family, community, or societal transitions. Healthy transitions are not only judged by the final outcome, such as mastery of roles, a sense of well-being, or well-being of relationships; they are also predicated on whether the processes themselves were healthy or unhealthy. Outcomes include the extent to which individuals who experience transition can freely define themselves with identity fluidity, for example, I am a cancer survivor and a professor—and not either one or the other.

Q2: How has your theory of "transition" evolved?

A2: My theoretical journey was first inspired by research findings from a master's-degree thesis that the health of informal caregivers of chronically ill patients and of their spouses was enhanced by their dialogue and clarity of interaction. My doctoral dissertation further reinforced that couples who can define each other's roles more accurately, hence having meaningful and productive dialogues and interactions that clarify those roles, tended to be more effective planners of their family's future. Subsequently, clinical experiences in caring for new parents highlighted the need for nurses to work with couples who are anticipating a first baby or whose lives have changed because of the birthing of first babies.

I became interested in transitions in the 1960s when I realized that nurses' major work was to prepare people for developmental, situational, and health–illness transitions and care for them to ensure that they cope well and emerge from a transition with well-being. I was interested in nurses' actions in developing interventions and defining outcomes, and my subsequent research focused on what happens to people who do not make healthy transitions and what interventions could facilitate people's healthy transitions.

Q3: What is the philosophical foundation of transition theory?

A3: I believe I was influenced early on in my theoretical journey by symbolic interactionism, which is a philosophical view of how people interact effectively and through which the dynamic self is formed as a result of a series of experiences and interactions. Role theory influenced my work on role supplementation and then, later on, feminist theories influenced my writings about the transition experiences. As I further developed transitions as a situation-specific theory, feminist postcolonialism triggered the inclusion of society and community as important conditions influencing how the marginalized and the socially vulnerable populations experience transitions and cope with them. Even the nursing therapeutics of who gets treated and who does not are influenced by sexism, homophobia, nationalism, and many other "isms." Therefore, my more recent writings are influenced by postcolonial feminism.

Q4: How would you discuss your theory in relation to research, practice, and education?

A4: Transitions theory is used and is helpful in practice, research, and education.

Let me start with education, first at the faculty level and then at the curriculum level. Knowing that there will be a transition experience and responses will be triggered by the resulting changes and events makes us as faculty pause to think about our students entering any program. This begs several questions: How do we make the students' transition most productive and are their behavior needs and responses the same at the onset of the event as compared to before the transition occurs or later on in the process? Therefore providing pretransition information gives opportunities to answer questions, clarify roles, and mobilize support for them. This may enhance their learning experience.

At the curriculum level, defining important developmental, health–illness, organizational, and situational events that trigger different patterns of experiences could be a framework for understanding the transition experience and offering the appropriate interventions. There are at least two teaching moments in using transitions as a framework for a curriculum. One is helping the student identify and reflect on her or his own transitions. The second is providing students with a curriculum that is cumulatively and progressively more complex, with well-defined milestones that lead from one stage of learning to a higher, more dynamic level. The curriculum would be built on such concepts as stages, milestones, turning points, experiences, and developmental, health and illness, organizational, and situational changes.

Transition as a middle-range theory has been used as a framework for developing situation-specific theories. Transition theory is used in some global graduate and undergraduate nursing programs. In the United States, transition theory was used as a curriculum framework in a number of colleges, including the School of Nursing at the University of Connecticut.

Finally, in addition to providing a framework for individual research projects, transitions theory has prompted me to strategize for the development of a research center that houses researchers whose investigations are focused on aspects of transition and health. Dr. Mary Naylor leads the Center. Her own collaborative program of research has been on testing transitional care models for elders and the chronically ill. The Center was established in 2007 and subsequently endowed and named The New Courtland Center for Transitions and Health.

Q5: What is your understanding of "nursing model of care"?

A5: There are many models of care. In the book *Caring for Women Cross-Culturally* (St. Hill, Lipson, & Meleis, 2003), I discussed one model of care. Another model of care was discussed in my 2007 theoretical nursing book (Meleis, 2007) in the chapter on middle-range theory in which I discussed transitions. In addition, there are general grand theories, middle-range theories, and situation-specific theories, all of which lend themselves to operationalization into several care models. A model of care is a conceptual framework that guides care. Please read my transitions literature, as they may help clarify the application of transitions to nursing models.

Q6: What do milestones mean in nursing interventions and how do you define milestones?

A6: A milestone in the transition theory means some important marker after which there is a turning point and new responses are manifested. A milestone may be the point at which self-care becomes more embodied, where an "aha" is achieved, or where a comfort level in a new role is attained.

Q7: I have just entered the nursing profession and am curious how someone like me could relate or use your theory to help a person with a chronic illness?

A7: Welcome to the best profession and the finest of disciplines! First of all, you need to read about the theory and review articles on its translation into practice. Then you need to think about your clients and their needs for health care at different points along their chronic-illness trajectory. One important point—a milestone occurs at the diagnosis phase, when the person has just learned that he or she is living with a chronic illness. What were the person's responses? What are the best nursing interventions at this important junction during his or her illness experience?

Transition theory can help you in defining the different milestones at which nursing care is needed, the nature of care needed, the appropriate teaching moments, and provide you with a framework for planning the most congruent intervention. The theory helps in defining for you some of the research questions that should be explored.

Q8: I teach ethics and have used your book, *Theoretical Nursing* (Meleis, 2007), as a reference resource for so many queries. I also have received a PhD in Philosophy and studied Aristotle's virtue ethics. I want to relate my own education and interest to health care ethics. I have developed a framework to relate Aristotle's concepts to health care with the idea that health care professionals in different fields may use it to care for patients. My question is, can my "model or theory" be a model for nursing if it is not exclusively for nurses?

A8: First, let me congratulate you on completing your PhD and on the subject matter you chose to study. We need people and nurses like you who spend time and effort in developing scholarship in ethics. So, thank you on behalf of our discipline.

Second, you have an organizing concept (the virtuous nurse/doctor) and I assume you define it, you discuss the antecedents and the context for becoming virtuous, the behaviors and the responses in the agent of virtuousness and in the recipients of virtuous care, and the consequences and outcomes that result from that care. I also assume you define the assumptions to each of these, on which you are building your arguments. If you have all that with supportive literature, you should call it a conceptual model. I prefer not calling it a theory because it is hard to differentiate between the two for the many reasons I mention in my book. Do not waste time on what to call it, invest time in developing it and disseminating it in the literature.

Q9: I am a third-year doctoral student in Thailand and have been interested in your theory since I was a first-year doctoral student. I have used your theory to explain the phenomenon of transition of premature infants' mothers and to establish the intervention of a transitional care program for premature infants' mothers. However, I am not clear if I am using your theory correctly so I have the following questions:

1. In my intervention, I will prepare mothers, the community, and the health care service as the facilitators for transitions. I will prepare mothers to begin to feel connected to their babies, their families, and health care providers; to interact with and become situated in their new role as mother, develop confidence in that role, and learn to cope with the challenges of caring for premature infants. Is the intervention correct?

2. If I would like to evaluate healthy transition, I can measure success from mastery of roles and self-care and the ability of those undergoing transition to have fluid integrative identities of the premature infants' mothers as outcome indicators. Is this approach correct?

3. The mastery of premature infants' mothers in their new role refers to the knowledge, skill, and behavior needed to care for an infant. And fluid integrative identities of premature infants' mothers refer to mothers who can care for babies correctly in everyday life. Is this correct? I am not clear about fluid integrative identities; please explain this concept in greater detail.

A9: I love your country and think highly of the progress made there in research and education. Here are the answers to your questions:

1. Yes, your intervention is correct but you need to clarify the mothers' roles, expectations, and concerns. You need to have a responsive team available for home visits, phone calls, or through other modes of communication.

2. Yes, it is correct to define and measure outcome indicators such as mastery of roles and self care and their skill in having different roles simultaneously and being fluid in integrating their different identities, including being a mother of a premature baby.

3. Yes, this is correct. "Fluid integrative identities" refers to having a defined role (I am a mother of a preemie and I know what that means and what to do about it) and being able to also live through other roles comfortably (I am also a mother of other kids, I am a teacher, a wife, etc.). It means that one role does not dominate and take over one's life.

Q10: I am a nurse and am currently working on my master's thesis at a university in Switzerland. The focus of my thesis will be qualitative phenomenological research about the experiences of patients at home who are starting to suffer from functional decline until their realization of impending death. I would like to use your theory but have the following questions: Is it possible to talk about transition from chronic illness toward end of life? Can death or the realization of approaching death be the other end of transition? What would be the positive outcomes?

A10: To answer your questions, yes, by all means it is possible to use "transitions" as a framework to describe the transitions that occur in a chronic illness as well as the transition of death. For either, the beginning and ending points are arbitrary and depend on the milestone to be discussed/researched. For example, the dying transition could be from diagnosis to acceptance of impending death or to really knowing one is dying. It could also be until a person is pronounced dead.

Realizing, becoming aware, accepting, and preparing for death could be ending points. Positive outcomes could be focusing on planning for death, inviting families to talk about death, planning your own funeral, being able to support your family, and so on. But I hope that is what you will find out.

Q11. I am doctoral student of nursing in Tehran, Iran. For my doctoral dissertation I am going to work on developing a "practice education model" to develop a partnership structure between academic and practice organizations. In this regard, I'm going to conduct a systematic literature review as the first step and as the deductive process. Next, I'm going to use the inductive process by conducting a qualitative study to determine what nurses perceive as their roles in the different settings. Finally, I plan to examine and refine the model in relation to the literature and based on the results of the qualitative study.

But, some methodological ambiguities exist for me and I could use your valuable advice regarding the following questions:

1. Is using such deductive and inductive processes correct or not?
2. Which strategy is the most appropriate one to use to develop this model?

A11: Yes, this is an excellent way to proceed. Here are the answers to your questions:

1. The deductive process will give you an opportunity to review the literature and critically assess existing models.
2. After you assess existing collaborative models, you may want to uncover existing models in Iran and find out if there has been any research conducted on these models.
3. Using a focus-group approach to review the evidence related to each model and to define priorities in Iran may be the Best way to develop your model.
4. I would then do a pilot study implementing the selected models to compare and contrast the outcomes as well as to describe the various intervention protocols. Start by operationalizing the concepts in each model and identifying ways to measure each variable.

Q12: I am a graduate student in Milwaukee, Wisconsin, studying health systems leadership pursuing a joint master's in business administration. This semester I am currently taking nursing theory and am doing a presentation on your theory of transitions.

I know that your theory has evolved over the years, exploring new avenues, and expanding knowledge through research to better understand transitions as a whole. I was just wondering if there is any advice or words of wisdom that you would have for me or my fellow peers as I present this theory?

A12: I am absolutely delighted you are studying the theory and I hope that you and your colleagues will use it in uncovering the responses and experiences of members of organizations undergoing change.

It is through difficult times such as we are facing now, with the economic meltdown, that knowing that transitions are processes that are dynamic and have a beginning, an ending, milestones and processes, is helpful. We could facilitate achieving healthy transitions and positive mastery outcomes by considering them from a coherent framework such as the Transition Theory.

Q13: I have some questions regarding the origin and philosophical foundations of Transitions Theory that maybe you could answer them for me. Is there any metatheoretical (philosophical) background in this theory? I understand that Dr. Turner's theory about Family Interactions guided you in the development of concepts for Transitions, but is there any Nursing Theory that also contributed as well such as Theory of Vulnerability? Is there any philosophical scientific movement (such as postmodernism) that could also have influenced this theory development when you decided to study the experiences of transitions? I would like to inform you how much I enjoyed analyzing transitions theory. Perhaps the fact that nurse anesthetists have been stereotyped as medically oriented nurses without touch and feeling, I have realized that we also deal with transitions day after day, from preop, intraop and postop, not only educating patients and family about anesthesia effects, but also how to plan their anesthesia and how to deal with their complications such as nausea and vomiting. We also assist families to learn their roles as caregivers for postanesthesia care.

A13: Thank you for your keen interest in the theory of transitions. The following are the responses to your questions:

1. No, there was not any additional nursing theory that contributed to the theory of transitions. However, I was influenced by Florence Nightingale's focus on environment, health and well-being. My overall thinking about transitions was deeply influenced by symbolic interactionism.
2. In hindsight, postmodernism and postcolonialist feminist theories guided my thinking and writing. However, that influence did not take shape until very recently and you could see that influence in the situation-specific theories that were subsequently developed.

Finally, I am very pleased that nurse anesthetists are thinking theoretically about their work. You have a great deal to contribute to advance nursing knowledge. Articulating what you do theoretically will move us forward. Keep doing it and keep me informed.

REFERENCES

Meleis, A. I. (2007). *Theoretical nursing: Development and progress* (4th ed.). Philadelphia: Lippincott Williams & Wilkins.

St. Hill, P., Lipson, J., & Meleis, A. I. (Eds.). (2002). *Caring for women cross-culturally: A portable guide*. Philadelphia: FA Davis.

Index

A
Acute care nurse practitioners, Taiwan, 430–439
  acute-care nurse practitioner, 439
  ambiguity phase, 433–434
  changed work model, 435
  data analysis, 433
  data collection, 433
  decision making, 435
  duty boundaries, 434
  ethical issues, 433
  gradually emerging work patterns, 434–435
  identified by patients, 435
  professional growth direction, 435
  research design, 432
  role-acquisition phase, 434–435
  role-implementation phase, 435–436
  sample, 432–433
  self-directed learning, 431
  staff recognition, 434
  work support system, 435
Adolescents, type 1 diabetes, 493–504
  child model, 499–500
  data analysis, 497
  data generation, 497
  dietetic advice, 497–499
  education, 497–499
  ethical issues, 496
  findings, 497
  literature review, 495
  method, 496
  participants, 497
  phases of transition process, 500–501
  recruitment, 496–497
  study, 496
Adult Attachment Scale, 136
Adult developmental theories, 88
African-American mothers, 53
Al-Somali, Shayda, 439
Alienation, 351–353
Altmiller, Geralyn M., 292
Altruism, 570
Alzheimer's disease, 571–579
  clarification, role, 576
  conceptual framework, 572–573
  driving, 578
  evaluation, 576–578
  family assessment, 573–574
  insufficiency, role, 572
  intervention, 576
  modeling, role, 5876
  nursing diagnosis, 574–575
  reference group interactions, 576
  rehearsal, role, 576
  repeated behaviors, 577–578
  role taking, 576
  role transition, 572
  supplementation, role, 572–573
Ancona, Janice, 153
Antecedents of transition to motherhood, 108–109
Anxiety, 541
Archer, Joanna, 153
Aroian, Karen, 232, 579
Arthritis, rheumatoid, women, 336–346
  analysis, 341–342
  awareness and perception, 339
  demographics, 341
  disconnectedness, 340
  health outcomes, 340, 344
  markers of transition process, 344
  nursing model, 339
  nursing support, 344
  patterns of response, 340
  procedures, 341
  process, 339
  sample, 340–341
  transition process, 342–344
    becoming aware, 342
    getting care, 342–343
    mastery, 344
Arvidsson, Barbro, 241
Asylum-seeking process, 245–247
Attitudes toward health, illness, 127
Australian nurses, critical incident stress debriefing, 603–612
  analysis, 605–606
  data collection, 605–606
  debriefing questionnaire, 605

B
Baccalaureate nursing students
  preceptored pregraduation practicums, 291–300
    liaison faculty observations, 297–298

preceptor observations, 298
student observations, 295–297
registered nurses to, 299–310
  assertiveness, 306–307
  beginnings, 305
  challenges, 307
  cornerstone courses, 305–306
  data analysis, 303–305
  description, 308
  empowerment, 306
  envisioning whole, 307
  expectations, 304–305
  procedure, 303
  recreating everyday practice, 307–308
  research design, 303
  sample, 303
Baird, Martha, 326
Baker, Katherine, 563
Beadle, Mary, 582
Being situated, 62
Bixby, M. Brian, 504
Boylstein, Craig, 170
Brackley, Margaret H., 531
Brazilian immigrant women, 251–271
  distrustful transnational border casualty, 266–267
  fluid transnational identities, 256–262
  gaining information, 262–263
  health, 267–268
  health resources, 268
  informal access, professional health care providers, 263
  multiple borders, crossing, 262
  participants and migration contexts, 252–253
  personal, communal health resources, 254–255
  personal responsibility, 259–260
  political resistance to tuberculosis prophylaxis, 264–266
  premigration health care practices, 253–254
  research methodology, 251–252
  transnational health, 255–257
  transnational resources, 253–257
  transnational syncretism, 259–260
  U.S. Health Care professionals, interfacing with, 263–267
Brennan, Graeme, 283
Brooten, Dorothy, 464, 479
Butler, Mollie, 439

C
Campbell, Roberta L., 479
Cancer, ovarian, recurrence of, 347–358
  alienation, 351–353
  data analysis, 349
  data collection, 349
  delay of cancer's advancement, hoping for, 351

ethical considerations, 349
findings, 349–351
responsibility, 353–354
settings, 349
structure-living in limbo, 354
trustworthiness, 356–357
Cancer patients, palliative care, 396–410
  data analysis, 400–402
  data collection, 398–399
  dwelling space, 403–404
  essential phenomenon, seeking, 405–406
  geographical space, 403
  lived body, 402–403
  lived other, 404–405
  lived space, 403
  lived time, 404
  sample, 397–398
  secure space, 403
Cardiac failure, 479–493, 504–512
  advanced practice nurse interventions, 506–507
  community resources, 507
  comorbid conditions, 508
  control group, 481
  cost analyses, 488
  death, 486
  effect persistence, 488
  family resources, 507
  functional status, 488
  intervention group, 481–483
  outcome measures, 483
  patient goals, 507
  patient-provider relationship, 507–508
  patient satisfaction, 488
  quality of life, 488
  readmissions, 486–488
  rehospitalization, 486
  statistical analysis, 483–486, 505
  study design, 480–481
  study sample, 480
Cardiac rehabilitation
  family-focused, 563–571
    altruism, 570
    cardiac rehabilitation, 564–565
    hope, instillation of, 569
    identifying need, 563–564
    imparting of information, 568–569
    protocol for group sessions, 565–568
    reference group, 569–570
    themes, 568–570
    therapeutic benefits, 568–570
    wellness, redefinition of, 569
  group counseling, 552–563
    compliance measures, 555
  hypotheses, 554

hypothesis testing, 557–560
preliminary data analyses, 556–557
procedures, 555–556
sample, 554–555
theoretical model, 553–554
Cardiac surgery, Taiwanese patients, 366–386
absence of concern, 377
analytical methods, 370
cardiac surgery, concerns regarding, 381–382
"caring about" type of concerns, 371
coping strategies used to manage concerns, 376–377
death, 373–375
empowerment of self, 380–381
"experiencing mortal fear" type of concerns, 375–376
financial needs, 374
hospital experiences, 373–375
implications, 382–384
instruments, 368–370
life goals, 371–373
limitations, 382–384
participant concerns at admission, 370–371
personhood, 378–379
poor quality of care, 375
procedures, 367–368
process of recovery, 371, 374–375
resuming normality, 379–380
sample, 367
seeking help from others, coping by, 376–377
trustworthiness, 370
turning to metaphysical resources, coping by, 377
uncertain concern, 375–376
unfinished responsibilities, 371–374
use of person-focused effort, coping by, 376
"worry about" type of concerns, 374–375
Care model, 459–464
Caregivers, parental, 531–539
experimental treatment, 534
instruments, 535–536
literature review, 532–533
sample, 534–535
Self-Rating Depression Scale, 535–536
Social Support Questionnaire, 535–536
statement of problem, 534
theoretical perspective, 533
Chang, Wei-Chin, 430
Change, transition, distinguished, 69
Change-related concepts, 32–33
Chick, Norma and Meleis, Afaf Ibrahim, 24
Clarification of role, 576
Clark, Suzanne, 552
Clyburn, Arline, 552
Collaboration, 446
Collaborative practice model, 430–439

acute-care nurse practitioner, 439
changed work model, 435
data analysis, 433
data collection, 433
decision making, 435
duty boundaries, 434
ethical issues, 433
gradually emerging work patterns, 433–435
professional growth direction, 435
research design, 432
role-acquisition phase, 434–435
role ambiguity phase, 432–434
role identified by patients, 435
role-implementation phase, 435–436
sample, 432–433
self-directed learning, 432
staff recognition, 434
work support system, 435
Community conditions, 60
Community resources, 507
Comorbid conditions, 505
Concept of role, 515–516
Condition of situational transition, rationale for using, 540–541
Conditions predisposing to problematic role transition, 15–16
Confidence, developing, 62
Conformity in geriatric sexuality, 145–152
case study for role supplementation, 151
conceptual scheme for intervention, 148–149
interventions at each level, 151–152
limited information, 151
permission, 151
role acceptance and rejection, 147
role conception, 147
role expectation, 146–147
role performance, 147–148
suggestions, 151–152
therapy, 149–151
intensive, 150–151
limited information, 149–150
permission, 149
suggestions, 150
Congregate living, independent, 182–187
late-life relocation, 182–184
readiness to move, assessment of, 184–186
Connaughton, Mary J., 449
Consequences of transition to motherhood, 109
Coping, 63
Coronary care, stress debriefing, 605
Costs, transition, 473–474
Counseling, cardiac rehabilitation, 557–568
compliance measures, 556
hypotheses, 554

hypothesis testing, 557–561
preliminary data analyses, 556–557
procedures, 555–556
sample, 554–555
theoretical model, 553–554
Couples' experiences, parental role, 527
Courtney, Mary, 439
Creation of healthy environment, 138
Critical incident stress debriefing
  Australian nurses, 603–612
    analysis, 605–606
    data collection, 605–606
    debriefing questionnaire, 605
  perianesthesia nurses, 612–616
    coping, 615
    critical incident stress debriefing, 614–616
    disengagement, 615–616
    emotional reactions, 615
    future planning, 615
    normalization, 615
    posttraumic stress, 613–614
Cultural beliefs, 59
Culture shock, 287–288

D
DAS. See Dyadic adjustment scale
Davies, Sue, 209
Debriefing, 587–621
  critical incident stress, 603–612
    analysis, 605–606
    data collection, 605–606
    debriefing questionnaire, 605
    perianesthesia nurses, 612–616
  midwife-led postnatal, 590–603
    background information questionnaire, 592
    dyadic adjustment scale, 593
    Edinburgh postnatal depression scale, 593
    efficacy of treatment, 595–598
    feedback, 598
    feedback after debriefing questionnaire, 594
    impact of events scale, 594
    intrapartum intervention scale, 594
    measures, 592–594
    parenting stress index short form, 594
    participants, 592
    perception of birth scale, 593–594
    procedure, 594–595
    state-trait anxiety inventory, 593
    symptom checklist 90-R, 592–593
  perianesthesia nurses
    coping, 605
    critical incident stress debriefing, 614–617
    disengagement, 615–616
    emotional reactions, 615
    future planning, 615
    normalization, 615
    posttraumic stress, 613–614
  postnatal, 582–590
    barriers to providing service, 586
    data analysis, 585
    ethical considerations, 585
    limitations, 586
    method, 583–585
    purpose of, 586
    sample, 585
    study, 583–585
Delaney, Colleen, 300
Dependent variable, transition as, 34–35
Desired Control Scale, 136
Developing countries, women's health, 200–202
Developmental transitions, 15, 38–39, 87–153
  future research, 92–93
  life-course perspective, 91–92
  markers of life, 88–89
  nonnormative development, 87–88
  normative development, 87–88
  parenthood transition, markers, 89–90
  retirement transition, markers, 90
  role theory, 90–91
  theories on adult development, 88
Diabetes
  adolescents, 493–504
    child model, 499–500
    data analysis, 497
    data generation, 497
    dietetic advice, 497–499
    education, 497–499
    ethical issues, 496
    findings, 497
    literature review, 495
    method, 496
    participants, 497
    phases of transition process, 500–501
    recruitment, 496–497
    study, 496
  Mexican immigrant women with, 326–338
    data analysis, 331
    design and measures, 330–331
    diabetes in Hispanic population, 327
    health-illness transition, 328–329
    Hispanic immigration trends, 327
    intervention, 329–330
    limitations, 336
    qualitative results, 333–335
    quantitative measures, 331
    quantitative results, 332–333
    sample, 332
    sample and recruitment, 330
    self-management, 327–328

Diagnostic transitions, 54
Dickson, Victoria Vaughan, 320
Discharge, 153–225
   care coordination, 159
   discharge teaching, 158–159
   hospital discharge, readiness for, 158
   hospitalization factors, 158
   limitations, 167–168
   outcomes of readiness for discharge, 161–164
   patient characteristics, 158
   postdischarge coping difficulty, 159
   predictors of readiness for discharge, 161
   procedures, 159–160
   support, 159–160
   theoretical framework, 154
   variables, 158
Disconnectedness, 26
Domain concepts, 28
Dorr, Mary T., 292
Douglas, Marilyn K., 271
Dracup, Kathleen, 552, 563
Driving, Alzheimer's disease, 58
Dyadic adjustment scale, 593

E
Early memory loss, 386–393
   avoiding, strategy of, 393
   clinical assessment, 387–389
   data analysis, 388–387
   data collection, 388
   discussion, 393–395
   forgetfulness, 389–395
   meaning, search for, 392–393
   memory loss as transition, 387
   normalizing, 390–391
   participants, 388
   watching, strategy of, 391–392
Edinburgh postnatal depression scale, 593
Edlefsen, Patricia, 563
Education, 282–319
Ekman, Inger, 359
Ekman, Sirkka-Liisa, 386
Ekwall, Ewa, 347
Emergency department critical incident stress debriefing, 605
Emotional well-being, importance of, 44–45
Empowerment, 279–280
Environment, 43–44, 461–479
   costs, 468–469
   costs for transitional care services, 468
   definitions, 464
   duration of services, 465
   entrepreneurial services, 472
   HMO follow-up services, 470–471
   home health care, 469–470
   home health care from community nursing services, 470
   hospital home care services, 470–471
   integrated health care systems, 473–475
   models of transitional care, 469–471
   nurse case management, 474
   providers of transitional care, 467–468
   quality cost model, 471–473
   research models of transitional services, 471–473
   subacute care units, 473
EPDS. *See* Edinburgh postnatal depression scale
Ephemeral state, transience as, 414–415
Eribes, Carmen, 271
Executive leadership, 452
Expanded model
   assessment component of, 115–117
   intervention component of, 117–119
   rationale for, 114–115
   scope of, 119
Expectations, 42
Expression of time, transience as, 413–414

F
FAD. *See* Feedback after debriefing questionnaire
Family assessment, Alzheimer's disease, 573–574
Family caregiving study, 56
Family conflicts, 247
Family-focused cardiac rehabilitation, 563–571
   altruism, 570
   cardiac rehabilitation, 564–565
   hope, instillation of, 569
   identifying need, 563–564
   imparting of information, 568–569
   protocol for group sessions, 565–568
   reference group, 569–570
   themes, 568–570
   therapeutic benefits, 568–570
   wellness, redefinition of, 569
Feedback after debriefing questionnaire, 594
Fluid integrative identities, 64
Forgetfulness, 389–395
Former management structure, 445–446
Fracture rehabilitation, 358–366
   autonomous, 361–362
   awareness, 362
   common traits, 362–363
   conceptions of, 361
   data analysis, 361
   future research, 365
   heedless, 362
   informants, 360
   interview, 360–361
   methods, 360
   relevance, 364–365
   shocking events, 362–363

study limitations, 364
zest for life, 363
Fridlund, Bengt, 242
Fulfillment of Meaning Scale, 136

G

Gaffney, Kathleen Flynn, 114
Gallegos, Gwen, 326
Geriatric Depression Scale, 136
Geriatric sexual conformity, 145–152
    case study for role supplementation, 151
    conceptual scheme for intervention, 148–149
    interventions at each level, 151–152
        limited information, 151
        permission, 151
        suggestions, 151–152
    role acceptance and rejection, 147
    role conception, 147
    role expectation, 146–147
    role performance, 147–148
    therapy, 149–151
        intensive, 150–151
        limited information, 149–150
        permission, 149
        specific suggestions, 150
Geriatrics, 129–144, 458–464. *See also* Alzheimer's disease
    Adult Attachment Scale, 136
    case study, 139–141
    cost, 464–465
    creation of healthy environment, 138
    critical incident stress debriefing, 605
    Desired Control Scale, 136
    Fulfillment of Meaning Scale, 136
    Geriatric Depression Scale, 136
    health, 132–135
    health care costs, 460
    health outcomes after discharge, 459–460
    healthy transition processes, 133–134
    Index of Activities of Daily Living, 136
    McGill Pain Questionnaire, 136
    Mini-Mental State Questionnaire, 136
    mobilization of resources, 138–139
    Multidimensional Functional Assessment, 136
    Mutuality Scale, 136
    nursing assessment, 135–136
    nursing therapeutics, 135–139
    patient satisfaction, 465
    preventable hospital readmissions, 459
    process indicators, 134–135
    reminiscence, 136–137
    research, 131–132
    research into practice, 461–462
    role supplementation, 137–138
    science advancement, 460–461

State/Trait Anxiety Inventory, 136
    transition, defining, 129–131
    transitional care model, 460
Governance, interdisciplinary, 445–454
    accountability, 452–453
    collaboration, 446
    disease center collaboration, 450–451
    executive leadership, 453
    former management structure, 446–447
    new governance model, 446–447, 451
Gresser, Susan, 153
Grief, unprocessed, 246
Gross, Anne H., 445
Group counseling, cardiac rehabilitation, 552–563
    compliance measures, 556
    hypotheses, 554
    hypothesis testing, 557–560
    preliminary data analyses, 556–557
    procedures, 555–556
    sample, 554–555
    theoretical model, 553–554

H

Hassinger, James, 445
Hattar-Pollara, Marianne, 87
Health, illness transitions, 320–423
Health care costs, 460
Health-illness transitions, 16, 40
Health outcomes after discharge, 459–460
Heart failure, 479–493, 504–512
    advanced practice nurse interventions, 506–507
    community resources, 507
    comorbid conditions, 508
    control group, 481
    cost analyses, 488
    death, 486
    effect persistence, 488
    family resources, 507
    functional status, 488
    intervention group, 481–483
    outcome measures, 483
    patient goals, 507
    patient-provider relationship, 507–508
    patient satisfaction, 488
    quality of life, 488
    readmissions, 486–488
    rehospitalization, 486
    self care, 319–326
        practice link, 324–325
        research, 322–324
        self-care, defining, 320
        situation-specific theory, 320–321
        theory link, 321–322
        statistical analysis, 483–484, 505

study design, 480–481
study sample, 481
Hinojosa, Melanie Sberna, 170
Hinojosa, Ramon, 170
Hip fracture rehabilitation, 358–366
   autonomous, 361–362
   awareness, 362
   common traits, 362–363
   conceptions of, 361
   data analysis, 361
   future research, 365
   heedless, 362
   informants, 360
   interview, 360–361
   methods, 360
   relevance, 364–365
   shocking events, 362–363
   study limitations, 364
   zest for life, 363
HMO follow-up services, 470–471
Holistic nurses, 310–319
   data analysis, 313
   data collection methods, 312–313
   design, 312
   findings, 313–316
   limitation, 312–313
   literature review, 310–311
   participants, 311
   recommendations, 316–317
   research questions, 313–316
Holmes, Sue Baird, 15
Hope, instillation of, 569
Hospital discharge, 153–170
   care coordination, 159
   discharge teaching, 158–159
   hospital discharge, readiness for, 158
   hospitalization factors, 158
   limitations, 167–168
   outcomes of readiness for discharge, 161–164
   patient characteristics, 158
   postdischarge coping difficulty, 159
   predictors of readiness for discharge, 161
   procedures, 159–160
   support, 159–160
   theoretical framework, 154
   variables, 158
Hu, Wen-Yu, 363
Huang, Guey-Shiun, 363

I
Iacono, Maureen, 612
IES. See Impact of events scale
IIS. See Intrapartum intervention scale
Im, Eun-Ok, 52, 121
Immigrant women, 226–282

Brazilian, 251–271
   distrustful transnational border casualty, 266–267
   fluid transnational identities, 256–262
   gaining information, 262–263
   health, 267–268
   health resources, 268
   informal access, professional health care providers, 263
   multiple borders, crossing, 262
   participants and migration contexts, 252–253
   personal, communal health resources, 254–255
   personal responsibility, 259–260
   political resistance to tuberculosis prophylaxis, 264–266
   premigration health care practices, 253–254
   research methodology, 251–252
   transnational health, 255–257
   transnational resources, 253–257
   transnational syncretism, 259–260
   U.S. Health Care professionals, interfacing with, 263–267
diabetes, 326–338
   data analysis, 334
   design and measures, 330–331
   diabetes in Hispanic population, 327
   health-illness transition, 328–329
   Hispanic immigration trends, 327
   intervention, 329–330
   limitations, 336
   qualitative results, 333–335
   quantitative measures, 331
   quantitative results, 332–333
   sample, 332
   sample and recruitment, 330
   self-management, 327–328
menopausal transition, 121–129
   attitudes toward health, illness, 127
   context, 126–127
   gender, 126
   interrelationships among transition conditions, 127
   management of symptoms, as indicator of health, 127
   menopausal transition, 123–125
   modifications in transition model, 125
   number, 125
   priority, 125
   seriousness, 125
   socioeconomic status, 125
   transition conditions, 125–127
needs of, 205–205
roles, 202–205
Impact of events scale, 594
Independent congregate living, 182–187

late-life relocation, 182–184
readiness to move, assessment of, 184–186
Independent living community, women, 187–198
　data analysis, 191–192
　data collection, 190
　design, 189–190
　emotional well-being, 190–191
　findings, 192–194
　late-life relocation, 188–189
　measures, 190
　person-environmental interactions, 191
　physical well-being, 190
　purpose, 189
　quality of life, 191
　setting, 189–190
　subjective well-being, 191, 193–194
　　integration, 194
　　quality of life, 193–194
　theoretical framework, 189
　transition conditions, 190, 192–193
　　emotional well-being, 193
　　person-environment interactions, 193
　　physical well-being, 192–193
Independent variable, transition as, 33
Index of Activities of Daily Living, 136
Indicators of healthy transitions, 45–46
Individual family visits, parental role, 524–525
Individual role modeling, parental role, 528–529
Inhibitors, 60–62
Insecure family having immigrant status, 245–246
Insufficiency of role, 572
Intensive care
　critical incident stress debriefing, 605
　neonatal, 104–113
　　analytical phase, 106
　　antecedents of transition to motherhood, 108–109
　　consequences of transition to motherhood, 109
　　fieldwork phase, 105–106
　　findings, 106–108
　　influencing factors, 109–111
　　motherhood transition, critical attributes, 108
　　psycho-emotional swirling, 108
　　research methodology, 105–106
　　theoretical phase, 105
　　time-dependent process, 108
Interdisciplinary governance, 445–454
　accountability, 452–453
　collaboration, 446
　disease center collaboration, 450–451
　executive leadership, 453
　former management structure, 446–447
　new governance model, 446–447, 451
　teamwork, 446
Internal instability, family with, 246

Interrelationships among transition conditions, 127
Interventions, 17–21
　communication, 20–21
　components, 17–18
　interaction, 20–21
　processes, 17–18
　reference group, 20
　role clarification, 18–19
　role modeling, 19
　role rehearsal, 19–20
　role taking, 19
　strategies, 17–18
Intrapartum intervention scale, 594
Involuntarily migrated families, 242–251
　analysis of data, 244–245
　being misunderstood, 246
　data collection, analysis, 244–245
　design, 244
　ethical issues, 244
　family health issues, 247–249
　family with internal instability, 246
　findings, 245–247
　grief, unprocessed, 246
　having family conflicts, 247
　insecure family having immigrant status, 245–246
　integration, lack of, 246–247
　mentally distressed family, 245–247
　methodological issues, 249
　participants, 244
　post-asylum reactions, living with, 246
　research, 249–250
　rights, living without, 245
　segregated family from society, 246
　setting, 244
　stable family, 247
　study, 244–245
　togetherness, living in, 247
　trauma, unprocessed, 246
　uncertainty, living in, 245
　well-functioning family, 247
　worthy life, living, 247

J
Jeavons, Sue, 603
Jones, Deloras, 514
Jones, Patricia S., 129

K
Kaas, Merrie J., 145
Karlsson, Jòn, 358
Kelley, Lisa Skemp, 571
Knafl, Kathleen A., 187
Koch, Tina, 493
Korean immigrant menopausal transition, 121–129
　　interrelationships among transition conditions, 127

INDEX   633

management of symptoms, as indicator of health, 127
menopausal transition, 123–125
modifications in transition model, 125
number, 125
priority, 125
seriousness, 125
transition conditions, 125–127
   attitudes toward health, illness, 127
   context, 126–127
   gender, 126
   socioeconomic status, 125
Kralik, Debbie, 72, 493

L
Lakin, Jean A., 571
Larkin, Philip J., 396, 410
Late-life relocation, 182–184
Level of knowledge/skill, 42–43
Level of planning, 44
Liaison faculty observations, 297–328
Life-course perspective, 91–92
Literature review, 72–83, 231–232, 284, 311–312, 414–416, 495, 532–533
defining of transition, 76–77
exclusion criteria, 74–75
findings, 75
literature, transition used in, 77
process, transition as, 78–79
search, 74
search methods, 74
terms describing transition process, 79–80
theoretical frameworks, 75–76
Lokken, Lisa, 153
Loss of memory, 386–396
avoiding, strategy of, 393
clinical assessment, 387–389
data analysis, 388–389
data collection, 388
discussion, 393–395
forgetfulness, 389–395
meaning, search for, 392–393
memory loss as transition, 387
normalizing, 390–391
participants, 388
watching, strategy of, 391–392
Lou, Meei-Fang, 366

M
Maislin, Greg, 479
Markers of life, 88–89
Maternal role, 94–104, 114–121
assessment component, expanded model, 115–117
expanded model, rationale for, 114–115
intervention component, expanded model, 117–119
scope of expanded model, 119

McCauley, Kathleen M., 479, 504
McEwen, Marylyn Morris, 326
McGill Pain Questionnaire, 136
McLachlan, Angus J., 594
McLaren, Suzanne, 594
McSherry, Rob, 283
Meanings, 41–42
Meleis, Afaf Ibrahim, 13, 38, 52, 65, 121, 129, 198, 241, 271, 366, 386, 514, 539, 552, 563
Memory loss, early, 386–396
analyzing, strategy of, 391–392
avoiding, strategy of, 393
clinical assessment, 387–389
data analysis, 388–389
data collection, 388
discussion, 394–395
forgetfulness, 389–395
meaning, search for, 392–393
memory loss as transition, 387
normalizing, 390–391
participants, 388
vigilance, strategy of, 393
watching, strategy of, 391–392
Menopausal transition, 53–54
Korean immigrant, 121–129
   attitudes toward health, illness, 127
   context, 126–127
   gender, 126
   interrelationships among transition conditions, 127
   management of symptoms, as indicator of health, 127
   menopausal transition, 123–125
   modifications in transition model, 125
   number, 125
   priority, 125
   seriousness, 125
   socioeconomic status, 125
   transition conditions, 125–127
Mentally distressed family, 245–247
Mercer, Ramona T., 94
Messias, DeAnne K. Hilfinger, 52, 226, 251, 271
Mexican women, 271–283
centrality of family, 279
coping strategies for maternal role, 276–277
data analysis, 274
data collection, 274
diabetes, 326–338
   data analysis, 331
   design and measures, 330–331
   diabetes in Hispanic population, 327
   health-illness transition, 328–329
   Hispanic immigration trends, 327
   intervention, 329–330

limitations, 336
    qualitative results, 333–335
    quantitative measures, 331
    quantitative results, 332–333
    sample, 332
    sample and recruitment, 330
    self-management, 327–328
  empowerment, 279–280
  maternal role, 275–277
  maternal role satisfiers, 275
  maternal role stressors, 275–276
  participants, 273
  role overload, 280–281
  spousal role, 277–278
    coping strategies for, 278
  spousal role satisfiers, 277
  spousal role stressors, 277–278
  study, 273–275
  valuation, 280–281
Middle-range theory, 52–65
  African-American mothers, 53
  attitudes, 59
  community conditions, 60
  cultural beliefs, 59
  diagnostic transitions, 54
  emerging framework, 55
  facilitators, 59–61
  family caregiving study, 55
  fluid integrative identities, 63
  health, 54–55
  inhibitors, 59–61
  knowledge, 60
  mastery, 63
  meanings, 59
  menopausal transition, 53–54
  migration, 54–55
  neglecting menopausal transition, 53–54
  outcome indicators, 62–63
  parents, diagnostic transitions, 54
  patterns of response, 61–62
    being situated, 62
    coping, 62
    developing confidence, 62
    feeling connected, 61
    interactions, 61–62
    location, 62
    process indicators, 61
  personal conditions, 59–60
  preparation, 60
  properties of transition experience, 57–59
    awareness, 57
    change, 57–58
    critical points, events, 58–59
    engagement, 57
    time span, 58
  societal conditions, 61
  socioeconomic status, 60
  studies, transitions as framework, 53–55
  work, 54–55
Midwife-led postnatal debriefing, 590–603
  background information questionnaire, 592
  dyadic adjustment scale, 593
  Edinburgh postnatal depression scale, 593
  efficacy of treatment, 595–598
  feedback, 598
  feedback after debriefing questionnaire, 594
  impact of events scale, 594
  intrapartum intervention scale, 594
  measures, 592–594
  parenting stress index short form, 594
  participants, 592
  perception of birth scale, 593–594
  procedure, 594–595
  state-trait anxiety inventory, 593
  symptom checklist 90-R, 592–593
Migration, 54–55, 226–231
  conditions of migration transitions, 229–230
  frameworks, 227
  health interventions, 230
  involuntary, 242–251
    analysis of data, 244–245
    asylum-seeking process, 245–247
    being misunderstood, 246
    data collection, analysis, 244–245
    design, 244
    ethical issues, 244
    family health issues, 247–249
    family with internal instability, 246
    findings, 245–247
    grief, unprocessed, 246
    having family conflicts, 247
    insecure family having immigrant status, 245–246
    integration, lack of, 246–247
    mentally distressed family, 245–247
    methodological issues, 249
    participants, 244
    post-asylum reactions, living with, 246
    research, 249–250
    rights, living without, 245
    segregated family from society, 246
    setting, 244
    stable family, 247
    study, 244–245
    togetherness, living in, 247
    trauma, unprocessed, 246
    uncertainty, living in, 245
    well-functioning family, 247
    worthy life, living, 247

models, 227
nature of migration transitions, 228–229
patterns of response, 230
resettlement, psychological adaptation, 232–241
    demographics, 235
    experience of migration, 235
    feeling at home, 237
    findings, 235–239
    future considerations, 239–240
    grief resolution, 237–239
    instruments, 233–234
    language, 236
    literature review, 232–233
    loss, 235–236
    novelty, 236
    occupation, 236
    procedure, 234–235
    sample, 233
    subordination, 236–237
transitions framework, 227–230
Mini-Mental State Questionnaire, 136
Mission of nursing, 65–72
  clinical example, 69–70
  redefining, 67–69
  transition *vs.* change, 69
Mobilization of resources, 138–139
Modeling parental role, 525–526
Moten, Julie, 590
Mu, Pei-Fan, 430
Multidimensional Functional Assessment, 136
Mutuality Scale, 136

N
Naylor, Mary D., 459, 464, 479, 504
Neonatal intensive care, 104–113
  analytical phase, 106
  antecedents, transition to motherhood, 108–109
  consequences, transition to motherhood, 109
  fieldwork phase, 105–106
  findings, 106–108
  influencing factors, 109–111
  motherhood transition, critical attributes, 108
  psycho-emotional swirling, 108
  research methodology, 105–106
  theoretical phase, 105
  time-dependent process, 108
Neurology critical incident stress debriefing, 605
New governance model, 446–447, 451
Nonnormative development, 87–88
Normative development, 87–88
Nursing home entry, 209–225
  data analysis, 214–215
  ethical considerations, 214
  findings, 215–222
  methods, 212–214
  rigour, 214
  study, 212–214
  theoretical perspectives, 210–211
  theory of nursing transitions, 210–212
Nursing therapeutics, 28–29
Nyström, Anne E. M., 358

O
O'Connor, Jillian, 603
Ollerenshaw, Alison, 590
Olsson, Lars-Eric, 358
Oncology, critical incident stress debriefing, 605
Operating theatre critical incident stress debriefing, 605
Organizational transitions, 40–41, 423–458
Ovarian cancer recurrence, 347–358
  alienation, 351–353
  data analysis, 349
  data collection, 349
  delay of cancer's advancement, hoping for, 351
  ethical considerations, 349
  findings, 349–351
  responsibility, 353–354
  settings, 349
  structure-living in limbo, 354
  trustworthiness, 356–357

P
Palliative care, 410–422
  cancer patients, 396–410
    data analysis, 400–402
    data collection, 398–399
    dwelling space, 403–404
    essential phenomenon, seeking, 405–406
    geographical space, 403
    lived body, 402–403
    lived other, 404–405
    lived space, 403
    lived time, 404
    sample, 397–398
    secure space, 403
  case studies, 415
  characteristics/attributes, identifying, 417
  concept definition, 414
  concept evaluation, 412–414
  conceptual boundaries, delineating, 418
  conceptual development, 411
  empirical study, 411
  ephemeral state, transience as, 414–415
  expression of time, transience as, 415–416
  findings, 414
  home, 416–417
  literature review, 414–416
  preconditions
    demonstrating, 417–418

        describing, 417–418
        search method, 412–414
        spatial phenomenon, transience as, 416
Parental caregivers, 531–539
    experimental treatment, 534
    instruments, 535–536
    literature review, 532–533
    sample, 534–535
    Self-Rating Depression Scale, 535–536
    Social Support Questionnaire, 535–536
    statement of problem, 534
    theoretical perspective, 535
Parental role, 523–531
    couples' experiences, 527
    families, 530
    group activities, purposes, 523–524
    individual family visits, 524–525
    individual role modeling, 528–529
    modeling, 525–526
    program assumption, premises, 527–531
    program evaluation, 530–531
    in reference group, 527–528
    rehearsal, 525–526
    role clarification, achieving, 529
    role mastery, 526–527, 529–530
    role rehearsal activity, 5329
Parenthood transition markers, 89–90
Parenting stress index short form, 594
Parents, diagnostic transitions, 54
Pasvogel, Alice, 326
Patient satisfaction, 460
Patterns of response, 27, 61–62
    being situated, 62
    coping, 62
    developing confidence, 62
    feeling connected, 61
    interactions, 61–62
    location, 62
    process indicators, 61
Pediatric critical incident stress debriefing, 605
Perception of birth scale, 593–596
Person-environmental interactions, 191
Personal conditions, 59–60
Piacentine, Linda B., 153
Piscopo, Barbara, 300
POBS. *See* Perception of birth scale
Ponte, Patricia Reid, 445
Pool nurses, 423–430
    facilitators, 427
    findings, 425–428
    inhibitors, 427
    limitations, 429
    nature, 425–427
    response patterns, 427–428

Post-asylum reactions, living with, 246
Postnatal debriefing, 582–590
    barriers to providing service, 586
    data analysis, 585
    ethical considerations, 585
    limitations, 586
    method, 583–585
    midwives, 590–603
        background information questionnaire, 592
        dyadic adjustment scale, 593
        Edinburgh postnatal depression scale, 593
        efficacy of treatment, 595–598
        feedback, 598
        feedback after debriefing questionnaire, 594
        impact of events scale, 594
        intrapartum intervention scale, 594
        measures, 592–594
        parenting stress index short form, 594
        participants, 592
        perception of birth scale, 593–594
        procedure, 594–595
        state-trait anxiety inventory, 593
        symptom checklist 90-R, 592–593
    purpose of, 586
    sample, 585
    study, 583–585
Postpartum reactions to supplementation of roles, 541
Prater, Marita, 579
Pregraduation practicums, baccalaureate nursing students, 291–300
    liaison faculty observations, 297–298
    preceptor observations, 298
    student observations, 295–297
Preventable hospital readmissions, 459
Preventive role supplementation, 514–523
    concept of role, 515–516
    reference groups, 516–517
    role clarification, 519–520
    role modeling, 520–521
    role rehearsal, 521–522
    role taking, 518–519
    significant others, 517–518
Process indicators, 61, 134–135
Professional socialisation, 283–292
    clinical issues, 289–290
    comfort zone, 288–289
    culture shock, 287–288
    emerging framework, 290–291
    entry issues, 285
    ethical considerations, 285
    formal/informal exposure to RGN role, 285
    framework for socialisation, 285–286
    literature review, 284
    procedures for data collection, 286

reality shock, 285
role identity, role confusion, 284
sample, 286
setting, 286
socialisation, defining, 284
techniques, 286
themes, identification of, 286–287
trustworthiness, 286–287
Properties of transition experience, 57–59
awareness, 57
change, 57–58
critical points, events, 58–59
engagement, 57
time span, 58
Protocol for group sessions, 565–568
PSI. See Parenting stress index short form
Psychiatric hospitalization, 579–581
therapeutic techniques, 580–581
transition entry group goals, 579–581
Psychiatry, stress debriefing, 605
Psycho-emotional swirling, 108
Psychological adaptation, migration, resettlement, 232–241
demographics, 235
experience of migration, 235
feeling at home, 237
findings, 235–239
future considerations, 239–240
grief resolution, 237–239
instruments, 233–234
language, 236
literature review, 232–233
loss, 235–236
novelty, 236
occupation, 236
procedure, 234–235
sample, 233
subordination, 236–237

R

Readiness to move, assessment of, 184–186
Recreating everyday practice, 307–308
Recurrence of ovarian cancer, 347–358
alienation, 351–353
data analysis, 349
data collection, 349
delay of cancer's advancement, hoping for, 351
ethical considerations, 349
findings, 349–351
responsibility, 353–354
settings, 349
structure-living in limbo, 354
trustworthiness, 356–357
Reference groups, preventive role supplementation, 516–517

Registered nurses, to baccalaureate nursing students, 299–310
assertiveness, 306–307
beginnings, 305
challenges, 307
cornerstone courses, 305–306
data analysis, 303–304
description, 307
empowerment, 306
envisioning whole, 307
expectations, 304–305
procedure, 303
recreating everyday practice, 307–308
research design, 303
sample, 303
Rehabilitation
cardiac, family-focused, 563–571
altruism, 570
cardiac rehabilitation, 564–565
hope, instillation of, 559
identifying need, 563–564
imparting of information, 568–569
protocol for group sessions, 565–568
reference group, 569–570
themes, 568–570
therapeutic benefits, 568–570
wellness, redefinition of, 569
hip fracture, 358–366
autonomous, 361–362
awareness, 362
common traits, 362–363
conceptions of, 361
data analysis, 361
future research, 365
heedless, 362
informants, 360
interview, 360–361
methods, 360
relevance, 364–365
shocking events, 362–363
study limitations, 364
zest for life, 363
Relocation, 153–225
data analysis, 191–192
data collection, 190
design, 189–190
emotional well-being, 190–191
findings, 192–194
late-life relocation, 188–189
measures, 190
person-environmental interactions, 191
physical well-being, 190
purpose, 189
quality of life, 191

setting, 189–190
subjective well-being, 191, 193–194
    integration, 194
    quality of life, 193–194
theoretical framework, 189
transition conditions, 190, 192–193
    emotional well-being, 193
    person-environment interactions, 193
    physical well-being, 192–193
Reminiscence, 136–137
Repeated behaviors, Alzheimer's disease, 527–528
Research potential, 32–34
Resettlement, psychological adaptation, 232–241
    demographics, 235
    disruption, 235–236
    experience of migration, 235
    feeling at home, 237
    findings, 235–239
    future considerations, 239–240
    grief resolution, 237–238
    instruments, 233–234
    language, 236
    literature review, 232–233
    loss, 235–236
    novelty, 236
    occupation, 236
    procedure, 234–235
    profiles, 235
    return visits, 237–239
    sample, 233
    subordination, 236–237
Retirement transition markers, 90
Review of literature, 72–83, 232–233, 284, 311–312, 414–416, 496, 532–533
    defining of transition, 76–77
    exclusion criteria, 74–75
    findings, 75
    literature, transition used in, 77
    process, transition as, 78–79
    search, 74
    search methods, 74
    terms describing transition process, 79–80
    theoretical frameworks, 75–76
Rheumatoid arthritis, women, 336–346
    analysis, 341–342
    awareness and perception, 339
    demographics, 341
    disconnectedness, 340
    health outcomes, 340, 344
    markers of transition process, 344
    nursing model, 339
    nursing support, 344
    patterns of response, 340
    procedures, 341

process, 339
sample, 340–341
transition process, 342–344
    becoming aware, 342
    getting care, 342–344
    mastery, 344
Rich, Victoria L., 423
Riegel, Barbara, 320
Rights, living without, 245
Rittman, Maude, 170
Robinson, Petra, 386
Rogers, Sandra, 198
Role insufficiency, 13–24
    communication, 20–21
    complementary nature, 16
    components, 17–18
    developmental transitions, 15
    health-illness transitions, 16
    interaction, 20–21
    nursing intervention, 17–21
    problematic role transition, conditions predisposing to, 15–16
    processes, 17–18
    reference group, 20
    relevance of role to nursing, 14–15
    role clarification, 18–19
    role insufficiency, 16–17, 22–23
    role mastery, 22–23
    role modeling, 19
    role rehearsal, 19–20
    role supplementation, 21–23
    role taking, 19
    situational transitions, 15–16
    strategies, 17–18
Role mastery, 22–23, 45
Role supplementation, 21–23, 137–138, 539–552
    anxiety, 541
    conceptual framework, 540
    condition of situational transition, rationale for using, 540–541
    data collection, 544
    experimental group, 543–544
    hypotheses, 542
    hypothesis, 548–550
    instruments, 545–548
    limitations, 550–551
    postpartum reactions, 541
    prenatal reactions, 541
    reference group, 543
    role modeling, 543
    role perceptions, 541
    role rehearsal, 543
    role supplementation, 543
    role supplementation visits, 544–545

sample, 542–544
setting, 542
study problems, 541–542
Role supplementation models, 514–581
Role theory, 90–91
Rossen, Eileen K., 182, 187
Rousseau, G. Kay, 145

S
Samarasinghe, Kerstin, 242
Saudi Arabia, 439–443
   advanced beginner, 441–442
   community, 442
   evaluation, 442–443
   expert, 442
   familiarizing with community, 440–442
   proficiency, 442
   recommendations, 444
   stages of transitional practice model, 440–442
   transitional practice model, 440
Sawyer, Linda M., 52
Schotsmans, Paul, 396, 410
Schumacher, Karen, 38, 52, 129
Schwartz, J. Sanford, 480
SCL 90-R. *See* Symptom checklist 90-R
SDS. *See* Self-Rating Depression Scale
Self-care, heart failure, 319–326
   defining, 321
   practice link, 324–325
   research, 323–324
   situation-specific theory, 320–321
   theory link, 321–323
Self-Rating Depression Scale, 535–536
Selkirk, Rosemary, 590
Sexual conformity, geriatric, 145–152
   case study for role supplementation, 151
   conceptual scheme for intervention, 148–149
   interventions at each level, 151–152
      limited information, 151
      permission, 151
      suggestions, 151–152
   role acceptance and rejection, 147
   role conception, 147
   role expectation, 146–147
   role performance, 147–148
   therapy, 149–151
      intensive, 150–151
      limited information, 149–150
      permission, 149
      suggestions, 150
Sharoff, Leighsa, 310
Shaul, Muriel P., 338
Shields, Linda, 552
Shih, Fu-Jin, 272, 366
Shin, Hyunjeong, 104

Significant others, preventive role supplementation, 517–518
Simpson, Elaine, 439
Situational transitions, 15–16, 39–40
   rationale for using, 540–541
Social Support Questionnaire, 535–536
Socialisation, professional, 283–292
   clinical issues, 289–290
   comfort zone, 288–289
   culture shock, 287–288
   emerging framework, 290–291
   entry issues, 285
   ethical considerations, 285
   framework for socialisation, 285–286
   literature review, 284
   procedures for data collection, 286
   reality shock, 282
   role identity, role confusion, 284
   sample, 286
   setting, 286
   socialisation, defining, 284
   techniques, 286
   themes, identification of, 286–287
   trustworthiness, 286–287
Societal conditions, 61
Socioeconomic status, 60, 125
Sorbe, Bengt, 347
Spinal care, critical incident stress debriefing, 605
Spousal role, coping strategies for, 277
SSQ. *See* Social Support Questionnaire
Stages of transitional practice model, 440–442
Staley, Marilyn, 552
State/Trait Anxiety Inventory, 136
Steele, Anne-Marie, 582
Stress debriefing, critical incident, 605
   perianesthesia nurses, 612–616
   coping, 615
   critical incident stress debriefing, 614–616
   disengagement, 615–616
   emotional reactions, 615
   future planning, 615
   normalization, 615
   posttraumic stress, 613–614
Stroke survivors, 170–181
   availability of others, 175
   bodily experiences, changes in, 173–174
   community integration, changes in, 177–179
   connectedness, changes in, 174–175
   contribution, ability to make, 176
   data analysis, 171–172
   data collection, 171
   description of stroke survivors, 172–173
   interaction with others, community, 176
   intimate relations, ability to engage in, 176–177

sample, 171
sense of self, changes in, 173–174
support from others, 175
Subjective well-being, 45
Supplementation of role, 13–24, 514–523, 539–552, 572–573
  anxiety, 541
  communication, 20–21
  complementary nature, 16
  components, 17–18
  concept of role, 515–516
  conceptual framework, 540
  condition of situational transition, rationale for using, 540–541
  data collection, 545
  developmental transitions, 15
  experimental group, 543–545
  health-illness transitions, 16
  hypotheses, 542
  hypothesis, 548–550
  instruments, 545–548
  interaction, 20–21
  limitations, 550–551
  nursing intervention, 17–21
  postpartum reactions, 541
  prenatal reactions, 541
  problematic role transition, conditions predisposing to, 15–16
  processes, 17–18
  reference group, 20, 543
  reference groups, 516–517
  relevance of role to nursing, 14–15
  role clarification, 18–19, 519–520
  role insufficiency, 16–17, 22–23
  role mastery, 22–23
  role modeling, 19, 520–521, 543
  role perceptions, 541
  role rehearsal, 19–20, 521–522, 543
  role supplementation, 22–23, 543
  role supplementation as independent variable, 21–22
  role supplementation visits, 544–545
  role taking, 19, 518–519
  sample, 542–543
  setting, 542
  significant others, 517–518
  situational transitions, 15–16
  strategies, 17–18
  study problems, 541–542
Surgery critical incident stress debriefing, 605
Swendsen, Leslee, 514, 539
Symptom checklist 90-R, 592–593
Symptom management, as indicator of health, 127

T
Taiwan, acute care nurse practitioners, 430–439
  acute-care nurse practitioner, 436
  changed work model, 435
  data analysis, 433
  data collection, 433
  decision making, 435
  duty boundaries, 434
  ethical issues, 433
  gradually emerging work patterns, 434–435
  professional growth direction, 435
  research design, 432
  role-acquisition phase, 434–435
  role ambiguity phase, 433–434
  role identified by patients, 435
  role-implementation phase, 435–436
  sample, 432–433
  self-directed learning, 431
  staff recognition, 434
  work support system, 435
Taiwanese patient cardiac surgery, 363–386
  absence of concern, 377
  analytical methods, 370
  cardiac surgery, concerns regarding, 381–382
  "caring about" type of concerns, 371
  coping strategies used to manage concerns, 376–377
  death, 373–375
  empowerment of self, 380–381
  "experiencing mortal fear" type of concerns, 375–376
  financial needs, 374
  hospital experiences, 373–374
  implications, 382–384
  instruments, 368–370
  life goals, 371–373
  limitations, 382–384
  participant concerns at admission, 370–371
  personhood, 378–379
  poor quality of care, 375
  procedures, 367–368
  process of recovery, 371, 374–375
  resuming normality, 379–380
  sample, 367
  seeking help from others, coping by, 376–377
  trustworthiness, 370
  turning to metaphysical resources, coping by, 377
  uncertain concern, 375–376
  unfinished responsibilities, 371–374
  use of person-focused effort, coping by, 376
  "worry about" type of concerns, 374–375
Ternestedt, Britt-Marie, 347
Theoretical development, 13–52
Togetherness, living in, 247
Toman, Sally, 153
Toy, Anne, 153
Trangenstein, Patricia A., 66
Transition conditions, 42, 125–127

Trauma, unprocessed, 246
Trustworthiness, 286–287, 356–357
Tsay, Shiow-Luan, 430

U
Uncertainty, living in, 245
Unprocessed grief, 246
Unprocessed trauma, 246

V
van Cleave, Janet, 458
van Loon, Antonia, 72
Vega-Stromberg, Teri, 153
Visentin, Kate, 72, 493

W
Wahlund, Lars-Olof, 386
Weiss, Marrianne E., 153
Well-being of relationships, 46
White-Traut, Rosemary, 104
Wieland, Diane M., 292
Winblad, Bengt, 386
Winer, Eric, 445
Wolf, Zane Robinson, 292
Women
  Brazilian immigrant, 251–271
    distrustful transnational border casualty, 266–267
    fluid transnational identities, 256–262
    gaining information, 262–263
    health, 267–268
    health resources, 268
    informal access, professional health care providers, 263
    multiple borders, crossing, 262
    participants and migration contexts, 252–253
    personal, communal health resources, 254–255
    personal responsibility, 259–260
    political resistance to tuberculosis prophylaxis, 264–266
    premigration health care practices, 253–254
    research methodology, 251–252
    transnational health, 255–257
    transnational resources, 253–257
    transnational syncretism, 259–260
    U.S. Health Care professionals, interfacing with, 263–267
  emotional well-being, 193
  Mexican, 271–283
    centrality of family, 279
    coping strategies for maternal role, 276–277
    data analysis, 274
    data collection, 274
    empowerment, 279–280
    maternal role, 275–277
    maternal role satisfiers, 275
    maternal role stressors, 275–276
    participants, 273
    role overload, 280–281
    spousal role, 277–278
    spousal role satisfiers, 277
    spousal role stressors, 277–278
    study, 273–275
    valuation, 279–280
  person-environment interactions, 193
  physical well-being, 192–193
  relocation to independent living community, 187–198
    data analysis, 191–192
    data collection, 190
    design, 189–190
    emotional well-being, 190–191
    findings, 192–194
    late-life relocation, 188–189
    measures, 190
    person-environmental interactions, 191
    physical well-being, 190
    purpose, 189
    quality of life, 191
    setting, 189–190
    subjective well-being, 191, 193–194
    theoretical framework, 189
    transition conditions, 190, 192–193
  rheumatoid arthritis, 336–346
    analysis, 341–342
    awareness, 342
    awareness and perception, 339
    demographics, 341
    disconnectedness, 340
    getting care, 342–343
    health outcomes, 340, 344
    markers of transition process, 344
    mastery, 344
    nursing model, 339
    nursing support, 343
    patterns of response, 340
    procedures, 341
    process, 339
    sample, 340–341
    transition process, 342–343
  subjective well-being
    integration, 194
    quality of life, 193–194
Work, 54–55
Worthy life, living, 247

Y
Yu, Po-Jui, 366